CLINICAL GUIDELINES
IN
ADULT HEALTH

Third Edition

Constance R. Uphold
PhD, ARNP-BC

Mary Virginia Graham
PhD, ARNP

2003

Barmarrae Books, Inc.

THIRD EDITION
Copyright © 2003 by Barmarrae Books, Inc.
Previous editions copyrighted 1994, 1999

All rights reserved. No part of this publication may be reproduced or transmitted in any form or by any means, electronic or mechanical, including photocopy, recording, or any information storage and retrieval system, without permission in writing from the publisher.

Barmarrae Books, Inc
3017 NW 62nd Terrace
Gainesville, Florida 32606

ISBN 0-9646151-8-5

Printed in the United States of America

PREFACE

In 1994, we published the first edition of *Clinical Guidelines in Adult Health*. Our original goal was to help clinicians quickly access up-to-date information regarding health maintenance and commonly occurring primary care problems. Over the decade we have been thrilled with the enthusiastic responses our book has generated. We have listened to our colleagues' comments and have added new topics and extensively updated and revised our original topics. Although the size of the book has grown to reflect the increasing complexities of patient care, the easy-to-follow format remains. We have worked to make this edition the best one to date. We have incorporated the latest advances in primary care to produce a comprehensive, yet practical and useful book for clinical practice.

A major challenge in writing this book was synthesizing the huge amount of research and literature related to primary care issues. Expert consensus or evidence-based practice guidelines developed by international, national, and professional advisory boards and organizations have grown exponentially. We have devoted extensive effort to include all the latest authoritative sources and best available evidence related to primary care in a clear and concise format.

In the third edition of *Clinical Guidelines in Adult Health* we made specific changes to improve our book. Each topic has been extensively updated to reflect current advances in the field. In particular, the management approaches in certain topics such as menopause, hormonal contraception, osteoporosis, HIV infection, chronic heart failure, atrial fibrillation, dyslipidemia, obesity, and rheumatoid arthritis have been completely reorganized to incorporate major scientific discoveries that have led to new and improved therapies. To mirror the growing recognition that many causes of death and disability can be prevented, the chapter on health maintenance has been extensively expanded and now includes an extensive section on cancer prevention. Throughout the book, prevention and patient education are emphasized. New topics such as restless legs syndrome, interstitial cystitis, plantar fasciitis, chronic fatigue, and age-related macular degeneration have been added. This edition has more emphasis on information access. Helpful web sites are listed to help clinicians find patient education tools and to keep abreast of healthcare advances and updates in clinical guidelines. Additional tables and illustrations have been added to help the reader quickly locate information.

Constance R. Uphold
Mary Virginia Graham

DEDICATION

To my mother, Myrtle Uphold, and my sister, Bonnie Marchi, and her family
In memory of my father, Charles Uphold
CRU

To my mother, Cecile T. King, the memory of my father, Ruben Randall King, my sister,
Madge King Cloud, and my brother, Durwood Wayne King
MVG

ACKNOWLEDGEMENTS

The authors would like to thank Sharren Gibbs for her preparation of this manuscript. She worked tirelessly, typing multiple drafts of each chapter and incorporating numerous revisions as we worked diligently to include the latest information before going to press.

A special thanks to Louis Clark, our talented artist/illustrator, who managed to produce every illustration that we requested, usually by the next day! In addition, Louis designed the cover and title page, and we feel very fortunate that he was willing to join us in this endeavor.

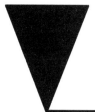

CONTRIBUTORS

Jean E. DeMartinis, PhD, FNP-BC
Cardiology and Prevention Nurse Practitioner
Consultant in Cardiology PC
Omaha, NE

J. Jordan Goodman, PhD, ARNP-BC
University of Florida
College of Medicine
Gainesville, FL

Mary Virginia Graham, PhD, ARNP
Family Nurse Practitioner
Gainesville, FL

Betsy Hernandez Warren, MSN, ARNP
Coordinator of Clinical Programs
University of Florida
Community Health and Family Medicine
Gainesville, FL

Tish Smyer, DNSc, RN
Associate Professor
Assistant Department Chair, Undergraduate Nursing
Project Director, Native American/Rural Nursing Grant
South Dakota State University College of Nursing
Brookings, SD

Constance R. Uphold, PhD, ARNP-BC
VA Research Career Development Awardee
North Florida/South Georgia Veterans Health System
Gainesville, FL

Sylvia Worden, MSN, RNCS, ARNP
Women's Health Nurse Practitioner
University of Florida Student Health Care Center
Gainesville, FL

REVIEWERS

The authors gratefully acknowledge the invaluable assistance provided by the following individuals who served as reviewers in the preparation of this edition of *Clinical Guidelines in Family Practice*.

Toni O. Barnett, PhD, FNP-C
MSN Coordinator, Family Nurse Practitioner Program
Department of Nursing, North Georgia College and State University
Dahlonega, Georgia

Madge K. Cloud, BA, MA
Consultant, Editorial Services
Elmhurst, IL

Rosemary Goodyear, EdD, RNC
Independent Consultant
Nurse Consultant Associates – www.ncassoc.org
Cardiff By The Sea, California

Lori Ann Hardcastle, MN, RNCS, FNP
Editorial Assistant
Gainesville, FL

Carol Massey Lavin, ARNP
Coordinator of Clinical Services
University of Florida Clinic at Fanning Springs
Gainesville, Florida

Anne A. Moore, MSN, RNC
Professor of Nursing
Women's Health Nurse Practitioner
Certified Nurse Colposcopist
Vanderbilt University
Nashville, TN

Grace Newsome, EdD, APRN, FNP-BC
Associate Professor
Department of Nursing, MSN/FNP Program
North Georgia College and State University
Dahlonega, Georgia   30597

Diane Stevens, MSN, APRN, FNP-BC
Clinical Coordinator
Family Nurse Practitioner Program
Husson College
Bangor, ME

TABLE OF CONTENTS

7 Skin Problems
MARY VIRGINIA GRAHAM

8 Problems of the Eyes
MARY VIRGINIA GRAHAM

9 Problems of the Ears, Nose, Sinuses, Throat, Mouth and Neck
CONSTANCE R. UPHOLD

10   Problems of the Upper Airways, Lower Respiratory System
BETSY HERNANDEZ WARREN and CONSTANCE R. UPHOLD

11   Cardiovascular Problems
JEAN E. DEMARTINIS, CONSTANCE R. UPHOLD and MARY VIRGINIA GRAHAM

12   Gastrointestinal Problems
MARY VIRGINIA GRAHAM

18 Neurologic Problems
MARY VIRGINIA GRAHAM

19 Hematologic Problems
MARY VIRGINIA GRAHAM

20 Minor Emergencies
CONSTANCE R. UPHOLD and MARY VIRGINIA GRAHAM

Index

Health Maintenance

MARY VIRGINIA GRAHAM

PERIODIC HEALTH EVALUATION FOR ADULTS

I.   Definition: Age-specific, evidence-based preventive services provided to *asymptomatic* adults by primary care clinicians within the context of routine care

II.   Overview of preventive health services and age-specific charts

    A.   The age-specific charts for adults developed by the US Preventive Services Task Force (USPSTF) are organized into three age groups: 11-24 years, 25-64 years, and 65 years and older
        1.   The USPSTF is in the process of reviewing, updating, and adding to the recommendations contained in the *Guide to Clinical Preventive Services* that was published in 1996; recommendations are being released as they are developed; all recommendations that have been released to date are contained herein
        2.   Recommendations for the care of pregnant women are not included here

    B.   Preventative services are divided into four categories: Screening tests, counseling interventions, immunizations, and chemoprophylaxis
        1.   *Screening tests* are those preventive services utilizing special tests or standardized examination procedures to identify patients requiring special intervention (Note: Screening tests are prioritized according to age group; for example, whereas blood pressure is ranked second on the list of screenings for the 11-24 year old age group, it is ranked first on the list for the two older age groups)
        2.   *Counseling interventions* involve the provision of information and advice to patients regarding personal behaviors (e.g., lap/shoulder belt use) that could reduce the risk of subsequent illness or injury (Note: Counseling areas are arranged in a priority listing in the age charts with a different priority given to each of the areas depending on the age group)
        3.   *Immunizations* include both vaccines and immunoglobulins (passive immunizations) given to persons with no evidence of infectious disease
        4.   *Chemoprophylaxis* refers to the use of drugs or biologics given to asymptomatic persons to reduce the risk of developing a disease (e.g., folic acid supplements for women of childbearing age) [in the third *Guide to Clinical Preventive Services*, which has not yet been completed, this category is called "chemoprevention"]

    C.   Preventive services for the general population are contained in each chart, according to age group
        1.   Interventions listed are based on leading causes of death as well as leading causes of morbidity in each age group
        2.   Potential effectiveness of each of the interventions in terms of improving clinical outcomes is a major factor in the determination of which interventions to include

    D.   Preventive services for members of high-risk groups are also included here

    E.   Leading causes of death by age group are listed at the top of each table
        1.   In the limited time allowed for counseling, clinicians are urged to consider the leading causes of mortality when establishing priorities for preventive counseling for a particular patient
        2.   For example, a 56-year old woman is considerably more likely to die from cardiac disease than from HIV, based on the leading causes of death for persons in her age group
        3.   Thus, in the few remaining minutes of an office visit, make the most of counseling interventions by being knowledgeable about the leading causes of death and morbidity in each age group

INTERVENTIONS CONSIDERED AND RECOMMENDED FOR THE PERIODIC HEALTH EXAMINATION AGES 11-24 YEARS

LEADING CAUSES OF DEATH
MOTOR VEHICLE/OTHER UNINTENTIONAL INJURIES
HOMICIDE
SUICIDE
MALIGNANT NEOPLASMS
HEART DISEASES

Interventions for the General Population

SCREENING
Height & weight
Blood pressure[1]
Papanicolaou (Pap)[2] test (females)
Chlamydia screen[3] (females <20 yrs)
Rubella serology or vaccination hx[4] (females >12 yrs)
Assess for problem drinking

COUNSELING
Injury Prevention
  ✓ Lap/shoulder belts
  ✓ Bicycle/motorcycle/ATV helmets*
  ✓ Smoke detector*
  ✓ Safe storage/removal of firearms*
Substance Use
  ✓ Avoid tobacco use
  ✓ Avoid underage drinking & illicit drug use*
  ✓ Avoid alcohol/drug use while driving, swimming, boating, etc.*
Sexual Behavior
  ✓ STD prevention: Abstinence*, avoid high-risk behavior*, condoms/female barrier with spermicide*
  ✓ Unintended pregnancy: Contraception

Diet and Exercise
  ✓ **Limit fat & cholesterol maintain caloric balance; emphasize grains, fruits, vegetables**
  ✓ Adequate calcium intake (females)
  ✓ **Regular physical activity***
Dental Health
  ✓ Regular visits to dental care provider
  ✓ Floss, brush with fluoride toothpaste daily

IMMUNIZATIONS
Tetanus-diphtheria (Td) boosters (11-16 yrs)
Hepatitis B[5]
MMR (11-12 yrs)[6]
Varicella (11-12 yrs)[7]
Rubella[4] (females >12 yrs)

CHEMOPROPHYLAXIS
Multivitamin with folic acid (females planning/capable of pregnancy)

(Note: Interventions that appear in bold have been revised. Please see revisions in table below: New Recommendations by the Third USPSTF: A Summary)

Interventions for High-Risk Populations

POPULATION	POTENTIAL INTERVENTIONS (see detailed high-risk definitions)
High-risk sexual behavior	RPR/VDRL (HR1); screen for gonorrhea (female) (HR2), HIV)HR3), **chlamydia** (female (HR4); hepatitis A vaccine (HR5)
Injection or street drug use	RPR/VDRL (HR1); HIV screen (HR3); hepatitis A vaccine (HR5); PPD (HR6); advise to reduce infection risk (HR7)
TB contacts: Immigrants; low income	PPD (HR6)
Native Americans/Alaska Natives	Hepatitis A vaccine (HR5); PPD 9HR6); pneumococcal vaccine (HR8)
Travelers to developing countries	Hepatitis A vaccine (HR5)
Certain chronic medical conditions	PPD (HR6); pneumococcal vaccine (HR8); influenza vaccine (HR9)
Settings where adolescents and young adults congregate	Second MMR (HR10)
Susceptible to varicella, measles, mumps	Varicella vaccine (HR11); MMR (HR12)
Blood transfusion between 1975-1985	HIV screen (HR3)
Institutionalized persons; healthcare/lab workers	Hepatitis A vaccine (HR5); PPD (HR6); influenza vaccine (HR9)
Family h/o skin cancer; nevi; fair skin, eyes, hair	Avoid excess/midday sun, use protective clothing* (HR13)
Prior pregnancy with neural tube defect	Folic acid 4.0 mg (HR14)
Inadequate water fluoridation	Daily fluoride supplement (HR15)

(Continued)

1) Periodic BP for persons aged ≥21 yrs; 2) If sexually active at present or in the past: Q ≤3 yrs. If sexual history is unreliable, begin Pap tests at age 18 yrs; 3) If sexually active; 4) Serologic testing, documented vaccination history, and routine vaccination against rubella (preferably with MMR) are equally acceptable alternatives; 5) If not previously immunized: current visit, 1 and 6 mos later; 6) If no previous second dose of MMR; 7) If susceptible to chickenpox; *) The ability of clinician counseling to influence this behavior is unproven

Source: US Preventive Services Task Force (1996). *Guide to clinical preventive services* (2nd ed.). Washington, DC: US Government Printing Office.

Access at www.ahrq.gov/clinic/cpsix.htm

INTERVENTIONS CONSIDERED AND RECOMMENDED FOR THE PERIODIC HEALTH EXAMINATION AGES 11-24 YEARS

(CONTINUED)

LEADING CAUSES OF DEATH
MOTOR VEHICLE/OTHER UNINTENTIONAL INJURIES
HOMICIDE
SUICIDE
MALIGNANT NEOPLASMS
HEART DISEASES

Detailed High-Risk Definitions

HR1 =   Persons who exchange sex for money or drugs, and their sex partners; persons with other STDs (including HIV); and sexual contacts of persons with active syphilis. Clinicians should also consider local epidemiology

HR2 =   Females who have: Two or more sex partners in the last year; a sex partner with multiple sexual contacts; exchanged sex for money or drugs; or a history of repeated episodes of gonorrhea. Clinicians should also consider local epidemiology

HR3 =   Males who had sex with males after 1975; past or present injection drug use; persons who exchange sex for money or drugs, and their sex partners; injection drug-using, bisexual, or HIV-positive sex partner currently or in the past; blood transfusion during 1978-1985; persons seeking treatment for STDs. Clinicians should also consider local epidemiology

HR4 =   Sexually active females with multiple risk factors including: History of prior STD; new or multiple sex partners; age under 25; nonuse or inconsistent use of barrier contraceptives; cervical ectopy. Clinicians should also consider local epidemiology of the disease in identifying other high-risk groups

HR5 =   Persons living in, traveling to, or working in areas where the disease is endemic and where periodic outbreaks occur (e.g., countries with high or intermediate endemicity; certain Alaska Native, Pacific Island, Native American, and religious communities); men who have sex with men; injection or street drug users. Vaccine may be considered for institutionalized persons and workers in these institutions, military personnel, and day-care, hospital, and laboratory workers. Clinicians should also consider local epidemiology

HR6 =   HIV positive, close contacts of persons with known or suspected TB, healthcare workers, persons with medical risk factors associated with TB, immigrants from countries with high TB prevalence, medically underserved low-income populations (including homeless), alcoholics, injection drug users, and residents of long-term facilities

HR7 =   Persons who continue to inject drugs

HR8 =   Immunocompetent persons with certain medical conditions, including chronic cardiac or pulmonary disease, diabetes mellitus, and anatomic asplenia. Immunocompetent persons who live in high-risk, environments or social settings (e.g., certain Native American and Alaska Native populations)

HR9 =   Annual vaccination of: Residents of chronic care facilities; persons with chronic cardiopulmonary disorders, metabolic diseases (including diabetes mellitus), hemoglobinopathies, immunosuppression, or renal dysfunction; and healthcare providers for high-risk patients (**this recommendation has been updated** – see p 18, *Influenza Vaccinations*)

HR10 =   Adolescents and young adults in settings where such individuals congregate (e.g., high schools and colleges), if they have not previously received a second dose

HR11 =   Health persons aged ≥13 years without a history of chickenpox or previous immunization. Consider serologic testing for presumed susceptible persons aged ≥13 years

HR12 =   Persons born after 1956 who lack evidence of immunity to measles or mumps (e.g., documented receipt of live vaccine on or after the first birthday, laboratory evidence of immunity, or a history of physician-diagnosed measles or mumps)

HR13 =   Persons with a family or personal history of skin cancer, a large number of moles, atypical moles, poor tanning ability, or light skin, hair, and eye color

HR14 =   Women with prior pregnancy affected by neural tube defect who are planning pregnancy

HF15 =   Persons aged ≤17 years living in area with inadequate water fluoridation (<0.6 ppm)

INTERVENTIONS CONSIDERED AND RECOMMENDED FOR THE PERIODIC HEALTH EXAMINATION AGES 25-64 YEARS

LEADING CAUSES OF DEATH
MALIGNANT NEOPLASMS
HEART DISEASES
MOTOR VEHICLE AND OTHER UNINTENTIONAL INJURIES
HUMAN IMMUNODEFICIENCY VIRUS (HIV) INFECTION
SUICIDE AND HOMICIDE

Interventions for the General Population

SCREENING
Blood pressure
Height and weight
Total blood cholesterol (men ages 35-65, women ages 45-65)
Papanicolaou (Pap)[1] test (women)
Fecal occult blood test[2] and/or sigmoidoscopy (≥50 yrs)
Mammogram +/- clinical breast exam[3] (women 50-69 yrs)
Assess for problem drinking
Rubella serology or vaccination hx[4] (women of childbearing age)

COUNSELING
Substance Use
✓ Tobacco cessation
✓ Avoid alcohol/drug use while driving, swimming, boating, etc
Diet and Exercise
✓ **Limit fat and cholesterol; maintain caloric balance; emphasize grains; fruits, vegetables**
✓ Adequate calcium intake (women)
✓ **Regular physical activity***
Injury Prevention
✓ Lap. shoulder belts
✓ Motorcycle/bicycle/ATV helmets

✓ Smoke detector*
✓ Safe storage/removal of firearms*
Sexual Behavior
✓ STD prevention: Avoid high-risk behavior*; condoms/female barrier with spermicide*
✓ Unintended pregnancy: Contraception
Dental Health
✓ Regular visits to dental care provider
✓ Floss, brush with fluoride toothpaste daily*

IMMUNIZATIONS
Tetanus-diphtheria (Td) boosters
Rubella[4] (women of childbearing age)

CHEMOPROPHYLAXIS
Multivitamin with folic acid (women planning or capable of pregnancy)
Discuss hormone prophylaxis (peri- and postmenopausal women)

(Note: Interventions that appear in bold have been revised. Please see revisions in table below: New Recommendations by the Third USPSTF: A Summary)

Interventions for High-Risk Populations

POPULATION	POTENTIAL INTERVENTIONS (See detailed high-risk definitions)
High-risk sexual behavior	RPR/VDRL (HR1); screen for gonorrhea (female) (HR2), HIV (HR3), **chlamydia** (female (HR4); hepatitis vaccine (HR5); hepatitis A vaccine (HR6)
Injection or street drug use	RPR/VDRL (HR1); HIV screen (HR3); hepatitis B vaccine (HR5); hepatitis A vaccine (HR6); PPD HR7; advice to reduce infection risk (HR8)
Low income; TB contact; immigrants; alcoholics	PPD (HR7)
Native Americans/Alaska Natives	Hepatitis A vaccine (HR6); PPD (HR7); pneumococcal vaccine (HR9)
Travelers to developing countries	Hepatitis B vaccine (HR5); hepatitis A vaccine (HR6)
Certain chronic medical conditions	PPD (HR7); pneumococcal vaccine (HR9); influenza vaccine (HR10)
Blood product recipients	HIV screen (HR3); hepatitis B vaccine (HR5)
Susceptible to measles, mumps, or varicella	MMR (HR11); varicella vaccine (HR12)
Institutionalized persons	Hepatitis A vaccine (HR6); PPD (HR7); pneumococcal vaccine (HR9); influenza vaccine (HR10)
Healthcare/lab workers	Hepatitis B vaccine IHR6); hepatitis A vaccine (HR6); PPD (HR7); influenza vaccine (HR10)
Family h/o skin cancer; nevi; fair skin, eyes, hair	Avoid excess/midday sun, use protective clothing* (HR13)
Previous pregnancy with neural tube defect	Folic acid 4.0 mg (HR14)

(Continued)

1) Women who are or have been sexually active and who have a cervix: Q ≤3 yrs; 2) Annually; 3) Mammogram Q 1-2 yrs, or mammogram Q 1-2 yrs with annual clinical breast examination; 4) Serologic testing, documented vaccination history, and routine vaccination (preferably with MMR) are equally acceptable alternatives; *) The ability of clinician counseling to influence this behavior is unproven

INTERVENTIONS CONSIDERED AND RECOMMENDED FOR THE PERIODIC HEALTH EXAMINATION AGES 25-64 YEARS

(CONTINUED)

LEADING CAUSES OF DEATH
MALIGNANT NEOPLASMS
HEART DISEASES
MOTOR VEHICLE AND OTHER UNINTENTIONAL INJURIES
HUMAN IMMUNODEFICIENCY VIRUS (HIV) INFECTION
SUICIDE AND HOMICIDE

Detailed High-Risk Definitions

HR1 = Persons who exchange sex for money or drugs, and their sex partners; persons with other STDs (including HIV); and sexual contacts of persons with active syphilis. Clinicians should also consider local epidemiology

HR2 = Women who exchange sex for money or drugs, or who have had repeated episodes of gonorrhea. Clinicians should also consider local epidemiology

HR3 = Men who had sex with men after 1975; past or present injection drug use; persons who exchange sex for money or drugs, and their sex partners; injection drug-using, bisexual, or HIV-positive sex partner currently or in the past; blood transfusion during 1978-1985; persons seeking treatment for STDs. Clinicians should also consider local epidemiology

HR4 = Sexually active women with multiple risk factors including: History of STD, new or multiple sex partners; nonuse or inconsistent use of barrier contraceptives; cervical ectopy. Clinicians should consider local epidemiology

HR5 = Blood product recipients (including hemodialysis patients), persons with frequent occupational exposure to blood or blood products, men who have sex with men, injection drug users and their sex partners, persons with multiple recent sex partners, persons with other STDs (including HIV), travelers to countries with endemic hepatitis B

HR6 = Persons living in, traveling to, or working in areas where the disease is endemic and where periodic outbreaks occur (e.g., countries with high or intermediate endemicity; certain Alaska Native, Pacific Island, Native American, and religious communities); men who have sex with men/ injection or street drug users. Consider for institutionalized persons and workers in these institutions, military personnel, and day-care, hospital, and laboratory workers. Clinicians should also consider local epidemiology

HR7 = HIV positive, close contacts of persons with known or suspected TB, healthcare workers, persons with medical risk factors associated with TB, immigrants from countries with high TB prevalence, medically underserved low-income populations (including homeless), alcoholics, injection drug users, and residents of long-term care facilities

HR8 = Persons who continue to inject drugs

HR9 = Immunocompetent institutionalized persons aged ≥50 yrs and immunocompetent persons with certain medical conditions, including chronic cardiac or pulmonary disease, diabetes mellitus, and anatomic asplenia

HR10 = Annual vaccination of: Residents of chronic care facilities; persons with chronic cardiopulmonary disorders, metabolic diseases (including diabetes mellitus), hemoglobinopathies, immunosuppression, or renal dysfunction; and health care providers for high-risk patients (**this recommendation has been updated** – see p 18, *Influenza Vaccinations*)

HR11 = Persons born after 1956 who lack evidence of immunity to measles or mumps (e.g., documented receipt of live vaccine on or after the first birthday, laboratory evidence of immunity, or a history of physician-diagnosed measles or mumps)

HR12 = Healthy adults without a history of chickenpox or previous immunization. Consider serologic testing for presumed susceptible adults

HR13 = Persons with a family or personal history of skin cancer, a large number of moles, atypical moles, poor tanning ability, or light skin, hair, and eye color

HR14 = Women with previous pregnancy affected by neural tube defect who are planning pregnancy

INTERVENTIONS CONSIDERED AND RECOMMENDED FOR THE PERIODIC HEALTH EXAMINATION AGES 65 YEARS AND OLDER

LEADING CAUSES OF DEATH
HEART DISEASES
MALIGNANT NEOPLASMS (LUNG, COLORECTAL, BREAST)
CEREBROVASCULAR DISEASE
CHRONIC OBSTRUCTIVE PULMONARY DISEASE
PNEUMONIA AND INFLUENZA

Interventions for the General Population

SCREENING
Blood pressure
Height and weight
Fecal occult blood test[1] and/or sigmoidoscopy
Mammogram +/- clinical breast[2] exam (women ≤69 yrs)
Papanicolaou (Pap) test[3] (women)
Vision screening
Assess for hearing impairment
Assess for problem drinking

COUNSELING
Substance Use
  ✓ Tobacco cessation
  ✓ Avoid alcohol/drug use while driving, swimming, boating, etc*
Diet and Exercise
  ✓ **Limit fat and cholesterol; maintain caloric balance; emphasize grains, fruits, vegetables**
  ✓ Adequate calcium intake (women)
  ✓ **Regular physical activity***
Injury Prevention
  ✓ Lap/shoulder belts
  ✓ Motorcycle and bicycle helmets

  ✓ Fall prevention*
  ✓ Safe storage/removal of firearms*
  ✓ Smoke detector*
  ✓ Set hot water heater to <120° F*
  ✓ CPR training for household members
Dental Health
  ✓ Regular visits to dental care provider*
  ✓ Floss, brush with fluoride toothpaste daily*
Sexual Behavior
STD prevention: Avoid high-risk sexual behavior*, use condoms*

IMMUNIZATIONS
Pneumococcal vaccine
Influenza[1]
Tetanus-diphtheria (Td) boosters

CHEMOPROPHYLAXIS
Discuss hormone prophylaxis (women)

(Note: Interventions that appear in bold have been revised. Please see revisions in table below: New Recommendations by the Third USPSTF: A Summary)

Interventions for High-Risk Populations

POPULATION	POTENTIAL INTERVENTIONS (see detailed high-risk definitions)
Institutionalized persons	PPD (HR1); hepatitis A vaccine (HR2); amantadine/rimantadine (HR4)
Chronic medical conditions; TB contacts; low income; immigrants; alcoholics	PPD (HR1)
Persons ≥75 yrs; or ≥70 yr with risk factors for falls	Fall prevention intervention (HR5)
Cardiovascular disease risk factors	Consider cholesterol screening (HR6)
Family h/o skin cancer; nevi; fair skin, eyes, hair	Avoid excess/midday sun, use protective clothing* (HR7)
Native Americans/Alaska Natives	PPD (HR1); hepatitis A vaccine (HR2)
Travelers to developing countries	Hepatitis A vaccine (HR2); hepatitis B vaccine (HR8)
Blood product recipients	HIV screen (HR3); hepatitis B vaccine HR8)
High-risk sexual behavior	Hepatitis A vaccine (HR2); HIV screen (HR3); hepatitis B vaccine (HR8); RPR/VDRL (HR9); advice to reduce infection risk (HR10)
Injection or street drug use	PPD (HR1); hepatitis A vaccine (HR2); HIV screen (HR3); hepatitis B vaccine (HR8); RPR/VDRL (HR9); advice to reduce infection risk (HR10)
Healthcare/lab workers	PPD (HR1); hepatitis A vaccine (HR2); amantadine/rimantadine (HR4); hepatitis B vaccine (HR8)
Persons susceptible to varicella	Varicella vaccine (HR11)

1) Annually; 2) Mammogram Q 1-2 yrs, or mammogram Q 1-2 yrs with annual clinical breast exam; 3) All women who are or have been sexually active and who have a cervix: Q ≤3 yrs. Consider discontinuation of testing after age 65 yrs if previous regular screening with consistently normal results; *) The ability of clinician counseling to influence this behavior is unproven

Source: US Preventive Services Task Force (1996). *Guide to clinical preventive services* (2nd ed.). Washington, DC: US Government Printing Office.

INTERVENTIONS CONSIDERED AND RECOMMENDED FOR THE PERIODIC HEALTH EXAMINATION AGES 65 YEARS AND OLDER
(CONTINUED)

LEADING CAUSES OF DEATH
HEART DISEASES
MALIGNANT NEOPLASMS (LUNG, COLORECTAL, BREAST)
CEREBROVASCULAR DISEASE
CHRONIC OBSTRUCTIVE PULMONARY DISEASE
PNEUMONIA AND INFLUENZA

Detailed High-Risk Definitions

HR1 = HIV positive, close contacts of persons with known or suspected TB, healthcare workers, persons with medical risk factors associated with TB, immigrants from countries with high TB prevalence, medically underserved low-income populations (Including homeless), alcoholics, injection drug users, and residents of long-term care facilities

HR2 = Persons living in, traveling to, or working in areas where the disease is endemic and where periodic outbreaks occur (e.g., countries with high or intermediate endemicity; certain Alaska Native, Pacific Island, Native American, and religious communities); men who have sex with men, injection or street drug users. Consider for institutionalized persons and workers in these institutions, and day-care, hospital, and laboratory workers. Clinicians should also consider local epidemiology

HR3 = Men who had sex with men after 1975; past or present injection drug use; persons who exchange sex for money or drugs, and their sex partners; injection drug-using, bisexual, or HIV-positive sex partner currently or in the past; blood transfusion during 1978-1985; persons seeking treatment for STDs. Clinicians should also consider local epidemiology

HR4 = Consider for persons who have not received influenza vaccine or are vaccinated late; when the vaccine may be ineffective due to major antigenic changes in the virus for unvaccinated persons who provide home care for high-risk persons, to supplement protection provided by vaccine in persons who are expected to have a poor antibody response; and for high-risk persons in whom the vaccine is contraindicated

HR5 = Persons aged 75 years and older; or aged 70-74 with one or more additional risk factors including: use of certain psychoactive and cardiac medications (e.g., benzodiazepines, antihypertensives); use of ≥ 4 prescription medications; impaired cognition, strength, balance, or gait. Intensive individualized home-based multifactorial fall prevention intervention is recommended in settings where adequate resources are available to deliver such services

HR6 = Although evidence is insufficient to recommend routine screening in elderly persons, clinicians should consider cholesterol screening on a case-by-case basis for persons aged 65-75 with additional risk factors (e.g., smoking, diabetes, or hypertension)

HR7 = Persons with a family or personal history of skin cancer, a large number of moles, atypical moles, poor tanning ability, or light skin, hair, and eye color

HR8 = Blood product recipients (including hemodialysis patients), persons with frequent occupational exposure to blood or blood products, men who have sex with men, injection drug users and their sex partners, persons with multiple recent sex partners, persons with other STDs (including HIV), travelers to countries with endemic hepatitis B

HR9 = Persons who exchange sex for money or drugs and their sex partners; persons with other STDs (including HIV); and sexual contacts of persons with active syphilis. Clinicians should also consider local epidemiology

HR10 = Persons who continue to inject drugs

HR11 = Healthy adults without a history of chickenpox or previous immunization. Consider serologic testing for presumed susceptible adults

NEW RECOMMENDATIONS BY THE THIRD US PREVENTIVE SERVICES TASK FORCE (USPSTF): A SUMMARY*

I. Screening Recommendations

Summary of Recommendations	Clinical Considerations
Screening for Chlamydial Infection – Update	
The USPSTF	
• Strongly recommends that clinicians routinely screen all sexually active women aged 25 and younger, and other asymptomatic women at increased risk for infection, for chlamydial infection	• Women and adolescents through age 20 years are at highest risk for chlamydial infection; age is the most important risk marker
• Makes no recommendations for or against	• Other patient characteristics associated with a higher prevalence of infection include being unmarried, African-American race, having a prior history of STDs, having new or multiple sexual partners, having cervical ectopy, and using barrier contraceptives inconsistently
✓ Routine screening of asymptomatic low-risk women in general population	
✓ Routine screening of asymptomatic men	
• Screening recommendations relating to pregnant women are not considered here	
Screening for Colorectal Cancer – Update	
The USPSTF	• Potential screening options for colorectal cancer include the following:
• Strongly recommends that clinicians screen all men and women 50 years of age or older for colorectal cancer	✓ Home FOBT, flexible sigmoidoscopy, the combination of home FOBT and flexible sigmoidoscopy, colonoscopy, and double-contrast barium enema
• Found fair to good evidence that several screening methods are effective in reducing mortality from colorectal cancer	✓ Each option has both advantages and disadvantages that may vary for individual patients and practice settings–clinicians should discuss with the patient the benefits, potential harms, and costs associated with each option before selecting a screening strategy
✓ Fair evidence that sigmoidoscopy alone or in combination with fecal occult blood testing (FOBT) reduces mortality	• The optimal interval for screening depends on the test
✓ Good evidence that periodic FOBT reduces mortality from colorectal cancer	✓ Annual FOBT offers greater reductions in mortality rates than biennial screening but produces more false-positive results
• Did not find direct evidence that screening colonoscopy is effective in reducing colorectal cancer mortality rates; however, efficacy of colonoscopy is supported by its integral role in trials of FOBT, and from extrapolation from sigmoidoscopy studies, and by the ability of colonoscopy to inspect the proximal colon	✓ A 10-year interval has been recommended for colonoscopy on the basis of evidence regarding the natural history of adenomatous polyps
• Concludes that double-contrast barium enema offers an alternative means of whole-bowel examination, but it is less sensitive than colonoscopy and there is no direct evidence that it is effective in reducing mortality rates	✓ Five year intervals have been recommended for flexible sigmoidoscopy and double-contrast barium enema because of the lower sensitivity of these methods
• Concludes that there are insufficient data to determine which screening strategy is best in terms of the balance of benefits and potential harms or cost-effectiveness	✓ Except for FOBT, there is no direct evidence with which to determine the optimal interval for colonoscopy, sigmoidoscopy, and double contrast barium enema
• Found insufficient evidence that newer screening techniques (e.g., computed tomographic colography) are effective in improving health outcomes	• The USPSTF recommends initiating screening at 50 years of age for men and women of average risk for colorectal cancer; however, in persons at higher risk (for example, those with a first-degree relative who receives a diagnosis of colorectal cancer before age 60), initiating screening at an earlier age is reasonable
	• The appropriate age at which colorectal cancer screening should be discontinued is not known; discontinuing screening is reasonable in patients whose age or comorbid conditions limit life expectancy
Screening for Depression – New	
The USPSTF	• Many formal screening tools are available (see section on DEPRESSION for more information). Asking two simple questions about mood and anhedonia may be as effective as using longer instruments
• Recommends screening adults for depression in clinical practices that have systems in place to assure accurate diagnosis, effective treatment, and follow-up	✓ "Over the past 2 weeks, have you felt down, depressed, or hopeless?"
• Makes no recommendations for or against routine screening of children or adolescents for depression	✓ "Over the past 2 weeks, have you felt little interest or pleasure in doing things?"
	• There is little evidence to support the choice of one screening method over another, so clinicians can select the method that best fits their personal preference, the patient population served, and the practice setting
	• All positive screening tests should trigger full diagnostic interviews using standard diagnostic criteria (i.e., those from the 4th edition of the *Diagnostic and Statistical Manual of Mental Disorders* [DSM-IV])

(Continued)

New Recommendations by the Third US Preventive Services Task Force: A Summary *(Continued)*

Summary of Recommendations	Clinical Considerations
Screening for Breast Cancer–Update	
The USPSTF	• The precise age at which the benefits from screening mammography justify the potential harms is a subjective judgment and should take into account patient preferences; clinicians should tell women that the balance of benefits and potential harms of mammography improves with increasing age for women between the ages of 40 and 70
• Recommends screening mammography, with or without clinical breast examination (CBE), every 1 to 2 years for women aged 40 and older	
• Concludes that the evidence is also generalizable to women aged 70 and older (who face a higher absolute risk of breast cancer) if their life expectancy is not compromised by comorbid disease	• The precise age at which to discontinue screening mammography is uncertain. Whereas older women face a higher probability of developing and dying of breast cancer, they also have a greater chance of dying of other causes. Women with comorbid conditions that limit their life expectancy are unlikely to benefit from screening
• Concludes that the evidence is insufficient to recommend for or against ✓ Routine CBE alone to screen for breast cancer ✓ Teaching or performing routine breast self examination	• Women who are at increased risk for breast cancer (e.g., those with a family history of breast cancer in a mother or sister, a previous breast biopsy revealing atypical hyperplasia, or first childbirth after age 30) are more likely to benefit from regular mammography than women at lower risk; the recommendation to begin screening in their 40s is strengthened by a family history of breast cancer having been diagnosed before menopause
	• The USPSTF did not examine whether women should be screened for genetic mutations (*BRCA1* and *BRCA2*) that increase the risk of developing breast cancer
	• Clinicians who advise women to perform BSE or who perform routine CBE to screen for breast cancer should understand that there is currently insufficient evidence to determine whether these practices affect breast cancer mortality and that they are likely to increase the incidence of clinical assessments and biopsies
Screening for Skin Cancer–New	
The USPSTF	• Benefits from screening are unproven, even in high-risk patients
• Concludes that the evidence is insufficient to recommend for or against routine screening for skin cancer using a total-body skin examination performed by a clinician for the early detection of cutaneous melanoma, basal cell cancer, or squamous cell skin cancer	• Clinicians should be aware that fair-skinned persons aged >65, persons with atypical moles, and those with >50 moles constitute known groups at substantially increased risk for melanoma
	• Clinicians should remain alert for skin lesions with malignant features noted in the context of physical examinations performed for other purposes

(Continued)

NEW RECOMMENDATIONS BY THE THIRD US PREVENTIVE SERVICES TASK FORCE: A SUMMARY (CONTINUED)

Summary of Recommendations	Clinical Considerations
Screening for Lipid Disorders–Update	
The USPSTF	• TC and HDL-C can be measured on nonfasting or fasting samples
• Strongly recommends that clinicians routinely screen men ≥35 years of age and women ≥45 years of age for lipid disorders and treat abnormal lipids in people who are at increased risk of CHD	• Screening is recommended for men aged 20 to 35 years and for women aged 20 to 45 years in the presence of any of the following
• Recommends that clinicians routinely screen younger adults (men aged 20 to 35 years and women aged 20 to 45 years) for lipid disorders if they have other risk factors for CHD	✓ Diabetes ✓ Family history of cardiovascular disease before age 50 in male relatives or age 60 in female relatives ✓ Family history suggestive of familial hyperlipidemia ✓ Multiple coronary heart disease risk factors (e.g., tobacco use, hypertension)
• Makes no recommendations for or against routine screening for lipid disorders in younger adults (men aged 20 to 35 years or women aged 20 to 45 years) in the absence of known risk factors for CHD	• Treatment decisions should take into account overall risk of heart disease rather than lipid levels alone and should also take into account costs and patient preferences
• Recommends that screening for lipid disorders include measurement of total cholesterol (TC) and high-density lipoprotein cholesterol (HDL-C)	• All patients, regardless of lipid levels, should be offered counseling about the benefits of a diet low in saturated fat and high in fruits and vegetables, regular physical activity, avoiding tobacco use, and maintaining a healthy weight
• Concludes that there is insufficient evidence to recommend for or against triglyceride measurement as a part of routine screening for lipid disorders	• An age to stop screening is not established
• Optimal interval for screening is uncertain	
✓ Reasonable options include every 5 years with shorter intervals for persons with lipid levels close to those warranting therapy and longer intervals for low-risk persons with low or repeatedly normal levels	
✓ Screening may be appropriate in older persons who have never been screened	
✓ Repeated screening is less important in older persons because lipid levels are less likely to increase after age 65	
Screening for Osteoporosis–Update	
The USPSTF	• The exact risk factors that should trigger screening in women in the 60 to 64 years of age group are difficult to specify based on evidence–lower body weight (weight <70 kg) is the single best predictor of low bone mineral density; there is less evidence to support the use of other individual risk factors (e.g., smoking, weight loss, family history, decreased physical activity, alcohol or caffeine use, or low calcium and vitamin D intake) as a basis for identifying high-risk women younger than 65 years of age
• Recommends that women ≥65 years of age be screened routinely for osteoporosis	
• Recommends that routine screening begin at 60 years of age for women at increased risk for osteoporotic fractures	• There are no data to determine the appropriate age to stop screening and few data on osteoporosis treatment in women older than 85 years of age; patients who receive a diagnosis of osteoporosis fall outside the context of screening but may receive additional testing for diagnostic purposes or to monitor response to treatment
• Makes no recommendation for or against routine screening in postmenopausal women who are younger than 60 years of age or in women 60 to 64 years of age who are not at increased risk for osteoporotic fractures	• At any given age, African-American women on average have higher bone mineral density than Caucasian women and are thus less likely to benefit from screening
• Optimal intervals for repeated screening have not been identified; a minimum of 2 years may be needed to reliably measure a change in bone mineral density–longer intervals may be adequate for repeated screening to identify new cases of osteoporosis	• Among bone measurement tests performed at various anatomic sites, bone density measured at the femoral neck by dual-energy x-ray absorptiometry is the best predictor of hip fracture and is comparable to forearm measurements for predicting fractures at other sites
	(Continued)

NEW RECOMMENDATIONS BY THE THIRD US PREVENTIVE SERVICES TASK FORCE: A SUMMARY (*CONTINUED*)

Summary of Recommendations	Clinical Considerations
Screening for Prostate Cancer–Update	
The USPSTF	• PSA testing and DRE can effectively detect prostate cancer in its early pathologic stages, but whether early detection improves health outcomes remains unknown
• Concludes that the evidence is insufficient to recommend for or against routine screening for prostate cancer using prostate-specific antigen (PSA) testing or digital rectal examination (DRE)	• The balance of potential benefits (reduction of morbidity and mortality from prostate cancer) and harms (false-positive results, unnecessary biopsies, and possible complications) of early treatment of the types of cancer found by screening, however, is uncertain
• Found good evidence that PSA screening can detect early-stage prostate cancer but mixed and inconclusive evidence that early detection improves health outcomes	• If early detection does improve health outcomes, the population most likely to benefit from screening will be men 50 to 70 years of age who are at average risk, and men >45 years of age who are at increased risk (African-American men and those with a first-degree relative with prostate cancer)
• Concludes that evidence is insufficient to determine whether the benefits outweigh the harms for a screened population	• Older men and men with other significant health problems who have a life expectancy of fewer than 10 years are unlikely to benefit from screening
	• PSA testing is more sensitive than DRE for detection of prostate cancer; using the conventional PSA cut-point of 4.0 ng/dL detects a large majority of prostate cancer; however, a significant percentage of early prostate cancer (10%-20%) will be missed
Screening for Type 2 Diabetes Mellitus in Adults—Update	
The USPSTF	• In the absence of direct benefits of routine screening for type 2 diabetes, the decision to screen individual patients is a matter of clinical judgment
• Concludes that the evidence is insufficient to recommend for or against routinely screening asymptomatic adults for type 2 diabetes, impaired glucose tolerance, or impaired fasting glucose	• Screening for diabetes in patients with hypertension or hyperlipidemia should be part of an integrated approach to reduce cardiovascular risk
• Recommends screening for type 2 diabetes in adults with hypertension or hyperlipidemia	• Three tests have been used to screen for diabetes: fasting plasma glucose (FPG), 2-hour post-load plasma glucose (2 hr PG), and hemoglobin A1c (HbA1c). The American Diabetes Association (ADA) has recommended the FPG test (>126 mg/dL) for screening because it is easier and faster to perform, more convenient and acceptable to patients, and less expensive than other screening tests
	• Regardless of whether the clinician and patient decide to screen for diabetes, patients should be encouraged to exercise, eat a healthy diet, and maintain a healthy weight, choices that may prevent or forestall the development of type 2 diabetes
	(Continued)

NEW RECOMMENDATIONS BY THE THIRD US PREVENTIVE SERVICES TASK FORCE: A SUMMARY *(CONTINUED)*

Summary of Recommendations	Clinical Considerations
Screening for Cervical Cancer--*Update*	
The USPSTF	• The goal of cytologic screening is to sample the transformation zone, the area where physiologic transformation from columnar endocervical epithelium to squamous (ectocervical) epithelium takes place and where dysplasia and cancer arise; the combined use of an extended tip spatula to sample the ectocervix and a cytobrush to sample the endocervix is recommended
• Strongly recommends screening for cervical cancer in women who have been sexually active and have a cervix	
• Found good evidence that screening with cervical cytology (Papanicolaou [Pap] smears) reduces incidence of and mortality from cervical cancer	• Optimal age to begin screening is unknown; however, data on the natural history of HPV infection and the incidence of high-grade lesions and cervical cancer indicate that screening can safely be delayed until 3 years after the onset of sexual activity, or until age 21—whichever comes first.
• Concludes that most of the benefit can be obtained by beginning screening within 3 years of onset of sexual activity or age 21 (whichever comes first) and screening at least every 3 years (see Clinical Considerations)	• There is little value in screening women who have never been sexually active; nonetheless, many US organizations recommend routine screening by age 18 or 21 for all women, based on the generally high prevalence of sexual activity by that age in the US and because clinicians may not always obtain accurate sexual histories
• Recommends against routinely screening women older than age 65 for cervical cancer if they have had adequate recent screening with normal Pap smears and are not otherwise at high risk for cervical cancer (see Clinical Considerations)	• Discontinuation of cervical cancer screening in older women is appropriate, provided women have had adequate screening with normal Pap results. Whereas the optimal age to discontinue screening is not clear, the risk of cervical cancer and the yield of screening decline steadily through middle age and the yield of screening is low in previously screened women after age 65. New American Cancer Society (ACS) recommendations suggest stopping cervical cancer screening at age 70
• Recommends against routine Pap smear screening in women who have had a total hysterectomy for benign disease	
• Concludes that the evidence is insufficient to recommend for or against the routine use of new technologies to screen for cervical cancer	• Screening is recommended in older women who have not been previously screened, when information about previous screening is unavailable, or when screening is unlikely to have occurred in the past
• Concludes that the evidence is insufficient to recommend for or against the routine use of human papillomavirus (HPV) testing as a primary screening test for cervical cancer	• There is no direct evidence that annual screening achieves better outcomes than screening every 3 years; however, because sensitivity of a single Pap test for high-grade lesions may only be 60-80%, most organizations in the US recommend that annual Pap smears be performed until a specified number (usually 2 or 3) are cytologically normal before lengthening the screening interval
	• Discontinuation of cytological screening after total hysterectomy for benign disease (e.g., no evidence of cervical neoplasia or cancer) is appropriate given the low yield of screening and the potential harms from false-positive results in this population. Clinicians should confirm that a total hysterectomy was performed (through surgical records or inspecting for the absence of a cervix)
	• Newer FDA-approved technologies, such as liquid-based cytology (e.g., ThinPrep) may have improved sensitivity over conventional Pap smear screening, but at a considerably higher cost and possibly with lower specificity. Liquid-based cytology permits testing of specimens for HPV, which may be useful in guiding management of women whose Pap smear reveals atypical squamous cells. HPV DNA testing for primary cervical cancer screening has not been approved by the FDA and its role in screening remains uncertain

(Continued)

13

NEW RECOMMENDATIONS BY THE THIRD US PREVENTIVE SERVICES TASK FORCE: A SUMMARY *(CONTINUED)*

Summary of Recommendations	Clinical Considerations
II. Counseling Recommendations	

Behavioral Counseling in Primary Care to Promote Physical Activity—*Update*

The USPSTF
- Concludes that the evidence is insufficient to recommend for or against behavioral counseling in primary care settings to promote physical activity

- Regular physical activity helps prevent cardiovascular disease, type 2 diabetes mellitus, obesity, and osteoporosis; it may also decrease all-cause morbidity and lengthen life span
- Whether routine counseling and follow-up by primary care clinicians result in increased physical activity among adult patients is unclear
- Multicomponent interventions combining provider counseling with behavioral interventions to facilitate and reinforce healthy levels of physical activity appear to be the most promising approaches. For example, interventions that include patient goal setting, written exercise prescriptions, individually tailored physical activity regimens, and mailed or telephone follow-up assistance provided by specially trained staff may enhance effectiveness of routine counseling

Behavioral Counseling in Primary Care to Promote a Healthy Diet—*New*

The USPSTF
- Concludes that the evidence is insufficient to recommend for or against routine behavioral counseling to promote a healthy diet in **unselected** patients in primary care settings
- Found good evidence that medium- to high-intensity counseling interventions can produce important changes in average daily intake of core components of a healthy diet (including saturated fat, fiber, fruit, and vegetables) among **adults at increased risk** for diet-related chronic disease

- Effective interventions combine nutrition education with behaviorally-oriented counseling to help patients acquire the skills, motivation, and support needed to alter their daily eating patterns and food preparation practices
- Two approaches appear promising to the general population of adult patients in primary care settings
  - ✓ Medium-intensity face-to-face dietary counseling (2-3 group or individual sessions) delivered by a specially trained primary care physician or nurse practitioner, a dietitian, or nutritionist
  - ✓ Lower-intensity interventions that involve 5 minutes or less of primary care provider counseling supplemented by self-help materials, telephone counseling, or other interactive health communications
  - ✓ Little is known about effective dietary counseling for children or adolescents in the primary care settings as research is lacking in that area

(Continued)

14

Summary of Recommendations	Clinical Considerations

III. Chemoprevention Recommendations

Use of Postmenopausal Hormone Replacement Therapy–Update

The USPSTF

- Recommends against the routine use of estrogen and progestin for the prevention of chronic diseases in postmenopausal women
- Found fair to good evidence that the combination of estrogen and progestin has both benefits and harms
  - ↑ Benefits include
    - ✓ Increased bone mineral density
    - ✓ Reduced risk for fracture
    - ✓ Reduced risk for colorectal cancer
  - ↑ Harms include increased risk for
    - ✓ Breast cancer
    - ✓ Venous thromboembolism
    - ✓ Coronary heart disease
    - ✓ Stroke
    - ✓ Cholecystitis
- Concludes that evidence was insufficient to assess the effects of hormone replacement therapy (HRT) on other important outcomes such as dementia and cognitive function, ovarian cancer, mortality from breast cancer or cardiovascular disease, or all-cause mortality
- Did not review the evidence for the use of HRT to relieve the symptoms of menopause, such as hot flashes, urogenital symptoms, and mood and sleep disturbances, as such a review was considered outside the scope of these recommendations
- Concludes that the evidence is insufficient to recommend for or against the use of unopposed estrogen for the prevention of chronic conditions in postmenopausal women who have had a hysterectomy

- Clinicians should develop a shared decision-making approach to preventing chronic diseases in perimenopausal and postmenopausal women with a focus on individual risk factors and patient preferences in selecting effective interventions for reducing the risk for fracture, heart disease, and cancer
- Refer to the section on MENOPAUSE for counseling women regarding the pros and cons of using HRT for the management of menopausal symptoms

Chemoprevention of Breast Cancer–New

The USPSTF

- Recommends against the routine use of tamoxifen or raloxifene for the primary prevention of breast cancer in women at low or average risk for breast cancer
- Recommends that clinicians discuss chemoprevention with women at high risk for breast cancer and at low risk for adverse effects of chemoprevention

- Risks for breast cancer include older age, a family history of breast cancer in a first-degree relative, a history of atypical hyperplasia on a breast biopsy are the strongest risk factors
- Risk factor information can be used to estimate the risk for breast cancer within the next 5 years by completing the US National Cancer Institute Breast Cancer Risk Tool (the Gail model, available at http://cancer.gov/bcrisktool)
- In general, the balance of benefits and harms of chemoprevention is more favorable for (1) women in their 40s who are at increased risk for breast cancer and have no predisposition to thromboembolic events, and (2) women in their 50s who are at increased risk for breast cancer with no predisposition to thromboembolic events, and who do not have a uterus

(Continued)

NEW RECOMMENDATIONS BY THE THIRD US PREVENTIVE SERVICES TASK FORCE: A SUMMARY (*CONTINUED*)

Summary of Recommendations	Clinical Considerations
Aspirin for the Primary Prevention of Cardiovascular Events–*Update*	• Decisions about aspirin therapy should take into account risk for CHD. Risk assessment includes asking about presence and severity of the following risk factors: age, sex, diabetes, elevated total cholesterol levels, low levels of HDL cholesterol, elevated blood pressure, family history (in younger adults) and smoking
The USPSTF	• Tools that incorporate information on multiple risk factors (http://www.intmed.mcw.edu/clincalc/heartrisk.html) provide more accurate estimation of cardiovascular risks than counting numbers of risk factors
• Strongly recommends that clinicians discuss aspirin chemoprevention with adults who are at increased risk for coronary heart disease (CHD)	• Men older than 40 years, postmenopausal women, and younger people with increased risk factors for coronary heart disease (e.g., hypertension, diabetes, or smoking) are at increased risk for heart disease and may wish to consider aspirin therapy
• The balance of benefits and harms is most favorable in patients at high risk of CHD (5-year risk ≥3%) but is also influenced by patient preferences	• Although the optimal timing and frequency of discussions related to aspirin therapy are unknown, reasonable options include every 5 years in middle-aged and older people or when other cardiovascular risk factors are detected
	• Optimal dose of aspirin for chemoprevention is not known–doses of approximately 75 mg per day appear as effective as higher doses (e.g., 100 mg per day or 325 mg every other day)
	• Enteric-coated or buffered preparations do not clearly reduce adverse gastrointestinal effects of aspirin; uncontrolled hypertension and concomitant use of other nonsteroidal anti-inflammatory agents or anticoagulants increase risk for serious bleeding

* The complete recommendations and rationale statements, evidence summaries, and the Systematic Evidence Reviews are also available at the US Preventive Services Task Force Web site (www.ahrq.gov/clinic/uspstfis.htm)

Recommended Adult Immunization Schedule, United States, 2002-2003

| | For all persons in this group | | Catch-up on childhood vaccinations | | For persons with medical / exposure indications |

Age Group ► / Vaccine ▼	19-49 Years	50-64 Years	65 Years and Older
Tetanus, Diphtheria (Td)*	1 dose booster every 10 years[1]		
Influenza	1 dose annually for persons with medical or occupational indications, or household contacts of persons with indications [2]	1 annual dose	
Pneumococcal (polysaccharide)	1 dose annually for persons with medical or occupational indications. (1 dose revaccination for immunosuppressive conditions) [3,4]		1 dose for unvaccinated persons[3] / 1 dose revaccination[4]
Hepatitis B*	3 doses (0, 1-2, 4-6 months) for persons with medical, behavioral, occupational, or other indications [5]		
Hepatitis A	2 doses (0, 6-12 months) for persons with medical, behavioral, occupational, or other indications [6]		
Measles, Mumps, Rubella (MMR)*	1 dose if MMR vaccination history is unreliable; 2 doses for persons with occupational or other indications [7]		
Varicella*	2 doses (0, 4-8 weeks) for persons who are susceptible [8]		
Meningococcal (polysaccharide)	1 dose for persons with medical or other indications [9]		

See Footnotes for Recommended Adult Immunization Schedule, United States, 2002-2003 on next page.

* Covered by the Vaccine Injury Compensation Program. For information on how to file a claim, call 800-338-2382 or visit http://www.hrsa.osp.gov/vicp. To file a claim for vaccine injury, write: US Court of Federal Claims, 717 Madison Place, N.W., Washington D.C. 20005 or call 202-219-9657.

This schedule indicates the recommended age groups for routine administration of currently licensed vaccines for persons 19 years of age and older. Licensed combination vaccines may be used whenever any components of the combination are indicated and the vaccine's other components are not contraindicated. Providers should consult the manufacturers' package inserts for detailed recommendations.

Report all clinically significant post-vaccination reactions to the Vaccine Adverse Event Reporting System (VAERS). Reporting forms and instructions on filing a VAERS report are available by calling 800-822-7967 or from the VAERS Website at www.vaers.org.

For additional information about the vaccines listed above and contraindications for immunization, visit the National Immunization Program Website at www.cdc.gov/nip/ or call the National Immunization Hotline at 800-232-2522 (English) or 800-232-0233 (Spanish).

Approved by the Advisory Committee on Immunization Practices (ACIP), and accepted by the American College of Obstectricians and Gynecologists (ACOG) and the American Academy of Family Physicians (AAFP).

1.   **Tetanus and diphtheria (Td)** – A primary series for adults is 3 doses: the first 2 doses given at least 4 weeks apart and the 3rd dose, 6-12 months after the second. Administer 1 dose if the person had received the primary series and the last vaccination was 10 years ago or longer. *MMWR* 1991; 40 (RR-10): 1-21. The ACP Task Force on Adult Immunization supports a second option: a single Td booster at age 50 years for persons who have completed the full pediatric series, including the teenage/young adult booster. *Guide for Adult Immunization.* 3rd ed. ACP 1004:20.

2.   **Influenza vaccination** – Medical indications: chronic disorders of the cardiovascular or pulmonary systems including asthma; chronic metabolic diseases including diabetes mellitus, renal dysfunction, hemoglobinopathies, immunosuppression (including immunosuppression caused by medications of by human immunodeficiency virus[HIV]) requiring regular medical follow-up or hospitalization during the preceding year; women who will be in the 2nd or 3rd trimester of pregnancy during the influenza season. Occupational indications: health-care workers. Other indications: residents of nursing homes and other long-term care facilities; persons likely to transmit influenza to persons a thigh-risk (in-home care givers to persons with medical indications, household contacts and out-of-home caregivers of children birth to 23 months of age, or children with asthma or other indicator conditions for influenza vaccination, household members and caregivers of elderly and adults with high-risk conditions); and anyone who wishes to be vaccinated. *MMWR* 2002; 51 (RR-3): 1-31.

3.   **Pneumococcal polysaccharide vaccination** – Medical indications: chronic disorders of the pulmonary system (excluding asthma), cardiovascular diseases, diabetes mellitus, chronic liver diseases including liver disease as a result of alcohol abuse (e.g., cirrhosis), chronic renal failure or nephritic syndrome, functional or anatomic asplenia (e.g., sickle cell disease or splenectomy), immunosuppressive conditions (e.g., congenital immunodeficiency, HIV infection, leukemia, lymphoma, multiple myeloma, Hodgkin's disease, generalized malignancy, organ or bone marrow transplantation), chemotherapy with alkylating agents, anti-metabolites, or long-term systemic corticosteroids. Geographic/other indications: Alaskan Natives and certain American Indian populations. Other indications: residents of nursing homes and other long-term care facilities. MMWR 1997; 47 (RR-8): 1-24.

4.   **Revaccination with pneumococcal polysaccharide vaccine** – One-time revaccination after 5 years for persons with chronic renal failure or nephritic syndrome, functional or anatomic asplenia (e.g., sickle cell disease or splenectomy), immunosuppressive conditions (e.g., congenital immunodeficiency, HIV infection, leukemia, lymphoma, multiple myeloma, Hodgkin's disease, generalized malignancy, organ or bone marrow transplantation), chemotherapy with alkylating agents, anti-metabolites, or long-term systemic corticosteroids. For persons 65 and older, one-time revaccination if they were vaccinated 5 or more years previously and were aged less than 65 years at the time of primary vaccination. MMWR 1997; 47 (RR-8): 1-24.

5.   **Hepatitis B vaccination** – Medical indications: hemodialysis patients, patients who receive clotting-factor concentrates. Occupational indications: healthcare workers and public-safety workers who have exposure to blood in the workplace, persons in training in schools of medicine, dentistry, nursing, laboratory technology, and other allied health professions. Behavioral indications: injecting drug users, persons with more than one sex partner in the previous 6 months, persons with a recently acquired sexually-transmitted disease (STD), all clients in STD clinics, men who have sex with men. Other indications: household contacts and sex partners of persons with chronic HBV infection, clients and staff of institutions for the developmentally disabled, international travelers who will be in countries with high or intermediate prevalence of chronic HBV infection for more than 6 months, inmates of correctional facilities. *MMWR* 1991; 40 (RR-13): 1-25. (www.cdc.gov/travel/diseases/hbv.htm)

6.   **Hepatitis A vaccination** – For the combined HepA-HepB vaccine use 3 doses at 0, 1, 6 months. Medical indications: persons with clotting-factor disorders or chronic liver disease. Behavioral indications: men who have sex with men, users of injecting and non-injecting illegal drugs. Occupational indications: persons working with HAV-infected primates or with HAV in a research laboratory setting. Other indications: persons traveling to or working in countries that have high or intermediate endemicity of hepatitis A. *MMWR* 1999; 48 (RR-12): 1-37. (www.cdc.gov/travel/diseases/hbv.htm)

7.   **Measles, Mumps, Rubella vaccination (MMR)** – Measles component: Adults born prior to 1957 may be considered to be immune to measles. Give 2 doses of MMR for adults with one or more of the following conditions and without vaccination history:

        ✓   adults born after 1956
        ✓   persons vaccinated with killed measles virus vaccine 1963-1969
        ✓   students in post-secondary education institutions
        ✓   healthcare workers
        ✓   susceptible international travelers to measles endemic countries

Mumps component: 1 dose of MMR should be adequate for protection. Rubella component: Give 1 dose of MMR to women whose rubella vaccination history is unreliable and counsel women to avoid becoming pregnant for 4 weeks after vaccination. For women of child-bearing age, regardless of birth year, routinely determine rubella immunity and counsel women regarding congenital rubella syndrome. Do not vaccinate pregnant women or those planning to become pregnant in the next 4 weeks. If pregnant and susceptible, vaccinate as early in postpartum period as possible. *MMWR* 1998; 47 (RR-8): 1-57.

8.   **Varicella vaccination** – Recommended for all persons who do not have reliable clinical history of varicella infection, or serological evidence of varicella zoster virus (VZV) infection; healthcare workers and family contacts of immunocompromised persons, those who live or work in environments where transmission is likely (e.g., teachers of young children, daycare employees, and residents and staff members in institutional settings), persons who live or work in environments where VZV transmission can occur (e.g., college students, inmates, and staff members of correctional institutions, and military personnel), adolescents and adults living in households with children, women who are not pregnant but who may become pregnant in the future, international travelers who are not immune to infection. **Note:** Greater than 90% of US born adults are immune to VZV. Do not vaccinate pregnant women or those planning to become pregnant in the next 4 weeks. If pregnant and susceptible, vaccinate as early in postpartum period as possible. *MMWR* 1996; 45 (RR-11): 1-36, *MMWR* 1999; 48 (RR-6): 1-5.

9.   **Meningococcal vaccine (quadrivalent polysaccharide for serogroups A, C, Y, and W-135)** – Consider vaccination for persons with medical indications: adults with terminal complement component deficiencies, with anatomic or functional asplenia. Other indications: travelers to countries in which disease is hyperendemic or epidemic ("meningitis belt" of sub-Saharan Africa; Mecca, Saudi Arabia for Hajj). Revaccination at 3-5 years may be indicated for persons at high risk for infection (e.g., persons residing in areas in which disease is epidemic). Counsel college freshmen, especially those who live in dormitories, regarding meningococcal disease and the vaccine so that they can make an educated decision about receiving the vaccination. *MMWR* 2000; 49)RR-7): 1-20.

Note: The AAFP recommends that colleges should take the lead on providing education on meningococcal infection and vaccination and offer it to those who are interested. Physicians need not initiate discussion of the meningococcal quadrivalent polysaccharide vaccine as part of routine medical care.

NUTRITION

I. Goals of nutrition are (1) to attain intakes of sufficient levels of essential dietary nutrients; (2) to consume a diet associated with reduced risk of chronic disease, and; (3) to maintain a balance between energy intake and physical activity

    A. A healthy weight for adults of both genders and all age groups is a BMI of 18.5 to 24.9

    B. More than 60% of adults in the US are classified as obese, making obesity the most serious and prevalent nutritional disorder in the US

II. The Food and Nutrition Board, Institute of Medicine, The National Academies, recently set forth reference values for specific nutrients with the development of Dietary Reference Intakes (DRIs), the collective term for four categories subsumed under the DRIs

    A. DRIs have been established using an expanded concept that includes indicators of good health and the prevention of chronic disease, as well as possible effects of overconsumption

    B. Thus, DRIs provide a more comprehensive approach to nutrition adequacy than the periodic reports called Recommended Dietary Allowances (RDAs) [now one of 4 categories encompassed by DRIs] set forth by the Food and Nutrition Board for over 50 years

    C. DRI categories are defined in the table below

DIETARY REFERENCE INTAKES

➡ Recommended Dietary Allowance (RDA): The average daily dietary nutrient intake level sufficient to meet nutrient requirement of nearly all (97% to 98%) healthy individuals in a particular life stage and gender group

➡ Adequate Intake (AI): The recommended average daily intake level based on observed or experimentally determined estimates of nutrient intakes by a group of healthy people that are assumed to be adequate–used when an RDA cannot be determined

➡ Tolerable Upper Intake Level (UL): The highest average daily nutrient intake level that is likely to pose no risk of adverse effects to almost all individuals in a general population

➡ Estimated Average Requirement (EAR): The average daily nutrient intake level estimated to meet the requirements of half the healthy individuals in a particular life stage and gender group*

---

*In the case of energy, an Estimated Energy Requirement (EER) is provided; it is the average dietary energy intake that is predicted to maintain energy balance in a healthy adult of a defined age, gender, weight, height, and level of physical activity consistent with good health

Adapted from Institute of Medicine, Food and Nutrition Board, The National Academies. (2002). *Dietary reference intakes: Energy, carbohydrate, fiber, fat, fatty acids, cholesterol, protein, and amino acids, part 2*. (Prepublication copy, unedited proofs). Washington, DC: National Academies Press.

III. Energy is required to sustain the body's various functions, including respiration, circulation, physical work, and protein synthesis; this energy is supplied by carbohydrates, proteins, and fats in the diet

    A. Carbohydrates (sugars and starches) provide energy to cells in the body, particularly the brain which is the only carbohydrate-dependent organ in the body

        1. RDA for carbohydrate is set at 130 g/day for adults based on the average minimum amount of glucose utilized by the brain (this level is typically exceeded to meet the energy needs while consuming acceptable levels of fat and protein)

        2. The median intake of carbohydrates is approximately 200 to 330 g/day for men and 180 to 230 g/day for women

        3. Because of a lack of sufficient evidence on the prevention of chronic diseases in generally healthy individuals, no recommendations based on glycemic index of carbohydrate-containing foods are made (see section on DIABETES MELLITUS for more information on the glycemic index)

        4. The current Food Pyramid–the food guide for the US–will be revised in 2003; some experts believe that the glycemic index (a quantification of the relative blood glucose response to carbohydrate containing foods) will be an important consideration in the placement of food groups within the new pyramid

B. Fats are a major source of fuel energy for the body and aid in the absorption of fat-soluble vitamins and other food components such as carotenoids

    1. For adults, neither AI nor RDA for fat has been set as there are insufficient data to determine a defined level of fat intake at which risk of inadequacy or prevention of chronic disease occurs (Acceptable Macronutrient Distribution Ranges [AMDRs], however, have been estimated for total fat and are contained in the box below)

    2. Saturated fatty acids, monounsaturated fatty acids, and cholesterol are synthesized by the body and are not required in the diet

C. Proteins form the major structural components of all the cells of the body; along with amino acids (dietary components of protein), they function as enzymes, membrane carriers, and hormones

    1. Nine amino acids are indispensable and thus dietary sources must be provided

    2. RDA for adults is 0.8 g/kg/day of good quality protein

D. Because carbohydrate, fat, and protein all serve as energy sources and can substitute for one another to some extent to meet caloric needs, the recommended ranges for consuming these nutrients should be useful and flexible for dietary planning; ranges for fat, carbohydrate, and protein illustrate the principle that these nutrients must be considered together

E. The Acceptable Macronutrient Distribution Ranges (AMDRs) for adults are estimated and represented as percent of energy intake

    1. These ranges represent the following: Intakes that are associated with reduced risk of chronic disease; intakes at which essential dietary nutrients can be consumed at sufficient levels, and intakes based on adequate energy intake and physical activity to maintain energy balance

    2. The AMDRs are contained in the box below

	Fat	Carbohydrate	Protein
Adults	20-35%	45-65%	10-35%

Adapted from Institute of Medicine, Food and Nutrition Board, The National Academies. (2002). *Dietary reference intakes: Energy, carbohydrate, fiber, fat, fatty acids, cholesterol, protein, and amino acids*, part 2. (Prepublication copy, unedited proofs). Washington, DC: National Academies Press.

IV. A growing body of evidence indicates that chronic consumption of a low-fat/high-carbohydrate or high-fat/low-carbohydrate diet may result in the inadequate intake of certain essential nutrients leading to adverse health effects

A. In the past few decades, the prevalence of overweight and obesity among both children and adults has increased at an alarming rate in the US

B. There are two issues to consider for the distribution of fat and carbohydrate in high-risk populations—distributions that predispose to the development of overweight/obesity, and those that worsen the metabolic consequences in populations that are already overweight or obese

---

Consequences of Low-Fat/High-Carbohydrate Diet (Outside the AMDRs) of Adults

➡ In isocaloric diets (energy intake is stable), when fat intakes are low and carbohydrate intakes are high, there is a reduction in plasma HDL cholesterol concentration, an increase in the plasma total cholesterol:HDL cholesterol ratio, and an increase in plasma triacylglycerol concentration; called the **atherogenic lipoprotein phenotype,** this pattern of intake is consistent with an increased risk of CHD

➡ In populations such as those in rural Asia and Africa that are routinely physically active and lean, the atherogenic lipoprotein phenotype is minimally expressed

➡ On the other hand, in sedentary populations that tend to be overweight or obese as in the US, very low-fat/high-carbohydrate diets clearly promote the development of this phenotype

Consequences of High-Fat/Low-Carbohydrate Diet (Outside the AMDRs) of Adults

➡ Individuals have a difficult time maintaining an isocaloric diet when fat intake is high for several reasons

➡ Foods containing high amounts of fat tend to be "energy dense"

➡ Taste is the primary influence for food choice, and high energy density foods are often more palatable than foods low in energy density and thus such foods tend to be overeaten, thereby promoting weight gain which increases risk for CHD

➡ Relationship between fat intake and CHD is related more to the quality of fat than to the quantity; populations that consume diets that are high in total fat and unsaturated fatty acids but low in saturated fatty acids have rates of CHD that are relatively low

➡ When fat is consumed in typical foods, it contains a mixture of saturated, polyunsaturated, and monounsaturated fatty acids; it is difficult to avoid high intakes of saturated fatty acids for most persons if total fat intake exceeds 35% of total energy

V.   The Food Guide Pyramid, which is the food guide for the US, translates recommendations on nutrient intake into recommendations for food intakes

A.   Encourage patients to use the Food Guide Pyramid to guide their food choices
1.   Remind patients to use plant foods as the foundation of meals
2.   Whereas there are many ways to create a healthy eating pattern, they all start with the three food groups at the base of the pyramid–grains, fruits, and vegetables

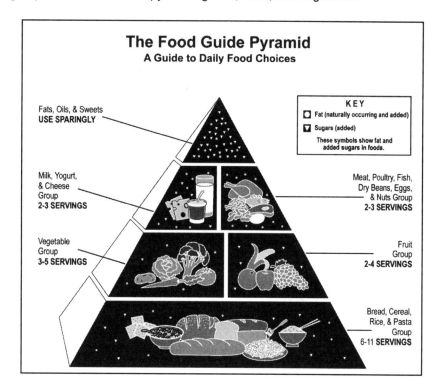

Figure 1.2. Food Guide Pyramid - Adults
Source: US Department of Agriculture/US Department of Health and Human Services. (2000). *Nutrition and your health: Dietary guidelines for Americans.* Washington, DC: Author, p. 15.

B.   The recommended ranges of daily servings from each of the five major food groups for both genders and all age groups are contained in the table below

HOW MANY SERVINGS ARE NEEDED EACH DAY?			
Food Group	Women, some older adults (about 1,600 calories)	Active women, most men (about 2,200 calories)	Active men (about 2,800 calories)
Grains Group: Bread, cereal, rice and pasta group – especially whole grain	6	9	11
Vegetable Group	3	4	5
Fruit Group	2	3	4
Milk Group: Milk, yogurt, and cheese – preferably fat free or low fat	2 or 3*	2 or 3*	2 or 3*
Meat and Beans Group: Meat, poultry, fish, dry beans, eggs and nuts – preferably lean or low fat	2, for a total of 5 ounces	2, for a total of 6 ounces	3, for a total of 7 ounces

* The number of servings depends on one's age. Adults >50 years need 3 servings daily. Others need 2 servings daily. During pregnancy and lactation, the recommended number of milk group servings is the same as for nonpregnant women

C. Point out to patients that most commonly available food portions exceed the USDA's standard portion sizes; this trend is part of the "supersizing" phenomenon first seen at fast food establishments. Unfortunately, there has also been a shift to larger portion sizes in the foods consumed at home—a shift that indicates marked changes in eating behavior in general

    1. Over the past two decades, food portion sizes have increased both inside and outside the home for the following categories: Salty snacks—increased from l.0 to 1.6 oz; soft drinks—from 13.1 to 19.9 fl oz; hamburgers—from 5.7 to 7.0 oz; french fries—from 3.1 to 3.6 oz, and; Mexican food—from 6.3 to 8.0 ounces

    2. Counsel patients that there is a marked trend toward larger portion sizes in the US, and to consider the impact of these increases in their attempts to maintain a healthy weight; the exact contribution of portion size changes to the increases in overweight and obesity in US has not yet been determined

    3. The quantity of food being consumed is just as important as what foods are consumed; use the table below *"What Counts As A Serving?"* to help guide patients in their choices and point out that standard portion sizes are quite small. For example, one serving of meat is about the size of a deck of cards

---

WHAT COUNTS AS A SERVING?

Grains Group: Bread, Cereal, Rice and Pasta – whole grain and refined:
- 1 slice of bread
- About 1 cup of ready-to-eat cereal
- 1/2 cup of cooked cereal, rice, or pasta

Vegetable Group:
- 1 cup of raw leafy vegetables
- 1/2 cup of other vegetables – cooked or raw
- 3/4 cup of vegetable juice

Fruit Group:
- 1 medium apple, banana, orange, pear
- 1/2 cup of chopped, cooked, or canned fruit
- 3/4 cup of fruit juice

Milk Group:* Milk, Yogurt and Cheese:
- 1 cup milk** or yogurt**
- 1 ½ ounces of natural cheese** (such as Cheddar)
- 2 ounces of processed cheese** (such as American)

Meat and Beans Group: Meat, Poultry, Dry Beans, Eggs, and Nuts:
- 2-3 ounces of cooked lean meat, poultry, or fish
- 1/2 cup of cooked dry beans[#] or 1/2 cup of tofu counts as 1 ounce of lean meat
- 2 ½-ounce soyburger or 1 egg counts as 1 ounce of lean meat
- 2 tablespoons of peanut butter or 1/3 cup of nuts counts as 1 ounce of meat

---

Note: Many of the serving sizes given above are smaller than those on the Nutrition Facts Label. For example, 1 serving of cooked cereal, rice, or pasta is 1 cup for the label but only ½ cup for the Pyramid

* This includes lactose-free and lactose-reduced milk products. One cup of soy-based beverage with added calcium is an option for those who prefer a non-dairy source of calcium

** Choose fat-free or reduced-fat dairy products most often

[#] Dry beans, peas, and lentils can be counted as servings in either the meat and beans group or the vegetable group. As a vegetable, ½ cup of cooked, dry beans counts as 1 serving. As a meat substitute, 1 cup of cooked, dry beans counts as 1 serving (2 ounces of meat)

Source: US Department of Agriculture/US Department of Health and Human Services. (2000). *Nutrition and your health: Dietary guidelines for Americans*. Washington, DC: Author, p. 14-15.

D. Assist patients/parents to increase their intake of whole grain foods by recommending liberal use of the foods in the table below

---

WAYS TO INCREASE INTAKE OF WHOLE GRAIN FOODS

Counsel patients/parents to choose foods that name one of the following ingredients first on the label's ingredient list

• Brown rice	• Oatmeal	• Whole oats
• Bulgur (cracked wheat)	• Popcorn	• Whole rye
• Graham flour	• Pearl barley	• Whole wheat

Encourage patients to try some of these whole grain foods: whole wheat bread, whole grain ready-to-eat cereal, low-fat whole wheat crackers, oatmeal, whole wheat pasta, whole barley in soup, tabouli salad

---

Adapted from US Department of Agriculture/US Department of Health and Human Services. (2000). *Nutrition and your health: Dietary guidelines for Americans*. Washington, DC: Author, p. 20.

E. Consuming a variety of fruits and vegetables each day provides essential vitamins, minerals, fiber, and other substances that are important to good health (most people eat fewer servings of fruits and vegetables than are recommended); assist patients/parents to select a variety of fruits and vegetables such as those featured in the box below

---

Which Fruits and Vegetables Provide the Most Nutrients?

Sources of vitamin A (carotenoids)
- Orange vegetables like carrots, sweet potatoes, pumpkin
- Dark-green leafy vegetables such as spinach, collards, turnip greens
- Orange fruits like mango, cantaloupe, apricots
- Tomatoes

Sources of vitamin C
- Citrus fruits and juices, kiwi fruit, strawberries, cantaloupe
- Broccoli, peppers, tomatoes, cabbage, potatoes
- Leafy greens such as romaine lettuce, turnip greens, spinach

Sources of folate
- Cooked dry beans and peas, peanuts
- Oranges, orange juice
- Dark-green leafy vegetables like spinach and mustard greens, romaine lettuce
- Green peas

Sources of potassium
- Baked white or sweet potato, cooked greens (such as spinach), winter (orange) squash
- Bananas, plantains, dried fruits such as apricots and prunes, orange juice
- Cooked dry beans (such as baked beans) and lentils

Adapted from US Department of Agriculture/US Department of Health and Human Services. (2000). *Nutrition and your health: Dietary guidelines for Americans.* Washington, DC: Author, p. 22.

F. Women and older adults have higher needs for some minerals, specifically calcium and iron
   1. Adults >50 years of age have an especially high need for calcium (most people need to eat plenty of good sources of calcium for healthy bones throughout life); see the box below for some sources of calcium to recommend to patients
   2. Women of childbearing age need enough good sources of iron; see the box below for recommendations

---

Some Sources of Calcium	**Some Sources of Iron**
• Yogurt	• Shellfish like shrimp, clams, mussels, and oysters
• Milk	• Lean meats (especially beef), liver, and other organ meats
• Natural cheeses such as Mozzarella, Cheddar, Swiss, and Parmesan	• Ready-to-eat cereals with added iron
• Soy-based beverage with added calcium	• Turkey dark meat (remove skin to reduce fat)
• Tofu, if made with calcium sulfate (read the ingredient list)	• Sardines
• Breakfast cereal with added calcium	• Spinach
• Canned fish with soft bones such as salmon, sardines	• Cooked dry beans (such as kidney beans and pinto beans), peas (such as black-eyed peas), and lentils
• Fruit juice with added calcium	• Enriched and whole grain breads
• Dark-green leafy vegetables such as collards, turnip greens	

Adapted from US Department of Agriculture/US Department of Health and Human Services. (2000). *Nutrition and your health: Dietary guidelines for Americans.* Washington, DC: Author, p. 17.

G. Encourage patients to choose a diet that is low in saturated fat and cholesterol and within the AMDR range; use recommendations based on content in boxes below to counsel patients
   1. Many experts believe that there should be a differentiation between the types of fats rather than lumping them together and placing them at the pinnacle of the Food Pyramid in the "use sparingly" category
   2. Revisions of the Food Pyramid are expected in 2003; unsaturated fats (from plant sources and some fish) may be removed from the "use sparingly" category and placed closer to the base in the new pyramid

Different Types of Fats

Saturated Fats
Foods high in saturated fats tend to raise blood cholesterol. These foods include high-fat dairy products (like cheese, whole milk, cream, butter, and regular ice cream), fatty fresh and processed meats, the skin and fat of poultry, lard, palm oil, and coconut oil. Intake of these foods should be kept low

Dietary Cholesterol
Foods that are high in cholesterol also tend to raise blood cholesterol—examples are liver and other organ meats, egg yolks, and dairy fats

Trans Fatty Acids
Foods high in *trans* fatty acids increase total and LDL cholesterol concentrations in the blood and therefore the risk of CHD; even very low intakes may increase risk. These foods include those high in partially hydrogenated vegetable oils, such as many hard margarines and shortenings. Foods with a high amount of these ingredients include many commercially fried foods and bakery goods (**Note**: The FDA recently mandated that *trans* fat [also known as *trans* fatty acids] be included on the Nutrition Facts Panel on food labels; it will be listed on a separate line from saturated fat on the nutrition label)

Unsaturated Fats
- Unsaturated fats (oils) do not raise blood cholesterol. Unsaturated fats occur in vegetable oils, most nuts, olives, avocados, and fatty fish like salmon. Unsaturated oils include both *monounsaturated fats* and *polyunsaturated fats*. Olive, canola, sunflower, and peanut oils are some of the oils high in monounsaturated fats. Vegetable oils such as soybean oil, corn oil, and cottonseed oil and many kinds of nuts are good sources of polyunsaturated fats
- Current dietary guidelines recommend consumption of fish high in omega-3 fatty acids twice weekly to prevent coronary heart disease. Good fish sources of omega-3s include salmon, bluefish, mackerel, arctic char, and sardines. For convenience, canned salmon, sardines, and herring can also be used as these products also contain high amounts of omega-3s (canned tuna contains lesser amounts)
- For an added bonus of calcium, encourage patients to eat the bones in canned sardines, salmon, and mackerel (bones are softened during cooking). For patients on salt-restricted diets, remind them that canned fish has ten times the amount of sodium as fresh fish and draining and rinsing fish in colander removes only a fair amount of salt

Food Choices Low in Saturated Fat and Cholesterol and Moderate in Total Fat

Advise patients to get most of their calories from plant foods (grains, fruits, vegetables). Counsel patients as follows:

Fats and Oils
- Choose vegetable oils rather than solid fats (meat and dairy fats, shortening)
- Decrease the amount of fat you use in cooking and at the table

Meat, Poultry, Fish, Shellfish, Eggs, Beans, and Nuts
- Choose 2-3 servings of fish, shellfish, lean poultry, other lean meats, beans or nuts daily. Trim fat from meat and take skin off poultry. Choose dry beans, peas, or lentils often
- Limit intake of high-fat processed meats such as bacon, sausages, salami, bologna, and other cold cuts. Try the lower fat varieties (check the Nutrition Facts Label)
- Limit intake of liver and other organ meats. Use egg yolks and whole eggs in moderation. Use egg whites and egg substitutes freely when cooking since they contain no cholesterol and little or no fat

Dairy Products
- Choose fat-free or low-fat milk, fat-free or low-fat yogurt, and low-fat cheese most often. Try switching from whole to fat-free or low-fat milk. This decreases the saturated fat and calories but keeps all other nutrients the same

Prepared Foods
- Check the Nutrition Facts Label to see how much saturated fat and cholesterol are in a serving of prepared food. Choose foods lower in saturated fat, cholesterol, and trans fats

Foods at Restaurants or Other Eating Establishments
- Choose fish or lean meats as suggested above. Limit ground meat and fatty processed meats, marbled steaks, and cheese
- Limit intake of foods with creamy sauces, and add little or no butter to food
- Choose fruit as dessert most often

Adapted from US Department of Agriculture/US Department of Health and Human Services. (2000). *Nutrition and your health: Dietary guidelines for Americans*. Washington, DC: Author, p. 28-29.

H. The Institute of Medicine has recently developed definitions for fiber (Dietary, Functional, and Total Fiber) and established Adequate Intakes (AI) for Total Fiber
1. Dietary Fiber is defined as nondigestible food plant carbohydrates and lignin (polymer found within "woody" plant walls) in which the plant matrix is largely intact; such sources of fiber also contain macronutrients (e.g., carbohydrate and protein such as in cereal brans) normally found in foods
2. Functional Fiber consists of isolated, nondigestible carbohydrates that have beneficial physiological effects in humans; included in this category are animal-derived carbohydrates such as connective tissue that are generally regarded as nondigestible
3. Total Fiber is the sum of Dietary and Functional Fibers
4. Benefits of fiber as well as the AI recommendations for Total Fiber are contained in the box below

Benefits of Fiber and Adequate Intake (AI) for Total Fiber
• Viscous fibers delay the gastric emptying of ingested foods into small intestine, which can result in a sensation of fullness (satiety)
• Delayed emptying effect also results in reduced postprandial blood glucose concentrations
• Viscous fibers can also interfere with the absorption of dietary fat and cholesterol as well as the enterohepatic recirculation of cholesterol and bile acids, which may result in reduced blood cholesterol concentrations
• Consumption of dietary and certain functional fibers, particularly those that are poorly fermented, is known to improve fecal bulk, laxation, and ameliorate constipation
• Relationship of fiber intake to colon cancer is the subject of ongoing investigation

Adapted from Institute of Medicine, Food and Nutrition Board, The National Academies. (2002). *Dietary reference intakes: Energy, carbohydrate, fiber, fat, fatty acids, cholesterol, protein, and amino acids, part 1.* (Prepublication copy, unedited proofs). Washington, DC: National Academies Press, p. 7-1.

Total Fiber AI Recommendations for Adults	
Group	Adequate Intake
Men	
19-50 years	38 g/day
51-70+ years	30 g/day
Women	
19-50 years	25 g/day
51-70+ years	21 g/day

Adapted from Institute of Medicine, Food and Nutrition Board, The National Academies. (2002). *Dietary reference intakes: Energy, carbohydrate, fiber, fat, fatty acids, cholesterol, protein, and amino acids, part 1.* (Prepublication copy, unedited proofs). Washington, DC: National Academies Press, p. 7-36, 7-38.

I.   Help patients select foods high in fiber from examples in the box below

Bulking Up on Fiber: Advise patients as follows:	
Keep beans handy–probably the best source of fiber	Instead of drinking juice, eat the orange, grapefruit, or tomato
• Cook a package of dried beans and freeze in usable quantities	
• Canned beans are also a good source of fiber	Eat fruits and nuts for snacks
o B & M Baked Beans Vegetarian (½ c = 7 g)	• Medium apple with skin = 3.7 g
o Kidney beans, red (1 c = 13.1 g)	• Medium banana = 2.7 g
o Lima beans (½ c = 6.6 g)	• Dates, dried (10) = 6.2 g
	• Medium orange = 3 g
Look for "100% whole wheat" of "whole-grain bread"	• Pears, canned/juice pack (1 c = 4 g)
• Aim for bread with 2 or 3 g of fiber per slice	• Prunes, dried (10) = 6 g
	• Peanuts, dry roasted (1 oz) = 2.3 g
Choose high-fiber breakfast cereals	
• Kellogg's Raisin Bran (1 c = 8 g) or Post 100% Bran (1/3 c = 8 g)	Vegetables
• For patients who don't like the high-fiber brands, suggest they mix some high-fiber brands with their preferred cereal each morning	• Broccoli (½ c = 2.3 g)
	• Campbell's Chunky Vegetable Soup (1 c = 4 g)
Eat berries, a great source of fiber (1 c blueberries = 3.9 g)	• Carrots, raw (1 medium = 2.2 g)
	• Baked potato with skin (1 medium = 3.4 g)
	• Cabbage, red (½ c = 1.5 g)

J.   Added sugars are defined as sugars and syrups added to foods in processing or preparation, not the naturally occurring sugars in foods like fruit and milk (see p. 29 regarding consumption of high-fructose corn syrup [HFCS], a liquid sweetener added to many foods that supplies nearly 10% of all calories consumed by Americans)

1. Increased consumption of added sugars can result in decreased intakes of certain micronutrients when energy dense, nutrient-poor foods are chosen

2. in addition, increased consumption of added sugars contributes to overweight and obesity

3. Foods containing sugars and starches can promote tooth decay; frequent consumption of sugary foods/beverages between meals is more likely to harm teeth than eating the same foods at meals and then brushing

4. Naturally occurring sugars are primarily consumed from fruits and dairy products that also contain essential micronutrients

5. Added sugars are listed on the "Nutrition Facts Label" of foods under "Total Carbohydrate" as "Sugars"

6. Counsel patients to limit consumption of added sugars in foods and beverages (**Note**: The number one source of added sugars in the US diet is soft drinks)

K. Counsel patients to choose and prepare foods with less salt
1. Healthy child adults need to consume only small amounts of salt to meet their sodium needs (no more than 2400 mg of sodium per day) [one teaspoon of salt provides about 2,000 mg of sodium]
2. Eating too little salt is not generally a concern for healthy people (lowering salt intake is safe)
3. Explain to patients that their preference for salt may decrease if they gradually add less salt or salty seasonings to food over a period of time
4. Foods that are high in convenience (frozen dinners and carry-out foods) are usually also high in sodium
5. Use information in the box below to counsel patients/parents about ways to decrease salt intake

---

Ways to Decrease Salt Intake

- Choose fresh, plain frozen, or canned vegetables without added salt most often
- Choose fresh or frozen fish, shellfish, poultry, and lean beef most often
- Read the Nutrition Facts label to compare the amount of sodium in processed foods – such as frozen dinners, packaged mixes, cereals, cheese, breads, soups, salad dressings, and sauces
- Leave the salt shaker in a cupboard

- Look for labels that say "low-sodium." They contain 140 mg (about 5% of the Daily Value) or less of sodium per serving
- If you salt foods in cooking or at the table, add small amounts. Learn to use spices and herbs, rather than salt, to enhance the flavor of food
- Go easy on condiments such as soy sauce, ketchup, mustard, pickles, and olives – they can add a lot of salt to your food

---

Adapted from US Department of Agriculture/US Department of Health and Human Services. (2000). *Nutrition and your health: Dietary guidelines for Americans.* Washington, DC: Author, p. 33.

L. Counsel patients who drink alcohol to do so in moderation (see ALCOHOL PROBLEMS for definition of drinking in moderation)
1. Drinking in moderation can lower risk for coronary heart disease, mainly among men over age 45 and women over age 55
2. However, there are other more important factors that reduce the risk of heart disease which should be emphasized including physical activity, a healthy diet, avoidance of smoking, and maintenance of a healthy weight

VI. Physical inactivity is a major risk factor for development of obesity in children and adults

A. *Healthy People 2010* set a goal of a minimum of 30 minutes of moderate intensity physical activity most days of the week but other experts have concluded that 30 minutes per day of moderate activity is insufficient to maintain body weight in the healthy range and to achieve health benefits associated with physical activity

B. The Institute of Medicine (2002) recommends that adults engage in 60 minutes of daily moderate intensity physical activity (e.g. walking/jogging at 4-5 mph) in addition to the activities required by a sedentary lifestyle
1. Maintaining an active lifestyle provides an important means for individuals to balance food energy intake with total energy expenditure
2. Consult the section on OBESITY for specific counseling recommendations relating to physical activity and exercise

VII. Whereas vitamin deficiency is encountered infrequently in the US, suboptimal vitamin status is fairly common, particularly among some subgroups of the population

A. Populations at risk for suboptimal vitamin intake include the elderly, who tend to absorb vitamin B_{12} poorly and are often deficient in vitamin D; persons who regularly consume one or two alcohol drinks per day; poor urban dwellers who may be unable to afford adequate intakes of vegetables and fruit; vegans, who require supplemental vitamin B_{12}, and women who might become pregnant

B. Inadequate intake of certain vitamins is associated with increased risk of chronic disease in adults including cardiovascular disease, cancer, and osteoporosis as well as an increased risk of neural tube defects in women of childbearing age

Review of the Role of Vitamins in Chronic Disease Prevention in Adults

- Folate, vitamin B_6 and B_{12} have joint effects on lowering homocysteine levels; elevated plasma total homocysteine level is a major risk factor for coronary disease (persons with the highest homocysteine levels have an estimated 2-fold increase in risk of CHD compared with those with the lowest risk levels, an effect that is independent of other known risk factors)
- Folate deficiency can cause a macrocytic anemia and suboptimal intakes of the vitamin can cause fetal neural tube defects; folate is also believed to reduce the risk of colon and breast cancer
- Vitamin E enhances immune function and is believed to prevent atherosclerotic disease both by antioxidant effects and also through inhibitory effects on smooth muscle proliferation and platelet adhesion
- It has been proposed that beta carotene supplementation (vitamin A) could prevent cardiovascular disease and cancer because of its antioxidant effects, but thus far results from research studies have been disappointing
- Vitamin D supplementation decreases bone turnover and increases bone mineral density; in the elderly, supplementation with vitamin D and calcium reduces bone loss and fracture rates
- Vitamin C has a strong antioxidant effect; presently, it does not appear to be strongly associated with reduction in cardiovascular disease risk but there is moderately strong evidence that diets high in vitamin C are associated with decreased risk of some cancers
- Vitamin K is essential for normal clotting; supplementation with this vitamin may prevent fractures, but the evidence for this is only moderate

Adapted from Fairfield, K.M,, & Fletcher, R.H. (2002). Vitamins for chronic disease prevention in adults. *Journal of the American Medical Association, 287*, 3116-3126.

    C.   Many experts recommend a daily multivitamin for adults that does not exceed the current Reference Daily Intakes (RDIs) of its component vitamins at a typical cost of $20 to $40 per year; the RDIs for vitamins are contained in the box below

        1.   Counsel patients that vitamin supplements do not substitute for a healthy diet and should be used to supplement a healthy diet that may be suboptimal in some areas

        2.   Nutrition counseling is always the first line approach to correct inadequacies in dietary intake

Current Reference Daily Intakes for Vitamins	
Vitamin	**Daily Value**
Vitamin A	1500 µg/L (5000 IU)
Vitamin C	60 mg
Vitamin D	10 µg/L (400 IU)
Vitamin E	20 mg (30 IU)
Vitamin K	80 µg/L
Vitamin B_6	2 mg
Vitamin B_{12}	6 µg/L
Folate	400 µg/L
Thiamin	1.5 mg
Riboflavin	1.7 mg
Niacin	20 mg

Source: http://www.cc.nih.gov/ccc/supplements. Accessed September 10, 2002.

VIII.   The American Cancer Society (ACS) has made recommendations on the role of nutrition in cancer prevention

    A.   The ACS guidelines are consistent with guidelines from the American Heart Association for the prevention of coronary heart disease (see chapter on CARDIOVASCULAR PROBLEMS for more information), from the National Heart, Lung, and Blood Institute—the *DASH diet* to control hypertension (see section on HYPERTENSION), as well as those of the Department of Health and Human Services for health promotion in adults—the *2000 Dietary Guidelines for Americans*, described above

    B.   The ACS recommendations are contained in the tables that follow

AMERICAN CANCER SOCIETY'S RECOMMENDATIONS FOR CANCER PREVENTION

Overview

For most Americans who do not smoke cigarettes, dietary choices and physical activity are the most important modifiable determinants of cancer risk; up to 35% of the half million cancer deaths that occur in the US each year can be attributed to diet and physical activity behaviors, with another third due to cigarette smoking

Thus, most of the variation in cancer risk across populations and among individuals is due to factors that are *not inherited*; thus, consuming a healthy diet, staying physically active, and abstaining from tobacco use can substantially affect one's risk of developing cancer

Recommendation: *Eat a variety of healthy foods, with an emphasis on plant sources*

   ✓   Eat five or more servings of a variety of vegetables and fruits each day in various forms—fresh, frozen, canned, dried, and juiced

   ✓   Fried vegetables such as French fries and snack chips should be consumed in only small amounts if at all

Benefits of Vegetables and Fruits

- Greater consumption of vegetables and fruits is associated with a lower risk of lung, oral, esophageal, and stomach cancer
- Evidence is less strong for cancers considered hormonal, such as breast and prostate
- Exact components of vegetables and fruits that are most protective against cancer remain unclear—these are complex foods, each containing more than 100 potentially beneficial vitamins, minerals, fiber, and other substances that may help to prevent cancer
- Until is more is known about specific food components, the best advice is to eat 5 or more servings of a variety of vegetables and fruits each day

Recommendation: *Choose whole grain rice, bread, pasta, and cereals and limit consumption of refined carbohydrates*

Benefits of Whole Grains

- Whole grains are an important source of many vitamins and minerals such as folate, vitamin E, and selenium that have been associated with a lower risk of colon cancer
- Whole grains are also high in fiber and although the association between fiber and cancer risk is uncertain, consumption of high fiber foods is still recommended; it is best to obtain fiber from whole grains—and vegetables and fruits—rather than from fiber supplements

Recommendation: *Limit consumption of red and processed meats, especially those high in fat*

   ✓   Choose fish, poultry, or beans as an alternative to beef, pork, and lamb

   ✓   Use meat as a side dish instead of a main dish; prepare meat by baking, broiling, or poaching rather than frying or charbroiling to reduce the overall fat content

   ✓   Beans are particularly rich in nutrients and fiber, and are a low-fat, high-protein alternative to meat

   ✓   Choose low-fat dairy products and substitute vegetable oils for butter or solid shortening

Benefits of Legumes

- Beans are legumes, a family of plants that include dried beans, pinto beans, lentils, and soy beans, among others; they are an excellent source of many vitamins and minerals, protein, and fiber
- Beans are especially rich in nutrients that may protect against cancer

Meat, Dietary Fat, and Cancer Risk

- Foods from animal sources remain major contributors to total fat, saturated fat, and cholesterol in the US diet—high fat diets have been associated with an increase in the risk of cancers of the colon and rectum, prostate, and endometrium
- It is uncertain whether the association between high-fat diets and various cancers is due to the total amount of fat, the particular type of fat—saturated, monounsaturated, or polyunsaturated—the calories contributed by fat, or some other factor associated with high-fat foods
- Saturated fat in red meats, omega-3 fatty acids in fish oils, and monounsaturated fats in olive oil likely differ in their effects on cancer risk, and current research studies are attempting to uncover and classify those risks
- Meats are good sources of high-quality protein and can supply many important vitamins and minerals; nonetheless, consumption of meat—especially red meats (beef, pork, and lamb)—has been associated with cancers in many studies, most notably those of the colon and prostate

(Continued)

Recommendation: *Adopt a physically active lifestyle*

✓ Engage in at least moderate activity for 30 minutes or more on at least 5 days of the week; 45 minutes or more of moderate to vigorous activity on 5 or more days a week may further enhance reductions in the risk of breast and colon cancer (Note: See the Institute of Medicine's (IOMs) recommendations regarding physical activity (VI.B. above) in which 60 minutes of daily moderate intensity physical activity is recommended)

✓ The IOM recommendation does not mean that 30 minutes of physical activity per day is not beneficial—for most people, cardiovascular and cancer prevention benefits can be reached with a half-hour of physical activity a day—this can be done with three 10-minute blocks of exercise any time during the day if 30 minutes at one time is not possible.

✓ The IOM recommendation of 60 minutes per day is directed to those adults who need to achieve and maintain a healthy weight, and with over 60% of adults in the US overweight or obese, that includes most adults

Benefits of Physical Activity

• Physical activity may reduce the risk of several types of cancer, including cancers of the breast and colon by both direct and indirect effects

• Colon cancer: Physical activity accelerates the movement of food through the intestine, thereby reducing the length of time the bowel mucosa is exposed to mutagens

• Breast cancer: Vigorous physical activity may decrease the exposure of breast tissue to circulating estrogen

• May also affect cancers of colon, breast, and other sites by improving energy metabolism and reducing circulating concentrations of insulin and related growth factors

Recommendation: *Maintain a healthy weight throughout life*

✓ Replacing dietary fat with foods that are high in calories from sugar and other refined carbohydrates does not protect against obesity

✓ In fact, the decrease in fat intake and increase in consumption of refined carbohydrates that occurred in the US between 1977 and 1995 coincided with an 85% increase in obesity prevalence

✓ Consumption of sugar is up by 50% over that of only 50 years ago—consumption of sucrose, the refined white granules made from cane or beets is actually down

✓ What is being overeaten is fructose—not from honey or fruit—but in the form of high-fructose corn syrup (HFCS) which as added to so many foods because it is sweeter, easier to blend with other ingredients, and much cheaper than sucrose. This liquid sweetener—made from corn starch and boosted with fructose via a special manufacturing process—supplies nearly 10% of all calories consumed by Americans with the figure actually closer to 20% for many people, especially children

✓ In addition to the calories that HFCS adds to the diet, the body uses fructose differently than it does other sugars; high levels of HFCS can boost triglycerides and possibly cholesterol and may have a negative effect on the body's ability to use calcium, chromium, and other minerals

Benefits of Maintaining a Healthy Weight

• Overweight and obesity are associated with increased risk for cancers at several sites: breast (among postmenopausal women), colon, endometrium, adenocarcinoma of the esophagus, gallbladder, pancreas, and kidney

Recommendation: *If alcoholic beverages are consumed, number of drinks per day should be limited*

✓ No more than 2 drinks per day for men and 1 drink per day for women (for all persons 65 years and older, no more than 1 drink per day). See section on ALCOHOL PROBLEMS for what constitutes a drink

Benefits of Limiting Alcohol Intake

• Alcohol consumption is an established cause of cancers of the mouth, pharynx, larynx, esophagus, liver, and breast

• Cancers of the mouth, larynx, and esophagus: Alcohol consumption combined with tobacco increases the risk of cancers of the mouth, larynx, and esophagus far more than the independent effect of either drinking or smoking

• Breast cancer: Regular consumption of even a few alcoholic beverages per week has been associated with an increased risk of breast cancer in women—mechanism of increased risk is uncertain but may be related to alcohol-induced increases in circulating estrogens or other hormones in the blood, reduction of folic acid levels, or to a direct effect of alcohol or its metabolites on breast tissue

• Complicating this recommendation by the ACS is the evidence that even moderate intake of alcoholic beverages may decrease the risk of CHD in both men and women

Adapted from Byers, T., Nestle, M. McTiernan, A., Doyle, C., Currie-Williams, A., Gansler, T., et al. (2002). American Cancer Society guidelines on nutrition and physical activity for cancer prevention: Reducing the risk of cancer with healthy food choices and physical activity. *CA: A Cancer Journal for Clinicians, 52*, 92-119.

BEST ADVICE TO REDUCE RISK FOR THE MOST COMMON CANCERS

Type of Cancer	Major Risk Factor	To Reduce Risk
Bladder	Smoking and exposure to certain industrial chemicals	Limited evidence suggests that consuming more vegetables and drinking more fluids may lower risk
Brain	No known nutritional risk factors	No known nutritional risk factors
Breast Most common cancer diagnosed in women; second only to lung cancer as a cause of cancer deaths in women	Nonmodifiable risk factors—menarche before 12 years of age, nulliparity or first child at 30 years or older, late age at menopause, and a family history of breast cancer	Limiting use of hormone replacement therapy, maintaining a healthy weight, breastfeeding, engaging in brisk physical activity at least 4 hours a week, avoiding or limiting alcoholic beverages
Colorectal Second leading cause of cancer death in men and women combined	Family history of colorectal cancer, use to tobacco products, and possibly excessive alcohol consumption Other factors associated with increased risk—obesity and diets high in red meat	Consumption of diets high in vegetables and fruits and vigorous physical activity which may have greater benefit in reducing risk that regular moderate exercise
Endometrial	Obesity and use of HRT after menopause	Maintaining a healthy weight through diet and exercise, and consumption of at least 5 servings of fruits and vegetables each day
Kidney	Overweight and obesity for unknown reasons	Maintaining a healthy weight
Leukemias and lymphomas	No known nutritional risk factors for these cancers	No known nutritional risk factors for these cancers
Lung Leading cause of cancer death in US	Smoking tobacco causes more than 85% of lung cancers	Avoiding tobacco use and exposure and by consuming at least 5 servings of fruits and vegetables each day
Mouth and esophagus	Tobacco use (including cigarettes, chewing tobacco, and snuff) and alcohol use; use of these substances combined increases the risk of these cancers far more than the independent effect of either drinking or smoking Obesity increases the risk of cancer of the lower esophagus, likely due to increased acid reflux	Avoiding all tobacco use, limiting alcohol intake, maintaining a healthy weight, and consuming at least 5 servings of vegetables and fruits each day
Ovarian	No well-established nutritional risk factors	Vegetable and fruit consumption may lower risk
Pancreatic Fifth leading cause of cancer death in US	Tobacco use, adult-onset diabetes, and impaired glucose tolerance Some evidence that obesity and physical inactivity (both factors strongly linked to abnormal glucose metabolism) may increase risk	Avoiding tobacco use, maintaining a healthy weight, being physically active, and consuming 5 or more servings of fruits and vegetables each day
Prostate Most common cancer among men and is clearly related to male sex hormones	High consumption of red meat and dairy products; some evidence that high calcium intake, mainly through supplements is also associated with increased risk	Limiting intake of animal-based products, especially red meats and high-fat dairy products, and by consuming 5 or more servings of fruits and vegetables each day (current research studies are investigating the possible protective effects of vitamin E, selenium, and lycopene)
Stomach Incidence continues to decrease worldwide, especially in US	Infection with *Helicobacter pylori* bacteria and consumption of a diet poor in vegetables and fruits	Consume 5 or more servings of fruits and vegetables each day

Adapted from Byers, T., Nestle, M., McTiernan, A., Doyle, C., Currie-Williams, A., Gansler, T., et al. (2002). American Cancer Society guidelines on nutrition and physical activity for cancer prevention: Reducing the risk of cancer with healthy food choices and physical activity. *CA: A Cancer Journal for Clinicians, 52*, 92-110.

IX.   Suggested resources relating to nutrition are contained in the box below

---

General Resources

Center for Nutrition Policy and Promotion, USDA
1120 20th Street, NW, Suite 200, North Lobby
Washington, DC   20036
Internet: www.usda.gov/cnpp

Centers for Disease Control and Prevention
1600 Clifton Road
Atlanta, GA   30333
Internet: www.cdc.gov

Food and Drug Administration
200 C Street, SW
Washington, DC   20204
Internet: www.fda.gov

US Department of Agriculture
Document Delivery Services Branch
National Agricultural Library
10301 Baltimore Ave., 6th Floor
Beltsville, MD   20705-2351
301-504-5755
http://www.nal.usda.gov/fnic
circinfo@nal.usda.gov

healthfinder – Gateway to Reliable Consumer Health Information
National Health Information Center
US Department of Health and Human Services
PO Box 1133
Washington, DC   20013-1133
Internet: www.healthfinder.gov

Food and Nutrition Information Center
National Agricultural Library, USDA
10301 Baltimore Boulevard, Room 304
Beltsville, MD   20705-2351
Internet: www.nal.usda.gov/fnic

International Food Information Council (IFIC) Foundation
1100 Connecticut Avenue, NW, Suite 430
Washington, DC   20036
http://ificinfo.health.org
email: foodinfo@ific.health.org

Annotated Nutrition Links for Healthcare Professionals
Arbor Nutrition Guide
http://www.arborcom.com

Special Dietary Needs

American Cancer Society
1599 Clifton Road, NE
Atlanta, GA   30329
800-ACS-2345
http://www.cancer.org

American Diabetes Association
National Service Center
1660 Duke Street
Alexander, VA   22314
800-232-3472
http://www.diabetes.org

American Heart Association
7272 Greenville Avenue
Dallas, TX   75231
800-AHA-USA-1
http://www.amhrt.org

National Heart, Lung, and Blood Institute (NHLBI) Information Center
PO Box 30105
Bethesda, MD   20824-0105
800-575-WELL
http://www,nhlbi.nih.gov/nhlbi/nhlbi.htm

National Cancer Institute
Office of Cancer Communications
31 Center Drive, MSC 2580
Building 31, Room 10A-29
Bethesda, MD   20892-2580
800-4-CANCER
http://cancernet.nci.nih.gov

OncoLink
Sponsor: University of Pennsylvania
http://www.cancer.med.upenn.edu

Osteoporosis and Related Bone Disease National Resource Center
1150 17th Street, NW, Suite 5000
Washington, DC   20036-4603
800-624-BONE
http://www.osteo.org

Vegetarian Resource Group
PO Box 1463
Baltimore, MD   21203
410-366-8343
Email: vrg@vrg.org
http://www.vrg.org

X.   Suggested readings relating to nutrition during childhood and adolescence are contained in the box below

---

- Nissenberg, K.K., Bogle, M.I., & Wright, A.C. (1995). *Quick Meals for Healthy Kids and Busy Parents: Wholesome Family Meals in 30 Minutes or Less.* New York, NY: John Wiley & Sons.
- Schlosser, E. (2002) *Fast Food Nation: The Dark Side of the All-American Meal.* New York: Perennial.
- US Department of Agriculture, Center for Nutrition Policy and Promotion. (1999). *Tips for Using the Food Guide Pyramid for Young Children 2 to 6 Years Old.* Washington, DC.

DENTAL HEALTH MAINTENANCE

I.   Tooth preservation is a lifelong process

   A.   Maintaining good oral hygiene is important throughout life because poor oral hygiene can lead to gingival recession, increased tooth mobility, and eventual tooth loss
      1.   Natural cleaning of the dentition in humans is considered to be almost non-existent; the natural physiological forces that clean the oral cavity are insufficient to remove all dental plaque
      2.   Plaque, to be controlled adequately, must be removed frequently by physical methods
      3.   Bacterial plaque on teeth is considered the direct cause of periodontal diseases and caries; in the absence of plaque, disease will not occur

   B.   Fortunately, there have been substantial improvements in dental care in the US over the past few decades
      1.   Among older adults in the population, there has been a general decline in edentulism
      2.   However, approximately 30% of noninstitutionalized persons age 65 and older are edentulous which exceeds the *Healthy People 2010* goal that no more than 20% of the population age 65 and older will be edentulous
      3.   New technologies have now made it possible to repair or replace damaged or missing teeth with substances or devices that often look and function like natural teeth

   C.   Adults are susceptible to dental caries and gum disease; factors that increase the risk of developing these oral conditions are the following
      1.   Lack of fluoridation of water supply (most effective when teeth are developing)
      2.   Diet inadequate in essential micronutrients (vitamins and minerals)
      3.   High intake of sugary foods and beverages, especially between meals
      4.   Genetics
      5.   Tobacco use; smokers are 7 times more likely to develop periodontal disease than are nonsmokers and smokeless tobacco is associated with gum recession and root damage

   D.   Aging risk factors are the following
      1.   Dry mouth or xerostomia—without adequate saliva to clean, disinfect, and re-mineralize teeth, development of caries and periodontal disease are likely
      2.   Diabetes mellitus, particularly if it is poorly controlled
      3.   Osteoporosis—there is a link between loss of bone mineral density that occurs with osteoporosis and periodontal disease
      4.   Diseases and conditions affecting self-care such as Alzheimer's or Huntington's disease
      5.   Medications that cause gingival hyperplasia such a phenytoin, cyclosporine, or calcium channel blockers
      6.   Wear and tear from a lifetime of use may cause even healthy gums to recede

   E.   Healthy teeth and gums are not a given; brushing, flossing, adequate fluoride, and having regular dental checkups are all important components of maintaining oral health

II.   Brushing and flossing: Counsel patients as follows regarding brushing and flossing so that they can get the most out of oral hygiene efforts

   A.   Brushing at margin of teeth and gums with a soft-textured, multi-tufted nylon bristle toothbrush is recommended after every meal or at least twice a day; use of a soft-bristled brush helps minimize wear and tear on gums (any soft bristled toothbrush will do—there is no evidence that a brush with rippled or angled bristles, tapered head, or angled handle is more effective than conventional brushes in removing plaque and keeping teeth clean)
      1.   Recommend placing brush on gumline at a 45° angle, and then brushing gums and teeth with an elliptical motion; proper brushing can disrupt or remove plaque from teeth and from the gingival sulcus groove between gums and teeth
      2.   Recommend that patient also lightly brush tongue, especially at the back, to remove additional bacteria from mouth
      3.   Stress that thoroughness, rather than vigor, is the key
      4.   Toothbrushes should be replaced every 3-4 months, or when the bristles become worn, bent, or frayed

5. For patients who have difficulty holding the toothbrush, toothbrush handle can be enlarged by inserting it into a sponge or tennis ball, or by wrapping the handle with foil or tape; an electric toothbrush may be easier to use for persons with dexterity problems that make brushing difficult

6. In recent years, a new generation of electric toothbrushes has become available; these brushes feature an oscillating, rotary action instead of the traditional side-to-side motion; such brushes may provide additional benefit compared with manual brushes

7. Use of fluoride-containing toothpaste in any age group speeds up remineralization, the process by which tooth enamel absorbs calcium and phosphorous

8. Tartar control or whitening toothpastes may cause gum or tooth sensitivity, and toothpastes for sensitive teeth can often lessen sensitivity

B. Flossing teeth after every meal can reduce plaque formation and may be even more important than brushing

1. Explain that waxed or unwaxed products are equally effective

2. For a better grip on dental floss, suggest use of a commercial dental floss holder

3. Tell patients to use a gentle sawing motion, and work the floss between teeth without snapping it into the gums

   a. At the gumline, hold floss taut, bend it into a "C" shape, and then move the floss up and down on side of each tooth

   b. The floss should go slightly below gumline until resistance is felt

C. For patients who cannot brush or floss after a meal, teach them to swish vigorously with a mouthful of water

1. Swishing with water washes away food particles and reduces mouth bacteria by 30%

2. In addition, swishing helps neutralize enamel-attacking acids

D. Persons with dentures should be counseled to do the following

1. Remove and rinse dentures after every meal and thoroughly clean with brush at least once a day

2. Thoroughly clean oral cavity (with dentures removed) daily, using soft toothbrush to brush all intraoral surfaces, especially those that underlie the dentures as well as the tongue

3. When cleaning dentures, do so over a water-filled sink to reduce risk of breakage if dropped in sink

III. Dental examinations: Counsel patients regarding timing and importance of regular check-ups

A. Regular visits to a dentist for evaluation and oral health counseling should be scheduled at least once a year

B. Because older persons are more likely to see a primary care provider than a dentist, a thorough oral exam must be performed as a routine part of health maintenance visits

1. All removable prostheses should be removed

2. A tongue depressor or a piece of gauze may be used to keep tongue out of the way during exam

IV. Additional counseling to promote oral health includes the following

A. Provide dietary counseling relating to adequate intakes of essential nutrients (see section on NUTRITION for recommendations); especially discourage intake of high sugar foods and beverages in the diet

B. Patients who use tobacco should be counseled in accordance with the recommendations contained in the section on TOBACCO USE AND SMOKING CESSATION

C. Provide treatment for dry mouth (xerostomia) based on the cause

1. If a medication is deemed responsible, consider modifying the dose if possible, or switch to another medication

2. Suggest that patient frequently sip water or a sugarless drink, chew sugarless gum, or suck on sugarless hard candy to increase saliva production

3. Patients should also be reminded to drink at least 64 ounces of water each day, to cut back on alcohol consumption, and to avoid alcohol-based mouthwashes

4. Patients who smoke should always be counseled to quit at every visit, whether or not dry mouth is a problem

REFERENCES

Byers, T., Nestle, M. McTiernan, A., Doyle, C., Currie-Williams, A., Gansler, T., et al. (2002). American Cancer Society guidelines on nutrition and physical activity for cancer prevention: Reducing the risk of cancer with healthy food choices and physical activity. *CA: A Cancer Journal for Clinicians, 52*, 92-119.

Centers for Disease Control and Prevention. (2002). Recommended adult immunization schedule—United States, 2002-2003. *Morbidity and Mortality Weekly Report, 51*, 904-908.

Fairfield, K.M., & Fletcher, R.H. (2002). Vitamins for chronic disease prevention in adults. *JAMA, 287,* 3116-3126.

Gluck, G.M., & Monganstein, W.M. (2003). *Jong's community dental health.* St. Louis: Mosby.

Institute of Medicine, Food and Nutrition Board, The National Academies. (2002). *Dietary reference intakes: Energy, carbohydrate, fiber, fat, fatty acids, cholesterol, protein, and amino acids, part 1.* (Prepublication copy, unedited proofs). Washington, DC: National Academies Press.

Institute of Medicine, Food and Nutrition Board, The National Academies. (2002). *Dietary reference intakes: Energy, carbohydrate, fiber, fat, fatty acids, cholesterol, protein, and amino acids, part 2.* (Prepublication copy, unedited proofs). Washington, DC: National Academies Press.

Nielson, S.J., & Popkin, B.M. (2003). Patterns and trends in food portion sizes, 1977-1998. *JAMA, 289*, 450-543.

US Preventive Services Task Force. (1996). *Guide to clinical preventive services* (2nd ed.). Washington, DC: US Printing Office.

US Department of Agriculture/US Department of Health and Human Services. (2000). *Nutrition and your health: Dietary guidelines for Americans.* Washington, DC: Author.

US Department of Health and Human Services. (2000). *Healthy people 2010.* McLean, VA: International Medical Publishing, Inc.

US Preventive Services Task Force. (2001). Screening for chlamydial infection: Recommendations and rationale. *American Journal of Preventive Medicine, 20*, 90-94.

US Preventive Services Task Force. (2002). Screening for colorectal cancer: Recommendation and rationale. *Annals of Internal Medicine, 137*, 129-131.

US Preventive Services Task Force. (2001). Screening for depression: Recommendations and Rationale. *Annals of Internal Medicine, 136*, 760-764.

US Preventive Services Task Force. (2002). Screening for breast cancer: Recommendations and rationale. *Annals of Internal Medicine, 137*, 344-346.

US Preventive Services Task Force. (2001). Screening for skin cancer: Recommendation and rationale. *American Journal of Preventive Medicine, 20*, 944-47.

US Preventive Services Task Force. (2001). Screening adults for lipid disorders: Recommendations and rationale. *American Journal of Preventive Medicine, 20*, 73-76.

US Preventive Services Task Force. (2002). Screening for osteoporosis in postmenopausal women: Recommendations and rationale. *Annals of Internal Medicine, 137*, 526-528.

US Preventive Services Task Force. (2002). Behavioral counseling in primary care to promote physical activity: Recommendation and rationale. *Annals of Internal Medicine, 137*, 205-207.

US Preventive Services Task Force. (2002). Postmenopausal hormone replacement therapy for primary prevention of chronic conditions: Recommendations and rationale. *Annals of Internal Medicine, 137*, 526-528.

US Preventive Services Task Force. (2002). Chemoprevention of breast cancer: Recommendations and rationale. *Annals of Internal Medicine, 137*, 56-58.

US Preventive Services Task Force. (2001). Aspirin for the primary prevention of cardiovascular events: Recommendations and rationale. *Annals of Internal Medicine, 136*, 157-160.

US Preventive Services Task Force. (2002). Screening for prostate cancer: Recommendation and rationale. *Annals of Internal Medicine, 137*, 915-916.

US Preventive Services Task Force. (2003). Behavioral counseling in primary care to promote a healthy diet. Retrieved January 3, 2003, from http://www.preventiveservices.ahrq.gov

US Preventive Services Task Force. (2003). Screening for cervical cancer: recommendations and rationale. Retrieved February 7, 2003, from http://www.ahcpr.gov/clinic/uspstfix.htm

US Preventive Services Task Force. (2003). Screening for type 2 diabetes mellitus in adults: recommendations and rationale. Retrieved February 7, 2003, from http://www.ahcpr.gov/clinic/uspstfix.htm

Van der Weijden, F., & Danser, M.M. (2000). Toothbrushes: benefits versus effects on hard and soft tissues. In M. Addy, G. Embery, W.M. Edgar, & R. Orchardson (Eds.), *Tooth wear and sensitivity* (pp. 217-225). London: Martin Dunitz.

General

CONSTANCE R. UPHOLD

Chronic Fatigue
Table: International Consensus Definition of Chronic Fatigue Syndrome

Fever
Table: Conversion of Temperature

Lymphadenopathy
Table: Palpable Lymph Nodes and Lymphatic Drainage

Pain
Table: Three Step Analgesic Ladder of the World Health Organization
Table: Nonsteroidal Anti-Inflammatory Drugs (NSAIDs)
Table: Controlled Drugs
Table: Website Resources

Weight Loss (Involuntary)

CHRONIC FATIGUE

I. Definition: A symptom that lasts at least six months and involves extreme, unusual tiredness, decreased physical performance, and excessive need of sleep

II. Pathogenesis

    A. Almost all illnesses can cause fatigue; in the following conditions, fatigue is prominent:
        1. Infectious diseases: HIV infection, mononucleosis, hepatitis, endocarditis, Lyme disease, cytomegalovirus infection, parasitic disease
        2. Endocrine and metabolic disorders: Addison's disease (adrenal insufficiency), hypothyroidism, diabetes mellitus, pituitary insufficiency, apathetic hyperthyroidism of the elderly, chronic renal failure, hepatocellular failure
        3. Rheumatologic conditions: Rheumatoid arthritis, fibromyalgia, polymyalgia rheumatica
        4. Hematologic and oncologic conditions: Cancer (especially pancreatic cancer), severe anemia
        5. Cardiopulmonary diseases: Congestive heart disease, chronic obstructive pulmonary disease
        6. Neurologic diseases: Parkinson's disease, multiple sclerosis, myasthenia gravis
        7. Psychological disorders: Depression, anxiety, somatization disorder
        8. Sleep disorders: Sleep apnea, narcolepsy, hypersomnia

    B. Medications (antidepressants, tranquilizers, hypnotics, antihypertensives, antihistamines, illicit drugs, alcohol, excessive coffee intake) and unhealthy lifestyles (poor eating habits, lack of exercise, insufficient sleep, excessive stress) may also result in fatigue

    C. Chronic fatigue syndrome (CFS) is a disabling systemic disease characterized by severe fatigue; unknown etiology, but many hypotheses have been proposed
        1. Although not universal, many patients have low levels of cortisol and a blunted adrenal response to stress, suggesting a problem in the hypothalamic-pituitary-adrenal axis
        2. Infections from Epstein-Barr virus, toxoplasmosis, and cytomegalovirus can precipitate long periods of fatigue, but it is unclear if these pathogens are causative agents or just triggers in predisposed persons
        3. Frequently considered a psychiatric condition because of the high prevalence of somatization disorder, depression, and increased risk of suicide; however, CFS patients usually do not have low self-esteem, anhedonia, guilt, and low motivation that typify most patients with psychiatric conditions
        4. CFS has similarities with other unexplained medical diagnoses (fibromyalgia, irritable bowel syndrome) leading some to believe that health beliefs and attributions play a major role

III. Clinical Presentation: One of the most common primary care complaints

    A. Clinicians often attribute fatigue to psychological problems, whereas patients usually fear that serious illnesses such as cancer or life-threatening infections are the causes

    B. Fatigue is usually associated with feelings of sleepiness, irritability, boredom, and decreased efficiency

    C. Chronic fatigue syndrome accounts for about 5-10% of all cases of chronic fatigue
        1. Peak prevalence is among individuals aged 20-50 years
        2. The 1994 case definition (see following table) is widely used for diagnosis
        3. Approximately 20-50% of adults have some improvement after one to two years, but few fully recover

INTERNATIONAL CONSENSUS DEFINITION OF CHRONIC FATIGUE SYNDROME*†	
Criteria	**Definition**
Major	Chronic or relapsing, unexplained severe fatigue for ≥6 months that is not the result of ongoing exertion; is not substantially alleviated by rest; and results in reduction in previous levels of occupational, educational, social or personal activities
Minor	✓ Impaired memory or concentration ✓ Sore throat ✓ Tender cervical or axillary lymph nodes ✓ Muscle pain ✓ Multijoint pain ✓ New headaches ✓ Unrefreshing sleep ✓ Postexertional malaise

*The major and four or more of the minor criteria are required for case definition
†Exclusionary clinical diagnoses are the following: (1) any active medical condition that could explain the chronic fatigue (2) any previously diagnosed medical condition whose resolution has not been documented and whose continued activity may account for chronic fatigue (3) psychotic major depression, bipolar affective disorder, schizophrenia, delusional disorders, dementias, anorexia nervosa, bulimia nervosa (4) alcohol or substance abuse within 2 years prior to the onset of chronic fatigue and any time thereafter

Adapted from Fukuda, K., Straus, S.E., Hickie, I., Sharpe, M., Dobbins., J., & Komaroll, A. (1994). The chronic fatigue syndrome: A comprehensive approach to its definition and study. *Annals of Internal Medicine, 121*, 953-959.

IV. Diagnosis/Evaluation

A. History; patients should be encouraged to share past experiences with medical personnel and frustrations they may have had with their previous care
1. Ask to describe the development and severity of fatigue
2. Question about associated symptoms
3. Inquire about sleep habits and quality of sleep
4. Ask about lifestyle behaviors such as eating habits, caffeine intake, exercising, use of alcohol, tobacco, and illicit drugs
5. A complete medical history is often needed; always ask about symptoms of depression, fever, dyspnea, muscular weakness, blood loss, weight loss, anorexia, and pain
6. Determine risk for HIV infection and sexually transmitted diseases
7. Obtain a family medical history
8. Obtain a medication history
9. Ask about stress, significant losses, crying spells, and suicidal ideations
10. Determine how fatigue has affected occupational, educational, recreational, social, and family activities
11. Inquire about travel to areas where parasitic infections are endemic

B. Physical Examination; a complete exam is needed to arrive at a definitive diagnosis and to assure the patient that his/her complaint of fatigue is being taken seriously
1. Measure vital signs, including postural pulse and blood pressure, temperature, and weight
2. Assess skin for moisture, texture, exanthems, pallor, jaundice, purpura, petechiae, and splinter hemorrhages
3. Perform a funduscopic examination, noting diabetic retinopathy; inspect sclera for icterus
4. Assess, noting petechial pharynx, a sign of mononucleosis
5. Perform a thyroid examination
6. Examine lymph nodes
7. Perform complete heart and lung examinations
8. Assess the abdomen, noting organomegaly, masses, ascites, and tenderness
9. Perform a rectal examination; check for occult blood
10. Assess the joints for signs of inflammation
11. Perform a complete neuromuscular examination, noting focal weakness, muscle atrophy, fasciculations of muscles, deep tendon reflexes, and tremors
12. Perform a mental status assessment

C. Differential Diagnosis
   1. In adults, approximately two thirds of cases of fatigue are related to depression or psychiatric conditions; one fourth are idiopathic, having some but not sufficient criteria to qualify for CFS; 5% meet criteria for CFS; and 3% have organic medical causes
   2. Great care must be taken to rule out underlying medical illness; most diseases have associated symptoms except for adrenal insufficiency in which fatigue is often the first and only presenting complaint
   3. Always consider unhealthy lifestyle behaviors as a possible cause

D. Diagnostic Tests; findings from the history and physical examination should guide selection of tests
   1. The basic screening evaluation usually includes a CBC with differential, renal function tests, liver enzymes, urinalysis, an erythrocyte sedimentation rate, and thyroid function tests
   2. In patients with recent onset of persisting fatigue and adenopathy, order a heterophile test for acute mononucleosis
   3. HIV testing should be done when diffuse adenopathy is present or when there is a history of high-risk behaviors
   4. Useful tests to rule out other diseases are glucose (diabetes), chest x-ray (cardiopulmonary problems), rapid cosyntropin test (adrenal insufficiency), rheumatoid factor (rheumatoid diseases), serologies for toxoplasmosis, Epstein-Barr, or cytomegalovirus (infectious diseases), and cerebral magnetic resonance imaging (for demyelination as occurs in multiple sclerosis)
   5. Diagnosis of CFS is based on clinical findings and eliminating other diagnoses

V. Plan/Management

A. Treat underlying cause of fatigue; treat medical or psychiatric conditions and provide symptomatic care such as pain medications and strategies to normalize sleep patterns

B. Treatment of chronic fatigue syndrome is variable and tailored to each patient
   1. Emphasis should be on rehabilitation rather than cure
   2. Patient education is important
      a. Acknowledge the reality of the illness and its associated symptoms while stressing that there is no underlying organic disease
      b. Reassure patients that CFS is not life-threatening and that most people are eventually able to return to work or school
   3. Continuous support and attention to symptomatic treatment are essential; focus on ameliorating the negative effects that fatigue is having on the patient's life; discuss the futility in continually searching for a cause and the importance of rehabilitation
   4. Cognitive-behavioral therapy helps the patient identify and reverse beliefs and coping behaviors that perpetuate disability and hinder recovery
      a. First explore the patient's beliefs about the illness and behaviors related to the illness
      b. Patients are encouraged to gain control of their illness and change behaviors of passivity and helplessness to active participation in their recovery
   5. Gradually increase activity; initially avoid intense exercise as this can lead to a pattern of overactivity and underactivity
   6. A targeted exercise program is effective
   7. A balanced diet and good sleep hygiene may improve symptoms
   8. Low-dose tricyclic antidepressants and/or selected serotonin reuptake inhibitors, combined with cognitive-behavioral therapy, may be beneficial
   9. Immunologic therapy, corticosteroids, supplements, massage, and transcutaneous electrical nerve stimulation are other therapies, but evidence of their effectiveness is limited

C. Follow Up
   1. Follow up is variable depending on the cause of fatigue
   2. After the first visits for evaluation and initiating treatment, patients with CFS should be scheduled for infrequent, but regular appointments

FEVER

I. Definition: Traditionally defined as body temperature greater than 38.0°C (100.4°F) rectally, 37.8°C (100°F) orally, or 37.2°C (98.9°F) axillary; more recently defined as early morning body temperature (measured orally) ≥37.2°C (≥98.9°F) or an afternoon temperature of ≥37.7°C (≥99.9°F) (see table that follows for conversion of temperature)

CONVERSION OF TEMPERATURE		
37°C	=	98.6°F
38°C	=	100.4°F
39°C	=	102.2°F
40°C	=	104.0°F

A. Fever without source (FWS): Unexplained fever (>38°C or >100.4°F, rectal temperature) of brief duration or lasting <5-7 days; source of acute febrile illness is not apparent after a careful history and physical examination

B. Fever of unknown origin (FUO): Fever (>101°F) persisting for 3 weeks and eluding one week of intensive diagnostic testing

II. Pathogenesis

A. Fever occurs when bacteria, viruses, toxins, or other agents are phagocytosed by leukocytes

B. Interluekin-1 and other chemical mediators (previously referred to as endogenous pyrogens) are then produced and activate the production of prostaglandins

C. Prostaglandins act on the thermoregulatory mechanism in the hypothalamus and upwardly readjust the body's thermostat

D. Raising the hypothalamic set-point initiates the process of heat production and conservation by increasing metabolism, triggering peripheral vasoconstriction, and less frequently by triggering shivering which increases heat production from the muscles

E. Infections (most common), neoplasms, and collagen-vascular diseases are the most common causes; most infections are viral in etiology

F. Other causes include the following:
1. Hypersensitivity to drugs
2. Recent immunizations with certain vaccines
3. Vascular occlusive and/or inflammatory events such as deep vein thrombophlebitis, pulmonary emboli, or myocardial infarction
4. Acute hemolytic episodes associated with acute autoimmune hemolytic anemia or sickle cell anemia
5. Central nervous system abnormalities

G. Common causes of fever of unknown origin
1. Systemic: Miliary tuberculosis, infective endocarditis, cytomegalovirus infection, toxoplasmosis, brucellosis, chronic meningococcemia
2. Localized: Hepatic infections (liver abscess, cholangitis), visceral infections (pancreatic, empyema of gallbladder), intraperitoneal infections (appendiceal, pelvic), urinary tract infections
3. Neoplasms, especially lymphomas, leukemias, and cancers metastatic to bone or liver
4. Collagen-vascular and other multisystem diseases: Temporal arteritis, systemic lupus erythematosus, rheumatoid arthritis, sarcoidosis

H. True fever must be differentiated from hyperthermia
  1. Hyperthermia occurs when there is increased body temperature but no alteration in the hypothalamic set point
  2. Hyperthermia may be due to increased metabolic heat (e.g., thyrotoxicosis), excessive environmental temperature (e.g., heat stroke), defective heat loss because of environmental conditions (e.g. high humidity, overdressing, sitting in unventilated, sunny car, exercise), or dermatologic disorder (e.g., ectodermal dysplasia)

I. Occasionally, a patient may have a factitious fever or a high reading on the thermometer which was artificially produced by the patient for secondary gains

III. Clinical Presentation

A. Fever, by itself, is not an illness; rather, a sign that the body is fighting an infection or reacting to a stimulus; normal temperatures are characterized by the following:
  1. Temperature is usually highest around 4 pm and lowest around 6 am
  2. Normal temperature deviations occur with physical activity, stress, ovulation, and environmental heat

B. Typical symptoms include malaise, fatigue, myalgias, and tachycardia (pulse rate is often elevated by about 10-15 beats per 1°C of fever)

C. Central nervous system symptoms may occur, ranging from mild changes in alertness to delirium, particularly in elderly patients and chronically-ill patients

D. Although each 1°F raises the basal metabolic rate by 7%, most patients can tolerate fevers well, with a few exceptions:
  1. Patients with underlying cardiac disease, chronic, debilitating disease, immunocompromised disease, history of intravenous drug abuse, implanted prosthetic devices, and those on corticosteroid or immunosuppressive therapy
  2. Small infants and the elderly are at a greatest risk for dehydration and other adverse events

E. Bacteremia, meningitis, and seizures are serious conditions related to fevers

IV. Diagnosis/Evaluation

A. History
  1. Inquire about onset, duration, and pattern of fever; ascertain that patient knows how to correctly measure temperature; inquire about type of thermometer used
  2. Inquire about associated symptoms such as anorexia, chills, headache, nasal congestion, earache, sore throat, cough, abdominal pain, vomiting, diarrhea, or painful urination
  3. Explore hydration status by asking about amount of fluid intake and frequency and amount of fluid output
  4. Ask about comfort level of patient
  5. Explore possibilities of heat illness (heat stroke) or other types of environmental exposure
  6. Ask whether patient started new medications, had a recent immunization, or had a recent transfusion
  7. Inquire about recent travel, dental or surgical procedures, illnesses, trauma, exposure to ticks, and insect or animal bites and scratches
  8. Ask about the consumption of raw or poorly cooked foods; ask about alcohol or drug use
  9. Ask whether other household members are ill or have fevers
  10. Obtain a complete past medical history; ask about medications, implanted prosthetic devices, previous illnesses and diseases, particularly any cardiac or chronically debilitating disorders
  11. Inquire about last dosage of an antipyretic and other self-treatment measures
  12. Explore social situation and home environment (e.g., adequacy of heat and water) of the family; assess availability of transportation, telephone, thermometer, and whether family is reliable
  13. A complete review of systems may be needed to uncover source of fever and to determine severity of debility due to elevated body temperature

B.   Physical Examination
1.   Measure temperature
a.   Always confirm initial temperature measurement
b.   Rectal temperatures are gold standard as they are accurate, reproducible, and not affected by environmental factors; rectal temperatures are approximately 1° higher than oral temperatures and 2 to 2.5° higher than axillary temperatures
c.   Oral temperatures are reliable with cooperative patient but may vary with rapid breathing and recent ingestion of hot or cold fluids
d.   The infrared ear thermometer estimates the temperature of the tympanic membrane (TM); improper placement and aiming, incomplete probe penetration into external ear canal, and obstruction/tortuosity of the external ear canal can lead to underestimating TM temperatures
e.   Skin and forehead measurements are inaccurate
2.   Measure respiratory rate, pulse, and blood pressure
3.   Pulse oximetry is a reliable predictor of respiratory problems
4.   Observe skin for color, rashes, petechiae or purpura; absence of petechial rash below the nipples makes meningococcemia less likely
5.   Assess for signs of dehydration such as skin turgor and capillary refill
6.   Assess neck for nuchal rigidity
7.   Check for lymphadenopathy
8.   Assess for swollen joints
9.   Perform neurologic exam, noting positive Kernig or Brudzinski signs
10. In most cases, perform a complete physical examination to find localized infection such as otitis media, pharyngitis, sinusitis, meningitis, cervical adenitis, pneumonia, urinary tract infection, arthritis, and osteomyelitis

C.   Differential Diagnosis
1.   Fevers almost always result in increases in pulse rates; absence of a pulse rate increase suggests factitious fever, mycoplasmal infection or typhoid fever
2.   It is important to differentiate true fever from hyperthermia

D.   Diagnostic Tests: Recommended diagnostic tests depend on patient's age, clinical presentation, and previous medical history
1.   In the majority of cases, the history and physical examination will uncover likely causes of the fever and suggest selective diagnostic tests
2.   For patients who look toxic, have an extremely elevated temperature, are immunodeficient, or have an underlying chronic disease, order the following:
a.   Urine analysis for specific gravity and the presence of ketones to determine hydration status
b.   CBC with differential and erythrocyte sedimentation rate (ESR) to determine likelihood of a bacterial etiology and/or an inflammatory process
c.   Blood cultures to rule out bacteremia and need for more aggressive treatments such as hospitalization and parenteral antimicrobial therapy; cultures are definitely needed if patient has a heart murmur, prosthetic heart valve, or other implantable device
3.   Consider other diagnostic tests
a.   Chest radiographs to detect infiltrates, effusions, masses, or nodes
b.   Abdominal x-rays to detect air-fluid levels in the bowel
c.   Plain films of bone to detect osteomyelitis
d.   Ultrasonography or computed tomography to detect mass lesions such as abscesses or tumors
e.   If there is a possibility of meningitis, a lumbar puncture is needed
f.   Liver function studies to detect obscure sources of fever such as occurs with hepatitis (elevation in transaminase levels)
g.   Microscopic evaluation of body fluids to detect infections
h.   Serologic tests are helpful in certain cases
(1) Antibody testing for HIV infection
(2) Skin tests for tuberculosis
(3) Antinuclear antibody and rheumatoid factor for vasculitis or rheumatoid disease
4.   Fevers of unknown origin (FUO) require an extensive diagnostic evaluation; consult an infectious disease specialist

V. Plan/Management

A. Hospitalize patients who are disoriented, delirious, or who have meningismus, petechiae, or purpura

B. Consider consultation and hospitalization for following patients:
1. Patients who are immunodeficient or have a history of cardiac or another serious disease
2. Very old patients
3. Patients who are taking corticosteroid or immunosuppressive therapy
4. Patients who have prosthetic devices
5. IV drug abusers
6. Patients who are dehydrated
7. Any patient who appears toxic (rigors, hypotension, oliguria, CNS abnormalities, leukocytosis or leukopenia, new, significant cardiac murmurs)
8. Any patient whose fever lasts longer than 7-10 days
9. Patient with extremely elevated temperatures

C. Treat cause of fever (i.e., antibiotics for bacterial infection)

D. Consider treatment with antipyretics
1. Reasons for NOT treating a low-grade or moderate fever in an otherwise well patient:
   a. Antipyretics cause side effects and toxicity and do NOT alter the course or duration of disease
   b. Antipyretics mask the signs and symptoms of a serious disease and confuse the clinical picture
2. However, most clinicians agree that antipyretics should be given in the following situations:
   a. When fevers are 103°F and higher
   b. In patients for whom side effects of fever may be harmful (e.g. patients with compensated cardiac diseases and chronic debilitating disorders, patients who become dehydrated rapidly, patients who are alcoholics)
   c. Patients who are uncomfortable and unable to rest
3. In hyperthermic states such as thyrotoxicosis, heat stroke and overdressing, the set point has not been changed and antipyretic medications are not effective because they act to lower set point
4. The drug of choice is acetaminophen (Tylenol); 325-650 mg every 4-6 hours (maximum dose is 4 g)
   a. Maximum effect at 2 hours
   b. Do not use in liver disease or transplant patients; strictly follow correct doses to prevent liver damage; typically safe in patients who drink <5 alcoholic beverages per day
5. Aspirin (325-650 mg every 4 hours) is a second choice for fever management
   a. Adverse effects: Gastric irritation and risk of bleeding
   b. Risk of asthma exacerbation and anaphylactic reaction, particularly in adults with history of asthma and nasal polyps
6. Ibuprofen (Motrin) is another therapeutic option
   a. Dosage is 400 mg every 4-6 hours
   b. Avoid in patients with aspirin allergies, ulcers, renal insufficiency, and bleeding disorders

E. Sponging may be performed but usually is unnecessary and may even be harmful because it can cause discomfort and chilling
1. If temperature is extremely high or if aggressive fever management is necessary, sponge patient after giving antipyretic
2. Sponging is an important part of the management plan in the following cases: Patients with severe liver disease who cannot take acetaminophen, neurologic problems in which temperature regulation mechanisms are abnormal, heat stroke, or in environments with excessive temperatures
3. When sponging, water should be lukewarm and should not cause the patient to shiver (colder temperatures are used for heat illness such as heat stroke)

F. Patient Education
1. Teach the correct method to assess temperature; keep thermometer in place for at least 2 minutes
2. Reinforce when to call a health care provider about an elevated temperature; call clinician when there is delirium (disorientation or confusion), seizures, stiff neck, petechial or purpural rash, and signs of dehydration (can teach how to assess capillary refill)
3. Teach when to administer antipyretics and the correct dosage of these medications

4. Remind patients to read labels and find "hidden" sources of acetaminophen that are often in over-the-counter cough and cold medications and can cause toxicity
5. Instruct to drink extra fluids; for patients who are dehydrated, teach to drink fluids every 15-60 minutes
6. Daily activities should be modified to provide for additional rest, light meals, and avoidance of strenuous activities depending on patient's condition
7. Remind patients to avoid overdressing when they have a fever
8. Tell patients to never use alcohol for sponging
9. Instruct that elevated temperatures are a normal body defense mechanism, not a disease; height of the temperature except when extremely high does not correlate well with serious diseases; assure everyone that there are almost always no adverse effects from fevers

G. Follow Up
1. Variable and depends on age, diagnosis, and clinical presentation of patient as well as the amount of friend and family support available
2. For the elderly and chronically-ill patients consider scheduling return visit for following morning or have telephone contact within 24 hours to assess condition
3. Instruct patients to return for further evaluation if fever persists for more than 2 or 3 days

LYMPHADENOPATHY

I. Definition: Lymph node enlargement (see also section on CERVICAL ADENITIS)

II. Pathogenesis

A. Following mechanisms result in lymphadenopathy
1. Proliferation in response to an antigen
2. Invasion of cells from cells outside the node such as malignant cells
3. Transformation of primary nodular tissue into neoplastic cells

B. Causes of generalized lymphadenopathy (mnemonic acronym "MIAMI" may aid recall)
1. **M**alignancies: Leukemia, lymphoma, immunoblastic lymphadenopathy, metastases
2. **I**nfections (most common cause)
   a. Viral: Human immunodeficiency virus (HIV), mononucleosis, cytomegalovirus, hepatitis B, measles, rubella, rubeola
   b. Bacterial: Group A β-hemolytic *streptococcus*, cat-scratch disease, secondary syphilis
   c. Mycobacterial: atypical mycobacterial infection, miliary tuberculosis
   d. Fungal: Histoplasmosis
   e. Protozoal: Toxoplasmosis
3. **A**utoimmune disorders: Systemic lupus erythematosus, rheumatoid arthritis, Sjögren's syndrome
4. **M**iscellaneous: Sarcoidosis, lipid storage disease, Kawasaki disease; hyperthyroidism, hypopituitarism, hypoadrenocorticism
5. **I**atrogenic states: Serum sickness, drug reactions (phenytoin and, less commonly, hydralazine, para-aminosalicylic acid, propylthiouracil, and allopurinol)

C. Causes of localized lymphadenopathy: due to local infection, tumor growth, or recent immunization in area drained by involved lymph node (also see table IV.B.1.)
1. Anterior auricular: Viral conjunctivitis, rubella, scalp infection
2. Submandibular or cervical (unilateral): Buccal cavity infection, pharyngitis, nasopharyngeal tumor, thyroid malignancy
3. Cervical (bilateral): Mononucleosis, sarcoidosis, toxoplasmosis, pharyngitis
4. Supraclavicular (right): Pulmonary, mediastinal, and esophageal malignancies
5. Supraclavicular (left): Malignancies (intra-abdominal, renal, testicular, ovarian), Hodgkin's disease
6. Axillary: Breast malignancy or infection, upper extremity infection
7. Epitrochlear: Syphilis (bilateral), hand infection (unilateral)
8. Inguinal: Syphilis, genital herpes, lymphogranuloma venereum, chancroid, lower extremity or local infection

9. Hilar adenopathy: Sarcoidosis, fungal infection, lymphoma, bronchogenic carcinoma, tuberculosis
10. Any region: Benign reactive hyperplasia, lymphomas, cat scratch disease, leukemia, sarcoidosis, malignancies

III. Clinical presentation: The following key factors are helpful in arriving at a diagnosis:

A. Generalized versus localized lymphadenopathy
    1. Generalized adenopathy is due to systemic disease
    2. Localized adenopathy is caused by local infection, tumor, or systemic disease

B. Location of node (see PATHOGENESIS, II.C.); left supraclavicular node, often called "sentinel" node, suggests Hodgkin's disease

C. Character of node
    1. Size: A large node (>1 cm) usually represents a specific pathology
    2. Metastatic cancer: Hard, painless, matted, fixed, often >3 cm
    3. Reactive: Discrete, mobile, rubbery, mildly tender
    4. Lymphadenitis: Tender, warm, red, fluctuant
    5. Infection: Firm, red, warm
    6. Lymphoma or leukemia: Firm or rubbery

D. Age of patient
    1. In patients <30 years, most cases are benign and caused by infection
    2. Benign reactive hyperplasia or transient node enlargement from unknown causes occurs frequently in young adults
    3. Palpable nodes in the anterior cervical triangle are common and usually normal, especially in young adults
    4. Posterior cervical node enlargement in young adults may be mononucleosis
    5. Risk of cancer increases with age

E. Onset and duration
    1. Nodes of acute onset and duration are typically due to viral or pyogenic infection
    2. Chronicity suggests neoplastic disease, sarcoidosis, tuberculosis, and fungal infections although lymphadenitis may take several months to resolve

F. Rate of change: Usually nodes that are rapidly growing are more pathologic than slow-growing nodes

G. Associated symptoms
    1. Low-grade fevers with night sweats and weight loss characterize lymphoma, HIV infection, or tuberculosis
    2. Fatigue and weight loss suggest systemic infection, cancer, or connective tissue disease
    3. Hilar lymph node enlargement may cause compression of thoracic structures and result in cough, dyspnea, and wheezing

H. Associated signs
    1. Splenomegaly: Mononucleosis, lymphoma, or leukemia
    2. Thyromegaly: Hyperthyroidism
    3. Tender, warm, or enlarged joints: Collagen vascular disease, leukemia, rheumatoid arthritis
    4. Rash: Viral disease, Kawasaki disease, collagen and vascular disease

I. Epidemiologic leads
    1. Recent exposure to cats is predisposing factor in cat-scratch disease
    2. History of multiple sexual partners and IV drug use may be associated with sexually transmitted disease or HIV infection
    3. Alcohol or tobacco abuse in elderly patient with cervical lymphadenopathy may represent head and neck carcinoma
    4. Occupational diseases such as silicosis or asbestosis may result in hilar and mediastinal lymphadenopathy
    5. Tick bite may be associated with Lyme disease
    6. Travel-related lymphadenopathy occurs

IV. Diagnosis/Evaluation

A. History
1. Ask about onset, duration, and rate of growth of all palpable nodes
2. Question about tenderness of node(s)
3. Ask about recent infections and trauma
4. Inquire about systemic symptoms such as fever, weight loss, night sweats, fatigue, diarrhea, rashes, and pain
5. Question about exposure to animals, travel to foreign countries, occupational hazards (silicon, beryllium), and explore other risk factors such as tobacco use, alcohol abuse, ultraviolet radiation, substance abuse, and sexual exposure
6. Ask about medications and immunization status
7. Explore past medical history and family history; especially ask about carcinomas

B. Physical examination
1. Assess all palpable nodes, noting size, location, consistency, tenderness, warmth, and fixation (see table that follows)

PALPABLE LYMPH NODES AND LYMPHATIC DRAINAGE	
Node	**Drainage Area**
Occipital	Posterior scalp, neck
Mastoid	Mastoid area
Submental	Apex of tongue and lower lip
Submaxillary	Buccal cavity, tongue, cheek, lips
Cervical	Head, neck, and oropharynx
Axillary	Greater part of arm, shoulder, superficial anterior and lateral thoracic and upper abdominal wall
Supraclavicular	Right: Inferior neck and mediastinum Left: Inferior neck, mediastinum, and upper abdomen
Epitrochlear	Hand, forearm, and elbow
Inguinal	Leg and genitalia
Femoral	Leg
Popliteal	Posterior leg and knee

   a. Normal, palpable nodes are discrete, freely mobile, and nontender
   b. Normal size of nodes is <1 cm with two exceptions:
      (1) Inguinal nodes are normal up to 1.5 cm
      (2) Epitrochlear nodes are abnormal if >0.5 cm
   c. To assess for an enlarged supraclavicular node, ask patient to perform Valsalva maneuver during palpation of supraclavicular fossa
2. For localized lymphadenopathy, carefully assess all body parts within the lymphatic drainage area (see preceding table)
3. For generalized lymphadenopathy a careful, comprehensive physical examination is needed

C. Differential Diagnosis
1. Other structures such as enlarged parotid glands, cervical hygromas, thyroglossal and brachial cysts, hemangiomas, abscesses, lipomas, and other tumors may be confused with enlarged lymph nodes (see figure COMMON LOCATION OF MASSES OF FACE AND NECK in topic CERVICAL ADENITIS in section on PROBLEMS OF EARS, NOSE, THROAT)
2. Potential causes range from simple and benign to complicated and serious
3. No specific cause is found in many cases (see PATHOGENESIS, II.A.B.C. for range of etiologies)
4. Persistent, generalized lymphadenopathy is defined as lymph node enlargement for at least three months in at least two extrainguinal sites; common causes are HIV infection, tuberculosis, syphilis, and lymphoma

D. Diagnostic Tests (if benign cause of lymphadenopathy is suspected, close observation is indicated); when the diagnosis is uncertain, stepwise testing with the following tests is needed:
   1. CBC
      a. Atypical lymphocytes: Mononucleosis or other viral syndromes
      b. Increased granulocytes: Bacterial infection
      c. Increased eosinophils: Hypersensitivity states
      d. Decreased red blood cells and platelets: Malignancy
      e. Pancytopenia: HIV infection and tumor
   2. Chest x-ray that will detect pulmonary disease and hilar adenopathy is needed for seriously ill patients and those with supraclavicular lymphadenopathy or respiratory complaints
   3. Serologic tests
      a. Monospot or Epstein-Barr virus: Mononucleosis
      b. VDRL: Syphilis
      c. HIV antibody: HIV infection
      d. Antinuclear antibody and rheumatoid factor: Collagen diseases
      e. Other serologic tests: Cytomegalovirus and toxoplasmosis infections
   4. Tuberculin skin test for mycobacterial disease and hilar adenopathy
   5. Cultures
      a. Throat for cervical adenopathy
      b. Urethral and cervical for inguinal adenopathy
      c. Aspirated lymph tissue for suspected fungal or mycobacterial infection
      d. Blood culture for suspected bacteremia
   6. Lymph node biopsy provides a definitive diagnosis; indicated when simple testing fails to provide a diagnosis or for cases when cancer, tuberculosis, or sarcoidosis are suspected
      a. The following characteristics suggest the need for an early biopsy:
         (1) Node >2 cm
         (2) Abnormal chest x-ray
         (3) Enlarged supraclavicular node
         (4) Associated signs and symptoms of weight loss and hepatosplenomegaly
         (5) Absence of respiratory tract symptoms
      b. Nodes that remain constant in size for 4-8 weeks and those that fail to resolve in 8-12 weeks need a biopsy
   7. Ultrasound and computed tomography are sometimes helpful in differentiating lymphadenopathy from nonlymphatic enlargement
   8. Bone marrow examination is needed for patients with severe anemia, neutropenia, thrombocytopenia, or peripheral smear for malignant blast cells

V. Plan/Management

A. Treatment depends on diagnosis; see sections on CERVICAL ADENITIS, KAWASAKI DISEASE, PHARYNGITIS, etc.

B. Consider consultation for patients suspected of having serious disease or one of the following:
   1. Undiagnosed adenopathy lasting longer than 2 months
   2. Firm, matted, rapidly enlarging, nontender nodes
   3. Associated signs and symptoms such as night sweats, weight loss, bone pain, hepatosplenomegaly, and fever of unknown etiology
   4. Associated CBC abnormality, positive PPD, or abnormal chest x-ray

C. Follow Up
   1. Diagnosis will determine when patient should return for follow-up
   2. Patients with benign clinical history, unremarkable physical examination, and no constitutional signs and symptoms can be re-evaluated in three weeks
   3. For other cases in which the cause of lymphadenopathy is uncertain, watchful waiting with follow up every 3-5 days for 2 weeks is appropriate

PAIN

I.   Definition: Unpleasant sensory and emotional experience related to actual or potential tissue damage

II.   Pathogenesis

    A.   Peripheral stimulation occurs when free nerve endings or nociceptors found in various parts of body (i.e., skin, blood vessels, viscera, muscles) are stimulated and then action potentials are transmitted along afferent nerve fibers to the spinal cord

    B.   Gate control theory further develops the pathophysiology of pain
        1.   The perception of pain is an interplay between the nociceptive pain fibers and the nonociceptive or non-transmitting neurons that synapse in the spinal cord
        2.   Clinically, this is important because certain treatments such as acupuncture, topical irritants, and transcutaneous electrical nerve stimulation (TENS) can stimulate the large nonociceptive neurons and produce an analgesic effect

    C.   Pain-initiated processes as well as other information are carried through the ascending spinal cord pathways (particularly the spinothalamic tract) to the brain

    D.   In the brain, pain is perceived as a partial summation of two processes:
        1.   Positive feedback is the nociceptive stimulus which activates pain transmission
        2.   Negative feedback is the brain's modulatory network composed of the endogenous opiate system (opiate receptors, endorphins) which inhibits pain

    E.   Other neurotransmitter substances such as acetylcholine, dopamine, norepinephrine, and serotonin play a role in pain transmission as well

    F.   The brain controls pain sensation through an organized descending or efferent pain transmission system

III. Clinical Presentation

    A.   Acute pain arises from injury, trauma, spasm, or disease of body parts
        1.   Usually is short-lived and decreases as damaged area heals
        2.   Associated with hyperactivity of the sympathetic nervous system resulting in the following: tachycardia, tachypnea, elevated blood pressure, diaphoresis, and dilated pupils

    B.   Persistent pain (previously called chronic pain)
        1.   Pain which lasts longer than 6 months is rarely accompanied with hyperactivity of sympathetic nervous system
        2.   Can be classified into 4 categories
            a.   Nociceptive pain may be visceral (located in abdomen or thorax) or somatic (initiated in muscles or connective tissue)
                (1)   Pain arises from tissue inflammation, mechanical deformation, ongoing injury, or destruction
                (2)   Responds well to traditional pain management strategies
            b.   Neuropathic pain results from a pathophysiologic process involving peripheral or central nervous system
                (1)   Examples include diabetic neuropathy and post-amputation phantom limb pain
                (2)   Responds to unconventional analgesics such as anticonvulsants and tricyclic antidepressants
            c.   Mixed or unspecified pain such as occurs with recurrent headaches and vasculitic pain syndromes; treatment often requires experimentation with different or combined approaches
            d.   Rare conditions in which psychologic disorders are cause of pain; psychiatry is needed
        3.   Persistent pain is commonly a result of one of the following:
            a.   Pain that persists beyond the normal healing time for an acute injury
            b.   Chronic disease pain
            c.   Pain without identifiable organic cause
            d.   Cancer pain
        4.   Depression often accompanies persistent pain; can lead to functional loss and social withdrawal

C. Pain is an important issue in the elderly population
1. Patients >65 years have more persistent pain but are less likely to obtain pain relief than younger patients; pain in older people often goes unrecognized by clinicians
2. Older patients often have an age-related sensitivity to opioid analgesics
3. Comorbid diseases and increased risk of adverse drug reactions complicate pain management

D. An individual's culture and belief system have a strong influence on pain perception and control

IV. Diagnosis/Evaluation

A. History: Patient's self-report of pain is the most accurate and reliable evidence of the existence of pain
1. Focus assessment on finding the cause of pain, determining characteristics of pain, and what factors are complicating the pain
2. The Joint Commission on Accreditation of Healthcare Organizations recommends that pain be considered the "fifth" vital sign and that pain should be assessed each time pulse, blood pressure, temperature, and respirations are measured
3. Mnemonic may be used to obtain patient's subjective description of pain
   a. P: palliative or precipitating factors such as stress, exertion
   b. Q: quality of pain such as sharpness, crushing, throbbing, burning
   c. R: region or radiation of pain
   d. S: subjective descriptions of severity of pain such as awakens at night or takes breath away
   e. T: temporal nature such as daytime, during meals; constant vs. intermittent
4. May use a visual analog scale to quantify pain or ask patient to relate where pain falls on a line from zero (no pain) to 10 (worst pain ever experienced)
5. Particularly in the elderly, ask about changes in cognition and behavior such as agitation and withdrawal; inquire about sleep alterations, bowel changes, depression, and gait problems
6. Inquire about current and prior pain medication use, efficacy, and prior adverse reactions
7. Ask about previous personal or family history of chronic pain
8. Assess patient's level of functioning in all spheres of living such as family relationships, social relationships, employment, and hobbies to help determine secondary gains
9. Assess patient's attitudes, beliefs, and knowledge about pain and its management
10. Complete review of systems to determine relationship of pain to other parts of body

B. Physical Examination
1. Assess vital signs
2. Observe general appearance, gait, and posture for signs of distress
3. Observe patient's affect
4. Inspect, palpate, percuss, and auscultate, as appropriate, all areas and surrounding structures which patient perceives as painful; assess pain referral sites
5. Assess for muscle spasms, trigger points, and areas sensitive to light touch
6. Perform complete musculoskeletal, neurologic, and mental status exams
7. Observe physical function, such as ability to perform activities of daily living

C. Diagnostic tests are variable depending of patient's condition

D. Differential Diagnosis
1. Malingering for ongoing litigation or secondary gains
2. Anxiety or depression

V. Plan/Management

A. General principles of pain management
1. Resist prescribing pain medications without a diagnosis
2. The psychosocial aspects of pain are as important as the biologic aspects
3. Cultivating a sense of control over the pain is important in both acute and chronic situations
4. Elderly patients often have increased sensitivity to the adverse effects of pain medications
5. Control of depression and other psychosocial factors facilitates pain management
6. In chronic situations, facilitate the patient's engagement in an active, productive life
7. Essential to involve the patient's family and friends in the management plan
8. Important to assess the patient's response to pain treatments at frequent intervals

B. Pharmacologic principles of treating pain
    1. Identify source of pain and treat as appropriate
    2. Use the least potent analgesic that is effective and has the fewest side effects
    3. Give analgesics for adequate trial time and properly titrate the dose, which means considering individual patient characteristics and needs
    4. For persistent pain use analgesics on a regular dosing schedule and not on a "prn" basis which promotes anxiety and contributes to future drug dependence
    5. Prevent persistent pain and relieve breakthrough pain; order rescue medication equivalent to half the standing dose to start on a prn basis
    6. Recognize and treat side effects; avoid excessive sedation
        a. Use neurostimulants to reduce sedative effects such as caffeine, dextroamphetamine (Dexedrine), methylphenidate (Ritalin)
        b. Regular laxative therapy with docusate sodium and sennosides (Senokot) twice a day is often needed to prevent constipation
    7. Use equianalgesic doses
    8. Use appropriate route of administration
        a. Use oral medications, if possible, because of ease of administration and cost effectiveness
        b. NSAID, ketorolac (Toradol), is available in IM preparation
        c. Fentanyl (Duragesic) is available as a transdermal patch
        d. Morphine and hydromorphone are available as rectal suppositories
        e. Subcutaneous or intravenous administration of morphine and hydromorphone may be needed; patient-controlled analgesia pumps can provide individualized pain relief
    9. Watch for development of tolerance; tolerance is unlikely to develop in patients with stable disease
    10. Depression and anxiety should be anticipated and treated along with other strategies; treatment of depression and anxiety should not be a substitute for pain management and vice versa

C. The Three-Step Analgesic Ladder of the World Health Organization; designed for chronic, cancer pain but can be used as a guide for all types of pain

THREE-STEP ANALGESIC LADDER OF THE WORLD HEALTH ORGANIZATION		
Step	**Oral Medications**	**Regimen**
Step 1	Acetaminophen 650 mg Q 4-6 hrs Salicylates: aspirin 325-650 mg Q 4 hrs NSAIDs (dosage in next table) Tramadol 50-100 mg Q 4-6 hrs	Nonopioid ± adjuvant
If pain persists, maximize nonopioid and add step 2 opioid		
Step 2	Codeine 30-60 mg Q 4 hrs Dihydrocodeine 16-32 mg Q 4 hrs Hydrocodone 5-10 mg Q 4-6 hrs Oxycodone 5 mg Q 6 hrs	Opioid: mild-to-moderate pain + nonopioid ± adjuvant therapy
If pain persists at step 2, increase dose of opioid or change to step 3 opioid		
Step 3	Morphine IR 15-30 mg Q 4-6 hrs Oxycodone 7.5-10 mg Q 4-6 hrs Hydromorphone 4 mg Q 4 hrs Fentanyl 50 µg/hr Q 72 hrs	Opioid: moderate-to-severe pain ± nonopioid ± adjuvant therapy

Adapted from WHO (1990). Cancer pain relief and palliative care: Report of WHO Expert Committee. *WHO Technological Report Service, 804*, 1-73.

D. Acetaminophen (Tylenol - APAP) is a nonnarcotic agent with antipyretic and analgesic effects; minimal anti-inflammatory effects; first drug to consider for mild to moderate pain of musculoskeletal origin
    1. Onset of 0.5-1 hour; duration 3-6 hours
    2. "Ceiling effect" exists, but many patients have greater pain relief from a single 1000 mg dose compared to single 650 mg dose
    3. Do not exceed 4 to 6 g per day to prevent liver damage
    4. Few adverse reactions; hepatotoxicity in overdose or in chronic alcoholics following therapeutic dosage; typically safe in patients who drink <5 alcoholic beverages per day

E. Acetylsalicylic acid (Aspirin - ASA) is a nonnarcotic agent with antipyretic, analgesic, and anti-inflammatory effects (see table on NSAIDs which follows)
1. Typically, not used for persistent pain because of dangers of gastrointestinal toxicity
2. Onset within 0.5 hours; duration 3-6 hours
3. "Ceiling effect" exists such that single doses greater than 650 mg do not result in greater degree of pain relief
4. Stop taking drug at least one week before surgery; single therapeutic dose irreversibly inhibits platelet function for the 7-day lifetime of platelet
5. Adverse reactions include Reye's syndrome, hypersensitivity reactions (asthmatic patients particularly), dyspepsia, indigestion, gastric ulcers, irreversible inhibition of platelet aggregation, tinnitus, renal effects, anemia
6. Check hematocrit and stool guaiac periodically; order plasma salicylate level determinations when patient is prescribed high dosages
7. Avoid in patients with asthma, thrombocytopenia, GI disorders

F. Other salicylic acid derivatives have a slower onset and longer duration than ASA, but are just as potent and cause fewer gastrointestinal and central nervous system side effects; good choice for older patients (see table on NSAIDs)

G. Nonsteroidal anti-inflammatory drugs (NSAIDs) are non-narcotic agents used for mild to moderate pain and have antipyretic, analgesic, and anti-inflammatory effects (see table on NSAIDs for dosing recommendations)
1. Useful for dental pain, rheumatoid arthritis, headaches, musculoskeletal pain, menstrual cramps, and bone pain with cancer; COX-2 inhibitors are preferred for older patients when acetaminophen or salicylic acid derivatives are ineffective; avoid nonselective NSAIDs in treating elderly patients who require long-term daily analgesic therapy
2. Dosing considerations:
    a. Patients have large variability in response to individual agents; Switch to another NSAID/class if one agent is ineffective; Do not switch until an adequate trial of efficacy has been undertaken (1-2 weeks depending on half-life of drugs)
    b. Always prescribe an adequate dosage (start with low dose and gradually increase to maximum dosage for patients in moderate pain)
    c. Do not use combination of different NSAIDs
    d. It is safe to combine an NSAID and acetaminophen, but there is no net gain in pain relief by combined use
3. Adverse effects
    a. GI distress (take with meals to lessen this effect), fluid retention, peripheral edema, hepatic problems, renal disorders, hypertension, and central nervous system effects such as dizziness and depression.
    b. For patients with gastritis and alcohol use, consider prophylaxis with misoprostol Cytotec), omeprazole (Prilosec), or sucralfate (Carafate); avoid piroxicam (Feldene)
4. Drug interactions
    a. Be careful in prescribing if patient is on other drugs; NSAIDs may enhance oral hypoglycemic agents and coumarin
    b. May impair diuretic function and antagonize the effects of antihypertensive medications by inhibiting renal prostaglandins
5. Cyclooxygenase-2 (COX-2 inhibitors) selective NSAIDs have a better safety profile (reduce but do not eliminate the risk of gastrointestinal bleeding and perforations) than nonselective NSAIDs and are not contraindicated with warfarin administration; renal toxicity, hypertension, and edema are possible adverse reactions
    a. Rofecoxib (Vioxx) is available in liquid and tablet form
        (1) Onset of action is more rapid and duration of effect longer than celecoxib (Celebrex)
        (2) Vioxx has higher risk of hypertension and myocardial infarctions than naproxen
    b. Celecoxib (Celebrex) is contraindicated for patients with allergies to sulfa; to date, when compared to nonselective NSAIDs, Celebrex had similar risk of cardiovascular adverse effects
    c. Valdecoxib (Bextra) has similar adverse effects as the older COX-2 inhibitors
6. Baseline tests for long-term therapy include hematocrit, liver function tests, urinalysis, blood urea nitrogen (BUN), serum creatinine; often these diagnostic tests are rechecked in first month after initiation and then at 6-month intervals

NONSTEROIDAL ANTI-INFLAMMATORY DRUGS (NSAIDs)

Class & Agent	Capsule/Tablet Size	Dose
FENAMATES		
Mefenamic Acid (Ponstel)	250	Initial: 500 mg, then 250 mg QID; max use 1 week
INDOLES		
Indomethacin (Indocin)	25, 50	25 mg BID or TID; max 200 mg daily
Sulindac (Clinoril)	150, 200	150 mg BID; max 400 mg/day
NAPHTHYLKANONE		
Nabumetone (Relafen)	500, 750	1 g/day QD or BID; max 2 g/day
OXICAMS		
Piroxicam Feldene)	10, 20	20 mg QD or 10 mg BID
PHENYLACETIC ACID		
Diclofenac sodium (Voltaren)	25, 50, 75, 100 ext. rel.	50-75 mg BID; max 200 mg/day 100 mg ext. rel. QD
PROPIONIC ACIDS		
Ibuprofen (Motrin)[†]	200, 400, 600, 800	200-600 mg Q 4-6 hrs; max 3.2 g/day
Naproxen (Naprosyn)*	250, 375, 500	250-500 mg initially, followed by 250 mg Q 6-8 hrs
PYRANOCARBOXYLIC ACID		
Etodolac (Lodine)	200, 300, 400, 500	200-400 mg Q 6-8 hrs; max 1200 mg/day
SALICYLATES		
Acetylsalicylic acid (ASA)	Varies	325-650 mg Q 4-6 hrs; max 4 g/day
Diflunisal (Dolobid)	250, 500	500-1000 mg initially, followed by 250-500 mg q 8-12 hrs
Choline magnesium trisalicylate (Trilisate)**	500, 750, 1000	500-1500 mg BID
COX-2 INHIBITORS		
Celecoxib (Celebrex)	100, 200	100-200 mg BID
Rofecoxib (Vioxx)	12.5, 25, 50	12.5 mg QD initially; max 25-50 mg QD
Valdecoxib (Bextra)	10, 20	10 mg QD

[†]Ibuprofen (Motrin Suspension, available 100 mg/5 mL)
*Naproxen (Naprosyn Suspension, available 125 mg/5 mL)
**Choline magnesium trisalicylate (Trilisate Liquid, available 500 mg/5 mL):

H.   Tramadol (Ultram), a central-acting analgesic, is sometimes used for treatment of mild-to-moderate pain; well suited when pain is not relieved by acetaminophen and the patient cannot tolerate NSAIDs and wishes to defer opioid therapy; use with caution in patients with seizure disorders

I.   Step 2 should be initiated when the patient continues to have mild-to-moderate pain despite taking a nonopioid analgesia; the following should occur at this step:
1.   Maximize the dose of the nonopioid analgesia - AND - add a step 2 opioid analgesia
2.   Step 2 opioids are restricted for the treatment of moderate pain because of their dose-limiting side effects or because they are prepared with fixed combinations of nonopioid analgesics (see table CONTROLLED DRUGS for classification)
    a.   Value of codeine (CIII) is limited because of increasing risk of side effects at doses above 1.5 mg per kg
    b.   Hydrocodone (Lortab) (CIII) and oxycodone (Percocet) (CII) are limited because of their combinations with acetaminophen; for example, do not exceed 6 g of acetaminophen per day; patients cannot take more than 15 mg of these opioids
3.   For episodic or noncontinuous pain prescribe opioids as needed rather than round the clock
4.   For continuous pain, prescribe long-acting or sustained-release preparations
5.   Identify and treat breakthrough pain with fast-onset, short-acting preparations
6.   Prevent constipation and opioid-related gastrointestinal symptoms
    a.   Assess bowel function before prescribing opioids and then at every follow-up visit
    b.   Begin a prophylactic bowel regimen when opioids are prescribed
    c.   Use bulking agents cautiously in immobile patients and those who may not be adequately hydrated
    d.   Encourage adequate fluid intake, exercise, frequent ambulation, and regular toileting habits
    e.   Prescribe a stimulant such as senna to provide regular bowel movements

7. Opioids often cause mild sedation and impaired cognitive performance, particularly in the elderly
   a. Monitor patient for profound sedation and respiratory depression
   b. For opioid antagonism, cautiously use naloxone by titrating with low incremental doses
8. Assess and treat nausea and fatigue that often accompany opioid therapy (see V.L.4.)

CONTROLLED DRUGS

CII:	High potential for abuse which may lead to severe psychological or physical dependence. Prescriptions must be written in ink or typewritten and signed by practitioner. Verbal prescriptions cannot be made.
CIII:	Use of these products may lead to moderate or low physical dependence or high psychological dependence. Prescriptions can be oral or written and may be redispensed.
CIV:	These drugs have a low abuse potential, use may lead to limited physical or psychological dependence. Prescriptions may be oral or written and may be redispensed up to 5 times within 6 months.
CV:	These drugs have a low abuse potential, may or may not require a prescription, and are subject to state and local regulation.

J. Step 3: If pain persists even when taking highest, safe dose of step 2 opioid, add a step 3 opioid to treat moderate to severe pain
   1. Morphine is first line agent; available in immediate release tablets (MSIR) (CII), sustained release tablets (MS Contin) (CII), extended release tablets (Avinza) (CII), rectal suppository, liquid, injection, and intravenous
   2. Other choices
      a. Oxycodone (OxyContin) (CII)
      b. Hydromorphone (Dilaudid) (CII)
      c. Fentanyl (Duragesic) (CII) transdermal patches can control pain for 72 hours; to avoid over-medication, remember that the drug continues to be delivered approximately 18 hours after removal of the patch
      d. Methadone (Dolophine) (CII) and levorphanol (Levo-Dromoran) are useful for severe pain, but because of long half-lives are not recommended for initial therapy

K. The following opioids are not recommended
   1. Meperidine (Demerol) has a short half-life and its metabolite, normeperidine, is toxic
   2. Propoxyphene (Darvon) has a long half-life and there is risk of accumulation of norpropoxyphene, a toxic metabolite
   3. Mixed narcotic agonist-antagonists such as pentazocine (Talwin) (CIV), butorphanol (Stadol) (CIV), and buprenorphine (Buprenex) (CIV) cause less constipation and biliary spasmodic activity but have the tendency to cause psychotomimetic responses

L. Adjuvant analgesics
   1. Tricyclic antidepressants (TCAs) such as amitriptyline (Elavil) (most frequently used, but has most side effects), imipramine (Tofranil), and desipramine (Norpramin) may be beneficial
      a. Have direct analgesic effects and may potentiate opiate analgesia
      b. Useful in treatment of pain due to nerve injury such as diabetic neuropathy
      c. Starting dose for TCA in elderly is 10mg; in other adults 25 mg; upwardly titrate; effective dose is 75 mg but some patients require maximum of 150mg
   2. Selective serotonin reuptake inhibitors (SSRIs) such as fluoxetine (Prozac) or sertraline (Zoloft) have fewer adverse effects than TCAs and may be beneficial
   3. Caffeine may increase analgesic effect when given with other pain medications
   4. Phenothiazines such as prochlorperazine (Compazine) 5-10 mg TID or promethazine (Phenergan) 25 mg BID are useful as antiemetics when used in combination with other pain medications
   5. Anticonvulsants are useful for management of brief lancinating pain in chronic neuralgia such as trigeminal neuralgia and postherpetic neuralgia; use one of following:
      a. Carbamazepine (Tegretol) 400-800 mg/day in two divided doses (begin with 100 mg BID) for pain in trigeminal neuralgia
      b. Gabapentin (Neurontin) 900-1200 mg/day in three divided doses (begin 300 mg HS for one day, then 300 mg BID for one, then 300 mg TID for one day and continue)
   6. Mexiletine (Mexitil) 150-300 mg TID is beneficial for neuropathic pain
   7. Corticosteroids are beneficial in patients with acute nerve compression, visceral distention, increased intracranial pressure, and soft-tissue infiltration
   8. Plain glucosamine sulfate reduces joint pain and may slow osteoarthritis progression

9. Topical local anesthetics can help reduce pain of the affected dermatome; prescribe capsaicin cream 0.025% (Zostrix), particularly for osteoarthritis and diabetic neuropathy. Apply 3-4 times daily; to diminish burning sensation, try a topical spray such as Solarcaine

10. Lidoderm (lidocaine 5%) patch is an option for postherpetic neuralgia; apply to skin, covering most of painful area; may apply up to 3 patches at once for up to 12 hours of a 24-hour period; do not apply to broken or inflamed skin

11. Vitamin D is helpful in certain cases
    a. Vitamin D deficiency is a potential cause of deep musculoskeletal pain or superficial light pressure pain, particularly in elderly homebound patients
    b. A single treatment of 100,000 I.U. (supplied as two 50,000 I.U. capsules) of vitamin D is likely to restore patient to normal vitamin D status

M. Treatment of metastatic bone pain includes radionuclides (strontium-89 and samarium-153 lexidronam) and bisphosphonates

N. A recent concept in acute pain therapy is preemptive analgesia that involves introducing an analgesic regimen prior to onset of noxious stimuli to prevent sensitization of the nervous system to subsequent stimuli that could amplify pain

O. Nonpharmacologic modalities to treat pain include meditation, relaxation, distraction, exercise, massage, imagery, aromatherapy, biofeedback, hypnosis, acupuncture, surgery (cordotomy), neuroablative blocks (chemical destruction of nerves), and nervous system stimulators such as dorsal column stimulators (DCS) and transcutaneous electrical nerve simulators (TENS)

P. Interdisciplinary pain management can reduce the patient's reliance on opiates through nonpharmacological methods such as biofeedback, visual imagery, and stress management

Q. Patient education; important to involve family members
    1. Research has shown that patient education alone can significantly improve pain management
    2. Provide information about nature of pain, medications, and non-pharmacological approaches
    3. Explain the difference between addiction that rarely occurs with chronic opioid use and dependence or tolerance that may occasionally occur
    4. Explain that patients typically develop tolerance to most adverse effects such as nausea, vomiting, and sedation
    5. When using opioid analgesics, instruct patient not to drive; patient and caregivers should be warned about potential for falls and accidents (precautions should be undertaken)
    6. Remind patients to carefully read labels of over-the-counter medications (especially cold, cough, fever, and headache drugs) because these drugs often have analgesic components (e.g., acetaminophen) that may cause over-medication, adverse reactions, and toxicity
    7. Warn patients that chewing or crushing continuous-release tablets destroys their controlled-release properties and may result in overdosage
    8. Cognitive coping strategies help patients understand that chronic pain is a chronic disease and goals of treatment are to improve functioning and quality of life rather than eliminate pain
    9. A physical activity program should be considered for all older patients
    10. Behavioral strategies such as controlling pain by relaxation methods, increasing pleasurable activities, and pacing their activities are beneficial
    11. Meditation which helps the patients accept their pain and distraction strategies (imagery, focal point, counting method) are also effective
    12. Website resources are available (see table WEBSITE RESOURCES)

WEBSITE RESOURCES	
American Academy of Hospice and Palliative Medicine	www.aahpm.org
American Academy of Pain Medicine	www.painmed.org
American Pain Society	www.ampainsoc.org
International Association for the Study of Pain	www.halcyon.com/iasp
International Hospice Institute and College	www.hospicecare.com
National Hospice Organization	www.nho.org
Worldwide Congress on Pain	www.pain.com

R. Follow up evaluation is important if patient is on a long-term pain management regimen
1. Regularly evaluate for drug efficacy
2. Carefully evaluate for side effects
   a. For patients on NSAIDs, monitor for gastrointestinal blood loss, renal insufficiency, edema, hypertension
   b. For patients on opioids, monitor for sedation, fatigue, confusion, constipation
   c. Monitor for drug-drug and drug-disease interactions
3. Periodically evaluate for inappropriate or dangerous drug-use patterns

WEIGHT LOSS (INVOLUNTARY)

I. Definition: Process that occurs when the number of calories available for utilization is below the patient's daily needs

A. In adults, loss of 5% of baseline body weight over 6 months is significant

B. The range of daily caloric intake for a moderately active adult is 2200-2800 calories for males and 1800-2100 calories for females who are not pregnant or lactating

II. Pathogenesis

A. Reduced food intake and/or anorexia can result in a calorie deficit from the following causes:
1. Psychological problems such as anorexia nervosa, depression, and anxiety
2. Physical and financial factors that limit purchasing, preparing, or eating food
   a. Poor dentition
   b. Immobility problems
   c. Dysphagia (Parkinson's disease, stroke)
3. Drug-related problems such as digitalis excess or amphetamine abuse
4. Gastrointestinal diseases (peptic ulcer disease, gallbladder disease, esophageal disease, hepatitis, constipation)
5. Infections such as human immunodeficiency virus (HIV) infection, tuberculosis, and fungal disease
6. Malignancy
7. Uremia
8. Hepatitis
9. Vitamin B deficiencies
10. Neurologic disorders, including trauma
11. Substance abuse and tobacco use
12. Competitive athletics (especially wrestling)

B. Calorie loss can occur because of malabsorption from the following conditions:
1. Crohn's disease
2. Pancreatic insufficiency
3. Cholestasis
4. Parasitic disease such as giardiasis
5. Blind loop syndrome

C. Calories can be lost in the urine or stool from the following illnesses:
1. Uncontrolled diabetes mellitus
2. Diabetes insipidus
3. Diarrhea and vomiting

D. Accelerated metabolism can contribute to weight loss in the following conditions:
1. Hyperthyroidism
2. Pheochromocytoma
3. Fever
4. Malignancy
5. Spastic states

III. Clinical presentation of common causes of weight loss

A. Patients with HIV infection often have chronic anorexia, nausea, vomiting, and diarrhea due to drugs or to infections of the hepatobiliary system

B. Malignancies, particularly of the gastrointestinal tract, pancreas, and liver, are a common cause
1. May be present without major signs and symptoms
2. Dramatic, rapid weight loss accompanied by aversion to food and later jaundice and abdominal pain characterizes pancreatic cancer

C. Uremia often presents initially with anorexia and subsequent weight loss

D. Uncontrolled diabetes mellitus has weight loss and increased food intake

E. Hyperthyroidism or thyrotoxicosis is the most common endocrine disease
1. Patients often have increased appetite, food intake, and motor activity
2. In the elderly, "apathetic" hyperthyroidism may be present; weight loss and weakness may predominate with little evidence of the typical symptoms of thyroid hormone excess (see section on HYPERTHYROIDISM)

F. In malabsorption syndrome, foul-smelling, bulky, greasy stools are typical

G. In the elderly population, cancer (lung and GI malignancies), depression, drugs (polypharmacy), neurologic diseases (Alzheimer's disease, stroke), cardiac disorders, benign GI diseases, and apathetic hyperthyroidism are common causes of weight loss

H. Signs and symptoms of malnutrition may occur with any illness if there is a loss of 10 to 20% of normal body weight
1. Typical complaints include fatigue, depressed immune function, increased susceptibility to infection, skin breakdown, and changes in emotional stability such as irritability and apathy
2. Laboratory tests: Serum albumin <3.4 g/dL and lymphocyte count <1,500 are indicative of malnutrition

IV. Diagnosis/Evaluation

A. History
1. Carefully ascertain amount of weight loss; ask about change in clothing size if unable to elicit number of pounds lost
2. Validate amount of weight loss from a family member or significant other
3. Obtain a 24-hour daily food intake
4. Determine whether patient has loss of appetite, normal appetite, or increased appetite; in patients with malignancies, depression, and adverse drug reactions, food often has an unappealing appearance, taste, and odor
5. Ask about abnormal or bad taste in mouth (occurs in hepatitis, drugs, sinusitis, vitamin B deficiencies, zinc deficiency, psychological disorders)
6. If decreased food intake is suspected, explore symptoms of depression, poor dentition, dysphagia, alcohol and drug use, pain, nausea, vomiting, fatigue, and symptoms of heart failure
7. Question about chewing or swallowing difficulties (occurs in neurologic, dental, oral, esophageal or pulmonary diseases)
8. If anorexia nervosa is suspected ask about eating habits, self-image and attitudes about weight control
9. If malabsorption is suspected determine character of stools, signs of jaundice, easy bruising, sore tongue, and paresthesias
10. If loss of calories in stool or urine is suspected, inquire about polyuria, polydipsia, nausea, and character of the stools
11. If accelerated metabolism is suspected inquire about fever, fatigue, melena, cough that has changed in character, and symptoms of hyperthyroidism such as tachycardia, nervousness, heat intolerance, menstrual disturbances, and palpitations
12. Obtain history of tobacco dependence, alcohol consumption, and drug use
13. Ask about medications
    a. Many medications have adverse effects on appetite (digitalis, theophylline, procainamide, cholestyramine, psychotropic medications, antibiotics, amphetamines, NSAIDs)
    b. Some medications interfere with absorption of nutrients

14. Inquire about participation in competitive athletics
15. Inquire about previous history of hepatitis exposure, renal disease, and endocrine problems
16. Determine family history, particularly noting any history of cancer in first-degree relatives

B. Physical Examination; assessment should focus on nutritional status as well as identification of the underlying cause of weight loss
   1. Measure height and weight, comparing with previous measurements (see OBESITY section for determining optimal weights for adults)
      a. A systematic investigation is needed for unexplained losses of >5% of usual body weight over 6 months
      b. Body weight measurement is not always a good indicator of weight loss; occasionally loss of body tissue is accompanied by equal gain in extracellular fluid such as ascites or edema; thus, it is important to observe face and limbs for loss of soft-tissue mass
   2. Assess for orthostatic hypotension which accompanies dehydration and malnutrition
   3. Observe general appearance for wasting such as sunken eyes, sallow complexion, and hair loss
   4. Assess for signs of depression such as inappropriate dress and dull affect
   5. Observe skin for pallor, ecchymosis, and jaundice
   6. Examine mouth for poor dentition, glossitis, and lesions
   7. Palpate neck for thyromegaly and lymphadenopathy
   8. Perform a complete cardiovascular examination
   9. Auscultate the lungs; obtain oxygen saturation level
   10. Inspect abdomen for shape, scars, and masses
   11. Auscultate abdomen for bowel sounds
   12. Palpate and percuss abdomen for tenderness, ascites, masses, and organomegaly
   13. Perform a rectal examination
   14. Assess extremities for edema, muscle wasting, and skin turgor
   15. Assess position and vibratory senses
   16. Assess deep tendon reflexes; check for prolonged relaxation phase of reflexes that often occurs with thyroid disorders

C. Differential Diagnosis; depression and psychological problems are the most common causes, especially in the elderly
   1. When weight loss occurs with increased food intake, consider diabetes, thyrotoxicosis, malabsorption, or possibly leukemia and lymphoma as the likely diagnosis
   2. When food intake is normal or decreased, consider psychological problems, malignancy, infection, renal disease, or endocrine problems as the likely diagnosis

D. Diagnostic Tests
   1. Diagnostic tests should be ordered based on the history and physical; an initial, recommended battery of tests includes three stool specimens for occult blood, CBC with differential, urinalysis, serum glucose, creatinine, albumin, and liver function tests and possibly chest x-ray and erythrocyte sedimentation rate
   2. Order thyroid stimulating hormone and T_4 in elderly patients because of the high incidence of thyroid disorders in this population; also order thyroid tests in patients who have not had reduced food intake with weight loss
   3. For patients with decreased intake consider ordering a serum calcium, potassium, and blood urea nitrogen
   4. If malnutrition is suspected, especially in the older patient, also order serum iron, transferrin, total iron-binding capacity, RBCs, folate, B_{12}, and zinc levels
   5. For patients with impaired absorption, a quantitative stool fat examination by means of a 72-hour stool collection or a breath test (definitive test); but screening for malabsorption can also be performed with Sudan stain of stool for fat and serum tests for carotenoids and folic acid
   6. Consider colonoscopy or flexible sigmoidoscopy, barium enema, upper endoscopy, or upper gastrointestinal series with small bowel follow-through, abdominal ultrasonography, computerized tomography of the abdomen, or magnetic resonance imaging if concerns of abdominal malignancy exist
   7. Order CBC and erythrocyte sedimentation rate if fever is present
   8. Erythrocyte sedimentation rate, chest x-ray, and mammogram are recommended if concerns of other types of cancer exist
   9. Consider serum amylase and lipase if a pancreatic disorder is suspected
   10. Stool for ova and parasites is ordered when giardiasis is suspected

11. To assess nutritional status consider the following: serum albumin concentration, grip strength, triceps skin-fold thickness, arm muscle circumference, total lymphocyte count, bioimpedance analysis, serum transferrin, and transthyretin (prealbumin) concentrations

V. Plan/Management

A. Treat underlying cause of weight loss (i.e., treat depression with antidepressant medications or pancreatic insufficiency with oral pancreatic enzyme preparations)

B. Consider hospitalization for any individual with weight loss of more than 10-20%

C. Vitamin supplementation may be needed; the fat soluble vitamins A, D, and K are most likely to be depleted in cases of malabsorption

D. Consultation with a dietitian/nutritionist is beneficial

E. Symptomatic therapy includes the following:
   1. Suggest patient eat small, frequent feedings (6 times per day) of foods with high-calorie density
   2. Suggest dietary supplements such as Ensure (see section on HIV INFECTION)
   3. Consider ordering vitamin supplementation
   4. Recommend community resources such as Meals on Wheels/senior center lunch programs
   5. For nausea, suggest salty foods, cool clear beverages, gelatin, popsicles; avoid sweet, greasy or high fat foods
   6. Eliminate unnecessary medications
   7. If possible eliminate symptom-producing medications
   8. Consider switching medications; for example, if patient has depression, consider use of mirtazapine that stimulates the appetite
   9. Appetite stimulants such as dronabinol (Marinol) and megestrol acetate (Megace) are recommended for AIDS patients, but are **not** FDA approved for unknown causes of weight loss

F. Follow Up
   1. Scheduling of subsequent visits will depend on underlying cause of weight loss and age of patient
   2. If the cause of weight loss is not evident, weight loss is not severe, and patient is without psychological and physical abnormalities, schedule return visit in 2 to 4 weeks; encourage patient to keep daily record of food intake, activity level, and symptoms

REFERENCES

Agency for Healthcare Research and Quality. (2001). *Defining and managing chronic fatigue syndrome.* (AHRQ Pub. No. 01-E061). Rockville MD: US Government Printing Office.

Agency for Health Care Policy and Research, Public Health Service, US Department of Health and Human Services. (1993). *Acute pain management in adults: Operative procedures.* (AHCPR Pub. No. 92-0019). Rockville, MD: US Government Printing Office.

American Geriatrics Society (AGS) Panel on Persistent Pain in Older Persons. (2002). The management of persistent pain in older persons. *Journal of the American Geriatrics Society, 50*(Suppl), S205-S224.

American Pain Society. (2002). *Guideline for the management of pain in osteoarthritis, rheumatoid arthritis, and juvenile chronic arthritis.* Glenview, IL: Author.

Bazemore, A.W., & Smucker, D.R. (2002). Lymphadenopathy and malignancy. *American Family Physician, 66,* 2103-2110.

Chodosh, J., Ferrell, B.A., Shekelle, P.G., & Wenger, N.S. (2001). Quality indicators for pain management in vulnerable elders. *Annals of Internal Medicine, 135,* 731-735.

Craig, T., & Kakumanu, J. (2002). Chronic fatigue syndrome: Evaluation and treatment. *American Family Physician, 65,* 1083-1090, 1095.

Ennis, B.W., Saffel-Shrier, S., & Verson, H. (2001). Diagnosing malnutrition in the elderly. *Nurse Practitioner, 26,* 52-65.

Fitzgerald, G.A., & Patrono, C. (2001). The coxibs, selective inhibitors of cyclooxygenase-2. *New England Journal of Medicine, 345,* 433-442.

Fainsinger, R.L. (2002). Symptomatic care pending diagnosis: Pain. In R.E. Rakel, & E.T. Bope (Eds.), *Conn's current therapy 2002.* Philadelphia: Saunders.

Fletcher, R. H. (1997). Lymphadenopathy. In L. Dornbrand, A.J. Hoole; & R.H. Fletcher (Eds.), *Manual of clinical problems in adult ambulatory care* (3rd ed.). Philadelphia: Lippincott-Raven.

Fukuda, K., Straus, S.E., Hickie, I., Sharpe, M., Dobbins, J., & Komaroll, A. (1994). The chronic fatigue syndrome: A comprehensive approach to its definition and study. *Annals of Internal Medicine, 121,* 953-959.

Gloth, F.M. III. (2000). Geriatric pain: Factors that limit pain relief and increase complications. *Geriatrics, 55,* 46-54.

Gloth, F.M. III. (2001). Pain management in older adults: Prevention and treatment. *Journal of the American Geriatrics Society, 49,* 188-199.

Gorman, T.E. (2000). Approach to the patient with chronic nonmalignant pain. In A.H. Goroll, & A.G. Mulley, Jr. (Eds.), *Primary care medicine.* Philadelphia: Lippincott.

Goroil, A.H., & Mulley, A.G. (2000). Evaluation of chronic fatigue. In A.H. Goroll & A.G. Mulley, Jr., (Eds.). *Primary care medicine: Office evaluation and management of the adult patient* (4th ed). Philadelphia: Lippincott.

Goroll, A.H., & Mulley, A.G. Jr. (2000). Evaluation of weight loss. In A.H Goroll, & A.G. Mulley, Jr. (Eds.), *Primary care medicine: Office evaluation and management of the adult patient* (4th ed). Philadelphia: Lippincott.

Gottschalk, A., & Smith, D.S. (2001). New concepts in acute pain therapy: Preemptive analgesia. *American Family Physician, 63,* 1979-1984.

Graham, D.B. (2002). Weight loss. In R.B. Taylor (Ed.). *Manual of family practice* (2nd edition). Philadelphia: Lippincott.

Huffman, G.B. (2002). Evaluating and treating unintentional weight loss in the elderly. *American Family Physician, 65,* 640-650.

Leff, B.A. (2003). Involuntary weight loss in the elderly. *Advanced Studies in Medicine, 3,* 31-38.

Levine, P.H. (1998). What we know about chronic fatigue syndrome and its relevance to the practicing physician. *American Journal of Medicine, 105,* 100S-109S.

Marcus, D.A. (2000). Treatment of nonmalignant chronic pain. *American Family Physician, 61,* 1331-1338.

Plaisance, K.I., & Mackowiak, P.A. (2000). Antipyretic therapy: Physiologic rationale, diagnostic implications, and clinical consequences. *Archives of Internal Medicine, 160,* 449-456.

Reid, S., & Wessely, S. (2002). Chronic fatigue syndrome. In R.E. Rakel & E.T. Bope (Eds.). *Conn's current therapy 2002.* Philadelphia: Saunders.

Rodriguez, R. (2002). The challenge of evaluating fatigue. *Journal of American Academy of Nurse Practitioners, 12,* 329-338.

Simon, H.B. (2000). Evaluation of fever. In A.H. Goroll, & A.G. Mulley, Jr. (Eds.), *Primary care medicine: Office evaluation and management of the adult patient* (4th ed). Philadelphia: Lippincott.

Simon, H.B. (2000). Evaluation of lymphadenopathy. In A.H. Goroll, & A.G. Mulley, Jr. (Eds.), *Primary care medicine: Office evaluation and management of the adult patient* (4th ed). Philadelphia: Lippincott.

Tan, E.M., Sugiura, K., & Gupta, S. (2002). The case definition of chronic fatigue syndrome. *Journal of Clinical Immunology, 22,* 8-12.

Welker, M.J. (2002). Symptomatic care pending diagnosis: Fever. In R.E. Rakel, & E.T. Bope (Eds.), *Conn's current therapy 2002.* Philadelphia: Saunders.

Wessely, S. (2001). Chronic fatigue: Symptom and syndrome. *Annals of Internal Medicine, 134,* 838-843.

WHO (1990). Cancer pain relief and palliative care: Report of WHO expert committee. *WHO Technological Report Service, 804,* 1-73.

ALCOHOL PROBLEMS

I.   Definition: Problems caused by alcohol that may be acute or chronic, may range from mild to severe and vary in their response to treatment; problems exist on a continuum of increasing severity ranging from at-risk use to alcohol abuse to alcohol dependence

II. Pathogenesis

    A.   Causes of alcohol problems are incompletely understood

    B.   Alcohol affects several brain neurotransmitters, including dopamine, γ-aminobutyric acid, glutamate, serotonin, adenosine, norepinephrine, and opioid peptides and their receptors

    C.   A dopaminergic pathway projecting from the ventral tegmental area to the nucleus accumbens mediates the pleasurable effects of alcohol

III. Clinical Presentation

    A.   **At-risk use** is a pattern of alcohol consumption that places person at risk for adverse consequences (level of consumption exceeds **general norms** for moderate use). See CRITERIA FOR AT-RISK DRINKING and WHAT IS MODERATE USE? in the tables below

CRITERIA FOR AT-RISK DRINKING	
Men	>14 drinks/ week or >4 drinks/occasion
Women	>7 drinks/week or >3 drinks/occasion

Source: National Institute on Alcohol Abuse and Alcoholism (1995)

WHAT IS MODERATE USE OF ALCOHOL?	
Although there is some inconsistency in definitions, the definitions used by the National Institute on Alcohol Abuse and Alcoholism (1995) are as follows:	
Moderate Drinking	No more than 2 drinks a day for men and 1 drink a day for women No more than 1 drink a day for all persons over age 65
Exceptions	Persons in the following categories must abstain from alcohol use entirely: Pregnant women, those under 21, those who take medications that interact with alcohol or who have medical conditions such as liver disease

    B.   **Alcohol abuse** is the continued use of alcohol in spite of adverse consequences (UCR mnemonic--*U*se, followed by adverse *C*onsequences, followed by *R*epetition). Consequences may be physical, social, or psychological (see CRITERIA FOR ALCOHOL ABUSE table)

CRITERIA FOR ALCOHOL ABUSE	
Pattern of alcohol use in which 1 (or more) of the following 4 criteria are present within a 12-month period	
Recurrent alcohol use resulting in	✓ Failure to fulfill major role obligations (home, work, school) ✓ Placing self and others in potentially hazardous situations (DUI) ✓ Legal problems (e.g., arrest for DUI)
Continued alcohol use despite	✓ Persistent or recurrent social/interpersonal problems due to effects of alcohol

Adapted from the American Psychiatric Association. (2000). *Diagnostic and statistical manual of mental disorders*, (4th ed.), Text Revision. Washington, DC: Author.

C. Alcohol dependence is a chronic disease characterized by impaired control over drinking, preoccupation with the drug alcohol, use of alcohol in spite of adverse consequences, and distortions in thinking, primarily denial (see CRITERIA FOR ALCOHOL DEPENDENCE table)

CRITERIA FOR ALCOHOL DEPENDENCE

Pattern of alcohol use in which 3 (or more) of the following 7 criteria are present within a 12 month period
- ✓ Physical tolerance (increased amounts are required for desired effect)
- ✓ Withdrawal symptoms when substance is discontinued
- ✓ Larger amounts of alcohol are used than intended
- ✓ Unsuccessful efforts to control use
- ✓ Much time and energy are spent in obtaining, using, and recovering from effects of alcohol
- ✓ Many social, work-related, and recreational activities are reduced because of alcohol use
- ✓ Continued use in spite of knowledge that alcohol causes physical and/or psychological problems

---

Adapted from the American Psychiatric Association. (2000). *Diagnostic and statistical manual of mental disorders*, (4th ed.), Text Revision. Washington, DC: Author.

D. Binge drinking is defined as the consumption of 5 or more alcoholic beverages on a single occasion
   1. Results in acute impairment and causes a substantial fraction of all alcohol-related deaths
   2. Adverse health consequences specifically associated with binge drinking include unintentional injuries, suicide, alcohol poisoning, hypertension, acute myocardial infarction, gastritis, pancreatitis, and poor control of diabetes
   3. Many sequelae of binge drinking have especially high social and economic costs including violence—homicide, rape, and domestic violence—as well as child neglect and lost productivity
   4. Reducing binge drinking among adults is a leading health indicator in *Healthy People 2010*; unfortunately, the prevalence of binge drinking along with its adverse health outcomes, has increased in recent years

E. Motor vehicle accidents resulting from driving under the influence of alcohol are the leading cause of death in the 15-24 year old age group

---

Facts about Alcohol-Related Traffic Deaths
- ➡ Alcohol-related traffic death rate in the US has dropped substantially in the last 20 years
- ➡ In 1982, the 60% of traffic deaths were related to alcohol compared with 41% in 2001 (most dramatic decreases have been among the youngest drivers)
- ➡ State with highest alcohol-related death rate: South Carolina, followed by Montana, Louisiana, and the District of Columbia
- ➡ State with the lowest rate: Utah, followed by Vermont, New York, Minnesota, New Jersey, and Massachusetts
- ➡ Men killed in traffic crashes are nearly 2 times as likely to be legally intoxicated as women
- ➡ Beer consumption is the cause of up to 80% of all alcohol-related crashes and fatalities
- ➡ In spite of the success of tougher drunk-driving laws, more than 17,000 persons still die each year in the US in alcohol-related crashes

---

F. Over 60% of all adults consume alcohol, and an estimated 10% of the adult population abuse alcohol

G. Alcohol abuse kills approximately 100,000 Americans annually and is the third leading preventable cause of death in the US. It is more prevalent in men than in women; excessive drinking accounts for almost a third of alcohol consumed in the US or over $34 billion of the total amount spent each year on alcohol
   1. Excessive drinking (consuming more than moderate amounts of alcohol) is linked to serious health problems including increased risk for motor vehicle crashes, other injuries, hypertension, stroke, violence, suicide, and certain types of cancer
   2. As much as half of violent crime, including murder, rape, assault, child molestation, and spouse abuse, is connected with concurrent alcohol abuse

H. About 5-10% of the population aged 65 and older are heavy alcohol users; alcohol problems in this age group go largely unrecognized in that psychosocial factors (spouse, job, and legal pressures, e.g., DUI) are not likely to be present as many older adults live alone, are retired, and no longer drive

IV. Diagnosis/Evaluation

A. History
1. Keep in mind that the history (including interview and use of questionnaires) is by far more sensitive and specific than are physical exam and laboratory findings
2. All patients should be screened for alcohol problems, beginning in early adolescence. **Ask 'Do you ever drink alcohol?"**
3. If patient **ever** drinks, ask **quantity-frequency** questions which deal with level of consumption, and can help distinguish moderate from at-risk drinking and identify binge drinking (see LEVEL OF CONSUMPTION and GENERAL EQUIVALENCIES OF ALCOHOLIC BEVERAGES tables)

LEVEL OF CONSUMPTION	
Frequency	How many days in a week do you usually have something to drink?
Quantity	On days that you drink, how many drinks do you have?
Maximum	What is the most you had to drink on any one day during the past month?
Last drink	When was your last drink? (Persons with a problem know exactly)
Scoring and interpretation	If quantity x frequency >7 drinks a week for women and >14 drinks for men, or if maximum per occasion is >3 for women and >4 for men, then patient exceeds criteria for low-risk drinking

Adapted from Bower, K.T., & Severin, J.D. (1997). Alcohol and other drug-related problems. In D.J. Knesper, M.B. Riba, & T.L. Schwenk (Eds.), *Primary care psychiatry*. Philadelphia: Saunders.

GENERAL EQUIVALENCIES OF ALCOHOLIC BEVERAGES*			
Hard liquor (80 proof spirits)		**Beer (4% to 5% alcohol)**	
1 shot or highball (1.5 ounces)	= 1 drink	1 12-ounce bottle or can	= 1 drink
1/2 pint of liquor	= ~5 drinks	1 40-ounce container	= ~3 drinks
1 pint of liquor	= ~10 drinks	1 .6-pack of beer	= 6 drinks
Wine (11% to 12% alcohol)		**Wine Coolers (5% alcohol)**	
1 glass of wine (5 ounces)	= 1 drink	1 wine cooler (12 ounces)	= 1 drink
1 bottle of wine (750 mL)	= 5 drinks		

* One drink contains approximately 12 g of alcohol

4. Follow quantity-frequency questions with the CAGE questions. See the following table

THE CAGE QUESTIONNAIRE	
C	Have you ever felt you ought to <u>C</u>ut down on your drinking?
A	Have people <u>A</u>nnoyed you by criticizing your drinking?
G	Have you ever felt bad or <u>G</u>uilty about your drinking?
E	Have you ever had a drink the first thing in the morning (<u>E</u>ye opener) to steady your nerves or get rid of a hangover?
Scoring and Interpretation	Person receives one point for each positive answer. One "yes" answer indicates hazardous drinking and two or more "yes" answers indicate alcohol abuse or dependence

Source: Bush, B., Shaw, S., Cleary, P., Delbanco, T.L., & Aronson, M.D. (1987). Screening for alcohol abuse using the CAGE questionnaire. *American Journal of Medicine, 82*, 231-235.

5. If patient answers "yes" to a CAGE question, prompt for more details
6. Patients who become angry and defensive with the CAGE questions have already responded positively to the second item in the questionnaire
7. If screening using quantity-frequency questions and CAGE questions indicates problems with alcohol, ask more specific questions based on criteria for alcohol abuse and dependence
8. Finally, carefully screen for use of other substances (high concomitant use of tobacco and other drugs by persons with alcohol problems)

9. Alternatives to the CAGE questionnaire are listed in table below

SCREENING TESTS FOR ALCOHOL PROBLEMS		
Test	Description	Source
AUDIT (Alcohol Use Disorders Identification Test)	Excellent and simple 10-question, self-administered questionnaire that assesses both levels of consumption and related problems	Saunders, J.B., Aasland, O.G., Babor, T.F., & Unreal, N. (1993). Development of the Alcohol Use Disorders Identification Test (AUDIT): WHO collaborative project on early detection of persons with harmful alcohol consumption. *Addiction, 88,* 791-804
MAST (Michigan Alcoholism Screening Test)	Contains 24 items and there are several versions and scoring protocols available, including the simpler 13-item Short MAST	Hedlund, J.L., & Vieweg, B.W. (1984). The Michigan Alcoholism Screening Test (MAST): A comprehensive review. *J. Operational Psychiatry, 15,* 55-65
MAST-G (MAST-Geriatric Version)	Also contains 24 items and is for use in older adults ≥55. Unlike the regular MAST, questions about fights, arrests, and work difficulties have been eliminated	Blow, F.C., Brower, K.J., Schulenberg, J.E., Demo-Dananberg, L.A., Young, J.P., & Beresford, T.P. (1992). The Michigan Alcoholism Screening Test--Geriatric Version (MAST-G): A new elderly-specific screening instrument. *Alcohol Clin Exp Res, 16,* 372
TACE	Contains 4 items and is based on the CAGE; for use with pregnant women	Russel, M., Martier, S.S., & Sokol, R.J., et al. (1994). Screening for pregnancy risk-drinking. *Alcohol Clin Exp Res, 18,* 1156-1161

B. Physical Examination
   1. Note that an absence of findings on physical exam does not indicate that the patient is free of alcohol problems (most early manifestations of alcohol abuse/dependence are psychosocial, not physical)
   2. Assess general appearance: weight loss, emaciated appearance are late findings in chronic alcoholism
   3. Examine skin for signs of chronic alcoholism (abnormal vascularization of the facial skin [spider angiomata] and jaundice when liver disease is present)
   4. Perform abdominal exam for hepatomegaly and right upper quadrant tenderness
   5. Male patients should be evaluated for gynecomastia, loss of axillary and pubic hair, and testicular atrophy
   6. Perform complete neurologic exam, including mental status exam, cranial nerves, gait, sensory, motor, reflexes, Romberg test
   7. During exam, note if patient smells of alcohol as alcohol on breath during primary care visit indicates that there is impaired control over drinking

C. Differential Diagnosis: Other mental disorders such as mood and anxiety disorders, psychosis, delirium, dementia; abuse of other psychoactive substances such as opioids, marijuana, hallucinogens, PCP, inhalants, and sedatives

D. Diagnostic Tests
   1. CBC (elevated mean corpuscular volume is a marker of excessive alcohol consumption; may be elevated due to other causes such as dietary deficiencies—B_{12}, folate—liver disease, smoking)
   2. Liver enzyme tests
      a. A γ-glutamyltransferase level that is 2 times the normal level in patients with an aspartate aminotransferase:alanine aminotransferase ratio of at least 2:1 strongly suggests a diagnosis of alcohol abuse
      b. Use of γ-glutamyltransferase level as a single test to diagnose alcohol abuse is not recommended because of its lack of specificity
   3. Carbohydrate-deficient transferrin can detect heavy drinking; may be useful for monitoring alcohol-dependent patients; this test is not yet readily available to most clinicians

V. Plan/Management

   A. Plan is determined by the **identification** and **confirmation** that the patient has problems with alcohol and by his/her **willingness to change** behavior

B. **Identification** of problem-drinking is determined primarily from screening using the CAGE and the Level of Consumption questions; the physical examination and the laboratory testing may provide additional evidence that a problem exists

C. **Confirmation** of the problem is based on the extent to which the patient meets the criteria for at-risk drinking, or for alcohol abuse or dependence and involves two important diagnostic issues
    1. What happens when the patient uses alcohol? (adverse consequences)
    2. What happens when the patient tries to stop? (impaired control, tolerance and withdrawal)

D. Diagnostic Issues
    1. **First diagnostic issue**. Assess problem areas first (adverse consequences) then link them to substance use. (Example: How are things going at home? At work? At school [for adolescents/college students]? In your social life? and so on. As the patient introduces problems, be empathetic, but ask patient "How do you think your use of alcohol fits in with this?")
    2. **Second diagnostic issue**
        a. Determine degree of **impaired control** by asking questions such as "Do you drink more than you intend to?" "Why do you think that happens?" "Do you ever make rules for your drinking?" "Are you able to follow those rules?"
        b. Assess **tolerance**. "Do you need more to get the same effect?"
        c. Ask about **withdrawal**. "Do you ever feel bad or sick when you try to stop drinking?"

E. **Motivation** for change on the patient's part is crucial to the success of any treatment plan. Appropriate questions to assess motivation are the following: "Are you concerned about your use of alcohol?" "Are you interested in changing?"; success of any intervention is dependent on the patient's willingness to participate in treatment goals

F. **Brief interventions have been demonstrated through research to be highly effective**
    1. Can be conducted in the office for the following groups of patients: At-risk and problem drinkers who are not alcohol-dependent (may be useful in motivating alcohol-dependent patients to enter alcohol treatment)
    2. Brief, nonspecific interventions by primary care clinicians often result in outcomes equal to more intensive interventions by highly trained specialists
    3. Use the *FRAMES* acronym to guide the intervention

FRAMES FOR BRIEF INTERVENTIONS	
Feedback	related to screening tests, history, physical examination and laboratory findings should be provided as well as the implications of the findings (e.g., your liver enzymes are elevated [show patient the lab report])
Responsibility	for changing alcohol use should be placed on the patient; success of treatment is up to patient
Advise	patient to cut down or abstain
Menu	of options should be presented to the patient in order to make the patient a partner in the decision-making process: Can attempt to stop on own; can attend AA meetings; can use self-help books
Empathic	approach is crucial; regardless of counseling methods, clinicians demonstrating empathy have the best outcomes
Self-efficacy	of the patient is encouraged by clinician's optimism relating to behavior change. Advise the patient to make a change--stop drinking altogether or, if controlled drinking is an option in your opinion, to limit drinking to no more than 2 drinks a day

Adapted from Miller, W.R., & Rollnick, S. (1991). *Motivational interviewing: Preparing people to change addictive behavior.* New York: Guilford Press.

G. Refer all patients and their families (at risk, problem drinkers, and alcohol-dependent) to self-help groups such as Alcoholics Anonymous (AA) for patients, Al-Anon for families. These groups are extremely effective in maintaining sobriety and helping patients and families to cope. Refer family even if patient declines to attend
    1. Help patients track down a nearby meeting at www.alcoholics-anonymous.org; this is a service your office must be ready and willing to perform
    2. Al-Anon Family Group Headquarters, Inc. 800-356-9996 or www.al-anon.org
    3. Alateen, 800-356-9996 or www.al-anon.alateen.org

H. Familiarize yourself with AA in your community by attending an open meeting
    1. With patient's permission, ask for an AA volunteer who is willing to act as sponsor to meet with patient in your office
    2. Sponsor should be same gender as patient

I.   Find a comprehensive listing of support groups for alcoholics and their families at
      www.mentalhelp.net/selfhelp

J.   For other information relating to alcoholism, see www.niaaa.nih.gov

K.   Recommend self-help books for both patients and family members (see table below)

SELF-HELP BOOKS FOR ALCOHOL PROBLEMS	
For the patient (author of book is a woman, so particularly useful for women patients)	Knapp, C. (1991). *Drinking: A love story.* New York: Doubleday Delacorte Press
For the patient (emphasis is on lifestyle as well as behavioral change)	Washington, A., & Boundy, D. (1990). *Willpower is not enough: Understanding and recovering from addictions of every kind.* New York: Harper-Perennial
For the school-age child (8-12) whose father has an alcohol problem	Black, C. (1982*). My dad loves me: My dad has a disease.* Denver: Mac Publishing
For parents of a patient with alcohol problems (written by former US Senator George McGovern)	McGovern, G. (1996). *Terry: My daughter's life and death struggle with alcoholism.* New York: Villard
For adult children of alcoholics and their risk issues	Black, C. (1981). *It will never happen to me: Children of alcoholics as youngsters-adolescents-adults.* New York: Ballantine

L.   Patients who are alcohol dependent usually need a two-phase treatment regimen: detoxification and
      rehabilitation
      1.   Detoxification ameliorates the symptoms of withdrawal
      2.   Rehabilitation helps the patient avoid future problems with alcohol
      3.   Refer alcohol dependent patients to residential treatment facilities, if possible
      4.   Residential treatment should be considered for patients who require supervision for medical or
            psychiatric safety, lack a home environment conducive to abstinence, work in highly safety-
            sensitive environments, or have failed previous inpatient treatments

M.   Be familiar with at least one specialized treatment facility in your area
      1.   Clinicians **must be ready with a plan** when the drinker is ready to quit
      2.   For a list of programs as well as a discussion of approaches, visit the American Society of
            Addiction Medicine at www.asam.org
      3.   Feedback from patients will help you learn which programs in your area are most effective
      4.   Referral for family therapy may be indicated when complex problems are present

N.   Pharmacologic treatment: The FDA has approved two drugs to treat alcohol dependence
      1.   Naltrexone (ReVia) is an opioid antagonist that blocks the alcohol-induced release of dopamine in
            the nucleus accumbens
            a.   Reduces the craving for alcohol
            b.   May deter patients who sample alcohol from progressing to relapse
            c.   Dosing is 50 mg once daily for 12 weeks
            d.   Consult PDR for prescribing information, contraindications, precautions, and adverse effects
      2.   Disulfiram (Antabuse) is an aversive drug which has been available for many years
            a.   Controlled clinical trials in recent years cast serious doubt on its efficacy
            b.   Nonetheless, some clinicians continue to prescribe it
            c.   Usual dose is 250 mg once daily (available in 250 and 500 mg tabs)
            d.   Consult PDR regarding dosing, contraindications, precautions, and adverse effects

O.   Another opiate antagonist that is currently in clinical trials in the US is acamprosate; based on clinical
      trials in Europe, this medication appears to be highly efficacious and should be available in 2003

P.   Patients who are alcohol dependent and who also have a psychiatric disorder should be referred for
      treatment for the underlying disorder as these patients are usually complex

Q.   Follow up is variable depending on type of treatment
      1.   Patients for whom brief intervention is conducted: Follow up in first few weeks with two or more
            visits/telephone contacts to monitor patient's progress and assess need for additional approaches
            (aim for 4 contacts in 6 weeks)

2. Patients who have been referred to alcohol treatment (residential) should be followed for ongoing support; the natural course of alcohol problems includes remission as well as relapse; these patients should be attending AA meetings on regular basis

3. For both groups of patients (brief intervention and residential treatment), supportive relapse visits should include the following

QUESTIONS/DISCUSSION FOR THE SUPPORTIVE RELAPSE VISIT	
Ask	"When was the date of the last drink?" "Have you used other drugs?" "Are you continuing with Alcoholics Anonymous/Narcotics Anonymous meetings?" "Do you have a sponsor?"
Discuss	Nutrition, exercise, sleep, sex, workplace attendance, and spiritual activities which are important to relapse prevention Problematic areas in early recovery - spousal and family relationships; spend time talking about this with the patient
Look for	Overconfidence Recurrence of negativity Declining interest in AA

ATTENTION DEFICIT/HYPERACTIVITY DISORDER

I. Definition: Descriptive category for cluster of symptoms that include inattention, impulsivity, and motor hyperactivity that are more frequent and severe than seen in persons of the same developmental level; this disorder is usually first diagnosed in childhood and can persist into adulthood

II. Pathogenesis

    A. Probably encompasses several distinct disorders involving multiple genetic, neurological, temperamental, and environmental factors

    B. Current research has found that certain brain regions might malfunction in persons with ADHD and that defective genes may also play a role in the expression of the disorder
        1. Several studies support involvement of the prefrontal cortex, part of the cerebellum, and two basal ganglia--the caudate nucleus and the globus pallidus
        2. Genes that dictate the way in which the brain uses dopamine have also been implicated (imaging studies have implicated frontostriatal circuitry [which is rich in dopaminergic innervation] in ADHD)

III. Clinical Presentation

    A. In adults, the symptoms of ADHD are seen in the workplace (or in the college classroom) as well as in the home (male to female ratio is about even in adulthood, although women may predominate)

    B. Once believed to largely resolve in childhood/adolescence, evidence now exists indicating that ADHD can persist into adulthood. **Important**: Not an acquired disorder of adulthood

    C. Presentation during adulthood (represents persistence from childhood):
        1. Despite a decrease in ADHD symptom intensity in adulthood, everyday life continues to become more complex as one assumes adult roles
        2. Symptoms take different forms in adults; disinhibition deficits in monitoring one's own behavior is often a central feature in adults
        3. Hyperactivity is the most likely symptom to remit with age so that this characteristic is often absent in adults; instead, feelings of restlessness and inability to relax are present
        4. Adults with inattention and distractibility seem unable to modulate their attention, often missing important information, overlooking details, and making mistakes in their social and family life and in the work-place; generally unable to complete started projects

5. Impulsivity is expressed by low tolerance for passive waiting (in lines, in traffic), by inability to wait turn in conversations (interrupting or finishing another's sentences)
6. Adults with persistent symptoms have completed less formal education, have lower status jobs, and have higher rates of antisocial personality

D. **Hyperactivity is no longer a required diagnostic criterion for ADHD at any age**

E. Diagnostic criteria for ADHD are contained in the following table
1. Note there are **two** dimensions, inattention and hyperactivity/impulsivity, with behaviors specific to each dimension
2. From these two dimensions, three subtypes are derived
   a. Predominantly inattentive type (criteria are met on inattention dimension, but **not** on the hyperactivity/impulsivity dimension)
   b. Predominantly hyperactive/impulsive type (criteria are met on hyperactive/impulsive dimension but **not** on the inattention dimension)
   c. Combined type (criteria are met for both dimensions)
3. The diagnostic criteria are meant to be age neutral but are much more applicable to children than to adults

ADHD DIAGNOSTIC CRITERIA

Either 1 or 2

1. Six or more symptoms of inattention have persisted for at least a 6 month period to the degree that is maladaptive and inconsistent with developmental level:

Inattention-- The person **often**	➡ Fails to pay close attention to details resulting in careless mistakes ➡ Has difficulty sustaining attention in activities (whether play or other tasks) ➡ Does not seem to listen when being spoken to ➡ Does not follow through on instructions and fails to complete schoolwork, chores, or duties in the workplace (not due to oppositional behavior or inability to understand directions) ➡ Has difficulty with organization ➡ Avoids, dislikes, or is reluctant to undertake activities that require sustained mental effort (such as schoolwork or homework) ➡ Loses items necessary for tasks or activities ➡ Becomes easily distracted by extraneous stimuli ➡ Is forgetful in daily activities

2. Six or more symptoms of hyperactivity-impulsivity have persisted for at least a 6 month period to a degree that is maladaptive and inconsistent with developmental level:

Hyperactivity-- The person **often**	➡ Fidgets with hands or feet or squirms in seat ➡ Leaves seat in situations where remaining in seat is expected ➡ Runs or climbs excessively in situations in which it is inappropriate to do so (in adolescents or adults, this may be limited to subjective feelings of restlessness) ➡ Has difficulty engaging in quiet play or leisure activities ➡ Is "on the go" or seems driven by a motor ➡ Talks excessively
Impulsivity-- The person **often**	➡ Blurts out answers before question has been asked ➡ Has difficulty waiting turn ➡ Interrupts or intrudes on others (butts into conversations or games)
In addition, the following must be true	➡ Some hyperactive-impulsive or inattentive behaviors were present **before** age 7 years ➡ Some impairment from the symptoms is present in two or more settings (home, school or work) ➡ Clear evidence of clinically significant impairment in social, academic, or work-related functioning must exist ➡ Symptoms may not better be accounted for by another mental disorder (e.g., mood, anxiety, personality, psychotic)

Adapted from American Psychiatric Association. (2000). *Diagnostic and statistical manual of mental disorders* (4th ed.), Text Revision, Washington, DC: Author

IV.   Diagnosis/Evaluation

    A.   History

HISTORY QUESTIONS

✓ Confirm that impairment was present in childhood (retrospective confirmation is required for the diagnosis) [determine age of onset]

✓ Determine if symptoms persistent since childhood (to establish duration) [for adults, old report cards can be helpful in documenting problems during childhood] symptoms do not wax and wane, nor are they episodic

✓ **Important:** Adults who report long periods in which they were symptom-free are unlikely to have ADHD

✓ Establish that impairment in function is global (impacting all areas of life--family, social, work/school) --rather than selective

✓ Use questionnaires developed for adults such as Wender Utah Rating Scale and Brown Attention-Activation Disorder Scale (see ADHD RATING SCALES table) [Consider referral of adults in whom ADHD is suspected to experts for diagnosis as this is a highly specialized area of practice]

✓ Determine if significant anxiety, depression, or substance abuse is present (see sections on ANXIETY DISORDERS, DEPRESSION, and ALCOHOL PROBLEMS)

✓ Obtain social history, development history, past and present medical history, and **current medications**

ADHD RATING SCALES

Wender Utah Rating Scale

    Source: Ward, M.F., Wender, P.H., & Reimherr, F.W. (1993). The Wender Utah rating scale: An aid in the retrospective diagnosis of childhood attention deficit hyperactivity disorder. *American Journal of Psychiatry*, 150, 885-890, and www.medal.org/ch18.html

Brown Attention-Activation Disorder Scale

    Source: Brown, T.E. (1992). *The Brown attention-activation disorder scale (BAADS)*. New Haven, CN: Yale U Press.

    B.   Physical Examination
        1.   Perform complete neurologic exam including gait, muscular strength and tone, deep tendon reflexes, sensory responses
        2.   Results of the PE are usually normal

    C.   Differential Diagnosis
        1.   Anxiety (suspect if symptoms present in only one setting, e.g., home, but not at work)
        2.   Substance abuse (suspect if patient exhibits symptoms uncharacteristic of previous behavior)
        3.   Mood disorders/depression (See DEPRESSION section)
        4.   **Note:** Most experts believe that adult ADHD is overdiagnosed and that anxiety, depression, or alcohol abuse are frequently the problem

    D.   Diagnostic Tests
        1.   Keep in mind that ADHD is a clinical diagnosis based primarily on history and secondarily on in-office observation and neuropsychological testing
        2.   Other diagnostic tests are not routinely indicated to establish the diagnosis of ADHD

V.   Plan/Management

    A.   Consult an expert in this area for recommendations regarding appropriate treatment

    B.   Refer adult patients for education and counseling related to ADHD
        1.   The aim of such counseling is to help patient develop compensatory strategies in the area of executive functioning (planning and organization) as this is very difficult for ADHD adults
        2.   Patients can also be given tips on ways to reduce distractions at home or in the workplace
        3.   Strategies to assist with time management and task completion are also needed by most patients
        4.   Recommend resources and books to patients such s the following: *Driven to Distraction: Recognizing and Coping with Attention Deficit Disorder from Childhood Through Adulthood* by E. Hallowell & J. Ratey. Published by Pantheon Books, New York, 1994 (especially good reference for diagnosis and treatment of ADHD in adults)

C. Providing there are no contraindications, the drugs of choice for patients with ADHD are psychostimulants—either methylphenidate or dextroamphetamine, which are class II (controlled) drugs
1. In general, the side effects are the same for both drugs
2. Adults have more complex lives, with more cognitively demanding tasks and longer days than children; therefore, it is important that medications with a longer duration of action are prescribed

---

Comparing Dextroamphetamine and Methylphenidate

- For both standard and sustained-release preparations, the peak plasma concentration and plasma half-life are higher and longer for dextroamphetamine than for methylphenidate

- For standard preparations of both drugs, the duration of maximal behavioral benefit parallels the absorption phase—1-2 hours for methylphenidate and 3-4 hours for dextroamphetamine

- Sustained-release preparations do not always provide more prolonged action than do the standard preparations, because the slower rates of absorption of the sustained-release preparations may delay their onset of action

- Because of their abuse potential, these drugs may not be appropriate for some patients

- Consult PDR or an expert in managing ADHD in adults for more information regarding the off-label use of these medications (approved for use in children, but not adults)

D. Alternatives to stimulants include tricyclic antidepressants (TCAs) (for example, desipramine, which is noradrenergic in its mechanism of action, and nortriptyline, a norepinephrine and serotonin reuptake inhibitor) or bupropion (Wellbutrin SR), an atypical antidepressant with more stimulant properties than the TCAs. Consult PDR for more information (off-label use for these drugs)

E. Atomoxetine (Strattera) is a non-stimulant drug recently approved by the FDA for treatment of ADHD in adults (also approved for use in children)
1. A selective, norepinephrine reuptake inhibitor, atomoxetine is the first FDA-approved treatment for ADHD that is not a controlled (class II) drug
2. Not associated with stimulant or euphoric effects, thus it avoids the abuse-potential of other FDA-approved treatments for ADHD (i.e., those approved for children), making it an attractive option for adults
3. In adults >70 kg, dosing is as follows:
    a. Initially, 40 mg/day; may be given once daily or in 2 evenly divided doses (in AM and late afternoon)
    b. Increase after at least 3 days to a target dose of about 80 mg/day (maximum dose is 100 mg/day)
    c. Available in 10, 18, 25, 40, and 60 mg caps
    d. Consult PDR for contraindications, precautions, interactions, and adverse reactions

F. Follow Up
1. Evaluation of patients suspected of having ADHD is a very time-consuming process; therefore, these patients are best managed in a specialized treatment center if one is available
2. Initial diagnosis and evaluation requires 2-3 visits (1-2 weeks apart); thereafter, follow-up schedule is variable depending on whether patient is being managed in a specialty treatment center or in a primary care setting
3. For all patients on medications, titration of dose to therapeutic level must be done at least weekly for first month or so, then monthly thereafter; very frequent monitoring for efficacy and for adverse events is essential

EATING DISORDERS

I. Definition: Symptomatic disturbances of eating behavior unique to the developed world, with anorexia nervosa (AN) and bulimia nervosa (BN) being the two major types

II. Pathogenesis

A. Eating disorders are best understood using a multidimensional model that encompasses biologic vulnerability, family issues, and societal pressure

B. Eating behavior is a complex integration of a person's attitude toward food and internal physiology resulting in individual concepts of hunger and satiety

C. Persons with AN tend to have perfectionistic, rigid, inflexible, and conforming personalities

D. Impact of family functioning on persons with AN and BN is difficult to determine, but family dynamics can influence both the development and the persistence of the disorder

E. A thin, unrealistic body size is idealized in today's society and concepts of beauty are highly related to body size in the media

III. Clinical Presentation

A. Disordered eating represents a spectrum of behavior that is unique to the developed world and is overwhelmingly a disease of young women; female athletes are at greater risk for developing eating disorders than are other young women of similar age

B. Female-to-male ratio of eating disorders is approximately 10:1; of the two disorders, males are much more likely to have BN, and overexercise is quite common

C. Because of the infrequency of this diagnosis in males, diagnosis and treatment may be more difficult

D. Using strict diagnostic criteria, the prevalence in the young female population, the group most often affected, is approximately 1% for AN and about 3% for bulimia

E. Using less stringent criteria, a much higher percentage of young women regularly engage in disordered eating including rigid dieting, binging, and purging, all behaviors that place them at risk for a number of sequelae

F. AN has the highest premature mortality rate of any psychiatric disorder; untreated, about 20% of AN patients die within 20 years with the most common causes of death being cardiac problems, renal failure, and suicide

G. Diagnostic criteria for AN according to *DSM-IV* (2000) are contained in the following table

---

DIAGNOSTIC CRITERIA FOR ANOREXIA NERVOSA

➡ Refusal to maintain weight at or above a minimally normal weight for age and height (body weight is less than 85% of expected)
➡ Intense fear of weight gain even though underweight
➡ Amenorrhea (in postmenarcheal females)
➡ Severe body-image disturbance in which weight has undue influence on feelings of self-worth; denial that current low body weight is problematic
➡ Types of anorexia nervosa:
  • Restricting Type: During current episode of AN, person has not regularly engaged in binge eating or purging behavior
  • Binge-Eating/Purging Type: During current episode of AN, person has regularly engaged in binge eating or purging behavior

---

Adapted from American Psychiatric Association. (2000). *Diagnostic and statistical manual of mental disorders* (4th ed.) Text Revision, Washington, DC: Author

H. Diagnostic criteria for BN according to *DSM-IV* (2000) are contained in the following table

---

DIAGNOSTIC CRITERIA FOR BULIMIA NERVOSA

➡ Recurrent episodes of binge eating which include **both** of the following
  - Eating, in a discrete time period, an amount of food substantially larger than most people would consume in the same time period
  - A sense of lack of control over eating during episode

➡ Recurrent inappropriate compensatory behavior to prevent weight gain such as laxative, diuretic, enema use, induced vomiting, fasting, excessive exercise

➡ The above two behaviors occur, on average, at least 2 times/week for 3 months

➡ Feelings of self-worth unduly influenced by weight

➡ Disturbance does not occur exclusively during episodes of AN

➡ Types of bulimia nervosa:
  - Purging Type: During the current episode of BN, person has engaged in self-induced vomiting, laxative, diuretic, or enema use on a regularly basis
  - Nonpurging Type: During the current episode of BN, person has used compensatory behaviors such as fasting or excessive exercise, but has not regularly engaged in self-induced vomiting, laxative, diuretic, or enema use

---

Adapted from American Psychiatric Association. (2000). *Diagnostic and statistical manual of mental disorders* (4th ed.) Text Revision. Washington, DC: Author

IV. Diagnosis/Evaluation

A. History
1. Obtain weight history including highest and lowest weights as adult (or adolescent), methods of losing weight, and how patient defines "ideal" weight; ask patient if she thinks she is too fat
2. Through appropriate questioning, establish the presence or absence of criteria for eating disorders (see DIAGNOSTIC CRITERIA FOR ANOREXIA AND BULIMIA NERVOSA in the preceding tables)
3. If possible, obtain additional information from family/friends as patient may lack the capacity to accurately describe own behavior
4. Inquire about other behaviors that can support the presence of an eating disorder such as preference for eating alone, severely limited food preferences, unusual eating habits (ritualistic patterns); ask how often vomiting is induced because of feeling uncomfortably full; ask patient if food dominates life
5. Obtain a careful diet history, with a focus on overall caloric intake and intake of specific nutrients such as calcium
6. In women, obtain a complete menstrual history
7. Question about exercise patterns (overexercise believed to be especially prevalent in males with eating disorders)
8. Ask what medications have been used or are currently being used to induce weight loss

B. Physical Examination
1. Measure weight with the patient undressed and gowned; measure height and calculate BMI (see OBESITY section for calculation of BMI and definition of "healthy weight")
2. Take vital signs including lying and standing blood pressure and pulse at initial evaluation and at all follow-up visits; pulse in patients with AN is often bradycardic (<60) and majority of ANs have hypotension with pressures <90/60
3. Perform complete physical examination, observing for the stigmata of vomiting which include parotid enlargement, soft palate lesions, dental erosions, and calluses on the dorsal surface of the hand (most frequently seen at the metacarpal-phalangeal joints)
4. Neurologic exam should include mental status, cranial nerves, motor and sensory systems, and cerebellar system

C. Differential Diagnosis
1. Numerous **medical conditions** can mimic presentation of eating disorders; however, persons with medical conditions that cause loss of appetite, weight loss, unexplained vomiting **lack the attitudinal features** of a primary eating disorder (obsession with thinness and body image distortion)
    a. Inflammatory bowel diseases (stool is often positive for blood; erythrocyte sedimentation rate is increased in IBD, and usually subnormal in eating disorders)
    b. Thyroid disease (physical findings of hyperthyroidism are usually present and laboratory findings confirm the diagnosis)

      c.   Diabetes mellitus (laboratory findings confirm the diagnosis) [eating disorders are almost twice as common in adolescent females with type 1 diabetes as in their non-diabetic peers]

      d.   Central nervous system lesions and occult malignancies anywhere in the body (appropriate imaging studies)

      e.   Chronic infections such as tuberculosis and acquired immunodeficiency

2.   Psychiatric disorders can also present with decreased appetite and weight loss

D. Diagnostic Tests

1. Initial laboratory evaluation should include CBC with differential, serum electrolytes, calcium, magnesium, and phosphorous levels, liver function tests, blood urea nitrogen (BUN) level, creatinine level, urinalysis, TSH, and electrocardiogram

2. Patients who have been underweight >6 months: consider evaluating for osteopenia and osteoporosis (DEXA, estradiol level, and testosterone level [in males])

3. Patients with atypical presentations should have laboratory evaluation based on history and physical examination in order to rule out other diagnoses

4. Serum amylase levels are elevated during active vomiting and return to normal within 72 hours after vomiting ceases (may be helpful in diagnosing bulimia or to follow treatment response [in patients with bulimia, serum amylase elevations are **almost always** caused by a salivary source and not by pancreatitis; can be confirmed by lipase measurement which is elevated in pancreatitis but normal in patients with amylase elevations due to a salivary source])

V. Plan/Management

A. Goals of treatment include restoring and maintaining normal weight, and management of physiologic and psychologic abnormalities; treatment at a specialty center is ideal

1. Weight gain is crucial for recovery; aim is a 2-3 pound per week gain in a structured treatment setting once patient has begun to cooperate with treatment (most outpatient programs find weight gain goals of 0.5-1 pound/week to be realistic)

2. The goal is to obtain ideal body weight (IBW) [defined as a BMI in the healthy weight range]; at a minimum, patient should obtain 90% of IBW for height; most experts believe that a healthy weight for women is one in which menstruation and ovulation are restored; in premenarcheal girls, a healthy goal weight is one at which normal physical and sexual development resumes

3. Because normalized weight is the best predictor of bone density, the restoration of weight and the avoidance of bone loss are important treatment goals; calcium and vitamin D supplementation are necessary, however

4. If the cycle of weight loss begins, return to a structured treatment setting may be necessary

B. In-patient versus outpatient management depends on the severity of the condition as well as availability of local resources and insurance status of the patient

1. Patients with hemodynamic instability, significant hypovolemia, arrhythmias, heart failure, or cardiomyopathy must be hospitalized

2. Failure of appropriate outpatient treatment is also a criterion for hospitalization

C. Most outpatient treatment for patients with eating disorders is managed by a decentralized team, with patients seeing a variety of providers (including a psychotherapist and nutritionist) who communicate with each other about the progress of the patient

D. Cognitive behavioral treatment is the treatment of choice for eating disorders

1. Objectives of cognitive techniques are to change faulty thought processes such as all-or-none thinking, judgmental thinking, and catastrophizing

2. Objectives of behavioral techniques are to break patterns of disordered eating through the use of food monitoring, thought monitoring, meal regularity, and nutritional monitoring

3. Family therapy is often an important component of treatment (for adolescents); individual therapy is more important for adults

E. Role of the primary care clinician

1. Identify patients with eating disorder and facilitate appropriate treatment

2. Refer for treatment (AN patients are much less likely to agree to treatment than are patients with BN)

3. Monitor the medical aspects of the condition (weekly weigh-ins, vital sign measurement, and periodic laboratory testing [CBC, serum electrolytes, and serum amylase levels])

4. Coordinate the efforts of the other professionals involved in care

F. Role of Medications
    1. In patients with AN, need for antidepressants is best assessed following weight gain when the effects of malnutrition are resolving
    2. In patients with BN, antidepressants are effective as one component of an initial treatment program
    3. For both groups of patients, selective serotonin reuptake inhibitors (SSRIs) are currently considered to be the safest antidepressants and may be especially helpful for patients with significant symptoms of depression, anxiety, and obsessive-compulsive tendencies

G. Risk for osteoporosis
    1. Peak bone mass achieved as a young adult is an important determinant of bone density and fracture risk later in the postmenopausal years
    2. Osteopenia and osteoporosis are among the most serious sequelae of amenorrhea and weight loss in young women with anorexia; AN is associated with markedly reduced bone density, particularly at the lumbar spine but also at the proximal femur and distal radius, increasing the long-term risk for any fracture almost 3-fold
    3. Osteopenia in AN is believed to be a low-turnover condition, associated with increased bone resorption and high serum cortisol levels, and thus is different from the osteopenia of postmenopausal women

H. Refer patients to the following resources

> ✓ The National Eating Disorders Organization, 6655 South Yale Avenue, Tulsa, OK 74136; 918-481-4044; http://www.laureate.com
> ✓ The American Anorexia/Bulimia Association, 293 Central Park West, Suite 1R, New York, NY 10024; 212-501-8351; http://members.aol.com/amanbu
> ✓ National Association of Anorexia Nervosa and Associated Disorders, Box 7, Highland Park, IL 60035; 847-831-3438

I. Follow Up: See V.E. above for role of the primary care clinician

OBESITY

I. Definition: Excessive accumulation of body fat

II. Pathogenesis

A. In all persons, obesity is caused by ingesting more energy than is expended over a long period of time

B. Multiple factors interact and contribute to development of overweight and obesity: a genetic predisposition combines with environmental factors to produce the disorder

C. The role of individual hormones and neurotransmitters in the etiology of obesity remains unknown; the recent discovery of the hormone leptin may revolutionize the field of obesity in the next few years

III. Clinical Presentation

A. Obesity has become pandemic in US—2 in 3 adults are classified as overweight (body max index [BMI] 25 to 29.9) or obese (BMI >30), compared with fewer than 1 in 4 in the early 1960s

B. Excess weight is a major risk factor for premature mortality, cardiovascular disease, type 2 diabetes mellitus, osteoarthritis, certain cancers, and other medical conditions—unfortunately, the general public continues to view obesity as more of a cosmetic than a health problem
    1. Obesity accounts for more than 280,000 death annually in the US and, if current trends continue, will soon replace smoking as the primary preventable cause of death
    2. Obesity is already associated with greater morbidity and poorer health-related quality of life than smoking, problem drinking, or poverty

C. Classifications for BMI are contained in the table

CLASSIFICATIONS FOR BMI	
	BMI
Underweight	<18.5
Normal weight	18.5 - 24.9
Overweight	25 - 29.9
Obesity (Class 1)	30 - 34.9
Obesity (Class 2)	35 - 39.9
Extreme obesity (Class 3)	≥40

Source: National Institutes of Health; National Heart, Lung, and Blood Institute, North American Association for the Study of Obesity. (2000). *The practical guide: Identification, evaluation, and treatment of overweight and obesity in adults.* Bethesda, MD: Author, p 1.

D. Waist circumference provides an independent predictor of risk over and beyond that of BMI; for women, waist circumference >35, and for men >40, places them at increased risk

E. Whereas 29% of men and 44% of women in US describe themselves at any given time as trying to lose weight, only about 20% report restricting caloric intake and increasing physical activity at the same time, in spite of recommendations that such an approach is effective

IV. Diagnosis/Evaluation:

A. History
   1. Weight milestones, including weight at birth, during early and late childhood, upon graduation from high school, college, and at marriage
   2. Diet history, including usual number of meals per day; type and number of snacks (questions about food consumption should be framed in a non-accusatory, matter-of-fact manner)
   3. Psychosocial history, to detect emotional stresses at home or work/school which may be aggravating problem
   4. Amount and type of physical activity engaged in each week
   5. Types and results of past dieting
   6. Past medical history for cardiovascular disease, diabetes mellitus, thyroid disease, hypertension, gout, emotional problems, orthopedic problems, and dermatitis
   7. Inquire about family history of overweight, dyslipidemia, diabetes, hypertension, premature CHD, or sudden death experienced by father or other male first degree relative at or before 55, or experienced by the mother or other female first-degree relative at or before 65 years of age
   8. Ask about symptoms of sleep apnea (very loud snoring, cessation of breathing during sleep which is often followed by a loud clearing breath, then brief awakening)
   9. Current medications and tobacco use

B. Physical Examination
   1. Measure blood pressure in both adults and children, taking care to use the correct size cuff (a common source of error is an incorrectly sized cuff)
   2. Assess for overweight and obesity

Note: Two surrogate measures are important to assess body fat in adults: Body mass index (BMI) and waist circumference
   ✓ BMI is a direct calculation based on height and weight, regardless of age or gender
   ✓ The primary classification of overweight is based on the assessment of BMI; see III.A. above for criteria for overweight and obesity
   ✓ BMI has some limitations: It can overestimate body fat in persons who are very muscular and underestimate it in persons who have lost muscle mass (e.g., many elderly)
   ✓ Waist circumference is the most practical tool a clinician can use to evaluate a patient's abdominal fat before and during weight loss treatment
   ✓ Fat located in the abdominal region is associated with a greater health risk than peripheral fat and appears to be an independent risk predictor when BMI is not markedly increased
   ✓ A high waist circumference is associated with an increased risk for type 2 diabetes, dyslipidemia, hypertension, and CVD in patients with a BMI between 25 and 34.9

See tables below for calculation of BMI (or consult BMI table on the following page) and for information on waist circumference measurement

WAIST CIRCUMFERENCE MEASUREMENT		CALCULATE BMI AS FOLLOWS

WAIST CIRCUMFERENCE MEASUREMENT

To measure waist circumference, locate the upper hipbone and the top of the right iliac crest. Place a measuring tape in a horizontal plane around the abdomen at the level of the iliac crest. Before reading the tape measure, ensure that the tape is snug, but does not compress the skin, and is parallel to the floor. The measurement is made at the end of a normal expiration.

High-Risk Waist Circumference
Men: >40 in (>102 cm)
Women: >35 in (>88 cm)

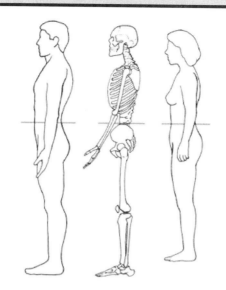

Measuring-Tape Position for Waist (Abdominal) Circumference in Adults

CALCULATE BMI AS FOLLOWS

$$BMI = \frac{weight\ (kg)}{height\ squared\ (M^2)}$$

If pounds and inches are used:

$$BMI = \frac{weight\ (pounds) \times 703}{height\ squared\ (inches^2)}$$

CALCULATION DIRECTIONS AND SAMPLE

Directions for calculating BMI. (Example: for a person who is 5 feet 5 inches tall weighing 180 lbs.)

1. Multiply weight (in pounds) by 703
   180 x 703 = 126,540

2. Multiply height (in inches) by height (in inches)
   65 x 65 = 4,225

3. Divide the answer in Step 1 by the answer in Step 2 to get the BMI.
   126,540 / 4,225 = 29.9
   BMI = 29.9

Source: National Institutes of Health; National Heart, Lung, and Blood Institute, North American Association for the Study of Obesity. (2000). *The practical guide: Identification, evaluation, and treatment of overweight and obesity in adults.* Bethesda, MD: Author, p. 9.

BODY MASS INDEX TABLE FOR BMIs 19-35

BMI	19	20	21	22	23	24	25	26	27	28	29	30	31	32	33	34	35
Height (inches)							Body Weight (pounds)										
58	91	96	100	105	110	115	119	124	129	134	138	143	148	153	158	162	167
59	94	99	104	109	114	119	124	128	133	138	143	148	153	158	158	168	173
60	97	102	107	112	118	123	128	133	138	143	148	153	158	163	168	174	179
61	100	106	111	116	122	127	132	137	143	148	153	158	164	169	174	180	185
62	104	109	115	120	126	131	136	142	147	153	158	164	169	175	180	186	191
63	107	113	118	124	130	135	141	146	152	158	163	169	175	180	186	191	197
64	110	116	122	128	134	140	145	151	157	163	169	174	180	186	192	197	204
65	114	120	126	132	138	144	150	156	162	168	174	180	186	192	198	204	210
66	118	124	130	136	142	148	155	161	167	173	179	186	192	198	204	210	216
67	121	127	134	140	146	153	159	166	172	178	185	191	198	204	211	217	223
68	125	131	138	144	151	158	164	171	177	184	190	197	203	210	216	223	230
69	128	135	142	149	155	162	169	176	182	189	196	203	209	216	223	230	236
70	132	139	146	153	160	167	174	181	188	195	202	209	216	222	229	236	243
71	136	143	150	157	165	172	179	186	193	200	208	215	222	229	236	243	250
72	140	147	154	162	169	177	184	191	199	206	213	221	228	235	242	250	258
73	144	151	159	166	174	182	189	197	204	212	219	227	235	242	250	257	265
74	148	155	163	171	179	186	194	202	210	218	225	233	241	249	256	264	272
75	152	160	168	176	184	192	200	208	216	224	232	240	248	256	264	272	279
76	156	164	172	180	189	197	205	213	221	230	238	246	254	263	271	279	287

Source: National Institutes of Health; National Heart, Lung, and Blood Institute, North American Association for the Study of Obesity. (2000). *The practical guide: Identification, evaluation, and treatment of overweight and obesity in adults.* Bethesda, MD: Author, p. 46.

3. Examination of the severely obese patient may be difficult (auscultation of the lungs and heart is compromised as is exam of the abdomen)

4. Skin over the neck may be hyperpigmented, thicker, and have a velvet appearance (acanthosis nigricans)

5. In women, observe for intertriginous dermatitis under breasts and abdominal panniculus

6. In men, examination of the genitalia may require that the prepubic fat tissue be lifted upward in order to visualize the penis which may be hidden by surrounding fat

C. Differential Diagnosis
   1. Most obesity is the result of overeating
   2. Major endocrine disorders that may manifest with obesity are the following:
      a. Pituitary and adrenal dysfunction
      b. Thyroid disease
      c. Polycystic ovary syndrome
      d. Hypothalamic disease

D. Diagnostic Tests: Obtain fasting lipid profile, fasting plasma glucose, and comprehensive chemistry profile

V. Plan/Management

A. Using the four-step process in the series of boxes below, identify the patient's risk status as a beginning point in formulating a treatment plan

---

Step 1. Determine the patient's **relative risk status** based on overweight and obesity parameters (BMI and waist circumference)

The table below presents a classification of overweight and obesity by BMI, waist circumference, and **relative** risk status (**Note:** Risk levels for disease depicted in this table are **relative**, i.e., they are relative to the risk at normal weight)

Classification of Overweight and Obesity by BMI, Waist Circumference, and Associated Disease Risk

	BMI (kg/m^2)	Obesity Class	Disease Risk* (Relative to Normal Weight and Waist Circumference)	
			Men ≤40 in (≤102 cm) Women ≤35 in (≤88 cm)	>40 in (>102 cm) >35 in (>88 cm)
Underweight	< 18.5		---	---
Normal**	18.5-24.9		---	---
Overweight	25.0-29.9		Increased	High
Obesity	30.0-34.9	I	High	Very High
	35.0-39.9	II	Very High	Very High
Extreme Obesity	≥40	III	Extremely High	Extremely High

* Disease risk for type 2 diabetes, hypertension, and CVD
** Increased waist circumference can also be a marker for increased risk even in persons of normal weight

---

Step 2. Identify patients at **very high absolute risk**

Patients with the following diseases have a very high absolute risk:

- <u>Established coronary heart disease</u> (CHD), including a history of myocardial infarction, angina pectoris (stable or unstable), coronary artery surgery, or coronary artery procedures

- Presence of <u>other atherosclerotic diseases</u>, including peripheral arterial disease, abdominal aortic aneurysm, or symptomatic carotid artery disease

- <u>Type 2 diabetes</u> (fasting plasma glucose ≥126 mg/dL or 2-h postprandial plasma glucose ≥200 mg/dL) is a major risk factor for CVD; its presence alone places a patient in the category of very high absolute risk

- <u>Sleep apnea</u>. Symptoms and signs include very loud snoring or cessation of breathing during sleep, which is often followed by a loud clearing breath, then brief awakening

---

Step 3. Identify patients with cardiovascular risk factors that impart a **high absolute risk**

Patients can be classified as being at high absolute risk for obesity-related disorders if they have 3 or more of the multiple risk factors listed in the chart below

Risk Factors

- Cigarette smoking
- Hypertension (systolic blood pressure of ≥140 mm Hg or diastolic blood pressure ≥90 mm Hg) or current use of antihypertensive agents
- High-risk low-density lipoprotein (LDL) cholesterol (serum concentration ≥160 mg/dL). A borderline high-risk LDL-cholesterol (130-159 mg/dL) plus two or more other risk factors also confers high risk

- Low high-density lipoprotein (HDL) cholesterol (serum concentration <35 mg/dL)
- Impaired fasting glucose (IFG) (fasting plasma glucose between 110 and 124 mg/dL). IFG is considered by many authorities to be an independent risk factor for cardiovascular (macrovascular) disease, thus justifying its inclusion among risk factors contributing to high absolute risk. IFG is well established as a risk factor for type 2 diabetes

- Family history of premature CHD (myocardial infarction or sudden death experienced by the father or other male first-degree relative at or before 55 years of age, or experienced by the mother or other female first-degree relative at or before 65 years of age)
- Age ≥45 years for men or age ≥55 years for women (or postmenopausal)

Step 4. Identify patients with **other risk factors** that deserve special consideration

The presence of two other risk factors heightens the need for weight reduction in obese patients

- <u>Physical inactivity</u> imparts an increased risk for both CVD and type 2 diabetes; in addition to exacerbating the severity of other risk factors, it also has been shown to be an independent risk factor for all CVD mortality
- <u>Elevated serum triglycerides</u> often accompany obesity; in the presence of obesity, high serum triglycerides are commonly associated with a clustering of metabolic risk factors known as the metabolic syndrome (atherogenic lipoprotein phenotype, hypertension, insulin resistance, glucose intolerance, and prothrombotic states)

Adapted from: National Institutes of Health; National Heart, Lung, and Blood Institute, North American Association for the Study of Obesity. (2000). *The practical guide: Identification, evaluation, and treatment of overweight and obesity in adults.* Bethesda, MD: Author, p. 10-13.

B.   Once the patient has been categorized according to BMI, waist circumference, and risk factors (relative, very high absolute, high absolute, or other), develop and implement a treatment plan based on recommendations in the following table

---

TREATMENT RECOMMENDATIONS FOR OVERWEIGHT AND OBESITY

Assessing a Patient for Treatment of Overweight and Obesity, Based on the Patient's Weight, Waist Circumference, and Presence of Risk Factors

➡ Those patients with a BMI between 25 and 29.9 **without** a high waist circumference and **with** one or no risk factors should work on maintaining their current weight at or below its present level, rather than embarking on a weight reduction program

➡ All patients who meet the following criteria should attempt to lose weight:

- BMI ≥30
- BMI 25 to 29.9 OR waist circumference >35 in (women) or >40 in (men) AND ≥2 risk factors

➡ Patients with overweight and obesity in the high absolute risk category need attention paid to cholesterol-lowering therapy and blood pressure management including smoking cessation, prudent diet, and increased physical activity

- **Note: Control of cardiovascular risk factors deserves the same emphasis as weight loss therapy**

➡ Patients with overweight and obesity in the very **high absolute risk** category need intense risk-factor modification and management of the disease(s) present (see sections on CARDIOVASCULAR PROBLEMS and DIABETES MELLITUS)

C.   Criteria for selecting treatment are summarized in the box below

A Guide to Selecting Treatment

Treatment	BMI Category				
	25-26.9	27-29.9	30-34.9	35-39.9	≥40
Diet, physical activity, and behavior therapy	With comorbidities	With comorbidities	+	+	+
Pharmacotherapy		With comorbidities	+	+	+
Surgery				With comorbidities	

✓ Prevention of weight gain with lifestyle therapy is indicated in any patient with a BMI ≥25 kg/m^2, even without comorbidities, while weight loss is not necessarily recommended for those with a BMI of 25-29.9 kg/m^2 or a high waist circumference, unless they have two or more comorbidities

✓ Combined therapy with a low-calorie diet (LCD), increased physical activity and behavior therapy provide the most successful intervention for weight loss and weight maintenance

✓ Consider pharmacotherapy only if a patient has not lost 1 pound per week after 6 months of combined lifestyle therapy

✓ The + represents the use of indicated treatment regardless of comorbidities

Source: National Institutes of Health; National Heart, Lung, and Blood Institute, North American Association for the Study of Obesity. (2000). *The practical guide: Identification, evaluation, and treatment of overweight and obesity in adults.* Bethesda, MD: Author, p. 25.

D. Management recommendations for weight loss are contained in the following tables and include dietary therapy, increased physical activity, and behavior therapy

---

TREATMENT STRATEGIES/MANAGEMENT RECOMMENDATIONS FOR WEIGHT LOSS

Step 1 Determine if the patient wants to lose weight; obviously this is the most crucial component of management and can be determined only through conversations with the patient

Step 2 If weight loss is desired, implement the three major components of weight loss therapy: Dietary therapy, increased physical activity, and behavior therapy

This 3-pronged approach should be tried for at least 6 months before pharmacotherapy is considered

Appropriate weight loss goals
- ✓ As initial goal for weight loss, experts recommend the loss of 10% of baseline weight at a rate of 1-2 pounds per week
- ✓ For individuals who are overweight versus obese, a weight loss of about 0.5 pounds per week may be more appropriate
- ✓ An average of 8% of body weight can be lost over 6 months
- ✓ After 6 months, most patients will equilibrate, with caloric intake balancing energy expenditure and thus will need an adjustment of their energy balance if they are to lose more weight

---

DIETARY THERAPY

- ✓ Goal is to achieve a slow, but progressive, weight loss with the centerpiece of therapy being a low calorie diet (LCD)
- ✓ In general, diets containing 1,000 to 1,200 kcal/day should be selected for most women and a diet between 1,200 and 1,600 kcal/day should be chosen for men
- ✓ Individually planned diet to help create a deficit of 500 to 1,000 kcal/day should achieve a weight loss of 1-2 pounds/week
- ✓ Composition of diet should be modified to minimize other cardiovascular risk factors (see section on ADULT NUTRITION); care should be taken to ensure that all of the dietary reference intakes (DRIs) are met; recommend use of a daily multivitamin
- ✓ Very low-calorie diets (VLCD) should be avoided except by weight management specialists because such diets require special monitoring and supplementation
- ✓ Adequate water intake should be emphasized (at least 64 ounces/day)

PHYSICAL ACTIVITY

Before Getting Started

- ✓ Counsel patient that physical activity should be an integral part of weight loss therapy and weight maintenance
- ✓ Advise patient that most weight loss occurs because of decreased caloric intake; sustained physical activity is most helpful in the maintenance of weight loss
- ✓ Based on the patient's age, symptoms, and concomitant risk factors, exercise testing for cardiopulmonary disease may be needed prior to the patient's embarking on a new physical activity regimen

Getting Started

- ✓ Physical activity should be started slowly, and intensity should be increased gradually
- ✓ A regimen of daily walking, which is safe and accessible, is an attractive form of physical activity for most people
  - Advise patient to begin by walking 10 minutes, 3 days a week, and then build to 60 minutes of more intense walking on most, if not all, days of the week
  - Over a 6-week period, patient should be encouraged to walk 2 miles daily faster than leisure-speed, interrupted as needed with brief intervals of slower walking until endurance is attained
  - When weather is bad, encourage patients to move their walk indoors – shopping malls are a popular alternative and many have walking clubs
  - The *Walking 10,000 Steps a Day* plan is becoming popular; encourage patients to purchase an inexpensive step-counter to help them keep track of how much they walk (average person takes less than 4,000 steps from routine daily activities) and encourage them to take 10,000 steps every day

Keeping It Up

- ✓ The most recent guidelines from the Institute of Medicine (2002) recommend that adults and children engage in 60 minutes of daily moderate intensity physical activity (e.g., walking/jogging at 4-5 mph) in addition to the activities required by a sedentary lifestyle
- ✓ Encourage patients to integrate physical activities into their lives by parking at the back of the parking lot and walking, taking the stairs instead of the elevator, and walking to destinations that are a few miles or less instead of driving
- ✓ Suggest that patients document their physical activity by keeping a diary and recording the activity, duration, and intensity of exercise

E. The third major component of weight loss therapy is behavior therapy, which is designed to overcome barriers to compliance with dietary therapy and increased physical activity

BEHAVIOR THERAPY: CLINICIAN STRATEGIES TO MAKE THE MOST OF EACH PATIENT VISIT

Consider patient's attitudes, beliefs, and history

- ✓ Communicate a nonjudgmental attitude that distinguishes between the weight problem and the patient with the problem
- ✓ Ask patient how obesity has affected his/her life
- ✓ Express your concern about health risks associated with obesity
- ✓ Examine your own attitudes and beliefs about obesity and obese people
- ✓ Remember that this is a chronic disease; compliance with most long-term treatment regimens that require behavior change is poor
- ✓ Keep your own expectations realistic regarding the ease, amount, speed, and permanence of weight change

Build a partnership with the patient

- ✓ Patient must actively participate in setting goals for behavior change
- ✓ Role of the clinician is to be a source of information, and to provide perspective and support; patient cannot be forced to meet goals he/she does not endorse

Set achievable goals

- ✓ A small number of goals that are specific should be selected on the basis of their likely impact on weight and health
- ✓ A goal to "exercise more" would become "walk for 30 minutes, 3 days a week for the next 2 weeks"
- ✓ Shaping is a behavioral technique that involves selecting a series of short-term goals that get closer and closer to the ultimate goal
- ✓ Progress over time from walking 30 minutes 3 times a week to 60 minutes on most days of the week
- ✓ Once goals have been set, help patient implement an action plan. This approach emphasizes that planning, not willpower, is the key to weight management
- ✓ Ask the patient:
  - What are the best days for you to take your walks?
  - What time of day is best for you?
  - What arrangements will you need to make for childcare?
  - Do you have a route in mind?
- ✓ Provide the patient with a written behavioral "prescription" listing the selected goals
- ✓ Consider developing a weight and goal record for each patient

(Continued)

BEHAVIOR THERAPY: CLINICIAN STRATEGIES TO MAKE THE MOST OF EACH PATIENT VISIT (CONTINUED)

Cultivate the partnership
- ✓ Follow-up visits to monitor health and weight status should be made on a regular basis, e.g. every 1-3 months for first year (rotate face-to-face visits with e-mails, telephone calls, and postcards)
- ✓ Imperfect goal attainment is often the norm
- ✓ Focus on the positive changes, and adopt a problem-solving approach toward the shortfalls
- ✓ Example: Instead of asking, "Did you meet your walking goal?" ask "How many days were you able to walk over the past 2 weeks?" If less than agreed upon, state "So even though you weren't able to walk 4 days each week, you did get out there at least twice a week. That's great!" Then try to help the patient problem-solve and figure out a way to come closer to the goal over the next 2 weeks. Ask, "What do you think interfered with your walking plans on the days you didn't walk?"
- ✓ **Emphasize that weight control is a journey, not a destination!**

Keep in touch
- ✓ Frequent contact is important; face-to-face encounters are not always necessary
- ✓ Patient can come to office each week for weight check with staff, to view educational videotapes, or perhaps to meet with other patients in the practice for a daily walk
- ✓ Can also use e-mail and telephone to keep in contact

Help the patient modify behaviors
- ✓ Explain the benefits of self-monitoring (patient keeping records of exercise, eating behaviors)
- ✓ Encourage patients to use rewards to help attain goals; numerous small rewards are preferable to bigger rewards that require a long, difficult effort
- ✓ Encourage the use of stimulus control (looking at which environment or social cues encourage undesired eating)

Focus on what matters
- ✓ Improvement of the patient's health is the goal of obesity treatment
- ✓ Simple clear records of body weight, relevant risk factors, other health parameters, and goal attainment should be kept as part of the patient record

Adapted from National Institutes of Health; National Heart, Lung, and Blood Institute, North American Association for the Study of Obesity. (2000). *The practical guide: Identification, evaluation, and treatment of overweight and obesity in adults.* Bethesda, MD: Author.

F. Pharmacotherapy may be used as an adjunct to non-pharmacologic approaches to weight loss in selected patients who have been unable to lose weight during a 6-month trial of dietary, physical activity, and behavioral therapies

> **Indications for the use of FDA approved weight-loss drugs are the following:**
> Patients with a BMI ≥30
> Patients with a BMI ≥27 in the presence of concomitant obesity-related risk factors or diseases

G. Drugs should be used only as part of a comprehensive program that includes healthy eating, physical activity, and behavior therapy

H. Weight loss drugs approved by the FDA for long-term use may be useful as an adjunct to diet and physical activity and are presented in the following table:

Weight Loss Drugs

Drug	Dose	Action	Adverse Effects
Sibutramine (Meridia)	5, 10, 15 mg caps 10 mg PO QD to start, may be increased to 15 mg or decreased to 5 mg	Norepinephrine, dopamine, and serotonin reuptake inhibitor	Increase in heart rate and blood pressure
Orlistat (Xenical)	120 mg caps 120 mg PO TID with fat-containing meals	Inhibits pancreatic lipase, decreases fat absorption	Decrease in absorption of fat-soluble vitamins; soft stools and anal leakage

National Institutes of Health; National Heart, Lung, and Blood Institute, North American Association for the Study of Obesity. (2000). *The practical guide: Identification, evaluation, and treatment of overweight and obesity in adults.* Bethesda, MD: Author, p. 36.

I. Weight loss surgery is an option for weight reduction in a limited number of patients with clinically severe obesity, i.e., BMIs ≥40 or ≥35 with comorbid conditions

J. Follow Up
  1. For patient on pharmacologic therapy:
      a. In 2-4 weeks for first return visit after initiation of medication
      b. Then monthly for 3 months
      c. Then every 3 months for the first year
      d. After first year, variable depending on clinician and patient preferences
      e. Purpose of visits is the following:
          ✓ To monitor weight, blood pressure, pulse
          ✓ To discuss side effects
          ✓ To conduct laboratory tests
          ✓ To answer patient's questions
  2. For follow-up of patients on nonpharmacologic therapy, refer to table above BEHAVIOR THERAPY: STRATEGIES TO MAKE THE MOST OF EACH PATIENT VISIT

TOBACCO USE AND SMOKING CESSATION

I. Definition: Destructive health behavior involving use of tobacco (cigarettes, chewing tobacco, and snuff)

II. Pathogenesis

  A. Tobacco smoke contains numerous substances which are toxic, mutagenic, or carcinogenic

  B. In addition to harmful volatile substances such as carbon monoxide, the particulate phase of cigarette smoke contains nicotine and tars

  C. The consequences of a product of combustion (smoke) being drawn into close contact with delicate pulmonary tissues are devastating

  D. The etiology of tobacco dependence is multidimensional with physiological, psychological, and social/behavioral factors
      1. Physiological factors include activation of the mesolimbic dopaminergic system ("reward circuit") and locus ceruleus (vigilance and arousal)
      2. Psychological factors evolve from positive feedback provided by pleasurable sensations
      3. Social/behavioral factors include the following: smoking becomes a habit or an automatic and intrinsic part of daily activities, and smoking can be used as self-medication to reduce unpleasant sensations that occur with tobacco withdrawal or stress

III. Clinical Presentation

  A. Tobacco use is the leading preventable cause of death in the US, responsible for more than 400,000 deaths annually, or 1 of every 5 deaths

  B. Presently, 23.5% of US adults smoke cigarettes
      1. Almost all smokers acknowledge that tobacco use is harmful to health, but tend to underestimate the risk to their **own** health
      2. Many smokers believe the benefits of smoking in the present outweigh the risk of disease in the future
      3. Half of regular smokers die prematurely of a tobacco-related disease

  C. The addictive nature of nicotine (it causes tolerance and physical dependence) is the primary physiological barrier to quitting tobacco use
      1. Withdrawal syndrome is characterized by symptoms of anxiety, irritability, anger, impatience, restlessness, difficulty concentrating, sleep disturbances, increased appetite and depressed mood
      2. Symptoms begin a few hours after the last cigarette, peak 2-3 days later, and then decline over a period of weeks or months

D. Psychological barriers to quitting include the fact that tobacco use is an integral part of the individual's daily routine
1. Smokers develop certain patterns of tobacco-use behavior such as smoking after meals, on breaks from work, and to relax at the end of the day
2. Smokers also frequently use tobacco to handle stress and negative emotions such as anxiety and anger

E. Tobacco addiction usually begins in childhood and adolescence; every day in the US, approximately 6000 young people start smoking and half of these youths will become daily smokers

F. In the US, 43% of children aged 2 to 11 are exposed to environmental tobacco smoke (ETS)
1. Consequences of ETS increase based on exposure; the more cigarettes smoked in the child's environment, the more particulate matter is discharged into the air
2. Children exposed to ETS have increased risk of growth disorders, sudden infant death syndrome, asthma, middle ear disease, pneumonia, cough, and upper respiratory infection

G. As with cigarette smoking, the use of smokeless tobacco, such as chewing tobacco and snuff, produces addiction to nicotine and has serious health consequences
1. Use of these products has increased in recent years, especially among white youth who live in the South and Midwest regions
2. Health risks from use of these products include gingival recession, periodontal bone loss, leukoplakia, oral cancer, and cardiovascular disease

H. Cigar smoking, which increased dramatically over the past decade, also poses serious health risks: smokers are at higher risk for coronary heart disease, COPD, lung and other cancers, with evidence of dose-dependent effects

I. Seventy percent of smokers report that they want to quit smoking completely
1. About 46% attempt to quit smoking each year, yet only about 20% of those seek help
2. Fewer than 10% of smokers who attempt to quit on their own are successful in the long term

J. Primary care clinicians have an unprecedented opportunity to reduce tobacco use rates in the US
1. More than 70% of smokers visit a health care setting each year where they could consistently receive effective tobacco interventions
2. Effective treatments now exist

K. Thirty-three states have established telephone quitlines to deliver cessation-counseling services to smokers who want to quit smoking

IV. Diagnosis/Evaluation

A. History
1. Inquire about smoking pattern, such as number of years of smoking, how much tobacco is used, and depth of inhalation
2. Ask how long after awakening the first cigarette is smoked
3. Ask about past attempts at quitting, including length of smoking cessation, problems encountered, and reasons for relapse
4. Explore smoke-related symptoms such as cough, sputum production, shortness of breath, recurrent respiratory infections
5. Review family history and personal medical history of tobacco-related diseases such as coronary heart disease, chronic obstructive pulmonary disease, and cancer

B. Physical Examination: Use the examination as an intervention, highlighting the damage that smoking can do to each body system which is assessed
1. Monitor vital signs, particularly blood pressure which adds an additional risk of heart disease if elevated
2. Examine ears, nose, sinuses, mouth, and pharynx, noting signs of inflammation due to irritation from tobacco
3. Perform complete exam of lungs
4. Perform complete exam of heart and peripheral vascular system

C. Diagnostic Tests
    1. Consider spirometry
        a. If normal, stress the benefits of smoking cessation before damage occurs
        b. If abnormal, stress the importance of cessation before further damage occurs
    2. Screen for lipid disorders to determine additional risk factors for heart disease

D. Differential Diagnosis: Not applicable

V. Plan/Management

A. Major intervention categories for treating tobacco use and dependence are as follows
    1. *Brief clinical interventions*--can be provided by any clinician but are most relevant to primary care clinicians who treat a wide variety of patients and who have severe time constraints; can be effectively implemented in 3 minutes and can increase cessation rates significantly
    2. *Intensive clinical interventions*--can be provided by any trained clinician who has the time and resources available; produce higher success rates and are most cost-effective in the long term than less-intensive interventions
    3. *Systems interventions*--involve healthcare delivery systems that institutionalize the consistent identification, documentation, and treatment of every tobacco user seen in the setting

B. ***Ask***–the first step in implementing an effective smoking cessation program for all patients in your practice is to implement an office-wide system to identify all tobacco users at every visit
    1. Expand vital sign section to include "tobacco use," with categories of "current," "former," or "never"
    2. As an alternative, put "tobacco use status" stickers on every chart
    3. If electronic charts used, incorporate into clinical reminder system
    4. **Note:** The rate at which clinicians provide advice on smoking cessation is now a standard measure for assessing quality of care delivered by health plans in US
    5. Evidence-based guidelines relating to tobacco use interventions at the systems (versus individual) level of healthcare delivery are available at http://www.thecommunityguide.org

C. ***Advise*** all smokers to stop
    1. *Be clear.* In a straightforward manner tell the patient that you believe it is important for him/her to quit smoking now, and that you can help; cutting down is not enough
    2. *Speak strongly.* Emphasize that quitting smoking is the single most important thing that patient can do for future health
    3. *Personalize advice.* Point out reasons that smoking cessation will improve the personal health as well as the health of loved ones exposed to ETS. See GOOD REASONS FOR YOUR PATIENT TO QUIT SMOKING in the table that follows

GOOD REASONS FOR YOUR PATIENTS TO QUIT SMOKING	
Teenagers	Bad breath, stained teeth, cost, potential decrease in athletic performance, frequent respiratory infections
Pregnant Women	Increased rate of spontaneous abortion, fetal death, low birth weight
Parents	Increased respiratory infections among children of smokers, poor role model for children
New Smokers	Easier to stop now
Asymptomatic Adults	Twice the risk of heart disease, six times the risk of emphysema, 10 times the risk of lung cancer, 5-8 year shorter life span, facial wrinkles
Symptomatic Adults	Upper respiratory infection, gum disease, dyspnea, ulcers, angina, claudication, osteoporosis, esophagitis, may not live long enough to enjoy retirement and grandchildren

Adapted from Glynn T, & Manley M. (1991). *How to help your patients stop smoking: A National Cancer Institute manual for physicians.* Bethesda, MD: National Institutes of Health.

D.   **Assess** willingness to make a quit attempt
  1.   Ask every patient if he/she is willing to make a quit attempt at this time (e.g., within the next 30 days)
  2.   Based on patient response, select an appropriate intervention

---

SELECT AN INTERVENTION BASED ON PATIENT RESPONSE TO "ARE YOU WILLING TO QUIT AT THIS TIME"?

If the answer is "**Yes, in the next 30 days**," go to V.E. through F. below
If the answer is "**Yes, but not now**," go to V.G. below
If the answer is "**No**," go to V.H. below

E.   **Assist** patient who is willing to quit now through a combination of *counseling* and *pharmacotherapy*; each approach is effective by itself, but the two in combination achieve the highest success rates
  1.   *Counseling*–Three types of counseling and behavioral therapies have been found to be especially effective and should be used with all patients who are attempting tobacco cessation
    a.   Provision of practical counseling
    b.   Provision of intratreatment social support (from clinician and staff)
    c.   Help in securing extratreatment social support (from family/coworkers, community resources)

COUNSELING TO ASSIST PATIENT WITH A QUIT PLAN

Advise the smoker to
  ➡   Set a quit date, ideally within 2 weeks
  ➡   Inform friends, family, and coworkers of plans to quit, and ask for support
  ➡   Remove cigarettes from home, car, and workplace
  ➡   Anticipate challenges, particularly during critical first few weeks, including nicotine withdrawal symptoms

Provide practical counseling (problem solving/skills training)
  ➡   Total abstinence is essential--not even a single puff
  ➡   Review previous quit attempts--what helped, what led to relapse
  ➡   Drinking alcohol is strongly associated with relapse
  ➡   Withdrawal typically peaks within 1-3 weeks after quitting
  ➡   Having other smokers in the household hinders successful quitting; patient should encourage housemates to quit or at least not smoke in his/her presence

Provide intratreatment social support
  ➡   Provide a supportive clinical environment while encouraging patient in his/her quit plan
  ➡   "My office staff and I are available to assist you"
  ➡   Use the telephone to deliver cessation-counseling services, thereby establishing an office "quitline"

Help patient obtain extratreatment social support
  ➡   Assist patient in development of social support for his/her quit attempt in environment outside of treatment
  ➡   "Ask your family, friends, coworkers to support you in your quit attempt"
  ➡   If there is a telephone quitline for smokers in the state, provide patient with contact information

Make culturally and educationally appropriate materials on cessation techniques readily available in your office
Such materials have little efficacy when used alone but may augment other interventions

---

Adapted from Fiore, M.C., Bailey, W.C., Cohen, S.J., Dorfman, S.F., Goldstein, M.G., Gritz, E.R., et al. (2000). Treating tobacco use and dependence. *Clinical practice guideline.*   Rockville, MD: USDHHS, Public Health Service.

Community Resources for Smoking Cessation Programs

American Cancer Society (ACS) offers FRESHSTART, a straightforward, no-nonsense program that consists of four, 1-hour sessions held during a 2-week period

- Works best for those who prefer the structure and support of a group
- Emphasizes quitting as a two-part process: stopping and staying stopped
- Meetings focus on the following:
  - ✓ Individual needs of smokers
  - ✓ Information and strategy
  - ✓ Understanding smoking as a chemical addiction, habit, and psychological dependency
  - ✓ Stress management
  - ✓ Weight control
- Also available on video and audiocassette for those unable to attend the sessions
- Refer patients to ACS at 800-ACS-2345

American Lung Association (ALA) offers Freedom From Smoking

- Within the Freedom From Smoking program, smokers can seek help in a group setting, individually with self-help materials (both written and audiotapes), and with materials that involve the entire family
- Refer patients to ALA at 800-LUNG-USA

2. *Pharmacotherapy*–There are six products to assist patient with smoking cessation
    a. The FDA has approved six products for smoking cessation: five nicotine-replacement products (transdermal patch, gum, lozenge, nasal spray, and vapor inhaler) and sustained-released bupropion
    b. Suggestions for the clinical use of these products are contained in the tables that follow

SUGGESTIONS FOR THE CLINICAL USE OF NON-NICOTINE THERAPY

Patient Selection	Appropriate as a first-line pharmacotherapy for smoking cessation: FDA-approved for this indication Behavioral/educational support is recommended with this therapy; should be especially considered in patients with a history of depression
Precautions	*Pregnancy:* Pregnant smokers should first be encouraged to attempt cessation without pharmacologic treatment. Bupropion SR should be used during pregnancy only if the benefits outweigh the risks. Similar factors should be considered in lactating women *Cardiovascular Diseases:* Generally well tolerated; infrequent reports of hypertension *Contraindications:* Contraindicated in individuals with a history of seizure disorder, a history of an eating disorder, who are using another form of bupropion (Wellbutrin or Wellbutrin SR), or who have used an MAO inhibitor in the past 14 days

Product	Daily Dose	Duration	Comments	Advantages	Disadvantages	Common Side Effects
Sustained-release bupropion (Zyban or Wellbutrin SR)	150 mg every morning for 3 days then 150 mg twice daily (begin treatment 1-2 weeks prequit)	7-12 weeks maintenance up to 6 months	May be used with nicotine replacement. Do not crush, chew, or divide tablets. Stop smoking within 1-2 weeks of starting drug. Avoid bedtime dosing. Do not use with other forms of bupropion	Easy to use (pill), no exposure to nicotine	Increases risk of seizure (≤0.1%)	Insomnia, dry mouth, agitation

SUGGESTIONS FOR THE CLINICAL USE OF NICOTINE-REPLACEMENT THERAPY

Patient Selection	Appropriate as first-line pharmacotherapy for smoking cessation; FDA-approved for this indication. Behavioral/educational support is recommended with this therapy
Precautions	***Pregnancy:*** Pregnant smokers should first be encouraged to attempt cessation without pharmacologic treatment. Nicotine-replacement therapy (NRT) should be used during pregnancy only if the benefits outweigh the risks. Similar factors should be considered in lactating women ***Cardiovascular Diseases:*** NRT is not an independent risk factor for acute myocardial events. NRT should be used with caution among particular cardiovascular patient groups: those within the immediate (within 2 weeks) postmyocardial infarction period, those with serious arrhythmias, and those with serious or worsening angina pectoris

Product	Daily Dose	Duration	Comments	Advantages	Disadvantages	Common Side Effects
Transdermal patch 24 hr (e.g., Nicoderm CQ)	21 mg/24 hrs* 14 mg/24 hrs 7 mg/24 hrs	4 weeks 2 weeks 2 weeks	Apply to clean, dry, nonhairy site on trunk or upper outer arm. Rotate sites. Remove after 16-24 hours	Provides steady level of nicotine; easy to use; unobtrusive; available without prescription	User cannot adjust dose if craving occurs; nicotine released more slowly than in other products	Local skin irritation, insomnia
16 hr (e.g., Nicotrol)	15-mg patch worn for 16 hrs	8 weeks	Apply to clean, dry, nonhairy site on hip or upper outer arm. Remove at bedtime. Rotate sites. Not for use in light smokers.			
Nicotine polacrilex gum (Nicorette)** 2 mg (<25 cig/day) 4 mg (≥25 cig/day)	1 piece/hr (<24 pieces/day)	Up to 12 weeks	▪ Proper chewing technique needed to avoid side effects and achieve efficacy** ▪ Instruct to chew gum on a fixed schedule (at least 1 piece/1-2 hrs) for 1-3 months may be more beneficial than *ad lib* use ▪ Use 4 mg strength for highly nicotine-dependent patients, or if failed with 2 mg	User controls dose; oral substitute for cigarettes; available without prescription	User cannot eat or drink while chewing the gum; can damage dental work; difficult for denture wearers to use	Mouth irritation, sore jaw, dyspepsia, hiccups
Nicotine polacrilex lozenge (Commit) 2 mg (if first cigarette smoked ≥30 min after waking) 4 mg (if first cigarette smoked ≤30 min after waking)	One lozenge every 1-2 hours (at least 9/day) for 6 weeks, then every 2-4 hours for 3 weeks, then stop (maximum dose is 20 lozenges/day)	12 weeks	Dissolve over 20-30 min; minimize swallowing	User controls dose; oral substitute for cigarettes; available without prescription Avoids sore jaw and dental work damage associated with gum	Cannot eat or drink for 15 minutes before and during use	Mouth and throat irritation
Vapor inhaler (Nicotrol Inhaler)	6-16 cartridges/day (delivered dose, 4 mg/cartridge)	3-6 months	20 minutes of active puffing releases 4 mg of nicotine (about 2 mg absorbed, equivalent to about 2 cigarettes)	User controls dose; hand-to-mouth substitute for cigarettes	Frequent puffing needed; device visible when used	Mouth and throat irritation; cough
Nasal spray (Nicotrol NS)	1-2 doses/hr (1 mg total; 0.5 mg in each nostril) (maximum 40 mg/day)	3-6 months	Do not sniff, swallow, or inhale spray. Nasal vasoconstrictors may delay absorption	Most irritating nicotine-replacement product to use; device visible when used	User controls dose; offers most rapid delivery and highest nicotine levels of all NRTs	Nasal irritation; sneezing, cough, teary eyes

* The starting dose is 21 mg/day unless the smoker weighs less than 45.5 kg (100 lb) or smokes fewer than 10 cigarettes per day, in which case the starting dose is 14 mg/day. The starting dose should be maintained for 4 weeks, after which the dose should be decreased every week until it is stopped

** Gum should be slowly chewed until a "peppery" taste emerges, then "parked" between cheek and gum to facilitate nicotine absorption. Gum should be intermittently "chewed and parked" for about 30 minutes. Acidic beverages (e.g., coffee, juices, soft drinks) interfere with the buccal absorption of nicotine, so eating and drinking anything except water should be avoided for 30 minutes before and during chewing

Adapted from Fiore, M.C., Bailey, W.C., Cohen, S.J., Dorfman, S.F., Goldstein, M.G., Gritz, E.R., et al. (2000). Treating tobacco use and dependence. *Clinical practice guideline.* Rockville, MD: USDHHS, Public Health Service.

F.   Follow up for patients who are attempting to quit at this time is outlined in the box below

> **Schedule follow-up contact either in person or by telephone (be proactive in your approach)**
> ➡ Timing
>   ✓ First follow-up contact within 2 weeks of quit date, preferably during first week
>   ✓ Second contact within the first month
>   ✓ Schedule further follow-up contacts as needed
> ➡ Actions during follow-up visits
>   ✓ Congratulate success
>   ✓ If a relapse occurred, obtain recommitment to abstinence
>   ✓ Remind patient that relapse can be used as learning experience
>   ✓ Identify problems encountered and anticipate challenges in the immediate future
>   ✓ Assess pharmacotherapy use and problems
>
> **Preventing relapse**
> ➡ Congratulate, encourage, and stress importance of abstinence at every opportunity
> ➡ Review benefits derived from cessation
> ➡ Inquire about problems encountered and offer possible solutions
> ➡ Anticipate problems or threats to maintaining abstinence
> ➡ Help patient identify sources of support
> ➡ Emphasize that beginning to smoke (even a puff) will increase urges and make quitting more difficult
> ➡ Assess pharmacotherapy use and problems
> ➡ Consider use or referral to more intensive treatment (group or individual counseling)
>
> **Referral for intensive tobacco dependence interventions**
> ➡ Appropriate for all tobacco users willing to participate in them
> ➡ Should not be limited to any subpopulation of tobacco users (e.g., heavily dependent smokers)
> ➡ Referral for group or individual counseling is appropriate for many patients and may be used in addition to the brief strategies to help patients that are clinician provided
> ➡ Effective when provided by trained counselors and includes repeated contacts over a period of at least 4 weeks
> ➡ Either individual or group counseling may be used; telephone counseling is also effective

G.   Brief clinical intervention for smokers who are willing to quit but at a later date (smokers who answer, "Yes, but not now," when asked "Are you willing to quit at this time?") are contained in the following table

> ### BRIEF CLINICAL INTERVENTIONS FOR PATIENTS WHO ARE WILLING TO QUIT SMOKING, BUT NOT AT THIS TIME
>
> - **Identify and address barriers to quitting in a nonjudgmental, supportive way**
>   ✓ Nicotine dependence
>   ✓ Fear of failure
>   ✓ Lack of social support
>   ✓ Lack of confidence
>   ✓ Concern about weight gain
>   ✓ Concurrent depression
>
> - **Identify reasons to quit smoking**
>   ✓ Health-related
>   ✓ Economic
>   ✓ Health of household members
>
> - **Follow up with patient at the next visit**

Adapted from Rigotti, N.A. (2002). Treatment of tobacco use and dependence. *New England Journal of Medicine, 346,* 508

H.   Brief clinical intervention for smokers who are not willing to quit smoking (Smokers who answer, "No," when asked "Are you willing to quit at this time?")
1.   Motivation is enhanced via use of the "5 Rs"-- *R*elevance, *R*isks, *R*ewards, *R*oadblocks, and *R*epetition
2.   See the table that follows for strategies to use with this intervention

BRIEF CLINICAL INTERVENTIONS FOR PATIENTS WHO ARE NOT WILLING TO QUIT

Why patient may be unwilling to quit:
Misinformation, concern about the effects of quitting and demoralization from previous unsuccessful quit attempts

Use of a motivational intervention: Use the "5R's," *Relevance, Risk, Rewards, Roadblocks,* and *Repetition*

Relevance: Encourage patient to tell you why quitting would be personally relevant to him/her	• Relevant to disease status or risk, family, social situation, work, etc • Ask to be as specific as possible
Risks: Ask the patient to identify potential negative consequences of tobacco use	• Acute risks: SOB, worsening of asthma, harm to pregnancy, impotence • Long-term risks: Heart attacks and strokes, lung and other cancers, COPD • Environmental risks: Exposure of family members (unborn children), and friends to environmental tobacco smoke (ETS)
Rewards: Ask the patient to identify potential benefits of stopping tobacco use (clinician may suggest and highlight those that seem most relevant to patient)	• Improved health • Food will taste better • Improved sense of smell • Save money • Feel better about self/feel better physically • Can stop worrying about quitting • Set a good example for children • Have healthier babies and children • Perform better in physical activities • Reduced wrinkling/aging of skin
Roadblocks: Ask the patient to identify barriers to quitting and note elements of treatment (problem-solving, pharmacotherapy) that could address barriers. Typical barriers might include:	• Withdrawal symptoms • Fear of failure • Weight gain • Lack of support • Depression • Enjoyment of tobacco
Repetition: Motivational intervention should be repeated every time an unmotivated patient visits the clinical setting; patients who have failed in previous attempts to quit should be reminded that most people make repeated attempts before they successfully quit	• Clinicians are most likely to use repetition when there is an office-wide system in place to identify all tobacco users at every visit • Without such a system, repeating the message to stop smoking is not likely to consistently occur

Adapted from Fiore, M.C., Bailer, W.C., Cohen, S.J., et al. (2000). Treating tobacco use and dependence. *Clinical practice guideline.* Rockville, MD: USDHHS. Public Health Service.

DEALING WITH PATIENT CONCERNS ABOUT WEIGHT GAIN

➡ Recommend starting or increasing physical activity

➡ Discourage "dieting"; instead, emphasize the importance of a healthy diet

➡ Reassure patient that some weight gain after quitting is common; usually limited to 10 pounds

➡ Encourage patient to tackle one problem at a time; quitting smoking should be the focus now

➡ Don't minimize patient's concern about weight gain; be empathetic, but help patient to re-focus

➡ Maintain the patient on pharmacotherapy known to delay weight gain (e.g., bupropion SR, NRTs, particularly nicotine gum)

➡ Refer patient to a specialist or program

I. Follow-Up
   1. For patients willing to quit at this time: See V.F. above
   2. For patients willing to quit, but not at this time: See V.G. above
   3. For patients who are not willing to quit: See V.H. above

REFERENCES

Alder, L.A., & Chua, H.C. (2002). Management of ADHD in adults. *Journal of Clinical Psychiatry, 63,* (Suppl. 12), 29-35.

American Academy of Pediatrics. (2001). Tobacco's toll: Implications for the pediatrician. *Pediatrics, 107,* 794-798.

American Gastroenterological Association, Clinical Practice Committee. (2002). AGA technical review on obesity. *Gastroenterology, 123,* 882-932.

American Psychiatric Association. (2000*). Diagnostic and statistical manual of mental disorders,* (4th ed.), Text Revision. Washington, DC. Author.

American Psychiatric Association. (2000). Practice guideline for the treatment of patients with eating disorders (revision). *American Journal of Psychiatry, 157*(Suppl. 1), 1-39.

Barnes, H.N., & Samet, J.H. (1997). Brief interventions with substance abusing patients. *Medical Clinics of North America, 81,* 867-880.

Blanck, H.M., Khan, L.K., & Serdula, M.K. (2001). Use of nonprescription weight loss products. *Journal of the American Medical Association, 286,* 930-935.

Brower, K.J., & Steverin, J.D. (1997). Alcohol and other drug-related problems. In D.J. Knesper, N.B. Riba, & T.L. Schwenk (Eds.), *Primary care psychiatry.* Philadelphia: Saunders.

Bush, B., Shaw, S., Cleary, P., Delbanco, T.L., & Aronson, M.D. (1987). Screening for alcohol abuse using the CAGE questionnaire. *American Journal of Medicine, 82,* 231-235.

Devlin, M.J. (2001). Binge-eating disorder and obesity. *Psychiatric Clinics of North America, 24,* 325-335.

Elia, J., Ambrosini, P.J., & Rapoport, J.H. (1999). Treatment of attention-deficit/hyperactivity disorder. *New England Journal of Medicine, 340,* 780-789.

Enoch, M., & Goldman, D. (2002). Problem drinking and alcoholism: Diagnosis and treatment. *American Family Physician, 65,* 441-449.

Fiore, M.C., Bailey, W.C., Cohen, S.J., Dorfman, S.F., Goldstein, M.G., Gritz, E.R., et al. (2000*). Treating tobacco use and dependence.* Clinical Practice Guideline. Rockville, MD: US Department of Health and Human Services.

Fontaine, K.R., Redden, D.T., Wang, C., Westfall, A.O., & Allison, D.B. (2003). Years of life lost due to obesity. *JAMA, 289,* 187-193.

Garbutt, J.C., West, S.L., Carey, T.S., Lohr, K.N., & Fulton, T.C. (1999). Pharmacological treatment of alcohol dependence: A review of the evidence. *Journal of the American Medical Association, 281,* 1318-1325.

Green, M., Wong, M., Atkins, D., Taylor, J., & Feinleib, M. (1999). *Diagnosis of attention-deficit/hyperactivity disorder.* Technical Review No. 3. AHCPR Publication No. 99-0050. Rockville, MD: Agency for Health Care Policy and Research.

Jadad, A.R., Boyle, M., Cunningham, C., Kim, M., & Schachar, R. (1999). Treatment of attention-deficit/hyperactivity disorder. Evidence Report/Technology Assessment No. 11. AHRQ Publication No. 00-E005. Rockville, MD: Agency for Healthcare Research and Quality.

Manson, J.F., & Bassuk, S.S. (2003). Obesity in the United States: A fresh look at its high toll. *JAMA, 289,* 229-230.

Naimi, T.S., Brewer, R.D., Mokdad, A., Denny, C., Serdula, M.K., & Marks, J.S. (2003). Binge drinking among US adults. *JAMA, 289,* 70-75.

National Institutes of Health; National Heart, Lung, and Blood Institute; & North American Association for the Study of Obesity. (2000). *The practical guide: Identification, evaluation, and treatment of overweight and obesity in adults.* Bethesda, MD: Author.

O'Connor, P.G. & Schottenfeld, R.S. (1998). Patients with alcohol problems. *New England of Medicine, 338,* 592-602.

Powers, P.S., & Santana, C.A. (2002). Eating disorders: a guide for the primary care physician. *Primary Care Clinics in Office Practice, 29,* 81-99.

Rigler, S.K. (2000). Alcoholism in the elderly. *American Family Physician, 61,* 1710-1716.

Rigorn, N.A. (2002). Treatment of tobacco use and dependence. *New England Journal of Medicine, 346,* 506-513.

Rosen, D.S., & Demitrack, M.A. (1997). Eating disorders and disordered eating. In D.J. Knesper, N.B. Riba, & T.L. Schwenk (Eds.), *Primary care psychiatry.* Philadelphia: Saunders.

Sadock, B.J., & Sadock, V.A. (2003*). Kaplan & Sadock's synopsis of psychiatry.* Philadelphia: Lippincott Williams & Wilkins.

Searight, H.R., Burke, J.M., & Rottnek, F. (2000). Adult ADHD: Evaluation and treatment in family medicine. *American Family Physician, 62,* 2077-2086.

Swift, R. (1999). Drug therapy for alcohol dependence. *New England Journal of Medicine, 340,* 1482-1490.

Szymanski, M.L., & Zolotor, A. (2001). Attention-deficit/hyperactivity disorder: Management. *American Family Physician, 64,* 1355-1362.

Tobacco Use and Dependence Clinical Practice Guideline Panel. (2000). A clinical practice guideline for treating tobacco use and dependence. *Journal of the American Medical Association, 283,* 3244-3255.

Treasure, J., & Serpell, L. (2001). Osteoporosis in young people: Research and treatment in eating disorders. *Psychiatric Clinics of North America, 24,* 359-367.

US Department of Health and Human Services. (2000). *Healthy people 2010.* McLean, VA: International Medical Publishing, Inc.

Whitaker, R.C. (2002). Understanding the complex journey to obesity in early adulthood. *Annals of Internal Medicine, 136,* 923-925.

Yanovski, S.Z., & Yanovski, J.A. (2002). Obesity. *New England Journal of Medicine, 346,* 591-602.

Zhu, S., Anderson, C.M., Tedeschi, G.J., Rosbrook, B., Johnson, C.D., Byrd, M., et al. (2002). Evidence of real-world effectiveness of a telephone quitline for smokers. *New England Journal of Medicine, 347,* 1087-1093.

Mental Health

TISH SMYER & MARY VIRGINIA GRAHAM

Anxiety Disorders
Table: Anxiety Disorders: Anxiety as a Primary Psychiatric Disorder
Table: Symptoms of Anxiety
Table: Medical Conditions/Medications that May Cause Anxiety
Table: Situations in Which Referral to a Specialist Is Indicated
Table: What Is Cognitive-Behavioral Therapy?
Table: Self-Help for Phobias
Table: Self-Help for Generalized Anxiety Disorder
Table: Self-Help for Obsessive Compulsive Disorder
Table: Self-Help for Post-Traumatic Stress Disorder
Table: Medications Useful in the Treatment of Anxiety Disorders in Primary Care

Depression
Table: Diagnostic Criteria for Major Depression
Table: Diagnostic Criteria for Dysthymic Disorder
Table: Diagnostic Criteria for Minor Depression
Table: Suicide Risk Assessment
Table: Brief Description and Source--BDI, Zung, GDS, and ODST
Table: Treatment for Depression: Selective Serotonin Reuptake Inhibitors (SSRIs)
Table: Treatment for Depression: Selected Tricyclic Antidepressants (TCAs)
Table: Selected Newer Antidepressants Commonly Used in Primary Care Settings
Table: Treatment with Antidepressants: Initiation, Monitoring, and Follow-Up
Table: Self-Help for Depression

Domestic Violence: Elder and Disabled Adult Abuse and Neglect
Table: SAFE Questions

Domestic Violence: Intimate Partner Violence
Table: SAFE Questions
Table: National Family Violence Resources

Grief
Table: Anticipatory Guidance
Table: Therapeutic Options for Dealing with Complicated Grief

Insomnia
Table: Sleep Hygiene: Patient Education
Table: Stimulus-Control Therapy
Table: Sleep Restriction Therapy
Table: Self-Help for Sleep Disorders
Table: Agents Commonly Prescribed to Treat Insomnia

ANXIETY DISORDERS

I. Definition: Symptoms of physiological arousal (e.g., palpitations, sweating) accompanied by a psychological mood of excessive worry that interferes with normal functioning and persists over time

II. Pathogenesis

    A. Several hypotheses have been formulated regarding pathophysiological processes involved in anxiety, with the same systems appearing to be invoked in "normal" and "disordered" anxiety

    B. Role of neurochemical systems (norepinephrine, serotonin, and gamma-aminobutyric acid [GABA]) has been uncovered through observations of the effects of pharmacologic agents, principally benzodiazepines, on anxiety
        1. Benzodiazepines appear to modulate anxiety by potentiating the action of GABA, the most prevalent inhibitory CNS neurotransmitter
        2. Receptors for benzodiazepine are coupled with receptors for GABA in the brain in both normal and disordered anxiety

    C. The central noradrenergic system, specifically norepinephrine-producing neurons located in the nucleus locus ceruleus, play an important role in anxiety dysregulation

III. Clinical Presentation

    A. Requests for "nerve pills" for feeling anxious or "nervous" are one of the most common chief complaints in primary care settings

    B. Patients with anxiety often present with somatic complaints and are high users of healthcare resources (frequent visits for multiple, unexplained symptoms; emergency department use; "doctor shopping")

    C. **Primary** anxiety disorders are psychiatric disorders with specific diagnostic categories and criteria as set forth by the American Psychiatric Association in the *Diagnostic and statistical manual of mental disorders, 4th edition, Text Revision (DSM-IV)* (2000)
        1. Using *DSM-IV* nomenclature, the nine primary anxiety disorders are panic disorder without agoraphobia; panic disorder with agoraphobia; agoraphobia without a history of panic disorder; specific phobia; social phobia; obsessive-compulsive disorder; post-traumatic stress disorder; acute stress disorder, and generalized anxiety disorder
        2. Clinical presentations for primary anxiety disorders are briefly summarized in the table on the following page (see table ANXIETY DISORDERS: ANXIETY AS A PRIMARY PSYCHIATRIC DISORDER) with several of the classifications grouped together to conserve space. **Note:** It is beyond the scope of this book to list all diagnostic criteria for all 9 classifications; thus, please consult the *DSM-IV* for a complete explication of the diagnostic classifications of anxiety, keeping in mind that many people with anxiety do not have a primary anxiety disorder

    D. Many patients have anxiety as a response to psychosocial or physical stressors (adjustment disorder with anxious mood); patient is anxious for good reason, but anxiety is excessive
        1. Very prevalent among patients in outpatient settings
        2. Should be suspected in patients who are experiencing a major psychosocial stressor (divorce or serious physical illness)

    E. Anxiety due to a medical condition or medication used to treat the condition occurs in a relatively small number of patients with certain conditions
        1. Essential feature is that anxiety is direct physiological consequence of medical condition or medication used in treatment
        2. Examples of conditions and medications that may cause symptoms are listed under IV. Differential Diagnosis

ANXIETY DISORDERS: ANXIETY AS A PRIMARY PSYCHIATRIC DISORDER

Disorder Category	Characteristics	Diagnostic Criteria
Panic Attacks (With or Without Agoraphobia) and Agoraphobia	**Panic attacks**: Sudden onset of intense fear or terror, with feelings of impending doom **Agoraphobia**: Anxiety about or avoidance of places/situations from which escape may be difficult in the event of a panic attack	Must have had 4 attacks within 4 weeks with at least 4 of the following symptoms present: shortness of breath, dizziness, faintness, palpitations, tachycardia, trembling, sweating, choking, nausea or abdominal distress, derealization, numbness or tingling sensations, hot flashes or chills, chest pain or discomfort, fear of dying, fear of going crazy or losing control
Phobias (both Specific and Social)	**Specific Phobia**: Excessive and persistent fear of certain objects/ situations so that exposure to the stimulus provokes an immediate anxiety response leading person to avoid the object/ situation or endure great anxiety when avoidance is not possible **Social Phobia**: Excessive anxiety provoked by certain types of performance/social situations such as giving a speech or dining in public places	Must have avoidant behavior that substantially interferes with occupational functioning, social and personal relationships
Generalized Anxiety Disorder	Excessive worry about several areas of life associated with a number of physical or psychological symptoms of anxiety; causes person great distress or impairment in social/occupational functioning	Must occur nearly every day and have persisted for at least 6 months. Three or more of the following 6 symptoms are predominant: restlessness/feeling keyed up, easily fatigued, difficulty concentrating, irritability, muscle tension, sleep disturbance
Obsessive-Compulsive Disorder	Characterized by distressing, consuming obsessions (recurrent or persistent intrusive thoughts), and/or compulsions which are repetitive behaviors or mental acts that person feels compelled to perform	Either obsessions or compulsions must be present *Obsessions* • Recurrent and persistent thoughts that are intrusive and inappropriate (not excessive worries about real-life problems) • Person tries to ignore or suppress thoughts • Person recognizes that thoughts are product of own mind (not imposed from without) *Compulsions* • Repetitive behaviors (hand washing, ordering) or mental acts (praying, counting) that person feels driven to perform • Behaviors or mental acts are aimed at preventing or reducing distress or preventing some dreaded event (no realistic relationship between behaviors/acts and events they are intended to prevent) At some point, the person has recognized that obsessions/ compulsions are excessive or unreasonable, cause marked distress, are time consuming (>1 hour/day) or interfere with person's normal routine, functioning, or usual social activities or relationships
Post-Traumatic Stress Disorder and Acute Stress Disorder	In both disorders, there is persistent re-experiencing of a traumatic event in the form of dreams, images, or feelings of reliving the event, often with intense psychological distress and physiological reactivity; there is avoidance of stimuli associated with the trauma and numbing of normal responsivity	Post-Traumatic Stress Disorder: Duration of disturbance must be longer than 1 month Acute Stress Disorder: Symptoms occur within 1 month of the traumatic stressor

F.   Substance abuse can also produce anxiety: (e.g., alcohol, caffeine, cannabis, cocaine, hallucinogens, inhalants). Accidental (or purposeful) exposure to volatile substances such as gasoline, paint, insecticides, and carbon monoxide can also produce anxiety

G.   Anxiety can also occur as part of the withdrawal from the following: alcohol, cocaine, sedatives, hypnotics, anxiolytics

H.   Anxiety associated with other psychiatric disorders (depression and alcohol dependence) is common
   1.   Discriminating between an anxiety disorder and a depressive illness is quite difficult because of the overlap in symptoms (e.g., sleep/appetite disturbances, difficulty concentrating, irritability, fatigue are characteristic of both anxiety and depression). See DEPRESSION section for more information about this disorder
   2.   Fifty to 75% of patients with social phobia, generalized anxiety disorder, or post-traumatic stress disorder have comorbid depression

IV.   Diagnosis/Evaluation

   A.   History
      1.   Inquire about onset, frequency, and duration of symptoms (acute or chronic)
      2.   Determine what specific events or situations are producing anxiety
      3.   Determine extent to which feelings of anxiety are interfering with daily functioning (home, work/school, leisure activities)
      4.   Patients who volunteer 1-2 symptoms of anxiety should be asked about presence of other physiological and psychological symptoms of anxiety listed in the SYMPTOMS OF ANXIETY table below
      5.   Ask about relieving factors

SYMPTOMS OF ANXIETY	
Physiological	Palpitations, shortness of breath, sweating, dry mouth, light-headedness, diarrhea, nausea, flushes or chills, feeling shaky, restless
Psychological	Excessive worry, disordered sleep, difficulty concentrating, irritable

      6.   Ask about caffeine intake, alcohol and illicit drug use
      7.   Obtain complete medication history including prescription, OTC drugs, as well as any supplements/herbal/complementary medicine remedies
      8.   Obtain complete past medical history, presence of any coexisting medical problems
      9.   Inquire about history of psychiatric illness, including treatments
      10. Always evaluate for suicide (see DEPRESSION for table on SUICIDE RISK ASSESSMENT)

   B.   Physical Examination: Exam should be directed toward ruling out disorders that may present as anxiety conditions (see C. below); a mental status exam should also be performed

   C.   Differential Diagnosis:
      1.   Anxiety as a primary psychiatric disorder: Does the patient meet criteria for one of the primary anxiety disorders? (see ANXIETY DISORDERS: ANXIETY AS A PRIMARY PSYCHIATRIC DISORDER table)
      2.   Anxiety as a response to psychological or physical stressors (adjustment disorder with anxious mood): Is the patient experiencing a major stress such as divorce, financial ruin, or a serious physical illness that might explain symptoms?
      3.   Anxiety due to a medical condition: Does the patient have a medical condition that produces anxiety as a symptom? See MEDICAL CONDITIONS/MEDICATIONS THAT MAY CAUSE ANXIETY table below

MEDICAL CONDITIONS/MEDICATIONS THAT MAY CAUSE ANXIETY	
Cardiovascular	Congestive heart failure, angina, arrhythmia
Endocrine	Hyperthyroidism, hypoglycemia, Cushing's syndrome
Neurological	Delirium, partial complex seizures, encephalitis
Respiratory	COPD, asthma, pneumonia
Medications	Theophylline, bronchodilators, amphetamines, anticholinergics, thyroid preparations, antidepressants, corticosteroids

      4.   Substance-induced anxiety: Is the anxiety due to the direct physiological effects of medications or toxins that the patient is taking/or being exposed to?

5. Anxiety associated with other psychiatric disorders: Does the patient have a history of depression, alcohol dependence, or psychosis? The condition diagnosed as the primary disorder should be treated first. See sections on DEPRESSION and ALCOHOL PROBLEMS to assist in discriminating between anxiety disorder and depressive illness or alcohol dependence

D. Diagnostic Tests: None indicated except to determine if anxiety is secondary to a medical condition

V. Plan/Management

A. General considerations in the treatment of anxiety disorders
1. Once a diagnosis has been made, determine if the disorder is appropriately treatable in a primary care setting

---

SITUATIONS IN WHICH REFERRAL TO A SPECIALIST IS INDICATED

- Significant diagnostic uncertainty
- Anxiety disorders that are often refractory, such as OCD and PTSD
- Anxiety disorders in which CBT is the treatment of choice, including specific phobias, social phobias, and agoraphobia
- Suicidal ideation (immediate emergency referral)
- Substance abuse
- Failure to respond to initial treatments
- **Any time the treatment modality exceeds the experience or interest of the clinician**

---

2. Educating the patient and family about the disorder and the availability of effective therapies should be provided whether or not the patient is referred to a specialist
3. A supportive, caring approach should be used as this can have a calming effect and reassure the patient that he/she is not "crazy"
4. If pharmacotherapy is initiated, the patient must be closely monitored until stable dosage and relief of symptoms are achieved

B. Patients with primary anxiety disorders are most responsive to pharmacotherapy or a combination of pharmacotherapy and psychotherapy by an expert in cognitive-behavioral therapy (CBT)

WHAT IS COGNITIVE-BEHAVIORAL THERAPY?

Therapy	Central Concept	Therapeutic Techniques
Cognitive	Psychological distress arises in part from self-defeating, irrational thoughts and beliefs; changing these thoughts and beliefs can reduce anxiety	➡ Helping patient see the link between the thoughts and the anxiety response ➡ Assisting patient to use "self-talk" to help deal with anxiety-provoking stressors ➡ Showing patient how to apply appropriate responses during stressful times, beginning with less stressful triggers and moving to more challenging ones ➡ Involves goal setting, activity assignments, and careful monitoring
Behavioral	Responses to certain cues are irrational; anxiety can be controlled through altering the behavioral response to anxiety provoking cues; most modern behavior therapy uses *exposure* as the central principle of treatment	➡ Exposure-based interventions involve the use of continuous exposure to the anxiety-provoking cue as the way to relieve anxiety (desensitization) ➡ Other techniques are the teaching of relaxation techniques and slow-breathing so that these become conditioned responses to cues ➡ Therapists also use participant modeling, or enacting a behavior then encouraging patient to repeat the behavior ➡ Involves goal setting, activity assignments, and careful monitoring

---

1. Panic attack (with or without agoraphobia) and agoraphobia
a. In most cases, CBT is the treatment of choice, but this approach may not be effective, available, or accessible
b. First-line pharmacologic treatment is use of the antidepressant medications-selective serotonin reuptake inhibitors (SSRIs) and tricyclics (TCAs); SSRIs are usually better tolerated and safer but are more costly than TCAs

2. Specific (simple) phobia
   a. CBT is the treatment of choice, with exposure therapy being the approach that is used most reliably
   b. Medications have no role in the management of specific phobias, although an occasional use of a benzodiazepine (BZ) may be justified (patient with fear of large crowds wants to attend son's graduation ceremony)
3. Social phobia
   a. CBT is treatment of choice, with exposure therapy being the most reliable approach
   b. Pharmacologic management is with SSRIs (**Note:** Only paroxetine is currently FDA approved for this indication)
   c. Beta blockers can also be used

SELF-HELP FOR PHOBIAS

Anxiety Disorders Association of America, 11900 Parklawn Drive, Suite 100, Rockville, MD 20852 for information on support groups or call 301-231-9350.

Go online to http://www.adaa.org

Recommend books for patients such as "Social Phobias: From Shyness to Stage Fright." New York: Basic Books, 1994

For brochures about phobias in English and Spanish go to: http://www.nimh.nih.gov/anxiety/socialphobiamenu.cfm

---

4. Generalized anxiety disorder (GAD)
   a. Pharmacologic therapy is the first-line treatment for patients with GAD
      (1) Antidepressants are effective for most patients with GAD, with about 70% of patients receiving benefit from this therapy
      (2) Venlafaxine, SSRIs, TCAs and Buspirone are all effective with agent selection based on safety, side effect profile, contraindications, and cautions, as well as cost
      (3) Benzodiazepines (BZs) are also effective (short course, only, for stabilization); clinicians should be cautious in the use of this class of drugs because long-term use (>2 weeks) carries the risk of dependence and withdrawal syndrome
      (4) Beta blockers are sometimes used to relieve the physiologic, but not the psychologic symptoms of anxiety; also useful for performance anxiety
   b. Traditional, insight-oriented psychotherapy (based on belief that self-understanding leads to cure) as well as CBT may be used
      (1) Unfortunately, response to insight-oriented psychotherapy and CBT is often disappointing
      (2) These modalities are not considered a principal therapy for GAD but may be supportive, with drug therapy being the first-line treatment

---

SELF-HELP FOR GENERALIZED ANXIETY DISORDER

Anxiety Disorders Association of America, 11900 Parklawn Drive, Suite 100, Rockville, MD 20852 for information on support groups or call 301-231-9350.

Go online to http://www.adaa.org

National Institute of Mental Health, 6001 Executive Boulevard, Rm 8184 MSC 9663, Bethesda, MD 20892, 301-443-4513; **Note:** Especially useful: "Anxiety Disorders," NIH-94-3879

For brochures about anxiety in English and Spanish go to: http://www.nimh.nih.gov/anxiety/gadmenu.cfm

---

5. Obsessive-compulsive disorder (OCD)
   a. Difficult to treat, even for specialists, because of complexity of therapy and poor patient response characterized by frequent relapses
   b. CBT is the mainstay, but this treatment is not as effective as it is for other anxiety disorders, with only about 20% of patients completing treatment and remaining symptom free
   c. Pharmacologic therapy is indicated for most patients with OCD, preferably as an adjunct to behavior therapy
      (1) SSRIs are effective and dosing is at the high end of the range
      (2) Sexual difficulties (impotence, decreased libido, difficulty achieving orgasm) caused by the SSRIs are the reason many patients discontinue the medication even though OCD is improved

(3)   Only about 60% of patients with OCD respond well to pharmacotherapy, and when the medication is stopped, almost all patients experience relapse

---

SELF-HELP FOR OBSESSIVE COMPULSIVE DISORDER

Obsessive-Compulsive Foundation (OCF) provides a forum for persons with OCD and for professionals, 203-315-2190 or email info@ocfoundation.org

Go online to: http://www.ocfoundation.org

Recommend self-help books such as "*Too Perfect: When Being in Control Gets Out of Control*" by A.E. Mallinger & J. DeWyze. New York. Clarkson Potter, 1992

For brochures about OCD in English and Spanish go to: http://www.nimh.nih.gov/publicat/ocdmenu.cfm

---

6.   Post-traumatic stress disorder (PTSD) and acute stress disorder
       a.   Psychotherapy should be the initial approach to treatment. Pharmacologic treatment with SSRIs may reduce intrusive thoughts. Use of BZs in PTSD patients is not recommended. Support groups may offer the most hope for helping patients manage the disorder. Persistent symptoms require referral
       b.   Patients with acute stress disorder are usually helped by supportive counseling; short-term (<1 week) use of BZs may also be effective

---

SELF-HELP FOR POST-TRAUMATIC STRESS DISORDER

Victims of rape, incest, or abuse may be referred to the Rape, Abuse, and Incest National Network (RAINN) at 800-656-HOPE, which automatically connects the caller to a support agency or go online to http://www.rainn.org

For brochures about PTSD in English and Spanish go to: http://www.nimh.nih.gov/anxiety/ptsdmenu.cfm

---

C.   Patients with adjustment disorders with anxious mood may be appropriately managed in primary care settings rather than specialty settings
       1.   Pharmacologic therapy using BZs for short-term (<2 weeks) can be very effective
       2.   Persistent anxiety symptoms require chronic treatment with an SSRI, TCA or Buspirone
       3.   Supportive counseling (by primary care provider or clergy) or in-depth therapy by a mental health specialist can be helpful; relaxation therapy may also be helpful

D.   Medications useful in the treatment of anxiety disorders are summarized in the table on the next page

E.   Patients with anxiety due to a medical condition require treatment of the underlying cause

F.   For patients with anxiety that is substance-induced
       a.   If medication that is being taken for another condition is the cause, consider switching to another class that may not produce anxiety
       b.   If licit or illicit drugs (e.g., cannabis, cocaine, hallucinogens, inhalants, or caffeine) are causing the anxiety, provide patient with counseling/referral to drug detoxification program

G.   Patients with anxiety associated with another psychiatric condition, most often depression, should be treated for the primary problem. See sections on DEPRESSION and ALCOHOL USE, ABUSE, AND DEPENDENCE for assistance in dealing with patients who have either of these problems. As stated above, most patients in this category should be referred to a specialist if possible

H.   Follow Up
       a.   Variable depending on diagnosis and involvement in treatment (e.g., if in-office counseling is being provided for an adjustment disorder, may need to be weekly for several weeks)
       b.   When pharmacotherapy is used, monitor the patient closely (every 2-3 weeks) until a stable dosage and relief of symptoms are achieved
       c.   Long-term use of medications is often required

MEDICATIONS USEFUL IN THE TREATMENT OF ANXIETY DISORDERS IN PRIMARY CARE*

Category, Generic and Trade Name	Initial Dose**	Therapeutic Range	Contraindications	Important Class Side Effects	Indications†
Selective serotonin-reuptake inhibitors (SSRIs) Escitalopram (Lexapro) Fluoxetine (Prozac) Paroxetine (Paxil) Sertraline (Zoloft)	10 mg daily 5-10 mg every morning 10 mg daily 25 mg daily	10-20 mg daily 10-80 mg every morning 10-50 mg daily 50-200 mg daily	Use of MAOIs within prior 21 days	Somnolence, agitation, sweating, nausea, anorexia, sexual dysfunction	OCD, PD/AG, SP, PTSD, GAD **OCD, PD/AG**, SP, PTSD, **GAD OCD, PD/AG, SP, PTSD, GAD OCD, PD/AG**, SP, **PTSD**, GAD
Tricyclic antidepressants (TCAs) Imipramine (Tofranil) Clomipramine (Anafranil)	10-25 mg at bedtime 25 mg at bedtime	150-300 mg daily 25-250 mg daily	Cardiac conduction abnormalities, glaucoma, suicide risk	Anticholinergic: dry mouth, constipation, blurred vision, orthostatic hypotension, weight gain, somnolence	PD/AG, GAD, PTSD **OCD**, PD/AG, PTSD,GAD
Serotonin- and norepinephrine-reuptake inhibitor Venlafaxine (Effexor XR)	37.5 mg daily	37.5-225 mg daily	Use of MAOIs within prior 21 days	Somnolence, agitation, sweating, nausea, anorexia, sexual dysfunction	**GAD**, PD/AG
Benzodiazepines (BZs) Alprazolam (Xanax) Clonazepam (Klonopin) Lorazepam (Ativan)	0.25 mg three x daily 0.25 mg twice daily 0.5 mg three x daily	0.25-4 mg daily 0.25-4 mg daily 1-6 mg daily	History of substance abuse; significant liver disease; narrow-angle glaucoma	Sedation, dizziness, lack of coordination, amnesia, headache	**GAD, PD/AG**, PTSD **PD/AG**, GAD, PTSD GAD, PD/AG, SP
Norepinephrine- and dopamine-reuptake inhibitor Buspirone (BuSpar)	5 mg twice daily	15-60 mg daily	Concomitant MAOIs	Dizziness, nausea	**GAD**
Beta-Blocker Propranolol (Inderal)	20 mg daily	20-160 mg daily	Asthma; heart disease/ conduction problems	Depression, sedation	Performance Anxiety

* Information in this table should be used as a general guide only. Always refer to package inserts and consult with pharmacists for dosing recommendations, precautions, and drug interactions

** Initial dose should be reduced in frail or elderly patients and in those with hepatic or renal dysfunction

† Bold indicates FDA approval for that indication at the time this book was published

OCD   Obsessive Compulsive Disorder
PD/AG   Panic Disorder/Agoraphobia
SP   Social Phobia
PTSD   Post-Traumatic Stress Disorder
GAD   Generalized Anxiety Disorder

DEPRESSION

I.   Definition: Unipolar mood disorders characterized by physical and psychological symptoms that cause significant distress and impairment in functioning and occur in the absence of elevated mood (mania or hypomania)

II. Pathogenesis

A.   Theories related to a biologic etiology of depression include the following:
   1.   Biogenic amine hypothesis: Occurs as result of depletion of levels of serotonin
   2.   Receptor suprasensitivity hypothesis: Results from suprasensitive catecholamine receptors in response to decreased levels of catecholamine in brain
   3.   Genetic predisposition plays a role in etiology as well as treatment. There is some evidence that patients will respond to an antidepressant medication that has been successful in a first-degree relative.

B.   Theories related to a psychosocial etiology of depression include the following:
   1.   Psychoanalytic: Mourning of symbolic object loss with rigid superego that leads one to feel worthless
   2.   Cognitive: Cognitive triad of (a) automatic negative thoughts and negative self-view, (b) negative interpretation of experience and pessimistic view of the world, and (c) negative view of future

III. Clinical Presentation

A.   Unipolar depressive disorders are psychiatric disorders with specific diagnostic categories and criteria as set forth by the American Psychiatric Association in the *Diagnostic and statistical manual of mental disorders (4th edition), Text Revision (DSM-IV)* (2000)
   1.   Using *DSM-IV* nomenclature, the three unipolar depressive disorders are major depression, dysthymic disorder, and minor depression (**Note:** Minor depression is the most common form of a diagnostic category called "depressive disorder, not otherwise specified," a category that includes several disorders)
      a.   Major depression is the most severe form of unipolar depression and consists of history of one or more major depressive episodes
      b.   Dysthymic disorder is a milder and chronic form of depression
      c.   Minor depression is characterized by fewer than five symptoms of major depression
   2.   Diagnostic criteria for each of the three disorders are summarized in the following tables

---

DIAGNOSTIC CRITERIA FOR MAJOR DEPRESSION

At least five of the following symptoms (one of which **must** be either [1] depressed mood or [2] loss of interest or pleasure) are present nearly every day during the same 2-week period

   ✓   Depressed mood (anhedonia)
   ✓   Loss of interest or pleasure in most activities
   ✓   Significant weight loss/gain or decreased/increased appetite
   ✓   Insomnia or hypersomnia
   ✓   Psychomotor agitation or retardation
   ✓   Loss of energy or fatigue
   ✓   Feelings of worthlessness or excessive/inappropriate guilt
   ✓   Diminished ability to think/concentrate or indecisiveness
   ✓   Recurrent thoughts of suicide or death
   ✓   Symptoms cause clinically significant distress or impairment in social, occupational or other important areas of functioning

---

DIAGNOSTIC CRITERIA FOR DYSTHYMIC DISORDER

Depressed mood (can be irritable mood in children/adolescents present for at least **one year**) for most of the day, for more days than not, for at least 2 years

During periods of depressed mood, at least two of the following additional symptoms are present:
- Appetite disturbance
- Insomnia or hyposomnia
- Low energy or fatigue
- Low self-esteem
- Poor concentration or difficulty making decisions
- Feelings of hopelessness

DIAGNOSTIC CRITERIA FOR MINOR DEPRESSION

- Presence of fewer than five symptoms of major depression
- Duration of symptoms (must include either depressed mood or loss of interest or pleasure in most activities) at least 2 weeks
- Disturbance does not occur exclusively during course of psychotic disorders

Previous three tables adapted from American Psychiatric Association. (2000). *Diagnostic and statistical manual of mental disorders* (4th ed.) Text revision. Washington, DC: Author.

B. **Depression** ranks second (behind hypertension) in terms of commonly occurring chronic conditions presenting in primary care
    1. Approximately 18.8 million American adults (about 9.5%) have a depressive disorder with a female to male ratio of 2:1
    2. Many patients with depression can be treated effectively in primary care settings; improvement in both depressive symptoms and functional status can be obtained through the use of antidepressants and depression-specific psychological treatments

C. **Major depression** is the fourth most important cause worldwide of loss in disability-adjusted life years; expected to be second only to heart disease as a cause of disability by 2020, according to World Health Organization (WHO)
    1. Disorder may develop at any age, but average age of onset is mid-20s
    2. Estimates are that 1 in 10 outpatients have this disorder; most cases are unrecognized or inappropriately treated
    3. See DIAGNOSTIC CRITERIA table above for clinical presentation description

D. **Dysthymia** occurs in approximately 5% of persons
    1. Most often begins in childhood, adolescence, or early adulthood
    2. Symptomatically less severe than major depression, but much more persistent (duration criterion of 2 years in adults)
    3. See DIAGNOSTIC CRITERIA table above for clinical presentation description

E. **Minor depression** is a diagnostic category for patients who have too few depressive symptoms to qualify for a diagnosis of major depression, and a duration too brief to fit into the dysthymic disorder category
    1. Associated with high use of health services
    2. See DIAGNOSTIC CRITERIA table above for clinical presentation description

F. Many patients who present with depressive symptoms in primary care settings do not meet the rigid diagnostic criteria for the above described disorders
    1. These patients use two or three times as many healthcare resources as patients without such symptoms
    2. Somatic complaints such as dizziness, diffuse systemic malaise, and pain (headache, pelvic, and low-back) are common complaints
    3. Complaints about emotional distress are usually not the chief complaint

G. Depression in the elderly may be difficult to distinguish from dementia (See section on ALZHEIMER'S DISEASE for more information)

H. Suicide is a definite risk in patients with depression; a recent review suggests that contact with healthcare services in the year prior to suicide is common
   1. Rates of contact are much higher for primary care providers relative to mental health specialists
   2. This suggests that interventions involving primary care professionals have the potential to significantly affect suicide rates

IV. Diagnosis/Evaluation

A. History: Keep in mind that depressive symptoms are evaluated along several continuums—intensity, duration, and impact on daily functioning
   1. Ask about onset, duration, and description of symptoms. Ask about symptoms that characteristically occur by referring to tables above that contain diagnostic criteria for major depression, dysthymic disorder, and minor depression or consider use of a brief screening tool for depression at this point in the history taking (see IV.D. below)
   2. Ask if these symptoms are new or if they have occurred before (current and past psychiatric history)
   3. Ask about the impact of these symptoms on daily functioning
      a. Does the patient have difficulty functioning at home/school/work?
      b. How are interpersonal relationships affected?
   4. Ask about presence of identifiable stressors using these three categories:
      a. Major discrete stressors: Ask about deaths, divorces, job losses
      b. Chronic stressors: Ask about marital conflict, abuse, on-going chronic illness in patient or family member
      c. Minor daily stressors: Ask about demands at work, home, that may be causing patient to feel overwhelmed
   5. Ask about mood swings (if present, consider bipolar disorder)
   6. Ask about alcohol/drug use
   7. Obtain past medical history and medication history (medications that may cause depression include steroids, antihypertensives, estrogen, NSAIDs, digoxin, and anti-Parkinson drugs)
   8. Always ask patients with depressive symptoms about suicidal thinking, impulses, and personal history of suicide attempts. (Suicidal risk factors are hopelessness, Caucasian race, male gender, age over 65, living alone, personal and family history of suicide attempts, personal and family history of alcohol/substance abuse; highest suicide rates are among elderly Caucasian males)

SUICIDE RISK ASSESSMENT

Initial and follow-up screening evaluations must include very specific questions
- Approach with a declaration such as: "It sounds as if you are having a really hard time," or "Sometimes when people feel down or depressed, they might think about dying"
- Then ask, "Do you ever think of hurting yourself or taking your own life?"
- If the answer is "Yes," ask, "When you have such thoughts, are you able to put them out of your mind, or do you find yourself dwelling on them?"
- Regardless of the answer, ask, "Do you feel that you might act on these thoughts?" or "Do you have a plan?"

Patients who have suicidal thoughts must be referred for emergency psychiatric evaluation

---

B. Physical Examination
   1. While completing history, part of mental status exam should be obtained:
      a. Observe general appearance and behavior (usual to see inattention to personal appearance, tearful, downcast, poor eye contact)
      b. Pay attention to affect (usually constricted, intense) mood (one of frustration, sadness), and speech (usually soft, low with little spontaneity)
      c. If inattention occurs during history taking, it should be documented during exam by testing ability to recall series of random numbers
   2. Physical exam should be directed toward ruling out an infectious, neoplastic, metabolic, or neurologic disorder

C. Differential Diagnosis
   1. Bipolar depression
   2. Psychotic disorders, particularly schizophrenia
   3. Bereavement
   4. Substance abuse
   5. Dementia

103

6. Anxiety disorder
7. Medical conditions such as thyroid dysfunction, other endocrine disorders, neurological problems, as well as medications that treat those disorders

D. Diagnostic Tests
1. The US Preventive Services Task Force recommends screening adults for depression using any one of several screening tools available (with one not recommended over another) or by asking two questions about mood and anhedonia: "Over the past 2 weeks, have you felt down, depressed, or hopeless?" and "Over the past 2 weeks, have you felt little interest or pleasure in doing things?"
2. The Beck Depression Inventory and the Zung Self-Rating Depression Scale have been used extensively in primary care research
3. The Geriatric Depression Scale (GDS) is an appropriate screening tool for assessing depression in the elderly (**Note:** Not valid in patients with cognitive impairment)
4. The Online Depression Screening Test (ODST) is a convenient screening test the patient can complete at home

BRIEF DESCRIPTION AND SOURCE--BDI, ZUNG, GDS AND ODST

Scale	Description	Source
Beck Depression Inventory II (BDI-II)	21 item self-report (also a 13 item version) Emphasis is on cognitive symptoms of depression All items apply to "the past 2 weeks"	This scale is available online at http://www.uea.ac.uk/~wp316/depression.pdf
Zung Self-Rating Depression Scale	20 items, rated by how much of the time each depressive symptom is present Zung describes scale as "depression thermometer"	For more information about this scale, consult the following publication: Zung, W.W.K. (1965). A self-rating depression scale. *Archives of General Psychiatry, 12*, 63-70. Also available on-line at http://www.wellbutrin-sr.com/hcp/depression/zung.html
Geriatric Depression Scale (GDS)	30 yes/no questions Takes 5-7 minutes to complete, is one page long, and easy to understand	This scale (public domain), is available online at GDS Long version: http://www.stanford.edu/~yesavage/GDS.english.long/html GDS Short version: http://www.stanford.edu/~yesavage/GDS.english.short.score.html
Online Depression Screening Test (ODST)	10 Likert type questions Easily completed by patient	New York University School of Medicine http://www.med.nyu.edu/Psych/screens/depres.html

5. All positive screening tests should trigger full diagnostic interviews that use standard diagnostic criteria, such as those from *DSM-IV*
6. Consider the following screening tests based on history/physical examination findings to rule out an organic cause or substance use: CBC, sedimentation rate, VDRL, chemistry profile, thyroid profile, folic acid, B_6 and B_{12}, and drug screen

V. Plan/Management

A. The following categories of patients should be referred to a specialist for treatment:
1. Those with high suicide risk (patients who admit to suicidal thinking, have a realistic plan, and have access to weapons, particularly guns [refer for emergency psychiatric evaluation])
2. Women who are pregnant or plan to become pregnant
3. Patients with no evidence of social support
4. Patients who are disabled by the depression (unable to function at work/school, unable to take care of day-to-day responsibilities)
5. Patients with comorbid conditions (primary anxiety disorder, substance abuse, dementia)
6. Children and adolescents with depressive disorders
7. Patients who fail to respond to one or two adequate trials of antidepressants

B.   Patients who are **not** in the above categories and who have (1) depression that has persisted for 2 weeks or longer, or (2) depression that is chronic and interferes with routine functions of family/work/school life are candidates for treatment with both pharmacologic and nonpharmacologic therapies

    1.   Pharmacotherapy: Mainstay of treatment by primary care providers is pharmacologic therapy; the two classes of drugs most commonly used are selective serotonin-reuptake inhibitors (SSRIs) and tricyclic antidepressants (TCAs) [equally efficacious]. Newer classes of antidepressants (in addition to SSRIs) are also equally efficacious

        a.   Medication selection can be guided mainly by adverse effect profile and clinical needs of the patient

        b.   Other factors to guide selection include patient's previous response to the medication and tolerance of and preference for different side effects

        c.   Cost is also a concern, particularly for patients who pay out-of-pocket (amitriptyline cost per month is ~$9; sertraline is ~$75)

    2.   Nonpharmacologic therapies: Include psychotherapy/counseling as well as other modalities such as exercise and behavior change

        a.   May be considered an alternative to medications in patients who are very reluctant to use pharmacotherapy

        b.   A more accurate concept of the role of this treatment modality is to support/augment medications rather than replace them

C.   Pharmacotherapy with antidepressants

    1.   Selective serotonin reuptake inhibitors (SSRIs) are often considered **first-line treatment** for depression based on excellent side effect profile and safety during overdose (generally less toxic than tricyclics)

        a.   Table below lists usual starting dose, target dose, and step-up dose

        b.   Most common side effects of this class of drugs are nausea, anorexia, weight loss, excessive sweating, nervousness, insomnia, sexual dysfunction, sedation, headache, and dizziness

TREATMENT FOR DEPRESSION: SELECTIVE SEROTONIN-REUPTAKE INHIBITORS (SSRIs)*

Medication	Initial Dose**	Target Dose†	Step-Up Dose‡
Fluoxetine (Prozac)	20 mg every morning	20 mg every morning	40-60-mg every morning
Sertraline (Zoloft)	50 mg every morning	100 mg every morning	150-200 mg every morning
Paroxetine (Paxil)	20 mg daily	20 mg daily	50 mg daily
Escitalopram (Lexapro)	10 mg daily	10 mg daily	20 mg daily

* Information in this table should be used as a general guide only. Always refer to package inserts and consult with pharmacists for dosing recommendations, precautions, and drug interactions
** Initial dose should be reduced in frail or elderly patients and in those with hepatic or renal dysfunction
† Target dose is dose likely to be effective for most patients.
‡ Step-up dose is the dose above which most patients would not derive any additional benefit

Adapted from Whooley, M.A., & Simon, G.E. (2000). Managing depression in medical outpatients. *New England Journal of Medicine, 343*, 1942-1950.

    2.   Tricyclic antidepressants (TCAs) are also effective but cause many side effects that reduce patient compliance

        a.   Side effects that are most common include sedation, anticholinergic effects (dry mouth, dry eyes, blurred vision, constipation, urinary retention, tachycardia, and confusion), postural hypotension, gastrointestinal upset, sexual dysfunction, and weight gain

        b.   Can have a significant effect on cardiac conduction through a quinidine-like effect and are **contraindicated** in patients with ischemic heart disease or known arrhythmias

        c.   Also **contraindicated** in patients with narrow-angle glaucoma and prostatic hypertrophy (See PDR for a full discussion of contraindications and precautions; **overdoses can be lethal!**)

        d.   With gradual dosage titration, most bothersome side effects of TCAs subside after a few weeks

        e.   Obtain an EKG in any patient over the age of 50 **before** prescribing these drugs and **after four weeks** of TCA treatment; **repeat** after any dose increase

        f.   Tables below list initial dose, target dose, and step-up dose of TCAs

TREATMENT FOR DEPRESSION: SELECTED TRICYCLIC ANTIDEPRESSANTS*
(SEROTONIN- AND NOREPINEPHRINE-REUPTAKE INHIBITORS)

Medication	Initial Dose**	Target Dose[†]	Step-Up Dose[‡]
Tricyclics (tertiary amines)			
Amitriptyline (Elavil)	25 mg at bedtime	100 mg at bedtime	150 mg at bedtime
Doxepin (Sinequan)	25 mg at bedtime	100 mg at bedtime	150-200 mg at bedtime
Imipramine (Tofranil)	25 mg at bedtime	100 mg at bedtime	150-200 mg at bedtime
Tricyclics (secondary amines)			
Desipramine (Norpramin)	25 mg at bedtime	100 mg at bedtime	150-200 mg at bedtime
Nortriptyline (Pamelor)	25 mg at bedtime	50-75 mg at bedtime	100-150 mg at bedtime

* Information in this table should be used as a general guide only. Always refer to package inserts and consult with pharmacists for dosing recommendations, precautions, and drug interactions
** Initial dose should be reduced in frail or elderly patients and in those with hepatic or renal dysfunction
[†] Target dose is dose likely to be effective for most patients.
[‡] Step-up dose is the dose above which most patients would not derive any additional benefit
Adapted from Whooley, M.A., & Simon, G.E. (2000). Managing depression in medical outpatients. *New England Journal of Medicine, 343,* 1942-1950.

3. Other categories of antidepressants (often called "newer" antidepressants) are contained in the following table
    a. Table below lists their initial dose, target dose, and step-up dose

SELECTED NEWER ANTIDEPRESSANTS COMMONLY USED IN PRIMARY CARE SETTINGS*

Medication	Trade Name	Initial Dose**	Target Dose[†]	Step-Up Dose[‡]
Norepinephrine- and dopamine-reuptake inhibitor				
Bupropion	Wellbutrin	75 mg twice a day	150 mg twice a day	150 mg three times a day
	Wellbutrin SR	150 mg every morning	150 mg twice a day	200 mg twice a day
Serotonin- and norepinephrine-reuptake inhibitor				
Venlafaxine	Effexor	37.5 mg twice a day	75 mg twice a day	100-150 mg twice a day
	Effexor XR	37.5 mg daily	75-150 mg daily	225 mg daily
Serotonin antagonist				
Mirtazapine	Remeron	15 mg at bedtime	30 mg at bedtime	45 mg at bedtime
Serotonin antagonists and reuptake inhibitor				
Trazodone[††]	Desyrel	50 mg at bedtime	200 mg at bedtime	200 mg at bedtime

* Information in this table should be used as a general guide only. Always refer to package inserts and consult with pharmacists for dosing recommendations, precautions, and drug interactions
** Initial dose should be reduced in frail or elderly patients and in those with hepatic or renal dysfunction
[†] Target dose is dose likely to be effective for most patients.
[‡] Step-up dose is the dose above which most patients would not derive any additional benefit
[††] Trazodone is too sedating at therapeutic doses for treatment of depression; best used in lower doses (50 mg at bedtime) as adjunctive for patients with insomnia
Adapted from Whooley, M.A., & Simon, G.E. (2000). Managing depression in medical outpatients. *New England Journal of Medicine, 343,* 1942-1950.

b. Lack significant cardiac effects and are relatively safe in overdose
c. Side-effect profile is variable, depending on particular agent
d. **Bupropion**: Most common side effects are agitation, dry mouth, insomnia, headache, nausea, vomiting, constipation, tremor; **contraindicated** in persons with seizure disorder or bulimia
e. **Venlafaxine**: May cause sustained increase in BP. Most common side effects are dry mouth, dizziness, nervousness, sweating, nausea, anorexia, constipation, and insomnia. Caution with history of MI and unstable heart disease

f. **Mirtazapine:** Most common side effects are related to H$_1$-receptor blocking activity and
~~increased~~ appetite, weight gain, dizziness, dry mouth, constipation; good
ion strategies as drug-drug interactions with other antidepressants

non side effects are drowsiness, dizziness, headache, nausea, and
, priapism in men (extremely rare but serious and is not dose related)
effective antidepressant but it is most often used in the management
with SSRI use. Dosing for this indication is 50 mg at bedtime]
s (MAOIs) are used primarily in treatment-resistant patients; patients
list for initiation of this class of antidepressants. Many serious and
associated with the MAOIs

fects **prior** to prescribing any antidepressant
ssants produce some side effects
ong drug classes
asses vary among patients
st commonly occurring adverse effects and emphasize that most side

ing him/her that most side effects resolve with time
er that most side effects are better than depression

SANTS: INITIATION, MONITORING, AND FOLLOW-UP

➡ **Initiating antidepressant therapy**

- Select medication and determine initial dose based on side effect profile and clinical needs of patient
- Instruct patient to increase dose gradually, approaching target dose (if different from initial dose) over period of 5-10 days
- Prescribe no more than one month supply initially (given potential for overdose)

➡ **Monitoring the patient** closely during first twelve weeks of treatment is crucial (minimum of three visits)

- In 2-4 weeks, schedule first follow-up visit; then schedule 2 more visits over next 8-10 weeks
  - At each visit, ask about adherence (about 50% of patients discontinue treatment during first month)
  - Advise patient that full therapeutic effect may not be evident for 4-6 weeks (some improvement may be apparent in 2-4 weeks, however)
- **If no improvement by 3-4 weeks**, and side effects are tolerable, increase dose to step-up dose (see tables for dosing)
- **If intolerable side effects occur and persist** at 3-4 weeks, consider a trial of an alternative medication
- **If step-up dose** (begun after 3-4 weeks of therapy) **produces little or no improvement** after trial of 3-4 weeks (total of 6-8 weeks of treatment), consider a trial of an alternative medication
- **Patients who fail to respond** to a medication or who have intolerable adverse effects may be switched to another medication as follows:
  - Switch to another medication within the same class
  - Switch to a different class of antidepressants
  - No washout period is required when switching among SSRIs and between this class and TCAs
  - **Abrupt** discontinuation of shorter-acting serotonergic drugs (examples are citalopram, paroxetine, sertraline, and venlafaxine) may cause discontinuation syndrome (tinnitus, vertigo, paresthesias)
- Antidepressant medications should be continued at least 6 months after symptoms are relieved to prevent relapse
- Patients at high risk of relapse (2 or more previous episodes of depression) should continue treatment for at least 2 years and perhaps indefinitely
- If trial of second medication is not successful or if symptoms worsen, refer to specialist (or obtain psychiatric consultation)

➡ **Follow-up visits** should be scheduled every 3-6 months after the initial 12-week period

E. **Nonpharmacologic therapies:** Cognitive and interpersonal therapies are probably the most efficacious forms of psychotherapy for patients with depressive disorders

1. Cognitive therapy is aimed at correcting the negative views of self, world, and future that many depressed persons hold
   a. Focus is on helping patient gain new skills, enhancing confidence, and broadening social circle
   b. Homework assignments are typically provided to help patient meet goals
2. Interpersonal therapy focuses on resolution of problematic interpersonal relationships or stressful events in patient's life
   a. Providing patient with opportunities to talk about conflicts and ways to problem-solve can be very therapeutic
   b. A common interpersonal deficit is social isolation; practical suggestions such as joining a social/religious group, or taking a class, or becoming a volunteer can help decrease isolation and promote feelings of being connected in the patient

3. Patients should be referred for cognitive and interpersonal therapies as most primary care providers lack the time and expertise for these approaches

F. **Nonpharmacologic therapies:** Exercise programs are low cost alternatives to psychotherapy and may be combined with antidepressants to potentiate the medication effects
   1. Exercise appears to have both direct and indirect effects on relief of depression
   2. Prescribe a 10-minute daily walk with a gradual increase in walking time to 30 minutes/day; write the exercise prescription on a prescription pad to demonstrate the value of the daily walk
   3. An organized exercise class may be helpful as it increases the likelihood that the patient will interact with others on a regular basis

G. **Nonpharmacologic therapies:** Recognize the value of helping the patient find pleasure in daily living
   1. "Doing better" may be a prerequisite to "feeling better"
   2. Prescribe a single pleasurable activity each day (e.g., buying self flowers, going to a movie)
   3. Encourage patient to continue in activity even though it may initially fail to elicit feelings of pleasure
   4. Have patient keep a log of activities to discuss at periodic visits, again as a way of demonstrating provider confidence in the therapeutic approach

H. **Nonpharmacologic therapies:** Support groups are another low-cost option for patients with depression
   1. Many no-cost support groups are available for depressed patients
   2. Groups that meet in many communities include Adult Children of Alcoholics, Overeaters Anonymous, bereavement groups, and incest survivors groups

---

SELF-HELP FOR DEPRESSION

- *"Feeling Good: The New Mood Therapy"* by David Burns. New York: Avon Books, 1980
- Contact National Foundation For Depressive Illness, Inc., P.O. Box 2257 New York, NY 10116 , phone 1-800-239-1265 or visit the website: http://www.depression.org
- Brochures are available from National Institute of Mental Health: http://www.nimh.nih.gov/publicat/depressionmenu.cfm

---

I. Follow-Up
   1. For patients on pharmacotherapy, see follow-up recommendations in table TREATMENT WITH ANTIDEPRESSANTS: INITIATING, MONITORING, AND FOLLOW-UP
   2. For patients on nonpharmacologic therapies, see patient minimum of 3 visits during acute phase (first 12 weeks) to determine adherence and progress; base schedule on patient needs after acute phase

---

DOMESTIC VIOLENCE: ELDER AND DISABLED ADULT ABUSE AND NEGLECT

I. Definition: The infliction of physical pain, injury, or mental anguish, unreasonable confinement, or willful deprivation of services which are necessary to maintain mental and physical health of a disabled adult or elderly person

II. Pathogenesis

A. Etiology is unclear, but a number of recurrent theories emerge

B. Dependency of the adult/elder arising from multiple medical illnesses or mental impairment is frequently encountered

C. Financial conditions also appear to play a role in the occurrence of abuse, with the abused person having limited resources and imposing a financial burden on the abuser

D. Alcoholism and drug dependency in a caregiver enhance the likelihood of abuse

III. Clinical Presentation

    A. Almost 2 million older adults (>60) are abused annually

    B. Victims of abuse are likely to be among the old-old, the mean age being 84

    C. Victim is usually a woman and perpetrator most often is spouse, or adult child, but paid and informal caregivers may also be responsible

    D. Almost 50% of abused adults have moderate to severe mental impairment

    E. Physical indicators of abuse:
        1. Unexplained fractures, burns, bruises, welts, bald spots, human bite marks
        2. Bruises or bleeding in external genitalia

    F. Behavioral indicators of abuse:
        1. Withdrawn, lethargic, wears clothes inappropriate to season to cover body
        2. Sleep disorders, poor appetite, depressed mood

    G. Physical indicators of neglect:
        1. Inappropriate dress, poor hygiene
        2. Unattended medical needs (lacking hearing aids, dentures, eyeglasses)

IV. Diagnosis/Evaluation

    A. History
        1. Obtain social history, including information about living arrangements, primary caregiver, and family functioning
        2. Screening for violence (with only the patient present) should be made a **routine part** of preventive care for elderly and disabled persons. One approach is to ask the SAFE questions

SAFE QUESTIONS	
Stress/Safety	What stresses do you have in your relationships? Do you feel safe in your relationship with (name family member/friend)?
Afraid	Are there situations in which you feel afraid? Have you ever been threatened or abused?
Friends/Family	If positive responses to items above: Ask "Are your friends/family aware that this is happening?" If negative responses to item above: Ask "Do you think you could tell them if it did happen?" "Would they help you?"
Emergency Plan	Do you have a safe place to go in an emergency situation? Would you like to talk with a social worker/counselor to help you develop a plan?
Any questions answered affirmatively should be followed with additional questions in order to determine the following: ✓ How and when mistreatment occurs ✓ Who perpetrates it ✓ How the patient copes with it	

Adapted from Ashur, M.L. (1993). Asking about domestic violence: SAFE questions (Letter to the editor). *JAMA 269*, 2367.

        3. If physical injury is present, ask detailed questions relating to time of occurrence and how it occurred
            a. Long interval between injury and seeking help is red flag
            b. Story that is inconsistent, contradictory, or fails to adequately explain injury is red flag
        4. If behavioral problems are evident, ask appropriate questions to determine etiology by asking direct questions such as the following:
            a. Are you alone a lot?
            b. Has anyone ever failed to help you take care of yourself when you needed help?
            c. Has anyone ever made you do things you did not want to do?
        5. Any positive responses should prompt asking how and when this occurs, who the perpetrator is, and how the patient copes with the mistreatment
        6. Question about past or present medical problems, current medications

7. Interview patient and complete a mental status exam
    a. Determine if the patient is cognitively impaired and unable to provide reliable information
    b. Patients who are cognitively impaired may require other data sources such as family members, neighbors, clergy, friends (in addition to the caregiver who may also be the perpetrator)
8. History should be carefully recorded as it may be part of a court case; stories that change over time are suggestive of abuse - thus, statements made as part of the initial disclosure take on added significance

B. Physical Examination
1. Record height, weight, and blood pressure, noting any decline in weight that may indicate poor nutritional status
2. Observe behavior during exam for fearfulness, listlessness, and withdrawn behavior
3. Inspect skin for hydration status, burns, bruises, bites, and lacerations
    a. Use measuring tape and record on anatomic diagrams on chart
    b. Accidental injuries usually occur on extensor surfaces; bruises or lacerations on other areas require more careful evaluation
4. Examine head, focusing on any patchy hair loss, Battle's sign (bruising over mastoid process behind ears) raccoon eyes, and blood behind the tympanic membranes. **Note:** Serious intracranial injuries caused by direct blows may have few or no external signs
5. Examine abdomen for signs of injury. **Note:** Cutaneous signs of abdominal injury are rare; blunt trauma to abdomen can cause serious injury difficult to detect with physical exam alone

C. Differential Diagnosis
1. Unintended injury
2. Poverty resulting in poor clothing/hygiene
3. Self-neglect due to cognitive/physical impairment

D. Diagnostic Tests: History and physical exam dictate tests

V. Plan/Management

A. Because of the associated trauma and pain, adult abuse is a health care issue; because it involves disturbed family relationships, it is a social service agency issue; because assault and abuse are involved, it is a criminal justice system issue

B. Once a case of adult abuse is identified, a multidimensional approach at intervention is important; **reporting requirements and procedures for elder abuse can be found at www.elderabusecenter.org which provides links to individual states**

C. While the intervention must be individualized, some generalizations can be made:
1. If the life of the adult is in jeopardy, Adult Protective Services (APS) must be notified; the patient must be removed from hostile environment and placed in safe place (this is the minority of cases)
    a. APS in each state has the legal responsibility for investigation/intervention when adult abuse/neglect suspected
    b. Mandatory reporting laws vary from state to state; know your responsibility as a healthcare provider in your state (see website in V.B. above)
2. If the adult is not in immediate danger, more comprehensive assessment can take place and implementation of supportive services aimed at alleviating some of the factors can be put into effect
    a. If risk factors for adult abuse or neglect are dealt with at an early stage, and if the caregiver is open to receiving assistance and support, prevention of abuse (or more severe abuse) may be possible
    b. Maintaining the independence and functional capabilities of both the abused person and the support system is the focus
    c. Institutionalization of the abused adult may be the best solution when needs for care outstrip the caregiver's ability to provide care
    d. Providing support in the abused adult's home in terms of homemaker services and Meals-On-Wheels may relieve tension
    e. Psychiatric/alcohol abuse counseling referral, and treatment for the perpetrator may be indicated

3.   Internet resources are contained in the box below

```
US Administration on Aging
http://www.aoa.gov
Offers information for healthcare and other professionals

National Aging Information Center
http://www.aoa.dhhs.gov/naic
A service of the Administration on Aging:  offers searchable
databases on AoA supported materials and reports

National Center on Aging Abuse
http://www.gwjapan.com/NCEA/
Links to publications, data, and resources related to elder abuse

National Citizen's Coalition for Nursing Home Reform
http://www.nccnhr.org
Provides information on federal and state regulatory and legislative
policy development and strategies to improve nursing home care and
life for residents
```

D.   Follow Up: Primary care clinicians have a responsibility to monitor the outcomes of all cases of adult abuse and neglect which have come to their attention

DOMESTIC VIOLENCE: INTIMATE PARTNER VIOLENCE

I.   Definition: Actual or threatened physical, sexual, psychological, or emotional abuse by a spouse, ex-spouse, boyfriend or girlfriend, ex-boyfriend or ex-girlfriend, or date; may include date rape, domestic abuse, spouse abuse, and battery. (**Note**: Although this definition refers to abuse by or to a man or woman, the focus of the discussion here is on female victims and male perpetrators since this is the pattern in 95% of all intimate-partner violence)

II.   Pathogenesis

    A.   Men who commit intimate partner violence (IPV) have no common set of traits and no consistent predictive personality characteristics

    B.   Alcohol and drug use can worsen violence, but has not been found to cause it

    C.   Many abusive partnerships are characterized by cycles of violence in which abuse occurs, the perpetrator repents, the couple reconciles, and then the whole cycle repeats

    D.   Men who are at risk of becoming violent are those who witnessed their mother being beaten by a male partner or who were victims of abuse as children

III.   Clinical Presentation

    A.   In the US, about 1.5 million women each year are raped, physically assaulted, or both by an intimate partner

    B.   Leading cause of injury to women 15 to 44 years of age – more common than automobile accidents, muggings, and rapes combined

    C.   Women who experience IPV are at increased risk of injury and death as well as a range of physical, emotion, and social consequences
        1.   Physical health problems include a 50% to 70% increase in gynecological, central nervous system, and stress-related problems
        2.   Mental and emotional health problems include depression, anxiety, suicidality, posttraumatic stress disorder, mood and eating disorders, substance dependence, antisocial personality disorders, and nonaffective psychosis

3. Abuse during pregnancy is associated with impairment in both mother and child—for the child, abuse can cause both direct harm (e.g., preterm birth caused by blow to woman's abdomen) and indirect harm (e.g., woman's reluctance to seek prenatal care)

D. The major risk factor for IPV is female gender; actions by men against women tend to be much more aggressive, more numerous, and more severe than actions by women against men

E. Data regarding partner violence against heterosexual men, gay men, and lesbians is largely lacking but clinical experience confirms that such violence does exist, but on a much smaller scale than violence against women men perpetrate

F. Physical indicators of abuse
1. Injuries to victims can be of many types, but most commonly involve the head, neck, and torso
2. Complaints such as chronic pain, headaches, sleep disturbances may be the presenting complaint when there has been an injury

G. Behavioral indicators of abuse
1. Most primary care visits by victims of abuse are for stress-related conditions rather than for physical trauma
2. Psychological symptoms that derive from abuse include depression, anxiety, and suicide attempts
3. Alcohol or drug abuse may also be present
4. Many times abuse begins or escalates during pregnancy

IV. Diagnosis/Evaluation

A. History
1. Obtain social history, including current living arrangements and significant relationships
2. Consider screening all women for IPV during routine history taking (probably justified on the basis of prevalence alone); women who present with symptoms or signs that could be associated with IVP should certainly be asked about abuse during the diagnostic evaluation
3. Screening can be conducted informally by asking direct questions relating to abuse, or formally by using a standardized screening instrument. Common sense dictates that the questions be asked in a private setting for patient safety and confidentiality
4. The SAFE questions are commonly used to screen for abuse and are contained in the table that follows

SAFE QUESTIONS	
Stress/Safety	What stresses do you have in your relationship with your partner? How do you handle disagreements? Do you feel safe in your relationship with (name spouse/partner)? Should I be concerned for your safety?
Afraid	Are there situations in which you feel afraid? Have you ever been threatened or abused? Has your partner forced you to have sexual intercourse that you did not want?
Friends/Family	If positive responses to items above: Ask "Are your friends/family aware that this is happening?" If negative responses to item above: Ask "Do you think you could tell them if it did happen?" "Would they help you?"
Emergency Plan	Do you have a safe place to go in an emergency situation? If you are in danger now, would you like me to help you find a shelter? Would you like to talk with a social worker/counselor to help you develop a plan?

Any questions answered affirmatively should be followed with additional questions in order to determine the following:
✓ How and when mistreatment occurs
✓ Who perpetrates it
✓ How the patient copes with it
✓ What she plans to do to protect herself (and children)

Adapted from Ashur, M.L. (1993). Asking about domestic violence: SAFE questions (Letter to the editor). *JAMA 269*, 2367.

3. If physical injury is present, ask detailed questions relating to time of occurrence and how it occurred
   a. Long interval between injury and seeking help is red flag
   b. Story that is inconsistent, contradictory, or fails to adequately explain injury is red flag
   c. Maintain a high index of suspicion when there is a discrepancy between injury and its explained mechanism
   d. Injuries sustained from battering are often attributed to household accidents, such as "I fell." In such case, ask for a more detailed description of how accident occurred
4. Question about past or present medical problems, current medications
5. History should be carefully recorded; stories that change over time are suggestive of abuse - thus, statements made as part of the initial disclosure take on added significance

B. Physical Examination
   1. Record height, weight, and blood pressure
   2. Observe behavior during exam for fearfulness, listlessness, and withdrawn behavior
   3. Inspect skin for burns, bruises, bites, and lacerations
      a. Use measuring tape and record on anatomic diagrams on chart
      b. Accidental injuries usually occur on extensor surfaces; bruises or lacerations on other areas require more careful evaluation
   4. Examine head, focusing on any patchy hair loss, Battle's sign (bruising over mastoid process behind ears) raccoon eyes, and blood behind the tympanic membranes. **Note:** Serious intracranial injuries caused by direct blows may have few or no external signs
   5. Examine abdomen for signs of injury. **Note:** Cutaneous signs of abdominal injury are rare; blunt trauma to abdomen can cause serious injury difficult to detect with physical exam alone

C. Differential Diagnosis
   1. Unintended injury
   2. Self-inflicted injury

D. Diagnostic Tests: History and physical examination dictate tests

V. Plan/Management

A. Competent adults who are experiencing abusive treatment may present for health care, but may refuse to leave their living situation or take legal action
   1. Victims of long-term abuse may not be psychologically or practically able to change their situation
   2. It is not helpful to insist that they do so, or to suggest that they "must like" the abuse

B. Whereas state laws require healthcare professionals to report suspected abuse or neglect involving children and elderly and disabled adults, reporting requirement involving competent adults who choose to stay in abusive relationships are less clear; **each healthcare provider, however, should learn the state law requirements regarding reporting physical abuse**
   1. Reporting of violence-inflicted injuries by unknown assailants is generally supported in all states in the US, but reporting injuries from domestic violence is much more controversial
   2. Opponents of mandatory reporting laws argue that such laws discourage the victim from seeking care, violate patient confidentiality and autonomy, and may accelerate violence by the perpetrator
   3. Proponents of mandatory reporting laws believe that such laws facilitate the provision of assistance for the victim, establish legal consequences for the perpetrator, and lift the burden of reporting off the victim
   4. Seven states specifically require reporting for injuries resulting from domestic violence
   5. For a state-by-state report card on reporting laws related to domestic violence, consult Family Violence Prevention Fund website (http://www.fvpf.org/statereport) or State Reporting Requirements at http://endabuse.org/statereport/list.php3

C. Referral to community resources is important because it gives the abused person a sense of hope; important telephone numbers of agencies should be given on plain paper (**Important**: Become familiar with local resources/reporting procedures and keep the information readily available!)

D.   National family violence resources are listed in the following table

┌───┐
| **NATIONAL FAMILY VIOLENCE RESOURCES** |

> National Domestic Violence Hot Line: 800-799-SAFE (TDD hearing impaired: 800-787-3224) or online at http://www.ndvh.org
> National Resource Center on Domestic Violence: 800-537-2238 or online at: http://www.pcadv.org
> Department of Justice Response Center: 800-421-6770 or online at: http://www.ojp.usdoj.gov/ovc/publications/infores/firstrep/welcome.html
> Centers for Disease Control and Prevention (domestic violence information) http://www.cdc.gov/ncipc/dvp/fivpt/spotlite/home.htm
> Family Violence and Sexual Assault Institute: 858-623-2777 or online at: http://www.fvsai.org
> National Center for Assault Prevention: 908-369-8972 or online at: http://www.ncap.org/aboutncap.htm
> National Coalition Against Domestic Violence: 303-839-1852 or online at: http://www.ncadv.org/
> National Council on Child Abuse and Family Violence: 202-429-6695 or online at: http://www.americancampaign.org/programs.htm
> Family Violence Prevention Fund (http://www.fvpf.org); national agency that focuses on prevention at all levels - primary, secondary, and tertiary
> Domestic Violence: A Practical approach for Clinicians: http://www.sfms.org/domestic.html
> Stop Abuse for Everyone (SAFE): http://www.safe4all.org/
> Same-Sex Domestic Violence: http://www.xq.com/cuav/domviol.htm

E.   Encouraging the victim to involve family members or friends who are sympathetic can help decrease the isolation that victims of abuse often experience

F.   A nonjudgmental, supportive attitude toward the victim must be maintained; such concern may eventually be pivotal in the patient's decision to take definitive action against the abusive partner

G.   The American Medical Association recommends making a safety plan with the input of the abused as the minimal intervention

H.   Follow Up
    1.   Confidentiality must be assured
    2.   Arrange for a safe way to follow up by telephone until situation has stabilized (at least for the present)
    3.   Ask for name of friend or family member who could be contacted if telephone contact with the patient is not possible

GRIEF

I.   Definition: Psychological, behavioral, social, and physical reactions to loss

II.   Pathogenesis

    A.   A full depressive syndrome that is a normal reaction to loss

    B.   Persons with uncomplicated bereavement regard the feeling of depressed mood as normal and transitory

III.   Clinical Presentation

    A.   Feelings of depression and associated symptoms of poor appetite, weight loss, and insomnia following loss

    B.   Feelings of guilt, if present, are usually related to things done or not done at time of death by the survivor (if the loss is via death)

C. Approximately 80% of persons are markedly improved in 10 weeks after the loss

D. Morbid preoccupation with feelings of worthlessness and prolonged functional impairment indicate abnormal grieving and the development of major depression

IV. Diagnosis/Evaluation

    A. History
       1. Determine when loss occurred, how person is accepting and coping with loss
       2. Prior experience with patient/family is crucial in making an assessment of adjustment
       3. Ask about functional status (if able to carry out usual activities)
       4. Ask about presence of support system
       5. Determine if patient is able to mourn
       6. Determine if patient is experiencing despair to the level of self-harm

    B. Physical Examination: Not indicated

    C. Differential Diagnosis: Major depression

    D. Diagnostic Tests: None indicated

V. Plan/Management

    A. **Interventions for acute grief**
       1. Encourage patient to mourn, and to express grief in ways that are consistent with the person's particular personality (people mourn differently). Message to patient should be "You have the right to mourn"
       2. Encourage family and small group of people who knew deceased to talk about him/her in presence of the grieving patient
       3. Emphasize that grief is normal, and the goal is not to get rid of it as quickly as possible
       4. Recognize that **your presence** is the most important comfort you have to offer
          a. Avoid the pressure to provide your own philosophy of death and loss (or to talk about your own losses)
          b. Don't worry about what to say; being present and listening are what the patient needs, not your advice
          c. Message should be, "I care"
       5. Provide patient tranquility but not sedation via medication (low dose lorazepam for 1-2 days may help with sleep which is always very disrupted during acute grief). Patients need to get some rest in order to cope with demands of dealing with arrangements that frequently must be made
       6. Don't use medications to interfere with the right to mourn, but to soothe, promote sleep, and relieve anxiety during the first hours after the loss
       7. Accept patient's grief for loss that conventional society may not acknowledge as very important (such as loss of pet)
       8. Make a condolence contact in the form of telephone call or handwritten note
       9. Recognize that clinicians are not equally capable of intervening effectively in situations of acute loss

    B. **Return to routines:** Encourage mourner to return to normal routines as soon as is practical (no more than 2 weeks between death and return to work/school)

    C. **Physical exercise:** Recommend daily exercise, which can be very beneficial in dealing with depression

    D. **Support groups:** Some families benefit from sharing with a group; others do not; prior knowledge about family functioning should guide referral

    E. **Anticipatory guidance:** The grieving person should not expect to adapt within a set time period, as each person grieves differently. Healthy mourning involves the process outlined in the following table

ANTICIPATORY GUIDANCE

The grieving person needs to:	The clinician can help by such questions/comments as:
Recognize the loss	"Tell me about (relative/friend's name) death." "How was it for you after he/she died?"
React to loss on an emotional level	"You've been through so much over the past few weeks." "How are things going for you now?"
Adjust to life (over time) without the deceased by seeking out other relationships/pursuits	"How has his/her death changed your life?" "Tell me how things are different for you now." "What have you done to help yourself cope with losing him/her?" "Have your friends/family been supportive of you during this difficult time?"
Learn to make accommodations in life because of the loss	"Is there anything that has been especially difficult for you in the past weeks since he/she died?"
Know that "acceptance" of loss and "recovery" are unrealistic goals	"Have you thought about getting back to (work/hobbies, etc) yet?"
Understand that loss and grief change people and a realistic goal is an altered life in which the person has adapted to the loss	"What are your plans for the future?"

Adapted from Casarett, D., Kutner, and Abrahm, J. (2001). Life after death: A practical approach to grief and bereavement. *Annals of Internal Medicine, 134,* 208-215.

    F.   Complicated grief, or failure to make some progress in readjustment over time, may occur in some patients
        1.   Difficult to identify because of great variation in how individuals experience grief
        2.   Two guidelines may be helpful
            a.   Some progress should be evident after about 2 months
            b.   By 4 months after the loss, patient should be experiencing clear improvement
            c.   If, at these two landmarks, there has been little or no improvement, grief may be complicated (estimates are that 17-27% of bereaved persons are clinically depressed in first year after loss)

THERAPEUTIC OPTIONS FOR DEALING WITH COMPLICATED GRIEF

Based on goals, needs, and preferences of the bereaved (as well as availability of services), offer options for treatment

→ Option that is most evidence-based is counseling: individual counseling by trained volunteer or professional peer-led support group; counseling by clergy
- Describe several options to patient
- Suggest that he/she try various types of counseling before making decision

→ Consider prescribing antidepressant therapy
- Evidence does not support use of pharmacotherapy in absence of depression
- Nonetheless, frequently prescribed and may be beneficial in persons with complicated grief
- Selective serotonin-reuptake inhibitors are a good choice because of their possible benefit and benign side effect profile. (See DEPRESSION section for dosing)

    G.   Follow Up: Once or twice by telephone/mail over the period of acute grief during first few weeks; more frequent follow-up required for complicated grief. Be alert for delayed grief reaction; these reactions may occur close to anniversary of a death (anniversary reaction)

INSOMNIA

I. Definition: Sleep that is unrefreshing or nonrestorative, as well as a persistent difficulty in falling or staying asleep

II. Pathogenesis

   A. Sleep disorders have been given the acronym DIMS (disorders of initiating and maintaining sleep)

   B. Insomnia is classified according to duration: transient (acute) or chronic insomnia
      1. Transient (acute) insomnia lasts 2 weeks or less and is generally due to situational stress, acute medical illness, jet lag, environmental disturbances such as noise, light and temperature, or self-medication
      2. Chronic insomnia lasts for >4 weeks and the etiology is multifactorial

   C. Generally, causes of insomnia can be categorized as follows:
      1. Drug-induced insomnia from both nonprescription drugs (alcohol, nicotine, decongestants, caffeine, recreational drugs) and prescription drugs (for example, thyroid hormones, β-agonists, β-blockers, SSRIs)
      2. Psychiatric disorders such as mood or anxiety disorders
      3. Acute or chronic stress such as associated with loss
      4. Medical conditions including gastrointestinal, cardiac, genitourinary, respiratory, endocrine, central nervous system, musculoskeletal conditions, as well as pain from any cause
      5. Disordered circadian rhythms, such as from jet lag, shift work
      6. Sleep disordered breathing, as may occur in obesity or obstructed breathing
      7. Nocturnal myoclonus, associated with restlessness of the legs
      8. Primary sleep disorder with difficulty initiating or maintaining sleep with no apparent underlying cause but contributing factors may be chronic stress, hyperarousal, poor sleep hygiene, and behavioral conditioning

III. Clinical Presentation

   A. Approximately 35% of adults in the US experience either transient or chronic insomnia, and about 20% of that group consult a clinician for the problem
      1. The primary consequences of transient insomnia are daytime sleepiness, irritability, and poor performance
      2. Patients with chronic insomnia suffer from fatigue, mood changes, trouble concentrating, and impaired functioning

   B. Each year in the US, motor vehicle accidents (MVAs) due to drivers falling asleep at the wheel number over 100,000 resulting in over 1500 deaths

   C. Divorced, separated, and widowed persons have insomnia more often than married persons

   D. Complaints about insomnia increase with age, so that up to 65% of the elderly suffer from insomnia at some point
      1. Alterations in the stages of sleep occur as a normal part of the aging process; older persons get less deep delta sleep and more lighter stage 1 sleep, and frequently return to consciousness during the night
      2. Elderly people spend more time in bed, take longer to fall asleep, have increased nocturnal wakefulness, and experience more sleepiness during the day than do younger adults

   E. Persons who abuse alcohol often have no difficulty in falling asleep but have early morning insomnia; in addition many patients who are moderate drinkers may use alcohol to help them get to sleep, but alcohol increases sleep disruption because it causes early morning awakening

   F. Patients with an underlying psychiatric disorder may complain about feeling irritable, having difficulty falling asleep, and being tired all the time; insomnia may be chief complaint in many psychiatric disorders

G. Diagnosis of chronic primary insomnia requires that the following be present:
  1. Difficulty in initiating or maintaining sleep or the presence of nonrestorative sleep (more than three nights per week for at least one month) that results in marked impairment in social or occupational functioning
  2. Disturbance is not due to another sleep or mental disorder, or the effects of a drug or medical condition
  3. A diagnosis of exclusion that is reached after more specific medical and psychiatric diagnoses have been ruled out

IV. Diagnosis/Evaluation

  A. History
    1. Ask about onset, duration of problem, and whether onset is linked with a specific event/situation. (Transient [acute] insomnia may be related to recent change in person's life; search for any recent changes at home or work, use of medications, use of substances such as caffeine, nicotine, or alcohol)
    2. Inquire about number of hours in bed each night; pattern of insomnia (determine if the problem is falling asleep, staying asleep, or both); if patient has problem falling asleep, ask how long it usually takes to get to sleep—a period known as sleep latency (sleep latency normally lasts up to 20 minutes; longer than 30 minutes is abnormal)
    3. Ask about daytime napping, occupation (shift work) and travel patterns
    4. Inquire whether inability to sleep affects daytime functioning
    5. Ask if he/she routinely feels sleepy at times when he/she needs to be alert, such as when driving (ask if he/she has ever fallen asleep at the wheel)
    6. Obtain past medical history and determine what medications are currently being taken
    7. Ask patient if pain or discomfort (such as with restless legs syndrome) is interfering with sleep
    8. With patient permission, interview appropriate family members for additional data (ask whether the patient snores loudly, wakes up gasping, behaves abnormally during sleep [e.g., confused, combative] or is excessively sleepy during day)

  B. Physical Examination: Should be focused based on history

  C. Differential Diagnosis: Causes of insomnia listed under II.C. above should be ruled out.

  D. Diagnostic Tests:
    1. Consider CBC, chemistry profile, TSH, B_{12}, and folate levels
    2. Other testing may be indicated based on the history and physical examination findings

V. Plan/Management

  A. Treat underlying causes when present
    1. When an underlying cause such as depression, alcohol or drug abuse, or a medical condition such as osteoarthritis causing pain is found, the underlying cause should be treated or referred for evaluation and management
    2. When insomnia is suspected of being drug-induced, treatment by eliminating the drug (if possible), reducing the dosage, or changing the timing of the dosing may be attempted (for example, caffeine intake might be limited to the early morning)
    3. If obstructive sleep apnea is suspected, or if severe daytime sleepiness is present, immediate referral to a sleep specialist is mandatory
    4. If any of the primary sleep disorders (for example, periodic limb movement) are suspected, polysomnography is required for diagnosis

B. When no underlying cause can be found, institute educational and behavioral interventions
   1. Reassure patient that most sleep difficulties are treatable and addressing them often leads to a better night's sleep
   2. Instruct patient to keep a sleep diary for 2 weeks which includes the following:

Sleep Diary		
Complete in morning	✓	Bedtime, and estimated time to fall asleep
	✓	Number of awakenings and total time awake, and rise time
	✓	Total number of hours slept and quality of sleep (good, fair, poor)
Complete at bedtime	✓	Naps (number, time, and duration)
	✓	Alcohol/caffeine drinks (number, timing, and amount)
	✓	Stresses during the day (if yes, list)
	✓	Rating of how felt during the day (in general) [wide awake, fairly alert, somewhat tired/sleepy, very tired/sleepy]

   3. Examine sleep log or diary after 2 weeks to assess sleep patterns and problems and develop a treatment based on one or more approaches

C. Basic educational counseling related to sleep hygiene is a good starting point for all patients

---

SLEEP HYGIENE: PATIENT EDUCATION

Advise patient to do the following

- ✓ Avoid use of alcohol in late evening. While it may facilitate sleep onset, alcohol can cause early awakening during the night
- ✓ Avoid stimulants such as nicotine and caffeine in the evening
- ✓ Avoid heavy meals. Choose a light snack instead
- ✓ Avoid exercise within 4 hours of sleep; exercise during the day or late afternoon
- ✓ Make sure bedroom is free of environmental sleep disturbers such as light, noise, alarm clocks, and excessive temperatures
- ✓ Wake up at the same time each day

Adapted from National Center on Sleep Disorders Research and Office of Prevention, Education and Control (1998) *Insomnia: Assessment and management in primary care.* NIH Publication No. 98-4088, p. 10.

D. Counseling directed at assisting patient to create a new association between the bed and bedroom and the rapid onset of sleep (called stimulus-control therapy) may also be helpful

---

STIMULUS-CONTROL THERAPY

Instruct patient as follows

- ✓ Go to bed only when sleepy
- ✓ Use bed only for sleeping (sex is the one exception)
- ✓ Do not read, eat, work, or watch television in bed
- ✓ If unable to go to sleep after 15-20 minutes in bed, get up, go into another room, and read with a dim light; do not watch television because the full-spectrum light produced by the TV has an arousing effect
- ✓ Do not return to bed until sleepy (goal is to re-establish the connection between the bed and sleep, rather than the bed and lying awake)
- ✓ Get out of bed at the same time each day, regardless of total hours of sleep
- ✓ Establishing a wake-up time helps to stabilize the sleep-wake schedule
- ✓ Minimize daytime napping; if absolutely necessary, a brief early-afternoon nap may be taken
- ✓ Avoid caffeine, nicotine, alcohol, and stimulating medications such as decongestants
- ✓ Continue to keep sleep diary

Adapted from Eddy, M. & Walbroehl, G.S. (1999). Insomnia. *American Family Physician, 59*(7), 1911-1916.

E.   A third approach is sleep restriction therapy, based on limiting time in bed to the actual time spent sleeping (sleep efficiency)

      1.   To use this method, first determine patient's present level of sleep efficiency, which is the percentage of time in bed that is spent sleeping (Example: patient who is in bed for 8 hours, 4 hours of which are spent in actual sleep has a sleep efficiency of 50%)

      2.   Use this baseline sleep-efficiency score to evaluate progress over time

      3.   Explain to patient how to calculate sleep-efficiency score so that he/she can chart progress each week

---

SLEEP RESTRICTION THERAPY

Advise patient to do the following

✓ Go to bed much later than usual

✓ Stay in bed only as long as sleeping, even if it is only 4-5 hours, then get up

✓ This allows a "sleep debit" to accrue which increases ability to fall asleep and stay asleep

✓ Incrementally, increase the amount of time spent in bed, by adding 15 minutes per week to start of each night's bed time

✓ Instruct the patient to continue to rise at the same time (when he/she awakes)

✓ The goal should be that at least 85% of the time spent in bed is spent sleeping

✓ A sleep debit must occur so that falling asleep and staying asleep will be likely

---

Adapted from Attarian, H.P. (2001). Helping patients who say they cannot sleep. *Postgraduate Medicine 107*(3), 127-141.

SELF-HELP FOR SLEEP DISORDERS

✓ Karvey, N.B. (1995). *Practical book of remedies: 50 ways to sleep better.* Lincolnwood, IL: Publication International. To order, call 800-745-9299

✓ National Center on Sleep Disorders, Research National Institutes of Health: General information about sleep disturbance http://www.nhlbi.nih.gov/about/ncsdr/index.htm

✓ National Sleep Foundation (NSF): Includes brochures and diaries http://www.sleepfoundation.org/about.html

---

F.   Consider prescribing medications that have a limited role in insomnia treatment

G.   General principles can guide the rational use of pharmacotherapeutic management of insomnia

      1.   Use the lowest effective dose

      2.   Prescribe for short-term use only (3-4 weeks)

      3.   Recommend that patient use every other night or every third night rather than nightly

      4.   Advise patient to discontinue gradually and be alert for rebound insomnia

      5.   Agents with a shorter half-life are preferred in order to decrease daytime sedation

H. Commonly prescribed sedative agents are contained in the following table

AGENTS COMMONLY PRESCRIBED TO TREAT INSOMNIA

Medication	Usual Therapeutic Dose (mg/day)		Time Until Onset in Minutes	Elimination Half Life (hours)	Comments
	Adult	Elderly >65			
Benzodiazepines					
Triazolam (Halcion)	0.125 - 0.25	0.125	15 - 30	1.5 - 5	Short acting and good for onset insomnia; withdrawal may occur
Temazepam (Restoril)	7.5 - 15	7.5	30	10 - 20	Intermediate acting and good for frequent wakening; less effective for sleep onset problems
Flurazepam (Dalmane)	15 - 30	Avoid using in elderly	15 - 45	30 - 250	Accumulation and daytime sedation are common
Estazolam (ProSom)	1 - 2	0.5 - 1	30 - 45	8 - 24	Newer agent with acceptable efficacy; daytime sedation is a problem
Quazepam (Doral)	7.5 - 15	7.5	45 - 60	40 - 75	Newer agent with acceptable efficacy; daytime sedation is a problem
Nonbendodiazepines					
Zolpidem (Ambien)	5 – 10	5	30	1.5 - 4.5	Low abuse potential and does not encourage tolerance or disturb sleep architecture
Zaleplon (Sonata)	5 - 10	5	<30	1	Useful in sleep initiation
Trazodone (Desyrel)	50 - 150	25 - 100	30 - 60	5 - 9	✓ Good for antidepressant-induced insomnia (e.g., fluoxetine) ✓ Use of this drug as a hypnotic agent is not an indication approved by FDA

I. In prescribing these drugs, adhere to the basic principles for rational pharmacotherapy for insomnia listed above

J. Caution: Do not prescribe these medications for use by pregnant women, persons with possible sleep apnea, and patients with renal or hepatic insufficiency

K. As with all medications, consult the PDR for specific prescribing recommendations, contraindications, and adverse reactions

L. Follow Up
1. In 2 weeks to examine sleep diary and in 1 month to re-evaluate usefulness of whichever educational and/or behavioral recommendation was prescribed
2. Suggest an alternate approach to the one already tried, and re-evaluate in 1 month
3. If no improvement, and other underlying causes have been ruled out, refer to sleep laboratory for evaluation if that is an option

REFERENCES

Ables, A.Z., Baughman, O.L. (2003). Antidepressants: Update on new agents and indications. *American Family Physician, 67*, 547-554.

Abramowicz, M. (2002). Escitalopram (Lexapro) for depression. *The Medical Letter, 44,* 83-84.

Abreu, A.C., & Filips, J.K. (2002). Anxiety disorders. In M.A. Graver & M.L. Lanternier (Eds.), *University of Iowa: The family practice handbook* (pp. 677-682). St. Louis: Mosby.

American Psychiatric Association. (2000). *Diagnostic and statistical manual of mental disorders* (4th ed.). Text Revision. Author.

American Medical Association. (1996). *Diagnostic treatment guidelines on domestic violence.* Chicago, IL.

Ashur, M.L. (1993). Asking about domestic violence. SAFE questions. *Journal of the American Medical Association, 269*, 2367.

Attarian, H.P. (2000). Helping patients who say they cannot sleep. *Postgraduate Medicine, 17,* 127-142.

Baldwin, D., Bobes, J., Stein, D.J. (1999). Paroxetine in social phobia/social anxiety disorder: Randomized, double blind placebo controlled study. *British Journal of Psychiatry, 175,* 120-126.

Blazer, D.G., Grossberg, G.T., & Pollock, B.G. (1998). Managing depression in the elderly. *Patient Care, May,* 73-97.

Blumenthal, J.A., Babyak, M.A., & Moore. K.A. (2000). Effects of exercise training on older patients with major depression. *Archives of Internal Medicine, 159,* 2349-2356.

Casarett, D., Kutner, J.S., & Abrahms, J. (2001). Life after death: A practical approach to grief and bereavement. *Annals of Internal Medicine, 124,* 208-215.

Doghramji, P. (2001). Detection of insomnia in primary care. *Journal of Clinical Psychiatry, 62*(Suppl. 10), 18-26.

Eddy, M. (1999). Insomnia. *American Family Physician, 59,* 1911-1916.

Erman, M.K. (2001). Sleep architecture and its relationship to insomnia. *Journal of Clinical Psychiatry, 62*(Suppl. 10), 9-17.

Eyler, A.E., Cohen, M., & Kershaw, M.O. (1997). Domestic violence and abuse. In D.J. Knesper, M.B. Riba, & T.L. Schwenk, (Eds.). *Primary care psychiatry.* Philadelphia: Saunders.

Fawcett, J. (2000). Predictors of early suicide: Identification and appropriate interventions. *Journal of Clinical Psychiatry, 49,* 7-8.

Gallo, J.J., & Coyne, J.C. (2001). The challenge of depression in late life. *Journal of the American Medical Association, 284,* 1570-1572.

Gelenberg, A.J. et al. (2000). Efficacy of venlafaxine extended-release capsules in nondepressed outpatients with generalized anxiety disorder: A 6-month randomized controlled trial. *Journal of the American Medical Association, 283,* 3082-3088.

Gundersen, L. (2002). Intimate-partner violence: The need for primary prevention in the community. *Annals of Internal Medicine, 136,* 637-640.

Hale, L. (2001). Treating transient insomnia in older patients. *Patient Care, 3,* 91-97.

Hooberman, R.E. (1998). Psychotherapy in the context of primary care. *The Female Patient, 23,* 23-28.

Houry, D., Sachs, C.J., Feldhaus, K.M., & Linden, J. (2002). Violence inflicted injuries: Reporting laws in 50 states. *Annals of Emergency Medicine, 39,* 56-60.

Kaplan, H.I., & Sadock, B.J. (2000). *Synopsis of psychiatry* (8th Ed.). Philadelphia: Williams & Wilkins.

Keller, M.B., McCullough, J.P., & Klein, D.N. (2000). A comparison of nefazodone, the cognitive behavioral-analysis system of psychotherapy, and their combination for the treatment of chronic depression. *New England Journal of Medicine, 241,* 1462-1470.

Lavie, P. (2001). Sleep disturbances in the wake of traumatic events. *New England Journal of Medicine, 345,* 1825-1832.

Luoma, J.B., Martin, C.E., & Pearson, J.L. (2002). Contact with mental health and primary care providers before suicide: A review of the evidence. *American Journal of Psychiatry, 159,* 909-916.

Lily, S. (2001). Evaluation and treatment of insomnia in primary care. *Family Practice Recertification, 23,* 37-55.

Mahowald, M.W. (2000). What is causing excessive daytime sleeping? *Postgraduate Medicine, 107,* 108-123.

Margolis, S., & Swartz, K. (2001). Depression and anxiety. *The Johns Hopkins White Papers.* New York: Medletter Associates.

Marshall, C.E., Benton, D., & Brazier, J.M. (2000). Elder abuse: Using clinical tools to identify clues to mistreatment. *Geriatrics, 55*, 42-53.

National Advisory Council on Violence Against Women. (2002). Ending violence against women-an agenda for the nation. Retrieved May 5, 2002, from http://www.4women.gov;violence/nations/htm

National Center on Sleep Disorders Research and Office of Prevention, Education, and Control. (1998). *Insomnia: Assessment and management in primary care*, NIH Publication NO. 98-4088. Washington DC: U.S. Department of Health and Human Services.

National Heart, Lung, and Blood Institute. Working Group on Insomnia. (1999). Insomnia: Assessment and management in primary care. *American Family Physician, 59*, 3029-3038.

Neufeld, B. (1996). SAFE questions: Overcoming barriers to the detection of domestic violence. *American Family Physician, 53*, 2575-2580.

Pennix, B.W. et al. (2000). Vitamin B_{12} deficiency and depression in physically disabled older women: Epidemiologic evidence from the Women's Health and Aging Study. *American Journal of Psychiatry, 157*, 715-721.

Pollack, M.H. (2001). Comorbid anxiety disorders in primary care. *Therapeutic Spotlight.* Clifton, NJ: Clinicians Group.

Rosenbaum, J.F., & Fava, M. (1998). Approach to the patient with depression. In T.A. Stern, J.B. Herman, & P.L. Slavin (Eds.). *The MGH guide to psychiatry in primary care.* New York: McGraw-Hill.

Rhodes, K.V., & Levinson, W. (2003). Interventions for intimate partner violence against women. *JAMA, 289*, 601-605.

Roy-Byrne, P.P, Stand, P., Wittchen, H.U., et al. (2000). Lifetime panic-depression comorbidity in the National Comorbidity Survey. Association with symptoms, impairment, course and help-seeking. *British Journal of Psychiatry, 176*, 229-235.

Schneider, R.K., & Levenson, J.L. (2002). Update in psychiatry. *Annals of Internal Medicine, 136*, 293-301.

Snow, V., Lascher, S., & Mottur-Pilson, C. (2000). Clinical guideline, part I: Pharmacologic treatment of acute major depression and dysthymia. *Annals of Internal Medicine, 132*, 38-742.

US Preventive Services Task Force. (2001). Screening for depression. Recommendations and rationale. *Annals of Internal Medicine, 136*, 760-764

Van Amerigen, M.A., Lane, R.M., Walker, J.R., et al. (2001). Sertraline treatment of generalized social phobia: A 20 week double blind, placebo-controlled study. *American Journal of Psychiatry, 158*, 275-281.

Weisman, A. (1998). The patient with acute grief. In T.A. Stern, J.B. Herman, & P.L. Slavin (Eds.). *The MGH guide to psychiatry in primary care.* New York: McGraw-Hill.

Wengel, S.P., & Burke, W.J. (2003). Escitalopram: What does it have to offer? *Primary Psychiatry, 10(1)*, 67-70.

Whooley, M.A., & Simon, G.E. (2000). Managing depression in medical outpatients. *New England Journal of Medicine, 343*, 1942-1950.

Williams, J.W., Barrett, J., Toxman, T., Frank, E., Katon, W., Sullivan, W., Cornell, J., & Sengupta, A. (2001). Treatment of dysthymia and minor depression in primary care: A randomized controlled trial in older adults. *Journal of the American Medical Association, 284*, 1519-1526.

Williams, J.W., Mulrow, C.D., Chiquette, E., Noel, P.H., Aguilar, C., & Cornell, J. (2000). A systematic review of new pharmacotherapies for depression in adults: Evidence report summary. *Annals of Internal Medicine, 132*, 743-756.

Williams, J.W., Noel, P.H., Cordes, J.A., Ramirez, G., & Pignone, M. (2002). Is this patient clinically depressed? *JAMA, 287*, 1160-1170.

Wu, L.R. (2002). Anxiety disorders in primary care. In R.E. Rakel & E.T. Bope (Eds.), *Conn's Current Therapy 2002* (pp 1124-1127) Philadelphia: Saunders.

Metabolic and Endocrine Problems

CONSTANCE R. UPHOLD & J. JORDAN GOODMAN

DIABETES MELLITUS

I. Definition: Group of metabolic diseases characterized by hyperglycemia from defects in insulin secretion, insulin action, or both

II. Pathogenesis and etiologic classification of diabetes mellitus (DM)

    A. Type 1 (formerly known as insulin-dependent [IDDM or juvenile-onset diabetes]): Due to β-cell destruction which usually results in absolute insulin deficiency

    B. Type 2 (formerly known as non-insulin dependent type [NIDDM or adult-onset diabetes]): A complex metabolic disorder characterized by resistance to the action of insulin and a relative or predominant impairment of insulin secretion

    C. Other specific types of diabetes
       1. Genetic defects in β-cell function
       2. Genetic defects in insulin action (type A insulin resistance, leprechaunism, lipoatrophic diabetes)
       3. Diseases of the exocrine pancreas (pancreatitis, trauma, infection, cancer)
       4. Endocrinopathies such as acromegaly, Cushing's syndrome, pheochromocytoma
       5. Drug or chemical-induced diabetes (steroids, thiazide diuretics, phenytoin, nicotinic acid, thyroid hormones, α-interferon)
       6. Infections such as congenital rubella or cytomegalovirus
       7. Immune-mediated diabetes ("stiff man" syndrome and anti-insulin receptor antibodies)
       8. Other genetic disorders such as Down's, Klinefelter's, and Turner's syndromes

    D. Gestational diabetes mellitus (GDM): Glucose intolerance with onset during pregnancy (will not be discussed further in this section)

    E. Impaired glucose tolerance (IGT) or impaired fasting glucose (IFG)
       1. Plasma glucose levels are higher than normal but are not diagnostic of diabetes mellitus
       2. Intermediate stage between glucose homeostasis and diabetes
       3. Insulin resistance syndrome or metabolic syndrome is associated with IGT and is a state in which insulin-sensitive tissues have a reduced sensitivity to effects of insulin on glucose uptake (see section on DYSLIPIDEMIA)

III. Clinical Presentation

    A. Criteria for diagnosing diabetes mellitus (see following table)

DIAGNOSTIC CRITERIA FOR DIABETES MELLITUS*

- Symptoms of diabetes (polydipsia, polyuria, and weight loss) plus casual plasma glucose concentration ≥200 mg/dl (11.1 mmol/l); "casual" is any time of day without regard to time since last meal
  OR
- Fasting plasma glucose (FPG) ≥126 mg/dl (7.0 mmol/l); "fasting" is no caloric intake for at least 8 hours
  OR
- 2 hour plasma glucose ≥200 mg/dl during an oral glucose tolerance test (OGTT); OGTT should be performed using a glucose load containing the equivalent of 75-g anhydrous glucose

*These criteria should be confirmed by repeat testing on a different day, except in the case of unequivocal hyperglycemia with acute metabolic decompensation

Adapted from American Diabetes Association. (2003). Report of the Expert Committee on the diagnosis and classification of diabetes mellitus. *Diabetes Care, 26*(Suppl. 1), S5-S20

    B. Criteria for diagnosing impaired fasting glucose (IFG) or IGT: FBG ≥110 mg/dl (6.1 mmol/l) and <126 mg/dl (7.0 mmol/l) or 2-hour glucose ≥140 mg/dl (7.8 mmol/l) and <200 mg/dl (11.1 mmol/l)

C. Type 1 diabetes
1. Occurs in approximately 10% of all persons diagnosed with diabetes
2. Can occur at any age with highest incidence in childhood and adolescence
3. Usually appears with acute onset of symptoms: polydipsia, polyphagia, polyuria, weight loss, blurred vision, and frequent infections, such as dermatologic fungal infections
4. After the initial presentation of symptoms, the newly diagnosed patient often undergoes a "honeymoon" period or remission phase which may last from several months to 2 years
5. In adults, diabetic ketoacidosis (DKA) rarely occurs due to good diagnostic testing; symptoms in severe cases include dehydration, Kussmaul respirations, fruity or acetone odor to breath, and impaired consciousness (see table DIAGNOSTIC CRITERIA FOR DKA AND HHS)

D. Type 2 diabetes in adults
1. Occurs mainly in adults >30 years of age
2. Frequently the patients are obese or have increased abdominal body fat
3. Gradual onset and slow progression of symptoms; many patients are asymptomatic and have had diabetes for numerous years and subsequent complications when they are diagnosed
4. Fatigue is a common symptom
5. Initially, these patients do not need insulin to survive, but approximately 50% of patients will eventually require insulin
6. Ketoacidosis rarely occurs except in times of stress, illness, or infection
7. Hyperosmolar hyperglycemic state (HHS) is more common in type 2 diabetes than in type 1 diabetes
   a. Characterized by blood glucose >600 mg/dl, minimal ketosis, serum osmolality ≥320 mOsm/kg, and profound dehydration (see table DIAGNOSTIC CRITERIA FOR DKA AND HHS)
   b. Often precipitated by hyperglycemic-inducing drugs (steroids, diuretics), therapeutic procedures (surgery, dialysis, hyperalimentation), chronic disease, and acute stress
8. Patients are at risk for coronary heart disease, stroke, peripheral vascular disease, dyslipidemia, and hypertension

DIAGNOSTIC CRITERIA FOR DKA AND HHS

	DKA Mild	DKA Moderate	DKA Severe	HHS
Plasma glucose (mg/dL)	>250	>250	>250	>600
Arterial pH	7.25-7.30	7.00-7.24	<7.00	>7.30
Serum bicarbonate (mEq/L)	15-18	10 to <15	<10	>15
Urine ketones*	Positive	Positive	Positive	Small
Serum ketones*	Positive	Positive	Positive	Small
Effective serum osmolality (mOsm/kg)**	Variable	Variable	Variable	≥320
Anion gap[†]	>10	>12	>12	Variable
Alteration in sensorial or mental obtundation	Alert	Alert/drowsy	Stupor/coma	Stupor/coma

* Nitroprusside reaction method
** Calculation: 2[measured Na (mEq/L)] + glucose (mg/dL)/18
[†] Calculation: $(Na^+) - (Cl^- + HCO_3^-)$ (mEq/L).
Source: American Diabetes Association. (2003). Hyperglycemia crisis in patients with diabetes mellitus. *Diabetes Care, 26*(Suppl), S109-S117.

E. Impaired glucose tolerance (IGT)
1. Patients are asymptomatic; at risk for developing coronary heart disease and diabetes
2. IGT is associated with insulin resistance syndrome, which is also known as the metabolic syndrome (syndrome X)

F. Macrovascular and microvascular complications occur in type 1 and type 2 diabetes of sufficient duration
1. Retinopathy is the leading cause of new adult blindness in US
   a. Background retinopathy or nonproliferative retinopathy involves microaneurysms and dot hemorrhages but does not impair vision unless it involves the macula
   b. Prevalence is related to the duration and type of diabetes; occurs in almost every patient with type 1 diabetes for 20 years or more and in >60% of patients with type 2 diabetes
   c. Proliferative retinopathy can lead to blindness and involves neovascularization (new vessels develop) with retinal detachment and vitreous hemorrhages

2. Nephropathy
   a. Develops in 35-45% of patients with type 1 and 20% with type 2 diabetes
   b. Progresses from the development of microalbuminuria to overt proteinuria and finally to end-stage renal disease (ESRD); this process may take as long as 23 years but once clinical albuminuria appears, the risk of ESRD is high in type 1 diabetes and significant in type 2 diabetes
   c. Diabetes is the most common single cause of ESRD in US
3. Neuropathy
   a. Most common manifestation is a peripheral, symmetric sensorimotor neuropathy which is usually only minimally uncomfortable
   b. A minority of patients have lancinating or burning pain
   c. Autonomic neuropathy may affect gastric or intestinal motility, erectile function, bladder function, cardiac function, and vascular tone
4. Cardiovascular disease: diabetes is a major risk factor
5. Other complications include an increased prevalence of infections, cognitive impairment, and contractures of digits (hammer toes, stiff fingers)

IV. Diagnosis/Evaluation

A. History
   1. To establish the diagnosis, explore the following:
      a. Ask about symptoms such as polyuria, polydipsia, polyphagia, weight loss, and fatigue
      b. Inquire about frequency of skin and other infections
      c. Ask about health practices such as eating and exercise patterns
      d. Explore family history of diabetes and other endocrine problems
      e. With adult females, ask about gestational history including the weight and condition of all babies and whether complications occurred during pregnancy or at the time of labor and delivery
   2. In patients who are already diagnosed, inquire about the following:
      a. Frequency, severity, and cause of hypoglycemia or ketoacidosis
      b. Symptoms and treatments of chronic eye, kidney, nerve, genitourinary (including sexual), bladder, gastrointestinal function, heart, peripheral vascular, foot, and cerebrovascular complications
      c. Prior or current infections
      d. Previous and current pharmacological, nutritional, and self-management treatment plans
      e. Patterns and results of glucose monitoring, laboratory tests, and special examinations such as ophthalmoscopic exams
      f. Dietary habits (especially amount of carbohydrates such as juices and soft drinks), nutritional status, and weight history
      g. Amount, intensity, and frequency of exercise
      h. Risk factors for atherosclerosis such as smoking, hypertension, obesity
      i. Contraceptive, reproductive, and sexual history
      j. Psychological, sociological and economic factors that may impact on management plan

B. Physical Examination; perform at diagnosis and then at least annually
   1. Measure height and weight (and compare to norms)
   2. Measure vital signs including orthostatic blood pressure to detect autonomic neuropathy
   3. Examine skin; inspect sites of previous insulin administration if applicable
   4. Complete a thorough ophthalmoscopic examination (best done with dilation)
   5. Perform thorough mouth and dental examinations
   6. Palpate thyroid
   7. Perform complete cardiac examination
   8. Palpate and auscultate pulses
   9. Perform abdominal examination; check for liver enlargement
   10. Assess hand, finger, and wrist, including mobility and presence of contractures
   11. Carefully examine feet; exam should include use of Semmes-Weinstein monofilament, tuning fork, palpation, and inspection
   12. Perform complete neurological exam
   13. May need to do a complete physical exam to exclude any sources of occult infection

C. Differential Diagnosis
   1. Glucosuria without hyperglycemia occurs in benign renal glucosuria or in renal tubular disease
   2. Diabetes insipidus presents with polyuria and polydipsia but not hyperglycemia

3. Transient hyperglycemia is present when patients have severe stress from trauma, burns or infection, or are on glucocorticoids
4. Salicylate intoxication mimics ketoacidosis

D. Diagnostic Tests
1. Screening tests to detect diabetes in asymptomatic, undiagnosed individuals (see table):

SCREENING CRITERIA

➡ Testing should be considered in all individuals ≥45 years and, if normal, it should be repeated at 3-year intervals (The American Association of Clinical Endocrinologists recommends screening for high risk individuals >30 years) (The US Preventive Services Task Force [2003] concludes there is insufficient evidence to recommend for or against routinely screening asymptomatic adults, but does recommend screening in adults with hypertension or hyperlipidemia)

➡ Testing should be considered at a younger age or be performed more frequently in individuals who
- are overweight (≥120% desirable body weight or a BMI ≥25 kg/m^2)
- have a first-degree relative with diabetes
- are members of a high-risk ethnic population (e.g., African-American, Hispanic-American, Native American, Asian-American, Pacific Islander)
- have delivered a baby weighing >9 lb or have been diagnosed with GDM
- are hypertensive (≥140/90 mm Hg)
- have an HDL cholesterol level ≤35 mg/dl (0.90 mmol/l) and/or a triglyceride level ≥250 mg/dl (2.82 mmol/l)
- on previous testing, had IGT or IFG
- have habitual inactivity
- have polycystic ovarian syndrome
- have history of vascular disease

➡ Fasting Plasma Glucose (FPG) is test of choice (fast for 8 hours prior to test)

➡ If FPG is ≥126 mg/dl, repeat test on different day to confirm diagnosis

➡ If FPG is <126 mg/dl and there is high suspicion for diabetes, an OGTT should be performed. A 2-hour postload in OGTT ≥200 mg/dl is a positive test and should be confirmed on an alternate day

---

Adapted from American Diabetes Association. (2003). Report of the Expert Committee on the diagnosis and classification of diabetes mellitus. *Diabetes Care, 26*(Suppl. 1), S5-S20

a. Random plasma glucose measurements can be made when food or drink has been ingested within 3 hours preceding test; ≥200 mg/dl is considered a positive screening test and the diagnosis of diabetes should be confirmed with an additional test, preferably a fasting plasma glucose (FPG) test
b. Screening for autoantibodies related to type 1 diabetes is not recommended outside the context of research studies
c. Consider screening lean new-onset adult diabetic patients for type 1 diabetes by measuring postprandial serum C peptide
2. Tests to determine the degree of glycemic control
a. Glycated hemoglobin (GHb) also referred to as glycohemoglobin, glycosylated hemoglobin, A1C, HbA1, or HbA1C
   (1) Reflects mean glucose levels for the preceding 2-3 months
   (2) Order at baseline and then at least every 6 months for well-controlled patients
   (3) Order more often (every 3 months) in diabetics with poor control or when beginning new therapies
   (4) Levels <7% should be the goal of treatment; usually need to change therapy regimens in patients with AIC results consistently >8%
   (5) Less stringent treatment goals may be acceptable for very young or older adults, individuals with hypoglycemic unawareness or limited life expectancy
   (6) Falsely low levels may occur in the presence of anemia and falsely elevated levels may occur in presence of uremia, alcoholism, and aspirin use
b. Glycemic control is best evaluated by combination of results of patient's self-monitoring of blood glucose (SMBG) and the current A1C
   (1) AIC also used to check accuracies of the patient's self-reported results and the patient's glucose meter
   (2) Following table shows correlation between A1C levels and mean plasma glucose levels
c. Glycated serum protein indicates glycemic control in a short period of time and needs to be performed monthly; currently this test is not recommended

CORRELATION BETWEEN A1C LEVEL AND MEAN PLASMA GLUCOSE LEVELS		
	Mean plasma glucose	
A1C (%)	mg/dl	mmol/l
6	135	7.5
7	170	9.5
8	205	11.5
9	240	13.5
10	275	15.5
11	310	17.5
12	345	19.5

From: American Diabetes Association. (2003). Standards of medical care for patients with diabetes mellitus. *Diabetes Care, 26*(Suppl. 1), S33-S50.

3. Tests helpful in defining associated complications and risk factors:
   a. Testing for diabetic retinopathy
     (1) Comprehensive eye examination by an ophthalmologist or optometrist should be completed within 3-5 years after onset of type 1 diabetes and shortly after diagnosis in type 2 diabetes
     (2) Assess annually or more often if retinopathy is progressing
   b. Order fasting lipid profile: total cholesterol, high-density lipoprotein (HDL) cholesterol, low density lipoprotein (LDL) cholesterol, and triglycerides
     (1) Order when diabetes is first diagnosed
     (2) Order annually; patients with borderline or abnormal values require additional testing
   c. Screening and diagnostic testing for coronary heart disease (CHD)
     (1) Annually assess for risk factors: Dyslipidemia, hypertension, smoking, family history of premature coronary disease, and presence of micro- or macroalbuminuria
     (2) Order electrocardiogram in patients with risk factors or cardiac symptoms
     (3) Order screening exercise stress (electrocardiogram [ECG]) testing in patients who have the following:
       (a) Typical or atypical cardiac symptoms
       (b) Abnormal resting ECG
       (c) History of peripheral or carotid occlusive disease
       (d) Sedentary lifestyle, age >35 years, and plans to begin a vigorous exercise program
     (4) Patients with abnormal exercise ECG and patients unable to perform an exercise ECG need additional or alternative testing such as stress nuclear perfusion and stress echocardiography (consultation with cardiologist is recommended for further diagnostic work-up)
   d. Order annual serum creatinine
   e. Order a urinalysis: ketones, glucose, protein, sediment
     (1) If protein is positive, a quantitative measure should be performed
     (2) If protein is negative, a test for the presence of microalbuminuria is necessary (see IV.D.3.f.), which immediately follows
   f. Testing for microalbuminuria
     (1) Test at the time of diagnosis; then, for patients with type 1 diabetes test annually if duration of diabetes is >5 years; test annually in patients with type 2 diabetes
     (2) Because of marked day-to-day variability in albumin excretion, at least two of three collections measured in a 3- to 6-month period should show elevated levels before arriving at a diagnosis
     (3) Testing for microalbuminuria can be performed by 3 methods
       (a) Assessment should first begin with measurement of the albumin-to-creatinine ratio in a random, spot collection
       (b) 24 hour collection with serum creatinine which allows for simultaneous measurement of creatinine clearance
       (c) Timed collection such as 4 hours or overnight
     (4) Microalbuminuria is defined in following table:

DEFINITIONS OF ABNORMALITIES IN ALBUMIN EXCRETION

Category	24-h Collection	Timed Collection	Spot Collection
Normal	<30 mg/24 h	<20 µg/min	<30 µg/mg creatinine
Microalbuminuria	30-299 mg/24 h	20-199 µg/min	30-299 µg/mg creatinine
Clinical albuminuria	≥300 mg/24 h	≥200 µg/min	≥300 µg/mg creatinine

Two of three specimens collected within a 3- to 6-month period should be abnormal before considering a patient to have crossed one of these diagnostic thresholds. Exercise within 24 hours, infection, fever, congestive heart failure, marked hyperglycemia, and marked hypertension may elevate urinary albumin excretion over baseline values

Adapted from American Diabetes Association. (2003). Diabetic nephropathy. *Diabetes Care, 26*(Suppl. 1), S94-S98.

g. In type 1 patients, order T_4 and thyroid stimulating hormone; order in type 2 patients if clinical presentation indicates a need

h. Some, but not all authorities, also suggest regular serum BUN and CBC tests

4. Testing for diabetic ketoacidosis and hyperosmolar hyperglycemic state

a. Order plasma glucose, blood urea nitrogen/creatinine, serum ketones, electrolytes (with calculated anion gap), osmolality, urinalysis, urine ketones by dipstick, initial arterial blood gases, complete blood count with differential, and electrocardiogram

b. If infection is suspected, order bacterial cultures of urine, blood, and throat

c. If indicated, order chest x-ray

d. Patients with hyperglycemic emergencies typically have leukocytosis, decreased serum sodium, and elevated serum potassium (also see table DIAGNOSTIC CRITERIA FOR DKA AND HHS, III.D.)

V. Plan/Management

A. Glycemic control: goals should be discussed with patients

1. Maintaining blood glucose values as close to normal as possible decreases the incidence of microvascular (retinopathy, nephropathy, and possibly neuropathy) complications

a. The Diabetes Control and Complications Trial (DCCT) found that type 1 diabetics with tight glycemic control had a significant reduction in their risk for developing retinopathy, nephropathy, and neuropathy when compared with the standard treatment groups

b. The United Kingdom Prospective Diabetes Study (UKPDS) enrolled 5,000 adults with newly diagnosed type 2 diabetes, and found that more intensive therapy (maintaining an A1C of 7% compared to 7.9%) reduced the overall microvascular complication rate by 25%

2. Degree of tight glycemic control must be individualized and balanced with the risk of developing hypoglycemia; elderly patients with significant atherosclerosis may be particularly vulnerable to permanent damage from hypoglycemia; use tight control cautiously

3. American Diabetes Association goals of glycemic control are shown in the following the table:

GLYCEMIC CONTROL FOR NONPREGNANT ADULTS

Measurement	Nondiabetic	Goal	Additional action suggested*
A1C (%)	<6	<7	>8
Plasma values[†]			
Preprandial glucose (mg/dl)	<110	90-130	<90 or >150
Bedtime glucose (mg/dl)	<120	100-150	<110 or >180
Postprandial (1-2 h)	<140	<180	
Whole blood values[‡]			
Preprandial glucose (mg/dl)	<100	80-120	<80 or >140
Bedtime glucose (mg/dl)	<110	100-140	<100 or >160

*Additional action must be individualized such as referral to endocrinologist, change in medications, self-management education, etc.
[†] Values calibrated to plasma glucose
[‡] Measurement of capillary blood glucose

Adapted from American Diabetes Association. (2004). Standards of medical care for patients with diabetes mellitus. *Diabetes Care, 26*(Suppl 1), S33-S50.

4. American College of Endocrinology and American Association of Clinical Endocrinologists recommends more stringent goals:
   a. A1C goal of <6.5%
   b. Fasting plasma glucose target of <110 mg/dl
   c. Postprandial (2-hour) glucose target of <140 mg/dl

B. Hospitalization should be considered for individuals with severe infection, dehydration, diabetic ketoacidosis (DKA), and hyperosmolar hyperglycemic state (HHS) (see VN.1 for treatment of DKA and HHS)

C. Consider hospitalization for the following patients with uncontrolled diabetes:
   1. Persistent refractory hyperglycemia associated with metabolic deterioration
   2. Recurring fasting hyperglycemia >300 mg/dl that is refractory to outpatient therapy or an A1C level greater than or equal to 100% above the upper limit of normal
   3. Recurring episodes of severe hypoglycemia (<50 mg/dl)
   4. Metabolic instability (swings between hypoglycemia and fasting hyperglycemia)
   5. Repeated absence from school or work due to severe psychosocial problems causing poor glycemic control

D. All diabetic patients benefit from medical nutritional therapy (MNT), exercise, and extensive patient education

E. Patient education is essential; education must be integrated with all aspects of the plan (also, see patient education in each of the following sections)
   1. Discuss basic pathophysiology
   2. Explain long-term complications, emphasizing that these complications can be prevented or delayed when blood glucose is well controlled
   3. Encourage patient to wear Medic-Alert tags
   4. Discuss contraception and emphasize the importance of glucose control before conception and during pregnancy in women of childbearing age
   5. See following table for good resources. The Small Steps•Big Rewards•Prevent type 2 Diabetes Campaign is first national diabetes prevention program. (See National Diabetes Education Program website for clinicians tool kit as well as tools for patients to determine if they are at risk for type 2 diabetes and a "game plan food and activity tracker" to help lose weight)

RESOURCES FOR PATIENTS	
Organization	**Website**
American Diabetes Association (ADA)	http:// www.diabetes.org
American Association for Clinical Endocrinologists	http://www.aace.com
ADA Diabetes Care & Educational Practice Group	http://www.eatright.org
National Diabetes Education Program	http://www.ndep.nih.gov

F. Nutritional recommendations or medical nutrition therapy (MNT)
   1. Collaboration or referral to a dietitian is beneficial; MNT should be individualized with respect to age, personal and cultural preferences, individual's wishes, and willingness to change
   2. Patients with type 1 diabetes:
      a. Cannot be treated with diet alone
      b. Monitor blood glucose levels and adjust insulin based on the amount of food usually consumed
         (1) Individuals on intensified insulin programs can make adjustments in rapid or lispro insulin to cover carbohydrate content of meals and/or snacks and for deviations from typical eating and exercising habits
         (2) For individuals on fixed insulin doses, day to day consistency in the amount of carbohydrate is needed
            (a) Plan meals to provide the amount of calories and nutrients that are expected to be metabolized when insulin is administered
            (b) Keep timing and amount of calories and nutrients in meals the same each day
         (3) Have a consistent, daily pattern of exercise and physical activity (may need supplemental snacks before and after exercise; may need to alter insulin dosage before activity)

    c.   Carbohydrate counting in which the patient takes insulin based on the amount of insulin consumed for a meal may be effective; approximately 1 unit of insulin will cover 10-15 grams of carbohydrate consumed

3.   Patients with type 2 diabetes can often improve blood glucose levels by moderate weight loss (5-9 kg or 10-20 lb) and hypocaloric diets (250-500 calories less than average daily intake as calculated from diet history) **alone**

    a.   Spacing of meals throughout day and regular exercise improve control

    b.   Portion control is important

    c.   For long-term weight loss, structured weight loss programs are often needed

4.   Dietary recommendations for both types of diabetics (see also DYSLIPIDEMIA section)

    a.   Carbohydrates and monounsaturated fats should make up approximately 60-70% of the total calories

        (1)   Unrefined carbohydrates (whole grains, vegetables [excluding potatoes], fruits, legumes, lowfat milk) and fiber should be eaten whenever possible; avoid refined starchy foods and concentrated sugar

        (2)   Select foods with a low glycemic index and low glycemic load (see following table)

            (a)   Glycemic index and glycemic load are systems for classifying carbohydrate-containing foods according to glycemic response

            (b)   High-glycemic foods produce an initial period of high blood glucose and insulin levels, followed in many persons by reactive hypoglycemia, counterregulatory hormone secretion, and increased serum free fatty acid concentration

            (c)   Regular consumption of high-glycemic meals results in higher average 24-hour blood glucose and insulin levels

GLYCEMIC INDEX AND GLYCEMIC LOAD VALUES FOR MAJOR CARBOHYDRATE SOURCES (RELATIVE TO WHITE BREAD)

Foods	Serving Size	Glycemic Index (%)	Carbohydrate (Grams)	Glycemic Load*
Potatoes, mashed	1 cup	104	37	38
Bread, white	1 slice	100	12	12
Orange juice	6 ounces	75	20	15
Banana	1 medium	88	27	23
Rice, white	1 cup	102	45	45
Pizza	2 slices	86	78	67
Pasta	1 cup	71	40	28
Coke	12 ounces	90	39	35
Apple	1 medium	55	21	12
Milk, skim	1 cup	46	12	5.4
Pancake	2 six-inch	119	56	66
Sugar, table	1 tsp.	84	4	3.4
Jam	1 tbsp.	91	14	13
Candy	1 ounce	99	27	27
Ice cream	½ cup	42	16	7
Carrots, raw	½ cup	131	4	5
Baked beans	1 cup	60	27	16
Cornflakes	1 cup	114	24	27
Cheerios	1 cup	106	22	23
Total	1 cup	109	32	35
Bran Flakes	1 cup	74	31	23
Oatmeal	1 cup	82	25	21

* Glycemic load calculated by multiplying grams of carbohydrate by glycemic index of bread (100%=1.0)

Glycemic index taken from: Jenkins, D.J.A., et al. (1981). Overview of implications in health and disease. *American Journal of Clinical Nutrition, 76*(Suppl.), 266S-273S.

Adapted from Willett, W.C. (2001). *Eat, drink, and be healthy: The Harvard Medical School guide to healthy eating.* New York: Simon & Schuster.

    b.   Protein intake should be the recommended dietary allowance for Americans or about 15-20% of daily calories

        (1)   Reduce intake if renal function is abnormal

        (2)   Choose healthy sources of protein (beans, nuts, fish, poultry, eggs)

     c.   Saturated fats (whole milk, ice cream, red meat, butter, coconut oil) should be restricted to <10% of total calories and cholesterol to <300 mg/day; unsaturated fats (olive, canola, corn, safflower oils, fish, peanuts) should replace saturated fats

         (1)   For individuals with LDL cholesterol ≥100 mg/dl, saturated fat intake should be <7% of calories and dietary cholesterol <200 mg/day

         (2)   When saturated fat is reduced, it can be replaced with carbohydrate and/or monounsaturated fat if weight loss is not an issue

         (3)   Intake of trans-fatty acids should be minimized

     d.   Patients can use nutritive and nonnutritive sweeteners

     e.   Excessive alcohol increases risks of hypertriglycemia and pancreatitis and contributes to hypoglycemia in persons with type 1 diabetes; in patients who choose to drink alcohol, intake should be limited to one drink per day for women and two drinks per day for men

     f.   Balance in salt is needed with upper limit of 6,000 mg/day of sodium chloride or 2,400 mg/day of sodium; a reduction in sodium lowers blood pressure

  5.   MNT in older adults

     a.   Energy requirements for older adults are less than for younger adults

     b.   Encourage physical activity

     c.   Undernutrition is more likely than overnutrition; use caution when recommending weight loss diets

G.   Physical activity is an integral component of diabetes management

  1.   Positive effects: increases metabolism and, over an extended period, reduces insulin resistance, reduces cardiovascular risk factors, improves weight loss, and promotes well being

  2.   Exercise program should be started after an appropriate health exam, which focuses on heart, blood vessels, eyes, kidneys and nervous system

  3.   A graded exercise test is needed for patients at high risk for cardiovascular disease

  4.   Patients who have complications of the eye, kidney, and autonomic neuropathy should avoid strenuous exercise

  5.   For patients on insulin therapy, the following guidelines are helpful:

     a.   Avoid exercising at times when insulin is at its peak action

     b.   Monitor blood glucose before and after exercise to identify when changes in insulin or food intake are necessary and to learn glycemic response to different exercise conditions

     c.   Avoid exercise if FPG levels are <80 mg/dl or >250 mg/dl and ketosis is present or if glucose levels are >300 mg/dl, regardless of whether ketosis is present

     d.   Ingest added carbohydrates if glucose levels are <100 mg/dl

     e.   Eat added carbohydrates as needed to avoid hypoglycemia; keep carbohydrate-based food available during and after exercise; in general, one serving of carbohydrates increases plasma glucose about 40 points

     f.   Avoid exercising extremities in which insulin has recently been injected

  6.   For patients with type 2 diabetes, exercise should be a high priority; benefit is probably greatest when it is begun early in course of disease

H.   Insulin therapy: Goals of normalized glycohemoglobin must be balanced with risks of hypoglycemia; insulin is required for management of type 1 diabetes and in some patients with type 2 diabetes

  1.   Consider type of insulin to use

     a.   If patients are on pork insulin, do not switch if they are well-controlled

     b.   Newly diagnosed diabetics should be on human insulin because of its lower incidence of insulin allergy, resistance, and lipoatrophy (see table VARIOUS HUMAN INSULIN PREPARATIONS for brand names of human insulin)

  2.   Persons without diabetes produce insulin continuously (basal insulin) in order to suppress hepatic glucose production, with increases or boluses of insulin at meal times to utilize prandial glucose; these same basal and postprandial patterns should be followed in persons with diabetes for insulin therapy to be effective

  3.   Insulin is commercially available in concentrations of 100 or 500 units/ml (designated U-100 and U-500, respectively); use U-100 insulin, as U-500 is used only in rare cases when patient requires extremely large doses

VARIOUS HUMAN INSULIN PREPARATIONS

Type	Onset (hours)	Peak (hours)	Duration (hours)
Rapid acting analog			
Humalog (Lispro)	<0.25	1	3.5-4.5
NovoLog (Aspart)	<0.25	0.75	3-5
Short acting			
Humulin R	0.5	2-4	6-8
Novolin R	0.5	2.5-5	8
Velosulin BR	0.5	1-3	8
Intermediate acting			
Humulin N (NPH)	1-2	6-12	18-24
Novolin N (NPH)	1.5	4-12	24
Humulin L (Lente)	1-3	6-12	18-24
Novolin L (Lente)	2.5	7-15	22
Long acting			
Humulin U (Ultralente)	4-6	8-20	24-48
Lantus (Glargine)	1.1	none	≥24
*Premixed: Insulin isophane suspension (NPH)/regular insulin (R)**			
Humulin 70/30	0.5	2-12	24
Humulin 50/50	0.5	3-5	24
Novolin 70/30	0.5	2-12	24
*Premixed: Lispro Protamine/Lispro**			
Humalog Mix 75/25	≤0.25	0.5-1.5	24
*Premixed: Aspart Protamine/Aspart**			
NovoLog 70/30	<0.25	1-4	24

***Do Not** use premixed with Type 1 diabetics as it severely limits flexibility

4. Initiating insulin therapy in adults with type 1 diabetes
   a. Give a total daily dose of 0.6 units per kg (others recommend 0.5-1.0 units)
   b. Both a basal (long or intermediate acting, usually comprising 40-60% of the total daily dose) and a rapid or short acting for meals is recommended
      (1) Insulin glargine provides 24 hour basal peakless coverage which aids in reducing hypoglycemia
      (2) Insulin lispro provides improved postprandial coverage from carbohydrate meals and less nocturnal hypoglycemia than regular or short-acting insulin
5. Honeymoon phase: after initial therapy is instituted this phase occurs and may last 12-18 months; insulin dosages may be reduced to 0.2-0.5 units/kg/day (important to tell patients about this phase to prevent false beliefs that the diabetes is partially cured)
6. Long-term insulin therapy
   a. Dosage: 0.6-0.8 units/kg/day
   b. Determine the pattern or regimen of insulin therapy (see table COMMON INSULIN REGIMENS)
7. Persons with type 2 diabetes vary considerably and may require small (5-10 units) to several hundred units per day

COMMON INSULIN REGIMENS

Regimen	Dosing	Comments
Single daily injection	Intermediate or long lasting at bedtime (usually start ~10 units)	• Only for type 2 • Use when daily doses are <30 units/day; for larger daily insulin doses, 2 or more injections are needed unless using Lantus (Glargine) • Suppresses hepatic glucose production • Often used in combination with daytime oral agent
2-injection -or- split/mix	2/3 of total daily dosing in AM* 1/3 of total daily dosing in PM* **THEN** AM 2/3 NPH + 1/3 rapid or short acting** PM 1/2 NPH + 1/2 rapid or short acting**	• Best in type 2 and early type 1 • Disadvantages: poor peaking of noon insulin and excess insulin at night (to resolve this problem, limit noon meal and eat a bedtime snack)
3-injection	Of total daily dose (approximate): AM* 20-30% NPH & ~25% rapid or short acting** PM* ~25% rapid or short acting** Bedtime 20-30% NPH **OR** AM* ~20-30% rapid or short acting** PM* ~20-30% rapid or short acting** Bedtime insulin glargine (~50%)	• Best in type 1 • Advantages: less risk of nighttime hypoglycemia and better control of dawn phenomenon or persistent AM hyperglycemia • Disadvantage: poor peaking of insulin at noon (to resolve this problem, limit noon meal)
4-Injection or prandial/basal	Of total daily dose (approximate): <u>Prandial insulin</u> (before each meal) ~15-20% rapid or short acting** (best to vary dose depending on food intake, i.e., higher dose at dinner) <u>Basal insulin</u> ~50% glargine at bedtime or ~25% NPH or ~25% lente in AM and bedtime	• Best in type 1 • Requires committed patient and care-provider, with frequent self-blood-glucose monitoring • Advantage: clear relationship between insulin dose and glucose level • Insulin glargine and lispro combination can lessen risk of hypoglycemia and result in a pattern that resembles endogenous insulin release
Continuous subcutaneous insulin infusion -or- insulin pump therapy	- Continually delivers rapid or short acting - Provides both basal insulin release and adjustable pre-meal bolus release	• Indications: inability to control glucose with 2 or more injections; recurrent, major hypoglycemia due to hypoglycemic unawareness, loss of counter-regulatory mechanisms or variable absorption of modified insulins • Prerequisites: patient must have intellectual & emotional abilities for self-care • Advantages: closely resembles endogenous insulin release; results in more predictable insulin absorption and fewer dosage errors • Disadvantages: expensive; blood glucose must be monitored 4 times/day

* AM is before breakfast: regular or short acting insulins should be taken 30-45 minutes before meal and rapid acting insulins should be taken within 15 minutes of meal; PM is before evening meal or supper
**Rapid acting insulins are often more convenient for patients because they can be injected immediately before (or after) meals and can lessen the likelihood of late post-prandial hypoglycemia and nocturnal hypoglycemia but they are more expensive and need more intensive monitoring than regular insulins

8. Adjusting insulin is based on daily blood glucose levels and on peak effect of a given insulin dose (patients should record their blood glucose and insulin doses with comments on a flow sheet)
   a. Self-monitoring of blood glucose is essential
      (1) Patients with type 1 diabetes should monitor 3-4 times a day
      (2) Patients with type 2 diabetes should monitor at various times such as some mornings, at bedtimes, and 1-2 hour after meals
   b. Calculating adjustments:
      (1) Adjust in 1-3 unit increments or decrements, especially in type 1
      (2) Larger adjustments can be made for type 2 patients
   c. Downward adjustments should be made the day following a "below range blood glucose" to avoid repeat hypoglycemia
   d. Upward adjustments should be delayed for 2 days to establish a pattern
   e. When increasing a long lasting or evening intermediate insulin, instruct patient to monitor blood glucose at 2-3 AM for hypoglycemia
   f. Consider timing and type of insulin when making adjustments (see following table):

ADJUSTING INSULIN THERAPY	
Insulin	**Affected Blood Glucose Value**
AM* Intermediate	Post-lunch Pre-supper
AM* Short or rapid acting	Post-breakfast Pre-lunch
PM** Intermediate	Early morning
PM** Short or rapid acting	Bedtime
Bedtime Intermediate or long acting	Early morning

*AM is before breakfast
**PM is before evening meal or supper

9. Tips on administering insulin therapy (see following table)

TIPS ON INSULIN THERAPY
• Insulin should approximate the natural release of insulin by the beta cell
• Administer Insulin to provide a basal amount in 40-60% of total daily dose as well as peaks after each meal
• One time a day insulin therapy is **not** sufficient for patients with type 1 diabetes
• Be careful in adjusting insulin with type 1 diabetics; they are very sensitive to adjustments because they have no endogenous insulin secretion
• Consider giving PM NPH at bedtime to reduce early morning hyperglycemia
• Combination insulin therapy of glargine and lispro insulins can lessen risk of hypoglycemia (however, do not mix insulin glargine in same syringe with other forms of insulin)
• Use NPH when there is a need to mix with another type of insulin
• Consider the following when blood glucose is not controlled with insulin: malignant insulin resistance, occult infection, noncompliance, poor coping skills

10. Patient education concerning the administering, storage, and disposal of insulin is essential (see following table)

PATIENT EDUCATION – INSULIN THERAPY

- Insulin in use can be kept at room temperature, for one month only, to limit local irritation at injection site; unopened insulin should be refrigerated
- Opened cartridges and prefilled pens can be kept for varying amounts of time (10-28 days) depending on the type
- When mixing insulin, the clear, rapid-acting and short-acting insulins should be drawn into syringe first
- Lantus (Glargine) and lente should not be mixed with other insulin
- Syringes can be prefilled and stored in a vertical position in the refrigerator for 3 weeks (do not allow if using rapid)
- Usually, regular or short-acting insulin should be given 30 minutes before eating; rapid should be given within 15 minutes of eating
- Subcutaneously inject insulin into upper arm, anterior and lateral aspects of thigh, the buttocks and abdomen (with exception of a circle with a 2-inch radius around the navel); do not frequently rotate to different anatomical sites, but do make injections in different areas of one anatomical site; absorption is most rapid and consistent from the abdomen
- Do not use clear insulin that is cloudy or discolored or any insulin that has sediment or other visible changes
- Dispose syringes in resistant disposal container and contact local public health unit or local trash-disposal authority for appropriate disposal provisions; avoid recapping, bending, or breaking needle to decrease risk of needlestick injury
- Proper procedure of syringe reuse involves cleaning needle after use and putting in refrigerator (only teach patients who have good cognitive and psychomotor functioning)
- Syringe alternatives such as jet injectors, pen-like devices, and insulin-containing cartridges are usually expensive but may be more convenient and improve technique of insulin injection
- Insulin syringes with engineered sharps injury protection (ESIP) are available

---

I. Special considerations of insulin therapy in older adults
   1. There are no long-term studies demonstrating the benefits of tight glycemic control in persons >65 years
   2. Older persons can be treated with insulin similarly to younger adults, but special care is required in dosing and monitoring
   3. Older persons may be more at risk to develop hypoglycemia than younger adults
   4. Use of insulin therapy requires good visual and motor skills as well as cognitive ability; for some older adults impairments in these systems may cause problems in self-injecting insulin; prefilled syringes may be helpful

J. Treatment of type 2 diabetes in adults is based on a step-wise plan
   1. **Patients with fasting blood glucose <250 mg/dl**: Initiate medical nutrition therapy (MNT) and exercise; if patient's glucose is not controlled within 3 months, advance to next step
   2. **Patients with fasting blood glucose ≥250 mg/dl and <400 mg/dl who do not have signs of dehydration, acidosis, or marked ketosis**: In addition to MNT and exercise, they should begin monotherapy with an oral antidiabetic agent (see table ORAL HYPOGLYCEMIC AGENTS); approximately 30-40% of patients do not satisfactorily respond to oral agents
      a. Patients with markedly elevated fasting blood glucose and ketonuria or ketonemia, or symptomatic patients may require insulin therapy initially to overcome glucose toxicity
      b. Precautions and contraindications for oral antidiabetic agents
         (1) Sulfonylureas: Use cautiously in persons with renal impairment, liver damage, alcohol abuse problems, sulfa allergy; contraindicated in pregnant women
         (2) Non-sulfonylurea secretagogues or meglitinides: Relatively safe, but use cautiously in persons with hepatic or kidney disease
         (3) Biguanides: Contraindicated in persons prone to lactic acidosis and those with renal disease; use cautiously in persons with liver dysfunction, heart failure, sepsis, alcohol abuse problems, dehydration, adrenal or pituitary insufficiency
            (a) Do not use if serum creatinine ≥1.4 mg/dl in women and ≥1.5 mg/dl in men
            (b) Temporarily discontinue if undergoing contrast studies or surgery
         (4) α-glucosidase inhibitors: Contraindicated in persons with cirrhosis and significant gastrointestinal problems; use cautiously in persons with renal dysfunction
         (5) Thiazolidinediones (TZDs): Use cautiously in persons with hepatic disease (monitor ALT values regularly). Contraindicated in persons with severe congestive heart failure

3. Dosing and selection of best oral antidiabetic agent for monotherapy (see ORAL HYPOGLYCEMIC AGENTS on next page)
   a. Metformin is often regarded as the best first-line therapy, especially in obese persons without contraindications
   b. Sulfonylureas are most effective when blood glucose is severely elevated; may also be first choice for lean persons who may have more pancreatic dysfunction than insulin resistance
   c. Thiazolidinediones are usually not the best monotherapy choice because they are expensive, require liver monitoring, and have adverse effects
   d. α-glucosidase inhibitors (meglitinides) may be most effective in persons with mild fasting hyperglycemia and who have predominantly postprandial hyperglycemia
   e. Begin slowly and increase dose every 1-2 weeks on the basis of self glucose monitoring until glucose is controlled; thiazolidinediones may take weeks or months for full glycemic effect so dose increasing should be done more slowly
   f. When glucose is controlled with a low dose, once a day dosing is recommended; when larger doses are needed to control glucose, doses are split and given twice a day
      (1) Dosages will depend on results of self glucose monitoring
      (2) Increase morning dose when the evening blood glucose is elevated; increase evening dose when the morning glucose is elevated
   g. Treatment should continue for 6-8 weeks before considering a change of regimens
4. The UKPDS demonstrated that type 2 diabetes is a progressive disease, and that most patients will not be controlled on monotherapy after several years
5. When patient fails to respond to first antidiabetic agent, add another agent(s) of a different class
   a. A logical approach is to add a drug which decreases insulin requirements with a drug that increases insulin availability; see table ORAL HYPOGLYCEMIC AGENTS for FDA approved combinations
   b. Addition of a third drug is an unlabeled use of oral agents and requires careful observation for drug interactions but may lower overall drug dosing, minimize adverse effects, and improve glycemic control
6. **If combination oral antidiabetic agent therapy fails**, add insulin or replace one of oral agents with insulin
   a. Add 10 units of intermediate acting or long lasting insulin at bedtime or calculate 0.25 units/kg of ideal body weight
   b. If postprandial glucose levels are high, a mixture of short or rapid acting insulin with long lasting or intermediate insulin may be useful
   c. Self blood glucose monitoring is needed
   d. Increase insulin 3-5 units every 3-4 days until desired fasting blood glucose is achieved
   e. In elderly, use insulin as last resort because of dangers of hypoglycemia
      (1) Keep insulin patterns simple
      (2) Use premixed insulin if possible to avoid errors
      (3) Consider use of prefilled insulin pens
   f. It is controversial whether oral antidiabetic agents should be continued indefinitely with insulin therapy or whether they should be slowly titrated downward and stopped
7. In patients with blood glucose ≥400 mg/dl or patients who have signs of dehydration, acidosis, or marked ketosis, begin insulin therapy
8. No consensus is available as to when to discontinue insulin therapy; some authorities advise tapering down or discontinuing insulin when blood glucose levels are controlled

ORAL HYPOGLYCEMIC AGENTS*

Drug	Usual Maintenance Range Per Day (in divided doses/day)	Mechanism of Action	Advantages	Major Adverse Reactions and Disadvantages	Food and Drug Administration Approval Status
Sulfonylureas (SUs) Glyburide (Micronase/DiaBeta) Glyburide, micronized (Glynase Pres Tabs) Glipizide (Glucotrol XL) Glipizide (Glucotrol) Glimepiride (Amaryl)	 1.25-20 mg (1-2) 0.75-12 mg (1-2) 5-10 mg (1) 5-40 mg (1-2) 1-4 mg (1)	↑ Pancreatic insulin secretion	• Well established • Decreases microvascular risk • Daily dosing	• Weight gain • Hypoglycemia	• Monotherapy • Combine with insulin, metformin, thiazolidinediones, α-glucosidase inhibitors
Non-Sulfonylurea Secretagogues Repaglinide (Prandin) Nateglinide (Starlix)	 0.5-4 mg take within 30 minutes before meals (2-4) 60-120 mg take 1-30 minutes before meals (3)	↑ Pancreatic insulin secretion	• Possibly less hypoglycemia and weight gain than SUs • Targets postprandial glycemia	• Hypoglycemia (skip dose if miss meal) • Weight gain • Complex dosing • No long-term data	• Monotherapy • Combine with metformin • Combine with thiazolidinediones
Biguanides Metformin (Glucophage) Metformin (Glucophage XR)	 500-2550 mg (2-3) 500-2000 mg (1-2)	↓ Hepatic glucose production ↑ Insulin action on muscle glucose uptake	• Well established • Weight loss • No hypoglycemia • Decreases microvascular and macrovascular risks • Decreases lipid levels • Increases fibrinolysis • Decreases hyperinsulinemia • Daily dosing	• Diarrhea and other GI effects • Lactic acidosis with incorrect dosing or renal disease • Many contraindications	• Monotherapy • Combine with insulin, SU, non-SU secretagogue, thiazolidinedione
α-Glucosidase Inhibitors Acarbose (Precose) Miglitol (Glyset)	 25-100 mg (3 x daily with meals) 25-100 mg (3 x daily with meals)	↓ Delays carbohydrate digestion	• Targets postprandial glucose • No hypoglycemia • Nonsystemic	• Complex dosing • GI effects • No long-term data	• Monotherapy • Combine with SU
Thiazolidinediones Pioglitazone (Actos) Rosiglitazone (Avandia)	 15-45 mg (1) 4-8 mg (1-2)	↑ Insulin action on muscle and fat glucose uptake	• Reverses prime defect of type 2 diabetes • Possible beta cell preservation • No hypoglycemia • Decreases lipid levels • Increases fibrinolysis • Decreases hyperinsulinemia • Improves endothelial function • Daily dosing	• Weight gain • Edema • Liver function test monitoring (especially with insulin, monitor every 2 months for first year) • Slow onset of action • Resumption of pre-menopausal ovulation in anovulating women (may result in pregnancy)	• Monotherapy • Combine with insulin, SU, metformin
Combination Sulfonylurea & Biguanide Glyburide & metformin (Glucovance) Glipizide & metformin (Metaglip)	 Initially 1.25 mg/250 mg (1-2 with meals) Initially 2.5 mg/250 mg (1)	See SU and biguanides above	See SU and biguanides above	See SU and biguanides above	See SU and biguanides above
Combination Thiazolidinedione & Biguanide Rosiglitazone & metformin (Avandamet)	 Initially 1 mg/500 mg (1)	See thiaz. and biguanides above	See thiaz. and biguanides above	See thiaz. and biguanides above	See thiaz. and biguanides above

* Begin at a low dose and gradually titrate upwards according to clinical effect (especially in elderly, malnourished, debilitated, or those with renal and/or hepatic dysfunction.)
Adapted from Inzucchi, S.E. (2002). Oral antihyperglycemic therapy for type 2 diabetes: Scientific review. *JAMA, 287,* 360-372.

K. Self-monitoring of blood glucose has replaced urine testing as a method to assess glucose control; however, type 1 patients need to check urine for ketones whenever their blood glucose levels are >300 mg/dl, during illness, stress, pregnancy, or when symptoms of ketoacidosis such as nausea, vomiting, or abdominal pain are present
   1. Frequent monitoring is essential when patients are on intensive insulin therapy or insulin pump therapy; monitor blood glucose three or more times, typically before meals, at bedtime and occasionally in the middle of night
   2. Less frequent monitoring may be appropriate for some patients, but even these patients should adhere to the following recommendations:
      a. When medications are altered should do the following:
         (1) Check blood glucose before each meal, at bedtime, and at 2-4 AM for 3 days
         (2) Next 7 days, check blood glucose before breakfast and dinner
      b. After glucose is initially controlled, check once a day at different times
      c. When glucose is stabilized, check 2-4 times per week at different times
   3. FDA has approved the GlucoWatch Biographer, a device that monitors patterns of glucose levels in adults without puncturing the skin; used as a supplement rather than a replacement for standard home glucose monitoring systems

L. Contingency plan for managing hypoglycemia (BG <70 mg/dl with or without symptoms)
   1. Teach patient and family the signs and symptoms of hypoglycemia such as shakiness, sweating, restlessness, hunger, headache, confusion, or seizures
   2. Instruct patient to carry source of oral glucose (glucose tablets, Lifesavers, raisins) with them at all times
      a. For BG 50-70 mg/dl, ~15 grams of carbohydrate (3-4 glucose tablets, 8 Lifesavers, 2 tablespoons of raisins, 4 oz. of fruit juice or soft drink, 8 oz milk) should raise BG 30-45 mg/dl
      b. For BG <50 mg/dl, ~30 grams should be taken
   3. Family or friends should be instructed in administering a subcutaneous or intramuscular injection of glucagon if patient is unresponsive or unable to swallow; if patient does not respond in 15 minutes, may give 1-2 more doses
      a. Adult or adolescent dose: 1 mg
      b. After consciousness is regained, patient should ingest oral carbohydrates to prevent further hypoglycemia
   4. Encourage patient to carry medical identification

M. Managing diabetes when the patient is ill; teach the following:
   1. Illnesses can be life-threatening and require careful monitoring
   2. Although difficult to predict, blood glucose usually increases; perform self-blood-glucose monitoring several times a day and check urine for ketones (twice a day)
   3. Imperative to call clinician in following circumstances:
      a. Vomiting with ketosis (may indicate diabetic ketoacidosis that requires immediate medical care to prevent complications and even death)
      b. Inability to drink fluids
      c. Blood glucose >240 mg/dL and urine positive for ketones
   4. Continue to take usual dose of insulin or oral agent; patients with oral agents may temporarily require insulin
   5. If patients are able to drink, increase intake of non-caloric fluids
   6. Drink small, continuous amounts of sugar-containing liquids such as juice, Gatorade or Coke in conjunction with the readings from their self-monitoring and if they are vomiting or nauseated

N. Management of associated problems and complications. There is growing recognition that tight glycemic control prevents or delays many of the following problems
   1. Treatment of hyperglycemic crisis
      a. Correct dehydration; typically IV isotonic saline is infused
      b. Unless the episode is mild, regular insulin by continuous intravenous infusion is usually recommended

c. To prevent hypokalemia, potassium replacement in the IV infusion is started after serum potassium levels fall below 5.5 mEq/L, assuming urine output is adequate

d. Assess need for bicarbonate therapy; bicarbonate may be beneficial in patients with a pH <6.9

e. To avoid cardiac and skeletal muscle weakness and respiratory depression due to hypophosphatemia, careful phosphate replacement may be indicated in patients with cardiac dysfunction, anemia, or respiratory depression and in those with serum phosphate concentration <1.0 mg/dl

f. Cerebral edema is a rare but frequently fatal complication of DKA and HHS; prevention involves gradual correction of glucose and osmolality as well as judicious use of isotonic or hypotonic saline depending on the sodium and the hemodynamic status of the patient

2. Diabetic retinopathy: refer to ophthalmologist; laser therapy and vitrectomy have been effective

3. Nephropathy

    a. Achieving normoglycemia and lowering blood pressure have proven to delay progression

    b. Both angiotensin-converting enzyme (ACE) inhibitors and angiotensin receptor blockers (ARB) can be used to treat albuminuria/nephropathy:

        (1) In type 1 diabetics (both normotensive and hypertensive) with any degree of albuminuria, ACE inhibitors are agent of choice

        (2) In hypertensive type 2 diabetics, ACE inhibitors and ARBs delay disease progression

        (3) In type 2 hypertensive patients with macroalbuminuria and renal insufficiency (serum creatinine >1.5 mg/dl) ARBs are recommended; irbesartan (Avapro) and losartan (Cosaar) are first approved drugs for these patients

        (4) Periodically monitor potassium levels to detect an adverse drug reaction of hyperkalemia

        (5) Periodically monitor urine albumin to document the effect of treatment and to detect the rare case of adverse effects of drug therapy

        (6) Target blood pressure for persons with diabetes and nephropathy is 125/75 mm Hg

    c. Consider use of non-dihydropyridine calcium channel blocker or beta-blocker in patients unable to tolerate ACE inhibitor or ARB

    d. Protein intake should be approximately the adult Recommended Dietary Allowance (RDA); protein restriction should be initiated when GFR starts to fall; meal plans should be developed by a registered dietitian

    e. Refer to a subspecialist in diabetic renal disease when GFR falls to <60 ml • min^{-1} • 1.73 m^{-2}, when serum creatinine is greater than 2.0 mg/dl, or there is difficulty managing hypertension or hyperkalemia

4. Cardiovascular disease; requires careful monitoring and intensive efforts to reduce risk factors and delay further progression of the disease

    a. Lipid abnormalities:

        (1) Often resolve when glycemic control is attained in type 1 diabetes

        (2) Goals for adults with type 2 diabetes are LDL <100 mg/dl (primary goal), HDL >40 mg/dl (men), HDL >50 mg/dl (women), and triglycerides (TG) <150 mg/dl

        (3) Treatment of LDL cholesterol is first priority for drug therapy (see following table); behavioral interventions such as weight loss, increased exercise, medical nutrition therapy (MNT), and education should be initiated (see section DYSLIPIDEMIA) when LDL is >100 mg/dl

        (4) Patients with coronary vascular disease or high LDL cholesterol levels (≥200 mg/dl) should be started on drug therapy simultaneously with behavioral therapy

        (5) Begin drug therapy (see table TREATMENT OF ADULT DIABETIC DYSLIPIDEMIA) after behavioral interventions, diet therapy, and glucose interventions in following patients:

            (a) Diabetic patients with coronary heart disease (CHD), peripheral vascular disease (PVD), or cardiovascular disease (CVD) and an LDL cholesterol >100 mg/dl (2.60 mmol/l)

            (b) Diabetic patients without pre-existing CHD, PVD or CVD and an LDL cholesterol ≥130 mg/dl (3.35 mmol/l)

            (c) Drug therapy is optional for patients with LDL between 100 mg/dl and 129 mg/dl

            (d) Diabetic patients with triglyceride levels >400 mg/dl (4.50 mmol/l)

            (e) Clinical judgment should be used in patients with triglycerides between 200 (2.30 mmol/l) and 400 mg/dl (4.50 mmol/l)

ORDER OF PRIORITIES FOR TREATMENT OF ADULT DIABETIC DYSLIPIDEMIA

LDL cholesterol lowering*

    First choice: HMG CoA reductase inhibitor (statin)

    Second choice: Bile acid binding resin (resin) or fenofibrate

HDL cholesterol raising

    Behavioral interventions such as weight loss, increased physical activity, and smoking cessation

    Difficult except with nicotinic acid, which is used with caution as may elevate blood glucose in higher doses, or fibrates

Triglyceride lowering

    Glycemic control first priority

    Fibric acid derivative such as gemfibrozil[†] or fenofibrate

    Statins are moderately effective at high dose in hypertriglyceridemic patients who also have high LDL

Combined hyperlipidemia

    First choice: Improved glycemic control plus high-dose statin

    Second choice: Improved glycemic control plus statin[††] plus fibric acid derivative[††] (fenofibrate has some LDL lowering activity)

    Third choice: Improved glycemic control plus resin plus fibric acid derivative **OR**

                    Improved glycemic control plus statin[††] plus nicotinic acid[††] (glycemic control must be monitored carefully)

*Decision for treatment of high LDL before elevated triglyceride is based on clinical trial data indicating safety as well as efficacy of the available agents.

[†]Gemfibrozil should not be started alone in patients with both elevated triglycerides and elevated LDL cholesterol.

[††]The combination of statins with nicotinic acid and especially with gemfibrozil may carry an increased risk of myositis.

Adapted from American Diabetes Association. (2003). Management of dyslipidemia in adults with diabetes. *Diabetes Care, 26*(Suppl 1), S83-S86.

    b.   Prescribe ACE inhibitor, if no contraindications, to patients >55 years with or without hypertension but who have another cardiovascular risk factor

    c.   Post myocardial infarction care: Cardioselective beta-blockers such as atenolol or metoprolol may decrease mortality even more in diabetics than in nondiabetics; new evidence is showing that these beta-blockers do not increase risk of serious hypoglycemia

    d.   Daily intake of aspirin (81-325 mg/day of enteric coated)

        (1)   Recommended for secondary prevention in patients with large vessel disease and as primary prevention in patients ≥40 years old with one or more other CV risk factors

        (2)   Do not use in persons <21 years of age

        (3)   Consider aspirin therapy for patients between 30-40 years of age with other cardiovascular risk factors

    e.   Smoking cessation: Advise all patients to stop smoking

    f.   Hypertension should be treated aggressively with goal to reduce arterial blood pressure (BP) to below 135/80 mm Hg

        (1)   Measure BP at every visit; if systolic blood pressure ≥130 mm Hg or diastolic blood pressure ≥80 mm Hg, BP measurement should be confirmed on a separate day

        (2)   Assess orthostatic BP at every visit

        (3)   In patients with a systolic BP of 130-139 mm Hg or diastolic BP of 80-89 mm Hg give lifestyle/behavioral therapy alone for maximum of 3 months, and then give pharmacological therapy if goals are not met

        (4)   In patients with systolic BP ≥140 mm Hg or diastolic BP ≥90 mm Hg give drug therapy in addition to behavioral therapy

        (5)   In elderly hypertensive patients lower BP gradually to avoid complications

        (6)   Initial drug therapy: ACE inhibitors, thiazide diuretics, and beta-blockers are preferred agents, but any drug class indicated for treatment of hypertension can be used; calcium channel blockers should not be used in patients who had recent coronary event (see following table for guidelines in selecting initial drug)

        (7)   Often patients will need two or more antihypertensive agents to reach target BP goal

    g.   Chronic heart failure (CHF): Metformin is contraindicated in patients with CHF. Cautiously prescribe thiazolidinediones as they are associated with fluid retention

CLINICAL TRIAL SUPPORT FOR INITIAL DRUG THERAPY OF HYPERTENSION

Characteristic	Preferred Drug Class*	Comment
Type 1 diabetes with or without hypertension, with any degree of albuminuria	ACE inhibitor	Delays progression to nephropathy
Type 2 diabetes with hypertension and microalbuminuria	ACE inhibitor or ARB	Delays progression to macroalbuminuria
Type 2 diabetes, hypertension, macroalbuminuria (>300 mg/day), nephropathy, or renal insufficiency	ARB	
>55 years of age, with or without hypertension, but with another cardiovascular risk factor	ACE inhibitor	Reduces risk of cardiovascular events
Microalbuminuria or overt nephropathy when ACE inhibitor or ARB is not well tolerated	Non-DCCB or beta-blocker	
Recent myocardial infarction	Beta-blocker should be considered as additional therapy	
African American	Consider thiazide diuretics	

* ACE inhibitor indicates angiotensin-converting enzyme inhibitor; ARB indicated angiotensin receptor blocker; Non-DCCB indicates non-dihydropyridine calcium channel blocker

5. Neuropathy
   a. Distal, sensorimotor type requires no treatment except education about foot care to prevent ulcer formation
   b. Painful neuropathy may respond to tricyclic antidepressants such as amitriptyline (Elavil) 25 to 150 mg at bedtime, gabapentin (Neurontin) 900 mg TID (start 300 mg QHS), carbamazepine (Tegretol) 400-800 mg/day in two divided doses, topical capsaicin 0.025% cream (Zostrix) TID or QID (also available in 0.075% cream); avoid narcotics

6. Autonomic nervous system problems
   a. Gastroparesis may respond to metoclopramide (Reglan) 10 mg or erythromycin 250 mg given 30 minutes before meals; diabetic diarrhea may respond to psyllium or clonidine
   b. Impotence may respond to oral medications (sildenafil [Viagra]), penile injections [papaverine, phentolamine or prostaglandin], or intraurethral drug suppositories (see section on ERECTILE DYSFUNCTION)
   c. Overflow incontinence (see section on INCONTINENCE) may respond to bethanechol

7. Immunizations
   a. Annual influenza immunization
   b. Pneumococcal immunization:
      (1) Provide at least one lifetime vaccine
      (2) A one-time revaccination is recommended for patients >64 years previously immunized when they were <65 years if the vaccine was given more than 5 years ago; revaccination also indicated for immunocompromised patients

8. Diabetic foot ulcers; patient education and prevention is important
   a. High-risk patients should perform daily foot inspections
   b. Teach how to maintain good foot hygiene, avoidance of injury or infection to feet (never go barefoot or wear sandals; wear well fitting shoes and clean socks), avoidance of factors that decrease circulation to feet (tight socks), necessity of smoking cessation and care when problems arise
   c. Diagnosis and treatment of foot ulcers
      (1) Refer high-risk patients to foot care specialist for preventive care and long-term surveillance
      (2) Refer patients with significant claudification for further vascular assessment and consider exercise and surgical options
      (3) Consider ordering x-rays and possibly other imaging studies to exclude subcutaneous gas, presence of foreign body, osteomyelitis, and Charcot's foot (presents with acutely swollen foot and no radiographic abnormalities; treatment is observation, rest, elevation, and immobilization as well as referral to specialist)
      (4) Consider obtaining a culture: irrigate necrotic tissue with sterile saline, followed by curettage of base of ulcer
      (5) Abscesses should be incised and drained; debride wound as needed
      (6) Minimize weight bearing on ulcer with bed rest, special shoes, casts

        (7)   Adequate nutrition is essential for healing
        (8)   May need surgical treatment
        (9)   If ulcer is infected, order Augmentin 500 mg PO TID
        (10)   Patients with slow healing ulcers may have decreased pulses and need Doppler studies to demonstrate that they are candidates for vascular reconstruction

9.   Hypothyroidism
    a.   About 10% of type 1 diabetic patients develop hypothyroidism
    b.   Periodically evaluate diabetic patients for abnormal TSH levels and goiters

O.   Follow Up: Scheduling of return visits will depend on type of diabetes, degree of glucose control, changes in therapeutic regimen, and presence of illnesses or complications of diabetes

1.   Patients beginning insulin or who are making a major change in their insulin program need frequent contact with the health team, possibly daily, until control is achieved and risk of hypoglycemia is low

2.   Patients beginning treatment with medical nutrition therapy or oral glucose-lowering agents may need weekly visits until control is achieved

3.   Most patients should be seen at least quarterly until their treatment goals have been achieved; thereafter, the frequency of visits can be decreased to every 6 months

4.   Increase visits if patients are involved in intensive insulin therapy, not meeting glycemic or blood pressure goals, or there is progression in microvascular/macrovascular complications

DYSLIPIDEMIA

I.   Definition: Elevation of one or more of the following: cholesterol, cholesterol esters, phospholipids, or triglycerides

II.   Pathogenesis

A.   Pathophysiology

1.   An elevated cholesterol level is an independent and significant risk factor for coronary heart disease (CHD)

2.   Blood lipid levels are regulated by lipoproteins or "carriers" which are a combination of lipids (fats) and proteins

3.   High-density lipoproteins (HDL), major carriers, are thought to prevent or delay atherogenesis because of their low fat content and their probable role in carrying lipids away from blood vessels to the liver for degradation

4.   The other major carriers, low density lipoproteins (LDL), are considered harmful lipoproteins because they keep cholesterol in the blood vessels, forming fatty deposits

5.   Chylomicrons transport triglycerides from the gut and are largest lipoproteins with the lowest density

6.   Very low density lipoproteins (VLDL) are triglyceride-rich lipoproteins produced by the liver and are associated with increased cardiovascular disease risk

B.   Etiology

1.   Primary hyperlipidemia results in defects in lipid metabolism and transport; occurs in individuals with specific inherited traits

2.   Several secondary factors can contribute to hyperlipidemia
    a.   Obesity
    b.   Low activity levels
    c.   High dietary saturated fat, cholesterol, carbohydrate, and calorie intake
    d.   Endocrine disorders such as diabetes mellitus, Cushing's syndrome, polycystic ovarian syndrome, hypothyroidism, lipodystrophies, anorexia nervosa, and acute intermittent porphyria
    e.   Renal disorders such as uremia and nephrotic syndrome,
    f.   Hepatic disorders such as obstructive liver disease, primary biliary cirrhosis, acute hepatitis, and hepatoma
    g.   Immunologic disorders such as systemic lupus erythematosus
    h.   Stress

      i.   Medications such as thiazide diuretics, loop diuretics, beta-blockers without intrinsic sympathomimetic activity, progestins, anabolic steroids, corticosteroids, and HIV protease inhibitors

      j.   Alcohol

III.   Clinical Presentation

A.   Empirical evidence is accumulating that atherosclerosis begins in childhood and that there is a relationship between childhood and adult cholesterol levels

B.   High levels of total cholesterol and LDL and low levels of HDL are major risk factors for CHD

C.   Most patients are asymptomatic, but symptoms arise with severe or longstanding dyslipidemia

    1.   In cases of hyperlipidemia due to specific inherited traits, cholesterol levels can reach as high as 1200 mg/dL and patients typically die of myocardial infarction before age 20; whereas patients with other types of hyperlipidemia do not develop symptoms of CHD until they are in their 60s or 70s

    2.   Dermatological manifestations can occur in severe cases; xanthomas (cutaneous or subcutaneous papules, plaques or nodules) may develop in the tendons, extensor surfaces of the extremities, buttocks, knees, skin folds, scars, and eyelids

    3.   Gastrointestinal problems may develop, particularly with hypertriglyceridemia

       a.   Severe abdominal pain associated with pancreatitis

       b.   Hepatomegaly or splenomegaly

    4.   Other clinical manifestations include premature arcus cornea, aortic stenosis, Achilles tendinitis, hyperinsulinemia, hyperuricemia, arthritis, and possibly cholelithiasis

D.   Metabolic syndrome affects over 40% of persons >60 years and increases risk of CHD

    1.   Also called dysmetabolic syndrome, syndrome X, and insulin resistance syndrome

    2.   Syndrome appears to enhance the atherogenic effects of low-density lipoprotein cholesterol

    3.   Syndrome is associated with prothrombotic and proinflammatory states

    4.   See following table for clinical identification of metabolic syndrome

---

METABOLIC SYNDROME CRITERIA

- Abdominal obesity (waist circumference >102 cm in men or >88 cm women)
- Atherogenic dyslipidemia (triglyceride ≥150 mg/dL, small LDL particles, HDL <40 mg/dL in men or <50 mg/dL in women)
- Hypertension (blood pressure ≥130/≥85 mm Hg)
- Fasting glucose ≥110 mg/dL

IV.   Diagnosis/Evaluation

A.   History

    1.   Ask about previous or present cardiovascular disease

    2.   Inquire about presence or absence of CHD risk factors (see table MAJOR RISK FACTORS in V.A.)

    3.   Explore past medical history including pancreatitis, renal disease, liver disease, vascular disease, diabetes mellitus, hypothyroidism, Cushing's syndrome, and immunologic disorders

    4.   Inquire about family history of premature cardiovascular disease or lipid disorders

    5.   Complete a medication history, focusing on drugs that elevate cholesterol levels (II.B.2.i.)

    6.   Explore amount of alcohol consumption

    7.   Determine amount and intensity of physical activity

    8.   Ask about occurrence of xanthomas and abdominal pain

    9.   If female, ask about menstrual history and type of hormone replacement therapy if applicable

    10.   Inquire about typical diet over a 24-hour period; to assess intake of LDL-raising nutrients, see table BRIEF DIETARY CAGE QUESTIONS

Adapted from National Institutes of Health. (2001). *Third report of the National Cholesterol Education Program (NCEP) Expert Panel on Detection, Evaluation, and Treatment of High Blood Cholesterol in Adults (Adult Treatment Panel III).* (NIH Publication 01-3670). Bethesda, MD: National Institutes of Health.

B.   Physical Examination
1.   Measure blood pressure
2.   Measure height and weight
3.   Observe skin for cutaneous xanthomas
4.   Palpate thyroid
5.   Perform complete heart and vascular exams
6.   Perform a complete abdominal exam; assess for hepatomegaly and splenomegaly

C.   Differential Diagnosis: rule out all secondary causes listed under pathogenesis

D.   Diagnostic Tests
1.   All adults ≥20 years of age need the following:
a.   A fasting (9-12 hours) lipid profile (total cholesterol, LDL cholesterol, HDL cholesterol and triglycerides) once every five years
b.   If non-fasting test is performed, only total cholesterol and HDL are useable; if total cholesterol is ≥200 mg/dL or HDL is <40 mg/dL, a follow-up fasting lipoprotein analysis is needed
2.   The following table presents the classification of cholesterol levels

ATP III CLASSIFICATION OF LDL, TOTAL, AND HDL CHOLESTEROL (MG/DL)

LDL cholesterol	
<100	Optimal
100-129	Near or above optimal
130-159	Borderline high
160-189	High
≥190	Very high
Total cholesterol	
<200	Desirable
200-239	Borderline high
≥240	High
HDL cholesterol	
<40	Low
≥60	High

Adapted from *Adult Treatment Panel III*

3.   Apolipoprotein (apo) B is considered the best measure to assess cardiac risk by some experts.
      a.   Apo B measures the number of LDL particles and their composition
      b.   May be a good measure to assess efficacy of statin therapy
      c.   Can be performed on nonfasting blood samples
      d.   Particularly useful inpatients who have hypertriglyceridemia, diabetes mellitus, type 3 dyslipoproteinemia, nephrotic syndrome, and liver disease.
      e.   Less useful to measure risk in patients with severe hypercholesterolemia

V.   Plan/Management

   A.   First step is to determine risk category
      1.   First category: persons with CHD or the following CHD risk equivalents:
         a.   Diabetes mellitus
         b.   Clinical atherosclerotic disease (peripheral arterial disease, symptomatic carotid artery disease, abdominal aortic aneurysm)
         c.   Multiple risk factors that confer a 10-year risk for CHD >20% (risk percentage for CHD can be determined in table FRAMINGHAM SCALE)
      2.   Second category: persons with both of the following:
         a.   Multiple (2+) risk factors (see table MAJOR RISK FACTORS to count risk factors)
         b.   10-year risk for CHD ≤20% (see table FRAMINGHAM SCALE to determine risk percentage for CHD)
      3.   Third category: persons having 0-1 risk factors

MAJOR RISK FACTORS (OTHER THAN LDL CHOLESTEROL) THAT MODIFY LDL GOALS*

Positive
- Cigarette smoking
- Hypertension (BP ≥140/90 mm Hg or on antihypertensive therapy)
- Low HDL cholesterol (<40 mg/dL)
- Family history of premature CHD (In first-degree relatives, CHD in males <55 years, in females <65 years)
- Age, years (men ≥45; women ≥55)

Negative**
- HDL Cholesterol ≥60 mg/dL

* Diabetes is regarded as a CHD equivalent
** Presence of "negative" risk factor removes 1 risk factor from the total count

Adapted from *Adult Treatment Panel III*

ESTIMATE OF 10-YEAR RISK FOR MEN
(Framingham Point Scores)

Age	Points
20-34	-9
35-39	-4
40-44	0
45-49	3
50-54	6
55-59	8
60-64	10
65-69	11
70-74	12
75-79	13

Total ** Cholester.	Points				
	Age 20-39	Age 40-49	Age 50-59	Age 60-69	Age 70-79
<160	0	0	0	0	0
160-199	4	3	2	1	0
200-239	7	5	3	1	0
240-279	9	6	4	2	1
≥280	11	8	5	3	1

	Points				
	Age 20-39	Age 40-49	Age 50-59	Age 60-69	Age 70-79
Nonsmoker	0	0	0	0	0
Smoker	8	5	3	1	1

HDL (mg/dL)**	Points
≥60	-1
50-59	0
40-49	1
<40	2

Systolic BP (mmHg)	If Untreated	If Treated
<120	0	0
120-129	0	1
130-139	1	2
140-159	1	2
≥160	2	3

Point Total	10-Year Risk %
<0	<1
0	1
1	1
2	1
3	1
4	1
5	2
6	2
7	3
8	4
9	5
10	6
11	8
12	10
13	12
14	16
15	20
16	25
≥17	≥30

10-Year risk _____%

ESTIMATE OF 10-YEAR RISK FOR WOMEN
(Framingham Point Scores)

Age	Points
20-34	-7
35-39	-3
40-44	0
45-49	3
50-54	6
55-59	8
60-64	10
65-69	12
70-74	14
75-79	16

Total ** Cholester.	Points				
	Age 20-39	Age 40-49	Age 50-59	Age 60-69	Age 70-79
<160	0	0	0	0	0
160-199	4	3	2	1	1
200-239	8	6	4	2	1
240-279	11	8	5	3	2
≥280	13	10	7	4	2

	Points				
	Age 20-39	Age 40-49	Age 50-59	Age 60-69	Age 70-79
Nonsmoker	0	0	0	0	0
Smoker	9	7	4	2	1

HDL (mg/dL)**	Points
≥60	-1
50-59	0
40-49	1
<40	2

Systolic BP (mmHg)	If Untreated	If Treated
<120	0	0
120-129	1	3
130-139	2	4
140-159	3	5
≥160	4	6

Point Total	10-Year Risk %
<9	<1
9	1
10	1
11	1
12	1
13	2
14	2
15	3
16	4
17	5
18	6
19	8
20	11
21	14
22	17
23	22
24	27
≥25	≥30

10-Year risk _____%

*Determine 10-year risk by summing points for each risk factor
** Total cholesterol and HDL-C values should be an average of at least two measurements
Adapted from *Adult Treatment Panel III*

B. Other factors are not included among the major risk factors for setting LDL goals but are targets for clinical intervention and can guide intensity of risk reduction therapy
   1. Lifestyle factors: obesity, inactivity, atherogenic diet
   2. Emerging risk factors: lipoprotein (a), homocysteine, prothrombotic and proinflammatory factors, impaired fasting glucose, and subclinical atherosclerotic disease
   3. Metabolic syndrome

C. Set treatment goals and begin therapy (see table LDL-C GOALS)
   1. Lowering LDL-C is the main goal of treatment
   2. Once the LDL-C goal is attained, other lipid and non-lipid risk factors can be treated
   3. Therapeutic lifestyle changes (TLC) are first-line therapies (see V.D.)
   4. Reserve drug therapy for higher risk patients
   5. **Always use** drug therapy along with TLC, **not** as a substitute for TLC

LDL-C GOALS				
	Risk Category	**LDL-C goal**	**LDL-C level to start TLC**	**LDL-C level to consider drug therapy**
1	CHD or CHD risk equivalent (10-year risk >20%)	<100 mg/dL	≥100 mg/dL	≥130 mg/dL 100-129 mg/dL: consider initiating or intensifying LDL-C lowering therapy, treat other risk factors, or use other lipid-modifying drugs (nicotinic acid or fibrates) if high TG or low HDL-C
2	2+ risk factors	<130 mg/dL	≥130 mg/dL	10-year risk 10-20%: ≥130* 10-year risk <10%: ≥160 * If baseline LDL-C is ≥130 mg/dL, TLC is initiated and maintained for 3 months before starting drugs
3	0-1 risk factor (10-year risk assessment not necessary)	<160 mg/dL	≥160 mg/dL	≥190 mg/dL 160-189 mg/dL: drug therapy optional; consider if single severe risk factor, multiple life-habits and/or emerging risk factors, or 10-year risk nearly 10%

D. Initiate therapeutic lifestyle changes (TLC) if LDL-C is above goal (see table LDL-C GOALS), regardless of whether drug therapy is started or not
   1. Nutrition: Recommend a Mediterranean-type diet (see table NUTRITION RECOMMENDATIONS)
      a. Total cholesterol intake <200 mg/dL
      b. Total fat may range from 25-35% of total calories, providing saturated fats are reduced to <7% of diet and *trans* fatty acids are kept low
         (1) Saturated fats are usually white, solid at room temperature, and derived from animals or tropical plants (coconut)
         (2) *Trans* fatty acids are hydrogenated or partially hydrogenated oils and found in most processed baked or fried foods and hard margarine
      c. Monounsaturated fats can provide up to 20% of calories and polyunsaturated up to 10%
         (1) A higher intake of monounsaturated fats (olive, peanut oil) can reduce LDL cholesterol relative to saturated fats
         (2) Polyunsaturated fats (most liquid vegetable oils) can reduce LDL when substituted for saturated fats in the diet
         (3) Omega-3 oils fatty acids reduce CHD risk as they have hypolipidemic, anti-inflammatory, antithrombotic, antiarrhythmic and vasodilatory properties
            (a) Eat variety of (preferably oily) fish twice a week
            (b) Include oils and foods rich in α-linolenic acid (flaxseeed, canola, and soybean oils; flaxseed and walnuts)
            (c) For patients with CHD, consume 1 gram of eicosapentaenoic acid (EPA) and docosahexaenoic acid (DHA) per day, preferably from oily fish; EPA + DHA supplements could be considered in consultation with the clinician
            (d) Patients needing triglyceride lowering therapy should take 2-4 grams of EPA + DHA per day provided as capsules under a clinician's care
      d. Carbohydrates should be 50-60% of total calories, mostly in the form of complex carbohydrates (whole grains, vegetables and fruits)

e.   Protein should be approximately 15% of total calories
     (1)   Soy protein can lower levels of total and LDL cholesterol
     (2)   Fish, especially cold water marine, are associated with reduced CHD
f.   The diet should be high in viscous (soluble) fiber (20-30 g/day); recommend psyllium, cereal grains, pectin-rich fruits, legumes, and vegetables such as broccoli, Brussels sprouts, and carrots
g.   Daily intake of plant sterols/stanols of 2-3 grams/day will lower LDL cholesterol
h.   Consider referral to a dietician
i.   Recommend patient access government-sponsored websites (see table GOVERNMENT-SPONSORED WEBSITES)

NUTRITION RECOMMENDATIONS

Food Items to Choose More Often	Food Items to Choose Less Often	Recommendation for Weight Reduction	Recommendations for Increased Physical Activity
Breads and Cereals ≥6 servings per day, adjusted to caloric needs Refined whole-grain breads and cereals, brown rice, dry beans, and peas **Vegetables** 3-5 servings per day fresh, frozen, or canned, without added fat, sauce, or salt **Fruits** 2-4 servings per day fresh, frozen, canned, dried **Dairy Products** 2-3 servings per day Fat-free, ½%, 1% milk, buttermilk, yogurt, cottage cheese; fat-free & low-fat cheese **Eggs** ≤2 egg yolks per week Egg whites or egg substitute **Fish, Meat, Poultry** ≤5 oz per day Fish, lean cuts loin; extra lean hamburger; cold cuts made with lean meat or soy protein; skinless poultry **Fats and Oils** Amount adjusted to caloric level Unsaturated fats: Olive oil, canola oil, peanut oil, vegetable oils, nuts, fish **TLC Diet Options** Stanol/sterol-containing margarines (Benecol); viscous fiber food sources; barley, oats, psyllium, apples, bananas, berries, citrus fruits, nectarines, peaches, pears, plums, prunes, broccoli, Brussels sprouts, carrots, dry beans, peas, soy products (tofu, miso)	**Breads and Cereals** Many bakery products, including doughnuts, biscuits, butter rolls, muffins, croissants, sweet rolls, Danish, cakes, pies, coffee cakes, cookies Many grain-based snacks, including chips, cheese puffs, snack mix, regular crackers, buttered popcorn **Vegetables** Vegetables fried or prepared with butter, cheese, or cream sauce **Fruits** Fruits fried or served with butter or cream **Dairy Products** Whole milk, 2% milk, whole-milk yogurt, ice cream, cream, cheese **Eggs** Egg yolks, whole eggs **Meat, Poultry, Fish** Higher fat meat cuts: ribs, t-bone steak, regular hamburger, bacon, sausage; cold cuts: salami, bologna, hot dogs; organ meats: liver, brains, sweetbreads; poultry with skin; fried meat; fried poultry; fried fish. **Saturated Fats** Coconut oil, butter, stick margarine	**Weigh Regularly** Record weight, BMI & waist circumference **Lose Weight Gradually** Goal: lose 10% of body weight in 6 months. Lose ½ to 1 lb per week **Develop Healthy Eating Patterns** ✓ Choose healthy foods (see Column 1) ✓ Reduce intake of foods in Column 2 ✓ Limit number of eating occasions ✓ Select sensible portion sizes ✓ Avoid second helpings ✓ Identify and reduce hidden fat by reading food labels to choose products lower in saturated fat and calories, and ask about ingredients in ready-to-eat foods prepared away from home ✓ Identify and reduce sources of excess carbohydrates such as fat-free and regular crackers; cookies and other desserts; snacks; and sugar-containing beverages	**Make Physical Activity Part of Daily Routines** ✓ Reduce sedentary time ✓ Walk, wheel, or bike-ride more, drive less; take the stairs instead of an elevator; get off the bus a few stops early and walk the remaining distance; mow the lawn with a push mower, rake leaves; garden; push a stroller; clean the house; do exercises or pedal a stationary bike while watching television; play actively with children; take a brisk 10-minutes walk before work, during your work break and after dinner **Make Physical Activity Part of Exercise or Recreational Activities** ✓ Walk, wheel, or jog; bicycle or use an arm pedal bicycle; swim or do water aerobics; play basketball; join a sports team; play wheelchair sports; golf (pull cart or carry clubs); canoe; cross-country ski; dance; take part in an exercise program at work, home, school or gym

Adapted from *Adult Treatment Panel III*

GOVERNMENT-SPONSORED WEBSITES	
Diet	www.nhlbi.nih.gov/chd www.nhlbi.nih.gov/subsites/index.htm -- then click Healthy Weight www.nhlbi.nih.gov/hbp www.nutrition.gov
Physical activity	www.fitness.gov
Body weight	www.nhlbi.nih.gov/subsites/index.htm -- then click Healthy Weight
Cholesterol	www.nhlbi.nih.gov/chd
Blood pressure	www.nhlbi.nih.gov/hbp
Smoking cessation	www.cdc.gov/tobacco/sgr_tobacco_use.htm

2. Stress weight reduction and patterns that promote weight loss (see table NUTRITION RECOMMENDATIONS)
   a. Discuss 10% weight loss goals
   b. Discuss portion control
3. Stress increased physical activity (see table NUTRITION RECOMMENDATIONS)
   a. Recommend 30 minutes/day of regular moderate intensity activity
   b. Give specific recommendations based on patient's age, cardiac status and how activity can be integrated into the patient's lifestyle
4. Government-sponsored website: www.surgeongeneral.gov/ophs/pcpfs.htm

E. For patients who did not meet LDL-C goals, but who were NOT started on drug therapy follow the steps in figure THERAPEUTIC LIFESTYLE CHANGES

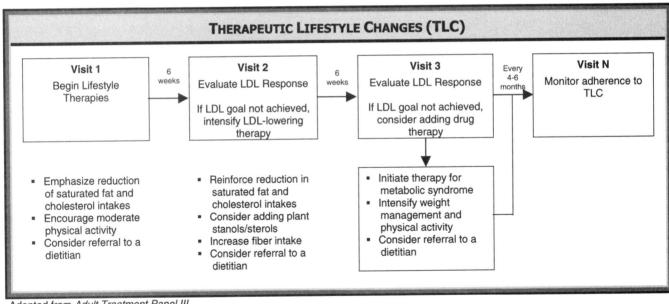

THERAPEUTIC LIFESTYLE CHANGES (TLC)

Visit 1	6 weeks	Visit 2	6 weeks	Visit 3	Every 4-6 months	Visit N
Begin Lifestyle Therapies		Evaluate LDL Response If LDL goal not achieved, intensify LDL-lowering therapy		Evaluate LDL Response If LDL goal not achieved, consider adding drug therapy		Monitor adherence to TLC

- Emphasize reduction of saturated fat and cholesterol intakes
- Encourage moderate physical activity
- Consider referral to a dietitian

- Reinforce reduction in saturated fat and cholesterol intakes
- Consider adding plant stanols/sterols
- Increase fiber intake
- Consider referral to a dietitian

- Initiate therapy for metabolic syndrome
- Intensify weight management and physical activity
- Consider referral to a dietitian

Adapted from *Adult Treatment Panel III*

F. Prescribe drug therapy for patients according to recommendations in table LDL-C GOALS (V.C.5.)
   1. Statins or the HMG-CoA reductase inhibitors produce the greatest LDL cholesterol lowering, are well-tolerated, and decrease mortality from CHD; considered drugs of choice for most patients (see following table)

SUMMARY OF STATINS (HMG-CoA REDUCTASE INHIBITORS)

Doses of available drugs

Atorvastatin (Lipitor)	Start 10 mg QD; max. 80 mg QD
Lovastatin (Mevacor)	Start 10-20 mg QD with evening meal; max. 80 mg in one or 2 divided doses
Simvastatin (Zocor)	Start 20 mg QD with evening meal; max 80 mg/day
Pravastatin (Pravachol)	Start 10-20 mg HS; max. 40 mg HS
Fluvastatin (Lescol)	Start 20-40 mg HS; max. 80 mg in 2 divided doses

Lipid/lipoprotein effects
- LDL decrease   18-55%
- HDL increase   5-15%
- TG   decrease   7-30%

Contraindications

Active or chronic liver disease

Use with caution

Concomitant use of cyclosporine, macrolide antibiotics, gemfibrozil, niacin, antifungal agents

Major adverse effects

Elevated hepatic transaminase, myopathy, upper and lower gastrointestinal complaints; use with anticoagulant may increase prothrombin time

Comments

Dosages should be adjusted at 6-week intervals
Order liver function tests at baseline, 12 weeks after starting, and periodically thereafter
Advise patient to stop therapy and order creatine kinase if patient reports muscle discomfort, weakness, or brown urine
Pravastatin metabolism is least affected by other drugs
Atorvastatin has the greatest LDL lowering effect
Do not take at same time as grapefruit juice
Generally, take at evening meal or at bedtime
In general, every doubling of dose lowers LDL by approximately 6%
Statins reduce the level of C-reactive protein (an inflammatory marker & emerging risk factor for CHD)

Adapted from *Adult Treatment Panel III*

2. Bile acid sequestrants are valuable in patients with moderately elevated LDL-C
   a. May be used as initial therapy in patients with hepatic disease, younger persons with elevated LDL, women considering pregnancy, or adolescents and children with marked hypercholesterolemia (see following table)
   b. May be added to a statin in patients if the LDL-C goal is not achieved

SUMMARY OF BILE ACID SEQUESTRANTS

Doses of available drugs

Cholestyramine (Questran Light)	Available in a 5 g packet or scoop (scoop is less expensive) Start 1 packet or scoop mixed with fluid or food 1-2 times/day; max. 4-6 packets or scoops in 2-3 divided doses
Colestipol (Colestid tablets)	Available in a 5 g packet or scoop or 1 g tablet Granules: 5-30 g daily once or in divided dose mixed with fluid Tablets: Start 2 g with adequate fluids 1-2 times/day; increase by 2 g 1-2 times/day at 1-2 month intervals; max. 16 g/day
Colesevelam (Welchol)	Available in 625 mg tablets; Take with meals, more easily tolerated than other sequestrants Monotherapy: 3 tabs twice daily or 6 tabs once daily; with statin: 4-6 tabs daily

Lipid/lipoprotein effects
LDL decrease 15-30%
HDL increase 3-5%
TG no change or increase

Contraindications
Familial dysbetalipoproteinemia
Triglycerides >400 mg/dL

Use with caution
Triglycerides >200 mg/dL

Major adverse effects
Gastrointestinal distress, constipation
Decreased absorption of other drugs (take other meds at least one hour before or four to six hours after the sequestrants)
Pancreatitis in patients with hypertriglyceridemia

Comments
To reduce GI complaints suggest the following:
- Take medicine slowly, reducing amount of swallowed air
- Increase fluid and fiber intake and drink with pulpier liquids such as orange juice
- May combine with psyllium hydrophilic mucilloid such as Metamucil

Adapted from *Adult Treatment Panel III*

3. Nicotinic acid is especially useful in patients with moderately elevated LDL-C, elevated triglycerides, and low HDL cholesterol (see following table)

SUMMARY OF NICOTINIC ACID

Doses of available drugs*	
Nicotinic acid derivative** (Niaspan)	>16 years: 500 mg HS for 4 weeks, then 1 g for weeks 5-8, then titrate to patient response and tolerance; do not increase by more than 500 mg in a 4 week period; max is 2 g/day
Crystalline (immediate release)	Start with 500 mg with food TID; adjust in increments of 500 mg at 2-4 week intervals; max. 4.5 g/day
Sustained (timed-release)	Usual dose 1-2 g/day, max is 2 g/d; greater risk of hepatotoxicity than other forms
Lipid/lipoprotein effects	LDL decrease 5-25% HDL increase 15-35% TG decrease 20-50%
Contraindications	Chronic liver disease, severe gout
Use with caution	High doses (>3 g/day) in type 2 diabetes mellitus; gout, or hyperuricemia
Major adverse effects	Flushing (less with Niaspan) and itching of skin, gastrointestinal distress, hepatotoxicity (especially sustained-release form); hyperglycemia, hyperuricemia or gout limit its use
Comments	Take enteric-coated aspirin before dose to lessen adverse effects Liver function should be evaluated before beginning niacin and 6-8 weeks after reaching a daily dose of 1,500 mg, 6-8 weeks after reaching the maximum daily dose, then at least annually Blood glucose and uric acid should be monitored initially, then 6-8 weeks after starting therapy, then annually or more frequently if indicated Lowers Lp(a), an emerging risk factor for CHD

* Many OTC preparations by various manufacturers for both crystalline and sustained-release nicotinic acid. The extended release preparation (Niaspan) is a prescription drug
** Swallow whole; take at bedtime with low-fat meal or snack. Avoid concomitant alcohol and hot beverage.
Adapted from *Adult Treatment Panel III*

4. Fibric acid derivatives or fibrates are effective for modifying atherogenic dyslipidemia, particularly lowering serum triglycerides (see following table)

SUMMARY OF FIBRIC ACID DERIVATIVES

Doses of available drugs	
Gemfibrozil (Lopid)	600 mg twice daily 30 minutes prior to morning and evening meals
Fenofibrate (Tricor)	54-160 mg daily; adjust at 6-8 week intervals; max is 160 mg/day
Clofibrate (Atromid-S)	1 g twice daily
Lipid/lipoprotein effects	LDL decrease 5-20% (may be increased in patients with high TG) HDL increase 10-20% TG decrease 20-50%
Contraindications	Severe renal disease Severe hepatic disease
Use with caution	Patients with history of gallstones; increased risk of rhabdomyolysis with statins; potentiates effects of anticoagulants
Major adverse effects	Gastrointestinal distress, cholesterol gallstones, myopathy
Comments	Fenofibrate appears to reduce LDL by a greater amount than other fibrates

Adapted from *Adult Treatment Panel III*

5. Ezetimibe (Zetia) differs from other classes of cholesterol-reducing compounds; ezetimibe acts on the brush border of the gut wall to prevent cholesterol absorption through the intestinal villi (see following table)

SUMMARY OF EZETIMIBE	
Doses of available drugs	10 mg daily as monotherapy or in combination with a statin; when used with statins measure liver enzymes prior to therapy and then periodically*
Lipid/lipoprotein effects	LDL decrease HDL increase
Contraindications	Hepatic insufficiency
Use with caution	Data unavailable
Major adverse effects	Upper and lower gastrointestinal complaints, myopathy, back pain
Comments	• Patients may take drug with or without food • Research is limited but recent studies found that ezetimibe is efficacious, safe, and that combination with statins is more effective than statin therapy alone

* Do not prescribe combination therapy to patients with altered enzymes

G. For patients on drug therapy, follow the steps in figure PROGRESSION OF DRUG THERAPY
   1. Ascertain that patient is adhering to therapy
   2. Most drugs can be combined, but some combinations should be used cautiously (see table DRUG SELECTION FOR COMBINATION THERAPY)
   3. Also, available is Advicor: each tablet contains 20 mg of lovastatin and one of the following 3 strengths of extended-release niacin (500, 750, and 1000 mg); starting dose is 500 mg niacin HS, increasing by no more than 500 mg of niacin every 4 weeks; maximum dose is 2000 mg/day of niacin

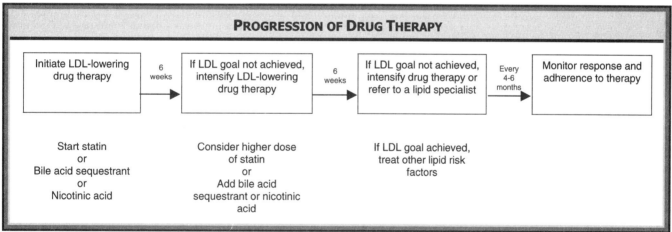

PROGRESSION OF DRUG THERAPY

Initiate LDL-lowering drug therapy → 6 weeks → If LDL goal not achieved, intensify LDL-lowering drug therapy → 6 weeks → If LDL goal not achieved, intensify drug therapy or refer to a lipid specialist → Every 4-6 months → Monitor response and adherence to therapy

Start statin or Bile acid sequestrant or Nicotinic acid

Consider higher dose of statin or Add bile acid sequestrant or nicotinic acid

If LDL goal achieved, treat other lipid risk factors

Adapted from *Adult Treatment Panel III*

DRUG SELECTION FOR COMBINATION THERAPY

Lipid Levels	Single Drug	Combination Drug
Elevated LDL-cholesterol and triglycerides <200 mg/dL	Statin Nicotinic acid (NA) Bile acid sequestrant (BAS)	Statin + BAS Statin + NA* NA + BAS
Elevated LDL-cholesterol and triglycerides 200-400 mg/dL	Statin Nicotinic acid	Statin + NA* Statin + fibrate[†] NA + BAS NA + fibrate[†]

*Possible increased risk of myopathy and hepatitis.
[†]Increased risk of myopathy. Must be used with caution.

Adapted from *Adult Treatment Panel III*

H. Identify metabolic syndrome and treat if syndrome is still present after 3 months of TLC (see III.D. for clinical characteristics)
1. Treat underlying causes: intensify weight management and increase physical activity
2. Treat lipid and non-lipid risk factors if they persist despite lifestyle changes
    a. Treat hypertension
    b. Use aspirin for CHD or CHD risk equivalent patients to reduce prothrombotic state
    c. Treat elevated triglycerides and/or low HDL (atherogenic dyslipidemia) (See V.I. & J.)

I. Treatment of elevated triglycerides (TG) (see table MANAGEMENT OF ELEVATED TG)
1. Elevated triglycerides are an independent CHD risk factor
2. Very low density lipoproteins (VLDL) are triglyceride rich lipoproteins and are the secondary target of therapy in persons with triglycerides ≥200 mg/dL; ATP III identifies the sum of LDL and VLDL cholesterol as non-HDL cholesterol (total cholesterol - HDL cholesterol)
3. Goal for non-HDL cholesterol in persons with high TG can be set at 30 mg/dL higher than that for LDL-C on the premise that a VLDL cholesterol level ≤30 mg/dL is normal
4. The following are non-HDL cholesterol goals for 3 risk categories:
    a. <130 mg/dL for patients in first risk category (CHD and CHD risk equivalent)
    b. <160 mg/dL for patients in 2nd risk category (2+ risk factors, 10 year-risk ≤20 years)
    c. <190 mg/dL for patients in 3rd risk category (0-1 risk factors)

MANAGEMENT OF ELEVATED TRIGLYCERIDES*		
The primary goal of therapy is to achieve the target goal for LDL-C		
Classification	Serum TG Level	In addition to achieving target LDL-C goal
Normal	<150 mg/dL	
Borderline-high	150-199 mg/dL	Reduce weight and increase physical activity
High	200-499 mg/dL	Non-HDL-C is secondary target (intensify LDL-C lowering therapy or add nicotinic acid or fibrate cautiously)
Very high	≥500 mg/dL	Initial aim is to prevent acute pancreatitis through TG lowering by using very low fat diets, weight reduction, increased physical activity, and a TG lowering drug (fibrate or nicotinic acid). After TG levels ≤500 mg/dL, focus on lowering LDL-C

* Recommend increased intake of omega-3 fatty acids. Supplements (2-4 g/day of eicosapentaenoic acid [EPA] and docosahexaenoic acid [DHA]) to augment diet are required
Adapted from *Adult Treatment Panel III*

J. Treatment of low HDL cholesterol
1. First reach LDL-C goal
2. Intensify weight management and physical activity
3. If triglycerides are 200-499 mg/dL, secondary priority goes to achieving the non-HDL-C goals (see V.I.4.)
4. If triglycerides <200 mg/dL (isolated low HDL), HDL raising drugs (nicotinic acid, fibrates) may be considered in persons with CHD or CHD equivalent

K. Treatment of elderly persons (men ≥65 years, women ≥75 years)
1. Most new CHD events occur in this age group
2. TLC is first line of therapy for primary prevention
3. No age restrictions are necessary for initiating LDL-lowering therapy

L. Special considerations for treatment in women aged 45-75 years
1. Hormone replacement therapy (HRT) did not lower CHD risk in recent studies
2. Cholesterol-lowering drugs such as statin therapy are preferable to HRT

M. Treatment of younger adults (men 20-35 years, women 20-45 years)
1. Early detection in young adulthood is needed to prevent premature CHD
2. Young adults with very high LDL-C (≥190 mg/dL) usually have genetic forms of hypercholesterolemia
    a. Family testing is needed to identify other relatives similarly affected
    b. Treatment usually involves combined drug therapy (statin plus bile acid sequestrant)

3.	For young adults with LDL-C ≥130 mg/dL, TLC should be started
4.	Young men who smoke and have LDL-C (160-189 mg/dL) are candidates for drug therapy

N.	Aggressively treat patients with diabetes and dyslipidemia (see section on DIABETES MELLITUS)

O.	In patients with chronic nephrotic syndrome, treat hypercholesterolemia (major lipid condition in this disease) with the statins

P.	Miscellaneous therapeutic approaches (research is limited on these approaches)
1.	Soy (proteins and isoflavones decrease total and LDL-C and TG); 25 g per day is needed to decrease lipid levels
2.	Cholestin (from red yeast extract); similar effect to low dose "drug statins"; 1,200 mg BID
a.	Available over the counter and may provide cost-saving option for patients without prescription drug plans
b.	Follow statin guidelines for monitoring liver function and creatine kinase

Q.	Follow Up
1.	Persons whose LDL-C levels are below goal at the first encounter should have repeat lipoprotein analysis
a.	<1 year if CHD or CHD risk equivalent and LDL-C <100 (should be on TLC)
b.	≤2 years if 2+ risk factors and LDL-C <130, or 0-1 risk factor and LDL-C 130-159
c.	≤5 years if 0-1 risk factor and LDL-C <130
2.	Persons on TLC who have reached goal LDL-C should be seen every 4-6 months to monitor adherence to TLC
a.	The patient can be counseled quarterly for the first year of long-term therapy and twice yearly after that; visits may be annual after the first year
b.	LDL-C is measured prior to each visit and results explained to patient
3.	Persons on TLC and drug therapy who have reached goal LDL-C are also seen every 4-6 months to monitor response and adherence to therapy
a.	Lipoprotein profiles should be assessed annually and preferably at each visit
b.	Regularly order liver function tests on persons taking statins or nicotinic acid
(1)	Statins require liver function tests initially, approximately 12 weeks after starting, then annually or more frequently
(2)	Nicotinic acid requires liver function tests initially, 6-8 weeks after reaching dose of 1500 mg, 6-8 weeks after reaching maximum dose, then at least annually
4.	Evaluate persons who do not reach goal LDL more frequently, such as every 6 weeks

HYPERTHYROIDISM

I.	Definition: Condition that results when tissues are exposed to an excess of thyroid hormone; clinical manifestation is termed thyrotoxicosis

II.	Pathogenesis

A.	Typically results from the uncontrolled secretion or release of thyroid hormones, thyroxine (T_4) and triiodothyronine (T_3), into the blood stream

B.	Etiology of hyperthyroidism in the general population
1.	Most common cause is Graves' disease, an autoimmune condition also referred to as diffuse toxic goiter caused by TSH receptor antibodies
2.	The second most common cause is toxic nodular goiter (Plummer's disease) which is due to a hyperfunctioning multinodular goiter
3.	Subacute thyroiditis has an unknown etiology (possibly viral)
4.	Silent (lymphocytic) thyroiditis often coexists with Graves' disease and may be an uncommon variant of Hashimoto's disease
5.	Postpartum (subacute lymphocytic) thyroiditis has possibly an immunologic etiology

6. Solitary, hyperfunctioning adenoma is less common and has an unknown etiology
7. Ingestion of or exposure to iodide-containing drugs (amiodarone) and contrast media and administration of exogenous thyroid preparations may be causative factors
8. Less commonly, other factors stimulate the thyroid to produce thyroid hormone:
   a. Thyroid-stimulating hormone (TSH) from a pituitary TSH-secreting tumor
   b. Human chorionic gonadotropin (hCG) from a choriocarcinoma
9. Subclinical hyperthyroidism is classified as endogenous (Graves' disease or nodular thyroid disease) or exogenous (treatment with levothyroxine)

III. Clinical Presentation (see table DIFFERENTIATING FEATURES OF CONDITIONS); elderly patients may have few symptoms and signs except for weight loss and cardiac abnormalities

A. Graves' Disease
   1. Condition is 8 times more common in females than males
   2. Often has an insidious onset; patients may be asymptomatic for months
   3. Elderly patients often present with less adrenergic symptoms (anxiety, tremor) and more cardiac dysfunction, dyspnea, atrial fibrillation, unexplained weight loss, and weakness
   4. Disease is occasionally self-limited, lasting 1-2 years
   5. Patients typically have one or more of the following complaints:
      a. Nervousness which manifests as irritability, inability to concentrate, emotional lability, or insomnia
      b. Weight loss may be present even though appetite is often increased
      c. Increase in bowel movements or diarrhea
      d. Heat intolerance is a common symptom
      e. Palpitations may be a troublesome, intermittent complaint
   6. The following are signs:
      a. Hair may be fine and silky; thinning of hair may occur
      b. Nails may develop onycholysis (irregular separation of the nail plate from the nail bed near its distal end), psoriasis (ridges in nail), or onychomycosis (thickening and yellowing of nail)
      c. Skin may have diffuse hyperpigmentation, particularly over the extensor surfaces of the elbows, knees, and small joints
      d. Pretibial myxedema that is characterized by erythematous, mildly scaly, indurated, nontender plaques on the skin of the ankles and pretibial areas may occur
      e. Eye changes include the following:
         (1) Ophthalmopathy and exophthalmos may cause diplopia, difficulty converging eyes, trouble in performing extreme movements of gaze, and in rare cases, blindness
         (2) Conjunctivitis
         (3) Lid lag
         (4) Lid retraction with increased scleral visibility above and below the iris often gives the patient the appearance of "staring"
      f. Thyroid may be visibly or palpably enlarged; thrill can sometimes be palpated or bruit can sometimes be auscultated
      g. Postural tremor, particularly of the hands, is commonly found
      h. Skeletal muscle wasting with proximal myopathy develops as the disease progresses
      i. Long-standing conditions may lead to osteoporosis and back pain
      j. In severe cases, signs of heart failure may be present

B. Thyroid storm, a life-threatening syndrome, occurs with decompensated hyperthyroidism
   1. Stressful events such as trauma and infection often precipitate an episode
   2. Symptoms such as nausea, vomiting, and abdominal pain may precede the storm
   3. Agitation, confusion, delirium, psychosis, or coma with high fever and diaphoresis may occur
   4. Tachycardia is always present; tachyarrhythmias may occur

C. Multinodular goiters (see section on THYROID NODULE)
   1. Usually affect older individuals who have long-standing goiters
   2. Often present with only subtle signs of hyperthyroidism such as weight loss, depression, anxiety, and insomnia

D. Subacute thyroiditis (also called painful thyroiditis or de Quervain's thyroiditis)
   1. Affected persons are usually aged 40 to 50 years; female to male ratio is 4:1
   2. Symptoms frequently develop after a respiratory or viral prodrome
   3. Severe pain in the thyroid area which often extends to ear on same side may occur

4. Low grade fever and symptoms of hypermetabolism are often present
5. With exception of exophthalmus and pretibial myxedema, presentation is similar to Graves' disease
6. Typically the erythrocyte sedimentation rate (ESR) is markedly elevated
7. As the disease progresses, patients may become mildly hypothyroid and eventually return to a euthyroid state with complete recovery within approximately 2-6 months

E. Silent thyroiditis (also called painless thyroiditis or subacute lymphocytic thyroiditis)
1. Many reported US cases occur in the Great Lakes region
2. Occurs between ages 30-40 years; female to male ratio is 4:1
3. Thyroid gland becomes enlarged and nontender
4. Half of all patients eventually develop hypothyroidism that lasts 1-4 months but occasionally hyperthyroidism persists

F. Postpartum thyroiditis
1. Develops in 5-10% of women within the first year after delivery
2. Typically has an initial hyperthyroid phase, followed by hypothyroidism, and eventually returns to euthyroid state; symptoms may persist for months

G. Solitary hyperfunctioning adenoma (see section on THYROID NODULE)
1. Elderly individuals are more likely to become thyrotoxic from the adenoma
2. Extent of patient's condition is positively related to mass of the nodule; nodules >4 cm in diameter often produce signs and symptoms of thyrotoxicosis

H. Transient thyroiditis may occur in association with subacute thyroiditis, lymphocytic thyroiditis, or Hashimoto's thyroiditis

I. Subclinical hyperthyroidism
1. Consistently low TSH (<0.1 microl U/mL) with normal free T_4 and T_3 levels
2. Some patients may have subtle signs and symptoms of thyrotoxicosis
3. Clinical significance is that condition may progress to overt hyperthyroidism and may have cardiac effects and cause a decrease in bone mineral density

DIFFERENTIATING FEATURES OF CONDITIONS CAUSING THYROTOXICOSIS

Cause	Thyroid Gland	FT_4I	TSH	RAIU
Graves' disease	Diffusely enlarged	↑	Suppressed	↑
Multinodular goiter	Nodular	↑	Suppressed	↑
Subacute thyroiditis	Tender, firm, nodular	↑	Suppressed	↓
Silent thyroiditis	Nontender, enlarged	↑	Suppressed	↓
Postpartum thyroiditis	Small, painless	↑	Suppressed	↓
Hyperfunctioning adenoma	Firm, enlarged	↑	Suppressed	↑
TSH-secreting pituitary tumor	Enlarged	↑	Normal or high	↑

FT_4I: free thyroxine index; TSH: thyroid stimulating hormone; RAIU: radioactive iodine uptake

J. Approximately 14-18% of patients taking amiodarone develop thyroid dysfunction (hyperthyroidism or hypothyroidism); obtain baseline TSH and at 6-month intervals during therapy

IV. Diagnosis/Evaluation

A. History
1. A complete review of systems is needed because symptoms may be subtle and involve every system of the body
2. Inquire about changes in weight
3. Obtain a complete medication history
4. Inquire about personal and family medical history; risk factors include previous thyroid dysfunction, goiter, surgery affecting thyroid gland, diabetes, vitiligo, pernicious anemia, leukotrichia (prematurely gray hair), and autoimmune diseases
5. Inquire about abnormal laboratory tests that suggest hyperthyroidism: hypercalcemia, elevated alkaline phosphatase, and elevated hepatocellular enzymes

B. Physical Examination
   1. Observe general appearance, paying particular attention to signs of nervousness or hyperactivity
   2. Measure blood pressure, resting pulse, temperature, and weight
   3. Inspect and palpate skin, noting pigmentation pattern, moistness, and turgor
   4. Inspect hair for texture and thickness, nails for ridges, discoloration or splitting
   5. Examine fingers and toes for thickening
   6. Examine eyes, noting exophthalmos, lid lag, and/or extraocular movements
   7. Test visual acuity
   8. Palpate for lymphadenopathy
   9. Observe the neck and palpate the thyroid, noting thrills, nodules, diffuse enlargement, firmness, and tenderness; measure size (see section on HYPOTHYROIDISM)
   10. Auscultate thyroid for bruits
   11. Auscultate the heart, noting murmurs and rate and rhythm
   12. Assess the abdomen for hepatomegaly and splenomegaly
   13. Do a complete neuromuscular exam, noting fast relaxation of tendon reflexes
   14. Evaluate for tremor (can place piece of paper on outstretched hand to observe for movement of paper with slight tremors)
   15. Test muscular strength; focusing on signs of proximal muscle weakness
   16. Assess lower extremities, noting pretibial myxedema

C. Differential Diagnosis
   1. Neoplasm is often suspected due to weight loss and weakness that typically accompanies hyperthyroidism
   2. Congestive heart failure and atrial fibrillation
   3. Psychological problems such as panic disorder and depression
   4. Tremors such as essential, physiological, cerebellar, and senile
   5. Suppressed TSH and elevated T_4 levels occur in conditions not associated with hyperthyroidism
      a. Estrogen administration or pregnancy raises thyroid binding globulin, resulting in high T_4 levels but normal free T_4 and sensitive TSH
      b. Glucocorticoids, amiodarone therapy, dopamine therapy, severe illness, and pituitary dysfunction may result in suppressed TSH in the absence of hyperthyroidism

D. Diagnostic Tests (see table DIFFERENTIATING FEATURES OF CONDITIONS in III.I. for typical test results with various types of hyperthyroidism)
   1. Screening: American Thyroid Association recommends that adults be screened for thyroid dysfunction with measurement of thyroid-stimulating hormone (TSH) at age 35 years and then every 5 years (see risk factors IV.A.4. & 5. to also guide screening)
   2. To diagnose hyperthyroidism accurately, order sensitive assay for TSH; expected value should be undetectable or lower than normal (0.02 or less microl U/mL)
   3. Consider ordering a free T_4 to confirm the diagnosis (expected values should be higher than normal); always order both T_4 and T_3 if pituitary problems are suspected
      a. Free T_4 measures unbound thyroxine in serum
      b. The alternative, second-line test, a total T_4, can be altered with estrogen and pregnancy
   4. If free T_4 levels are normal, order T_3 level because approximately 5% of hyperthyroid patients have normal T_4 levels
   5. Consider ordering 24-hour radioiodine uptake (RAIU) test in two situations
      a. To determine the correct dosage of radioactive iodine to treat Graves' disease or toxic multinodular goiter
      b. To differentiate Graves' disease and multinodular goiter from subacute thyroiditis and silent thyroiditis (in both types of thyroiditis the RAIU test will be low; whereas in Graves' disease and multinodular goiter it is elevated); test probably not needed to confirm diagnosis of Graves' disease if patient has ophthalmopathy, clinical hyperthyroidism, and diffusely enlarged thyroid
   6. Thyroid autoantibodies including TSH receptor antibody (TSI, TSHRab or TRab): not ordered routinely except in selected cases such as pregnancy
   7. Thyroid scan (either ^{123}I or technetium-99m) particularly useful in assessing the functional status of palpable thyroid irregularities or nodules related to a toxic goiter
   8. In females, consider performing a urine pregnancy test
   9. Computed axial tomography (CAT scan) or magnetic resonance imaging (MRI) of the orbit is often recommended for patients with exophthalmos, particularly those patients with unilateral eye signs
   10. Consider electrocardiogram for elderly patient or those with cardiac arrhythmias
   11. Consider dual energy radiographic absorptiometry to determine osteoporosis

V. Plan/Management

A. Three treatments (radioactive iodine, antithyroid drugs, and surgery) are available for acquired hyperthyroidism; patients and/or parents should be advised of risks and benefits of each treatment and collaborate in making decisions about their plan of care

B. Radioactive iodine (sodium iodide, I^{131}, Iodotope) is treatment of choice for most adults and adolescents who have Graves' disease and severe symptoms of thyrotoxicosis with multinodular goiter and single hyperfunctioning adenoma; increasingly recommended by specialists for children as well
   1. Many experts recommend an ablative dose of radioactive iodine whereas some prefer to render the patient euthyroid with smaller doses
   2. Radioactive iodine works slowly; most patients become euthyroid in 8-26 weeks
      a. In the days or weeks after administration, increased release of thyroid hormone may worsen hyperthyroidism; one of the following may be helpful:
         (1) Adjunctive therapy with β-blockers (see V.D.)
         (2) Others prescribe antithyroid drugs (see V.C.) before and sometimes after radioiodine therapy to deplete stores of thyroid hormone and prevent exacerbation of hyperthyroidism (particularly beneficial for elderly patients who are more at risk for serious heart disease); discontinue antithyroid drugs for at least 3 days before and three days after radioiodine therapy
      b. Monitor free T_4 and T_3 every 6-8 weeks; most patients become hypothyroid and require lifelong thyroid replacement therapy; therapy with levothyroxine is started when patient becomes either euthyroid or hypothyroid (see section on HYPOTHYROIDISM)
   3. Other considerations include the following:
      a. Ophthalmopathy may worsen with therapy
      b. Therapy contraindicated in pregnant women; always order pregnancy testing in patients who are scheduled for this therapy
      c. Women should use birth control 6 months after therapy, even though studies have not found teratogenic effects from therapy
      d. Breast-feeding is contraindicated

C. Antithyroid drugs, propylthiouracil (PTU) and methimazole (Tapazole)
   1. Although used extensively in the past as first-line drugs, today these drugs are reserved for patients with mild Graves' disease, small goiters, or to temporarily regress the thyroid sufficiently for thyroid ablation with either radioiodine or surgery in adults and adolescents; often preferred initial treatment for children, pregnant women, and patients scheduled for surgery
   2. Elderly and cardiac patients may be given antithyroid drugs before and after radioactive therapy (see V.B.2.a.)
   3. Drugs will control excessive production of thyroid hormone, but about half of patients will have a remission if no other treatment is instituted
   4. One of the following drugs is usually prescribed:
      a. Methimazole (Tapazole) is often first choice because it is long-acting; initial adult dosage is 15-60 mg daily in three divided doses depending on severity of disease (available in 5 and 10 mg tablets); when patient is euthyroid use maintenance therapy of 5-10 mg QD
      b. Propylthiouracil (PTU) has the most rapid onset with initial adult dosage of 100-150 mg every 8 hours (available in 50 mg tablets); when patient is euthyroid use maintenance therapy of 50-100 mg BID
   5. May need to give both these drugs at higher dosages if patient is severely ill
   6. It takes 4-6 weeks for patients taking methimazole and 6-12 weeks for patients taking PTU to reach euthyroid state; monitor with thyroid tests every 6 weeks
   7. Patients usually remain on drugs for 1-2 years, then drug is gradually withdrawn with the hope of permanent remission
   8. Instruct patient to call provider if severe sore mouth, sore throat, or fever develops (signs of agranulocytosis, a rare side effect of both drugs)
   9. Order WBC count before initiating therapy and then periodically during the first 3 months of treatment; however, agranulocytosis occurs so rapidly that periodic monitoring is not considered cost-effective by some experts
   10. A transient rash may occur; symptomatically treat with an antihistamine

D.   Adjunctive therapy:
1.   β-blockers may be initiated before or in conjunction with radioactive iodine therapy
     a.   Provide symptomatic relief, stabilize the patient with all types of hyperthyroidism, and reduce the signs and symptoms of thyrotoxicosis
     b.   Propranolol (Inderal LA) 160 mg daily with maximum of 720 mg or cardioselective agent such as atenolol (Tenormin) 50-100 mg daily with maximum of 200 mg
     c.   Teach patient to monitor pulse several times daily with a goal of ~80 beats per minute
2.   Patients who cannot tolerate β-blockers may be prescribed a calcium channel blocker such as diltiazem
3.   Gradually discontinue adjunctive therapy as soon as the patient is euthyroid

E.   Surgical therapy is a less frequently considered option due to potential complications such as hypoparathyroidism and vocal cord paralysis

F.   Thyroid storm, a medical emergency, requires prompt therapy
1.   Antithyroid drugs are often recommended and coadministered with corticosteroids, beta-adrenergic blockers and iopanoic acid (Telepaque)
2.   Other supportive measures include fluids, nutritional support, and electrolyte corrections

G.   Ophthalmopathy
1.   For mild cases prescribe eye lubricants such as artificial tears, petrolatum, or mineral oil ocular ointment (Lacri-Lube), apply 1/4" as needed; local mechanical therapies such as sunglasses, elevation of head of bed, bedtime diuretics, and eye protectors during sleep are helpful
2.   When condition progresses, refer to specialist and consider use of high-dose prednisone, orbital irradiation, or surgical decompression of the orbit

H.   Patients with multinodular goiter
1.   If patient has elevated T_4 levels and symptoms, treatment of choice is radioactive iodine, especially in older patients
2.   Patients who are euthyroid do not require pharmacological treatment unless the gland is cosmetically disfiguring or causing obstruction
3.   Baseline and follow up ultrasounds are useful for assessing changes in size

I.   Subacute thyroiditis is a self-limiting condition and does not require permanent therapy
1.   Nonsteroidal anti-inflammatory agents may be prescribed to relieve the pain; occasionally oral prednisone 20-40 mg per day in divided doses and tapered over two to four weeks is needed to control pain
2.   May prescribe β-blockers or anti-thyroid drugs when patient has thyrotoxic symptoms

J.   Silent thyroiditis does not require pharmacological treatment, however thyroid hormone levels must be monitored periodically as approximately 50% of these patients develop hypothyroidism
1.   Advise patient that condition will usually disappear in 4-10 weeks
2.   If symptoms are bothersome, β-blockers may be given

K.   Postpartum thyroiditis
1.   Acute symptoms are treated with β-blockers
2.   Antithyroid drugs are not indicated because the symptoms are caused by release of preformed T_3 and T_4 from the damaged gland
3.   When patient's symptoms are severe or longstanding in the hypothyroid phase, replacement of the thyroid hormone is indicated

L.   Treatment of single, hyperfunctioning adenoma is radioactive iodine

M.   Subclinical hyperthyroidism
1.   Treatment of endogenous subclinical hyperthyroidism is controversial but generally experts recommend monitoring TSH, T_4, and T_3 every 6 months; if patient has sustained TSH suppression (<0.1 microl U/mL) then therapy is usually recommended in following cases:
     a.   Subclinical hyperthyroidism associated with toxic goiter, toxic adenoma, and multi-nodular goiter
     b.   Elderly patients with atrial fibrillation or at high risk for atrial fibrillation
     c.   Patients with unexplained weight loss
     d.   Patients with osteopenia, osteoporosis, or menopausal women not taking estrogen replacement who are at high risk for bone loss

2. Treatment of choice for endogenous subclinical hyperthyroidism is often antithyroid drugs (low-dose is often recommended), but radioactive iodine and surgery are sometimes recommended, especially in patients with goiters and adenomas

3. For patients with exogenous subclinical hyperthyroidism, reduce dose of levothyroxine

N. Amiodarone-induced hyperthyroidism
1. In patients with type 1 amiodarone-induced hyperthyroidism (similar to iodine-induced hyperthyroidism) consider stopping amiodarone
2. For type 2 cases (resembles destructive thyroiditis) corticosteroid therapy is recommended; some patients require surgical removal of thyroid

O. Immediate referral for patients with a pituitary tumor

P. Patient education
1. Recommend a supplemental multivitamin; additional calcium and vitamin D may rebuild bone density lost during period of hyperthyroidism; remind patients that increased thyroid hormone is a risk factor for osteoporosis
2. Successful treatment of hyperthyroidism may be followed by serious depression; warn patient and family of this potential risk and frequently monitor mental health

Q. Follow Up
1. Patients treated with radioactive iodine
   a. Order free T_4 levels every 4-8 weeks until patient becomes euthyroid or hypothyroid and thyroid hormone replacement is needed
   b. Once patients are stable, schedule visits at 3 months, then 6 months, and then annually
2. Patients on antithyroid drugs
   a. Free T_4 level should be measured after a month of treatment and every 2-3 months thereafter
   b. Order WBC after several weeks of therapy and after any changes in drug doses
   c. Order liver enzymes every 3-6 months when patient is stable
3. Patients on β-blockers should be initially followed every 1-3 months, and then periodically depending on symptoms
4. Patients who are not treated with medications should be followed periodically based on their diagnosis and clinical presentation (i.e., every 3-12 months)

HYPOTHYROIDISM

I. Definition: Condition in which serum thyroid hormone levels are not sufficient to maintain normal intracellular hormone levels

II. Pathogenesis of acquired hypothyroidism

A. Primary hypothyroidism, the most common form, is the result of a defect in the thyroid gland causing it to produce insufficient thyroid hormone
1. Frequent cause is Hashimoto's thyroiditis (also called chronic thyroiditis)
2. Idiopathic hypothyroidism is most likely an autoimmune disease
3. Post-therapeutic hypothyroidism occurs after treatment (usually for Graves' disease) with radioactive iodine, surgery, or thioamide drugs
4. Transient hypothyroidism is often associated with acute or subacute thyroiditis which may have a viral etiology
5. Hypothyroidism can occur after hyperthyroidism in women following pregnancy (postpartum thyroiditis)
6. Less common causes include iodine ingestion, neck irradiation, and certain medications such as lithium or para-aminosalicylic acid
7. Subclinical hypothyroidism may progress to overt hypothyroidism; most common cause of subclinical hypothyroidism is Hashimoto's thyroiditis

B. Secondary hypothyroidism is due to the failure of the pituitary gland to stimulate the thyroid to produce sufficient T_4 levels; often occurs from postpartum pituitary infarction, granulomatous disease, or cranial mass lesion

C. Tertiary hypothyroidism is due to the malfunctioning of the hypothalamic-pituitary axis as a result of deficient secretion of thyroid releasing hormone (TRH) from the hypothalamus or lack of thyroid stimulating hormone (TSH) from the pituitary

III. Clinical Presentation

A. Severity of acquired hypothyroidism depends on the duration and extent of hormone deficiency; symptoms range from subtle symptoms to severe, multisystem problems with myxedema
1. Early symptoms have an insidious onset and consist of fatigue, dry skin, nail changes, slight weight gain, cold intolerance, constipation, and heavy menses
2. As disease progresses, following symptoms present: dry skin, yellow skin, coarse hair, hair loss of lateral eyebrows, eyelid edema, decreased sweating, slight alopecia, hoarseness, weight gain, cognitive changes, slow speech, forgetfulness, depression, and hypersomnia
3. Myxedematous changes occur in the later stage with thickened, scaly and "doughy" skin, enlarged tongue, muscle weakness, joint complaints, hearing impairment, bradycardia, possibly cardiac enlargement, pleural effusion, and ascites
4. Signs and symptoms of hypothyroidism may be similar to normal aging changes, making it difficult to detect the disease in elderly patients
5. Myxedema coma is an infrequent sequelae of long-standing disease
    a. Usually occurs in the elderly and is precipitated by intercurrent illness
    b. Symptoms, in addition to obtundation or coma, include hypothermia, bradycardia, respiratory failure, and possibly cardiovascular collapse
6. Patients with acquired hypothyroidism due to Hashimoto's thyroiditis have variable symptoms and typically experience transient hyperthyroidism that progresses to hypothyroidism whereas others remain euthyroid; in rare cases, the patient may change from hypothyroid to euthyroid or hyperthyroid

B. "Subclinical" hypothyroidism (sometimes termed "mild hypothyroidism")
1. Occurs in about 1-10% of adults with increased prevalence in women, elderly persons, and persons who have high dietary iodine intake
2. Patients have nonspecific complaints, normal levels of serum thyroid hormone but an elevation of TSH; may have an enlarged thyroid
3. Strong predictor of progression to overt hypothyroidism; progression is most likely in patients with goiters, thyroid antibodies, or both

C. With malfunctioning of the hypothalamic-pituitary axis, there may be loss of axillary and pubic hair, amenorrhea, and postural hypotension; low levels of TSH and T_4 will be present

D. Goiter or thyroid nodules are common in patients with hypothyroidism; sudden enlargement of thyroid gland raises concern of thyroid lymphoma (see section on THYROID NODULE)

E. The following groups of individuals are at high risk for developing hypothyroidism
1. Patients with a strong family history of thyroid disease
2. New mothers in the postpartal period
3. Persons over the age of 65 years
4. Individuals with autoimmune diseases (e.g., type 1 diabetes, Addison's disease)
5. Patients exposed to certain medications (lithium carbonate, iodide, amiodarone)

F. Hypothyroidism and other comorbidities
1. Diabetes mellitus
    a. About 10% of patients with type 1 diabetes mellitus develop chronic thyroiditis during their lifetime
    b. Periodically examine diabetic patients for development of goiters
    c. Sensitive TSH measurements should be obtained regularly, particularly if patient has goiter or other autoimmune disorder
    d. Postpartum thyroiditis develops in up to 25% of women with type 1 diabetes
2. Patients with infertility problems or menstrual irregularities often have subclinical or clinical hypothyroidism; in some patients with elevated TSH levels, levothyroxine therapy may normalize menstrual cycle and restore normal fertility

3. Depression
   a. Depression should alert clinician to possibility of subclinical or clinical hypothyroidism and need for evaluation and measurement of TSH
   b. Patients on lithium need periodic evaluation as lithium may induce goiter or hypothyroidism

IV. Diagnosis/Evaluation

A. History
   1. A complete review of systems is needed because symptoms are subtle and may involve every system of the body
   2. Ask about pain and swelling or enlargement in the neck
   3. Ask about history of radiation to the neck
   4. Inquire about previous endocrine problems in past or family medical history
   5. Obtain a complete medication history
   6. In women, determine date, characteristics, and duration of last menstrual period
   7. If patient was previously diagnosed with thyroid disease, ascertain past symptoms, treatments, and responses; in past, patients were frequently treated with medications for reasons that are unacceptable by today's standards

B. Physical Examination
   1. Observe overall appearance, noting slow movements and dull facies
   2. Measure height and weight
   3. Measure blood pressure, resting pulse, temperature, and weight
      a. Diastolic pressure may be increased
      b. Heart rate may be low or normal
   4. Perform a complete dermatologic examination
   5. Inspect head for coarseness and thinning of hair, thinning of eyebrows, thickened tongue
   6. Perform a complete eye examination
   7. Assess for lymphadenopathy
   8. Inspect the neck; fully extend neck and observe from front and side; observe for prominences and scars (evidence of previous surgery)
   9. Palpate neck and thyroid for the following:
      a. Tenderness
      b. Consistency (i.e., firmness, fluctuance)
      c. Measure size of gland
      d. Note whether there is a focal nodule or diffuse growth
   10. Auscultate thyroid for bruits
   11. Determine point of maximal impulse (PMI) as an indirect method for uncovering dilation and hypertrophy of the heart
   12. Auscultate heart, noting rate, rhythm, and murmurs
   13. Do a complete lung exam
   14. Palpate for splenomegaly
   15. Auscultate the abdomen, noting bowel sounds which may be diminished in hypothyroidism
   16. Perform a complete neurological exam; tendon reflexes may have a brisk contraction and a prolonged relaxation period in hypothyroidism
   17. Perform a musculoskeletal examination
   18. Perform a mental status examination

C. Differential Diagnosis: The following conditions mimic certain characteristics of hypothyroidism
   1. Ischemic heart disease
   2. Nephrotic syndrome
   3. Cirrhosis
   4. Depression

D. Diagnostic Tests
   1. Screen for thyroid disease in the following individuals:
      a. All symptomatic individuals
      b. Females >50 years, because of the high prevalence of hypothyroidism
      c. Past history of medically or surgically treated thyroid disease (screen annually)
      d. Past history of receiving supervoltage x-ray therapy to neck for nonthyroid cancer
      e. Patients with other autoimmune diseases and those with cognitive dysfunction, unexplained depression, and hyperlipidemia
      f. Patients on lithium therapy

g. Patients with type 1 diabetes; 10% of these patients develop hypothyroidism in their lifetimes; obtain sensitive TSH levels at regular intervals, particularly if a goiter develops

h. Consider screening for patients with infertility problems, repeated pregnancy losses, menstrual irregularities, and a family history of thyroid disease

i. The American Thyroid Association recommends that all adults have serum TSH at 35 years and every 5 years thereafter

2. Diagnostic testing for acquired hypothyroidism includes the following: (all tests may be normal in patients with chronic thyroiditis and certain medications [corticosteroids, dopamine] as well as illnesses and starvation may interfere with results of thyroid function tests)

a. A sensitive thyroid-stimulating hormone (TSH) assay (normal TSH concentration is 0.02 micro U/mL or less)

(1) TSH is elevated in hypothyroidism

(2) If serum TSH is normal, there is no need for additional thyroid tests as 98% of the time T_4 is normal when TSH is normal

b. Free T_4 assay in following circumstances:

(1) When TSH is elevated, a low free T_4 level will confirm the diagnosis of acquired hypothyroidism

(2) When hypothyroidism associated with pituitary or hypothalamic failure is suspected

(a) TSH may be normal, low, or mildly elevated (TSH does not rise proportionally to low T_4)

(b) Further evaluation is needed with results suggesting secondary or tertiary hypothyroidism: neuroradiologic studies, measurement of serum prolactin, and assessment of pituitary-adrenal and pituitary-gonadal function are indicated

c. If autoimmune thyroiditis is suspected, order either antimicrosomal antibody (anti-TPO antibody) which is test of choice or antithyroglobulin antibody; positive in 95% of patients with Hashimoto's thyroiditis

d. Thyroid scan or sonogram may be needed to evaluate suspicious structural thyroid abnormalities

e. The free thyroxine index provides an indirect estimate of free T_4 and is rarely ordered today

3. Consider ordering the following:

a. Serum electrolytes, blood urea nitrogen, creatinine, glucose, calcium, PO_4, and albumin

b. Urine pregnancy test

c. Urinalysis to detect proteinuria

d. Lipid studies for hyperlipidemia which often occurs with hypothyroidism

V. Plan/Management

A. Consult specialist when patient is myxedemic, has significant cardiac disease, has secondary or tertiary hypothyroidism, or is chronically ill or hospitalized with abnormal thyroid function tests

B. Pharmacological treatment with levothyroxine is the recommended first-line therapy for acquired hypothyroidism; prescribe a high-quality brand preparation of levothyroxine (Synthroid, Levothroid, Levoxyl) and always prescribe the same brand throughout treatment

1. Usual starting dose of levothyroxine is 50-100 micrograms (0.05-0.10 mg) per day, which may be started in young, otherwise healthy adults; increase by 25 micrograms QD every 4-6 weeks based on clinical condition and laboratory values; average dose is 125 micrograms (0.125 mg) QD and maximum dose is 300 micrograms (0.30 mg)

2. In elderly patients and patients at risk for exacerbation of heart disease the starting dose should be 12.5-50 micrograms (0.0125-0.050 mg); dose should be gradually increased every 2-6 weeks as tolerated until the optimal dose of 75-150 micrograms (0.075-0.150 mg) is reached

3. Continually monitor response to medication

a. TSH assay should be ordered every 6-8 weeks until concentration is normalized (keep in mind that TSH levels may remain elevated for several months despite effective treatment; rapid increase in medication based on TSH levels should be avoided because of the risk of thyrotoxicosis or excessive thyroid hormones)

b. Ask patient about symptoms of thyrotoxicity such as tachycardia, nervousness, tremor and evaluate with diagnostic tests

(1) If hyperthyroidism is confirmed the current dose of levothyroxine should be withheld for one week and restarted at a lower dose

(2) Some patients remain asymptomatic even with elevated free T_4 and/or TSH abnormalities; these patients should have their doses reduced until TSH concentration is normalized to prevent development of osteoporosis which may occur with levothyroxine over-replacement

      c.   Signs and symptoms of hypothyroidism should improve within 2 weeks and resolve within 3-6 months

    4.   Maintenance treatment is lowest dosage required to maintain euthyroidism with a nonelevated serum TSH and a normal or slightly elevated T_4

    5.   Drug interactions
        a.   Drugs such as cholestyramine, ferrous sulfate, calcium, sucralfate, and aluminum hydroxide antacids may interfere with levothyroxine absorption from the stomach; space levothyroxine at least 4 hours from these medications
        b.   May need to increase dose of levothyroxine when used with phenytoin, carbamazepine, sertraline hydrochloride, and rifampin as they increase the metabolism of thyroxine
        c.   Women on estrogen may need a higher dose as estrogen increases serum thyroxine binding globulin

C.   Triiodothyronine (T_3) is the active form of thyroid hormone
    1. T_3 or liothyronine sodium (Cytomel) is rarely used as an alternative medication
    2.   Low doses have been used in combination with levothyroxine (T_4) as T_3 may improve mood and neuropsychological function

D.   Treatment of subclinical hypothyroidism
    1.   Levothyroxine therapy is usually recommended in the following cases:
        a.   If thyroid autoantibodies are positive and TSH is ≥10 microl U/L
        b.   Patients with TSH levels between 5 and 10 microl U/mL in conjunction with goiter or positive anti-thyroid peroxidase antibodies or both
        c.   Pregnant women and women with ovulatory dysfunction with infertility
        d.   Patients with symptoms of mild hypothyroidism and hypercholesterolemia
    2.   The adverse effects of levothyroxine must be weighed against benefits
        a.   May improve subtle abnormalities, prevent goiter growth, forestall the development of frank hypothyroidism, and make the patient feel better
        b.   Therapy decreases LDL cholesterol and total cholesterol in some patients
        c.   Elderly or cardiac patient with only a slight TSH elevation may do better without levothyroxine treatment
    3.   Do not treat this condition with too high doses of levothyroxine which may cause subclinical hyperthyroidism and result in osteoporosis or cardiac dysfunction
        a.   Initial dose of 0.025 to 0.075 mg per day is usually sufficient; patients with coronary artery disease should receive 0.0125 to 0.025 mg per day
        b.   Measure TSH 6-8 weeks after starting therapy and adjust dose as necessary; target TSH level should be between 0.3 and 3.0 microl U/mL
        c.   Important to decrease dosage if TSH is suppressed below the normal range
    4.   Once a stable TSH is achieved, annual assessment is recommended
    5.   Patients who are not treated should be re-evaluated every 6-12 months

E.   Transient, sub-acute hypothyroidism
    1.   Usually condition is self-limited and symptoms resolve in 2-3 months
    2.   Therapy is not needed if symptoms are minimal; pain can be treated with relatively large doses of non-steroidal anti-inflammatory drugs
    3.   If symptoms are significant and hypothyroidism is prolonged, therapy should be started; re-evaluate these patients every 6-8 weeks

F.   Follow Up
    1.   When beginning medication therapy, patient's therapeutic response should be monitored every 4-6 weeks until TSH is normalized
    2.   After medication dosage is stabilized, schedule visits every 6-12 months and order serum TSH assays and consider ordering T_4
    3.   If drug dosage is changed, patient should have repeat TSH in 2-3 months
    4.   Values within normal limits imply adequate treatment
    5.   Undetectable TSH levels suggest over-treatment and medications should be decreased; over-treatment increases the risk of osteoporosis
    6.   Elevated TSH indicates under-treatment or noncompliance; after ascertaining that patient is taking medication, increase dose

THYROID NODULE

I. Definition: Thyroid nodule or nodules in an individual whose thyroid gland is otherwise normal

II. Pathogenesis

    A. Mechanism underlying thyroid nodule formation and growth is unknown

    B. Solitary nodules include the following types:
        1. Most palpable solitary nodules are actually the largest of poorly demarcated, multiple colloid nodules that merge with surrounding tissue in a small, multinodular goiter
        2. Benign adenomas are common and usually grow slowly; most patients are euthyroid but those with large adenomas may be hyperthyroid
        3. Follicular adenomas arise spontaneously from follicular epithelium and have well-developed fibrous capsules
        4. Thyroid cysts (15-25% of all nodules); may resolve after the diagnostic fine needle aspiration

III. Clinical Presentation

    A. Asymptomatic neck mass is the major clinical finding

    B. Singular nodules are more common in following individuals: Women, elderly individuals, persons exposed to ionizing radiation, and persons living in areas endemic for iodine deficiency

    C. Patients who actually have multinodular goiters may present with symptoms of thyrotoxicosis; however, as the nodules age, there is gradual loss of glandular function and they eventually become hypothyroid

    D. Malignant thyroid nodules must be differentiated from other nodules
        1. Fewer than 5% of all nodules are malignant; however, incidence is increasing
        2. Death due to malignant nodules is uncommon due to early detection and effective therapy
        3. Risk factors include extremes in age (<30 years and >60 years), history of head and neck irradiation, family history of medullary thyroid carcinoma occurring either alone or with multiple endocrine neoplasia type II (MEN II)
        4. Malignant nodules are usually large, fixed, nontender, firm, irregular and fail to move with swallowing
            a. Patients with malignant nodules do not usually have symptoms of hypothyroidism or hyperthyroidism
            b. Symptoms of local invasion raise probability of cancer
        5. Patients often have hoarseness and enlarged cervical lymph nodes

IV. Diagnosis/Evaluation

    A. History
        1. Ask about symptoms suggesting local invasion such as hoarseness, dysphagia, and obstruction
        2. Ask whether neck is tender or painful
        3. Inquire about symptoms that typically accompany both hypothyroidism and hyperthyroidism
        4. Inquire about history of external irradiation to head, neck, or chest, or exposure to nuclear fallout
        5. Inquire about family history of thyroid problems
        6. Ask about medication history
        7. Ascertain that patient is not pregnant

    B. Physician Examination
        1. Palpate nodule (see physical examination in section on HYPOTHYROIDISM)
            a. Determine whether nodule is single or multinodular
            b. Note tenderness, consistency, size, and whether nodule is fixed or movable
        2. Check for cervical adenopathy
        3. Check for signs of hypothyroidism and hyperthyroidism which require a complete physical with emphasis on the skin, eyes, heart, and musculoskeletal and nervous systems (see sections on HYPERTHYROIDISM & HYPOTHYROIDISM)

C. Differential Diagnosis: essential to differentiate malignant from benign nodules (see clinical presentation)

D. Diagnostic Tests
   1. Fine-needle aspiration biopsy has become the initial test in most patients with palpable nodules larger than 1.5 cm because it is safe, inexpensive, and results in a better selection of patients who are in need of surgery than other tests
   2. Order serum thyroid-stimulating hormone concentration to determine whether patient is euthyroid, hypothyroid, or hyperthyroid; if TSH is low, order a free T_4 to determine the extent of thyroid hypersecretion
   3. Radionuclide scans measure the amount of iodine trapped within the nodule and are useful in patients with indeterminate cytologic results; hot (hyperfunctioning) nodules have increased uptake and are benign in 98% of cases whereas cold nodules have decreased uptake and have the highest risk of malignancy
   4. Ultrasonography
      a. Can determine if nodule is a cyst or multinodular
      b. Cannot distinguish benign from malignant nodules but can be beneficial in determining rate of growth in subsequent visits
   5. Order serum calcitonin in patients who have a family history of medullary thyroid carcinoma or other components of MEN II

V. Plan/Management (usually refer patient to endocrinologist)

A. Patient can be followed without surgery or pharmacologic therapy if he/she has a negative fine needle biopsy and is euthyroid
   1. In past, asymptomatic patients with benign nodules were often treated with levothyroxine suppressive therapy to shrink the nodule
   2. Due to potential risks of osteoporosis and heart disease, today most experts carefully follow patients without levothyroxine treatment
   3. Nodules which increase in size should be biopsied again; if nodule is benign and enlarging, modest suppressive therapy is recommended

B. Patients who have abnormal thyroid hormone levels should be treated based on clinical guidelines presented in HYPOTHYROIDISM and HYPERTHYROIDISM sections

C. Main indications for surgery are malignancy, indeterminate cytologic features, disabling symptoms, or neck disfigurement

D. Patient Education: Instruct patient to call provider if there is change in nodule size, development of lymphadenopathy, pain, dysphagia, hoarseness, or new or worsening symptoms of hypothyroidism and hyperthyroidism

E. Follow Up
   1. Patients who have benign nodules and who are euthyroid require semi-annual to annual office visits to determine nodule's size and hormonal output
   2. Follow up ultrasonography is useful for assessing changes in size
   3. Patients with benign nodules but abnormal thyroid hormone levels and clinical manifestations need more frequent monitoring
   4. Follow up for patients with malignant nodules is variable

GYNECOMASTIA

I. Definition: Proliferation of glandular component of male breast

II. Pathogenesis: Due to an imbalance between serum estrogen and androgen levels with an excess of estrogens resulting in breast duct proliferation

   A. Physiologic causes: In adults, breast enlargement is due to normal or increased conversion of androgens to estrogens in extraglandular tissues

   B. Pathological causes
      1. Carcinomas: testicular, adrenal, pituitary, breast, lung, pancreas, colon
      2. Chronic diseases: liver disease, renal disease and dialysis, pulmonary disease, congestive heart failure, nervous system damage
      3. Malnutrition
      4. Hyperthyroidism or hypothyroidism
      5. Adrenal disorders
      6. Primary gonadal failure
      7. Secondary hypogonadism
      8. Drugs such as hormones (i.e., androstenedione), anti-infectives (e.g., isoniazid, ketoconazole, metronidazole), antiulcer drugs, cardiovascular drugs (e.g., digoxin, verapamil, captopril, spironolactone), psychoactive agents (e.g., diazepam, tricyclic antidepressants, phenothiazines), drugs of abuse (e.g., alcohol, amphetamines, heroin, marijuana), protease inhibitors for HIV infection, finasteride, phenytoin, and penicillamine
      9. Enzymatic defects of testosterone production
      10. Androgen-insensitivity syndromes
      11. Idiopathic gynecomastia
      12. Familial gynecomastia

   C. The most common type is idiopathic gynecomastia; drugs and alcohol, cirrhosis, malnutrition, and primary hypogonadism are common causes

   D. The following are risk factors for developing gynecomastia: Klinefelter's syndrome, obesity, testicular failure, recovery from prolonged severe illness associated with malnutrition and weight loss, positive family history, Peutz-Jeghers syndrome, male pseudohermaphroditism, and alcoholism

III. Clinical Presentation

   A. Physiological: Occurs in about 40-60% of men 50 years of age and older

   B. Pathological
      1. Tumors: Risk of breast cancer in males is proportional to the amount of breast tissue present; increased risk in patients with substantial gynecomastia
      2. Familial gynecomastia may be an X-linked recessive or sex-linked autosomal dominant trait
      3. Patients with other pathological causes present with variable signs and symptoms

IV. Diagnosis/Evaluation

   A. History
      1. Carefully determine the age of onset of gynecomastia, and its course and duration
      2. Ask about pain and discharge from breast
      3. Ask whether the breast(s) is(are) growing or shrinking
      4. Inquire about medication history; inquire about use of androstenedione
      5. Inquire about alcohol use and illegal drug use
      6. Obtain a complete nutrition history
      7. Determine whether patient is active in athletics and/or lifts weights to identify breast enlargement due to pectoral muscle hypertrophy

8.   Inquire about family history of breast enlargement
9.   Inquire about previous medical history including liver, renal, pulmonary, nervous, adrenal, pituitary, and endocrine disorders
10.   Ask about changes in libido
11.   Inquire about any recent weight loss or gain
12.   Explore the impact of the gynecomastia on the patient's lifestyle and self-image

B.   Physical Examination
1.   Obtain measurements of height, weight, and arm span to detect Klinefelter's syndrome
2.   Assess general health and observe for evidence of feminization, such as lack of male hair distribution and a eunuchoid body habitus
3.   Assess skin for signs of hepatocellular failure (jaundice, spider angiomata, palmar erythema) and hyperthyroidism (warm, sweaty)
4.   With patient lying supine, grasp breast between thumb and forefinger and gently bring the 2 fingers toward the nipple; a disk-like mound of tissue is often felt with gynecomastia
    a.   Measure dimensions of glandular tissue and areolae
    b.   Note consistency, tenderness, and mobility of any lesion or mass; squeeze nipple and note any discharge
    c.   Asymmetry and nodules deserve special attention
5.   Palpate for axillary lymphadenopathy
6.   Check for signs of thyroid hormone excess such as thyromegaly, tachycardia, diaphoresis, and exophthalmus
7.   Perform a cardiopulmonary examination for signs of congestive heart failure
8.   Check for signs of liver dysfunction such as hepatomegaly
9.   Deeply palpate upper abdomen for tumor of the adrenal glands or kidney
10.   Perform complete testicular examination
    a.   Measure size of testes (small, firm testes are characteristic of Klinefelter's syndrome)
    b.   Palpate for masses or tumor

C.   Differential Diagnosis: Gynecomastia may be a normal physiologic phenomenon or a result of a pathologic condition
1.   Pseudogynecomastia presents with smooth, fatty enlargement of breasts without glandular proliferation; more common in obese males
2.   In patients with Klinefelter's syndrome, gynecomastia occurs around puberty and patients have long limbs and small, firm testes
3.   Patients with cirrhosis and gynecomastia have loss of libido, loss of body hair, and testicular atrophy
4.   Breast cancer, uncommon in males, is characterized by a unilateral, hard or firm mass which is fixed to the underlying tissues and may be associated with dimpling of the skin, ulceration, retraction or crusting of the nipple, nipple discharge or bleeding, or axillary lymphadenopathy
5.   Neurofibromas, lipomas, and dermoid cysts are other breast masses that may present like gynecomastia

D.   Diagnostic Tests: ordered on the basis of patient's clinical presentation
1.   Order mammogram or fine-needle aspiration biopsy if breast enlargement is not characteristic of typical physiologic gynecomastia
2.   When the following characteristics exist, there is a need for further evaluation:
    a.   Males with genital abnormalities such as small testes with penile enlargement, hypospadias, or incomplete testicular descent
    b.   Gynecomastia that persists beyond 2 years or is unusually prominent
    c.   Males >18 years with recent onset of enlarging and tender breasts
    d.   Males who have physical abnormalities of unknown etiology
    e.   Breast masses which are large (>4 cm in diameter)
3.   Consider the following workup for the above mentioned group of males who need further evaluation (consultation with a specialist is recommended)
    a.   Begin with measurement of luteinizing and follicle-stimulating hormone
        (1)   High concentrations are associated with testicular failure, Klinefelter's syndrome, and hCG-secreting tumors
        (2)   Low concentrations may result from use of exogenous steroid such as androstenedione or may be more worrisome and due to autonomous androgen or estrogen production

b. Next, consider ordering the following tests:
  (1) Free testosterone to detect testicular failure and carcinomas
  (2) Serum estradiol; elevated in interstitial-cell tumors and feminizing adrenal tumors
  (3) Serum β-hCG level (may be elevated in carcinomas)
c. Consider the following additional tests in special cases:
  (1) Dehydroepiandrosterone (may be abnormal in adrenal diseases)
  (2) Prolactin (may be elevated in pituitary tumors)
  (3) Thermography and testicular ultrasound should be considered when patient has a suspected testicular tumor
  (4) Chest film to screen for pulmonary tumors and metastatic lesions
  (5) Thyroid, liver function tests, BUN, and creatinine, if indicated
  (6) Chromosomal karyotype (if both testes are small)

V. Plan/Management

A. Consultation with an endocrinologist is recommended

B. Postpubertal males who have had a thorough negative evaluation will also need assurance that the breast enlargement is not pathological

C. Males that have residual fibrous tissue may benefit from referral to a surgeon if they are embarrassed or emotionally distressed by the breast enlargement

D. Medical approaches to treating gynecomastia have included use of antiestrogens (i.e., clomiphene, tamoxifen), testosterone, nonaromatizable androgens, danazol, and diethylstilbestrol (DES)

E. Follow up will vary depending on patient's clinical diagnosis

REFERENCES

AACE Thyroid Task Force. (2002). American Association of Clinical Endocrinologists medical guidelines for clinical practice for the evaluation and treatment of hyperthyroidism and hypothyroidism. *Endocrine Practice, 8,* 457-469.

Alexander, E.K., Hurwitz, S., Heering, J.P., Benson, C.B., Frates, M.C., Doubilet, P.M., et al. (2003). Natural history of benign and solid thyroid nodules. *Annals of Internal Medicine, 138,* 315-318.

ALLHAT Officers and Coordinators for the ALLHAT Collaborative Research Group. (2002). Major outcomes in moderately hypercholesterolemic, hypertensive patients randomized to pravastatin vs usual care: The Antihypertensive and Lipid-Lowering treatment to prevent Heart Attack Trial (ALLHAT-LLT). *JAMA, 288,* 2998-3007.

American Association of Clinical Endocrinologists and American College of Endocrinology. (1995). AACE clinical practice guidelines for the evaluation and treatment of hyperthyroidism and hypothyroidism. *Endocrine Practice, 1,* 56-62.

American Association of Clinical Endocrinologists. (2000). AACE medical guidelines for clinical practice for the diagnosis and treatment of dyslipidemia and prevention of atherogenesis. *Endocrine Practice, 6,* 162-213.

American Association of Clinical Endocrinologists. (2001). AACE Consensus Conference guidelines for glycemic control. *Endocrine Practice.*

American Association of Clinical Endocrinologists. (2002). Medical guidelines for the management of diabetes mellitus: The AACE system of intensive diabetes self management – 2002 update. *Endocrine Practice, 8*(Suppl. 1), 41-82.

American Diabetes Association. (2003). Aspirin therapy in diabetes. *Diabetes Care, 26*(Suppl. 1), S87-S88.

American Diabetes Association. (2003). Evidence-based nutrition principles and recommendations for the treatment and prevention of diabetes and related complications. *Diabetes Care, 26*(Suppl. 1), S51-S61.

American Diabetes Association. (2003). Hyperglycemic crisis in patients with diabetes mellitus. *Diabetes Care, 26*(Suppl. 1), S109-S117.

American Diabetes Association. (2003). Hospital admission guidelines for diabetes mellitus. *Diabetes Care, 26*(Suppl. 1), S118.

American Diabetes Association. (2003). Immunization and the prevention of influenza and pneumococcal disease in people with diabetes. *Diabetes Care, 26*(Suppl. 1), S126-S128.

American Diabetes Association. (2003). Implications of the United Kingdom prospective diabetes study. *Diabetes Care, 26*(Suppl. 1), S28-S32.

American Diabetes Association. (2003). Insulin administration. *Diabetes Care, 26*(Suppl. 1), S121-S124.

American Diabetes Association. (2003). Management of dyslipidemia in adults with diabetes. *Diabetes Care, 26*(Suppl. 1), S83-S86.

American Diabetes Association. (2003). Report of the Expert Committee on the diagnosis and classification of diabetes mellitus. *Diabetes Care, 26*(Suppl. 1), S5-S20.

American Diabetes Association. (2003). Screening for diabetes. *Diabetes Care, 26*(Suppl. 1), S21-S24.

American Diabetes Association. (2003). Standards of medical care for people with diabetes mellitus. *Diabetes Care, 26*(Suppl. 1), S33-S50

American Diabetes Association. (2003). Tests of glycemia in diabetes. *Diabetes Care, 26*(Suppl. 1), S106-S108.

American Diabetes Association. (2003). Treatment of hypertension in adults with diabetes. *Diabetes Care, 26*(Suppl. 1), S80-S82.

American Diabetes Association. (2003). Diabetic nephropathy. *Diabetes Care, 26*(Suppl. 1), S94-S98.

American Heart Association. (2001). Summary of the scientific conference on dietary fatty acids and cardiovascular health. *Circulation, 103,* 1034-1039.

Arafah, B. M. (2001). Increased need for thyroxine in women with hypothyroidism during estrogen therapy. *New England Journal of Medicine, 344,* 1743-1749.

Biondi, B., Palmieri, E.A., & Fazio, S. (2000). Endogenous subclinical hyperthyroidism is not a benign process. *Journal of Clinical Endocrinology and Metabolism, 85,* 4701-4705.

Biondi, B., Palmieri, E.A., Lombardi, G., & Fazio, S. (2002). Effects of subclinical thyroid dysfunction on the heart. *Annals of Internal Medicine, 137,* 904-914.

Brown, A.B. (2001). Individualizing insulin therapy for optimum glycemic control. *Patient Care, 35,* 35-47.

Brown, B. G., Zhao, X.Q., Chait, A., Fisher, L.D, Cheung, M.C., Morse, J.S., Dowdy, R.D., Marino, E.K., Bolson, E.L., Alapovic, P., Frohlich, J., & Albers, J.J. (2001). Simvastatin and niacin, antioxidant vitamins, or the combination for the prevention of coronary disease. *New England Journal of Medicine, 345,* 1583-1592.

Bunevicius, R., Kazanavicius, G., Zalinkevicius, R., & Prange, A.J. (1999). Effects of thyroxine as compared with thyroxine plus triiodothyronine in patients with hypothyroidism. *New England Journal of Medicine, 340,* 424-470.

Burman, K.D. (2001). Hyperthyroidism. In K.L. Becker (Ed.), *Principles and practice of endocrinology and metabolism* (3rd ed.). Philadelphia: Lippincott.

Cooper, D.S. (2001). Subclinical hypothyroidism. *New England Journal of Medicine, 345,* 260-265.

Deblinger, L, Colwell, J.A., & Feinglos, M.N. (2001). Using insulin in type 2 diabetes. *Patient Care, 35,* 36-48.

DeFronzo, R.A. (1999). Pharmacologic therapy for type 2 diabetes mellitus. *Annals of Internal Medicine, 131,* 281-303.

Diabetes Prevention Program Research Group. (2002). Reduction in the incidence of type 2 diabetes with lifestyle intervention or metformin. *New England Journal of Medicine, 346,* 393-403.

Dujovne, C.A., Ettinger, M.P., McNeer, J.F., Lipka, L.J., LeBeaut, A.P., Suresh, R., et al. (2002). Efficacy and safety of a potent new selective cholesterol absorption inhibitor, ezetimibe, in patients with primary hypercholesterolemia. *American Journal of Cardiology, 90,* 1092-1097.

Feldman, E.L., Stevens, M.J., Russell, J.W., & Greene, D.A. (2001). Diabetic neuropathy. In K.L. Becker (Ed.), *Principles and practice of endocrinology and metabolism* (3rd ed.). Philadelphia: Lippincott.

Ford, E.S., Giles, W.H., & Deitz, W.H. (2002). Prevalence of the metabolic syndrome among US adults: Findings from the Third National Health and Nutrition Examination Survey. *JAMA, 287,* 356-359.

Goroll, A.H., & Mulley, A.G. (2000). Approach to the patient with hyperthyroidism. In A.H. Goroll & A.G. Mulley. *Primary care medicine: Evaluation of the adult patient* (4th ed.). Philadelphia: Lippincott.

Goroll, A.H., & Mulley, A.G. (2000). Approach to the patient with hypothyroidism. In A.H. Goroll & A.G. Mulley. *Primary care medicine: Evaluation of the adult patient* (4th ed.). Philadelphia: Lippincott.

Goroll, A.H., & Mulley, A.G. (2000). Evaluation of gynecomastia. In A.H. Goroll & A.G. Mulley. *Primary care medicine: Evaluation of the adult patient.* (4th ed.). Philadelphia: Lippincott.

Goroll, A.H., & Mulley, A.G. (2000). Evaluation of thyroid nodules. In A.H. Goroll & A.G. Mulley. *Primary care medicine: Evaluation of the adult patient* (4th ed.). Philadelphia: Lippincott.

Harper, C.R., & Jacobson, T.A. (2001). The fats of life: The role of omega-3 fatty acids in the prevention of coronary heart disease. *Archives of Internal Medicine, 161,* 2185-2192.

Hermus, A.R., & Huysmans, D.A. (1998). Treatment of benign nodular thyroid disease. *New England Journal of Medicine, 338,* 1438-1447.

Hever, D., Yip, I., Ashley, J.M., Elashoff, D.A., & Go, V.L. (1999). Cholesterol-lowering effects of a proprietary Chinese red-yeast -rice dietary supplement. *American Journal of Clinical Nutrition, 69,* 231-236.

Holmboe, E.S. (2002). Oral antihyperglycemic therapy for type 2 diabetes: Clinical applications. *JAMA, 287,* 373-376.

Hueston, W.J. (2001). Treatment of hypothyroidism. *American Family Physician, 64,* 1717-1724.

Inzucchi, S.E. (2002). Oral antihyperglycemic therapy for type 2 diabetes. *JAMA, 287,* 360-372.

Jackson, I.M., & Hennessey, J.V. (2001). Thyroiditis. In K.L. Becker (Ed.), *Principles and practice of endocrinology and metabolism* (3rd ed.). Philadelphia: Lippincott.

Jenkins, D.J.A., Kendall, C.W.C., Augustin, L.S.A., Franceschi, S., Hamidi, M., Marchie, A., et al. (2002). Glycemic index: Overview of implications in health and disease. *American Journal of Clinical Nutrition, 76*(Suppl.), 266S-273S.

Knopp, R.H. (1999). Drug treatment of lipid disorders. *New England Journal of Medicine, 341,* 498-511.

Kris-Etherton, P.M., Harris, W.S., Appel, L.J. for Nutrition Committee. (2002). Fish consumption, fish oil, omega-3 fatty acids, and cardiovascular disease. *Circulation, 106,* 2747-2757.

Ladenson, P.W., Singer, P.A., Ain, D.B., Bagchi, N., Bigos, S.T., Levy, E.G., Smith, S.A., & Daniels, G.H. (2000). American Thyroid Association guidelines for detection of thyroid dysfunction. *Archives of Internal Medicine, 160,* 1573-1575.

Ludwig, D.S. (2002) The glycemic index: Physiological mechanisms relating to obesity, diabetes, and cardiovascular disease. *JAMA, 287,* 2414-2423.

Luna, B., & Feinglos, M.N. (2001). Oral agents in the management of type 2 diabetes mellitus. *American Family Physician, 63,* 1747-1756.

Mahley, R.W. (2001). Biochemistry and physiology of lipid and lipoprotein metabolism. In K.L. Becker (Ed.), *Principles and practice of endocrinology and metabolism* (3rd ed.). Philadelphia: Lippincott.

Mazzaferri, E. L. (2001). Thyroid cancer. In K.L. Becker (Ed.), *Principles and practice of endocrinology and metabolism* (3rd ed.). Philadelphia: Lippincott.

Morelli, V., & Zoorkob, R.J. (2000). Alternative therapies: Part II. Congestive heart failure and hypercholesterolemia. *American Family Physician, 62,* 1325-1330.

Nathan, D.M. (2002). Clinical practice. Initial management of glycemia in type 2 diabetes mellitus. *New England Journal of Medicine, 347,* 1342-1349.

National Cholesterol Education Program. (1997). *Cholesterol lowering in the patient with coronary heart disease.* (NIH Publication No. 97-3794). Bethesda, MD: National Institutes of Health, National Heart, Lung, and Blood Institute.

National Institutes of Health. (2001). *Third Report of the National Cholesterol Education Program Expert Panel on Detection, Evaluation, and Treatment of High Blood Cholesterol in Adults (Adult Treatment Panel III).* (NIH Publication 01-3670). Bethesda, MD: National Institutes of Health.

Neuman, J.F. (1997). Evaluation and treatment of gynecomastia. *American Family Physician, 55,* 1835-1844.

Sandeep, V., & Hayward, R.A. (2003). Treatment of hypertension in type 2 diabetes mellitus: Blood pressure goals, choice of agents, and setting priorities in diabetes care. *Annals of Internal Medicine, 138,* 593-602.

Saunders, C.S., Keane, W.F., & Nelson, R.G. (2001). Advances in slowing the progress of diabetic nephropathy. *Patient Care, 35,* 28-41.

Schaeffer, E.J. (2001). Lipoprotein disorders. In K.L. Becker (Ed.), *Principles and practice of endocrinology and metabolism* (3rd ed.). Philadelphia: Lippincott.

Schwetz, B.A. (2001). New diabetes glucose test. *JAMA, 285,* 56.

Shapiro, L.E., & Surks, M.I. (2001). Hypothyroidism. In K.L. Becker (Ed.), *Principles and practice of endocrinology and metabolism* (3rd ed.). Philadelphia: Lippincott.

Slatosky, J., Shipton, B., & Haney, W. (2000). Thyroiditis: Differential diagnosis and management. *American Family Physician, 61,* 1047-1054.

Smallridge, R.C. (2000). Postpartum thyroid disease: A model of immunologic dysfunction. *Clinical and Applied Immunology Reviews, 1,* 89-103.

Sniderman, A.D. (2002). How, when, and why to use apolipoprotein B in clinical practice. *American Journal of Cardiology, 90*(Suppl), 48i-54i.

Snow, V., Weiss, K.B., Mottur-Pilson, C. for the Clinical Efficacy Assessment Subcommittee of the American College of Physicians. (2003). The evidence base for tight blood pressure control in the management of type 2 diabetes mellitus. *Annals of Internal Medicine, 138,* 587-592.

Toft, A.D. (2001). Subclinical hyperthyroidism. *New England Journal of Medicine, 345,* 512-516.

Tuomilehto, J., Lindstrom, J., Ericksson, J.G., Valle, T.T., Hamalainen, H., Ilanne-Parikka, P., et al. (2001). Prevention of type 2 diabetes mellitus by changes in lifestyle among subjects with impaired glucose tolerance. *New England Journal of Medicine, 344,* 1343-1350.

US Preventive Services Task Force (USPSTF). (2003). Screening for type 2 diabetes mellitus in adults: Recommendations and rationale. *Annals of Internal Medicine, 138,* 212-214.

Veterans Health Administration & Department of Defense. (2001). *VHA/DoD Clinical practice guideline for the management of dyslipidemia in primary care.* Washington DC: Author.

Vijan, S., & Hayward, R.A. (2003). Treatment of hypertension in type 2 diabetes mellitus: Blood pressure goals, choice of agents and setting priorities in diabetes care. Annals of Internal Medicine, 138, 593-602.

Wartofsky, L., & Ahmann, A.J. (2001). The thyroid nodule. In K.L. Becker (Ed.), *Principles and practice of endocrinology and metabolism* (3rd ed.). Philadelphia: Lippincott.

Weir, G.C. (2001). Insulin therapy and its complications. In K.L. Becker (Ed.), *Principles and practice of endocrinology and metabolism* (3rd ed.). Philadelphia: Lippincott.

Welker, M.J. & Orlov, D. (2003). Thyroid nodules. *American Family Physician, 67,* 559-566, 573-574.

White, J.R., Campbell, R.K., & Yarborough, P.C. (2001). Diabetes management therapies. In M.E. Franz (Ed.). *A core curriculum for diabetes educators* (4th ed.). Chicago: American Association of Diabetes Educators.

Willett, W.C. (2001). *Eat, drink, and be healthy.* New York: Simon & Shuster.

Infectious Disease

CONSTANCE R. UPHOLD

Cat Scratch Disease

Fifth Disease (Erythema Infectiosum)

Influenza
>   *Table: Websites for Information on Influenza*
>   *Table: Selection of an Antiviral Drug for Treatment*
>   *Table: Properties of Antiviral Drugs*
>   *Table: Target Groups for Influenza Vaccine*
>   *Table: Dose and Schedule for Influenza Vaccine*
>   *Table: Persons for Whom Chemoprophylaxis Is Indicated*

Lyme Disease
>   *Table: Recommended Treatment of Lyme Disease*

Mononucleosis, Infectious

Rocky Mountain Spotted Fever

Rubella (German Measles)

Rubeola (Measles)

Varicella (Chickenpox)
>   *Table: Clinical Features that Distinguish Chickenpox from Smallpox*

CAT SCRATCH DISEASE

I. Definition: Infection causing unilateral regional adenitis, usually due to scratch of a cat

II. Pathogenesis

   A. *Bartonella henselae* (previously *Rochalimaea)* is the causative pathogen in most cases

   B. Pathogen enters the body through a break in the skin, primarily caused by the scratch of a cat (usually cats are immature and not ill); dogs, monkeys, and fleas are other possible transmitters; no evidence of person-to-person transmission

   C. Period of communicability is unknown

III. Clinical Presentation

   A. Diagnosis of cat scratch disease (CSD) is based on the presence of 3 out of 4 of the following criteria:
      1. History of animal (usually cat) contact, with presence of a scratch or inoculation lesion of the eye, skin, or mucous membrane
      2. Positive cat scratch disease skin test
      3. Regional lymphadenopathy (predominant sign) with normal laboratory results for other causes of lymphadenopathy
      4. Biopsied lymph node that has characteristic histopathologic features

   B. Natural history:
      1. Cat scratch occurs and produces a primary cutaneous lesion 7-12 days later; lesion typically begins as a macule, progresses to a papule, then to a vesicle
      2. Nodes that drain the site of inoculation enlarge in 1-2 weeks after lesion appears
         a. Node is usually singular, but may present in a cluster; typically node measures between 1.5-5.0 cm
         b. Area around affected node is usually tender, warm, erythematous, and indurated

   C. In most cases, the illness is self-limited with minimal malaise, headaches, and generalized aching; approximately 30% of cases have fever and mild systemic symptoms

   D. Lymphadenopathy usually regresses within 2-4 months, but may persist for more than a year

   E. Occasionally, Parinaud oculoglandular syndrome develops
      1. Soft granuloma or polyp develops on palpebral conjunctiva
      2. Preauricular lymphadenopathy is usually present
      3. Patient typically does not recall cat scratch; hypothesized that pathogen is transmitted in saliva left on cat's fur; patient pets cat, rubs eye, and transmits organism to conjunctiva

   F. Rare complications include encephalitis, splenomegaly, and hepatic granulomata

IV. Diagnosis/Evaluation

   A. History
      1. Ask about onset and duration of all symptoms
      2. Determine whether patient lives in household with a cat (particularly kitten) or other animals
      3. Carefully determine whether patient saw scratch or bite of any animal
      4. Specifically ask whether any skin lesion was noticed within the last 2-3 months
      5. Ask about symptoms which typically accompany CSD such as low-grade fever and myalgia
      6. Ask about symptoms which are related to other illnesses that present with lymphadenopathy such as pharyngitis (mononucleosis), weight loss and fatigue (malignancy), exanthem (Kawasaki disease), cough (tuberculosis), ear pain (otitis media), facial tenderness (sinusitis), mouth pain (dental abscess)
      7. Inquire about symptoms which would denote complications of CSD such as abdominal pain, neurological complaints, conjunctivitis

B. Physical Examination
    1. Obtain vital signs, noting temperature
    2. Carefully examine skin for inoculation lesion, which may be hidden in the interdigital webs of fingers, eyelids, or scalp
    3. Observe skin for exanthem
    4. Palpate all areas where lymph nodes are present, noting any node enlargement, erythema, or tenderness (see section on LYMPHADENOPATHY)
    5. If a node is enlarged, assess the area that the node drains for signs of infection
    6. Inspect eyes for signs of conjunctivitis
    7. Perform complete examinations of ears, eyes, nose, and throat to rule out infection
    8. Auscultate heart and lungs
    9. Palpate abdomen for organomegaly, masses, and tenderness
    10. Perform a neurological examination to rule out complications

C. Diagnostic Tests: usually no tests are needed
    1. Indirect fluorescent antibody test for detection of serum antibody to antigens of *Bartonella* species is useful for diagnosis (available through the Centers for Disease Control and Prevention)
    2. Polymerase chain reaction assays are available in some commercial laboratories
    3. A stain (Warthin-Starry silver impregnation stain) can identify the pathogen if lymph node, skin, or conjunctival tissue is available; test is not specific for *Bartonella henselae*
    4. Pathologic and microbiologic examinations are useful to exclude other diseases

D. Differential Diagnosis: (see sections on LYMPHADENOPATHY and CERVICAL ADENITIS)

V. Plan/Management

A. Management is usually symptomatic (e.g., pain management); complete resolution occurs without medications in 2-4 months

B. Antibiotic therapy may be beneficial in immunosuppressed patients and other patients who are severely ill but is <u>NOT</u> recommended for healthy patients
    1. Oral antibiotics (rifampin [Rifadin], trimethoprim-sulfamethoxazole [Bactrim], ciprofloxacin [Cipro], azithromycin [Zithromax], or intramuscular gentamicin [Garamycin]) are possible choices
    2. Therapy is discontinued when enlarged node has decreased in size (about 10 mm), the patient has no systemic symptoms, and has been afebrile for at least one week

C. Node aspiration is done when nodes are tender and fluctuant to relieve symptoms; node excision is generally unnecessary

D. Patient Education
    1. Animals do not need to be destroyed or removed from the house
    2. No person-to-person transmission so patients do not need to be isolated
    3. Instruct patients to always thoroughly cleanse animal scratches and bites to prevent CSD
    4. Persons with immune deficiencies should avoid contact with cats that scratch or bite
    5. Recommend that care of cats should include flea control

E. Follow-up: None needed if patient's condition remains stable

FIFTH DISEASE (ERYTHEMA INFECTIOSUM)

I. Definition: Mild viral disease with an erythematous eruption

II. Pathogenesis

A. Causal agent is human parvovirus B19

B. Mode of transmission probably is through contact with infected respiratory secretions or blood and from vertical transmission between mother and her fetus

C. Incubation period is 4-14 days from acquisition of infection to onset of initial symptoms

D. Period of communicability: Greatest before onset of rash; probably not communicable after onset of rash; patients with aplastic crises are contagious from before the onset of symptoms and at least through the week after onset

III. Clinical Presentation

A. Parvovirus B19 infections are ubiquitous and cases can occur as a community outbreak or sporadically in the late winter and early spring

B. >50% of individuals have serologic evidence of past infection by age 15 years and are immune; young children are usually susceptible to infection

C. First manifestation is typically a rash which usually appears without fever or other symptoms; in some cases there may be a mild prodrome with fever, headache, conjunctivitis, coryza, and pharyngitis; about 20% of infected individuals are asymptomatic

D. Rash is characteristic and may be pruritic
   1. First erupts as a bright, erythematous rash on cheeks and forehead with circumoral pallor; adults often do not have rash on face
   2. A maculopapular rash on the trunk occurs next
   3. Rash gradually spreads, leaving a lacelike appearance as it clears; this stage lasts 2-4 days
   4. In third stage, rash appears transiently when skin is traumatized by pressure, sunlight, or extremes of hot and cold

E. Complications
   1. Although uncommon in children, arthritis and arthralgia occur frequently in adults, especially in women; usually resolve in one or two weeks, but may last for several months
   2. Thrombocytopenia and neutropenia may occur
   3. Chronic bone marrow failure may occur in immunocompromised patients, and aplastic crisis may occur in patients with hemolytic anemia

F. Infection during pregnancy can result in fetal hydrops and death (risk of fetal death is <10% after proven maternal infection in first half of pregnancy and even less in second half of pregnancy)

IV. Diagnosis/Evaluation

A. History
   1. Question about degree, onset, and duration of fever or prodromal symptoms
   2. Ask patient to describe progression of rash
   3. Ask whether rash becomes more visible when patient is in sunlight or becomes overheated
   4. Determine whether there are other accompanying symptoms
   5. Determine whether other family or household members have similar symptoms
   6. Inquire about symptoms which would denote complications such as joint pain and stiffness
   7. Determine medication use
   8. Inquire about present and past health history of patient and other household members; specifically question about immunosuppression and pregnancy in women

B. Physical Examination
   1. Measure vital signs
   2. Assess general appearance
   3. Carefully inspect skin; apply pressure to skin noting whether rash becomes more visible
   4. To rule out other viral exanthems, may need to perform examinations of the head, eyes, ears, nose, throat and mouth
   5. Assess neck for nuchal rigidity and adenopathy
   6. Auscultate heart and lungs
   7. Assess joints for tenderness, swelling, and range of motion

C. Differential Diagnosis: "Slapped cheek" appearance, lacy rash, and transient nature of rash with heat, cold, and pressure are characteristic of fifth disease and lead to diagnosis; consider other conditions such as rubella, enteroviral diseases, and drug rashes, but these typically have different rash patterns

D.   Diagnostic Tests
1.   No tests are needed unless diagnosis is uncertain or when treating immunosuppressed patients or pregnant women
2.   Assay for serum B19-specific IgM antibody is available for confirming recent infection; serum IgG antibody indicates previous infection and immunity
3.   If exposure is highly suspicious in pregnant woman, additional testing is needed; consult specialist who will typically order IgG and IgM titers and then alpha-fetoprotein (MSAFT) levels if titers are positive; serial ultrasonography is needed if MSAFT is elevated
4.   Tests such as nucleic acid hybridization assay or polymerase chain reaction assay are available; typically ordered to determine chronic infection in immunocompromised patients

V.   Plan/Management

A.   Treatment is symptomatic for healthy persons; usually the condition is benign and self-limited

B.   Patients with aplastic crisis may need blood transfusions

C.   For immunosuppressed patients with chronic infection, intravenous immunoglobulin therapy is effective

D.   Control procedures
1.   Precautions for pregnant women:
a.   Routine exclusion from the workplace where disease is occurring is not recommended due to the high prevalence of B19, the low incidence of ill effects on fetus, and the fact that avoidance of child care or teaching classrooms can only reduce but not eliminate the risk of exposure
b.   Explanation of the relatively low potential risk and option of serologic testing should be given to pregnant women who have been in contact with patients in the incubation period of disease or who were in aplastic crisis; fetal ultrasound can be offered to assess damage to the fetus
2.   Good hand washing and disposal of facial tissues containing respiratory secretions lessen transmission of infection

E.   Follow Up: None needed unless complications develop

INFLUENZA

I.   Definition: Acute viral disease of the respiratory tract

II.   Pathogenesis

A.   Causal agents: Influenza A (accounts for 99.5% of cases) and influenza B cause epidemic human disease

B.   Mode of transmission: Spread from person to person by inhalation of small particle aerosols, by direct contact, by large droplet infection, or by articles recently contaminated with nasopharyngeal secretions

C.   Incubation period: Ranges from 1- 4 days with an average of 2 days

D.   Period of communicability: Patients are most infectious in the first 24 hours before onset of symptoms and during the period of peak symptoms; viral shedding in nasal secretions usually stops within 7 days of onset of infection

III.   Clinical Presentation

A.   In the US, influenza with associated pneumonia was the sixth leading cause of death in 1995; persons >65 years accounted for >90% of deaths

B.   Influenza virus infection occurs in epidemics that last approximately 5-6 weeks and may be associated with attack rates as high as 10-20% of population

C.	Reason for continuing problems with epidemic influenza is the phenomenon of antigenic variation in which there are alterations in the structure of antigens, leading to variants against which the general population has little or no resistance

D.	Antigenic shift is primarily due to changes in the viral hemagglutinin and results in widespread and lethal pandemics; occurs at irregular intervals of 10 or more years

E.	Characterized by abrupt onset of fever, malaise, diffuse myalgia, headache, anorexia, rhinitis, and nonproductive cough
1.	Less common symptoms are sore throat, nasal congestion, and sneezing
2.	Cough is usually the most frequent and troublesome symptom and may be associated with substernal discomfort
3.	Symptoms usually last about 3-4 days, but cough and malaise may persist for 1-2 weeks

F.	Nausea, vomiting, and diarrhea occur in children, but are less common in adults

G.	Influenza can affect metabolism of certain medications such as theophylline; toxicity from high serum concentrations may occur

H.	Complications include primary influenza pneumonia, secondary bacterial pneumonia, myositis (calf tenderness), myocarditis, pericarditis, Reye's syndrome, and central nervous system problems; influenza can exacerbate underlying medical conditions such as cardiopulmonary disease

IV.	Diagnosis/Evaluation

A.	History
1.	Inquire about onset, duration, and character of symptoms
2.	To assess for complications, ask about chest pain, hemoptysis, severe muscle pain, and central nervous system manifestations such as confusion
3.	Determine whether household members or close contacts of patient are ill
4.	Determine history of previous influenza vaccinations
5.	Obtain a medication history; especially ask about use of theophylline

B.	Physical Examination
1.	Measure vital signs
2.	Observe general appearance for lassitude and distress
3.	Assess hydration status
4.	Perform complete eyes, ears, nose, and throat examinations
5.	Palpate sinuses for tenderness
6.	Examine neck for nuchal rigidity and cervical adenopathy
7.	Auscultate heart
8.	Perform complete lung exam
9.	Always perform abdominal and neurological exams in patients with severe cases

C.	Differential Diagnosis: Difficult to differentiate influenza from other respiratory infectious diseases
1.	Onset of symptoms is more abrupt in influenza than the common cold
2.	Sore throat, nasal congestion, and sneezing are less common in influenza than the common cold
3.	Myalgia and malaise are predominant symptoms in influenza, but may not be present in other respiratory infectious diseases; fever, anorexia, headache, fatigue, and chest discomfort are more common in patients with influenza than patients with common colds
4.	Always consider illnesses associated with biological warfare: Inhalational anthrax, smallpox, inhalational tularemia, pneumonic plague, and hemorrhagic fever (such as would be caused by Ebola or Marburg viruses)

D.	Diagnostic Tests
1.	Epidemiologic data are usually sufficient to make diagnosis in uncomplicated cases (when it is known that a certain influenza type is prevalent in a community, most persons with acute, febrile, respiratory symptoms and myalgia can safely be assumed to have influenza); epidemiologic information can be obtained from health departments as well as websites (see table that follows)

2. Consider cultures of nasopharyngeal secretions; must collect within the first 72 hours of illness
3. Rapid diagnostic kits are available commercially to detect antigens from nasopharyngeal secretions; sensitivity and specificity varies
   a. Order rapid tests for all patients hospitalized with acute respiratory infection during an epidemic period
   b. Not necessary for initiating treatment in outpatient settings but provides reassurance that therapy is appropriate and permits clinician to withhold antibiotics with confidence
   c. Be aware that CDC estimates that up to 30% of samples may produce false-negative results
4. Change in antibody titer between acute and convalescent sera using complement fixation, hemagglutination inhibition, neutralization, or enzyme immunoassay tests can help confirm diagnosis retrospectively
5. Consider CBC and urinalysis

V. Plan/Management

A. Antiviral drugs for treatment
   1. Consider treatment for the following persons:
      a. All high-risk individuals regardless of vaccination status
      b. Persons with severe influenza
      c. Consider for others to shorten duration of illness
      d. Potential benefit of treatment is the reduction in transmission to household members
   2. Start therapy as soon as possible; treatment is effective only when begun within first 2 days of symptom onset; however, zanamivir and oseltamivir may reduce risk of complications in high-risk persons on the third or fourth day of their illnesses
   3. Selection of an antiviral drug (see table that follows): Zanamivir and oseltamivir are preferred because they have lower complication rates, lower risks of drug resistance, and are effective against influenza B

SELECTION OF AN ANTIVIRAL DRUG FOR TREATMENT				
	Cost	Complication Rate	Risk of Drug Resistance	Effective against Influenza B
Amantadine (Symmetrel)	Low	High*[†]	High	No
Rimantadine (Flumadine)	Low	Moderate[†]	High	No
Zanamivir (Relenza)	High	Low	Low	Yes
Oseltamivir (Tamiflu)	High	Low[†]	Low	Yes

* Incidence of CNS-related (anxiety, depression, insomnia, etc.) adverse effects highest when amantadine is used; adverse effects are more common in patients with seizure disorders, psychiatric disorders, and renal insufficiency
[†] Amantadine, rimantadine and oseltamivir occasionally cause nausea, vomiting, and dyspepsia

   4. Duration of therapy: 2-5 days or for 24-48 hours after patient becomes asymptomatic; immunocompromised patients may require longer course (do not exceed 10 to 14 days, regardless of patient's status)
   5. See table PROPERTIES OF ANTIVIRAL DRUGS for prescribing medications

6. Adverse effects of antiviral drugs
   a. Amantadine: Insomnia, lightheadedness, nervousness, difficulty concentrating, delirium, hallucinations, and seizures
   b. Rimantadine has CNS effects but they are less prevalent than with amantadine
   c. Zanamivir: Cough, nasal and throat discomfort, headache, and in patients with asthma, bronchospasm
   d. Oseltamivir: Nausea, vomiting, headache

PROPERTIES OF ANTIVIRAL DRUGS				
		Daily Dose		
Drug	Route	Adults	Elderly	Available Form
Amantadine	Oral	100 mg BID‡	100 mg QD‡	Tablets and syrup
Rimantadine	Oral	100 mg BID‡	100 mg QD‡	Tablets and syrup
Zanamivir	Oral inhalation	10 mg (2 inh) BID*	10 mg (2 inh) BID*	Powder for an inhaler
Oseltamivir	Oral	75 mg BID‡	75 mg BID‡	Capsules

‡ The dose should be reduced in persons with renal insufficiency
* Is not generally recommended in patients with COPD, asthma, or other underlying airway disease
Adapted from Couch, R.B. (2000). Prevention and treatment of influenza. *New England Journal of Medicine, 343*, 1778-1787.

B. Patient Education
   1. Symptomatic treatment of fever, myalgia, and cough may be needed
   2. Recommend rest and increased fluids
   3. Encourage cessation of smoking in household
   4. Instruct patient to return to clinic if chest pain, dyspnea, hemoptysis, wheezing, increased temperature, agitation, behavioral changes, or confusion occur
   5. Instruct patient who is taking amantadine to be cautious of concurrent medications that affect the central nervous system, such as antihistamines and anticholinergic drugs

C. Control Measures
   1. Consider annual influenza vaccine for certain groups of individuals (see following table, TARGET GROUPS FOR INFLUENZA VACCINE)
   2. Administer influenza vaccine in the fall (optimal time is October to November), before the start of the influenza season (see following table DOSE AND SCHEDULE OF INFLUENZA VACCINE)
      a. Vaccine prevents influenza illness in 70-90% of healthy persons <65 years; elderly persons and persons with certain chronic diseases may develop lower postvaccination antibody titers than healthy, young adults but vaccine is still effective in preventing secondary complications and reducing risk of death in this age group
      b. Do **not** administer vaccination to persons known to have anaphylactic hypersensitivity to eggs or other components of the vaccine without consulting an expert in infectious disease
      c. Do **not** vaccinate adults with acute febrile illnesses until their symptoms have abated; minor illnesses with or without fever should not contraindicate use of vaccine
      d. Adverse reactions include soreness at site of vaccination; severe reactions are rare (concern about Guillain-Barré syndrome should not deter persons from receiving vaccine)

TARGET GROUPS FOR INFLUENZA VACCINE

Groups at Increased Risk for Influenza-Related Complications

- ✓ Persons ≥50 years of age
- ✓ Residents of nursing homes or chronic-care facilities
- ✓ Adults and children with chronic disorders of the pulmonary or cardiovascular system, including children with asthma
- ✓ Adults and children who required regular medical care during preceding year because of chronic metabolic diseases, renal dysfunction, hemoglobinopathies or immunosuppression (including immunosuppression caused by medications or by HIV)
- ✓ Children (6 months-18 years) receiving long-term aspirin therapy who might be at risk for developing Reye's syndrome
- ✓ Women who will be in the second or third trimester of pregnancy during the influenza season

Groups That Can Transmit Influenza to Persons at High Risk

- ✓ Health care providers in both hospitals and outpatient settings, including emergency response workers
- ✓ Employees of nursing homes and chronic-care facilities who have contact with residents
- ✓ Providers of home care to persons at high risk
- ✓ Household members (including children) of persons in high risk groups including high risk infants

Special Groups

- ✓ Persons with HIV infection: vaccine is effective in persons with mild AIDS-related symptoms and high CD4+ T-lymphocyte counts; may not produce protective antibody titers in patients with advanced HIV disease and low CD4+ T-lymphocytes
- ✓ Breast-feeding is not contraindicated for vaccination
- ✓ Persons traveling to foreign countries: risk of exposure to influenza varies depending on season and destination; if persons traveling were not vaccinated the previous fall or winter, encourage vaccine
- ✓ General population: administer to any person who wishes to receive; especially encourage persons who provide community services and students or other persons living in institutional settings
- ✓ Children aged 6-23 months are at increased risk for hospitalizations related to influenza; vaccination for this age group is encouraged when feasible

Adapted from Advisory Committee on Immunization Practices. (2002). Prevention and control of influenza: Recommendations of Advisory Committee on Immunization Practices (ACIP). *MMWR, 51*(RR-3), 1-31.

DOSE AND SCHEDULE FOR INFLUENZA VACCINE *[†]

Age Group	Product	Dosage	# Doses
Adults	Whole or split virus	0.50 mL	1

* The recommended site of vaccination is the deltoid muscle
[†] Dosages are those recommended in recent years; refer to product circular each year for correct dosage

Adapted from Advisory Committee on Immunization Practices. (2002). Prevention and control of influenza: Recommendations of Advisory Committee on Immunization Practices (ACIP). *MMWR, 51*(RR-3), 1-31.

D. Chemoprophylaxis with antiviral drugs is an adjunct for influenza vaccine for control and prevention of influenza; antiviral drugs are **not** a substitute for vaccination
　　1. Chemoprophylaxis in vaccinated persons may provide additional protection and does not interfere with the immune response, particularly useful for high-risk persons if influenza outbreak occurs before or <2 weeks after vaccination (see following table)
　　2. For maximal effectiveness of prophylaxis, drug must be taken each day for duration of influenza activity in community; to be cost effective, prophylaxis should only be prescribed during period of peak influenza activity; typically prophylaxis is continued up to 6-8 weeks

Adapted from Advisory Committee on Immunization Practices. (2001). Prevention and control of influenza: Recommendations of Advisory Committee on Immunization Practices (ACIP). *MMWR, 50*(RR04), 1-46.

3. Prophylactic doses
    a. Amantadine (Symmetrel)
       (1) Adults <65 years: Amantadine 100 mg BID
       (2) Persons ≥65 years should not exceed 100 mg per day and for certain elderly persons and persons with renal insufficiency the dose should be further reduced
    b. Rimantadine (Flumadine)
       (1) Adults: Rimantadine 100 mg BID
       (2) Consider reducing dose to 100 mg/day for persons ≥65 years, particularly for those with side effects; in persons with renal insufficiency and hepatic dysfunction, the dose should be reduced to 100 mg/day or below 100 mg/day
    c. Oseltamivir (Tamiflu) 75 mg QD is approved for chemoprophylaxis of influenza; zanamivir (Relenza) is waiting for approval for prophylaxis

E. Influenza surveillance information is available at http://www.cdc.gov/ncidod/diseases/flu/weekly.htm

F. Follow Up: None needed unless symptoms persist >7-10 days

LYME DISEASE

I. Definition: Infection caused by *Borrelia burgdorferi*, a member of the family of spirochetes or corkscrew-shaped bacteria

II. Pathogenesis

A. Ticks of the *Ixodes ricinus* complex usually transmit the disease during the nymph stage when they are small in size and are likely to feed unnoticed on individuals for 2 or more days

B. Small mammals, particularly rodents, are important hosts of ticks and critical for maintenance of *B. burgdorferi* in nature; deer are hosts for the adult tick

C. Adult ticks are less likely to transmit disease because they are readily noticed and removed; transmission of the disease is unlikely if tick attachment is less than 48-72 hours

D. Incubation period is 3-31days (typically 7-14 days); late manifestations occur months to years later

III.   Clinical Presentation

    A.   Epidemiology
        1.   Leading vector-borne disease in US
        2.   Incidence is increasing and there has been an expansion of the affected geographic area
        3.   Occurs in the Northeast from Maine to Maryland, in the Midwest, especially Wisconsin and Minnesota, and in the West, particularly northern California and Oregon
        4.   Most human infections occur during late spring and early summer months
        5.   Less than 50% of all patients with Lyme disease remember receiving a tick bite

    B.   Case definition for the national surveillance of Lyme disease (Centers for Disease Control and Prevention, 1990)
        1.   Erythema migrans observed by clinician; to be counted for surveillance purposes, a solitary lesion must reach a size of at least 5 cm; however, recent studies have found that some patients with Lyme disease do not present with erythema migrans but rather have only systemic symptoms such as fever, chills, malaise, and occipital headaches
        2.   At least one manifestation and laboratory confirmation of infection
            a.   Nervous system: lymphocytic meningitis, cranial neuritis, radiculoneuropathy, or rarely, encephalomyelitis
            b.   Cardiovascular system: acute-onset, high-grade (2nd or 3rd degree) atrioventricular conduction defects that resolve in days or weeks
            c.   Musculoskeletal system: recurrent, brief attacks (lasting weeks to months) of objectively confirmed joint swelling in one or a few joints
            d.   Laboratory evidence: isolation of *B. burgdorferi* from tissue or body fluid, or detection of diagnostic levels of antibody against the spirochete by the two-test approach of enzyme-linked immunosorbent assay and Western blotting

    C.   First stage is called early localized and is characterized by the following:
        1.   Erythema migrans (EM) is a lesion that starts as a red macule or papule at the site of a recent tick bite and enlarges over days or weeks to form a large, round lesion, often with central clearing; occurs in about 80% of patients with Lyme disease in the US
        2.   Patient may not have erythema migrans or may have a rash that mimics cellulitis (erythematous plaque); rash may have a vesicular center
        3.   Fever, malaise, headache, neck stiffness, and arthralgia may occur with rash; these symptoms may be intermittent over several weeks

    D.   Second stage is called early disseminated disease and presents as the following:
        1.   Multiple erythema migrans lesions typically develop 3 to 5 weeks after tick bite and appears as annular erythematous lesions which are smaller but similar to primary lesion
        2.   Other common manifestations are palsies of cranial nerves, meningitis, conjunctivitis, and systemic symptoms such as arthralgia, myalgia, headache, and fatigue; carditis, which presents as various degrees of heart block, is a rare occurrence

    E.   Third stage is called late disease and signs and symptoms in this stage may not present until months or years after tick bite; characterized by following:
        1.   Recurrent arthritis which is pauciarticular and affects large joints, particularly the knees
        2.   Central nervous system manifestations include subacute encephalopathy and polyradiculoneuropathy
        3.   Third stage occurs infrequently in children treated with antibiotics in early stages of disease

    F.   After an episode of appropriately treated Lyme disease, some persons have subjective complaints (such as myalgia, arthralgia, fatigue) and have been classified as having "chronic Lyme disease" or "post-Lyme disease syndrome"; there is insufficient data to regard this syndrome as a separate diagnostic entity and repeated or prolonged courses of antibiotics have been ineffective

IV.   Diagnosis/Evaluation

    A.   History
        1.   Ask about possible exposure to tick bites such as recent camping trip, frequent yard work, and pets who are outside in vegetation
        2.   Ask patient to describe the duration, characteristics, and course of any skin lesion
        3.   Question about fatigue, headache, fever, myalgias
        4.   Inquire about late manifestations such as arthritis and neurologic and cardiac problems

B. Physical Examination
   1. Carefully inspect the skin
   2. Palpate for lymphadenopathy
   3. Perform a thorough cardiac exam
   4. Inspect joints for swelling, tenderness, or erythema
   5. Perform a neurological examination

C. Differential Diagnosis
   1. Infectious diseases such as Reiter's syndrome, Rocky Mountain spotted fever, acute rheumatic fever, tularemia, viral syndrome, or meningitis/encephalitis
   2. Rheumatoid arthritis
   3. Systemic lupus erythematosus
   4. Bell's palsy

D. Diagnostic Tests; accurate identification of the tick is useful and is often available free of charge from health departments
   1. Serologic testing at time of tick bite is usually **not** recommended; antibodies to *B. burgdorferi* do not have sufficient time to develop at time of tick bite
   2. Patients who meet case definition for Lyme disease (III.B.), who have rash resembling erythema migrans, or who have a history of characteristic rash and a previous tick bite should have empiric antibiotic therapy; no diagnostic tests are needed
   3. Closely monitor persons who remove attached ticks for signs and symptoms of Lyme disease for up to 30 days, specifically assessing for skin lesion at site of bite or temperature >38°C
   4. Carefully assess and consider testing and therapy for any person who develops skin lesion or clinical symptoms within one month of removing tick; **Patients with singular symptoms of arthralgias, myalgia, headache, fatigue, or palpitations** have a low chance of having Lyme disease and **should not be tested**
   5. Although the Infectious Disease Society of America does not recommend testing for tick-borne infectious organisms, some clinicians obtain serologic tests for antibodies, especially for those persons who live in communities with high incidence of Lyme disease; tests should be performed in a reference rather than a commercial laboratory
      a. First, order an enzyme-linked immunosorbent assay (ELISA) or an immunofluorescence assay (IFA); these tests often have false positive results
      b. For specimens that give positive or equivocal ELISA or IFA results, order a Western immunoblot to test for antibodies
   6. Other diagnostic tests are not usually ordered but may be beneficial:
      a. In persons with suspected early disease and a negative serologic test, changes in antibody levels in paired acute-phase (close to time of tick bite) and convalescent-phase (6-8 weeks later) serum samples may help diagnose disease, but published data are not yet available to determine the clinical utility of this approach
      b. Seek consultation with a specialist on testing of patients with suspected central nervous system involvement; antibody testing of cerebrospinal fluid may be recommended
      c. Investigational tests such as polymerase chain reaction (PCR) are more sensitive and specific, but their clinical usefulness is unproven
   7. To establish or exclude diagnosis in patients who have received the recombinant outer surface protein A (rOspA) vaccine, order the Western immunoblot test

V. Plan/Management

A. Treat the following patients with antibiotics (see following table on RECOMMENDED TREATMENT)
   1. Patients with erythema migrans
   2. Consider treatment for any person who develops skin lesion or clinical symptoms (i.e., temperature >38°C) within one month of removing tick; Patients with singular symptoms of arthralgias, myalgia, headache, fatigue, or palpitations have a low chance of having Lyme disease and should not be treated
   3. Consider treatment for patients who live in high incidence area and who have positive results from the two-test protocol (ELISA or IFA and Western blot)

B. Do not treat patients whose only evidence of Lyme disease is a positive immunologic test; the risks of empiric antibiotic treatment outweigh the benefits

RECOMMENDED TREATMENT		
Disease Category	Drug/Duration	Dosage
Early Localized Disease*	Doxycycline (Vibramycin) 14-21 days	100 mg BID
	Amoxicillin (Amoxil) 14-21 days	500 mg TID
Early Disseminated and Late Disease		
• Multiple erythema migrans	Same as early disease except duration is 21 days	
• Isolated facial palsy	Same as early disease, except duration is 21-28 days[‡]	
• Arthritis	Same as early disease except duration is 28 days	
• Persistent or recurrent arthritis[§] • Carditis • Meningitis or encephalitis	{ Ceftriaxone (Rocephin) IV or IM for 14-21 days	2 g QD or 1 g BID
	OR	
	Penicillin G IV for 14-21 days	20 million units in 4 divided doses

*Cefuroxime axetil is alternative drug for patients allergic to penicillin; other alternatives are erythromycin or penicillin
[†]Do not give corticosteroids
[‡]Antibiotics do not affect resolution of nerve palsy; purpose is to prevent late disease
[§]Considered persistent when there is objective evidence of synovitis for at least 2 months after treatment is initiated. Some experts use a second course of an oral agent before using an IV antibiotic

Adapted from American Academy of Pediatrics. (2000). In L.K. Pickering (Ed.). *2000 Red Book: Report of the Committee on Infectious Diseases* (25th ed.). Elk Grove Village, IL: American Academy of Pediatrics.

C.   Prevention
    1.   Patient education
        a.   Avoidance of tick-infested areas is the most important preventive measure
        b.   Keep grass mowed and remove leaves, brush, tall grass, and woodpiles from around houses and at the edges of gardens
        c.   Always inspect body carefully after being outdoors; pay special attention to exposed hairy regions of the body
        d.   Daily inspect pets and remove ticks
        e.   Wear lightly colored clothing so that ticks can be seen more easily
        f.   Prevent ticks from getting under clothing; tuck pant legs into socks or tape area where pants and socks meet, and tuck shirt into pants
        g.   Wear a hat and long-sleeved shirt
        h.   Avoid overhanging grass and brush by walking in the center of trails
        i.   Spray permethrin on clothing or treat clothes with permethrin which kills ticks on contact and prevents tick attachment
        j.   Spray insect repellent containing n,n-diethyl-m-toluamide (DEET) on all exposed skin other than face, hands, and abraded skin (must reapply every 1-2 hours); use DEET sparingly because of rare reports of serious neurologic complications after use (wash treated skin with soap and water after being outdoors)
        k.   Remove clothing and wash and dry it in high temperature after outdoor exposure
    2.   Remove attached ticks with fine tweezers or blunt, medium-tipped angled forceps as close to skin as possible; pull tick straight back with a slow steady force; remove tick completely, including the mouth part; disinfect skin before and after tick is removed; do not use nail polish, alcohol, or matches to remove tick
    3.   Routine use of antimicrobial agents to prevent disease is not recommended because therapy is associated with potential risks and costs and is not efficacious; however, a recent study found that a single, 200 mg dose of doxycycline prevented infection after a nymphal tick bite, particularly when duration of attachment was prolonged
    4.   Lyme disease vaccine was removed from market in 2002 due to poor sales

D.   Follow Up
1.   Patients treated with oral antibiotics should be reevaluated at the end of treatment
2.   Patients with severe symptoms should be seen more frequently based on their clinical condition

INFECTIOUS MONONUCLEOSIS

I.   Definition: Acute viral syndrome with classic triad of fever, pharyngitis, and adenopathy

II.   Pathogenesis

    A.   Causal agent is the Epstein-Barr virus (EBV)

    B.   Spread person-to-person by the oropharyngeal route (via saliva); rarely via blood transfusion

    C.   Incubation period is from 30 to 50 days

    D.   Period of communicability is indeterminate but may be prolonged
        1.   Respiratory tract viral excretion may persist for many months or more after illness
        2.   Asymptomatic carriage is common

III.   Clinical Presentation

    A.   Common infection in college-age adults and adolescents living in group settings such as educational institutions

    B.   Spectrum of disease is variable; patients may be asymptomatic or suffer from fatal infection

    C.   Common signs and symptoms include the classic triad of fever, exudative pharyngitis, adenopathy (particularly posterior cervical), as well as fatigue, eyelid edema, headache, pain behind eyes, and a palatal petechial rash

    D.   Atypical lymphocytosis often accompanies disease and approximately 95% of adults will have abnormal liver function tests

    E.   Splenic enlargement may occur; usually resolves within the first month of the illness

    F.   Duration of the illness is variable with the average, uncomplicated illness lasting 3-4 weeks; some patients have a low level of fatigue for 6-12 months

    G.   Complications occur more often in patients <10 years, >50 years, and those who are immunocompromised; complications include central nervous system (CNS) disorders such as aseptic meningitis, encephalitis, and the Guillain-Barré syndrome; rare complications include splenic rupture, thrombocytopenia, agranulocytosis, myocarditis, hemolytic anemia

    H.   The definition of "chronic" mononucleosis is controversial

IV.   Diagnosis/Evaluation

    A.   History
        1.   Ask about onset, pattern, and character of symptoms
        2.   Ascertain that patient does not have trouble breathing or severe swallowing difficulty
        3.   Question about severe headaches, weakness, and confusion (CNS complications of mononucleosis)
        4.   Question about recent history of exposure to others with mononucleosis

    B.   Physical Examination
        1.   Observe general appearance
        2.   Measure vital signs

3.   Observe skin for exanthems
4.   Perform complete ears, nose, and throat examinations
5.   Auscultate the heart
6.   Auscultate the lungs, making certain that the patient does not have upper airway obstruction from enlarged tonsils and lymphoid tissue
7.   Palpate abdomen for organomegaly
8.   Perform a neurological examination to rule out CNS complications

C.   Differential Diagnosis
1.   Streptococcal or viral pharyngitis (posterior cervical adenopathy and splenomegaly help distinguish pharyngitis of infectious mononucleosis from other types of pharyngitis)
2.   Viral syndromes
3.   Hepatitis
4.   HIV infection
5.   Cytomegalovirus infection
6.   Toxoplasma infection
7.   Secondary syphilis

D.   Diagnostic Tests
1.   Order complete blood count with differential; absolute lymphocytosis in which more than 10% of cells are atypical is characteristic
2.   Order nonspecific serologic tests for heterophil antibody (Paul-Bunnell test and slide agglutination reaction are most widely available)
    a.   Will identify 90% of cases
    b.   Early in the course of this illness, some infected persons will have a negative test because the level of antibodies in the blood has not reached sufficient levels; if patient continues to have symptoms repeat test in 7-10 days
    c.   A positive result may remain positive for up to a year after the initial illness
3.   Multiple specific serologic antibody tests for EBV are available
    a.   Most commonly used test is for IgG and IgM antibodies against viral capsid antigen (VCA); particularly useful for evaluating patients who have heterophil-negative infectious mononucleosis (testing for other viral agents such as cytomegalovirus is needed for these patients)
    b.   Testing positive for IgM antibodies indicates recent infection
    c.   Positive IgG antibodies with findings of negative IgM antibodies, indicates past infection
4.   Consider obtaining throat swab and perform rapid strep test. If the rapid strep test is negative (3-30% of patients with mononucleosis also have streptococcal infection) send a throat culture
5.   Consider ordering liver function tests

V.   Plan/Management

A.   Patients with uncomplicated acute mononucleosis require only symptomatic therapy

B.   For patients with more severe symptoms, consult specialist and consider the following:
1.   Corticosteroid therapy is considered only for patients with complications such as obstructive tonsillar enlargement, hemolytic anemia, aplastic anemia, encephalitis, myocarditis, and massive splenomegaly; prescribe prednisone 1mg/kg/day orally for 7 days and then taper
2.   Acyclovir is not currently recommended

C.   If patient has concomitant streptococcal pharyngitis treat with erythromycin (see section on PHARYNGITIS); Do not prescribe ampicillin or amoxicillin-containing agents because they cause a rash; infrequently, penicillin can also cause a rash

D.   Patient Education
1.   Help patient plan a realistic schedule of rest with modification of work and/or school responsibilities depending on patient's condition
2.   Increased fluid intake may be beneficial
3.   Instruct patient to immediately report pain in left upper area of abdomen or in shoulder, as this could be a sign of splenic rupture
4.   Isolation is not needed, but good hand washing technique, avoidance of sharing eating or drinking utensils with others, and avoidance of kissing or sharing oral secretions are important
5.   Avoid contact sports, heavy lifting, and strenuous activity for at least one month or until resolution of splenomegaly because an enlarged spleen is susceptible to rupture

6. Avoid alcohol consumption for at least a month to decrease the work of the liver
7. Instruct patient with a recent history of mononucleosis to avoid donating blood
8. Avoid ampicillin or amoxicillin during course of disease as a drug-related rash may develop
9. Inform patient that recovery is typically in 2 to 4 weeks, but that some patients have a slow recovery of 2 to 3 months

E. Follow Up: every 1-2 weeks until symptoms resolve for uncomplicated cases

ROCKY MOUNTAIN SPOTTED FEVER

I. Definition: Systemic, small vessel vasculitis with characteristic rash that results from bite of infected tick

II. Pathogenesis

A. Infectious agent is *Rickettsia rickettsii*

B. Mode of transmission
1. Tick must attach and feed on blood for approximately 4-6 hours to become infectious in humans
2. No person-to-person transmission

C. Incubation period ranges from 2-14 days

III. Clinical Presentation

A. Primarily occurs in children <15 years of age during the months of April through October

B. Most cases are in south Atlantic, southeastern, and south central states; other areas include the upper Rocky Mountain States, Canada, Mexico, and South and Central America

C. Patient typically presents with sudden onset of moderate to high fever (which persists if untreated for 2-3 weeks), severe headache, myalgia, conjunctival injection, nausea, and vomiting

D. Characteristic maculopapular rash usually appears before the sixth day of illness
1. Rash spreads from wrists and ankles to trunk, neck, and face
2. In untreated patients, the lesions become petechial in about 4 days, then purpuric and coalesced

E. Thrombocytopenia develops in most patients; anemia is present in about 30% of cases

F. Disease can persist for 3 weeks and can be severe with CNS, cardiac, pulmonary, gastrointestinal, and renal involvement as well as disseminated intravascular coagulation which can lead to shock and ultimately to death; death is uncommon when diagnosis and treatment are prompt

IV. Diagnosis/Evaluation

A. History
1. Inquire about onset, duration, and characteristics of all symptoms
2. Ask patient to describe characteristics and progression of any rashes or skin lesions
3. Inquire about possible exposure to tick bites such as a recent camping trip or frequent yard work
4. May need to do a complete review of systems to detect complications from the infection

B. Physical Examination
1. Measure vital signs, noting fever
2. Observe general appearance for signs of distress and lethargy
3. Carefully inspect skin for rashes and lesions
4. Inspect eyes for conjunctival injection
5. Palpate for lymphadenopathy
6. Perform complete heart, lung, and neurological examinations to rule out complications

C. Differential Diagnosis
   1. In advanced disease, bacterial sepsis, meningitis, and meningococcemia are parts of differential diagnosis
   2. Cutaneous anthrax as a result of bioterrorism
      a. Rash occurs primarily on exposed areas of hands, arms, or face
      b. An area of local edema develops into a painless, pruritic macule or papule that enlarges and ulcerates after 1-2 days
      c. Subsequently, a painless, depressed black eschar develops
      d. Lymphangitis and painful lymphadenopathy are often present
      e. Without antibiotic treatment (ciprofloxacin, doxycycline), mortality can reach 20%
   3. Other illnesses caused by intentional release of biologic agents such as smallpox and hemorrhagic fever due to Ebola or Marburg viruses

D. Diagnostic Tests
   1. Consider ordering acute and convalescent sera, group-specific serologic tests (a fourfold rise in antibody titer is diagnostic of the disease)
      a. Titers can be determined by indirect fluorescent antibody, enzyme immunoassay, complement fixation, latex agglutination, indirect hemagglutination, or microagglutination
      b. Never delay initiation of antimicrobial treatment to confirm diagnosis
   2. Consider ordering a CBC with differential, BUN, serum albumin, serum electrolytes, and liver function studies

V. Plan/Management (consult specialist)

A. Important to treat patients with antimicrobial therapy early in the course of disease; mortality sharply increases when therapy is delayed until the fifth day of illness

B. Doxycycline (Vibramycin) is the drug of choice
   1. Dose is doxycycline 100 mg BID after a loading dose of 200 mg
   2. Therapy is continued until patient is afebrile for at least 2-3 days; usual course is 7-10 days

C. Patients who have any signs of complications should have a specialist consult and probably be admitted to the hospital because of the dangers of vascular collapse

D. Prevention: Teach patient about measures to avoid tick bites (see section on LYME DISEASE)

E. Follow Up
   1. Because of the possible dangerous complications, close monitoring is needed
   2. Teach patients to return to clinic if any danger signs such as alterations in mental status, stiff neck, severe headache, prolonged nausea and vomiting, shortness of breath, decreased urine output, high fever, severe weakness, and dizziness occur
   3. Patients should return to clinic within 24-48 hours of initial visit; and patient should be re-evaluated at the end of the antimicrobial therapy

RUBELLA (GERMAN MEASLES)

I. Definition: Febrile viral disease with diffuse maculopapular rash; postnatal rubella is usually mild and congenital rubella is associated with high incidence of congenital anomalies

II. Pathogenesis

A. Causal agent is rubella virus which is a RNA virus

B. Postnatal rubella is spread by direct or droplet contact with secretions of nose and throat

C. Incubation period ranges from 14-21 days

D. Period of communicability
   1. One week before and 5-7 days after onset of rash
   2. Infants with congenital rubella may shed virus for months after birth

III. Clinical Presentation

   A. Epidemiology
      1. Importance of this viral illness is not the morbidity of the disease itself, but rather the consequences that can occur to a fetus during a maternal infection (congenital defects, mental retardation, growth retardation, neurologic disorders, respiratory problems, and cardiovascular conditions)
      2. Before the use of vaccines, rubella was a wide-spread disease; today the incidence of disease has declined by more than 99% from the prevaccine era
      3. Most cases today occur in young, unvaccinated adults and outbreaks in colleges and occupational settings; approximately 10% of young adults are susceptible to rubella

   B. Clinical presentation
      1. Mild disease with rash, impressive lymphadenopathy (suboccipital, postauricular, cervical), and slight fever; rarely involves complications
      2. Exanthem is typically a pink, maculopapular eruption which begins on the face and spreads downward to the trunk and extremities
         a. Rash is usually completely cleared by third or fifth day after initial presentation
         b. Lesions remain discrete and pink which contrasts with the rash of rubeola which is deep red and becomes confluent
      3. Transient polyarthralgia and polyarthritis are common in adolescents and adults; rare in children

IV. Diagnosis/Evaluation

   A. History
      1. Inquire about duration and occurrence of rash, fever, and enlarged lymph nodes which indicate rubella as well as other symptoms such as cough, coryza, conjunctivitis, and pharyngitis which are associated with other exanthematous diseases
      2. Ask about recent exposure to persons with a rash
      3. Ask about medication and drug use
      4. Inquire about history of rubella illness and/or illnesses with exanthems (history of rubella illness is not a reliable indicator of immunity; identification of immune status is based on the presence of demonstrable antibody)

   B. Physical Examination
      1. Measure vital signs
      2. Inspect skin, noting characteristics of exanthem
      3. To eliminate other exanthematous diseases as the diagnosis, examine the following:
         a. Eyes, noting signs of conjunctivitis
         b. Head, ears, nose, and throat
         c. Mouth for signs of Koplik's spots which indicate measles, not rubella
         d. Neck, noting nuchal rigidity and adenopathy
         e. Heart, noting murmurs associated with Kawasaki syndrome

   C. Differential Diagnosis
      1. Infectious diseases such as rubeola, roseola, Rocky Mountain spotted fever, scarlet fever, Kawasaki syndrome, infectious mononucleosis
      2. Enteroviral infections are a common cause of exanthems
         a. Enteroviruses consist of different strains of echoviruses, coxsackieviruses, and polioviruses that typically cause infection in summer and fall
         b. Patients typically have a nonspecific febrile illness with rhinitis, pharyngitis, pneumonia, vomiting, diarrhea, abdominal pain, or conjunctivitis
         c. Patients infected with coxsackievirus A16 or enterovirus 71 may have hand, foot, and mouth syndrome; papulovesicular lesions occur in mouth, palms, fingers, soles, and occasionally on buttocks
         d. Severe cases may have aseptic meningitis, encephalitis, paralysis, hepatitis, acute hemorrhagic conjunctivitis, myopericarditis
         e. Treatment is symptomatic for most cases; consult specialist for serious cases
      3. Drug reaction

D. Diagnostic Tests
1. The virus can be isolated from nasal specimens by inoculation of appropriate cell culture; notify laboratory personnel that rubella is suspected, because additional testing is required
2. Throat swabs, blood, urine, and cerebrospinal fluid can also be used to detect the virus, particularly in congenitally infected infants
3. A fourfold or greater rise in antibody titer or seroconversion between acute and convalescent sera is indicative of infection
4. Detection of specific rubella IgM antibodies indicates a recent postnatal or congenital infection
5. Congenital infection can also be confirmed by stable or increasing levels of rubella-specific IgG over several months
6. Serologic screening tests include latex agglutination, fluorescence immunoassay, passive hemagglutination, hemolysis-in-gel, or enzyme immunoassay

V. Plan/Management

A. Treatment: Only symptomatic treatment (such as rest and increased fluid intake) is needed

B. Treatment of exposed persons
1. Pregnant women need blood specimens tested for rubella antibody; consult specialist for further treatment of exposed pregnant women; routine use of immune globulin is not recommended and only considered if termination of pregnancy is not an option
2. Live rubella vaccine given within 3 days after exposure to nonpregnant persons does not theoretically prevent the disease, but may be indicated, and will provide protection against developing rubella in the future

C. Control procedures
1. All cases of rubella and congenital rubella should be reported to the local public health unit
2. In institutions such as hospitals, patients suspected of having rubella should be isolated
3. Patients should not go to work or school for 5-7 days after onset of rash; patients with congenital rubella should be considered contagious until they are one year old, unless nasopharyngeal and urine cultures after 3 months of age are repeatedly negative
4. Efforts should be made to identify and counsel all pregnant females who had contact with patient with infection

D. Follow up is not needed except for cases in which convalescent titers after 2-3 weeks of initial illness are required

RUBEOLA (MEASLES)

I. Definition: Acute, highly communicable viral disease consisting of fever, rash, and presence of cough, coryza, or conjunctivitis

II. Pathogenesis

A. Causal agent is the measles virus which is an RNA virus

B. Transmitted by direct contact with infectious droplets, or less frequently, by airborne spread

C. Incubation period is 8-12 days from exposure to onset of symptoms

D. Period of communicability: Patient is infectious 1-2 days before onset of symptoms and 3-5 days prior to rash to approximately 4 days after rash

III. Clinical Presentation

A. Epidemiology
1. One of most serious exanthematous diseases
2. Prior to widespread immunization, measles were common in childhood; effective immunization programs have reduced rate by 99%
3. Most recent cases result from importations rather than indigenous spread

B.   Center for Disease Control's clinical case definition is as follows:
1.   Generalized rash lasting 3 or more days
a.   Deep, macular rash on face and neck that spreads down trunk and extremities
b.   Begins as discrete lesions, but later becomes confluent and salmon-colored
c.   When fever subsides, around sixth day, a faint brown stain on the skin remains and desquamation of skin often begins
2.   Fever greater than 38.3°C (100.9°F)
3.   At least one of the following symptoms: Cough, coryza, and conjunctivitis (sometimes referred to as the 3 "C"s); symptoms typically last 1-4 days and patient is usually very ill

C.   Koplik's spots are pathognomonic for measles; this enanthem presents as tiny, bluish white spots on an erythematous base which cluster adjacent to the molars on the buccal mucosa

D.   Most patients recover after the first 3-4 days

E.   Complications are common and include otitis media, pneumonia, croup, and encephalitis

IV.   Diagnosis/Evaluation

A.   History
1.   Ask about occurrence and duration of rash, cough, conjunctivitis, coryza, and Koplik's spots
2.   Inquire about other symptoms that denote complications such as chest pain, ear pain, and confusion
3.   Ask about immunization status
4.   Ask about recent exposure to persons with a rash
5.   Inquire about medical history (immunosuppressed patients may need different treatment regimens; patients who are chronically ill often develop life-threatening symptoms)
6.   Ask about medication use

B.   Physical Examination
1.   Measure vital signs
2.   Inspect skin, noting characteristics of exanthem
3.   Examine eyes, noting signs of conjunctivitis
4.   Examine head, ears, nose, and throat because complications often involve these areas
5.   Examine mouth for signs of Koplik's spots
6.   Examine neck for adenopathy and nuchal rigidity
7.   Carefully perform heart, lung, neurological, and mental status examinations

C.   Differential Diagnosis
1.   Infectious diseases such as rubella, roseola, Rocky Mountain spotted fever, scarlet fever, infectious mononucleosis, secondary syphilis, enterovirus, or Kawasaki syndrome
2.   Drug reaction
3.   Illnesses caused by release of intentional biologic agents: Anthrax, smallpox, and hemorrhagic fever caused by Ebola or Marburg viruses

D.   Diagnostic Tests:
1.   Usually none are needed
2.   Detection of measles specific IgM antibodies (present 3-4 weeks after rash) or a significant rise in IgG antibody concentrations between acute and convalescent sera confirms the diagnosis

V.   Plan/Management

A.   Symptomatic treatment: Rest, fluids, and avoidance of bright lights to lessen photosensitivity

B.   Treatment of exposed persons
1.   Give live measles vaccine if exposure was within 72 hours; recommended dose is 0.5 mL, given subcutaneously
2.   In addition to vaccine, give immune globulin (IG) within 6 days of exposure to susceptible household contacts, particularly immunocompromised contacts, contacts <1 year of age, and pregnant women
a.   Induces passive immunity and prevents or modifies symptoms
b.   Recommended dose is 0.25 mL/kg/dose IM (immunocompromised patients should receive 0.5 mL/kg). Maximum dose is 15 mL

C.   Primary prevention of measles (see immunization schedules in HEALTH MAINTENANCE section)

D.   Outbreak control procedures; prevention of disease spread depends on prompt immunization of exposed and potentially exposed persons who cannot provide documentation of measles immunity, including date of vaccination

E.   Follow Up
       1.   Clinical assessment (can be performed by nurse) is needed daily during acute phase to rule out complications
       2.   Patient should then be seen in the clinic about 3-4 days after onset of rash for full-examination

VARICELLA (CHICKENPOX)

I.   Definition: Viral disease with a pruritic, vesicular exanthem that appears in crops

II.   Pathogenesis

       A.   Causal agent is varicella-zoster virus (VZV), a member of the herpesvirus family

       B.   Transmission (highly contagious disease):
              1.   Primary mechanism is airborne spread from respiratory tract secretions
              2.   Direct contact with patients with varicella or zoster (shingles)
              3.   Contact with fluid from vesicles

       C.   Incubation period is 10-21 days with an average of 14-16 days

       D.   Patient is communicable one to two days before the rash is apparent until all the vesicles have crusted, typically 5 days after onset of rash

III.   Clinical Presentation

       A.   Number of cases has significantly declined due to increased vaccination coverage rates

       B.   Most cases in US occur in children <10 years

       C.   Often adults have a severe prodrome of high fever and malaise, and course of disease is prolonged

       D.   A few hours to days after the prodrome, a rash on the scalp, neck, or upper trunk emerges:
              1.   Exanthem occurs in stages: begins as macules, but then turns to papules, and then to vesicles, all within 12-24 hours
              2.   When vesicles begin to resolve, crusts develop
              3.   Rash spreads centrifugally (away from center) and lesions may occur on mucous membranes of mouth, conjunctivae, esophagus, trachea, rectum, and vagina
              4.   Usually patient has little scarring unless infection of skin occurs

       E.   Certain groups of patients have more severe cases
              1.   Neonates and patients with leukemia may suffer severe, prolonged, or fatal chickenpox
              2.   Adults often have prolonged and severe illness
              3.   HIV-infected patients may develop chronic chickenpox
              4.   Severe and **fatal varicella has occurred in healthy individuals receiving intermittent courses of corticosteroids**

       F.   Complications are uncommon but may include the following:
              1.   Secondary bacterial skin infection, cerebellar ataxia, meningoencephalitis, thrombocytopenia, glomerulonephritis, and pneumonia (rare in normal children, but the most common complication in older patients)
              2.   Reye's syndrome was more common in the past due to salicylate therapy
              3.   Compared to children, adults have a 25-fold increased risk of mortality

G.   Varicella reinfections may occur and are more common than previously thought

H.   The virus remains in a latent form after the primary infection; zoster or shingles occurs with reactivation

IV.   Diagnosis/Evaluation

A.   History
    1.   Inquire about recent exposure to chickenpox
    2.   Ask patient to specifically describe when and where the first lesion occurred
    3.   Ask about the spread, characteristics, and changes in the lesions
    4.   Ask about prodromal symptoms
    5.   Question about associated symptoms or potential complications such as pulmonary and neurological problems
    6.   Obtain a medication history; especially noting use of corticosteroids
    7.   Ask about any self-treatments
    8.   Determine whether patient is immunocompromised or has any other risk factors
    9.   Ask whether any household contacts lack immunity to varicella and if there are immunocompromised individuals who were exposed to infected patient

B.   Physical Examination
    1.   Observe skin and describe types of lesions, location of lesions, arrangement of lesions
    2.   Palpate for adenopathy
    3.   Auscultate heart and lungs
    4.   Perform a focused neurological examination

C.   Differential Diagnosis
    1.   Scabies or insect bites
    2.   Skin disorders such as herpes simplex, folliculitis, impetigo, contact dermatitis
    3.   Viral exanthems such as coxsackievirus and echovirus have vesicles, but these vesicles do not usually crust as occurs in chickenpox
    4.   Drug eruptions
    5.   Secondary syphilis
    6.   Smallpox, a bioterrorism agent (see table below that distinguishes smallpox from varicella)

CLINICAL FEATURES THAT DISTINGUISH CHICKENPOX FROM SMALLPOX

	Chickenpox	Smallpox
Pruritus	Yes	No
Lesion location	More central and involve the scalp; palms and soles are not involved	More on face and extremities; affects palms and soles
Development of lesions	Appears in crops or groups over several days	Synchronous in their stages of development
Depth of lesions	More superficial, thin-walled, and easily ruptured	Deeply embedded in dermis

Adapted from Relman, D.A., & Olson, J.E. (2002). Smallpox: A brief overview. *Consultant, 177-178.*

D.   Diagnostic Tests: Usually none needed
    1.   Virus can be isolated from scrapings of the vesicle base and vesicle scrapings during the first 3 days of eruption; can use tissue cultures, DFA, or Tzanck smears
    2.   Acute and convalescent titers by standard serologic assays can retrospectively confirm diagnosis (significant increase in serum varicella IgG antibodies confirms diagnosis)

V.   Plan/Management

A.   Oral acyclovir is recommended, if it can be initiated **within the first 24 hours (or possibly 48 hours) after the onset of rash**
    1.   Prescribe oral acyclovir 80 mg/kg/day in 4 divided doses for 5 days; maximum dose is 3200 mg/day; patient should be well hydrated
    2.   Intravenous acyclovir is recommended treatment of immunocompromised patients
    3.   In the pregnant woman with uncomplicated varicella, oral acyclovir therapy is not recommended

B. Measures to control pruritus:
1. Calamine or Cetaphil lotion to lesions
2. Prescribe hydroxyzine (Atarax). Dosage is 25 mg TID/QID
3. Alternatively, prescribe diphenhydramine HCl (Benadryl). Dosage is 25-50 mg TID/QID
4. Bathe with baking soda or Aveeno and cut nails to prevent bacterial superinfection

C. Symptomatic treatment to reduce fever and discomfort: Use acetaminophen (Tylenol); NSAIDs may increase risk of more severe varicella

D. Control measures: Patients may return to school/work after all the lesions are crusted which may be several days in mild cases to several weeks in severe cases

E. Care of exposed persons: Potential therapies for susceptible persons exposed to varicella include varicella vaccine **or** varicella-zoster immune globulin (VZIG)
1. Administer varicella vaccine (one dose) to susceptible persons within 72 hours and possibly up to 120 hours after exposure
2. Administer varicella-zoster immune globulin (VZIG) within 96 hours after exposure to varicella to susceptible persons at high risk for severe varicella
   a. Obtain VZIG from American Red Cross Blood Services or FFF Enterprises (telephone number is 1-800-843-7477)
   b. VZIG should be given to the following persons if they have had significant exposure such as residing in same household, indoor face-to-face contact, hospital contact:
      (1) Immunocompromised children without history of varicella
      (2) Immunocompromised adults and adolescents
      (3) Susceptible, pregnant women
      (4) Newborns whose mothers had onset of varicella within 5 days before or within 2 days after delivery
      (5) Hospitalized premature infants
         (a) ≥28 weeks gestation whose mother has no history of varicella or seronegativity
         (b) <28 weeks of gestation or ≤1000 g regardless of maternal history or serostatus
   c. Dosage: One vial VZIG containing 125 units is given intramuscularly (IM) for each 10 kg of body weight; maximum dose is 625 units or 5 vials
3. Consider a 7-day course of acyclovir to susceptible adults beginning 7-9 days after varicella exposure if vaccine is contraindicated or to adults with late presentations

F. Active or primary immunization (see immunization schedule in HEALTH MAINTENANCE section)

G. Follow Up
1. Teach patients to identify potential complications such as secondary skin infections, central nervous system problems, and pneumonia
2. In uncomplicated cases, no follow up is needed

REFERENCES

American Academy of Pediatrics. (2000). In L.K. Pickering (Ed.). *2000 red book: Report of the Committee on Infectious Diseases* (25th ed.). Elk Grove Village, IL: Author.

American Academy of Pediatrics, Committee on Infectious Diseases. (2000). Prevention of Lyme disease. *Pediatrics, 105,* 142-146.

Breman, J.G., & Henderson, D.A. (2002). Diagnosis and management of smallpox. *New England Journal of Medicine, 346,* 1301-1304.

Centers for Disease Control and Prevention. (1990). Case definition for public health surveillance. *MMWR, 39(RR-13),* 1-43.

Centers for Disease Control and Prevention, Advisory Committee on Immunization Practices. (1999). Recommendations for the use of Lyme disease vaccine. *MMWR, 48(RR07),* 1-17.

Centers for Disease Control and Prevention. (2001). Control and prevention of rubella: Evaluation and management of suspected outbreaks, rubella in pregnant women, and surveillance for congenital rubella syndrome. *MMWR, 50(RR12),* 1-23.

Centers for Disease Control and Prevention. 2002. Measles – United States 2000. *MMWR, 51*(06), 120-123.

Centers for Disease Control and Prevention, Advisory Committee on Immunization Practices. (2002). Prevention and control of influenza: Recommendations of Advisory Committee on Immunization Practices (ACIP). *MMWR, 51(RR-3),* 1-31.

Chin, J. (Ed.). (2000). *Control of communicable diseases manual* (17th ed.). Washington DC: American Public Health Association.

Colgan, R., Michocki, R., Greisman, L, & Moore, T.A.W. (2003). Antiviral drugs in the immune competent host: Part II. Treatment of influenza and respiratory syncytial virus infections. *American Family Physician, 67,* 763-766.

Couch, R.B. (2000). Prevention and treatment of influenza. *New England Journal of Medicine, 343,* 1778-1787.

Gammons, M., & Salam, G. (2002). Tick removal. *American Family Physician, 66,* 63-64.

Hall, S., Maupin, T., Peterson, C., Goldman, G., Mascola, L, Seward, J., et al. (2002). The second varicella infections: Are they more common than previously thought? *Pediatrics, 109,* 1068-1073.

Hanson, C.M. (2001). Fifth disease. *American Journal for Nurse Practitioners, 5,* 35-40.

Iglesias, E.A., & Fisher, M. (2002). Infectious mononucleosis. In R.E. Rakel, & E.T. Bope (Eds.), *Conn's current therapy 2002.* Philadelphia: Saunders.

Ingelsby, T.V., O'Toole, T., Henderson, D.A., et al. (2002). Anthrax as a biological weapon, 2002: Updated recommendations for management. *JAMA, 287,* 2236-2252.

Montalto, N.J. (2003). An office-based approach to influenza: Clinical diagnosis and laboratory testing. *American Family Physician, 67,* 111-118.

Montalto, N.J., Gum, K.D., & Ashley, J.V. (2000). Updated treatment of influenza A and B. *American Family Physician, 62,* 2467-2476.

Nadelman, R.B., Nowakowski, J., Fish, D., Falco, R.C., Freeman, K., McKenna, D., et al; Tick Bite Study Group. (2001). Prophylaxis with single-dose doxycycline for the prevention of Lyme disease after an *Ixodes scapularis* tick bite. *New England Journal of Medicine, 345,* 79-84.

Relman, D.A., & Olson, J.E. (2002). Smallpox: A brief overview. *Consultant,* 177-178.

Reef, S.E., Frey, T.K., Theall, K., Abernathy, E., Burnett, C.L., Icenogle, J., et al. (2002). The changing epidemiology of rubella in the 1990s: On the verge of elimination and new challenges for control and prevention. *JAMA, 287,* 464-472.

Seward, JF., Watson, B.M., Peterson, C.L., Mascola, L., Pelosi, J.W., & Zhang, J.X. (2002). Varicella disease after introduction of varicella vaccine in the United States, 1995-2000. *JAMA, 287,* 606-611.

Shapiro, E.D. (2001) Doxycycline for tick bites – Not for everyone. *New England Journal of Medicine, 345,* 113-114.

Sood, S.K. (2003). Lyme borreliosis. *Advanced Studies in Medicine, 3,* 22-26.

Steere, A.C. (2001). Lyme disease. *New England Journal of Medicine, 345,* 115-125.

Steere, A.C., Dhar, A., Hernandez, J., Fischer, P.A., Sikand, V.K., Schoen, R.T., et al. (2003). Systemic symptoms without erythema migrans as the presenting picture of early Lyme disease. *American Journal of Medicine, 114,* 58-62.

Thanassi, W. D., & Schoen, R.T. (2000). The Lyme disease vaccine: Conception, development, and implementation. *Annals of Internal Medicine, 132,* 661-668.

Wormser, G.P., Nadelman, R.B., Dattwyler, R.J., Dennis, D.T., Shapiro, E.D., Rush, T.J., et al. (2000). Practice guidelines for the treatment of Lyme disease: Guidelines from the Infectious Disease Society of America. *Clinical Infectious Diseases, 31*(Suppl 1), S1-S14.

Skin Problems

MARY VIRGINIA GRAHAM

Fungal and Yeast Infections

Candidiasis

Dermatophyte Infections

Tinea Versicolor

Infestations and Bites

Scabies

Pediculosis (Lice Infestation)

Cutaneous Larvae Migrans (Creeping Eruption)

Papulosquamous Disorders

Psoriasis

Pityriasis Rosea
Lichen Planus

Disorders of Pigmentation

Pityriasis Alba

Viral Infections

Herpes Simplex

Herpes Zoster

Molluscum Contagiosum
Warts

CARE OF DRY AND OILY SKIN

I. Definition: Care aimed at preserving or restoring the normal physiologic state of the skin

II. Pathogenesis

   A. Dry skin results from reduced water content of the stratum corneum and may occur because of genetic influences and/or environmental factors such as exposure to irritating substances (household/industrial chemicals), decreased humidity (optimal humidity for skin is ≥70%; during winter, indoor humidity can get as low as 10%), and frequent or prolonged exposure to water

   B. Oily skin is a result of excess sebum production by sebaceous glands that are largest and most numerous on face, chest, and upper back

III. Clinical Presentation

   A. Dry skin presents as scaly, dry appearing skin that feels dry to touch, and is most often located on the hands and extensor surfaces of legs and arms

   B. Dry skin may appear at any age, but is more common among the elderly, with the legs being the most commonly affected in this age group

   C. Dry skin is sensitive (that is, easily irritated) and usually pruritic

   D. Oily skin presents as moist appearing, shiny skin which feels oily to touch and is most often located on face, chest, and upper back

   E. Oily skin may occur at any age, but is most common among adolescents

IV. Diagnosis/Evaluation

   A. History
       1. Inquire about distribution, onset, duration
       2. Ask about skin cleansing practices, occupational, and household exposures
       3. Ask about treatments tried and results

   B. Physical Examination
       1. Examine entire skin surface
       2. For patients complaining of dry skin, focus on legs, extensor surfaces, and hands, where drying is likely to be worse
       3. For oily skin, focus on face, upper back, and chest

   C. Differential Diagnosis
       1. Atopic dermatitis
       2. Contact dermatitis
       3. Ichthyosis
       4. Dyshidrotic eczema

   D. Diagnostic Tests: None indicated

V.   Plan/Management

A.   For dry skin, provide the following recommendations:

ADVICE FOR PATIENTS WITH DRY SKIN

➡ Keep skin well hydrated by daily baths or showers in water no warmer than 90°

➡ Use mild, super-fatted soaps such as Dove, Keri, Basis, Caress, or Eucerin; use soap in the axilla and groin area and avoid rubbing over entire body; avoid over-aggressive use of wash cloth that can exfoliate and remove the stratum corneum (avoid Ivory Soap which tends to be drying)

➡ A waterless liquid cleanser such as Cetaphil or Aquanil may also be used, especially for washing face

➡ Omit use of bubble baths and bath oils which pose hazard (falls)

➡ After bath, brush away excess water with hands, then pat or blot skin with towel

➡ Apply moisturizers from the list below immediately after bathing, while skin is somewhat moist to seal in moisture

➡ **Note:** Lotions are the least moisturizing but the most acceptable to patients; ointments are the most moisturizing and should always be recommended to patients with very dry skin

Moisturizing Lotions	**Moisturizing Creams**	**Moisturizing Ointments**
Petrolatum-based	Petrolatum-based	Petrolatum-based
Dermasil	Purpose Dry Skin Cream	Vaseline Pure Petroleum Jelly
DML Lotion	Cetaphil Cream	(Fragrance, preservative, and
Moisturel Lotion	Keri Cream	lanolin free)
Replenaderm		
Mixtures of lanolin and petrolatum	Mixtures of lanolin and petrolatum	Mixtures of lanolin and petrolatum
Eucerin Lotion	Eucerin Creme	Aquaphor Natural Healing Ointment
Lubriderm Lotion		(Fragrance and preservative free)
Nivea Moisturizing		
Without lanolin or petrolatum	Without lanolin or petrolatum	
Corn Huskers Lotion	Neutrogena Norwegian Formula	
Cetaphil Lotion	Hand Cream	

B.   Consult the box below for a listing of relatively inexpensive moisturizers that were given high ratings for moisturizing effectiveness by *Consumer Reports* (**Note:** Efficacy in skin care products does not necessarily correlate with cost; cheaper products are often as good as, if not better than, more expensive ones)

MOISTURIZERS RATED BEST BY *CONSUMER REPORTS*

Face
L'Oreal Plenitude Active Daily Moisture SPF15
Pond's Nourishing Moisturizer SPF15

Body
Vaseline Intensive Care Advanced Healing with Skin Protection Complex
Curel Therapeutic Moisturizing Original Formula

Hands
Curel Soothing Hands Moisturizing with Chamomile
Neutrogena New Hands Restorative SPF15

Adapted from Editors (2000). The skin game. *Consumer Reports*, January 2000, 38-41

C.   Agents containing lactic acid or urea should be used judiciously as these products draw water from the environment and thus don't work well unless the surrounding humidity is relatively high; they are also very irritating to dry skin and make the skin more sensitive to the sun; burning and stinging limit the usefulness of these products

1.   Strictly speaking, such agents are not moisturizers

2.   They enhance shedding of superficial cells and this exfoliation results immediately in a smoother, more uniform surface

---

Urea Creams and Lotions
- Cream 10% (Aquacare, Nutraplus)
- Cream 20% (Carmol 20)
- Lotion 10% (Aquacare, Carmol 10)

Lactic Acid-Containing Lotions
- 5% (LactiCare)
- 12% (Lac-Hydrin) [Rx product]

D.   For oily skin, provide the following recommendations:

ADVICE FOR PATIENTS WITH OILY SKIN

➡ Use a deodorant soap such as Dial or Safeguard containing an antibacterial or a mildly drying soap (Ivory)
➡ Avoid using preparations containing oils
➡ Use an astringent or toner on face
➡ For women, use cosmetics such as those listed below

COSMETICS FOR WOMEN WITH OILY SKIN

Allercreme
    Matte-Finish Makeup (waterbase, oil free)
Charles of the Ritz
    T-Zone Controller
Clinique
    Pore Minimizer Makeup (fragrance and oil free)
    Stay True Oil-Free (for sensitive skin, SPF 15)
Covergirl
    Fresh Complexion, 100% oil-free
Esteé Lauder
    Tender Matte Makeup (fragrance and oil free)
    Simply Sheer
    Lucidity Makeup

Lancome
    Maquicontrol, Oil-Free Liquid Makeup
L'Oreal
    Mattique Illuminating Makeup
Monteil
    Habitat Natural Light Makeup
Max Factor
    Shine-Free Makeup
Revlon
    Spring Water Matte Makeup
Shisheido
    Pureness Oil-Control Makeup
Ultima II
    The Nakeds: The Foundation Oil-Free Formula

E.   Use every opportunity to discuss the role of sun exposure in photoaging (see section on BENIGN SKIN LESIONS for recommendations relating to sun avoidance counseling)

F.   Follow-up: None indicated

BENIGN SKIN LESIONS

I.   Definition: Cutaneous growths with no malignant potential

II.   Pathogenesis: Variable depending on lesion

III.   Clinical Presentation

BENIGN SKIN LESIONS: CLINICAL PRESENTATION

Seborrheic keratosis	✓ Common benign skin tumors of varying coloration, generally seen beginning in middle age ✓ Most people develop at least one in their lifetime; can arise at any site except palms and soles ✓ Sharply circumscribed, flat or raised lesions 0.2 to 2 cm in size that vary in color from light brown to jet black; surface may be smooth, velvety, or verrucous; most have a waxy, stuck-on appearance, with a surface that crumbles when picked
Stucco keratosis	✓ A variant of seborrheic keratosis; small hypopigmented to white papules found commonly on lower extremities of older Caucasians; a marker of aging ✓ Papules are white-gray, dry, and keratotic and are most often concentrated on the dorsa of the feet, ankles and on the lower legs; often numerous in number ✓ Usually 1.0-10.0 mm in size; may rub off but often recur
Dermatosis papulosa nigra	✓ A variant of seborrheic keratosis commonly found on African-Americans and Asians ✓ Numerous 1-2 mm dark brown keratotic papules concentrated around eyes and on malar cheeks ✓ May be called "moles" by patients who have them; a marker of aging
Cherry angioma	✓ Punctate, mature, vascular neoplasm found on nearly all people >30 years of age ✓ Appear in early adulthood and increase in number with aging ✓ Discrete, 0.5 to 5.0 mm, smooth, dome-shaped papules with color varying from cherry red to deeper purple as lesions increase in size; found in greatest density on trunk ✓ Number of lesions can range from a few to hundreds
Sebaceous hyperplasia	✓ Small tumors composed of enlarged sebaceous glands; appear as soft, skin-colored to pale yellow papules that are 1-2 mm in size and minimally elevated ✓ Occur on face (usually forehead) of older persons ✓ Over time, lesions become yellow, dome-shaped, and umbilicated ✓ A marker of aging and associated with sun damage ✓ May be confused with basal cell carcinoma
Solar lentigo	✓ Appear as lightly pigmented tan macules with irregular borders in sun-exposed areas ✓ About 75% of Caucasians >60 years of age have one or more lesions caused by sun exposure ✓ Commonly called liver spots ✓ Increase in number and size with advancing age

IV. Diagnosis/Evaluation

    A. History
        1. Inquire about onset, and growth rate of lesions
        2. Ask about new or recently changing lesions
        3. Inquire about personal and family history of skin tumors
        4. Ask about sun exposure and use of sun protection strategies

    B. Physical Examination
        1. Examine entire skin surface noting hallmark characteristics of lesions
        2. Use exam to teach patient skin self-exam for malignant lesions
        3. Determine patient skin type and sun sensitivity and use this information to reinforce education about sun avoidance and sunscreen use

SKIN TYPES AND SUN SENSITIVITY

Skin Type	Description
I	Fair skin, always burns, never tans
II	Fair skin, usually burns, sometimes tans
III	Lightly pigmented, usually tans, sometimes burns
IV	Pigmented, always tans, never burns
V	Moderately pigmented, never burns
VI	Heavily pigmented (black) skin

    C. Differential Diagnosis
        1. Sebaceous hyperplasia: Basal cell carcinoma (has pearly surface rather than dull yellow surface of senile sebaceous hyperplasia)
        2. Seborrheic keratosis, solar lentigines: Benign intradermal nevus (mole), basal cell carcinoma, malignant melanoma, squamous cell carcinoma

    D. Diagnostic Tests: None indicated when lesions are characteristic; questionable lesions should be evaluated via biopsy

V.   Plan/Management

A.   Provide reassurance that lesions are benign and explain that no treatment is required for these very common lesions

B.   Counsel about sun exposure and need for skin self-exam on regular basis
1.   Discuss sun protection noting that the three keys to sun protection (from the most effective to the least effective) are avoidance, use of protective clothing, and use of sunscreen; advise patients as follows:
a.   Explain to patient that there are no safe, healthy tans and no safe tanning devices
b.   Avoid sun exposure between 10 AM and 4 PM except during late fall and winter months
c.   Use protective clothing (broad brimmed hat to shield face and ears, long-sleeved shirt and pants); special protective clothing is available from Sun Precautions, 2815 Wetmore Avenue, Everett, WA 98201, www.sunprecautions.com
d.   Wear sunglasses with at least 99% protection against both ultraviolet A and ultraviolet B sunlight
e.   Use sunscreen with a SPF ≥30; apply 30 minutes before sun exposure and reapply every hour as it is washed off with sweating and swimming
2.   Teach patients how to carefully examine skin each month using the guide below

---

HOW TO EXAMINE YOUR SKIN: A GUIDE FOR PATIENTS

- To perform a self-examination, have a hand-held mirror available and stand naked in front of a full-length mirror in a well-lighted room
- Start by learning where your birthmarks, moles, and blemishes are and what they usually look like
- Search for anything new: a change in the size, texture, or color of a mole or a sore that does not heal
- Look at the front and back of your body in the mirror. Raise your arms and look at both sides of your body
- Bend your elbows and look at your palms, tops and undersides of your forearms, and your upper arms
- Examine the back and front of your legs. Look between your buttocks and around the genital area
- Sit and examine your feet, including the soles and the spaces between the toes
- Look carefully at your face, neck, and scalp. A comb or a blow dryer to move your hair may be helpful
- If you find anything unusual, see your clinician as soon as possible

---

Adapted from National Cancer Institute. (2000). What you need to know about skin cancer. Available at: nttp://www.cancernet.nci.nih.gov/wyntk_pubs/skin.htm. Accessed July 14, 2002.

C.   Refer for removal for cosmetic purposes if patient desires

D.   Treatment of solar lentigines can usually be done without referral using **one** of the following

---

TREATMENT OF SOLAR LENTIGO

✓   Hydroquinone solutions and azelaic acid cream can reduce hyperpigmentation over weeks to months
  - Hydroquinone: Eldoquin Forte, 4% cream; Apply to affected areas BID; maximum 2 months; supplied in 15 g and 30 g tubes
  - Azelaic acid: Azelex cream; Apply to affected areas BID; may decrease to 1x daily for maximum of 2 months; supplied in 30 g tube

✓   Use of liquid nitrogen on lesions for 10 seconds or less is also usually effective
  - Melanocytes are very sensitive to liquid nitrogen
  - Easily destroyed with very small amounts and short exposure times
  - Lesions may heal with hypopigmentation

E.   Patients can be referred to The Skin Cancer Foundation website for patient education handouts including color pictures

Skin Cancer Foundation Website:
http://www.derm-infonet.com/Moles.html

F.   Follow Up: None required unless changes in lesions occur

CANCERS OF THE SKIN
(BASAL CELL, SQUAMOUS CELL, AND MELANOMA)

I. Definition: Malignant cutaneous neoplasms found in humans

II. Pathogenesis

   A. Basal cell carcinoma (BCC)
      1. Cells of BCC resemble those of basal layer of epidermis
      2. BCC grows by direct extension and requires surrounding stroma to support growth
      3. Major etiologic factor is solar radiation

   B. Squamous cell carcinoma (SCC)
      1. Atypical squamous cells originate in epidermis and proliferate
      2. Cells then penetrate the epidermal basement membrane and proliferate into the dermis producing SCC

   C. Melanoma
      1. Arises from cells of the melanocyte system; begins either de novo or develops from a pre-existing lesion
      2. Initially grows superficially and laterally, confining itself to epidermis and papillary dermis
      3. Vertical growth then occurs with penetration of reticular dermis and subcutaneous fat

   D. Malignant tumors are a result of cumulative cellular effects of ultraviolet radiation and inability of skin to mount a defense to ultraviolet light

   E. Fair skin and sun exposure are important predisposing factors

III. Clinical Presentation

CANCERS OF THE SKIN: CLINICAL PRESENTATION	
Basal cell carcinoma	✓ The most common skin cancer; locally destructive and slow growing tumor ✓ More common after age 40, but may occur at any age; fair skinned person are at greatest risk; less common among Asian-Americans and rare among African-Americans ✓ Commonly found on the head and neck; less often on sun-exposed areas of trunk/extremities ✓ Fair-skinned persons, persons living in sunny climates, and elderly persons are at increased risk ✓ Are rarely, if ever, life threatening; metastases virtually never occur ✓ Tumor takes many forms. Most common is the nodular form—a pearly colored nodule with fine telangiectasia over the surface and a depressed center or rolled edge
Squamous cell carcinoma	✓ Accounts for about 20% of all skin cancers; is far more aggressive than previously believed ✓ Occurs most often in middle-aged and elderly population; incidence doubles with each 8-10 degree decline in latitude ✓ Most common in sun-exposed areas; 80% to 90% occur on head, neck, and hands; also arises in skin damaged by thermal burns or chronic inflammation but the majority are caused by ultraviolet light exposure ✓ Tumors may metastasize via the lymphatics to local lymph nodes ✓ Usual appearance is a firm irregular papule with a scaly, keratotic, bleeding, and friable surface appearing on a background of sun-damaged skin characterized by atrophy, telangiectasias, and blotchy hyperpigmentation *(Continued)*

CANCERS OF THE SKIN: CLINICAL PRESENTATION *(CONTINUED)*

Melanoma	✓ The 8th most common malignancy in US, accounting for 4% of all cancers in men and 3% in women; mortality rate (among cancers) is second only to lung cancer
	✓ Incidence continues to rise faster than that of any other type of cancer
	✓ Frequently affects young people; median age is early 40s
	✓ Risk factors include fair skin; presence of atypical nevi in both sun-exposed and sun-protected areas; and intermittent heavy sun exposure (history of blistering sunburn); episodic heavy exposure appears to be more of a risk factor than constant mild exposure
	✓ Most common early signs include an increase in nevus size and change in color or shape; most common early symptom is itching; later symptoms include tenderness, bleeding, and ulceration
	✓ Has ability to metastasize to any organ, including brain
	✓ Melanomas tend to have Asymmetry, Border irregularity, Color variegation, and Diameter greater than 6 mm

IV. Diagnosis/Evaluation

    A. History
        1. Question regarding any skin changes/new growths
        2. Question regarding family and personal history of skin cancer
        3. Question about history of acute blistering sunburns, chronic sun exposure, and use of sun protection strategies
        4. Question about prior radiation, thermal injury, cigarette smoking

    B. Physical Examination
        1. Examine entire surface of skin for suspicious lesions
        2. Use magnifying glass to assist in visualization of surface characteristics
        3. All pigmented lesions should be carefully evaluated
        4. A hair dryer is helpful in examining the scalp; can also use cotton-tipped applicator to examine scalp

    C. Differential Diagnosis
        1. Actinic keratosis
        2. Leukoplakia
        3. Common nevus
        4. Seborrheic keratosis
        5. Solar lentigo

    D. Diagnostic Tests: Skin biopsy should be performed for all lesions suggestive of malignancy

V. Plan/Management

    A. Patients suspected of having skin cancer should be referred to a dermatologist or surgeon for biopsy

    B. Early diagnosis and intervention are crucial (see BENIGN SKIN LESIONS for recommendations about patient teaching); refer patients to the following web site for good information about skin cancer and prevention

American Academy of Dermatology Website: http://www.AAD.org

    C. Educate patients about importance of sun exposure protection (see section on BENIGN SKIN LESIONS)

ROSACEA

I.   Definition: Chronic, cutaneous disorder primarily of the convexities of the central face (cheeks, chin, nose, and central forehead), characterized by remissions and exacerbations

II. Pathogenesis

    A.   Causes of rosacea are unknown; there are no histologic or serologic markers

    B.   Most experts believe that it is primarily a vascular disorder; *Helicobacter pylori* may also play a role in the disorder

III. Clinical Presentation

    A   Syndrome is quite common and is most frequently observed in patients with fair skin; has also been diagnosed in Asians and African Americans

    B.   Occurs in both men and women; may occur at any age; onset is typically at any time after age 30

    C.   Characteristically, affected individuals have facial flushing, especially with increases in skin temperature, ingestion of hot or spicy food, and alcohol consumption

    D.   Over time, the flushing frequently develops into persistent erythema of the face and fine telangiectases develop as a result of the continual vascular engorgement
        1.   Edema, papules, and pustules appear, most often on the central portion of the face
        2.   Skin of upper and lower eyelids, skin below the eyes, and above the nasolabial folds becomes edematous, giving the areas a "baggy" look

    E.   In the final stages of the disease, erythema of the face is deep and persistent, there are numerous telangiectatic blood vessels, particularly in the paranasal area, and pustules, papules, and nodules are prominent; in addition, edema and enlarged pores, especially of the nose, are evident
        1.   Rhinophyma, the red, bulbous nose of rosacea, occurs almost exclusively in men
        2.   It is the end result of increase in connective tissue of the nose due to chronic inflammation, vascular dilation, and sebaceous gland hyperplasia

    F.   Almost 60% of patients with rosacea have some eye involvement including blepharitis and conjunctival injection; the **most common** type of eye involvement, however, is dry eye syndrome

    G.   Diagnostic criteria for rosacea based on a provisional classification system are contained in the table that follows

---

DIAGNOSTIC CRITERIA FOR ROSACEA

Primary Features: Presence of at least one of the following signs with a central face distribution is diagnostic. These signs are commonly transient, and each may occur independently:

➡ Flushing. Transient erythema
➡ Nontransient erythema. Persistent redness–most common sign of rosacea
➡ Papules and pustules. Comedones should be considered part of an acne process not rosacea
➡ Telangiectasia. Common but not a necessary sign

Secondary Features: Following signs and symptoms often present with one or more of primary features above:

➡ Burning or stinging. Occurs with or without scaling or dermatitis, especially on malar skin
➡ Plaque. Elevated red plaques occur without changes in surrounding skin
➡ Dry appearance. Central facial skin may be dry appearing with scale
➡ Edema. May accompany or follow prolonged facial erythema
➡ Ocular manifestations. Common; range from symptoms of itching/burning to conjunctival hyperemia and lid inflammation
➡ Peripheral location. Frequency and occurrence of this are ill-defined
➡ Phymatous changes. Can include patulous follicles, skin thickening, and a bulbous appearance

---

Adapted from Wilkins, J., et al. (2002). Standard classification of rosacea: Report of the National Rosacea Society Expert Committee on the Classification and Staging of Rosacea. *Journal of the American Academy of Dermatology, 46,* 584-587.

H. In addition to the primary and secondary features of rosacea contained in the above table, there are four subtypes and one variant that occur less frequently. It is beyond the scope of this book to consider those here; see above reference for additional information

IV. Diagnosis/Evaluation

    A. History
        1. Inquire about onset, initial symptoms, and progression of symptoms over time
        2. Using the diagnostic criteria listed in the table above, determine if patient meets the criteria under either primary or secondary features
        3. Ask what makes the condition worse; specifically, ask about the effects of hot ambient temperatures, effects of eating hot or spicy foods, or ingesting alcohol
        4. Ask about treatments tried and results

    B. Physical Exam
        1. Examine facial skin for characteristic distribution (central facial area) and for characteristic erythema, papules, pustules, plaque, dry appearing skin, edema, telangiectasia, and phymatous changes
        2. Examine eyelids for scaling or erythema, and sclera and conjunctiva for hyperemia

    C. Diagnostic Tests: Diagnosis can be made based on whether the diagnostic criteria are met using clinical data obtained during history and physical examination

    D. Differential Diagnosis: Acne (no comedones in rosacea), lupus erythematosus (obtain biopsy to rule out lupus, if suspected)

V. Plan/Management

    A. Provide patient with information about the disorder and emphasize that control rather than cure is the goal of treatment

    B. Counsel patient to cleanse the face twice daily with a soapless cleanser such as Aquanil or Cetaphil
        1. Patient should avoid use of soaps, scrubs, astringents, and toners that often cause burning and stinging
        2. Women should use makeup that is hypoallergenic and should avoid products that may cause irritation (see table containing examples of hypoallergenic cosmetics in section on ACNE)

    C. Treatment of choice is **combination** therapy with a systemic antibiotic and a topical antibiotic
        1. Systemic antibiotics are effective for treating inflammatory lesions, papules, pustules, as well as flushing, erythema, and telangiectases

2. Topical antibiotics are effective for reducing erythema, resolving inflammatory papules and pustules and allow for long-term control without subjecting the patient to systemic effects caused by oral antibiotics
3. Topical and systemic antibiotics should be started at the same time with the aim of tapering off the systemic antibiotic over a period of 3-4 months and continuing to use the topical antibiotic for maintenance

D. Choose one of the oral antibiotics from the following table

SYSTEMIC ANTIBIOTICS USEFUL IN TREATMENT OF ROSACEA		
Generic (Trade) Name	**Dosing**	**Comment**
Tetracycline (Sumycin)	500 mg BID x 4-6 weeks (Available as 250, 500 mg caps)	✓ Reduce dose to 500 mg QD (AM or PM) as soon as significant improvement occurs ✓ Then, continue treatment for next 4-6 weeks ✓ If remission continues, decrease the dose to 250 mg QD for an additional 4-6 weeks ✓ If skin is clear after treatment, discontinue systemic treatment at this point ✓ If flares occur, return to lowest dose (250 mg) QD
Erythromycin (Ery-Tab)	500 mg BID x 4-6 weeks (Available as 250 mg tabs)	✓ Follow the same pattern as Tetracycline (above) [decreasing dose every 4-6 weeks]
Doxycycline (Vibramycin)	100 mg BID tapering to QD, then every other or every 3rd day (Available as 50, 100 mg caps)	✓ Follow the same pattern as with Tetracycline (above) [decreasing dose every 4-6 weeks]
Minocycline (Minocin)	100 mg BID tapering to QD, then every other or every 3rd day (Available as 50, 100 mg caps)	✓ Follow the same pattern as with Tetracycline (above) ✓ [decreasing dose every 4-6 weeks]

Monitor blood, renal, and hepatic function in long-term use ($\geq$4 weeks) for all drugs listed in table

E. Choose one of the topical antibiotics from the following table

TOPICAL AGENTS USEFUL IN THE TREATMENT OF ROSACEA	
Metronidazole, 0.75% gel or cream (MetroGel, MetroCream, and Noritate) **(Note**: Recently became available in 1% concentration which can be dosed QD)	✓ Apply BID ✓ Use gel for patients with oily skin and cream for patients with dry skin ✓ Women may apply makeup over the medication ✓ Supplied as gel—30, 45 g; cream—45 g
Sulfacet--R lotion	✓ Apply BID ✓ Especially useful for oily skin; available tinted or tint-free ✓ Supplied as 25 g

F. Provide counseling to patient in terms of what to expect and the need for continuing therapy in most cases; provide patient with resources such as those contained in the following box

---

The National Rosacea Society
800 S. Northwest Highway, Suite 200
Barrington, IL 60010
1-888-NO BLUSH (662-5874)

Materials provided include educational information for healthcare providers and patients
Newsletter called "Rosacea Review" is also published by the society
Call the toll free number for more information or visit the web site at www.rosacea.org

---

G. Environmental and lifestyle factors may trigger flares
1. Identification of the factors is an individual process
2. Factors that cause problems in one patient may not in another
3. Among common triggers are sun, stress, heat, alcohol, spicy foods, exercise

4. Provide patient with counseling regarding how to deal with common triggers identified above (e.g., avoiding sun exposure between 10 AM and 4 PM, wearing protective clothing, wide brim hat, and sunscreen with an SPF of 30 or greater; refer for stress management techniques, etc.)
5. Men should consider use of electric shaver that is less irritating than safety razor

H. Patients with dry eye syndrome can relieve symptoms with use of lubricant eyedrops
   1. Advise patient to use drops as soon as eyes begin feeling dry or before engaging in activities that are drying to eyes such as looking at computer screen or jogging outdoors
   2. Product examples, all preservative-free, are Bion Tears, HypoTears PF, and Duratears Naturale

I. Patients with blepharitis can be treated as described in section on BLEPHARITIS

J. Patients with moderate to severe telangiectasia and rhinophyma may require surgical intervention and should be referred for treatment

K. Follow up: Every 2-4 weeks when initiating therapy, then less frequently once the condition is controlled

ACNE

I. Definition: A disease of the pilosebaceous unit that is most intense in areas where sebaceous glands are numerous

II. Pathogenesis

A. A number of factors and events work in concert to make the pathogenesis of acne multifactorial in nature

B. Excessive sebum produced by the androgen-dependent sebaceous glands, combined with excessive numbers of desquamated cells from the walls of the sebaceous follicles cause obstruction of the follicles (which are located primarily on the face and trunk)

C. As a consequence of this obstruction, microcomedones are formed that may eventually evolve into either comedones or inflammatory lesions

D. A resident anaerobic organism, *Propionibacterium acnes* (found in very low numbers on normal skin) finds the environment created by the excessive sebum and desquamated follicular cells very conducive to growth and produces chemotactic factors and proinflammatory mediators that may lead to inflammation

III. Clinical Presentation

A. Acne is the most common skin disorder, affecting almost 80% of persons at some point in their lives, most often between the ages of 11 and 30
   1. Acne begins in the pre-pubertal period when the adrenal glands begin secreting increased amounts of adrenal androgens which leads to increased production of sebum
   2. Androgen production and sebaceous gland activity are further stimulated with gonad development during puberty

B. Most patients with acne are probably hyper-responsive to androgens rather than overproducers of androgens; androgen excess, however, has been implicated in the development of acne

C. **Comedonal acne** represents the **earliest** clinical expression of acne, occurring in the pre-teen and early teenage years
   1. Characteristic lesions are noninflammatory comedones located on central forehead, chin, nose, paranasal area
   2. Comedones are open (blackheads) or closed (whiteheads)
   3. Colonization with *P. acnes* has not yet occurred; thus, no inflammatory lesions are present

D. **Mild inflammatory acne** usually develops in teenagers **after the first phase** of non-inflammatory comedonal acne; also occurs in adult women in their 20s
   1. Characterized by scattered small papules or pustules with a minimum of comedones and rarely results in scarring
   2. Arises from microcomedones in which two factors are present
      a. Abnormal desquamation of epithelial cells in the follicles
      b. Proliferation of *P. acnes*

E. **Inflammatory acne** represents the **final** phase in the evolution of acne from noninflammatory comedonal acne, to small numbers of inflammatory lesions on the face, to a more generalized eruption, first on the face, and then on the trunk
   1. Most patients with acne have inflammatory acne, with comedones, papules, and pustules on the face and trunk
   2. In a minority of patients, large, deep inflammatory nodules (called cysts) develop reflecting the presence of a very destructive type of inflammation
   3. Cystic acne requires prompt attention since ruptured cysts may result in scar formation

IV. Evaluation/Diagnosis

   A. History
      1. Question regarding onset, type of lesions, distribution
      2. In females, question about history of cyclic menstrual flares, use of oral contraceptives
      3. Inquire about types of cleansers and lubricants used on face
      4. Document previous treatments and results

   B. Physical Examination
      1. Examine skin to determine form of acne:
         a. Comedonal acne—noninflammatory comedones
         b. Mild inflammatory acne—scattered small papules or pustules with a minimum of comedones
         c. Inflammatory acne—comedones, papules, and pustules on the face and trunk
         d. Inflammatory acne with large, deep inflammatory nodules
      2. Determine areas of involvement and document in patient record

   C. Differential Diagnosis
      1. Rosacea
      2. Steroid rosacea
      3. Molluscum contagiosum
      4. Folliculitis

   D. Diagnostic Tests: None indicated

V. Plan/Management

   A. Explain the mechanism of acne and treatment plan to the patient
      1. Emphasize that little improvement may be evident for 2-3 months
      2. Use written patient education materials to reinforce teaching

   B. Counsel patient regarding the following general measures:
      1. Cleanse affected areas gently with mild soap (Purpose, Basis) or cleansers such as Cetaphil lotion no more than 2-3 x day (emphasize that use of topical agents such as soaps and astringents have no effect on sebum production but only remove sebum from the surface of the skin which has little therapeutic value)
      2. Avoid picking at lesions as it may cause scarring
      3. Avoid oil-based cosmetics, hair styling mousse, and face creams that have no effect on sebum production but do increase the amount of oil on the face

4.   Use nonacnegenic moisturizers such as Moisturel, and cosmetics from the table that follows

NONACNEGENIC COSMETICS FOR WOMEN	
Allercreme ✓ Matte-Finish Makeup (Waterbase, oil free) **Charles of the Ritz** ✓ T-Zone Controller **Clinique** ✓ Pore Minimizer Makeup (Fragrance and oil free) ✓ Stay True Oil-Free (For sensitive skin, SPF 15) **Covergirl** ✓ Fresh Complexion, 100% Oil-Free **Esteé Lauder** ✓ Tender Matte Makeup (Fragrance and oil free) ✓ Simply Sheer Fresh Air Makeup Base, Oil-free	**Lancome** ✓ Maquicontrol, Oil-Free Liquid Makeup **Mary Kay Cosmetics** ✓ Oil-Free Foundation (Fragrance and oil-free) **Max Factor** ✓ Shine-Free Makeup **Revlon** ✓ Spring Water Matte Makeup **Shisheido** ✓ Pureness Oil-Control Makeup

5.   Dietary factors have no effect on sebum production, and patient should be counseled to eat a well-balanced diet

C.   Consider whether patient is a candidate for oral contraceptive use (see section on Contraception in GYNECOLOGY chapter); the FDA has approved several OCs (e.g., Ortho Tri-Cyclen and Estrostep Fe) for acne therapy in women without contraindications who desire contraception (not considered a first-line drug for acne)

D.   Treatment of acne using both topical and oral agents is outlined in the following table

TREATMENT OF ACNE

Treatment Aims	Treatment	Comments

Comedonal Acne
 	
• Reduce or counteract abnormal desquamation of follicular epithelium
	Topical comedolytic agents are the treatment of choice
	Select a comedolytic agent from the following list of topical agents
	
	Tretinoin
	(Retin-A) available as cream, gel, or liquid
	  Cream: 0.025%, 0.05%, and 0.1%, supplied as 20 g, 45 g
	  Gel: 0.01%, 0.025%, supplied as 15 g, 45 g
	  Liquid: 0.05%, supplied as 28 mL
	(Retin-A Micro) sustained release delivery system, available as 0.1% aqueous gel, supplied as 20 g, 45 g
	(Avita) available as cream, gel (0.025%), supplied as 20 g, 45 g
	Apply QD at bedtime, beginning with a lower concentration of the cream, gel, or liquid and increasing if local irritation does not occur
	(**Note:** Considered the standard against which all other comedolytics are judged)
	
	Adapalene *(Differin)*, a naphthoic derivative with retinoid activity, available as cream, gel, solution, and pledgets
	  Cream and Gel: 0.1%, supplied as 15 g, 45 g
	  Solution: 0.1%, supplied as 30 mL
	  Pledgets: 0.1%, supplied as 60 pledgets
	Apply QD at bedtime, beginning with a lower concentration of the solution or gel, and increasing if local irritation does not occur
	(**Note:** Causes less irritation than topical tretinoin and is often effective in patients who cannot tolerate topical tretinoin)
	
	Azelaic acid *20% (Azelex)* has both comedolytic and antibacterial effects, available as cream (one concentration only); supplied as 30 g
	Apply BID, in the morning and evening to clean dry skin
	(**Note:** May cause less irritation than tretinoin and often causes hypopigmentation which may be desirable for some patients)
		⬆ Advise patient to apply thin layer of the topical agent to the entire face, not just the individual lesions
		
		⬆ Warn about increased photosensitivity – patient must apply sunscreen daily for any sun exposure
		
		⬆ Gels are usually preferred in hot/humid climates and creams in cold/dry climates
		
		⬆ Several months may be necessary to achieve good results
		
		⬆ Treatment should be continued until no new lesions are developing

Mild Inflammatory Acne • Reduce or counteract abnormal desquamation of follicular epithelium • Prevent proliferation of *P. acnes*	*Topical therapy with a combination of a comedolytic **and** an antibiotic is the treatment of choice* **Select a comedolytic agent from the list below** **Select an antibiotic agent from the list below** (**Note:** When used in combination, **once** daily dosing for the comedolytic and the antibiotic is acceptable; each product should be used at separate times of day: Use comedolytic in AM and antibiotic in PM. **The BID dosing schedule for both comedolytic and antibiotic agents in the lists given here are the dosing recommendations when the agents are used alone!**) **Topical Antibiotics** *Benzoyl peroxide, (Benzac)* available as a gel with alcohol-base in 5%, 10% concentrations; also available as aqueous-base gel (Benzac-W) in 2.5%, 5%, 10% concentrations Both products supplied as 60 g Apply QD to clean, dry skin (**Note:** Very effective anti-*P. acnes* agent; major disadvantage is irritation which can be minimized by using lower concentrations and water-base form)	⬆ Most patients respond to treatment after 2-4 weeks ⬆ Treatment should be continued until no new lesions develop, then slowly discontinued ⬆ Many products available, some of which are generic and less expensive *(Continued)*

Treatment Aims	Treatment	Comments
Mild Inflammatory Acne (*Continued*)		
	Erythromycin, 2% solution and alcohol-base gel (A/T/S) Supplied as solution—60 mL, and gel—30 g Apply BID to clean, dry skin	↑ Many products available, some of which are generic and much less expensive
	Clindamycin, 1% (Cleocin-T) available as solution, pledgets, lotion, and alcohol-base gel Supplied as solution—30 mL, 60 mL; pledgets—boxes of 60; lotion—60 mL; gel—30 g, 60 g Apply BID to clean, dry skin	
	*Benzoyl peroxide **plus** erythromycin (Benzamycin)*, contains 3% erythromycin and 5% benzoyl peroxide in gel form (alcohol base) Supplied as gel—23.3 g, 46.6 g Apply BID to clean, dry skin (**Note:** Considered by many to be the **most effective** topical antibiotic therapy against *P. acnes*)	
Inflammatory Acne		
• Reduce or counteract abnormal desquamation of follicular epithelium • Prevent proliferation of *P. acnes* and the resultant inflammation produced by the organism	*Topical therapy with comedolytic **and** systemic antibiotic therapy (all acne begins with follicular impaction)* **Select a comedolytic agent from the list above** **Select an antibiotic from the following list**	↑ Deciding between topical and systemic antibiotics should be guided by two factors: Extent of skin involvement and severity of inflammation
	Oral antibiotics	↑ **Do not use tetracycline derivatives** in pregnant women, nursing mothers, or children under the age of 12
	Doxycycline (Vibramycin), available as 50 mg, 100 mg caps 100 mg BID x 1 day, then 50 mg BID; dose can be reduced to 50 mg QD after improvement	↑ Patients treated with oral antibiotics may also be given topical antibiotics once the oral dose is reduced to a maintenance level
	Minocycline (Minocin), available as 50 mg, 100 mg caps 50 mg BID; dose can be reduced to 50 mg QD after improvement	
	(**Note:** Above two agents are more lipid-soluble than tetracycline and erythromycin and are generally considered to be more effective than tetracycline and erythromycin)	
	Tetracycline (Achromycin V), available as 250 mg, 500 mg caps 1 g/day in 2 divided doses, then 125-500 mg/day with further reduction after improvement	
	Erythromycin (E-Mycin), available as 250 mg, 333 mg tabs 500 mg BID or 333 mg BID, with reduction after improvement	

E.   Refer patients with widespread, nodular cystic lesions to a dermatologist for treatment aimed at therapy to suppress sebum production

F.   Follow Up: Three follow up visits (over 8-10 weeks) are generally needed to establish a successful treatment program
1.   For patients with comedonal and mild inflammatory acne on topical agents:
a.   Use chart to document location, type, and number of lesions to determine treatment response on each visit
b.   Adjust strength and frequency of topical agents depending on irritation and effectiveness
c.   If skin dryness is a problem that interferes with compliance, suggest use of a nonacnegenic moisturizer such as Moisturel, Purpose lotion, or Neutrogena Moisture after application of gel, or switch to a cream preparation
2.   For patients with inflammatory acne using **topical** comedolytics as well as **oral** antibiotics:
a.   Do a., b., and c. in F.1. above.
b.   Begin tapering oral antibiotic dose after 4-6 weeks of treatment (depending upon when development of new inflammatory lesions ceases); once the oral dose is reduced to a maintenance level, can add topical antibiotics to provide control
c.   Most patients require prolonged courses (months) or frequent, intermittent courses before complete and final remission occurs. **Consult PDR regarding need to monitor blood, renal, and hepatic function in patients on long-term antibiotic use!**
3.   For patients who are not on a successful treatment program after a total of 10-12 weeks of therapy, referral to a dermatologist is indicated

ATOPIC DERMATITIS

I.   Definition: Extremely pruritic skin disorder involving cutaneous hypersensitivity

II.   Pathogenesis

A.   A hereditary disorder whose exact pathogenesis is unknown

B.   Recently, factors involved in both epidermal barrier function and immunity (such as the serine protease inhibitor SPINK-5 and interleukin-4 mutations) have been implicated in the pathogenesis

III.   Clinical Presentation

A.   Generally, begins in infancy/childhood, has periods of remission, exacerbation, and resolves by age 30. Highest incidence is among children

B.   Abnormally dry skin and lowered threshold for itching are significant factors

C.   Itching occurs in paroxysms and may be severe, especially in evenings

D.   Once itch-scratch cycle is established, characteristic lesions are created secondary to trauma cause by scratching

E.   Patterns of inflammation begin with severe pruritus and erythema. As skin changes are produced by trauma from scratching, skin becomes dry and scaly (xerosis)

F.   Several patterns of lesions may be produced: erythematous papular lesions that become confluent; diffuse erythema and scaling; lichenification (thickening of dermis with accentuation of skin lines)

G.   Involvement of the eyelids is common in all phases of atopic dermatitis

H.   Atopic dermatitis is divided into 3 phases that are outlined in the following table

ATOPIC DERMATITIS	

Infant phase
(birth to 2 years)
	Usually appears at about 3 months of age especially during cold, dry weather
	    Erythema and scaling of cheeks, chin with sparing of perioral and paranasal areas is
	        frequently seen and there is sparing of the diaper area as well. May have generalized
	        eruption of papules that are erythematous and scaly
	    Exudative lesions (oozing, weeping) are typical in infancy

Childhood phase
(2-12 years)
	Characteristic appearance at this age is flexural area involvement; perspiration produced by act
	of flexing and extending stimulates itching and itch-scratch cycle
	    Erythematous papules coalesce into plaques and scratching produces lichenification
	    Foot dermatitis is common in school-age children as well as in adolescents
	    Exudative lesions are seen less frequently

Adult phase
(12 years to adult)
	New onset as adult is rare
	    Onset of puberty may be associated with exacerbation
	    Localized inflammation of flexural areas with lichenification is most common pattern
	    Hand dermatitis occurs much more frequently in the adult phase

IV.   Diagnosis/Evaluation

    A.   History
          1.   Inquire about personal or family history of atopy—allergic rhinitis, asthma, atopic dermatitis--and age of onset
          2.   Question about itching, appearance and distribution of lesions, if dermatitis is chronic or chronically relapsing
          3.   Question regarding hand dermatitis
          4.   Ask about routine skin care at home including frequency of bathing and products used

    B.   Physical Examination
          1.   Have patient disrobe completely
          2.   Examine the skin methodically and determine the extent of the eruption and its distribution
          3.   Determine the primary lesion and the nature of the secondary lesions
          4.   Examine flexural areas for erythema and scaling but also look for lichenification in these areas
               a.   Examine the hands. Look for erythema and scaling on dorsal aspects of hands
               b.   Look for dry, fissured fingertip pads

    C.   Differential Diagnosis
          1.   Contact dermatitis, irritant or allergic
          2.   Seborrheic dermatitis
          3.   Nummular dermatitis
          4.   Scabies
          5.   Tinea

    D.   Diagnostic Tests: Not routinely indicated

V.   Plan/Management

    A.   Patients with acute, severe dermatitis should be referred to an expert for management

    B.   For patients with less acute and less severe forms of the disorder, emphasize that this is a chronic condition and exacerbating factors must be controlled for successful management

    C.   Dry skin is a constant feature of atopic dermatitis; counsel patient/family how to control exacerbating factors using guidelines in the following table

KEYS TO REDUCING OR ELIMINATING FACTORS THAT PROMOTE DRYNESS AND INCREASE DESIRE TO SCRATCH

➡ Keep environment slightly cool and well humidified (home or office humidifiers)

➡ Avoid frequent hand washing; wear plastic gloves for wet work

➡ Keep skin well hydrated by daily baths in water no warmer than 90 degrees and soak for 10 minutes; always use a mild cleansing bar such as Dove, Basis, Eucerin to wash in axilla and groin areas; use plain water on other parts of body

➡ Avoid over-aggressive use of wash cloth which can exfoliate and remove the stratum corneum

➡ Skin should be patted dry after bath and moisturizers applied immediately to still-moist skin (see table below)

➡ Wear loose-fitting 100% cotton clothing; avoid wool

➡ Use fragrance-free laundry products such as Ivory Snow Flakes, Cheer-Free

➡ Recognize that emotional stress can worsen (by possibly increasing desire to scratch) but not cause the disorder

D. Lubrication of the skin done daily on a consistent basis is the key to control
   1. Bathing should always be followed by immediate use of emollients applied after patting the skin dry
   2. Remind patient to moisturize skin throughout the day if the skin feels dry; more frequent lubrication is necessary during winter months
   3. Recommend moisturizers from the table below
   4. In terms of moisturizing, ointments are the most moisturizing but leave a greasy feel to the skin; creams are thicker and more lubricating than lotions; very dry skin benefits the most from ointments and patients should always be encouraged to use ointments at least at night

RECOMMENDED MOISTURIZERS

Moisturizing Lotions	Moisturizing Creams	Moisturizing Ointments
Petrolatum-based ✓ Dermasil ✓ Moisturel Lotion ✓ Replenaderm Lotion	Petrolatum-based ✓ Purpose Dry Skin Cream ✓ Cetaphil Cream ✓ Keri Cream	Petrolatum-based ✓ Vaseline Pure Petroleum Jelly (Fragrance, preservative, and lanolin free)
Mixtures of lanolin and petrolatum ✓ Eucerin Lotion ✓ Lubriderm Lotion ✓ Nivea Moisturizing Lotion	Mixtures of lanolin and petrolatum ✓ Eucerin Creme Without lanolin or petrolatum ✓ Neutrogena Norwegian Formula Hand Cream	Mixtures of lanolin and petrolatum ✓ Aquaphor Natural Healing Ointment (Fragrance and preservative free)
Without lanolin or petrolatum ✓ Corn Huskers Lotion ✓ Cetaphil Lotion		

E. Pharmacologic therapy: Mainstays of therapy are topical steroid ointments and oral antihistamines
   1. To reduce inflammation, it is often necessary to use topical steroid preparations applied thinly 2x/day until controlled (up to 14 days)
      a. Triamcinolone acetonide ointment 0.1% (Aristocort ointment 0.1%, supplied as 15, 60 g)
      b. In milder cases, may use steroid cream instead of ointment; ointments leave a greasy feel to the skin which many patients dislike
      c. Lubricants can also be applied to the skin not being treated with the steroid ointment; (lubricant creams/ointments should **not** be applied over the steroid ointment)
      d. Once inflammation is controlled, substitute lubricants for the steroid ointments to improve skin barrier function
      e. Use the topical corticosteroid of the lowest potency that will control the condition
   2. Pruritus control with the use of antihistamines and topical antipruritics is the other mainstay of pharmacologic therapy (see following table); focus is on relief of itching so that patient is not constantly fighting the urge to scratch

PRURITUS CONTROL USING PHARMACOLOGIC INTERVENTIONS

Oral Antihistamines (Second-Generation H₁-Receptor Blockers)

Fexofenadine (Allegra), supplied as 60 mg caps and 30, 60, 180 mg tabs
Dosing: 60 mg BID or 180 mg once/day

Loratadine (Claritin), supplied as 5 mg/5 mL syrup, 10 mg tabs, and 10 mg disintegrating (Reditabs)
Dosing: 10 mg once/day

Desloratadine (Clarinex), supplied as 5 mg tabs
Dosing: 5 mg once/day

Cetirizine (Zyrtec), supplied as 1 mg/mL syrup, and 5, 10 mg tabs
Dosing: 5-10 mg once/day

➡ Of the second-generation H₁-receptor blockers above, Allegra seems to offer the best combination of effectiveness and safety (see Abramowicz, M., (2001). Newer antihistamines. *Medical Letter, 43,* 35-36.)
➡ Any of the H₁-receptor blockers listed above is preferred over first-generation H₁-receptor blockers which can impair psychomotor performance even in the absence of sedation

Oral Antihistamines (First-Generation H₁-Receptor Blockers)

Hydroxyzine (Atarax), supplied as 10 mg/5 mL syrup and 10, 25, 50, 100 mg tablets
Dosing: 25-50 mg/dose TID PRN
A single dose at bedtime is frequently all that is necessary

➡ A good choice for use at bedtime; cost is much less than the second-generation antihistamines (loratadine will be generic and thus will also be somewhat more affordable by the end of 2002)

Topical Antipruritic Agents

Sarna lotion, Prax lotion, and *Itch-X gel* are all OTC products

Cetaphil with menthol 0.25% and phenol 0.25% is an Rx product

Doxepin HCL cream 5% (Zonalon) may be used only for short-term (**<8 days**)
Supplied as 30 g, 45 g

➡ Apply QID PRN in addition to topical steroid cream (do not use over ointments as may produce too much occlusion)
➡ May cause drowsiness and contact dermatitis

Topical agents may be used in addition to or instead of oral antihistamines

---

F. Counsel patient to avoid exposure to chemicals, and to use gloves for protection when engaging in "wet work"

G. Patients who do not respond to conventional therapies after a 2-4 week trial should be referred to a specialist for management or the use of a topical immunomodulator may be considered (see below)

H. Tacrolimus (Protopic) and pimecrolimus (Elidel) are new prescription products—the first in a new class of topical immunomodulators
   1. Tacrolimus, an ointment, has been approved by the FDA for short-term and intermittent long-term therapy for patients with **moderate to severe** atopic dermatitis in whom the use of conventional therapies is inadvisable, ineffective, or not tolerated
      a. Use either 0.03% or 0.1% formulation; continue for one week after resolution
      b. Apply BID in thin layer to affected areas; do not occlude or apply to wet skin
      c. Consult PDR for prescribing information, precautions, contraindications, and adverse reactions before prescribing this or any other medication
   2. Pimecrolimus, a cream, has been approved by the FDA for short-term or intermittent long-term treatment of **mild to moderate** atopic dermatitis when conventional therapies are inadvisable, ineffective, or not tolerated
      a. Available in 1% cream formulation
      b. Apply BID to affected areas; do not occlude
      c. Consult PDR for prescribing information, precautions, contraindications, and adverse reactions before prescribing this or any other medication

I. Follow up
1. The first follow-up visit should be within 2-4 weeks to determine the effectiveness of therapy
   a. Ask patient to bring in the steroid ointment/cream that is being used
   b. Have patient demonstrate how it is being applied to determine if appropriate amount is being used
2. Monthly visits are appropriate until patient is using lubricants only; then every 3-6 months
3. Patient should understand that this is a chronic, recurrent disorder and should be offered practical counseling on each visit regarding ways to deal with the disorder
4. Reliable patients should be given ample refills of topical corticosteroids so that they can control the condition themselves (if there is not a concern about overuse/inappropriate use)

CONTACT DERMATITIS

I. Definition: Skin inflammation due to irritants (irritant contact dermatitis) or allergens (allergic contact dermatitis)

II. Pathogenesis

A. Irritant contact dermatitis
1. Damage to one of the components of the water-protein-lipid matrix of the outer layer of the epidermis of the skin caused by irritants including chemicals, dry, cold air, and friction
2. An eczematous response in the skin is produced that is nonallergic in origin

B. Allergic contact dermatitis
1. A form of cell mediated immunity that occurs in 2 phases
2. The sensitization phase which occurs when allergens penetrate the epidermis and produce proliferation of T lymphocytes (sensitization phase; can take days or months)
3. In the elicitation phase, the antigen-specific T lymphocytes present in the skin combine with the subsequent exposures to the allergen to produce inflammation

III. Clinical Presentation

A. Irritant contact dermatitis
1. About 80% of cases of contact dermatitis involve irritants rather than allergens
2. In adults, the hands are by far the most commonly affected
3. Intensity of inflammation is related to the concentration of the irritant, the exposure time, and the state of the epidermal barrier
4. Acute irritant contact dermatitis is characterized by papules and/or vesicles on an erythematous patchy background with weeping and edema; burning usually predominates over itching
5. Persistent, chronic dermatitis is characterized by lichenification, patches of erythema, and fissures in the skin
6. Frequent hand washing is a very common cause in adults; jobs involving repeated wet work such as food service, childcare, healthcare, and hair styling predispose workers to irritant contact dermatitis

B. Allergic contact dermatitis
1. Much less common than irritant contact dermatitis
2. A genetically predisposed hypersensitivity reaction
3. May correspond exactly to contactant (e.g., fabric treatments, clothing, nickel in jewelry, latex in gloves, ingredients in cosmetics or topical medications)
4. Hands, forearms, and face are common sites
5. Skin findings include vesicles, edema, erythema, and pruritus
6. Poison ivy, oak, and sumac are by far the most common causes in the US
   a. In classic presentation, vesicular lesions on erythematous base are in a linear distribution on exposed skin caused from leaves brushing skin or from streaking oleoresin when scratching
   b. Extreme pruritus is usually present
   c. Diffuse patterns may occur when oleoresin is contacted from contaminated pets or smoke from burning plants

C. Distribution often provides clues to diagnosis
    1. Scalp and ears: Hair care products, jewelry
    2. Eyelids: Cosmetics, contact lens solution
    3. Face/neck: Cosmetics, cleansers, medications, jewelry
    4. Trunk/axilla: Clothing, deodorants
    5. Arms/hands: Poison oak, ivy, sumac, soaps, detergents, frequent hand washing, jewelry, rubber gloves
    6. Legs/feet: Clothing, shoes
    7. Preservatives in OTC and prescriptive topical products may produce dermatitis at area of application

D. Older persons usually have relatively little vesiculation or inflammation and instead have scaling as a prominent feature of the eruption

E. The most common causes of allergic contact dermatitis in the elderly are topical medications, including neomycin, Furacin, vitamin E, lanolin, and adhesives in transdermal medications

IV. Diagnosis/Evaluation

A. History
    1. Question regarding location of eruption, time and rate of onset (abrupt or insidious), and associated symptoms such as pruritus; ask if others in household have similar symptoms
    2. Ask about occupation and recreational pursuits
    3. Question regarding exposures to such substances as chemicals, detergents, medications, poison plants, lubricants, cleansers, and rubber gloves, both at home and at work or in recreational pursuits
    4. Obtain family history, personal history of allergies, treatments tried and results

B. Physical Examination
    1. Examine skin to determine the location of the inflammation
    2. Determine the primary lesion
    3. Determine the distribution of the eruption as a clue to diagnosis

C. Differential Diagnosis
    1. Atopic dermatitis: Usually more chronic, occurs in flexural distribution, onset in childhood
    2. Scabies: Usually begins in finger webs, wrists, spreading to groin, axilla and itching is prominent; other household contacts are symptomatic
    3. Nummular dermatitis: Discrete, coin-shaped, erythematous, scaling plaques
    4. Dermatitis herpetiformis: Usually localized to elbows, knees, buttocks, posterior scalp

D. Diagnostic Tests: None indicated

V. Plan/Management: Irritant contact dermatitis

A. The most common type of irritant contact dermatitis involves the hands

B. The first step in management is to identify the offending agent and eliminate or at least limit further exposure (preventive measures)

C. For patients with hand involvement who must engage in wet work
    1. Suggest the wearing of cotton gloves under vinyl gloves which may reduce need to wash hands as frequently
    2. Use mild soap when washing hands
    3. Appropriate protective gloves should be worn for specific solvent or chemical exposures
    4. Frequent application of occlusive ointments such as Vaseline or Aquaphor should be used (remind patient that ointments should not be applied over steroid ointments or creams if also using as this creates too much occlusion)
    5. Topical steroid ointment applied BID can help in reducing erythema
        a. Triamcinolone acetonide 0.1% (Aristocort A) ointment
        b. Supplied as 15, 60g
        c. Use for 10-14 days then use lubricant only

VI.   Plan/Management: Allergic contact dermatitis

A.   Avoidance of allergens is necessary for recovery and to prevent recurrences

B.   If poison ivy, oak, sumac are identified as the source, advise patient as follows:
1.   Wash skin immediately with soap and water to remove oleoresin—must be done within 15 minutes of exposure, so this is information most useful in preventing future episodes rather than dealing with the present episode
2.   Apply cold, wet compresses to affected areas—can use Burrow's solution or tap water 3-4 times daily for 20 minutes during acute phase (vesicles present) to suppress inflammation and reduce itching
3.   Bathing with Aveeno may be helpful
4.   Use of calamine lotion may be helpful and is drying which makes it beneficial for exudative inflammation; avoid use of topical products containing diphenhydramine
5.   Other topical antipruritic agents include Prax (pramoxine), PrameGel (pramoxine and menthol), and Sarna (menthol, camphor, and phenol)

C.   Prescribe topical steroids to clear the dermatitis and decrease discomfort
1.   Refer to V.C.5. above for use on hands, arms, legs, and trunk
2.   Use lower potency for face and groin area (hydrocortisone 2.5% cream)

D.   Also prescribe oral antihistamines for pruritus control (see table *Pruritus Control* in section on ATOPIC DERMATITIS) for products and dosing information or prescribe topical antipruritic agents such as Sarna lotion, Prax lotion (OTC products), or Cetaphil with menthol 0.25% and phenol 0.25% (Rx)

E.   When skin involvement is extensive, the face and/or groin areas are involved, and pruritus is poorly controlled with oral and topical therapies, use of an oral corticosteroid may be indicated (consider referral to an expert for management)
1.   Prednisone (taper dose): 50 mg/day x 2 days, 45 mg/day x 2 days, 40 mg/day x 2 days, 30 mg/day x 2 days, 20 mg/day x 2 days, 10 mg/day x 2 days, and 5 mg/day x 2 days for a total of 14 days of treatment
2.   Dose packs are usually inadequate but are convenient to prescribe
3.   Follow up in 3-4 days for moderate dermatitis requiring topical or oral corticosteroid treatment

F.   Follow Up
1.   None indicated if dermatitis is mild
2.   In 3-4 days for moderate to more severe dermatitis requiring topical or oral corticosteroid use

KERATOSIS PILARIS

I.   Definition: An eruption consisting of follicle-based, scaling papules most commonly on the posterolateral aspects of the upper arms, anterior thighs, and the buttocks that is common in person with atopic dermatitis

II.   Pathogenesis

A.   Results from mild follicular plugging and peri-follicular inflammation

B.   Exact mechanism of pathogenesis is unknown, but may be caused by a disorder in keratinization so that follicular plugging with keratin debris occurs

C.   May also represent a response to drying of the skin surface; the scaling produced is trapped in follicular opening

III.   Clinical Presentation

A.   Commonly occurs in individuals with atopic dermatitis with children, adolescents, and young adults most often affected; occurrence peaks in adolescence

B. Appears as small, pinpoint, follicular papules and pustules on the extensor aspects of the extremities, and the buttocks—a "gooseflesh" appearance

C. The affected skin surface feels rough and dry; hair in the center of the papule/pustule confirms a follicular location

D. Condition is aggravated by cold, dry climates, and is usually associated with extremely dry skin

IV. Diagnosis/Evaluation

A. History
1. Ask about location of eruption, onset, duration, and appearance of lesions
2. Determine if there is a history of atopic dermatitis
3. Ask if condition gets better or worse at any time of the year
4. Question about associated symptoms (there should be none)

B. Physical Examination
1. Examine skin, focusing on areas typically affected—extensor aspects of arms, legs, and the buttocks
2. Touch affected areas for rough skin texture; examine all skin surfaces for signs of dryness

C. Differential Diagnosis
1. Microcomedones of acne (distribution of acne is face, chest, upper back)
2. Molluscum contagiosum (lesions are waxy-appearing with central umbilication)
3. Drug eruption (drug eruption usually has acute onset and keratosis pilaris is chronic)

D. Diagnostic Tests: None indicated

V. Plan/Management

A. Mild forms: Recommend application of lubricants applied to moist skin immediately after bathing (see CARE OF DRY AND OILY SKIN for table of moisturizers)

B. Moderate to severe forms
1. Recommend/prescribe products containing alpha hydroxy acids (glycolic, lactic, and citric acids)
2. A property of all alpha hydroxy acids is that they enhance shedding of surface corneocytes and the exfoliation of the dried out corneocytes results in a smoother, more uniform surface
3. Lactic acid 12% cream (Lac-Hydrin) applied BID usually controls the condition
4. Advise patient to continue to use lubricants (recommended under V.A. above)
5. Patient should be advised to use cautiously on face and to avoid sun exposure to treated skin

C. Advise patient to soak 3-4 x per week for 10 minutes in tepid water, to use cleansers such as Dove, Purpose, or Basis, and to apply moisturizers after bathing while skin is still damp after having been patted dry (**Note:** Persons who shower typically use hotter water than those who take tub baths—brief soaking in tepid water (bathing) may be a good alternative to help keep skin hydrated)

D. Follow up: None indicated

POMPHOLYX

I. Definition: A disease of unknown etiology that disrupts the skin of the palms and soles

II. Pathogenesis: Recurrent eczematous dermatitis of unknown etiology; also referred to as dyshidrosis or dyshidrotic eczema

III. Clinical Presentation

A. Condition is characterized by sudden eruptions of itchy vesicles on the palms, or on lateral fingers, or on the plantar feet (acute phase)

B. Waves of vesiculation may occur; vesicles are 1-5 mm in size, are symmetrical in distribution, and are filled with clear fluid making the eruption look like tapioca

C. Moderate to severe itching usually precedes the emergence of the vesicles

D. Over 1-3 weeks vesicles slowly resolve, and are replaced by scaling, redness, and lichenification (chronic phase)

IV. Diagnosis/Evaluation

A. History
   1. Question about location of lesions, onset, duration, and changes in lesions over time
   2. Ask about associated symptoms
   3. Inquire about skin allergies
   4. Ask about treatments tried and results

B. Physical Examination
   1. Examine lesions looking for vesicles, or if the acute process has ended, exfoliation of skin revealing a red, cracked base
   2. Examine all skin surfaces to determine if vesicles are located in areas other than palms and soles

C. Differential Diagnosis
   1. Contact dermatitis
   2. Tinea
   3. Atopic dermatitis
   4. Pustular psoriasis of palms and soles (with this disease, vesicles are cloudy with purulent fluid; pain rather than itching is the chief complaint); referral is needed

D. Diagnostic Tests: None indicated

V. Plan/Management

A. Initial treatment consists of use of cold, wet compresses and application of topical corticosteroids
   1. Cold wet compresses: Apply cold, sopping wet compresses (using either cold tap water or Burrow's solution) twice a day to affected area; leave in place at least 30 minutes
   2. Follow wet dressings with application of triamcinolone acetonide cream, 0.025% (Aristocort A cream, 0.025%) to affected areas BID x 7-10 days

B. For severe flares, short course of oral corticosteroids tapered over one week could be considered; **should not be used on a chronic basis**; prescribe Medrol Dosepak

C. Oral antihistamines can be prescribed to relieve pruritus (see section on ATOPIC DERMATITIS for table of medications and dosing recommendations)

D. Follow up: None indicated

SEBORRHEIC DERMATITIS

I. Definition: A common, chronic, inflammatory skin disorder with a characteristic pattern for different age groups

II. Pathogenesis

A. The yeast *Pityrosporum ovale* is believed to play a role in the etiology

B. Both genetic and environmental factors seem to influence onset and course of disease

III.	Clinical Presentation

A.	Affects adults of all ages, particularly those with coexisting neurologic diseases or who are HIV+

B.	Mild seborrheic dermatitis presents as fine, dry, white or yellow greasy scale, on an inflamed base

C.	More severe eruptions appear as dull, red plaques with thick, white or yellow scale in a diffuse distribution

D.	Occurs in seborrheic areas: Scalp, scalp margins, eyebrows, base of lashes, paranasal, nasolabial folds, external ear canals, posterior auricular fold, presternal areas, and upper back

E.	Seborrheic dermatitis is one of the most common early cutaneous manifestations of HIV infection

F.	White scaling that adheres to the eyelashes and lid margins is characteristic of seborrheic blepharitis (see section on BLEPHARITIS)

IV.	Diagnosis/Evaluation

A.	History
1.	Question regarding onset, duration, and location of lesions
2.	Inquire about personal or family history of seborrheic dermatitis
3.	Determine if immunosuppressed
4.	Ask about treatments tried and results

B.	Physical Examination
1.	Examine skin for characteristic lesions: fine, dry, white or yellow scale on inflamed base or dull, red plaques with thick white or yellow greasy appearing scale
2.	Determine distribution

C.	Differential Diagnosis
1.	Psoriasis (lesions are usually on elbows/knees and consist of thick, silvery scale; facial involvement is less common; psoriasis of scalp may be difficult to differentiate from seborrheic dermatitis)
2.	Tinea capitis/faciale (fungal culture/KOH prep can help differentiate; tinea faciale is usually unilateral)
3.	Acne rosacea (central facial erythema and a significant flushing component are present with this condition; also telangiectasia and inflammatory papules may be present)

D.	Diagnostic Tests: None indicated if typical lesions, distribution

V.	Plan/Management

A.	Treatment of seborrheic dermatitis is described in the table that follows

---

TREATMENT OF SEBORRHEIC DERMATITIS

For scalp involvement that is mild, use of a medicated shampoo to remove and control mild scale is usually effective
✓	Selenium sulfide: Exsel, Selsun Blue, and Reme-T (OTC)
✓	Sulfur and salicylic acid combination: Sebulex (OTC)
✓	Coal tar: Denorex, T/Gel, Tegrin (OTC)
✓	Above shampoos must be left on a minimum of 5-10 minutes before rinsing
✓	Ketoconazole: Nizoral (Rx): Use 2-3 x/week x 1 month; may need to use once a week for maintenance

For scalp involvement that is more extensive, (or for milder cases in which initial treatment [above] was not successful), treatment involves the removal of some of the scale prior to use of the medicated shampoo
✓	Instruct patient to apply warm peanut oil or olive oil to the scalp at bedtime to loosen scale; in AM, shampoo hair with one of the medicated shampoos listed above

For facial involvement, dermatitis usually responds to ketoconazole (Nizoral Topical 2% cream) [apply BID up to 4 weeks]; alternative is antidandruff shampoo diluted with water and used daily as a facial wash
✓	For more severe facial involvement, prescribe ciclopirox (Loprox Gel) applied once daily for up to 2 weeks

For intertriginous involvement, hydrocortisone 2.5% cream (Hytone cream 2.5%) should be used for 7 days; ointments should not be used on intertriginous areas (opposition of two skin surfaces greatly enhances absorption)

For chest involvement, medicated shampoos may be used on chest skin; may also use triamcinolone 0.1% lotion BID OR topical ketoconazole (Nizoral 2% cream) BID until clear; then use once or twice weekly

B.   Recalcitrant cases should be referred to a specialist for management

C.   Follow up: Not indicated except in treatment failures

IMPETIGO AND ECTHYMA

I.   Definition: Bacterial skin infection caused by invasion of the epidermis by pathogenic *Staphylococcus aureus* or *Streptococcus pyogenes,* or a combination of these organisms

II.   Pathogenesis

A.   Most skin microorganisms in healthy persons are nonpathogenic

B.   Microscopic breaks in the epidermal barrier allows penetration by the two major pathogens found on the skin—*S. aureus* and/or *S. pyogenes*

C.   The depth of invasion in impetigo is superficial; the entire epidermis is involved in ecthyma

D.   Poststreptococcal glomerulonephritis may follow skin infections involving strains of nephritogenic streptococci; rheumatic heart disease is not a sequela of this infection

III. Clinical Presentation

A.   Impetigo begins as small (1-2 mm) superficial vesicles with fragile roofs that are quickly lost; vesicles rupture leaving erosions covered by moist, honey-colored crusts

B.   Multiple lesions are usually present, and face and extremities are the **most common** sites of involvement

C.   The terms bullous and nonbullous impetigo have been used to describe two patterns of infection with bullous impetigo suggesting staphylococcal origin and nonbullous, streptococcal origin. The preferred term presently is simply, "impetigo," since differentiation is difficult based on appearance, and both organisms cause many infections

D.   In ecthyma, ulcers form with a dry, dark crust, and surrounding erythema; lesions are usually found on legs

E.   Both ecthyma and impetigo may occur simultaneously

F.   Both infections occur most frequently in children but also occur in adults

G.   Enhanced by poor hygiene and warm, moist climates; disease is self-limiting

IV.   Diagnosis/Evaluation

A.   History
      1.   Question about location of lesions, onset, duration, and any associated symptoms
      2.   Ask if other family members are affected; treatments tried and results

B.   Physical Examination
      1.   Determine if febrile
      2.   Examine skin (focus on areas of typical involvement—face, arms, legs) looking for erosions covered by moist, honey-colored crusts that characterize impetigo, and firm, dry, dark crusts with surrounding erythema that characterize ecthyma
      3.   Check for regional lymphadenopathy

C. Differential Diagnosis
1. Tinea (with tinea, there is central clearing, and KOH test is positive)
2. Herpes simplex infections (HSV is characterized by clusters of lesions, and can be confirmed via fluorescent antibody testing of smears from intact vesicles)
3. Second-degree burn may be confused with ecthyma (careful history is important; Gram stain for bacteria should be negative unless burn site contaminated with bacteria)
4. Allergic contact dermatitis (itching is prominent symptom in allergic contact dermatitis)
5. Cutaneous anthrax may be confused with ecthyma; bacterial culture would be needed

D. Diagnostic Tests: None required as clinical features are so characteristic; if uncertain about diagnosis, perform Gram stain on fluid from intact vesicle/pustule looking for gram-positive cocci in clusters (*S. aureus*) or chains (*S. pyogenes*); see IV.C. above for other diagnostic tests

V. Plan/Management

A. For multiple lesions, systemic antibiotics are the preferred therapy and there are several options

> Dicloxacillin, supplied as suspension, 62.5 mg/5 mL, and caps, 250, 500 mg
> Dosing: 250 mg QID x 10 days, OR
>
> Cephalexin (Keflex), supplied as suspension (250 mg/5 mL), caps (250, 500 mg) and tabs (250, 500 mg)
> Dosing: 500 mg BID x 10 days
> Note: Better compliance with this drug than with dicloxacillin

B. If only a few lesions are present, consider use of topical mupirocin ointment (Bactroban) which has been shown to be as efficacious as oral cephalexin for mild infections
1. Apply to affected areas TID x 7-10 days or until all lesions have cleared
2. Re-evaluate if no response in 3-5 days

C. Gentle washing of lesions to remove loose crusts may be helpful and must be done if mupirocin is used; scrubbing of lesions with antibacterial soaps has not been shown to be effective and is not recommended

D. Good hand washing and personal hygiene are recommended to reduce likelihood of spread; use of a mild antibacterial soap such as Lever 2000 for hand washing and bathing may be helpful

E. Highly contagious nature of the infection should be emphasized

F. Follow up: In one week to determine response to treatment

CELLULITIS

I. Definition: An acute, diffuse inflammation of the skin and subcutaneous structures characterized by hyperemia, edema, and leukocytic infiltration

II. Pathogenesis

A. Invasion of bacteria (usually pathogenic streptococci) into the dermis and subcutaneous fat with subsequent spread through the lymphatics

B. Many other bacteria are causative agents including *Staphylococcus aureus* and *Haemophilus influenzae* (less common in US since introduction of the *Haemophilus influenzae*, Type B [Hib] vaccine)

C. May develop in apparently normal skin, but more often trauma to the skin provides a portal of entry for invading organisms

III.   Clinical Presentation

    A.   Erythema, warmth, edema, and pain are usual clinical features; the erythematous plaque is usually tender-to-painful to touch without a sharply demarcated border and may cover a small to large area of the skin

    B.   Fever, chills, malaise, and lymphadenopathy are frequently present

    C.   The most susceptible populations are those with diabetes mellitus, cirrhosis, renal failure, malnutrition, and HIV+

    D.   Typically, there is a preceding wound or trauma to the skin which compromises lymphatic drainage

    E.   Findings that signal an emergent condition are listed in the following table

INDICES OF AN EMERGENT CONDITION
✓ Extensive, rather than limited, localized cellulitis
✓ Fever, or other signs and symptoms of septicemia (toxic presentation)
✓ Diminished arterial pulse in a cool, swollen, infected extremity
✓ Presence of cutaneous necrosis
✓ Closed space infections of the hand
✓ Periorbital cellulitis because of proximity to brain
✓ Immunosuppressed or diabetic host

    F.   Erysipelas, a distinctive type of superficial cellulitis is virtually always caused by group A streptococci

    G.   In erysipelas, infection is more superficial, with margins that are more clearly demarcated from normal skin than in cellulitis

    H.   Lower legs, face, and ears are most frequently involved in erysipelas

    I.   Lymphatic involvement ("streaking") is prominent in erysipelas which also differentiates it from other types of cellulitis

IV.   Diagnosis/Evaluation

    A.   History
        1.   Question about location, onset, duration, degree of spread, and presence of pain
        2.   Ask if there was a pre-existing wound or trauma to involved area
        3.   Determine if systemic symptoms are present (fever, chills, malaise)

    B.   Physical Examination
        1.   Vital signs and BP to determine if febrile, and to evaluate cardiovascular status
        2.   Examine involved area of skin to determine how extensive infection is, degree of erythema, presence of purulent discharge, presence of necrotic tissue
        3.   Examine adjacent skin/lymph nodes to determine presence of "streaking," degree of lymphadenopathy

    C.   Differential Diagnosis
        1.   Pressure erythema
        2.   Contact dermatitis
        3.   Swelling over septic joint

    D.   Diagnostic Tests
        1.   Obtain Gram stain and culture and sensitivity of wound before treatment is instituted
        2.   Obtain CBC and blood cultures if cellulitis is extensive or associated with systemic toxicity and refer for emergent care

V. Plan/Management

    A. Treatment of erysipelas and cellulitis depends on the patient's condition and underlying risk factors

    B. Refer all patients who meet criteria for emergent conditions (see table above) for expert care

    C. Patients with nontoxic presentation and localized and limited skin involvement can be treated empirically with oral antibiotics aimed at staphylococcal and streptococcal organism

    D. For uncomplicated cases, choose ONE of the following antibiotics, and **treat for 10-14 days** (except for Zithromax which has a treatment course of 5 days):

Dicloxacillin
    Dosing: 500 mg QID, **OR**
Cephalexin (Keflex) supplied as caps, 250, 500 mg; tabs, 250, 500 mg
    Dosing: 500 mg BID, **OR**
Amoxicillin/clavulanic acid (Augmentin) supplied as tabs, 250, 500, 875 mg; chewable tabs, 125, 200, 250, 400 mg
    Dosing: 500 mg TID **OR**
Azithromycin (Zithromax) supplied Z-Pak (6 tabs)
    Dosing: 500 mg on day 1, then 250 mg/day on days 2-5

    E. In all cases, antibiotic therapy may require changing based on culture results and clinical response

    F. Local measures such as immobilization, elevation, application of moist heat (3-4 x day for 15-20 minutes) should be used with all patients to provide symptomatic relief and speed resolution of the infection

    G. Follow up in 24-48 hours to determine response to therapy

FOLLICULITIS, FURUNCLES, AND CARBUNCLES

I. Definition: Bacterial invasion of the follicular wall

II. Pathogenesis

    A. Most commonly due to *Staphylococcus aureus*

    B. Other organisms may be involved, and, in general, the microbiology of cutaneous infection reflects the microflora of the part of body involved

III. Clinical Presentation

    A. Folliculitis is inflammation of the hair follicle caused by infection, chemical irritation, or injury

    B. Furuncle (abscess or boil) is a deep folliculitis, consisting of a walled-off, pus filled mass that is painful, firm, or fluctuant; fever is uncommon
        1. Furuncle may appear at any site
        2. Most often occurs in areas of friction (waistline, groin, buttocks, axilla)

    C. Carbuncles are aggregates of infected, abscessed follicles located deep in dermis; it points and drains through multiple openings
        1. Very painful and systemic signs such as chills, fever may be present
        2. Occur in areas with thick dermis (back of neck, lateral aspect of thigh)

    D. Furuncles and carbuncles are uncommon in children

IV. Diagnosis/Evaluation

    A. History
        1. Ask about location, appearance of lesion, onset, duration, and if purulent drainage is exuding from surface
        2. Inquire about associated symptoms of pain and systemic symptoms of fever and chills
        3. Inquire about frequency of occurrence

    B. Physical Examination
        1. Take temperature to determine if systemic involvement
        2. Inspect lesion(s) for signs of local inflammation (erythema, swelling, and pustular surface)
        3. Palpate surface of lesion for fluctuance, which indicates accumulation of purulent matter; palpate adjacent lymph nodes

    C. Differential Diagnosis
        1. Acne pustules
        2. Epidermal cyst
        3. Hidradenitis suppurativa

    D. Diagnostic Tests: Wound culture should be done to verify antibiotic choice

V. Plan/Management

    A. For folliculitis in which skin involvement is limited, treatment with topical antibiotics is usually sufficient; use **one** of the following
        1. Mupirocin (Bactroban) cream may be used: Apply small amount TID to affected area x 7-10 days
        2. Erythromycin 2% solution (A/T/S) BID x 7-10 days
        3. Clindamycin solution (Cleocin T) BID x 7-10 days

    B. For folliculitis in which skin involvement is more extensive, oral antistaphylococcal antibiotics are indicated (see V.D. below for antibiotic choices and dosing information)

    C. For carbuncles and furuncles, frequent warm, moist compresses provide relief and promote localization and spontaneous draining

    D. Incision and drainage is commonly required for carbuncles and furuncles

---

Systemic antistaphylococcal antibiotics should be used to treat furuncles and carbuncles
- ✓ Treatment of choice is dicloxacillin supplied caps, 250, 500 mg
  - Dosing: 250 mg QID x 10 days
- ✓ Alternative treatment is cephalexin (Keflex) supplied as caps, 250, 500 mg
  - Dosing: 500 mg BID x 10 days

    E. Refer patients with cutaneous abscesses located on face, scalp, and neck

    F. Culture recurrent abscesses and refer patients for evaluation for diseases that may underlie recurrent furunculosis: Immunodeficiency, diabetes mellitus, alcoholism, malnutrition, and severe anemia

    G. Patients with recurrent abscess formation who are otherwise healthy may benefit from mupirocin 2% ointment (Bactroban Nasal); apply 0.25 g to inside of each nostril BID for 5 days in order to eradicate nasal carriage of *S. aureus*

    H. To prevent recurrence, stress role of good hygiene to patient and family. <u>Most useful: frequent hand washing and daily skin cleansing</u> with an antibacterial soap such as Dial or Hibiclens antimicrobial skin cleanser

    I. Follow Up: None indicated if patient is responding to treatment

CANDIDIASIS

I.   Definition: Skin and mucous membrane infections caused by the yeast-like fungus, *Candida albicans*

II.   Pathogenesis: *C. albicans* is part of the normal flora of skin and mucous membranes; invasion of the epidermis occurs when moisture, warmth, and breaks in epidermal barrier allow overgrowth

III. Clinical Presentation

A.   **Oral** cavity: In immunocompromised patients, tongue is almost always involved; may spread into trachea, esophagus, and angles of mouth, and become chronic processes

B.   **Intertriginous** areas: Occurs most often in obese individuals (inframammary, axillary, neck, and inguinal body folds). Presents as red, moist, glistening plaque or moist red papules and pustules

C.   **Vagina**: Appears as a cheesy discharge with white plaques on erythematous base. External genitalia become red, swollen, with some skin erosions (see GYNECOLOGY section for discussion of vulvovaginal candidiasis)

D.   **Male genitalia**: Occurs mainly in uncircumcised but also occurs in circumcised. Multiple, round red erosions on glans and shaft (candida balanitis); usually painful. Often involves scrotum whereas tinea spares scrotum

E.   **Nails**: Tender erythema and swelling at cuticle area (paronychia)

F.   Pain, discomfort usually symptoms regardless of site. Itching usually occurs with vulvovaginitis

IV.   Diagnosis/Evaluation

A.   History
      1.   Inquire about location of lesions, medications used (e.g., inhaled steroids or oral corticosteroids) and underlying chronic conditions (diabetes, HIV+)
      2.   If genitalia involved, ask about associated symptoms of discharge, itching, and burning

B.   Physical Examination
      1.   Examine skin, mucous membranes, and nails for characteristic lesions
            a.   White plaques on erythematous base (oral); red moist plaques with satellite lesions (intertriginous)
            b.   Red erosions on glans, shaft (penis); non-tender erythema of nail margins (nail)
            c.   For vulvovaginal candidiasis, see under GYNECOLOGY
      2.   Palpate adjacent lymph nodes

C.   Differential Diagnosis is outlined in the box below

Oral:	Intertriginous areas:	Vaginal:	Male genitalia:	Nails:
Geographic tongue	Miliaria	See GYNECOLOGY section	Bacterial	Bacterial
Aphthous stomatitis	Bacterial		Psoriasis	Tinea
Leukoplakia			Tinea	

D.   Diagnostic Tests
      1.   None indicated when typical lesions present
      2.   Potassium hydroxide (KOH) wet mount that is positive for pseudohyphae and budding spores confirms the diagnosis

V.   Plan/Management

A.   Oral candidiasis: For the majority of patients, topical treatments are effective

---

TREATMENT FOR ORAL CANDIDIASIS

Topical treatment is preferred for limited disease in normal hosts
  ➡ Nystatin (Mycostatin) oral suspension (100,000 U/mL) QID x 10 days
      • 4-6 mL (1/2 dose in each side of mouth)
      • Medication should be retained in mouth as long as possible before swallowing
  ➡ Alternative treatment for patients with thrush or angular cheilitis: 10 mg clotrimazole (Lotrimin) buccal troches, dissolve 1
      PO 5x day for 2 weeks
Systemic therapy is necessary for moderate to severe disease that occurs in immunocompromised persons (see HIV/AIDS
section for treatment recommendations)

B.   For candidal vaginitis, see GYNECOLOGY section

C.   Candidal balanitis: For limited disease, select one of the topical agents from the table

---

TREATMENT FOR CANDIDAL BALANITIS

➡ Nystatin cream, 2-3 x day for 10 days
➡ Miconazole (Monistat-Derm) or clotrimazole (Lotrimin) cream 2 x day for 10 days
➡ Econazole (Spectazole) cream, BID x 10 days
➡ Relief occurs quickly once treatment begins; remind patient to use for 10 days even though discomfort
   is gone

D.   Candidal intertrigo: Select one of the topical agents from the table

---

TREATMENT FOR CANDIDAL INTERTRIGO

➡ Miconazole (Monistat Derm) cream applied BID x 10-14 days
➡ Econazole (Spectazole) cream; apply QD x 14 days
➡ Clotrimazole (Lotrimin) cream, solution, lotion; apply BID x 10 days
➡ Oxiconazole (Oxistat) cream; apply QD or BID x 14 days
➡ Counsel regarding weight reduction and elimination of conditions leading to maceration of skin
➡ If there is maceration, use wet Burrow's compress 3-4 x day for 15-20 minutes to promote drying
➡ Advise patient to expose areas to light and air several times a day to promote drying
➡ Once infection has resolved, recommend use of absorbent powder such as Zeasorb which acts as a dry
   lubricant in intertriginous areas

E.   Candida paronychia (chronic): The following treatment is recommended

---

TREATMENT FOR CANDIDAL PARONYCHIA

➡ 3% thymol in 95% ethanol (must be compounded by pharmacist) TID
➡ **In addition, select one** of the following to be used BID 2-4 weeks
    • Clotrimazole (Lotrimin) solution
    • Ciclopirox (Loprox) lotion
    • Mycostatin (Nystatin) cream
➡ Advise patient to avoid excess exposure to water
➡ For refractory cases, refer to specialist

F.   Treat predisposing factors. Rule out HIV+ and diabetes mellitus in patients with recurring infection

G.   Follow up is not indicated; patient should return if no improvement after 2 weeks and cause for the
      treatment failure should be determined

DERMATOPHYTE INFECTIONS

I. Definition: Infections by a group of fungi that have the ability to infect and survive only on keratin

II. Pathogenesis

    A. Causative organisms belong to 3 genera: *Microsporum, Trichophyton*, and *Epidermophyton*

    B. Predisposing factors include debilitating diseases, poor nutrition, poor hygiene, tropical climates, and contact with infected persons or animals

III. Clinical Presentation

    A. Tinea capitis, fungal infection of the scalp
        1. *Trichophyton tonsurans* infection accounts for 95% of all tinea capitis in US
        2. Rarely occurs in adults
        3. Erythema and scaling of the scalp with patchy hair loss are characteristic
        4. Usually asymptomatic unless kerion, a tender, boggy, lesion representing a hypersensitivity reaction to the fungal infection is present

    B. Tinea corporis, fungal infection of the body and face (excluding beard area in men)
        1. Occurs in all age groups; more common in warm climates
        2. Lesion is generally circular, erythematous, well demarcated with a raised, scaly, vesicular border
        3. The central area becomes hypopigmented, and less scaly as the active border progresses outward
        4. Pruritus is common

    C. Tinea cruris, fungal infection of the groin and upper thighs
        1. Frequent in males, usually obese ones; rare in females
        2. Eruption is sharply demarcated, scaling patches; usually extremely pruritic
        3. Involvement of the scrotum is uncommon (unlike candidal infections in which scrotal involvement is common)

    D. Tinea pedis, fungal infection of the foot
        1. Common infection in adolescents and adults (uncommon in prepubertal children)
        2. Lesions are fine, vesiculopustular or scaly and usually itch
        3. Any area of the foot may be involved, but likely to occur on the instep or between the toes

    E. Tinea unguium, fungal infection of the nails (onychomycosis)
        1. Occurs in adolescents and adults; rare in children
        2. May occur simultaneously with hand or foot tinea or present independently
        3. Usually involves only 1 or 2 nails; toenails more often than fingernails
        4. Distal thickening and yellowing of the nail plate are characteristic features

IV. Diagnosis/Evaluation

    A. History
        1. Question regarding onset, duration, distribution, morphology of lesions, and presence of symptoms
        2. Question regarding contact with others (or infected dogs, cats) with similar lesions, symptoms
        3. Ask about predisposing conditions—sweaty feet, occlusive footwear
        4. Inquire about treatments used and outcomes

    B. Physical Examination
        1. Examine skin to determine type, distribution of lesions
        2. Use of Wood's light may aid in exam as some species cause tinea to fluoresce (pale or brilliant green). The most common fungus infecting the scalp, *T. tonsurans* **does not** fluoresce. Lint, scales, serum exudate, and hair preparations containing petrolatum fluoresce a bluish or purplish color, which may be confusing

C.   Differential Diagnosis
1.   Seborrheic dermatitis
2.   Psoriasis
3.   Alopecia areata
4.   Atopic dermatitis
5.   Contact dermatitis

D.   Diagnostic Tests

DIAGNOSTIC TESTS FOR DERMATOPHYTE INFECTIONS

Microscopic examination for fungus
- ➡ Scrape the border of lesion with a sterile scalpel blade (No. 15) moistened with tap water to contain scales; can also "pluck" 2 or 3 hairs using a hemostat. Transfer specimen to slide with a small droplet of plain water
- ➡ Add 1 or 2 drops of KOH solution, put on coverslip and warm the slide carefully for 15-30 seconds with a flame
- ➡ Examine the specimen under low power with minimal illumination
- ➡ Identify hyphae—thin, often branching strands of uniform diameter; switch to high dry (43X) objective to confirm finding
- ➡ While a positive exam establishes the diagnosis, a negative test does not rule out the disease

Dermatophyte test medium (DTM) for diagnosis of tinea capititis
- ➡ Using a hemostat, remove 5-10 hairs from a scaling area or rub a moistened 2 x 2 gauze (or previously sterilized toothbrush) [a painless technique for the patient] vigorously over an area of scaling and alopecia
- ➡ Inoculate the plucked hair/scrapings from the gauze directly onto the culture medium, breaking the agar surface, and incubate at room temperature (with cap on loosely)
- ➡ After 1-2 weeks, phenol red indicator in agar will turn from yellow to red in area surrounding dermatophyte colony

---

V.   Plan/Management

A.   Treatment for tinea capitis is contained in the table below

---

TREATMENT FOR TINEA CAPITIS

Tinea capitis requires systemic antifungal therapy

Griseofulvin microsize (Grifulvin V), supplied as 250, 500 mg tabs; 125 mg/5 mL suspension
- ➡ 500 mg/day in a single daily dose x 4-8 weeks
- ➡ Take with high fat food such as whole milk, peanut butter, or ice cream to enhance absorption
- ➡ Treat for up to 12 weeks
- ➡ Continue medication for 2 weeks after clinical resolution

Selenium sulfide, 2.5% shampoo or ketoconazole 2% (Nizoral) shampoo used 2 x week for 2 weeks may reduce fungal shedding
- ➡ If kerion present, a short course of oral steroid therapy to reduce inflammation and prevent scarring of scalp may be needed
- ➡ Prednisone, 25-50 mg once daily for 10-14 days is recommended
- ➡ Taper dose over last half of therapy
- ➡ Advise patient that hair regrowth is slow

Laboratory monitoring for 12 week course of this medication is not necessary
Repeat fungal culture after treatment ends to document clearance

---

B.   Selected topical treatments for tinea corporis, pedis, and cruris are contained in the table below; all of these products are by prescription only

SELECTED TOPICAL TREATMENTS FOR TINEA CORPORIS, PEDIS, AND CRURIS

Topical Antifungal Agents	Supplied As	Dosing	Duration of Treatment
Miconazole (Monistat-Derm)	Cream, 15 g, 1 oz, 3 oz	BID	Tinea corporis, cruris - 2 wks Tinea pedis - 4 wks
Terbinafine (Lamisil) Solution	Solution, 30 mL Pump-spray	QD for tinea corporis, cruris; BID for tinea pedis	1 week
Econazole (Spectazole)	Cream, 15, 30 g	QD	Tinea corporis, cruris - 2 wks Tinea pedis - 4 wks
Ciclopirox (Loprox)	Cream, 15, 30, 90 g Lotion, 30, 60 mL	BID	Up to 4 weeks
Ketoconazole (Nizoral)	Cream, 15, 30, 60 g	QD	Tinea corporis, cruris - 2 wks Tinea pedis - 6 wks
Oxiconazole (Oxistat)	Cream, 15, 30 g Lotion, 30 mL	QD or BID	Tinea corporis, cruris - 2 wks Tinea pedis - 4 wks
Sulconazole (Exelderm)	Cream, 15, 30, 60 g Solution, 30 mL	BID for tinea pedis (use cream only) QD or BID for tinea corporis, cruris	Tinea pedis - 4 wks Tinea corporis, cruris - 3 wks
Butenafine 1% (Mentax)	Cream, 15, 30 g	BID or QD for tinea pedis QD for corporis, cruris	Tinea pedis - 1 wk (BID) **OR** 4 wks (QD) Tinea pedis, cruris - 2 wks

C. General measures: Advise patient as follows:
1. **T. pedis**: If moist lesions, soak affected foot/feet in Burrow's solution BID until skin has dried. Expose feet to air as much as possible by going barefoot—wearing sandals is next best. Wear synthetic socks which wick away moisture; change socks during the day in hot weather. Air out shoes between use and do not wear the same pair day in, day out. Use strand of lamb's wool (Dr. Scholl's Lamb's Wool) between toes, if there is interdigital/toe web involvement. May apply powder such as Zeasorb to dry feet after infection has resolved. Avoid the use of powders containing cornstarch that may actually promote fungal growth
2. **T. cruris and corporis**: If moist lesions, apply wet compresses using Burrow's solution BID until skin has dried; apply Zeasorb powder after infection has resolved

D. For resistant infections, refer to expert for management

E. Treatment for onychomycosis is outlined in the table below; select **one** of the following (see F.3. below for monitoring requirements)

ORAL AND TOPICAL AGENTS FOR TREATMENT FOR ONYCHOMYCOSIS

Medication	Fingernail	Toenail
Oral		
Terbinafine	250 mg/d for 6 weeks	250 mg/d for 12 weeks
Itraconazole (continuous)	200 mg/d for 6 weeks	200 mg/d for 12 weeks
Itraconazole (pulse)	200 mg twice daily for 1 week on and 3 weeks off, repeated for 2 pulses	200 mg twice daily for 1 week on and 3 weeks off, repeated for 3 pulses*
Topical		
Ciclopirox nail lacquer 8%	Daily application for 48 weeks	Daily application for 48 weeks

* Not FDA approved for this indication

F. Follow Up
1. For mild cases of T. corporis, cruris, no follow up is required unless there is a treatment failure
2. For T. capitis, a visit in 2-4 weeks to evaluate the effectiveness of the griseofulvin therapy; repeat KOH examination, and culture to determine need for increasing length of therapy; if lesions are KOH and culture negative, a total of 6 weeks of therapy may be all that is required
3. For onychomycosis, need to monitor CBC, ALT, and AST levels before initiating oral treatment, at 4 weeks into treatment, and then monthly for duration of treatment

TINEA VERSICOLOR

I. Definition: Common non-inflammatory fungal infection of the skin caused by lipophilic yeast

II. Pathogenesis

   A. Fungal infection of skin caused by *Pityrosporum orbiculare*

   B. *P. orbiculare* is part of normal flora; overgrowth occurs for unknown reasons

III. Clinical Presentation

   A. Occurs at any age, but most likely to occur in adolescence and young adulthood

   B. Presents as multiple small, circular macules of various colors—white, pink, or brown—(color is uniform in each patient)—thus the name "versicolor"; fine scale is present on surface of macules which can be appreciated by scraping lightly with a #15 surgical blade

   C. Infection is limited to the outermost layers of the skin

   D. Upper trunk most commonly affected, rarely located on face (except in children); may itch, but usually asymptomatic; may be contagious

   E. Proliferation exacerbated by heat, humidity, pregnancy, corticosteroid therapy, oral contraceptives, and immunosuppression

   F. Infection is most evident in summer because the organism produces azelaic acid, a substance that inhibits pigment transfer to keratinocytes

IV. Diagnosis/Evaluation

   A. History
       1. Ask about location, onset, duration, and appearance of lesions
       2. Inquire if associated symptoms present
       3. Ask if any medications, including oral contraceptives are being taken
       4. Determine if patient is immunocompromised

   B. Physical Examination
       1. Examine skin for characteristic lesions
       2. Use Wood's light to look at skin. While not useful as a diagnostic aid (because fluorescence is not predictably present) can demonstrate extent of the infection better than ordinary light

   C. Differential Diagnosis
       1. Vitiligo
       2. Tinea corporis
       3. Seborrheic dermatitis
       4. Pityriasis alba

   D. Diagnostic Tests
       1. Microscopy of KOH-cleared scrapings
       2. Short, curved hyphae and clusters of round yeast cells ("spaghetti and meatballs") pattern are diagnostic

V. Plan/Management

A. For limited disease, **topical** therapies are usually effective. Select **one** from the following table

> ### TREATMENT FOR TINEA VERSICOLOR USING TOPICAL THERAPIES
>
> Selenium sulfide 2.5% lotion (Selsun), supplied as 4 oz
> ➡ Apply daily x 7 consecutive days; rinse off after 10 minutes
> ➡ Advise patient to apply Selsun from neck down
> ➡ Allow skin to repigment for one month; if not cleared in one month, have patient repeat above treatment
> ➡ Repeat the treatment monthly until satisfactory result obtained; treatment is cheap and usually effective
>
> Ketoconazole (Nizoral) 2% shampoo
> ➡ Apply to damp skin in affected area with wide margins
> ➡ Lather, and leave in place for 5 minutes before rinsing
> ➡ May be used as a single application or used daily for 3 days

B. Use **oral therapies** for extensive or recalcitrant infection (poor response to topical therapy)
   1. Ketoconazole (Nizoral) 400 mg PO x 1 dose. Small risk of liver toxicity with this drug **OR**
   2. Fluconazole (Diflucan) 300 mg PO as an initial dose; repeat this dose (300 mg) after 2 weeks
   3. Sweating may improve transfer of these drugs to skin surface
   4. Advise patient not to bathe for 12 hours after treatment with oral medication to allow accumulation of drug on skin

C. Tell patients that clearing may be temporary, since an inhabitant of normal skin causes infection

D. Recommend prophylactic monthly use of selenium sulfide lotion (especially during summer) to prevent recurrences

E. Advise that treatment does not repigment the skin; once the infection is cleared up, the skin will normally repigment itself, but it will take 2 months or longer

F. Follow Up: In one month to evaluate therapy

SCABIES

I. Definition: Skin infestation of the mite, *Sarcoptes scabiei*

II. Pathogenesis

A. A fertilized female mite excavates a burrow in the stratum corneum and deposits eggs and fecal pellets

B. The larvae hatch and reach maturity in about 14 days, mate, and repeat the cycle

C. Humans are the source of infestation with transmission occurring most often by prolonged, close personal contact (a mild self-limited infestation can be acquired from dogs)

D. A hypersensitivity reaction rather than a foreign-body response is responsible for the intense pruritus

E. Incubation period in persons without previous exposure is 4-6 weeks

III. Clinical Presentation

A. Occurs mainly in children, young adults; also among institutionalized persons of all ages (e.g., elderly in nursing homes)

B. Primary lesions are serpiginous burrows, vesicles, and papules
1. Burrows appear as gray or skin-colored ridges up to a few centimeters in length; scratching destroys burrows, so they may be difficult to find
2. Vesicles are isolated, pinpoint, and filled with serous fluid; may contain mites
3. Papules are small, isolated, represent a hypersensitivity reaction, and rarely contain mites

C. Secondary lesions with erythema and scaling caused by scratching are present in more chronic cases

D. Common sites are hands (90%), especially finger webs, flexor aspects of the wrists, belt line, thighs, navel, intergluteal cleft, penis, areola, and axillae

E. Main symptom is intense itching, which is usually worse at night, and the diagnosis should be considered with widespread pruritus presenting primarily with skin excoriation

F. Although uncommon, a generalized urticarial rash may occur in debilitated, immunodeficient, or malnourished persons; called Norwegian scabies, this condition is the result of penetration of the underlying epidermis by hundreds of mites and results in widespread, crusted, hyperkeratotic lesions

IV. Diagnosis/Evaluation

A. History
1. Question regarding onset, duration, morphology, and location of lesions
2. Ask if itching is present, and if it is worse at night
3. Ask about exposures to friends or family members with similar symptoms
4. Inquire what treatments have been tried and their effectiveness

B. Physical Examination
1. Examine the skin for typical burrows
2. Pay particular attention to the hands, especially the finger webs and wrists (flexor aspect), axillary folds, belt line, navel, penis, areas surrounding the areolae
3. A magnifying glass and good lighting are essential

C. Differential Diagnosis
1. Atopic dermatitis
2. Allergic and irritant contact dermatitis
3. Papular urticaria
4. Pediculosis

D. Diagnostic Tests
1. Microscopic identification of mite, ova, or feces proves the diagnosis. Two ways to do this:
   a. Locate tiny black dot at end of burrow; insert a 25-gauge hypodermic needle at dot. Mite, ova, or feces (dot) will stick to it and can be transferred to immersion oil on slide; cover with slip and examine under low power
   b. Slice off whole burrow with sterile scalpel blade (# 15) held parallel to skin; put slice on slide, add immersion oil, cover with slip, and examine under low power
2. If no burrows are found, no diagnostic test indicated

V.   Plan/Management

A.   Use a scabicide from the following table

TREATMENT OF SCABIES

Recommended regimen is 5% permethrin (Elimite) cream
➡ Apply cream over the entire body from the neck down
➡ Remove by bathing in 8-14 hours
➡ Of drugs available to treat scabies, this drug is safest for use in pregnant and lactating women

Alternative regimens:
➡ Lindane (Kwell, Scabine) lotion (1 oz) or cream (30 g)
  • Apply as for permethrin cream above except remove in 8 hours
  • *Caution: Lindane should not be used in pregnant and lactating women; should not be used immediately after a bath or shower, and should not be used by persons who have extensive dermatitis*

➡ Ivermectin 200 µg/kg orally, repeated in 2 weeks
  • Not recommended for pregnant and lactating women

Adapted from Centers for Disease Control and Prevention. (2002). Sexually transmitted diseases treatment guidelines. *MMWR, 51* (RR-6), 68-69.

B.   Appropriate treatment of crusted scabies (Norwegian scabies) remains unclear; substantial treatment failure might occur with single topical scabicide or oral ivermectin treatment
1.   Some experts recommend combined treatment with a topical scabicide and oral ivermectin or repeated treatments with ivermectin
2.   Lindane should be avoided because of risks of neurotoxicity with heavy applications and denuded skin
3.   Consult infectious disease specialist for treatment of patients with this variant of scabies

C.   To control itching that can be intense, prescribe hydroxyzine (Atarax) which also provides sedation at night [the time of day when itching is most intense] and recommend topical agents to control pruritus
1.   Hydroxyzine (Atarax): Available as syrup, 10 mg/5 mL and tabs, 10, 25, 50, 100 mg
  a.   25-50 mg at bedtime for 5-7 days
  b.   TID use is safe, but patient should be warned about sedation and impaired psychomotor performance that could interfere with normal activities
  c.   A better choice for daytime use is fexofenadine (Allegra): 60 mg BID
2.   Sarna lotion, Prax lotion and Itch-X are available without prescription; instruct patient to use as directed on label
3.   Advise patient that pruritus may continue for up to 2 weeks after treatment because of the hypersensitivity reaction created by the mite

D.   If secondary bacterial infection of lesions is present, prescribe topical or oral antibiotics (see section on IMPETIGO AND ECTHYMA for treatment recommendations)

VI.   Control Measures

A.   Prophylactic therapy recommended for household members; therefore all household members should be treated simultaneously to prevent reinfection
1.   Launder all clothing and bedding in hot water and hot drying cycle
2.   Clothing that cannot be laundered should be placed in plastic storage bags for at least a week; parasites cannot survive off the skin for longer than 3-4 days

B.   Follow up
1.   Some experts recommend re-treatment after 1-2 weeks for patients who remain symptomatic
2.   Others recommend re-treatment only if live mites are observed
3.   Patients who do not respond to the recommended treatment should be re-treated with an alternative regimen

PEDICULOSIS

I. Definition: Infestation with one of the three species of lice that infest humans

   A. *Pediculus humanus* var. *capitis* (head louse)

   B. *Pediculus humanus* var. *corporis* (body louse)

   C. *Pthirus pubis* (pubic or crab louse)

II. Pathogenesis

   A. Transmission of head lice occurs by direct contact with infested persons or through hats, brushes, and combs; head lice cannot jump or fly and pets are not vectors

   B. Fomites play a major role in transmission of body lice, but almost no role in transmission of pubic lice, which are transmitted through sexual contact

   C. Ova hatch in a week; lice feed on human blood

   D. Incubation period from laying of eggs to hatching of first nymph is 6-10 days; mature lice (capable of reproducing) do not appear until 2-3 weeks later

III. Clinical Presentation

CLINICAL PRESENTATION OF LICE

Pediculosis capitis (head lice)
➡ Most common in girls between the ages of 5 and 11; all socioeconomic groups affected; rare in blacks
➡ Eggs are initially translucent and attached to a hair shaft close to scalp
➡ After hatching, the 1mm long empty egg cases (nits) become white and more visible; nits remain firmly attached to hair shaft, moving away from scalp as hair grows
➡ Distance of nits from scalp is measure of age (1 cm = 1 month)
➡ Additional information can be found at www.headlice.org

Most infestations involve fewer than 10 lice (mostly small nymphs 1-2 mm long); adults are about the size of a sesame seed (3-4 mm long)
➡ Lice most commonly seen in hair on back of the head near nape of neck
➡ Head lice can survive only 1-2 days away from the scalp
➡ Excoriation from scratching, secondary bacterial infections, and cervical adenopathy are common

Pediculosis corporis (body lice)
➡ Generally found on persons with poor hygiene; lice cannot survive away from blood source for longer than 10 days
➡ Body lice are vectors of disease including typhus, trench fever, and relapsing fever
➡ Excoriation and secondary bacterial infection are common
➡ Body lice and nits may be found in seams of clothing

Pediculosis pubis (pubic lice)
➡ Highly contagious; chance of acquiring from one exposure is about 90%
➡ Common in adolescents and young adults; African-Americans and other racial groups are affected with same frequency
➡ Pubic hair is most common site of infestation, but can also infest hair on chest, abdomen, and thighs
➡ Infested adults may spread pubic lice to eyelashes of children
➡ Eyelash infestation is seen almost exclusively in children
   • Acquired from other children or adult infested with pubic lice
   • May be a sign of sexual abuse in children
➡ Frequently coexists with other sexually transmitted diseases

IV. Diagnosis/Evaluation

A. History
1. Determine if nits or lice have been visualized and when they were first noticed
2. Ask if itching present, especially nocturnal; determine if itching is generalized or localized
3. Question if nits, lice present in close contacts

B. Physical Examination
1. For head lice, the following approach is recommended

STEPS IN EXAMINING HAIR AND SCALP FOR LICE AND NITS

➡ First, comb or brush hair to remove tangles
➡ Using a fine-toothed "nit" comb (teeth of comb should be 0.2 to 0.3 mm apart to trap lice) insert the comb near the crown touching the scalp
➡ Draw comb firmly down the length of the hair
➡ Repeat the process with small sections of the hair until the entire head of hair has been systematically combed at least twice
➡ After each stroke, examine the comb for lice
➡ Usually takes approximately one minute to find the first louse
➡ Combing wet hair is probably more sensitive than combing dry hair but is impractical for routine clinical use

Adapted from Roberts, F.J. (2002). Head lice. *New England Journal of Medicine, 346*, 1645-1650.

---

2. Check eyelashes closely
3. Examine skin of infested site for excoriation secondary to scratching
4. If body lice suspected, examine seams of clothing for lice

C. Differential Diagnosis: Scabies, neurotic excoriation

D. Diagnostic Tests
1. Identification of eggs, nymphs, and lice with naked eye or magnifying glass
2. Microscopic exam usually unnecessary

V. Plan/Management

A. The following products are recommended for the treatment of head lice; **select one**

TREATMENT OF HEAD LICE

Permethrin 1% cream rinse (Nix) OTC
➡ Apply cream rinse to shampooed, rinsed, and towel dried hair (and scalp)
➡ Leave on for 10 minute; rinse
➡ A single treatment is usually adequate, but some experts recommend retreatment 7-10 days after the initial treatment

Malathion 0.5% lotion (Ovide) Rx
➡ Apply to dry hair until scalp and hair are wet and thoroughly coated (bedtime application is most convenient)
➡ Allow hair to dry naturally and after 8-12 hours, shampoo hair thoroughly
➡ Repeat application is not routinely recommended; a second treatment may be given in 7 days if crawling lice are still found after treatment

Pyrethrins 0.33% shampoo or mousse (RID) OTC
➡ Apply to area until thoroughly wet, massage in, wait 10 minutes, add water to form lather, shampoo, and rinse thoroughly

---

B. To remove nits for aesthetic reasons (not necessary to prevent spread)
1. Soak hair with white vinegar; then wrap damp towel soaked in the vinegar around head for 30-60 minutes
2. Use fine-tooth comb to mechanically remove nits
3. There are numerous nit removal aids available; product examples include Clear Lice Egg Remover, Pronto Crème, and Rid Lice Egg Loosener Gel
4. With heavy involvement, a haircut may be preferable to tedious nit removal (child should not be forced to have hair cut, however, if he/she would find it humiliating)

C. Combs and brushes should be soaked in hot water with pediculicide shampoo for 15 minutes

D.   Treatment of pubic and body lice is described below

RECOMMENDED REGIMENS FOR TREATMENT OF PUBIC LICE

Pubic Lice:
Permethrin 1% creme rinse (Nix) [OTC] applied to affected areas and washed off after 10 minutes
OR
Lindane 1% shampoo (Kwell) [Rx] applied to the affected areas and then thoroughly washed off after 4 minutes; this regimen is not recommended for pregnant or lactating women
OR
Pyrethrins 0.33% shampoo, or mousse (A-200, RID) [OTC] applied to the affected area and washed off after 10 minutes

Other management considerations: The recommended regimens should not be applied to the eyes. Sex partners within the last month should be treated. Patients who do not respond to one of the recommended regimens should be re-treated with an alternate regimen. Patients should be evaluated for other sexually transmitted diseases

For infestation of eyelashes or eyebrows, apply occlusive ophthalmic ointment (such as Lacri-Lube (OTC) which contains petrolatum and mineral oil) to the eyelid margins twice a day for 10 days

Body Lice
For the treatment of body lice, pediculicides are not necessary
✓   Treatment consists of improving hygiene and laundering clothing
✓   Infested clothing should be washed and dried at very hot temperatures to kill lice

---

E.   Household and other close contacts should be examined and treated if they have head or body lice; bed mates should be treated prophylactically (**Note:** Head lice do not live on pets; thus pets should not be treated!)

F.   Clothing, bedding should be laundered in hot soapy water and dried on hot cycle or dry cleaned; combs, brushes should be washed in hot (130 degree) soapy water; floor and furniture should be vacuumed

G.   Use of insecticides to disinfect furnishings is not recommended

H.   Provide patients with good written information such as the CDC Division of Parasitic Diseases fact sheet available at http://www.cdc.gov/ncidod/dpd/parasites/lice/

I.   Follow Up: Unnecessary unless treatment failure

CUTANEOUS LARVAE MIGRANS

I.   Definition: A skin disease caused by infected larvae of cat and dog hookworms with *Ancylostoma braziliense* and *Ancylostoma caninum* the usual causes; often referred to as creeping eruption

II.   Pathogenesis

A.   Ova of *A. braziliense* or *A. caninum* are deposited in cat or dog feces

B.   Larvae in soil or sand penetrate human skin that contacts soil

III.   Clinical Presentation

A.   A disease of persons likely to come into contact with sandy soil contaminated with cat/dog feces (e.g., children, gardeners, sunbathers, outdoor workers)

B.   Disease is most prevalent in the southeastern part of the US

C.   Classically presents as pruritic, erythematous, thread-like (or serpiginous) lesions that advance about one cm/day

D.   Lesions are usually located on feet, hands, buttocks, or upper thighs; excoriation may obscure the otherwise typical serpiginous lesion

IV. Diagnosis/Evaluation

    A. History
        1. Inquire about location, onset, duration, and if pruritus is present
        2. Ask if sitting or playing in soil/sand has occurred recently

    B. Physical Examination: Examine skin for typical serpiginous, thread-like lesions; look for signs of scratching

    C. Differential Diagnosis
        1. Tinea
        2. Urticaria
        3. Erythema chronicum migrans
        4. Scabies

    D. Diagnostic Tests: None indicated

V. Plan/Management

    A. Drugs recommended for treatment of hookworm infection (nonpregnant adults only) are the following: (**Note:** All three of the drugs listed are approved drugs, but considered investigational for this indication by the FDA)
        1. Albendazole, 400 mg PO daily x 3 days **OR**
        2. Ivermectin, 200 mcg/kg PO daily x 1-2 days **OR**
        3. Thiabendazole suspension, apply topically to affected areas x 5-7 days

    B. If itching is bothersome, prescribe hydroxyzine (Atarax) and/or recommend OTC topical products
        1. Hydroxyzine: 25-50 mg/dose (supplied as 10, 25, 50 mg tabs)
        2. Sarna lotion, Prax lotion, and Itch-X gel are all OTC

    C. Patient Education: Should be advised not to sit, lie, or walk barefoot on wet soil or sand in areas where cats or dogs are likely to deposit feces

    D. Follow Up: None indicated

PSORIASIS

I. Definition: A chronic, relapsing hyperproliferative inflammatory disorder of the skin of unknown cause

II. Pathogenesis

    A. A complex cascade of events within the skin begins with antigen presentation and T-cell activation that result in the release of cytokines and chemoattractants; these local chemical mediators create a hyperproliferative state in the epidermis and increased vascularity in the dermis

    B. In addition to the obvious genetic component, numerous initiating factors are postulated as causing the T-cell deficit including local trauma, infection, stress, and use of certain medications including β-blockers, lithium, and antimalarials

III. Clinical Presentation

    A. Affects 1-3% of persons throughout the world, with the mean age of onset between 20-30 years
        1. Fewer than 10% of patients have onset during childhood
        2. About 60% of patients develop lesions before age 35

    B. Males and females are equally affected and about 30% of patients have a family history of the disorder
        1. Patients are likely to have history of chronic dandruff, and chronic scaling of ears
        2. Past medical history of many patients is positive for other autoimmune diseases

C. Several distinct clinical variants of psoriasis exist, but the most common form is the localized plaque-type

D. Plaque-type lesions are distinctive; begin as purplish red, scaling papules that coalesce to form plaques with adherent silvery-white scale that are easily distinguishable from normal skin
   1. Scale reveals bleeding points when removed (called Auspitz sign)
   2. Most common sites are extensor surfaces of the elbows and knees
   3. Scalp, umbilicus, intergluteal cleft are also common sites
   4. Bilateral symmetrical involvement of the extremities is a consistent feature (**Note**: Scalp psoriasis is typically asymmetrical, probably due to habitual scratching or picking at one area rather than another)

E. Other variants are characterized by involvement of the palms, soles, or fingernails
   1. Nail pitting (small pits or yellow-brown spots--called oil spots in the nail bed) is the best-known nail abnormality
   2. Distal separation of the nail plate from the bed, producing a whitish to yellowish discoloration of the nail plate, is also a sign of the disorder

F. Guttate psoriasis is a less common variant that presents with scaly papules on the trunk more so than on the extremities and is usually in response to T-cell stimulus by streptococcal antigens

G. Pruritus can contribute to patient discomfort and appearance of the lesions may be altered by scratching or picking at the lesions

H. About 5-8% of patients with psoriasis will develop psoriatic arthritis, a distinct form of arthritis in which rheumatoid factor is negative; distal interphalangeal (DIP) joint disease is the most common expression

I. Disease is often severe when associated with immunodeficiency

IV. Diagnosis/Evaluation

A. History
   1. Inquire about location and appearance of lesions, onset, and duration; if there are bleeding points when thick scale is removed
   2. Ask if nail pitting, arthritis, particularly in DIP joints of fingers or toes
   3. Ask about past history of chronic dandruff, scaling of external ear and canal
   4. Ask about recent streptococcal infection (pharyngitis) and determine if patient is at risk for HIV infection
   5. Ask about treatments tried and results
   6. Review past medical history, particularly presence of other autoimmune disorders
   7. Assess the impact of the disease on the patient's quality of life
   8. Ask about family history of psoriasis in first-degree relatives

B. Physical Examination
   1. Examine entire body surface beginning with the scalp and including the soles of the feet
   2. Look for characteristic lesions, particularly on extensor surfaces, keeping in mind that symmetry of distribution and classic silvery scale are the hallmarks of the plaque-form of the disease (which is by far the most common)
   3. Use tongue blade to scrape over a lesion surface to elicit the fine pinpoint bleeding referred to as Auspitz sign
   4. Quantify the extent of the disease by using the guidelines below (see ESTIMATING BODY SURFACE AREA)
   5. Examine nails for pitting and joints in fingers and toes for inflammatory changes

C. Differential Diagnosis
   1. Seborrheic dermatitis
   2. Nummular dermatitis
   3. Atopic dermatitis
   4. Pityriasis rosea

D. Diagnostic Tests
1. When diagnosis is uncertain, a biopsy should be performed
2. If joint inflammation present, order rheumatoid factor levels, erythrocyte sedimentation rate, and uric acid levels
3. If guttate psoriasis is suspected (scaly papules on trunk), obtain throat swab for culture and antistreptolysin-O antibody titers

V. Plan/Management

A. Education of the patient and the family is the first step in management
1. Emphasize that psoriasis is a chronic condition that can certainly be controlled, but not cured
2. Reassure patient that the disorder is not contagious (patients are often treated as though it were by others, even family members and friends)
3. Most patients believe that psoriasis adversely affects their lives; provide patient with opportunities to discuss feelings in this area
4. Counsel patient regarding elements of a healthy lifestyle, including well-balanced diet, good skin care, frequent exercise, moderate alcohol intake, and avoidance of all tobacco products
5. Discuss the role of stress (from acute illnesses such as respiratory tract infections and from psychosocial sources such as family difficulties, work related problems)
6. Shaving (face in men, armpits and legs in women) should be done very cautiously to avoid trauma to the skin; moisturizers should be applied afterwards
7. Provide patient with information about the National Psoriasis Foundation (NPF), a nonprofit organization that can be a major resource for patient education

> **National Psoriasis Foundation**
> 6600 SW 92nd Avenue, Suite 300
> Portland, Oregon 97223-7195
> 800-723-9166
> http://www.psoriasis.org

B. Good skin care, with an emphasis on keeping the skin well hydrated, is one of the cornerstones in the treatment of psoriasis and can have a sustainable impact on the patient's well being
1. Dry skin, the most common cause of itching, can cause much discomfort
2. Daily lubrication and moisturization of the skin is of paramount importance
3. See recommendations regarding care of dry skin in section CARE OF DRY AND OILY SKIN

C. Treatment for psoriasis is divided into three major categories: topical therapy, phototherapy, and systemic therapy

D. Determine degree of body surface involvement as a guide to selection of the appropriate therapy from the three categories

---

ESTIMATING BODY SURFACE AREA (BSA) IN ORDER TO QUANTIFY THE DISEASE

➡ The palm of the patient's hand represents approximately 1% BSA
➡ Using that diameter as a guide, estimate the degree of involvement
➡ Involvement of no more than 15% (see V.E. and F. below for exceptions) indicates that this patient is a candidate for topical therapy alone (at least initially) and management in a primary care setting is probably appropriate

---

E. Patients with psoriatic involvement of greater than 15% of body surface area (BSA) or with moderate to severe disease should be referred to a dermatologist for management; many of these patients are candidates for phototherapy and/or systemic therapy

F. Most patients with localized plaque involvement involving the trunk and extremities can be treated with topical therapy alone (**Note**: This generalization does not apply to forms of psoriasis such as hand and foot psoriasis which may have less than 15% of BSA involvement but which can be very disabling)

G. Recommendations below are for localized plaque psoriasis involving the trunk and extremities in which less than 15% of body surface is affected
1. Aim of treatment is to bring the psoriasis into remission or an inactive state
2. Selected residual lesions on some parts of the body may need to be left rather than treated aggressively

H.   Topical preparations are most frequently used for treatment of localized plaque psoriasis; the following table lists these preparations

---

TOPICAL THERAPY FOR BODY AND EXTREMITIES

➡ **Initial therapy** with a high potency topical corticosteroid cream or ointment (**Note**: This is different from recommendations in previous years in which the least potent agents were tried first, and then more potent agents were used when treatment failures occurred)

- **Choose one** of the following:
  - ✓ Betamethasone dipropionate 0.05% (Diprolene AF) emollient cream **OR**
  - ✓ Triamcinolone acetonide 0.5% (Aristocort A) cream or ointment

- **Instruct patient** on appropriate use of topical corticosteroids
  - ✓ Apply BID and apply no more often than this
  - ✓ Use only the amount that will easily rub into skin in less than a minute
  - ✓ Apply gently and confine application to the plaque
  - ✓ Always wash hands after application so that medication is not inadvertently applied to other areas such as face or groin
  - ✓ Use for 1-2 weeks which should induce significant clearing

➡ **Maintenance Therapy:** After 1-2 weeks of topical therapy with a high potency agent, a long-term maintenance program should be started that involves the use of calcipotriene cream or ointment and intermediate potency topical corticosteroids for flares

- Use the nonsteroidal calcipotriene as maintenance therapy
  - ✓ Calcipotriene (Dovonex) is a synthetic vitamin B_3 analogue that is believed to reduce epidermal differentiation and T-lymphocyte proliferation
  - ✓ Dovonex is available as a cream or ointment and should be applied once or twice a day as tolerated in amounts up to 100 g/week
  - ✓ Patients may prefer to use the cream during the day since it is more cosmetically acceptable and the ointment at bedtime
  - ✓ Advise patient to confine application to the plaque
  - ✓ This agent avoids the complications of skin atrophy and telangiectasia seen with topical corticosteroids
  - ✓ Rare complication of calcipotriene is hypercalcemia
- Use intermediate potency topical corticosteroids for flares (pulse therapy)
  - ✓ Prednicarbate 0.1% (Dermatop emollient cream), supplied as 15, 60 g
  - ✓ Desonide 0.05% (Tridesilon cream), supplied as 15, 60 g
  - ✓ Steroids become less effective with continued use; therefore, advise patients to **use only with flares, not continually**
- Continue to emphasize to patient the importance of good skin care

---

I.   Recently topical tazarotene (Tazorac), a topical receptor-selective retinoid, has been approved by the FDA for treatment of psoriasis; it is available as either a gel or a cream
   1.   Patients who have failed the regimen contained in the table above may benefit from topical tazarotene
   2.   Instruct the patient to apply daily to affected areas (no more than 15% of BSA) and to apply a topical corticosteroid at night to control irritation
   3.   Once irritation is controlled, steroids should be used for flares only

J.   Topical therapy for scalp depends on the degree of scalp involvement as well as the degree of patch thickening; treatment of the scalp is outlined below

---

TREATMENT OF THE SCALP

The scalp is often one of the most difficult areas to treat
- ➡ For moderate scalp involvement, instruct patient to apply peanut oil or olive oil to scalp at bedtime in order to loosen scale; in AM, patient should shampoo hair with a medicated shampoo containing a keratolytic agent such as salicylic acid (T/Sal) or tar (T/Gel, Reme-T, Pentrax); patient should repeat this process several times a week until scalp is clear; also prescribe a topical corticosteroid solution such as fluocinolone acetonide (Synalar) 0.01% solution to be applied BID for erythema and pruritus (not to be used continuously, but PRN) [supplied in 20, 60 mL bottles, and for use after shampooing]
- ➡ For more severe (dense) scalp lesions, a medium-potency topical steroid oil, fluocinolone acetonide (Derma-Smoothe/FS Topical Oil) 0.01% oil, under occlusion with a shower cap at bedtime may be used for 5-6 days

---

K.   Topical therapy for face, flexural folds, and genitalia is described in table below

TOPICAL THERAPY FOR FACE, FLEXURAL FOLDS, AND GENITALIA
➡ Should be with low potency agents such as hydrocortisone 1% cream
• Treatment should be BID
• Treat for no longer than 2 weeks
• Explain to patient that pulse therapy (once or twice a week) should be used for maintenance
➡ Daily and regular sunlight exposure is beneficial to 4 out of 5 psoriasis patients; advise patients to avoid sunburn (short time in sun with no sun exposure during 10 AM until 4 PM); do not recommend sun exposure to patients with increased skin cancer risk (fair skin, easily burned, history of skin cancer or irradiation)

L.   Follow Up: In 2-3 weeks in all patients in whom therapy has been initiated; then monitor for side effects every 2-3 months

PITYRIASIS ROSEA

I.   Definition: A common, benign, often asymptomatic, self-limiting skin eruption of unknown etiology

II.   Pathogenesis: Unknown, but some evidence suggests it is viral in origin

III.   Clinical Presentation

   A.   Most commonly seen in children, adolescents and young adults (75% of cases are in persons 10-35 years of age)

   B.   May be preceded by a prodrome of pharyngitis, lymphadenopathy, headache, and malaise, but in most cases, no history of these symptoms is given

   C.   In its typical form, a 2-10 cm scaly, round-to-oval plaque (the herald patch) appears on the trunk
   1.   Precedes the appearance of the generalized eruption by 7-14 days
   2.   Herald patch, unlike the subsequent lesions, usually has central clearing

   D.   The herald patch is followed by a generalized eruption consisting of multiple, pink (in Caucasians) to dark brown (in African Americans) macules progressing to plaques which enlarge and become oval; a peripheral rim of fine scale is present

   E.   Long axes of oval lesions tend to run parallel to each other, creating a "Christmas tree" distribution on trunk

   F.   Lesions usually fade over 4-6 weeks and mild to intense itching is common

IV.   Diagnosis/Evaluation

   A.   History
   1.   Question regarding recent occurrence of herald patch and location and presence of other lesions
   2.   Question regarding medications currently taking
   3.   Question if symptoms such as pruritus are present

   B.   Physical Examination
   1.   Examine skin for characteristic lesions; look specifically for herald patch which is usually on trunk
   2.   Determine distribution of lesions, looking to see if long axes of oval-shaped lesions are parallel to each other
   3.   Check the mucous surfaces, palms, and soles which are spared by pityriasis rosea

C. Differential Diagnosis
   1. Tinea corporis
   2. Tinea versicolor
   3. Viral exanthems
   4. Drug eruptions
   5. Syphilis

D. Diagnostic Tests: **Always** order VDRL or RPR as syphilis can mimic this disorder

V. Plan/Management

A. No therapy is required, but symptomatic management of pruritus may be indicated (see section on ATOPIC DERMATITIS for prescribing information)

B. Sunlight exposure to the point of minimal erythema will hasten disappearance of lesions and decrease itching; caution against sunburn

C. Follow Up: Usually unnecessary except for follow-up on syphilis serology

LICHEN PLANUS

I. Definition: A chronic, inflammatory cutaneous and mucous membrane reaction pattern of unknown etiology

II. Pathogenesis

A. Cause is unknown; possibly due to cell-mediated immune response to epidermal cell antigens

B. Genetic factors may play a role in etiology; familial cases are more severe

III. Clinical Presentation

A. Age of onset is usually between 30-70 years; rare in children <5 years of age; more common in women than men

B. Primary lesion is a 2-10 mm flat-topped papule with an irregular polyangular border; new lesions are white to pink, but with time become purple

C. Close inspection of the surface of lesion reveals a lacy, reticulated pattern of whitish lines (called Wickham's striae)

D. Clinical features of lichen planus (the 5 Ps): pruritic, planar (flat-topped), polyangular, purple, papules or plaques

E. Number of lesions varies from a few chronic lesions to a generalized eruption

F. Oral mucous membrane lichen planus can occur without cutaneous disease
   1. Lesions may be on tongue, lips, but most common site is buccal mucosa
   2. Mucous membrane involvement may consist only of the lace-like lesions

G. Five to ten percent of patients have nail changes ranging from minor dystrophy to total nail loss

H. Anti-hepatitis C virus antibodies are detected in approximately 16% of patients with cutaneous and 30% of patients with the oral form

IV.   Diagnosis/Evaluation

    A.   History
        1.   Question about appearance and location of lesions, onset, duration (whether a chronic or acute process)
        2.   Ask if lesions are pruritic
        3.   Question about presence of lesions in mouth
        4.   Ask if any first-degree relatives have a similar eruption

    B.   Physical Examination
        1.   Examine the involved skin, looking for flat-topped, polyangular, purple papules
        2.   Use a magnifying glass to inspect the surface of lesions for reticulated pattern of whitish lines
        3.   Examine oral cavity, particularly the buccal mucosa, the most common site; look for Wickham's striae on the buccal mucosa

    C.   Differential Diagnosis
        1.   Drug eruption
        2.   Psoriasis
        3.   Aphthous stomatitis
        4.   Leukoplakia
        5.   Thrush

    D.   Diagnostic Tests: Consider antibody assays for anti-HCV (hepatitis C infection has been associated with lichen planus, particularly the oral form)

V.   Plan/Management

    A.   Mouth lesions: Triamcinolone acetonide 0.025% cream in an adhesive base (Orabase) BID for 1-2 weeks; medication should be carefully placed on oral lesions and not rubbed in, as rubbing in disrupts adhesive properties of Orabase; inhaled corticosteroids (for example, triamcinolone [Azmacort]) may be used as an alternative; spray on lesion BID for 1-2 weeks (not FDA approved for this indication)

    B.   Body lesions (not mucous membrane): Triamcinolone acetonide 0.1% cream (Aristocort, supplied as 15, 60 g) applied 2-3 x day for 1-2 weeks (caution patient about steroid atrophy)

    C.   Prescribe antihistamines for pruritus, if present (see section on ATOPIC DERMATITIS for prescribing information)

    D.   Follow up: None

PITYRIASIS ALBA

I.   Definition: A disorder of pigmentation that may be a form of atopic dermatitis, but it occurs without the features of atopic dermatitis

II.   Pathogenesis

    A.   Cause of hypopigmentation is unknown

    B.   Likely related to inflammatory mediators that inhibit melanocyte function

III.   Clinical Presentation

    A.   Occurs primarily in children before puberty; up to 40% of children are affected

    B.   Presents as multiple oval, scaly, hypopigmented patches on the face, extensor surfaces of upper arms, and on neck

C. Lesions range in size from 5-10 mm in diameter with 10-20 lesions commonly seen

D. Lesions are asymptomatic but are cosmetically bothersome to child and parents

IV. Diagnosis/Evaluation

    A. History
       1. Inquire about location, onset, duration, and any symptoms of lesions
       2. Ask about treatments tried and results

    B. Physical Examination: Examine skin for characteristic lesions

    C. Differential Diagnosis
       1. Tinea versicolor
       2. Vitiligo (dead white appearing; does not scale)

    D. Diagnostic Tests: KOH exam to exclude tinea versicolor

V. Plan/Management

    A. There is no satisfactory treatment for this skin disorder; emphasize the chronic, recurrent nature of this benign disorder; reassure patient/parent that condition gradually improves after puberty

    B. Triamcinolone acetonide, 0.025% (Aristocort A) cream applied BID x 7-10 days may be prescribed so long as the patient/parent understands that this treatment has limited efficacy and does not affect pigmentation

    C. After 7-10 day course of topical steroids, apply moisturizers such as Moisturel at bedtime to control scaling

    D. Emphasize the importance of good skin care (see information on managing dry skin in the section CARE OF DRY AND OILY SKIN)

    E. Use this opportunity to discuss sun avoidance, use of protective clothing, and use of sunscreen with an SPF >30

    F. Follow Up: None indicated

HERPES SIMPLEX

I. Definition: Cutaneous infections with herpes simplex viruses that are enveloped, double-stranded, DNA viruses of two types that have major genomic and antigenic differences

    A. HSV-1 is usually associated with orolabial infections

    B. HSV-2 is usually associated with genital infections (genital herpes is considered under SEXUALLY TRANSMITTED DISEASES)

II. Pathogenesis

    A. HSV-1 and HSV-2 are epidermotropic viruses with infection occurring within keratinocytes

    B. Transmission is only by direct contact with active lesions, or by virus-containing fluid such as saliva or cervical secretions in persons with no evidence of active disease

    C. Inoculation of the virus into skin or mucosal surfaces produces infection, with an incubation period of 2 days to 2 weeks

D. About 48 hours after entering the host, the virus transverses afferent nerves to find host ganglion
    1. The trigeminal ganglia are the target of the oral virus—primarily HSV-1
    2. The sacral ganglia are the target of the genital virus—most often HSV-2

E. Upon reactivation, the virus retraces its route, causing recurrence in the cutaneous area affected by the same nerve root, but not necessarily in the original site

F. Generally HSV-1 is associated with orolabial infection and HSV-2 with the genitalia (see SEXUALLY TRANSMITTED DISEASES section for a full discussion of this topic)

G. An increasing number of genital herpes cases are attributable to HSV-1

III. Clinical Presentation

A. Two clinical stages define the course of herpes viruses: primary infection after which the virus becomes established in a nerve ganglion, and recurrent infection

B. During the first stage--primary infection with HSV-1 virus--the following usually occurs:
    1. Lesions may appear 2-14 days following inoculation; lesions are typically grouped vesicles on an erythematous base, usually affecting the orolabial area (herpes labialis), and commonly known as "cold sores" or "fever blisters"
    2. Vesicles rupture, leaving erosions that slowly form crusts; crusting signals the end of viral shedding; lesions are intraepidermal and usually heal without leaving a scar
    3. There may be tenderness, pain, mild paresthesia, or burning prior to and during the eruption of lesions; person may also have fever, myalgia, malaise, or cervical lymphadenopathy
    4. In addition to orolabial infection, another clinical variant of herpes simplex that commonly occurs is herpes gladiatorum that can occur on the torso of wrestlers (or other athletes) with frequent skin-to-skin contact
    5. Nearly 30% of infected persons are entirely asymptomatic during the primary infection state

C. During the primary infection stage, the virus enters nerve endings in the skin below the lesions and travels through peripheral nerves to the dorsal root ganglia, and remains dormant

D. During the recurrent infection, or second clinical stage, the virus is reactivated and travels down peripheral nerves to the site of the initial infection, causing the characteristic focal infection; recurrent infection is not inevitable and may be triggered by one or more of the following:
    1. Local skin trauma
    2. Sunlight exposure
    3. Systemic changes such as menses, fatigue, or fever

IV. Diagnosis/Evaluation

A. History
    1. Question regarding location, onset, duration, and appearance of lesions; ask if pain, burning, or paresthesia present prior to eruption
    2. Ask about associated symptoms of fever, myalgia, malaise
    3. Ask regarding previous occurrence of similar lesions, symptoms
    4. Inquire about exposures to infected persons

B. Physical Examination
    1. Examine lesions for characteristic location, distribution, and appearance
    2. Check for cervical lymphadenopathy

C. Differential Diagnosis: Erythema multiforme, pemphigus

D. Diagnostic Tests
    1. Premier type-specific HSV-1 IgG test (Meridian Diagnostics, Research Triangle Park, North Carolina) is a rapid ELISA test available for the diagnosis of HSV-seropositivity
    2. Viral culture is also an option, but the results are not immediate
        a. Unroof vesicle and scrape the material with Dacron-tipped swab
        b. Place swab in viral transport media
        c. Viral detection usually requires 1-3 days after inoculation

V. Plan/Management

  A. Reassure patient that infections resolve without treatment
    1. Base treatment decisions on needs of each patient
    2. Several oral antiviral drugs and topical agents are available for the treatment or primary and recurrent herpes orolabial infection and are listed in the table that follows

TREATMENT OF HERPES LABIALIS			
Oral Therapy (Therapy must be initiated within 48 hours of the onset of signs and symptoms)			
Primary/recurrent orolabial infections	Acyclovir (Zovirax)* Famciclovir (Famvir)* Valacyclovir (Valtrex)	400 mg PO 5 times a day x 5 days **OR** 500 mg PO BID x 7 days **OR** 2 g PO Q 12 hrs x 1 day	$52.81** $103.27 $25.98
Topical Therapy (can also be used in lieu of oral antiviral agents, but oral treatment is usually more efficacious)			
✓	Penciclovir cream 1% (Denavir), applied every 2 hours while awake x 4 days reduces the duration of herpes labialis by about half a day		$23.09
✓	Docosanol cream 10% (Abreva), applied 5 x/day until healed and is available without a prescription		$13.75
✓	Tetracaine cream 1.8% (Cepacol Viractic Cream) reduces healing time of recurrent herpes labialis lesion by about 2 days and is available without a prescription		$12.50
✓	Lips should be protected from sun exposure with agents such as zinc oxide or with lip balm containing sun-blocking agents		
✓	Compresses with cool water decrease erythema and help to débride the lesion		

* Not FDA approved for this indication (Famvir is approved for use in HIV-infected patients)
** Cost of one course of treatment with oral drug or tube of cream in 2002

  B. Immunocompromised patients with persistent intraoral or extralabial lesions
    1. Acyclovir, 200 mg PO 5 x/day x 7 days OR
    2. Valacyclovir, 500 mg PO BID x 5 days
    3. If suppressive therapy is indicated, prescribe acyclovir, 200-400 mg PO BID

  C. Follow Up: None indicated

HERPES ZOSTER (SHINGLES)

I. Definition: A cutaneous viral infection, usually involving skin of a single dermatome but may involve one or two adjacent dermatomes

II. Pathogenesis

  A. Varicella-zoster virus causes two distinct syndromes
    1. Primary infection presents as varicella or chickenpox, a contagious but usually benign illness that occurs in childhood
    2. Subsequent reactivation of latent varicella-zoster virus in dorsal-root ganglia results in an eruption known as herpes zoster or "shingles"

  B. The risk of herpes zoster increases with declining virus-specific cell-mediated immune responses which occur naturally as a result of aging or can be induced by immunosuppressive illness or medical treatments

III. Clinical Presentation

  A. Over 90% of adults in the US have serologic evidence of varicella-zoster virus infection and are at risk for herpes zoster

  B. Increasing age is a key risk factor for the development of the disease

  C. The other well-defined risk factor is altered cell-mediated immunity (e.g., persons with neoplastic diseases, those receiving immunosuppressive drugs, including corticosteroids, and organ-transplant recipients)

D. Persons who are seropositive for human immunodeficiency virus (HIV) have higher occurrence rates than those who are seronegative

E. Prodrome of local tingling, burning, pain, and hyperesthesia often begins along the dermatome several days before the eruption appears (see Figure 7.1.)

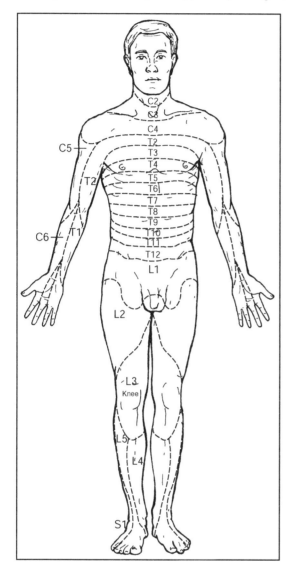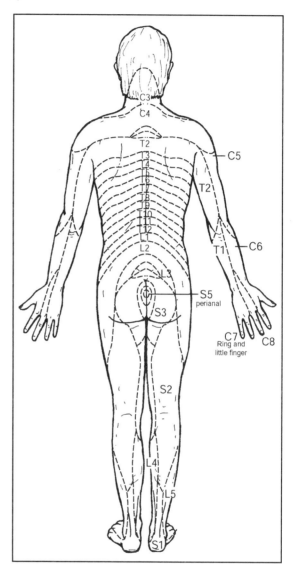

Figure 7.1. Dermatomes

F. Headache, photophobia, and malaise may also precede the eruption; fever is rare

G. Eruption begins with an erythematous maculopapular rash and the distribution is dermatomal and unilateral (does not cross the midline)
    1. Clear vesicles arise in clusters from the erythematous base
    2. Successive crops continue to form for 3-5 days and evolve through stages of pustulation, ulceration, and crusting
    3. Over a period of 2-4 weeks, healing occurs; often, there is scarring and permanent changes in pigmentation
    4. The presence of a few skin lesions outside the primary or adjacent dermatome is not unusual in immunocompetent patients

H. The cervical and thoracic dermatomes are most commonly affected; recurrences occur in the same dermatome almost half the time (**Note:** Only 5% of persons will experience more than one episode of herpes zoster [HZ])

I.   If the ophthalmic branch of the trigeminal nerve is involved, there is a significant risk for severe and permanent eye damage

J.   Infection usually resolves over 2-4 weeks, but elderly or debilitated persons may have a prolonged and difficult course

K.   Postherpetic neuralgia (pain that persists more than 30 days after the onset of rash or after cutaneous healing) occurs frequently in the elderly and can be debilitating; both incidence and duration of postherpetic neuralgia are directly correlated with the patient's age

L.   HZ may be an early clinical sign of HIV infection and should be suspected when the disease occurs in otherwise asymptomatic adults younger than 50 years of age, or when a case is protracted, recurrent, or involves more than one dermatome

IV.   Diagnosis/Evaluation

A.   History
      1.   Inquire when the eruption began and ask about appearance and distribution of the lesions
      2.   Question if there was preeruptive pain, itching, or burning in the affected dermatome several days before the eruption
      3.   Ask about history of prior varicella infection
      4.   Question regarding immunosuppressed status

B.   Physical Examination
      1.   Examine skin for characteristic lesions and distribution (grouped vesicles on an erythematous base in a dermatomal distribution with unilateral involvement)
      2.   Be aware that location or appearance of the lesions may be atypical in immunocompromised patients
      3.   Determine if there is ophthalmic involvement

C.   Differential Diagnosis
      1.   Varicella
      2.   Herpes simplex
      3.   Poison ivy
      4.   Cellulitis

D.   Diagnostic Tests
      1.   Most rapid and sensitive confirmatory test for HZ is the direct immunofluorescence assay performed on scrapings from base of a vesicle
      2.   If patient is a younger adult (under age 50), or if this is a recurrent, protracted case, consider HIV testing

V.   Plan/Management

A.   Patients with involvement of the ophthalmic branch of the trigeminal nerve require **immediate** referral for ophthalmologic evaluation and aggressive antiviral treatment because of the high risk for severe and permanent damage to the eye

B.   Goals of therapy are to decrease pain, inflammation, vesicle formation, and viral shedding during the acute phase and to limit and/or treat postherpetic neuralgia (if it occurs) after the acute phase has resolved
      1.   Treatment of HZ with oral antiviral agents is indicated to reduce pain, hasten resolution of the exanthem, reduce viral shedding and possibly shorten the duration of postherpetic neuralgia
      2.   Treatment is most effective when initiated within the first 48 hours of the development of prodromal symptoms (or outbreak of the eruption if there is no prodrome); reasonable to use antiviral therapy in patients more than 48 hours after vesicles appear if lesions are not completely crusted

3. The following table contains the recommended drugs and dosages

RECOMMENDED ORAL DRUGS FOR THE TREATMENT OF HERPES ZOSTER		
Drug	**Dosage**	**Comments**
Valacyclovir (Valtrex)	1 g PO TID x 7 days	In immunocompetent adults >50 years of age with HZ, valacyclovir produces more rapid resolution of zoster-associated pain and shorter duration of postherpetic neuralgia than acyclovir
Famciclovir (Famvir)	500 mg PO TID x 7 days	Administration of famciclovir to immunocompetent patients >50 years of age with HZ within 72 hours after onset of rash decreases the duration of postherpetic neuralgia but not its incidence
Acyclovir (Zovirax)	800 mg PO 5 x/day x 7-10 days	Acyclovir is generally well tolerated; intravenous (IV) acyclovir is drug of choice for treatment of serious infections caused by varicella zoster virus

Adapted from Abramowicz, M. (2002). Drugs for non-HIV viral infections. *The Medical Letter, 44*, 9-16.

C. The following recommendations can be made for symptomatic relief during the acute phase
   1. Use of cool tap water (or Domeboro soaks) applied for 20 minutes several times a day
   2. A sterile, nonocclusive, nonadherent dressing placed over the involved dermatome will protect the lesions from contact with clothing
   3. Antihistamines at bedtime: hydroxyzine (Atarax) 25, 50 mg PO at HS
   4. See section on *Pain* in GENERAL chapter (Chapter 2) for recommendations regarding effective pain management. Scheduled short-acting narcotics should be prescribed for acute pain. For persistent pain, long-acting, controlled-release opioids (oral or transdermal) are preferred

D. Antiviral drugs do not reliably prevent postherpetic neuralgia; chronic neuropathic pain will develop (unpredictably) in certain patients even with appropriate antiviral treatment

E. The following table contains a listing of topical and oral medications that may provide some relief for some patients with postherpetic neuralgia

TOPICAL AND ORAL MEDICATIONS USED FOR PAIN RELIEF IN PATIENTS WITH POSTHERPETIC NEURALGIA
Topical Products
✓ Capsaicin cream (Zostrix, Zostrix HP) [OTC]; apply to affected area 3-4 x/day; apply only to healed, intact skin; advise patient to avoid eyes and wash hands thoroughly after application
✓ Lidocaine 2.5%, Prilocaine 2.5% (EMLA cream) [Not FDA approved for this indication]; apply in thick layer to intact skin; may use plastic wrap for occlusion to increase efficacy; also available in patch form (lidocaine 5% patch); consult PDR for more information
Oral Medications
✓ Tricyclic antidepressants (e.g., nortriptyline, 10-25 mg at bedtime) [not FDA approved for this indication]
✓ Gabapentin (Neurontin) was recently FDA approved for this indication; is as effective as tricyclics and is often better tolerated; prescribe 300 mg/day on Day 1, 300 mg BID on Day 2, 300 mg TID on Day 3; then titrate to 600 mg TID if needed (no evidence that higher doses are more effective, and they cause more side effects) [consult PDR for precautions, contraindications, need for monitoring, and side effects]
✓ See section on *Pain* in GENERAL chapter for prescribing recommendations for pain management

F. Treatment of postherpetic neuralgia is complex; patients who do not respond to treatment after an adequate trial should be referred to an expert in pain control for management

G. Adults who are HIV+ with HZ infection are managed with acyclovir, 10 mg/kg IV Q 8 hours x 7 days

H. For secondarily infected lesions, apply mupirocin (Bactroban) cream TID for 10 days (**Note:** Cream formulation is recommended for secondary infections)

I. Isolate patient from neonates, pregnant women, and immunosuppressed persons since the active lesions are potentially infectious, though this is rare—patient with HZ can **only** infect someone who is seronegative for varicella-zoster virus (VZV)

J. Follow up in 3-5 days after diagnosis; then again in 7-10 days; for patients with postherpetic neuralgia, follow up for support and evaluation of response to pain control management should be based on patient need

MOLLUSCUM CONTAGIOSUM

I. Definition: A benign, usually asymptomatic viral disease of the skin characterized by discrete, flesh-colored to translucent dome-shaped papules

II. Pathogenesis

   A. Caused by a poxvirus (sole member of the genus Molluscipoxvirus) that induces epidermal cell proliferation

   B. Humans are the only known source of the virus and infectivity is relatively low

   C. Spreads by direct contact, including sexual contact, or by fomites such as towels

   D. Incubation period varies between 2-7 weeks and may be up to 6 months

III. Clinical Presentation

   A. More common in children and adolescents, but may affect any age group

   B. Tiny (2-5 mm), early lesions are shiny, flesh-colored to translucent, dome-shaped discrete papules with a firm, waxy appearance that often occur in groups
      1. As lesions mature, the centers become soft and umbilicated
      2. Usual number of lesions ranges from 2-20
      3. Commonly occur on the face, trunk, and extremities and in genital area in adults; an eczematous reaction may encircle the papules in about 10% of patients

   C. Self-limiting; usually spontaneously clears in 6-9 months

   D. A common, cutaneous manifestation of HIV infection

IV. Diagnosis/Evaluation

   A. History
      1. Inquire about location, appearance of lesions, onset and duration
      2. Ask about past medical history, determine if patient is immunocompromised

   B. Physical Examination
      1. Examine skin for characteristic lesions
      2. Magnification may assist in seeing central umbilication in more mature lesions
      3. Palpate the lesions to reveal their solid versus fluid-filled nature (wear gloves)

   C. Differential Diagnosis
      1. Basal cell carcinoma
      2. Epidermal cyst
      3. Wart
      4. Herpes simplex

   D. Diagnostic Tests: Usually based on clinical appearance of lesions; biopsy of lesion is recommended in persons who are immunocompromised

V. Plan/Management

   A. For small number of asymptomatic lesions that are stable (not spreading), observe for spontaneous resolution over next few months; advise patient that there is a small risk of scarring with all removal modalities

   B. Genital lesions should be treated to prevent spread via sexual contact (see D. below)

C. Removal using a curette works well when there are just a few lesions; removal of the umbilicated core (evisceration) can be done simply with the use of a hollow needle and this results in resolution of the lesion(s) when there are just a few

D. Liquid nitrogen therapy is also an option that is often used with genital lesions
1. Papule is touched lightly with the nitrogen-bathed probe until the advancing, white, frozen border progresses down the side of the lesion to form a 1 mm halo on the normal skin surrounding the lesion
2. Process is very rapid (around 5 seconds)
3. Excessive freezing can cause scarring, hypopigmentation, or hyperpigmentation

E. Other options involve use of one of the following topical agents
1. Salicylic acid 17% (Duofilm liquid), available as 15 mL with applicator; apply thin layer daily up to 12 weeks (not FDA approved for this indication) **OR**
2. Podofilox 0.5% gel (Condylox topical gel), available as 3.5 g; apply BID x 3 days (not FDA approved for this indication) **OR**
3. Imiquimod 5% cream (Aldara), available as 12 single use packets; apply a thin layer 3 times a week at bedtime and remove with soap and water after 6-10 hours for up to two weeks (not FDA approved for this indication) **OR**
4. Tretinoin gel 0.01% (Retin-A-Gel), (available as 15 g); apply sparingly at bedtime for up to two weeks (not FDA approved for this indication)
5. With all of these topical agents, protection of surrounding skin with petrolatum is recommended
6. Prescribe medications for off-label use cautiously!

F. Follow Up: In 2-4 weeks to evaluate treatment efficacy

WARTS

I. Definition: Virus-induced proliferation of keratinocytes resulting in tumors of the skin and mucous membranes

II. Pathogenesis

A. Human papillomaviruses (HPVs) produce epithelial tumors of the skin and mucous membranes

B. HPVs are members of the Papovaviridae family and are DNA viruses

C. More than 70 types have been identified; a small number of HPV types account for most warts

D. HPV types causing nongenital warts generally are distinct from those causing anogenital infections

III. Clinical Presentation

A. Cutaneous warts occur much less commonly in adults than in school-age children who have prevalence rates as high as 50%

B. Warts are transmitted by touch and commonly appear at sites of trauma on the hands, periungual regions from biting, and on plantar surfaces from weight bearing

C. Most warts resolve in 12-24 months without treatment

D. Generally, warts are asymptomatic except for plantar warts that may be painful

E. Presentation is variable depending on type:
1. Common warts (*verruca vulgaris*) may arise anywhere on body (often on hands) and appear as solitary flesh-colored papules with scaly, irregular surface; usually are asymptomatic and multiple
2. Filiform warts are usually seen on face (lips, nose, eyelids) and appear as thin projections on a narrow stalk
3. Flat warts (*verruca plana*) are usually located on face and extremities and appear in groups as flat-topped, skin-colored papules

4. Plantar warts occur on weight-bearing areas of the feet; papule is pushed into skin and verrucous surface appears level with skin surface (characterized by marked hyperkeratosis and sometimes with black dots [black dots appear in warts when small dermal vessels become thrombosed])
5. Anogenital warts are considered under SEXUALLY TRANSMITTED DISEASES section

IV. Diagnosis/Evaluation

A. History
1. Question about location, onset, duration, and if any symptoms are present
2. Ask about treatments tried and results

B. Physical Examination
1. Examine lesion looking for characteristic appearance
2. Use hand lens to aid in visualizing surface characteristics

C. Differential Diagnosis
1. Calluses (have smooth rather than rough irregular surface)
2. Lichen planus (look for Wickham's striae)
3. Seborrheic keratosis (have stuck-on appearance with horn cysts visible on close inspection)

D. Diagnostic Tests: Most are easily diagnosed based on clinical appearance

V. Plan/Management

A. Counsel patient that most nongenital warts eventually regress without treatment but may persist for weeks or months

B. Optimal treatment for warts that do not resolve spontaneously has not been identified; nonetheless, many patients desire treatment and some success has come from methods that rely on chemical or physical destruction of the infected epithelium

C. Common wart: Topical salicylic acid preparations applied at bedtime for 6-8 weeks
1. Examples of 17% concentrations are Occlusal HP, DuoPlant, Compound W, Duofilm, Wart-Off; all are OTC and in liquid form
2. An example of a 15% solution in karaya gum base patches for use on isolated thicker lesions is Trans Ver Sal (40 patches of varying size with securing tapes and emery file)
3. May use liquid nitrogen in cooperative patients

D. Filiform wart: Refer for removal by snip excision

E. Flat wart: Refer for removal; these warts are resistant to treatment and are usually located in cosmetically important areas

F. Plantar wart: Use 40% salicylic acid plasters; examples are Mediplast and Duofilm Patch
1. Plaster is cut to size of wart and applied over wart
2. Plaster is removed in 24-48 hours and pliable dead white keratin is removed with pumice stone
3. Process is repeated every 24-48 hours until wart is removed (usually 6-8 weeks)
4. Pain relief occurs early because a large part of wart is removed in first few days of treatment

G. Follow Up: In 2-4 weeks to evaluate response to treatment (if any treatment was initiated)

REFERENCES

Abramowicz, M. (2002). Drugs for non-HIV viral infections. *The Medical Letter, 44,* 9-16.

Abramowicz, M. (2002). Desloratadine (Clarinex). *The Medical Letter, 44,* 27-28.

Abramowicz, M. (2002). Topical pimecrolimus (Elidel) for treatment of atopic dermatitis. *The Medical Letter, 44,* 48-50.

Abramowicz, M. (2002). Tazarotene (Tazorac) for acne. *The Medical Letter, 44,* 52-53.

American Academy of Pediatrics. (2000). Cutaneous larva migrans. In L.K. Pickering (Ed.), *2000 red book: Report of the Committee on Infectious Diseases* (25th ed., pp. 225-226). Elk Grove Village, IL: Author.

American Academy of Pediatrics. (2000). Herpes simplex. In L.K. Pickering (Ed.), *2000 red book: Report of the Committee on Infectious Diseases* (25th ed., pp. 309-318). Elk Grove Village, IL: Author.

American Academy of Pediatrics. (2000). Hookworm infections. In L.K. Pickering (Ed.), *2000 red book: Report of the Committee on Infectious Diseases* (25th ed., pp. 321-322). Elk Grove Village, IL: Author.

American Academy of Pediatrics. (2000). Molluscum contagiosum. In L.K. Pickering (Ed.), *2000 red book: Report of the Committee on Infectious Diseases* (25th ed., pp. 403-404). Elk Grove Village, IL: Author.

American Academy of Pediatrics. (2000). Pediculosis capitis (head lice). In L.K. Pickering (Ed.), *2000 red book: Report of the Committee on Infectious Diseases* (25th ed., pp. 427-429). Elk Grove Village, IL: Author.

American Academy of Pediatrics. (2000). Pediculosis corporis. In L.K. Pickering (Ed.), *2000 red book: Report of the Committee on Infectious Diseases* (25th ed., pp. 429-430). Elk Grove Village, IL: Author.

American Academy of Pediatrics. (2000). Pediculosis pubis. In L.K. Pickering (Ed.), *2000 red book: Report of the Committee on Infectious Diseases* (25th ed., pp. 430-431). Elk Grove Village, IL: Author.

American Academy of Pediatrics. (2000). Scabies. In L.K. Pickering (Ed.), *2000 red book: Report of the Committee on Infectious Diseases* (25th ed., pp. 506-508). Elk Grove Village, IL: Author.

American Academy of Pediatrics. (2000). Tinea capitis (ringworm of the scalp). In L.K. Pickering (Ed.), *2000 red book: Report of the Committee on Infectious Diseases* (25th ed., pp. 569-570). Elk Grove Village, IL: Author.

American Academy of Pediatrics. (2000). Tinea corporis (ringworm of the body). In L.K. Pickering (Ed.), *2000 red book: Report of the Committee on Infectious Diseases* (25th ed., pp. 570-572). Elk Grove Village, IL: Author.

American Academy of Pediatrics. (2000). Tinea cruris (jock itch). In L.K. Pickering (Ed.), *2000 red book: Report of the Committee on Infectious Diseases* (25th ed., pp. 572-573). Elk Grove Village, IL: Author.

American Academy of Pediatrics. (2000). Tinea pedis (athlete's foot). In L.K. Pickering (Ed.), *2000 red book: Report of the Committee on Infectious Diseases* (25th ed., pp. 573-574). Elk Grove Village, IL: Author.

American Academy of Pediatrics. (2000). Tinea versicolor. In L.K. Pickering (Ed.), *2000 red book: Report of the Committee on Infectious Diseases* (25th ed., pp. 574-576). Elk Grove Village, IL: Author.

American Academy of Pediatrics. (2000). Varicella-zoster infections. In L.K. Pickering (Ed.), *2000 red book: Report of the Committee on Infectious Diseases* (25th ed., pp. 624-637). Elk Grove Village, IL: Author.

Centers for Disease Control and Prevention. (2002). Sexually transmitted diseases treatment guidelines 2002. *MMWR, 51* (RR-6), 1-84.

Dahl, M.V. (2002). Contact dermatitis. In R.E. Rakel, & E. T. Bope (Eds.), *Conn's current therapy* (pp. 852-853). Philadelphia: Saunders.

Dzubow, L., & Levit, E.K. (2002). Cancer of the skin. In R.E. Rakel, & E. T. Bope (Eds.), *Conn's current therapy* (pp. 777-780). Philadelphia: Saunders.

Eichenfield, L.F., Lucky, A.W., Boguniewicz, M., Langley, R.G., Cherill, R., Marchall, K., Bush, C., et al. (2002). Safety and efficacy of pimecrolimus (ASM 981) cream 1% in the treatment of mild and moderate atopic dermatitis in children and adolescents. *Journal of the American Academy of Dermatology, 46,* 495-504.

Gnann, J.W., & Whitley, R.J. (2002). Herpes zoster. *New England Journal of Medicine, 347,* 340-346.

Habif, T.P., Campbell, J.L., Quitadamo, M.J., Zug, K.A. (2001). *Skin disease: Diagnosis and treatment.* St. Louis: Mosby.

Hainer, B.L. (2003). Dermatophyte infections. *American Family Physician, 67,* 101-108.

Hwogn, H., & Levy, M.L. (2002). Atopic dermatitis. In R.E. Rakel, & E. T. Bope (Eds.), *Conn's current therapy* (pp. 843-845). Philadelphia: Saunders.

Jackson, A.D. (2002). Warts and their management. In R.E. Rakel, & E. T. Bope (Eds.), *Conn's current therapy* (pp. 801-804). Philadelphia: Saunders.

Landau, J.W. (2002). Warts and molluscum contagiosum. In. F.D. Burg, J.R. Ingelfinger, R.A. Polin, & A.A. Gershon (Eds.), *Gellis and Kagan's current pediatric therapy* (pp. 873-876). Philadelphia: Saunders.

Lebwohl, M., & Ali, S. (2001). Treatment of psoriasis. Part 1. Topical therapy and phototherapy. *Journal of the American Academy of Dermatology, 45,* 487-498.

Leyden, J.J. (1997). Therapy for acne vulgaris. *New England Journal of Medicine, 336,* 1156-1162.

Liao, D.C. (2003). Management of acne. *Journal of Family Practice, 52,* 43-51.

Luba, M.C., Bangs, S.A., Mohler, A.W., & Stulberg, D.L. (2003). Common benign skin tumors. *American Family Physician, 67,* 729-738.

Pardasani, A.G., Feldman, S.R., & Clark, A.R. (2000). Treatment of psoriasis: An algorithm-based approach for primary care physicians. *American Family Physician, 61,* 725-736.

Podczaski, E., & Cain, J. (2002). Cutaneous malignant melanoma. *Clinical Obstetrics and Gynecology, 45,* 830-843.

Roberts, F.J. (2002). Head lice. *New England Journal of Medicine, 346,* 1645-1650.

Rockwell, P.G. (2001). Acute and chronic paronychia. *American Family Physician, 63,* 1113-1116.

Rogers, P., & Bassler, M. (2001). Treating onychomycosis. *American Family Physician, 63,* 663-672.

Russell, J.J. (2002). Topical tacrolimus: A new therapy for atopic dermatitis. *American Family Physician, 66,* 1899-1902.

Schwetz, B.A. (2001). New treatment for eczema. *Journal of the American Medical Association, 285,* 1874-1876.

Shenefelt, P.D. (2002). Parasitic diseases of the skin. In R.E. Rakel, & E. T. Bope (Eds.), *Conn's current therapy* (pp. 824-827). Philadelphia: Saunders.

Webster, G. (2002). Acne vulgaris and rosacea. In R.E. Rakel, & E. T. Bope (Eds.), *Conn's current therapy* (pp. 771-773). Philadelphia: Saunders.

Weinberg, J.M. (2002). Fungal diseases of the skin. In R.E. Rakel, & E. T. Bope (Eds.), *Conn's current therapy* (pp. 827-829). Philadelphia: Saunders.

Wilkerson, M.D. (2002). Bacterial diseases of the skin. In R.E. Rakel, & E. T. Bope (Eds.), *Conn's current therapy* (pp. 815-817). Philadelphia: Saunders.

Wilkin, J., Dahl, M., Detmari, M., Drake, L., Feinstein, Al, Odom, R., et al. (2002). Standard classification of rosacea: Report of the National Rosacea Society Expert Committee on the Classification and Staging of Rosacea. *Journal of the American Academy of Dermatology, 46,* 584-587.

Zic, J.A. (2002). Papulosquamous diseases. In R.E. Rakel, & E. T. Bope (Eds.), *Conn's current therapy* (pp. 784-788). Philadelphia: Saunders.

Problems of the Eyes

Mary Virginia Graham

AGE-RELATED MACULAR DEGENERATION

I.   Definition: Age-dependent alterations of the sensory retina, retinal pigment epithelium, and choriocapillaris complex in the central retina (macula)

II. Pathogenesis: Causes of age-related macular degeneration (ARMD) are unknown

III. Clinical Presentation

    A.   ARMD is the leading cause of significant, irreversible, central visual loss in patients over 50 years of age in the US

    B.   Incidence of the disease is age-dependent, with an increase in prevalence among persons who are 55 years of age and older, approximately 2% of persons in their 50s develop the disease and 20% of those 75 years of age and older

    C.   Risk factors in addition to increasing age include the following: Caucasian race, smoking, ultraviolet light exposure, hypertension, and family history of the disease
        1.   Persons with light skin color and blue eyes seem to be somewhat more at risk, and the condition occurs in women slightly more than in men
        2.   Ongoing research is examining the relationship between low consumption of vegetables and fruits (high in antioxidants) and ARMD

    D.   The condition has a dry and a wet form

> **Dry ARMD**
> - This is by far the most common form, accounting for about 90% of cases but is responsible for only about 10-20% of severe vision loss
> - Characterized by drusen, pigmentary changes, and atrophy
> - Drusen are the hallmark of dry ARMD and represent the most common and earliest finding in dry ARMD
> - Represent metabolic byproducts of retinal pigment epithelial cell metabolism
> - Clinically, drusen appear as yellow deposits deep to the retina
> - Unless the center of the macula is involved with geographic atrophy, visual loss is usually mild in dry ARMD
>
> **Wet ARMD**
> - Much less common than dry ARMD, but accounts for the vast majority of severe vision loss
> - Characterized by exudative changes including hemorrhage (bright red subretinal blood, and dark gray subretinal pigment epithelial blood) and hard exudates
> - Vascular changes and/or fluid under the sensory retina and retinal pigment epithelium (RPE) cause the detachment of the retina and RPE from the underlying structures
> - Eyes with wet ARMD lose central vision fairly rapidly, compared with eyes affected by dry ARMD

    E.   Symptoms of ARMD include visual blurring (may describe vision as dim, fuzzy, or less sharp than usual vision), central scotomas (isolated areas in visual field in which vision is absent or depressed and does not go away over time), and metamorphopsia (visual distortion in which images may appear smaller [micropsia] or larger [macropsia] than they really are)
        1.   Patients may state that reading requires more light than in the past
        2.   Often, the first symptom of wet ARMD is that straight lines (e.g., the edge of the newspaper, ceramic tiles on floor or wall, telephone poles, or other straight-edge surfaces) appear wavy

IV.   Diagnosis/Evaluation

   A.   History
      1.   Determine onset, duration, and course of symptoms
      2.   Ask specifically about any visual blurring, loss of central vision, and distorted vision (ask if straight lines seem wavy)
      3.   Ask is more light is needed for reading
      4.   Ask about previous eye problems and treatments
      5.   Obtain past medical and medication history

   B.   Physical Examination
      1.   Use the Amsler grid to test patient's central vision (see Amsler grid on next page, and instructions for testing). **Teach patient how to use the grid in order to self-test at home for vision problems**
      2.   Perform ophthalmoscopy examination of the eyes; satisfactory exam can usually be through an undilated pupil provided that the media (aqueous, lens, vitreous) are clear
      3.   Fundus lesions should be measured using the disk diameter as a reference size
      4.   Drusen occur as scattered small yellow lesions in the peripheral fundus
      5.   Observe for hemorrhages and exudates around the retinal arteries and veins

   C.   Differential Diagnosis: Other degenerative diseases of the macula including central serous choroidopathy, pigment epithelial detachments, and cystoid macular edema

   D.   Diagnostic Tests: Fluorescein angiography, a photographic test used in the diagnosis of ARMD, will be performed by the ophthalmologist in patients who demonstrate signs and symptoms of the disease in order to identify and localize abnormal vascular processes

V.   Plan/Management

   A.   Immediate referral to an ophthalmologist for evaluation and management is indicated when patients demonstrate signs and symptoms of ARMD

   B.   Follow up: By ophthalmologist to whom the patient is referred

Figure 8.1. The Amsler Grid
The Amsler Grid was developed by Marc Amsler to help in the early detection of macular degeneration, the leading cause of vision impairment for people over 65. The grid was developed to allow patients to test their own central vision for early signs of macular degeneration, so it may be treated sooner

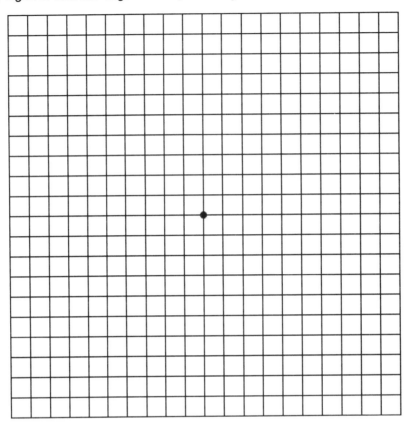

Procedure for Using the Amsler Grid

Patients who normally wear reading glasses or corrected lenses for near vision should wear them for the test

1. Ask the patient to hold the grid about 12 inches away from eyes at normal reading distance
2. Instruct patient to keep both eyes open and focus on the dot at the center of the grid
3. Then, occlude the patient's left eye and ask the following questions:
   - ✓ Can you see all four corners of the grid?
   - ✓ Are any of the lines blurry, wavy, distorted, bent, gray, or missing?
   - ✓ Are there any large holes or pieces of the grid missing?
4. Finally, cover the patient's right eye and repeat the process

Provide the patient with a copy of the grid and instruct him/her to test self once or twice a week, keeping the grid at the same distance from eyes each time. The grid can be placed on the side of the refrigerator or some other convenient location to remind the patient to use regularly each week

The grid may be accessed at http://www.mnssb.org/allages/vision-loss/amsler_grid.html

BLEPHARITIS

I.   Definition: Inflammation of the eyelid margins

II.   Pathogenesis:

      A.   Often due to colonization of eyelash follicles and the meibomian glands with staphylococci

      B.   Allergic disorders and dermatologic diseases (usually seborrheic dermatitis or rosacea) are also common causes

III. Clinical Presentation

      A.   A common, chronic problem that often begins in childhood and continues throughout adulthood

      B.   Characterized by hypertrophy and desquamation of the epidermis near the lid margin that results in erythema and scaling of the lid border

      C.   Main complaint is redness of the eyelid margin but sensation of foreign body, burning, and eye discomfort may be additional symptoms

      D.   Severe and chronic cases may produce purulent discharge and over time permanent changes in the eyelid structure can occur (misdirection and lost eyelashes and distortion of lid contour)

      E.   Patient usually has a history of recurrent chalazia and hordeola

IV.   Diagnosis/Evaluation

      A.   History
            1.   Determine onset and duration of symptoms
            2.   Ask about presence of flaking, crusting at lid margins, frequency of eye rubbing
            3.   Inquire about eye pain, visual disturbances, dry eyes and tearing
            4.   Obtain ocular history including prior eye disease, injuries, surgery, or other treatments and medications
            5.   Inquire about previous and present skin problems, particularly of the face and scalp
            6.   Ask about chronic exposure to irritants such as smoke, cosmetics, and chemicals

      B.   Physical Examination
            1.   Determine visual acuity
            2.   Perform a complete eye examination, paying particular attention to the following components:
                  a.   Inspect eyelid margins (with magnifying glass if necessary) for crusting, scaling, erythema, and erosions
                  b.   Examine sclera and conjunctiva for abnormalities
                  c.   Palpate lid margins and lid for masses
            3.   Palpate for preauricular adenopathy
            4.   Examine skin of face and scalp for characteristic findings of seborrheic dermatitis and rosacea (see sections on SEBORRHEIC DERMATITIS and ROSACEA)

      C.   Differential Diagnosis: Chalazion, hordeolum, conjunctivitis, and keratitis

      D.   Diagnostic Tests: None are usually indicated

V.   Plan/Management:

      A.   If an underlying source of the lid irritation can be identified, it is important to treat the source as the first step in management
            1.   If seborrheic dermatitis of the scalp and face is present, institute appropriate treatment (see section on SEBORRHEIC DERMATITIS for treatment recommendations)

2. If rosacea is present, institute treatment (see section on ROSACEA for treatment recommendations)
3. If dry eyes are present, advise patient to use ocular lubricants such as Cellufresh or Bion Tears

B. Treatment for blepharitis is outlined below
   1. Instruct patient in lid hygiene as follows
      a. Apply warm, wet facecloth compresses for two minutes, 2-4 times a day to the lids to increase circulation, mobilize meibomian secretions, and help cleanse crusting debris on lid margins
      b. After a compress application, gently scrub eyelids once a day with fingertips (or cotton-tipped applicator) using baby shampoo diluted 1:1 with clean water (or commercial cleansing pads such as Eye Scrub or Lid Wipes SPF) in order to remove crusts and scale
      c. Blepharitis associated with seborrhea is often improved by use of a dandruff shampoo on scalp and eyebrows
   2. For flares, topical antibiotic therapy may also be helpful: Adults and children: Prescribe erythromycin 0.5% (Ilotycin or generic) ophthalmic ointment BID x 7 days OR sulfacetamide sodium 10% (Bleph-10) available as ophthalmic solution or ointment (solution: 1-2 drops Q3H during day; ointment: QID and at HS) x 7 days

C. Because most cases of blepharitis are chronic and require long-term therapy, they are best managed by an ophthalmologist

D. Follow Up
   1. None needed for mild cases
   2. Refer recurrent cases to ophthalmologist for management

CATARACT

I. Definition: A decrease in the transparency of the crystalline lens to the degree that vision is disturbed

II. Pathogenesis

A. Protein coagulations form opaque areas in the crystalline lens of the eye for unknown reasons; when transparency of the crystalline lens decreases enough to disturb vision, a clinically significant cataract exists

B. Occurs most often as a natural process of aging

III. Clinical Presentation

A. Age-related cataracts are the most common cause of decreased visual acuity in adults; 95% of persons >65 years of age have some degree of lens opacity

B. Approximately 1 million cataract extractions are done each year in the US; worldwide, cataracts account for more than 15 million cases of treatable blindness

C. **Decreased Vision.** A gradual, painless, progressive loss of vision occurs over time, and many patients are unaware of vision problems until the image blur interferes with indoor activities such as reading

D. **Glare.** One of the symptomatic manifestations of light scattering and is experienced when person looks at a point source of light and sees a diffusion of bright white and colored light which reduces visual acuity; glare interferes with night driving and is an early sign of cataract

E. **Distortion.** Makes straight edges appear wavy or curved; patient may complain of double vision (double vision caused by cataract is usually monocular versus binocular)

F. **Altered Color Perception.** Yellowing of lens nucleus alters color perception so that colors are seen differently (loss of contrast sensitivity)

G. Unilateral cataract occurs in only one eye (monocular) or may mature more rapidly in one eye than in the other

H. Factors that influence the risk of adult-onset cataract include excessive ultraviolet B radiation exposure, diabetes mellitus, corticosteroid therapy (including inhaled), tobacco and alcohol use, and (possibly) low antioxidant vitamin use

IV. Diagnosis/Evaluation

A. History
1. Inquire regarding present status of visual function (patient's self-assessment of visual status); determine if there have been any changes in vision, onset of such changes, and if one or both eyes are involved
2. Ask about increased problems with glare and if changes in ways colors are seen have occurred in recent months
3. Inquire about presence of risk factors (see III.H. above)
4. Obtain medication and past medical history including **ocular** history (prior eye disease, eye injuries, surgery, treatments, and medications)

B. Physical Examination
1. Measure visual acuity at both near and far distances with and without current spectacle correction (**Note**: Most common objective finding associated with cataracts is decreased visual acuity)
2. Check pupillary reaction to light (**Note**: Pupillary reaction is unaffected by cataract)
3. Observe for leukokoria (white pupil) seen in mature cataracts
4. Assess visual fields by confrontation (**Note**: This is a very gross measurement, but visual fields should be full or only mildly limited)
5. Examine the red reflex with the ophthalmoscope set on +4 (black) diopters at about 20 cm from patient (**Note**: Examination will reveal a black lens opacity against the red-orange pupillary light reflex)

C. Differential Diagnosis
1. Age-related macular degeneration
2. Diabetic retinopathy

D. Diagnostic Tests: Additional testing should be done by the ophthalmologist to whom the patient is referred (**Note**: Cataracts are best evaluated by slitlamp biomicroscopy; in addition, A-scan and B-scan ultrasonography are used for measuring the thickness and location of a cataract)

V. Plan/Management

A. Ophthalmology referral for evaluation
1. Decision to obtain cataract surgery is based on degree of functional impairment
2. Patient should weigh the risks and benefits associated with surgery
3. Most common technique is phacoemulsification (ultrasound fragmentation of lens with aspiration; artificial lens implants are then put in place)

B. Nonsurgical management by the ophthalmologist includes changing lens prescription, use of strong bifocals or magnification, and appropriate illumination

C. Patient should be informed that cataract does not need to be removed unless there is impairment of normal activities

D. Progression of cataract formation may be slowed by decreasing amount of sun exposure (wearing of hat and dark glasses when outdoors), smoking cessation, and increasing antioxidant vitamin ingestion (diets high in the antioxidant vitamin A may be helpful)
1. Wearing a hat with a brim reduces ocular exposure to UVB by 50%
2. Using a UV coating or UV screener incorporated into spectacle lenses virtually eliminates UVB ocular exposure

E. Follow Up: By ophthalmologist

CHALAZION

I. Definition: Focal chronic inflammation of a meibomian gland

II. Pathogenesis

   A. Chronic granuloma from obstructed meibomian gland

   B. May occur as a result of a chronic hordeolum (a focal acute infection of meibomian gland)

   C. Secondary infection of the surrounding tissues may develop

III. Clinical Presentation

   A. Usually hard, non-tender nodule is found on midportion of the tarsus, away from the lid border; may develop on lid margin if the opening of the duct is involved and can present with lid tenderness, pain, and swelling

   B. Chalazia that become infected result in painful swelling of the entire lid

   C. Small chalazia may resolve spontaneously without treatment

   D. History of chronic hordeolum and prior excision of chalazia are often present

IV. Diagnosis/Evaluation

   A. History
      1. Determine onset and duration of symptoms
      2. Inquire about pain or tenderness of the lid
      3. Inquire about any changes in visual acuity level
      4. Ask about past episodes and previous treatments

   B. Physical Examination
      1. Assess visual acuity
      2. Perform a complete eye examination, paying particular attention to the following components
         a. Inspect eyelids for inflammation and masses
         b. Palpate eyelids for masses and tenderness
         c. Evert the eyelid and examine inner surface for pointing
         d. Inspect sclera and conjunctiva for abnormalities
      3. Palpate for preauricular adenopathy

   C. Differential Diagnosis
      1. May be associated with a hordeolum and blepharitis
      2. Sebaceous cell carcinoma is a rare condition that should be considered

   D. Diagnostic Tests: None indicated

V. Plan/Management

   A. Small, asymptomatic, chronic chalazia do not require treatment and usually disappear spontaneously within a few months

   B. If chalazia are large or if there is secondary infection, treatment is needed
      1. Apply warm, moist compresses for several minutes throughout the day
      2. Prescribe erythromycin ointment 0.5% (Ilotycin or generic), small amount to affected eye, BID-QID x 7 days OR polymyxin B-trimethoprim drops (Polytrim), 1-2 drops to affected eye, BID-QID x 7 days

C. If the chalazion does not respond to conservative therapy, patient should be referred to an expert for injection of the lesion or incision and curettage

D. Follow Up
1. Small chalazia do not require follow up
2. Follow up for chalazia that do not respond to conservative therapy should be with ophthalmologist

CONJUNCTIVITIS

I. Definition: Inflammation of the conjunctiva characterized by vascular dilation, cellular infiltration, and exudation

II. Pathogenesis

A. **Viral conjunctivitis**
1. Usually caused by adenovirus
2. May develop during or after an upper respiratory tract infection

B. **Bacterial conjunctivitis**
1. Caused by a wide range of gram-positive and gram-negative organisms, but gram-positive organisms predominate
2. *Staphylococcus aureus* is probably the most common cause of bacterial conjunctivitis, particularly in adults
3. *Streptococcus pneumoniae* (more commonly a causative organism in children rather than adults)
4. *Haemophilus influenzae* (more commonly a causative organism in children rather than adults)

C. **Hyperacute bacterial conjunctivitis**
1. Most commonly caused by *Neisseria gonorrhoeae* and less often by *Neisseria meningitidis*
2. Occurs via autoinoculation from infected genitalia

D. **Chlamydial conjunctivitis**: Ocular chlamydial infections are of two types
1. Trachoma is associated with serotypes A through C and causes a chronic keratoconjunctivitis which frequently results in blindness; this condition is rare in the US but occurs in rural areas of developing countries, particularly Africa, Asia, and the Middle East
2. Inclusion conjunctivitis is associated with serotypes D through K and is a common, primarily sexually transmitted disease

E. **Allergic conjunctivitis**
1. Seasonal allergic conjunctivitis (SAC), a type I, IgE-mediated hypersensitivity to certain allergens (e.g., grass and tree pollens in the spring and ragweed pollen in the fall) is most common form of ocular allergy
2. Perennial allergic conjunctivitis (PAC), is similar to SAC but symptoms are less severe; tends to occur year round because of the nonseasonal nature of the antigens, e.g., animal dander, house mite feces, mold, and dust
3. Conjunctivitis medicamentosa is an allergic response that occurs as a reaction to use of ocular medications

III. Clinical Presentation

A. **Viral conjunctivitis** (presumably adenoviral)
1. Leading cause of conjunctivitis; highly contagious
2. Usual modes of transmission are contaminated fingers and swimming pool water
3. Characterized by conjunctival hyperemia, edema, and a watery discharge; onset is usually acute
4. Vision is unaffected; watery discharge can cause some transient blurring; photophobia is uncommon
5. Usually self-limited but treatment with a topical antibiotic shortens its course

B. **Bacterial conjunctivitis**
   1. Characterized by acute onset of ocular irritation and tearing
   2. Develops in one eye initially, and then spreads to the other eye within 48 hours
   3. Within one or two days, a mucopurulent or purulent discharge develops
   4. Eyelids are often edematous with a collection of debris at base of lashes and matting of the eyelashes upon awakening
   5. Diffuse hyperemia of the bulbar and tarsal conjunctiva is usually prominent
   6. Lymphadenopathy is generally minimal

C. **Hyperacute bacterial conjunctivitis**
   1. A severe, rapidly progressing sight-threatening ocular infection most often affecting sexually active young adults; organism is transmitted from genitalia to hands, and then to eyes
   2. Characterized by an abrupt onset of copious yellow-green purulent discharge that is bilateral, with lid edema, erythema, and chemosis
   3. Preauricular adenopathy often present
   4. Because of rapid onset, progression, and severity of signs and symptoms, patient often seeks care before infection has spread to both eyes

D. **Chlamydial conjunctivitis**
   1. Usually presents in young sexually active urban dwellers between the ages of 18 and 30, and is often initially unilateral
   2. Transmission occurs most often via autoinoculation from infected genital secretions
   3. Typically, an indolent infection that is characterized by a thin, mucoid discharge
   4. Patient may have photophobia and enlarged, tender preauricular nodes
   5. Subacute or chronic in nature, with patients presenting with symptoms that have been present for as long as 6 months

E. **Allergic conjunctivitis**
   1. Itching is the hallmark of this condition; often accompanied by tearing and nasal congestion, and mucoid discharge
   2. SAC symptoms are itchy, watery eyes, often with rhinitis or allergic pharyngitis; eye signs are mild lid edema, fine papillary hypertrophy, and bulbar conjunctival hyperemia; corneal involvement is rare
   3. PAC symptoms are itching, burning, and tearing in normal-appearing eyes (symptoms are less severe in PAC than in SAC)
   4. Conjunctivitis medicamentosa is characterized by bilateral dilatation of the conjunctival blood vessels, with eyelid edema, erythema, and scaling in a patient using a topical ophthalmic medication

IV. Diagnosis/Evaluation

A. History
   1. Inquire regarding onset and duration of symptoms (is the condition acute, subacute, chronic, or recurrent?)
   2. Determine if condition is unilateral or bilateral; ask about the type and amount of discharge
   3. Determine if ocular pain, photophobia, or blurred vision (that fails to clear with a blink) are present
   4. Ask if itching and other symptoms of allergy are present
   5. Ask about contact with a person with "pink-eye"
   6. Inquire about personal and family history of hay fever, allergic rhinitis
   7. Obtain past medical and medication history, specifically asking about use of any ocular medications (including OTCs); ask about allergies

B. Physical Examination
   1. Determine visual acuity, visual fields, pupillary function, and extraocular movements
   2. Examine eyelids for inflammation or tenderness
   3. Examine sclera and conjunctiva for hyperemia and edema; check cornea for clarity
   4. Determine type of discharge
   5. Palpate for regional lymphadenopathy

C.   Differential Diagnosis: Patients typically present with the main complaint of red eye; there is need to distinguish conjunctivitis from other conditions causing red eye
1.   In conjunctivitis, redness of the conjunctiva is diffuse, pain is minimal (except in hyperacute bacterial conjunctivitis), and vision, pupil size, and reactivity are normal
2.   Acute angle-closure glaucoma presents with redness of the eye, moderate-to-severe pain, headache, and blurred vision; the redness is most pronounced in the area adjacent to the limbus (circumcorneal injection); frequently presents in evening when reduced ambient light provokes dilatation of the pupil, initiating a cascade of events that eventuate in blockage of the narrow angle, thereby preventing the outflow of aqueous humor
3.   Acute anterior uveitis, inflammation of the iris and ciliary body, usually occurs in young or middle aged adults; the pupil is constricted, irregular, and poorly reactive to light
4.   Lacrimal duct obstruction presents with pain, redness, and edema around lacrimal sac; pressure over lacrimal sac will express mucopurulent material from the upper and lower canaliculi
5.   Blepharitis may have similar presentation as conjunctivitis with burning and itching of the conjunctiva, but with blepharitis there also is inflammation of lid margins and it is almost always a chronic, recurring condition
6.   Corneal abrasions usually have a history of trauma with mild to moderate bulbar injection and a foreign-body sensation

D.   Diagnostic Tests

In Most Cases
Culture of discharge is usually not recommended for mild conjunctivitis with a suspected viral, bacterial, or allergic origin

Exceptions
If there is severe inflammation as occurs with hyperacute conjunctivitis, or if the condition is unresponsive to initial treatment, culture and sensitivity are indicated

Nonculture tests for chlamydia can be used in adolescents/adults to diagnose ocular infections

---

V.   Plan/Management

A.   **Viral conjunctivitis**
1.   Usually self-limited, but some evidence indicates that treatment with a topical antibiotic shortens its course
2.   One rationale for treatment is that it prevents bacterial superinfection
3.   Prescribe broad-spectrum topical eyedrops: Polymyxin B-trimethoprim combination (Polytrim), one or two drops QID x 7 days
4.   Topical antiviral drugs are not administered
5.   See Patient Education under V.G., below for recommendations regarding patient counseling

B.   **Bacterial conjunctivitis**: If treatment is based on clinical evaluation alone (which occurs in the majority of cases), select a broad spectrum topical antibiotic such as ONE of the following, administered 4 times daily for 7-10 days
1.   Gentamicin solution (0.3%) [Garamycin, Genoptic, generic]
2.   Tobramycin solution (0.3%) [Tobrex, generic]
3.   The topical fluoroquinolones, ciprofloxacin and ofloxacin, are also highly effective but should be reserved for <u>severe</u> infections
4.   **Note:** Empiric treatment is highly effective and adverse consequences are infrequent

C.   **Hyperacute bacterial conjunctivitis**: Immediate referral to an ophthalmologist is required for aggressive management to prevent serious complications; systemic antibiotics (as well as topical antibiotics) are required (systemic antibiotics given for the conjunctivitis will be effective against the genital reservoir of the disease)

D.   **Chlamydial conjunctivitis**: Prescribe systemic antibiotics—doxycycline (Vibramycin) 100 mg BID for 14 days
1.   Once a diagnosis has been established, a genital work-up of the patient and sexual partner is indicated
2.   Pregnant and lactating women: Use erythromycin 250 mg QID x 21 days
3.   Diagnosis of chlamydial disease should prompt investigation for other sexually transmitted diseases, including syphilis, gonorrhea, hepatitis B, and HIV infection

E. **Allergic conjunctivitis**
  1. A simple and inexpensive treatment is to remove the offending allergen when possible or diluting it by instilling artificial tears every two or three hours during the acute phase
  2. Prescribe topical and systemic antihistamines to relieve itching
      a. **Topical agent:** Levocabastine hydrochloride (0.05%) [Livostin] drops; One drop in both eyes QID OR olopatadine hydrochloride (0.1%) [Patanol] solution—combination antihistamine and mast cell stabilizer; one drop in affected eye(s) BID
      b. **Systemic agent:** Fexofenadine (Allegra) tabs, 60 mg BID
  3. Consider prescribing a topical mast-cell stabilizer for chronic conditions such as perennial allergic conjunctivitis. Prescribe cromolyn sodium (Crolom) ophthalmic solution: 1-2 drops 4 times a day

F. Refer the patient for emergent management by an expert if any of the following occur
  1. There is no improvement in 24 hours
  2. Patient has moderate to severe ocular pain, decreased visual acuity, abnormal eye exam
  3. Infection from herpes simplex virus
  4. Hyperacute bacterial conjunctivitis

G. Patient Education
  1. Instruct patient to instill medication in the inner aspect of the lower eyelid
  2. Teach patient that infection is easily spread to unaffected eye and to other household members
  3. The role of frequent handwashing in limiting the spread of ocular infections cannot be overemphasized
  4. Discuss with patient that eye secretions are contagious for 24 to 48 hours after therapy begins
  5. Patient with viral infection should be instructed that the ocular infection is contagious for at least 7 days after the onset

H. Follow Up
  1. If no improvement in 24 hours, or if condition worsens, patient should return for referral for expert care
  2. No follow up is indicated for mild cases that resolve without problems

DRY EYES

I. Definition: Dry eyes, or keratoconjunctivitis sicca (KCS) is a condition in which the precorneal tear film is deficient and cannot fulfill its normal function of lubricating the anterior surface of the cornea, causing chronic, low-grade irritation of the eyes

II. Pathogenesis

  A. Precorneal tear film is a fluid layer measuring approximately 6 to 10 microns in thickness that is adherent to the corneal epithelium

  B. Consists of three components
     1. Outer layer is composed of a thin lipid layer produced by the meibomian glands, the openings of which are along the margins of the upper and lower lids
     2. Middle layer is the predominant component and is composed of aqueous tears derived from the lacrimal glands
     3. Innermost layer is a mucin layer attached to outer epithelial cell surface and is responsible for keeping the aqueous layer attached to the corneal surface; the mucin is derived mainly from conjunctival goblet cells, but can be produced by corneal and conjunctival epithelial cells

  C. With aging, reflex tearing is reduced producing lacrimal aqueous and meibomian lipid layer insufficiency—and dry eyes are the result

  D. While many patients with dry eyes have no systemic disease or other ocular disease to account for the lacrimal insufficiency, conditions that can interfere with the normal functioning of the precorneal tear film are lupus erythematosus, ocular pemphigoid, Sjögren syndrome, erythema multiforme, scleroderma, diabetes mellitus, HIV, hepatitis B and C, rosacea, and seventh nerve palsy

E. Drug-induced tear hyposecretion can also commonly occur with a variety of drugs including phenothiazines, antihistamines, antihypertensives, antidepressants, antiulcer agents, anticholinergics, nasal decongestants, and anti-muscle spasmodics

III. Clinical Presentation

A. Condition may be seen in all age groups, but is much more common after 60 years of age; women are more likely than men to develop dry eyes later in life, probably because of varying estrogen levels in postmenopausal women—the group in whom the condition is most likely to occur

B. In younger patients who develop dry eyes, there may be an underlying collagen vascular disorder present and dry eyes may be the earliest manifestation of the disorder

C. Patients with dry eyes usually complain of irritation, foreign body sensation, a sensation of sand in the eye, and light sensitivity; symptoms are usually absent in the morning on awakening (especially in mild cases) and become more bothersome in the afternoon or evening

D. Patients who are regularly exposed to environmental irritants such as air pollution, dust, and dry air are more symptomatic than those without such exposures

E. Patients may also have associated symptoms of eyelid inflammation and blepharitis

IV. Diagnosis/Evaluation

A. History
   1. Inquire regarding onset and duration of symptoms
   2. Ask about treatments tried and results
   3. Ask about the presence of any associated symptoms—eye pain, visual disturbances, tearing, itching
   4. Ask about the presence of risk factors (see II. D. above) and acute/chronic exposures to irritants such as smoke, cosmetics, and chemicals
   5. Obtain past medical and medication history (see II.E. above for medications commonly associated with dry eye syndrome), including ocular history (prior eye disease, eye injuries, surgery, treatments, and ocular medications)

B. Physical Examination
   1. Measure visual acuity (distant and near, with and without corrective lenses)
   2. Inspect the eyelids and lashes for the presence of inflammation, scaling, and the lashes for orientation
   3. Inspect the sclera and conjunctiva for abnormalities
   4. Perform an ophthalmoscopic examination

C. Differential Diagnosis
   1. Blepharitis
   2. Seasonal/perennial allergic conjunctivitis (SAC/PAC)
   3. Rosacea

D. Diagnostic Tests
   1. Patient can be referred to ophthalmologist for evaluation of tear film adequacy; there are several tests available to measure tear quantity (e.g., Schirmer test), tear quality (e.g., qualitative mucous assay), and tear film stability (e.g., test of tear film breakup time [TFBUT])
   2. Based on history and physical examination, other testing may be indicated if an underlying condition is suspected

V. Plan/Management

A. Patients found to have an underlying medical condition as the cause of dry eyes should be treated appropriately or referred for further evaluation

B. Patients who are taking medications that are believed to cause dry eyes should be evaluated in terms of possibly discontinuing the medication (usually not possible) or to changing to another medication that may not have tear hyposecretion as a side effect

C.	For many patients with chronic, low-grade keratoconjunctivitis sicca, the condition is idiopathic—that is, there is no systemic disease or other ocular disease to account for the lacrimal insufficiency; the following sequence of therapy is indicated to provide symptomatic relief for patients with dry eyes whether or not an underlying cause can be established

---

Lid hygiene to stabilize the tear film
Advise patient to apply warm, wet facecloth compresses to eyelids for two minutes, 2-4 times/day
Once daily (after the final compress application for the day), instruct patient to apply baby shampoo lather with the fingertips and clean and rinse the lash line

Tear replacement therapy
Frequency of use of artificial tears depends on patient's level of discomfort
  ✓ *With minimal involvement*, advise patient to use product 4-8 times a day (usually sufficient to relieve symptoms in mild cases); use may increase or decrease based on symptoms
  ✓ *For moderate symptoms*, artificial tears must be used every 2 hours, or even every hour for comfort; when air is very dry, or when air pollutants are present, use of artificial tears must but increased

---

PRODUCTS TO RECOMMEND

Recommend products that are preservative-free

Patients who are sensitive to preservatives or who must use artificial tears frequently are likely to benefit by using products without preservatives

The disadvantage of nonpreserved tears is that they are unit dose-packaged and must be discarded at the end of the day, making them more expensive than larger quantities of artificial tears that contain preservatives, but their ease of use and comfort may compensate for the cost

Preservative-free drops include the following (all OTC)
  ✓ Bion Tears
  ✓ Duratears Naturale
  ✓ Tears Naturale Free

Preservative-free ointments (a good choice for bedtime use) are the following (also OTC)
  ✓ Lacri-Lube NP
  ✓ Refresh PM

D.	Follow Up
	1.	Not necessary unless symptoms persist with lid hygiene measures and consistent use of artificial tears
	2.	Patients who do not respond to conservative therapy should be referred to an ophthalmologist for further evaluation and management

GLAUCOMA

I.	Definition: A group of ocular disorders characterized by elevation of intraocular pressure (IOP) accompanied by characteristic optic nerve damage and/or visual field loss via capillary microinfarction causing optic nerve ischemia

II.	Pathogenesis

A.	Glaucoma can be generally classified into two categories: Open-angle, and angle-closure glaucoma (**Note**: The two primary types of glaucoma—open-angle and angle-closure glaucoma—are classified according to the anatomy of the anterior chamber angle)

B.	Primary Open-Angle Glaucoma (POAG)
	1.	An abnormality in the trabecular angle tissue causing resistance to fluid flow
	2.	Condition is not secondary to another condition

C.   Primary Angle-Closure Glaucoma
    1.   Relative pupillary block is the mechanism of angle closure
    2.   Resistance to fluid flow of aqueous humor between posterior iris surface and lens related to their close approximation at the pupil

III.   Clinical Presentation

A.   Glaucoma is the third leading cause of blindness is the US, after cataract and age-related macular degeneration; approximately 1.25 million persons have the diagnosed condition, and about another one million are affected but are unaware of it

B.   Risk factors include high IOP, older age, African-American race, family history of glaucoma, myopia, diabetes, and hypertension

C.   Primary open-angle glaucoma (POAG) is by far the most prevalent form of the disorder
    1.   Onset of the disorder is slow and insidious, with gradual loss of peripheral vision; usually there are no other symptoms; central visual acuity, usually bilateral, is affected late in course
    2.   Signs include elevated IOP and increased cup-to-disc ratio as well as other signs that are detectable through slitlamp examination
    3.   A significant number of patients with open-angle glaucoma have intraocular pressure below 21 mm Hg (as measured by tonometry), a condition which is referred to as normal tension glaucoma
    4.   Intraocular pressure **alone** is not the primary determinant for diagnosis

D.   In primary angle-closure glaucoma (a relatively rare condition), manifestations of angle closure depend on the extent and reversibility of the pupillary block
    1.   Angle-closure glaucoma is most likely to occur in persons of Asian descent
    2.   Patients may complain of unilateral headache (same side as affected eye), visual blurring, nausea, and photophobia
    3.   Angle-closure glaucoma is an ophthalmologic emergency as irreversible eye damage can occur if left untreated

E.   Present standard for determining visual loss in glaucoma is the visual-field test, an automated examination that is reserved for the ophthalmologist's office

IV.   Diagnosis/Evaluation

A.   History
    1.   Inquire about onset and duration of symptoms, and if one or both eyes are affected
    2.   Ask about difficulties with peripheral vision, and if symptoms of headache, photophobia, visual blurring are present
    3.   Inquire about family history of eye disease
    4.   Obtain complete medical and medication history

B.   Physical Examination
    1.   Quickly examine external eye for swelling, ptosis, injection of conjunctiva, tearing, and corneal clarity
    2.   If emergent condition not suspected, visual acuity testing should be performed (may be normal in persons with glaucoma)
    3.   Measurement of intraocular pressure using a hand-held device such as the Schiötz tonometer is a useful screening approach (provides gross measurement only)
        a.   Normal intraocular pressure is 10-20 mm Hg (IOP >22 mm Hg should be considered abnormal and more precise testing is indicated)
        b.   Women have slightly higher normal pressures than men
    4.   Asians may normally have higher intraocular pressures than African-Americans and Caucasians
    5.   Estimate peripheral vision using direct confrontation (provides gross measurement of visual fields)
    6.   Ophthalmoscopic exam may reveal notching of the cup and a difference in cup-to-disc ratio between the two eyes

C.   Differential Diagnosis
    1.   Conjunctivitis
    2.   Acute uveitis
    3.   Age-related macular degeneration

D. Diagnostic Test: None except those described under Physical Examination. Further evaluation should be performed by the ophthalmologist who bases diagnosis on the appearance of the optic nerve [i.e., color and contour], applanation tonometry, and findings on visual field examination

V. Plan/Management

A. Angle-closure glaucoma is an ocular emergency; if this condition is suspected, immediate referral to an ophthalmologist is indicated

B. All patients who present with complaints of ocular pain, photophobia, visual blurring, or sudden loss of vision should be immediately referred for emergency care by an ophthalmologist

C. If primary open-angle glaucoma suspected based on physical examination, refer to ophthalmologist for evaluation

D. Follow Up: By ophthalmologist

HORDEOLUM (STYE)

I. Definition: Focal, acute infection of the eyelid margins

II. Pathogenesis: An acute infectious process involving the meibomian glands or other glands of the eyelid margins usually caused by *Staphylococcus aureus*

III. Clinical Presentation

A. More common in children and adolescents than adults

B. Patient often presents with sudden onset of localized tenderness, redness, and swelling of the eyelid

C. May occur in crops because the infecting pathogen may spread from one hair follicle to another

D. May point to the conjunctival side of the lid (posterior hordeolum involving the meibomian glands) or may involve the lid margin (anterior hordeolum involving the sebaceous or sweat glands)

IV. Diagnosis/Evaluation

A. History
   1. Determine onset and duration of symptoms
   2. Inquire about pain and visual disturbances
   3. Ask about past episodes and previous treatments

B. Physical Examination
   1. Assess visual acuity
   2. Inspect eyelids for inflammation, swelling, and discharge
   3. Palpate eyelids for induration and masses
   4. Evert the eyelid and examine inner surface for pointing
   5. Examine sclera and conjunctiva for abnormalities
   6. Palpate for preauricular adenopathy

C. Differential Diagnosis
   1. Chalazion
   2. Blepharitis

D. Diagnostic Tests: None indicated

V. Plan/Management

    A. Apply warm, moist compresses for 15 minutes throughout the day

    B. Prescribe erythromycin 0.5% (Ilotycin or generic) ophthalmic ointment BID-QID x 7 days OR polymyxin B-trimethoprim (Polytrim) drops, 1-2 drops in affected eye BID-QID x 7 days

    C. Cleanse eyelids daily with a neutral soap (e.g., Johnson's Baby Shampoo) in a 1:1 solution with clean water

    D. If not responsive to medical therapy, refer to expert for incision and drainage

    E. If crops of styes occur, diabetes mellitus must be excluded and patient should be told not to rub eyes; some authorities recommend a course of tetracycline to stop recurrences

    F. Patient Education
        1. Advise patient that good lid hygiene may help prevent recurrence (see section on BLEPHARITIS for description)
        2. Advise female patients to abstain from wearing eye makeup until clear and disposing of all old make up as it may be contaminated

    G. Follow Up: None indicated

VISUAL IMPAIRMENT

I. Definition: A decline in vision in one or both eyes

II. Pathogenesis

    A. Etiology of impaired vision can be divided into two general categories
        1. Refractive errors or those problems that can be improved by glasses (common causes: myopia, hyperopia, presbyopia, anisometropia, and astigmatism)
        2. Non-refractive errors (retinal abnormalities, glaucoma, cataract, retinoblastoma, eye muscle imbalance, and systemic disease with ocular manifestations) that cannot be corrected by glasses alone

    B. For clear vision, light must focus precisely on the retina
        1. In nearsightedness, or myopia, light is focused in front of the retina and the person sees near objects best
        2. In farsightedness, or hyperopia, light is focused behind the retina and the person sees far objects best

    C. **Myopia** is a condition in which objects can be seen clearly if held close enough to the eye (the person is "nearsighted"); person typically has no problem with reading or close work but distance vision is blurred

    D. **Hyperopia** is called farsightedness, and means that the individual cannot see near objects

    E. **Presbyopia** develops as part of the aging process; the lens becomes less resilient, does not thicken as readily, and poor near vision (presbyopia) occurs
        1. In an attempt to compensate for this decrease in vision, the person holds reading material farther away to aid in accommodation
        2. Eventually, reading glasses become necessary

    F. **Anisometropia** is a state in which there is a difference in the refractive error of the two eyes; condition may be congenital or acquired (due to asymmetric age changes or disease)

G.   **Astigmatism** is a condition in which curvature variations of the optical system result in unequal light refraction and impaired vision

H.   Pathophysiology of conditions causing non-refractive errors is dependent on the condition

III.   Clinical Presentation

A.   Refractive errors remain the most common cause of decreased visual acuity in adults

B.   Adults with refractive errors most often complain about difficulty with near vision (hyperopia)
1.   They may also complain of headache, fatigue, and blurred vision when doing tasks requiring extended use of eyes for near vision
2.   Onset is usually slow with a gradual decline in ability to see near objects well
3.   Almost 100% of adults require glasses by age 60 in order to see well for both far and near circumstances

C.   **Presbyopia** usually begins in middle-age (45-55); symptoms of presbyopia include the following
1.   Longer reading distance required (objects less than 20 cm away cannot be brought into focus)
2.   Inability to focus on close work and excessive illumination required
3.   Greater difficulty with close work occurs as day progresses

D.   **Astigmatism** can begin in either childhood or adulthood and can be easily corrected if it causes blurred vision or eye discomfort

E.   Adults with non-refractive errors have impaired vision at both near and far distances
1.   Open-angle glaucoma usually causes few symptoms until neural damage has occurred; visual dysfunction in glaucoma is first expressed in the mid-peripheral field of vision (central vision functions such as acuity remain relatively intact until late in the disease process)
2.   Patients with cataract complain of poor visual acuity and problems with glare
3.   Retinal detachment may cause flashes of light and abrupt vision loss
4.   Uveitis causes pain of the globe and photophobia
5.   Patients with age-related macular degeneration may complain of blurred and gradual loss of vision

F.   Visual acuity correctable by glasses or contact lenses to 20/200 or less in both eyes, or visual fields in both eyes less than 10 degrees centrally, constitutes legal blindness in the US

IV.   Diagnosis/Evaluation

A.   History
1.   Determine if vision in one or both eyes is impaired and if both near and far vision are affected
2.   Ask if there are associated symptoms of eye discomfort, increased tearing, cloudy vision, or flashing lights
3.   Ask about chronic or past eye problems, previous treatments, and response
4.   Ask if there is a family history of eye disease

B.   Physical Examination
1.   Examine external eye for swelling, ptosis, injection of the conjunctiva, and corneal clarity
2.   Determine extraocular movement
3.   Measure peripheral vision (recognizing that this is only a very gross assessment of visual fields)
4.   Elicit red reflex and perform ophthalmoscopic exam
5.   Perform visual acuity testing

C. Differential Diagnosis
  1. Refractive errors
  2. Non-refractive errors (common causes: glaucoma, cataract, retinal detachment, uveitis, macular degeneration)

D. Diagnostic Tests: None indicated other than those described under IV.B. above

V. Plan/Management

A. Indicators requiring further evaluation of visual acuity are outlined in the table below

---

PATIENTS REQUIRING FURTHER EVALUATION

- ➡ Patients with visual acuity of 20/30 or worse
- ➡ More than a **one-line** difference between eyes

B. If the cause of the impaired vision is not believed to be a refractive error, refer to ophthalmologist for further evaluation

C. Patients with acute onset of impaired vision need immediate referral for emergency care

D. Patients requiring visual acuity determination for purposes of legal blindness or disability determination or for any medicolegal cases should be referred to an ophthalmologist

E. Follow Up: By ophthalmologist or optometrist

References

Azar, D.T. (2002). The crystalline lens and cataract. In D. Pavan-Langson (Ed.), *Manual of ocular diagnosis and therapy* (pp. 140-165). Philadelphia: Lippincott Williams & Wilkins.

Centers for Disease Control and Prevention. (2002). Sexually transmitted diseases treatment guidelines. *MMWR, 51* (No. RR-6): 1-82.

Gault, J.A., & Friedman, D.S. (2002). Visual fields. In J.F. Vander & J.A. Gault (Eds.), *Ophthalmology secrets* (pp. 47-52). Philadelphia: Hanley & Belfus, Inc.

Goroll, A.H., & Mulley, A.G. (2002). *Primary care medicine recommendations.* Philadelphia: Lippincott Williams & Wilkins.

Laibson, P.R. (2002). Dry eyes. In J.F. Vander & J.A. Gault (Eds.), *Ophthalmology secrets* (pp. 103-107). Philadelphia: Hanley & Belfus, Inc.

Lanternier, M.L. (2002). Ophthalmology. In M.A. Graber & M.L. Lanternier (Eds.), *University of Iowa: The family practice handbook* (pp. 699-711). St. Louis: Mosby.

Leibowitz, H.M. (2000). The red eye. *New England Journal of Medicine, 343,* 345-351.

Pavan, P.R., & Pavan-Langston. (2002). Retina and vitreous. In D. Pavan-Langston (Ed.), *Manual of ocular diagnosis and therapy.* Philadelphia: Lippincott Williams & Wilkins.

Pavan-Langson, D. (2002). Cornea and external disease. In D. Pavan-Langson (Ed.), *Manual of ocular diagnosis and therapy* (pp. 67-129). Philadelphia: Lippincott Williams & Wilkins.

Pavan-Langson, D. (2002). Ocular examination techniques and diagnostic tests. In D. Pavan-Langson (Ed.), *Manual of ocular diagnosis and therapy* (pp. 1-20). Philadelphia: Lippincott Williams & Wilkins.

Pavan-Langson, D. & Grosskreutz, C.L. (2002). Glaucoma. In D. Pavan-Langson (Ed.), *Manual of ocular diagnosis and therapy* (pp. 251-285). Philadelphia: Lippincott Williams & Wilkins.

Rubin, P.A. (2002). Eyelids and lacrimal system. In D. Pavan-Langson (Ed.), *Manual of ocular diagnosis and therapy* (pp. 47-55). Philadelphia: Lippincott Williams & Wilkins.

US Preventive Services Task Force. (1996). *Guide to clinical preventive services.* (2nd ed.). Baltimore: Williams & Wilkins.

Problems of the Ears, Nose, Sinuses, Throat, Mouth, and Neck

CONSTANCE R. UPHOLD

FOREIGN BODY IN EAR

I. Definition: Presence of object(s) in the external auditory canal

II. Pathogenesis

   A. Intentional placement of object into ear usually due to curiosity, boredom, or imitation of others

   B. Accidental entry of foreign body; insects may fly into ear

III. Clinical presentation

   A. Symptoms depend on depth of object, nature and composition of object, and duration in the canal
       1. Nonreactive substances such as plastic do not usually cause any symptoms
       2. Insects usually cause discomfort, erythema, and sometimes drainage
       3. Vegetable matter may cause itching and minor pain
       4. Alkaline batteries may leak acid and result in pain, swelling, and discharge
       5. Decreased hearing may occur if the object is large or causes swelling

   B. Complications are uncommon; otitis media, perforation of tympanic membrane, and development of cholesteatoma may occur

IV. Diagnosis/Evaluation

   A. History
       1. Inquire about onset, duration, and character of symptoms
       2. Determine if there is a history of placing objects in ear

   B. Physical Examination; perform a thorough examination of the ear
       1. If foreign body is suspected, but cannot be visualized, instill water to fill the medial half of the external canal; this may allow visualization of the tympanic sulcus in which objects often become lodged
       2. Inspect auditory canal and tympanic membrane for signs of inflammation and injury

   C. Differential Diagnosis
       1. Otitis externa
       2. Otitis media

V. Plan/Management

   A. Removal of nonreactive foreign bodies
       1. Stabilize patient's head
       2. Use alligator forceps under direct visualization with an operating head otoscope to remove object; pulling the pinna superiorly and laterally will facilitate removal
       3. Gentle irrigation with warm water may also be used if tympanic membrane (TM) is intact and there is no inflammation in the external canal
       4. Direct stream around the object and position patient such that gravity will help drainage
       5. **Do not irrigate if foreign body is vegetable matter** as these objects tend to swell when water is applied
       6. Frazier tip suction can also be used to retrieve objects

   B. For round, smooth objects, place a curette with a curved end behind object and gently pull out

   C. Live insects should be killed by instilling mineral oil into ear before extraction with suction or alligator forceps

   D. Alkaline batteries should be removed immediately; magnets may facilitate removal

E.	Following removal of object perform the following:
1.	Carefully inspect tympanic ear and external auditory canal
2.	If there are any signs of inflammation or injury and TM is intact; instill 2% acetic acid otic solution (VoSoL Otic) 5 drops QID X 5-7 days or polymyxin B sulfate, neomycin, hydrocortisone (Cortisporin Otic suspension); 3-4 drops in canal, QID x 7 days

F.	Refer to otorhinolaryngologist if foreign body cannot be removed after several attempts, if moderate or severe injury to ear has occurred, if patient has severe pain, or if patient cannot remain still and needs general anesthesia for removal

G.	Follow Up: Evaluate patient in 2-3 days if there are signs of inflammation or injury to the ear, otherwise no follow up is needed unless patient has problems

HEARING LOSS

I.	Definitions:	Reduction in a person's ability to perceive sound

A.	Hearing loss is measured according to hearing thresholds (the softest tone heard by patient at a given frequency) during pure tone audiometric testing
1.	Normal hearing: 0 to 25 dB
2.	Mild impairment: 26 to 40 dB
3.	Moderate impairment: 41 to 55 dB
4.	Moderately severe: 56 to 70 dB
5.	Severe: 71 to 90 dB
6.	Profound: 91 dB and above

B.	Conductive hearing loss occurs when sound is inadequately conducted through the external or middle ear to the sensorineural apparatus of the inner ear; conductive hearing loss occurs when there is interference with the mechanical reception or amplification of sound

C.	Sensorineural hearing loss occurs when sound is normally carried through the external and middle ear but there is a defect within the inner ear or eighth cranial nerve which results in sound distortion

II.	Pathogenesis

A.	Common causes of conductive hearing loss
1.	Impacted cerumen
2.	Foreign bodies
3.	Otitis externa
4.	Benign tumors of middle ear
5.	Carcinoma of external auditory canal and/or middle ear
6.	Eustachian tube dysfunction
7.	Otitis media
8.	Perforation of the tympanic membrane
9.	Serous otitis media with effusion
10.	Otosclerosis
11.	Cholesteatoma
12.	Tuberculosis of the temporal bone

B.	Common causes of sensorineural hearing loss
1.	Presbycusis due to atrophy of the basal end of the organ of Corti, a loss in number of auditory receptors, vascular changes, and stiffening of the basilar membranes
2.	Noise exposure
3.	Ménière's disease (see DIZZINESS section)
4.	Acoustic tumors (see DIZZINESS section), tumor of eighth cranial nerve
5.	Opportunistic infections of the temporal bone may occur in patients with acquired immunodeficiency syndrome

6. Other diseases
   a. Syphilis
   b. Paget's disease
   c. Collagen diseases
   d. Endocrine disease such as diabetes mellitus or hypothyroidism
   e. Bacterial meningitis
   f. Tuberculosis of the temporal bone
7. Basilar migraines
8. Viral illnesses such as mumps, cytomegalovirus, and herpes zoster
9. Demyelinating processes such as multiple sclerosis
10. Drug ototoxicities
    a. Antibiotics such as streptomycin, neomycin, gentamicin, erythromycin, and vancomycin
    b. Diuretics such as ethacrynic acid and furosemide
    c. Salicylates
    d. Antineoplastic agents such as cisplatin and vincristine sulfate
11. Trauma such as skull fracture or tympanic membrane perforation

III. Clinical presentation of common causes of hearing loss

A. Epidemiology and clinical consequences
   1. About 4% of persons <45 years and 29% of those >65 years have a handicapping hearing loss; third most prevalent chronic condition in older Americans
   2. Even moderate hearing loss can seriously impact one's quality of life; depression is strongly correlated with hearing loss
   3. Hearing loss may be erroneously diagnosed as dementia or behavioral problems in the elderly

B. In conductive hearing loss, sensitivity to sound is diminished, but clarity is unchanged; if volume is increased to compensate for loss, the hearing is normal
   1. Serous otitis media
      a. Most frequent cause in children and an important factor of hearing loss in adults
      b. Patient usually has fullness and decreased hearing in one or both ears
   2. Otosclerosis is associated with slow, progressive hearing loss (usually bilateral) beginning in second or third decade of life; in women, hearing loss is often first noticed during pregnancy
      a. Most common cause of progressive conductive hearing loss in young adults
      b. Hereditary condition of unknown etiology in which there is an irregular ossification in the bony labyrinth of the inner ear, particularly of the stapes
      c. Patients have tinnitus and hearing loss which may progress to deafness
      d. On physical examination, the tympanic membrane (TM) is normal
   3. Cholesteatoma
      a. Benign, slowly growing lesion in the middle ear or mastoid that destroys bone and normal ear tissue
      b. Chronic drainage that fails to resolve with antibiotics is typical presentation

C. Sensorineural hearing loss results in decreased sound sensitivity to high frequencies
   1. Presbycusis (most common cause of hearing loss in US) is a slowly progressive problem in persons >65 years
      a. Frequently patients are unaware of their hearing problems
      b. Typically is bilateral and characterized by high-frequency hearing loss
      c. Results in a decrease in speech discrimination (cannot understand speech even when spoken loudly)
      d. Tinnitus and hypersensitivity to noise occur
   2. Noise-induced hearing loss (second most common cause) is due to excessive noise exposure in the workplace or during recreation
      a. Loss is permanent and not fully treatable, but is 100% preventable
      b. Early in condition there is isolated pure tone loss at 4000 Hz unilaterally or bilaterally
      c. Pure tone loss progresses to other frequencies with increased exposure
   3. Acoustic neuroma presents with tinnitus, unilateral, unexplained hearing loss, and disequilibrium (see DIZZINESS section)
   4. Ménière's disease is characterized by episodic vertigo, fluctuating sensorineural hearing loss, and roaring tinnitus (see DIZZINESS section)

IV.   Diagnosis/Evaluation

A.   History
   1.   Question about nature of the hearing loss (unilateral vs. bilateral; rapid or slow progression; acute vs. chronic; fluctuating vs. constant)
   2.   Determine what sounds the patient has most trouble hearing; difficulty understanding spoken words suggests sensorineural hearing loss
   3.   Inquire about associated symptoms such as fever, ear pain, discharge from ear, vertigo, tinnitus, and neurologic disturbances
   4.   Explore predisposing factors such as trauma, barotrauma (air plane travel or diving), antecedent infections, and medication use
   5.   Ask about excessive noise exposure; for adults, ask if patient must shout at work to converse with someone at arm's length (indicates a potentially harmful noise level)
   6.   Obtain a thorough past medical history
   7.   Ask about family history of hearing loss and neoplastic diseases
   8.   Ask whether hearing problems cause embarrassment or frustration when talking to others
   9.   Question patient about the impact of the hearing loss on activities of daily living

B.   Physical Examination
   1.   Examine the nasopharynx
   2.   Perform visual examination of TM and external auditory canal
   3.   Perform pneumatic otoscopy to determine mobility of TM
   4.   Perform clinical hearing test: whispered voice should be done with the patient using a finger to occlude the opposite ear to prevent crossover
   5.   Perform Weber and Rinne tests (see table that follows)

TUNING FORK TESTS		
	Weber Test	Rinne Test
Procedure	Strike fork and hold in middle of forehead or apex of skull and ask patient to localize sound	Strike fork, then place firmly on mastoid tip (measure of bone conduction [BC]); ask patient to raise hand when sound is no longer present; then move fork so that it resonates beside ear (measure of air conduction [AC])
Conductive Loss	Sound louder in ear in which patient perceives the hearing loss	In affected ear, sound is louder when on mastoid tip than beside ear (BC>AC)
Sensorineural Loss	Sound louder in unaffected ear	In normal ear and ear with sensorineural hearing loss, the sound is louder beside the ear than on the mastoid tip (AC>BC)

   6.   Complete head, neck, and cranial nerve examinations are often indicated

C.   Differential Diagnosis: See common causes of hearing loss under pathogenesis; important to determine the following:
   1.   Is hearing loss acute versus chronic? (acute hearing loss almost always requires immediate intervention such as removal of cerumen or treatment with antibiotics for otitis media)
   2.   Is hearing loss conductive versus sensorineural?

D.   Diagnostic Tests
   1.   Hearing screening is recommended periodically for older adults by several professional organizations (see table that follows)

RECOMMENDATIONS FROM PROFESSIONAL ORGANIZATIONS FOR SCREENING FOR HEARING LOSS					
Professional Organization	**Population**	**Frequency of Screening**	**Question Patient About Hearing**	**Otoscopic Examination and Audiometric Testing**	**Other Tests**
US Preventive Services Task Force (http://www.ahcpr.gov /clinic /uspstfix.htm)	Older adults	Periodically at clinician's discretion	Recommended	Recommended for patients with evidence of impaired hearing	AudioScope testing discussed but no recommendation given
Canadian Task Force on Preventive Health Care (http://www.ctfphc.org)	Elderly adults	During periodic health examination	Recommended	Not discussed	AudioScope testing and Whispered Voice test recommended
American Academy of Family Physicians (http://www.aafp.org/exam.xml)	Adults >60 years of age	During periodic health examination	Recommended	Not discussed	None
American Speech-Language-Hearing Association (http://www.asha.org /hearing/testing)	Adults >50 years of age	Every 3 years	Recommended	Recommended	None

Adapted from Yueh, B., Shapiro, N., MacLean, C.H., & Shekelle, P.G. (2003). Screening and management of adult hearing loss in primary care: Scientific review. *JAMA, 289*, 1976-1985.

2. An AudioScope can be used as a screening tool for hearing loss
   a. Hand-held combination of otoscope and audiometer
   b. Held directly in the external auditory canal (probe tip seals canal) and AudioScope delivers a 25- to 40-dB pure tone at 500 Hz, 1000 Hz, and 4000 Hz
   c. In addition to screening for hearing loss, the AudioScope enables the clinician to directly inspect ear canal
   d. If patient cannot hear predetermined series of tones refer for formal audiometry testing
3. Other tests used for diagnosis or to evaluate the extent of hearing loss:
   a. Puretone audiometry should be used in older children and adults; it characterizes the extent of impairment; air-conduction and bone-conduction measurements are made for sounds of varying intensity (decibels) and frequency (Hertz or cps): Indicated for all cases of chronic hearing loss and in cases of acute hearing loss with uncertain etiology
      (1) Presbycusis: higher frequency loss at 8000 than at 4000 cycles
      (2) Noise-induced hearing loss: high frequency loss, greatest at 4000 cycles and improvement at 8000 cycles
      (3) Conductive hearing loss: low frequency hearing loss (125-500 cycles)
   b. Vestibular testing should be considered if there are symptoms of tinnitus and vertigo: electronystagmometry, rotational tests, and posturography are useful adjuncts
   c. Computerized tomography should be considered if tumors and bony lesions are suspected
   d. If acoustic neuroma is suspected, order magnetic resonance imaging
   e. Order fluorescent treponemal-antibody-absorption test if there is a possibility of late latent syphilis
   f. Tympanometry should be considered to assess TM stiffness
   g. Impedance audiometry evaluates middle ear function by testing tympanic membrane compliance and acoustic reflex thresholds

V. Plan/Management

A. Referral to otolaryngologist is needed for patients with acute hearing loss who do not have an apparent diagnosis or for patients with apparent treatable acute or chronic causes for hearing loss who do not improve with standard treatments

B. Referral to audiologist is needed for patients with chronic deficits who may benefit from a hearing device and other audiology services

C. Many patients with hearing loss can be helped by surgical procedures; for example, in patients with profound sensorineural hearing loss (defined as >80 dB of loss in the better ear) or true deafness, cochlear implantation is often beneficial

D. Aural rehabilitation is often beneficial for patients with sensorineural hearing loss
    1. Hearing aids are the mainstay of therapy
    2. Inexpensive auditory amplifiers are available and include telephone receiver amplifiers and radio and television earphones
    3. Cochlear implants stimulate the eighth cranial nerve directly and can provide sound awareness for patients with severe hearing loss
    4. Lip reading and sign language may be helpful
    5. Tinnitus may be relieved by masking it with background music or with "tinnitus retraining therapy" (sound therapy such as hearing aids combined with skilled counseling)

E. Patient education
    1. Discuss ways to enhance communication such as facing patient, obtaining his/her attention before speaking, speaking slowly, using gestures, and only speaking louder or moving closer if the patient states that it is helpful
    2. The older patient often has some difficulty in discriminating consonants; take time to carefully enunciate all words to patient
    3. Because many patients are embarrassed about wearing a hearing aid, emphasize that today's hearing aids are small, less noticeable, and more efficient
    4. Discuss prevention of hearing loss
        a. Ear plugs or fluid-filled ear muffs with tight seal may reduce noise by 10-30 dB
        b. People vary in their susceptibility to noise-induced trauma, but typically if sound causes pain, tinnitus, or temporary blocking of ear, extended exposure to this noise will cause permanent hearing loss
        c. Limit exposure to loud noise; prolonged or repeated exposure to any noise above 85 dB can cause hearing loss; most lawn mowers, motorcycles, chain saws, and powerboats produce noise >85 dB; personal stereos, rock concerts, and firecrackers may produce noise at 140 dB or more
    5. Sources of patient information (see following table)

WEBSITE RESOURCES ON HEARING LOSS AND TINNITUS	
Organization	**Website**
American Academy of Audiology	www.audiology.org
American Academy of Otolaryngology-Head & Neck Surgery	www.aao-hns.org
American Speech-Language-Hearing Association	www.asha.org
American Tinnitus Association	www.ata.org
National Campaign for Hearing Health	www.hearinghealth.net/pages/home
National Institute on Deafness and Other Communication Disorders (National Institutes of Health)	www.nidcd.nih.gov
Self Help for Hard of Hearing People, Inc.	www.shhh.org

F. Follow up is dependent on the type and cause of the hearing loss

IMPACTED CERUMEN

I. Definition: Obstruction of the ear canal by cerumen (earwax)

II. Pathogenesis

A. Cerumen is produced by the ceruminous glands in the outer portion of the canal and is a naturally occurring lubricant and protectant of the external ear canal

B. While cerumen is normally cleared from the ears through the body's natural mechanisms, excessive accumulation may occur and partially or totally occlude the canal

III. Clinical Presentation

    A. Commonly occurs in the elderly and industrial workers

    B. Ear pain may be present if cerumen hardens and touches the tympanic membrane, or if the external canal is irritated by build up of hardened cerumen

    C. Symptoms may include pain, itching, and sensation of fullness on the affected side; conductive hearing loss may also be present with total occlusion of the canal

IV. Diagnosis/Evaluation

    A. History
        1. Ask about onset, and if ear discomfort or a feeling of fullness is present
        2. Ask patient how ears are usually cleaned (are cotton-tipped swabs used?)
        3. Ask if wax removal has been required in the past
        4. Determine if patient has history of previous ear surgery with resultant scarring and increased risk of perforation (procedure is **contraindicated** if patient responds positively)

    B. Physical Examination
        1. Examine both ear canals
        2. Attempt to visualize the tympanic membranes around the wax to ascertain intactness
        3. Test hearing to determine if the affected ear is the only hearing ear (if so, referral to a specialist is indicated)

    C. Differential Diagnosis
        1. Foreign body
        2. Otitis media
        3. Otitis externa

    D. Diagnostic Tests: None indicated

V. Plan/Management

    A. Removal of cerumen may be necessary in the following situations
        1. Accumulation is causing decreased hearing, tinnitus, feeling of fullness, vertigo, or ear discomfort
        2. Accumulation is obstructing the examiner's view of the tympanic membrane

    B. Contraindications to removal of impacted cerumen: large perforation of tympanic membrane; severe ear trauma; irregular, sharp foreign body; very hard wax; inability to fully immobilize the patient; cholesteatoma; tumors

    C. Removal of cerumen using either the curette or irrigation technique is usually successful (see tables that follow)

    D. The irrigation technique takes longer than the curette technique and is usually implemented when the curette technique fails or is poorly tolerated by patient; irrigation technique rarely fails

REMOVAL USING CURETTE TECHNIQUE

Equipment needed/types of curette	Metal and plastic Metal curettes are either rigid or flexible Plastic are either the flex-loop ear curette or infant ear scoop
Positioning patient	Place in supine position and restrain head carefully or seat comfortably on exam table and explain procedure and the importance of remaining still
Visualize cerumen	Using otoscope, look into the canal using posterior traction on helix
Select the appropriate curette	Gently remove the impacted cerumen, working through the otoscope or by direct vision (after having identified where the impaction is and keeping in mind the anatomy of the external auditory canal)
If hard wax is encountered	Stop the procedure and instill a few drops of mineral oil into the canal to soften for 10 minutes and then resume removal
If wax appears to be adherent to the tympanic membrane itself	Removal must be via gentle irrigation
Immobilization	**Absolutely necessary** to avoid risk of perforation and trauma to the ear canal!
If removal is via direct vision	Use the otoscope to assess progress during procedure

REMOVAL USING IRRIGATION TECHNIQUE

Equipment needed	• Use a soft-tipped syringe such as a 22-gauge butterfly intravenous catheter tubing with needle and butterfly removed and a 20 to 50 cc syringe, or • A bulb syringe, or • A water jet device such as Water-Pik
Irrigate with lukewarm water	• **Caution**: Use of cold or hot water may lead to dizziness and nausea! • Squirt water on your wrist to verify that temperature is correct
Positioning patient	• Place in supine position, or seat comfortably on exam table • Cover the patient's shoulder with towel • Instruct the patient to tilt head toward side being irrigated and place a small kidney-shaped basin under the ear to catch water (patient can hold basin)
Visualize cerumen	• Use otoscope to determine location
Place the tip of the tubing or syringe just inside the canal	• Infuse the water with a moderately strong and steady force • If the water jet irrigator is used, set at **lowest** setting to reduce risk of perforation
Direct the jet of water superiorly toward the occiput; aim stream of water at the superior gap or interface between the wax plug and the canal wall	• Allow for space in the canal for the return of water and cerumen • **Do not** direct the stream of water onto the tympanic membrane • Try to direct the stream of water past the plug of cerumen so as to create outward pressure on it • Take care not to touch the canal as this can produce cough and pain
Evaluate the effluent	• Sometimes an intact plug of cerumen is expelled and at other times the effluent will be tinted yellow but no obvious plug will be seen
Reassess progress using the otoscope	• It will be necessary to dry the external canal with gauze for good visualization and to reduce risk of infection
If pain or bleeding occur	• **STOP!**
If the irrigation is not successful after a few minutes	• Terminate the procedure
Instruct the patient to	• Instill 1-2 drops of baby oil in the affected ear twice a week to soften wax, or • Use 3 drops of hydrogen peroxide and water solution (1:1 solution) in affected ear 2-3 times a week
Ask the patient to return	• In one week for evaluation and removal of cerumen

E.   Cerumen solvents that are commercially available are not recommended because they frequently make the condition worse

F. If recurrences are a problem, instruct patient to apply 1 or 2 drops of baby oil in each ear once or twice weekly to help soften wax; patient may also use a squeeze bulb syringe filled with lukewarm water to gently irrigate canals every month or so (best to do about 10 minutes after oil has been instilled into canals)

G. Patient education
1. Instruct to avoid the use of cotton-tipped applicators that can impact cerumen
2. Inform that cerumen is a normal bodily secretion that protects the ear canal and does not usually need removal

H. Follow Up:
1. None indicated unless cerumen removal fails
2. Contact office if decreased hearing, vertigo, dizziness, drainage, or pain occurs

OTITIS EXTERNA

I. Definition: Inflammation of the external auditory canal

II. Pathogenesis

A. Predisposing factors
1. Frequent exposure to moisture (e.g., swimming; humid, warm climates), aggressive cleaning of the canal, or trauma
2. Allergies or skin conditions such as psoriasis or seborrhea

B. Pathogens
1. Bacterial: *Pseudomonas aeruginosa* (most common), *Staphylococcus aureus* (common), and less frequently *Proteus* species and anaerobes
2. Fungal (account for 9% of cases): *Candida* and *Aspergillus*

C. Secondary fungal otitis externa (OE) may develop following treatment of OE with topical antibiotics

III. Clinical Presentation

A. Ear pain (occurs in approximately 85% of cases) may begin gradually or suddenly; increases when pressure is placed on the tragus or when the pinna is moved

B. Sensation of fullness or obstruction of the ear occurs early in the process

C. Itching may occur and it is the predominant symptom with fungal infections

D. Otorrhea (discharge in or coming from the external auditory canal) is common
1. Acute bacterial OE typically has white mucus that is usually scant but may be thick
2. Chronic bacterial OE often has a bloody discharge, particularly in the presence of granulation tissue
3. Fungal OE has fluffy, white discharge or discharge may be black, gray, bluish-green, or yellow

E. If there is sufficient swelling to occlude the external auditory canal, hearing loss may occur

F. Systemic symptomatology such as fever or chills is uncommon

G. An uncommon, serious complication is malignant or necrotizing external otitis which can lead to cranial neuropathies and infection of the temporal bone
1. Characterized by deep-seated nocturnal pain and granulation tissue at the bony-cartilaginous junction
2. Most common in elderly male diabetics and immunocompromised persons

IV.   Diagnosis/Evaluation

    A.   History
        1.   Ask about the location of pain/discomfort and time of onset
        2.   Ask about the occurrence of itching and bleeding/purulent exudate
        3.   Question about hearing loss
        4.   Ask about location and frequency of swimming
        5.   Obtain history of recent ear trauma; ask type of ear cleaning method
        6.   Ask if there is a history of previous episodes and risk factors such as diabetes and immunosuppression

    B.   Physical Examination
        1.   Determine if febrile
        2.   Carefully inspect the skin as many dermatological conditions can cause OE
        3.   Assuming the ear is extremely tender, carefully examine the external canal with the otoscope; the following are signs of otitis externa:
            a.   Erythema and edema of the canal
            b.   Weeping secretions, purulent otorrhea, and exudate or crusting of the skin
        4.   Apply pressure to the tragus and move the pinna, noting degree of tenderness
        5.   If possible, observe the tympanic membrane which is usually normal; edema may impede observation
        6.   Palpate the infra-auricular cervical lymph nodes for signs of lymphadenitis and lymphadenopathy

    C.   Differential Diagnosis
        1.   Furunculosis
        2.   Otitis media
        3.   Mastoiditis
        4.   Foreign body

    D.   Diagnostic Tests: Culture should be performed if resistance to initial management occurs

V.   Plan/Management

    A.   Referral is recommended whenever malignant otitis externa cannot be ruled out or for severe, recalcitrant infections, and recurrent otitis externa

    B.   Before treatment, remove all exudative and epidermal debris (meticulous clearing of the canal is the cornerstone of effective treatment) (see section CERUMEN REMOVAL)
        1.   Can use either curette or irrigation technique
        2.   Irrigation should not be done if perforation of tympanic membrane cannot be ruled out

    C.   If swelling prevents the passage of topical medications, insert cotton wick
        1.   Insert by gently twisting the wick into the canal
        2.   Place drops on wick for first two days, then remove wick and place drops directly in ear

    D.   If it is unknown whether the tympanic membrane (TM) is perforated or intact, prescribe a nonototoxic quinolone antibiotic such as ofloxacin 0.3% solution (Floxin Otic)

    E.   For routine cases of OE with intact TM, 2% acetic acid otic solution (VoSoL Otic) is usually effective; prescribe 5 drops QID for 5-7 days; also available with hydrocortisone (VoSoL HC Otic) to decrease inflammation, and with aluminum acetate (Otic Domeboro)

    F.   Other effective agents are available:
        1.   Polymyxin B sulfate, neomycin, hydrocortisone (Cortisporin Otic suspension); 3-4 drops in canal, QID x 7 days
        2.   Tobramycin, dexamethasone (TobraDex) suspension, 4 gtts in canal, TID or QID x 7 days

    G.   For fungal infections prescribe one of the following otic medications for 7 days:
        1.   Acetic acid, aluminum acetate solution (Otic Domeboro) 5 drops QID
        2.   Propylene glycol solution of acetic acid (VoSoL) 5 drops QID
        3.   Clotrimazole (Lotrimin) solution 3 drops BID

H. Duration of treatment for all topical medications is three days beyond cessation of symptoms (typically 5-7 days); for more severe cases, duration is extended to 10-14 days

I. Systemic oral antibiotics are rarely needed, but should be used when OE is persistent, associated with acute otitis media, when patient has systemic symptoms such as fever and lymphadenopathy, or when patient is immunocompromised; prescribe Ciprofloxacin (Cipro) 500 mg BID

J. Patient education
1. Advise patient to keep moisture out of ear for 4-6 weeks. May bathe or shower but plug ear with cotton impregnated with petroleum jelly. Swimming is not permitted for 7-10 days
2. When using topical medications, suggest the following:
   a. Particularly with ofloxacin, warm the bottle in hands before instilling to minimize dizziness
   b. Insert a small cotton plug moistened with drops if patient cannot lie still long enough to allow absorption
3. Teach patients to prevent recurrence of infection
   a. Advise to instill 2-3 drops of 1:1:1 solution of vinegar/isopropyl alcohol/water after each contact with water; solution is also beneficial for patients with persistent OE
   b. Use ear plugs while swimming, showering, or shampooing
   c. Instruct in proper way to clean ears; avoid using cotton-tipped applicators or other devices such as hairpins

K. Follow Up
1. If properly treated, otitis externa should resolve in 7 days; mild cases do not require follow-up
2. Moderate and severe cases should return to office in 3 days and 24 hours, respectively

OTITIS MEDIA, ACUTE

I. Definitions: Otitis media is an inflammation in the middle ear without reference to etiology

A. Acute otitis media (AOM): Presence of middle ear effusion in conjunction with rapid onset of one or more signs or symptoms of inflammation of the middle ear; other terms used in the past and synonymous with AOM include suppurative otitis media, acute bacterial otitis media, and purulent otitis media

B. Persistent AOM: Persistence of symptoms and signs of middle ear infection following 1 to 2 courses of antibiotic therapy

C. Recurrent AOM: Three or more separate episodes of AOM in a 6-month time span or 4 or more episodes in a 12-month time span

D. Middle ear effusion (MEE) is liquid in the middle ear and can occur with AOM or otitis media with effusion

II. Pathogenesis

A. Most important factor is eustachian tube dysfunction that prevents effective drainage of middle ear fluid
1. Typically, patient has an antecedent event such as an infection or allergy which results in edema and congestion of the mucosa of the nasopharynx, eustachian tube, and middle ear
2. The congestion of the eustachian tube impedes the flow of middle ear secretions
3. Negative pressure often increases, which further pulls fluid into the middle ear
4. As middle ear secretions increase microbial pathogens grow, resulting in otitis media; common pathogens are as follows:
   a. *Streptococcus pneumoniae* (predominant)
   b. *Haemophilus influenzae*
   c. *Moraxella catarrhalis*
   d. Viruses
   e. Other bacteria such as *Streptococcus pyogenes* and *Staphylococcus aureus*

5. Due to overuse and/or inappropriate use of antibiotics as a result of overdiagnosis of AOM, pathogens of this condition are becoming increasingly resistant
   a. Drug-resistant *S. pneumoniae* (DRSP) is becoming a major health problem (particularly in persistent and recurrent AOM)
   b. The rates of infections due to beta-lactamase producing organisms *(M. catarrhalis* and *H. influenzae)* are also increasing

B. Risk factors for recurrent otitis media:
   1. An episode of AOM during first 6 months of life
   2. Passive and active smoking
   3. Male gender
   4. Congenital disorders such as cleft palate and trisomy 21
   5. History of enlarged adenoids, tonsillitis, or asthma
   6. Family history of otitis media

III. Clinical Presentation

A. Occurs most frequently in winter months; commonly seen following a viral upper respiratory infection

B. Symptoms (see table CONSENSUS DEFINITION OF ACUTE OTITIS MEDIA)

CONSENSUS DEFINITION OF ACUTE OTITIS MEDIA
AOM is defined as

1. Presence of MEE as demonstrated by the actual presence of fluid in the middle ear as diagnosed by tympanocentesis or the physical presence of liquid in the external ear canal as a result of TM perforation or indicated by limited or absent mobility of the TM as diagnosed by pneumatic otoscopy, tympanogram, or acoustic reflectometry with or without the following:
    a. opacification, not including erythema
    b. a full or bulging TM
    c. hearing loss
AND
2. Rapid onset (over the course of 48 hours)
OF
3. One or more of the following signs or symptoms:
    a. otalgia
    b. otorrhea
    c. fever

Adapted from Rosenfeld, R.M., Casselbrant, M.L., and Hannley, M.T. (2001). Implications of the AHRQ evidence report on acute otitis media. *Otolaryngology-Head and Neck Surgery, 125*, 440-448.

C. Complications include hearing loss, perforation of eardrum, cholesteatoma, acute mastoiditis, bacteremia, meningitis, and epidural abscess

IV. Diagnosis/Evaluation

A. History
   1. Determine onset and duration of symptoms
   2. Ask about ear pain, fever, irritability
   3. Inquire about hearing loss, tinnitus, and dizziness
   4. Ask about drainage from ear
   5. Inquire about associated symptoms such as nasal congestion, headache, sore throat, or cough
   6. Carefully document the number and, if possible, dates of previous occurrences; ask about successes and failures of previous treatments
   7. Determine whether an upper respiratory infection preceded the fever or ear pain
   8. Inquire about history of allergies and other risk factors such as active or passive smoking and congenital disorders such as cleft palate

B. Physical Examination
   1. Measure vital signs
   2. Inspect conjunctivae, pharynx, and nasal mucosa
   3. Palpate sinuses
   4. Palpate for auricular and cervical adenopathy
   5. Examine auricle and external auditory canal

6. Carefully examine tympanic membranes (TM) bilaterally for position, color, degree of translucency, and mobility (important to remove cerumen if TM is partially occluded)
   a. Position: Process of the malleus should be visible but not prominent through the membrane; retraction and bulging indicate effusion
   b. Color: Normal TM is gray; an amber color often indicates an effusion; erythema may indicate infection but also may be due to crying, severe coughing, or vascular engorgement
   c. Translucency: Middle ear or bony landmarks should be visible through the TM; air fluid level, bubbles, and inability to visualize middle ear landmarks suggest effusion
   d. Mobility: Normal ear will move with pneumatic otoscopy; **to be diagnosed with AOM there must be presence of fluid in middle ear; this can only be detected with pneumatic otoscopy, tympanogram, or acoustic reflectometry**
   e. Distorted light reflex and bullae between layers of TM are suggestive of AOM
7. Perform a lung examination
8. When a healthy adult has ear pain and the examination of the ear is completely normal, a more thorough evaluation of the head and neck is essential
   a. Examine mouth and teeth for dental disorders
   b. Assess functioning of temporomandibular joint
   c. Assess nose and pharynx for nasopharyngeal carcinoma
   d. Assess cranial nerves to detect neurological problems that could be associated with intracranial neoplasms

C. Differential Diagnosis (health care providers can generally detect OM 90% of time when it is present, but over diagnosis frequently occurs [as high as 40%])
   1. Otitis externa
   2. Transient middle ear effusion may result with flying or traveling in high altitudes (barotrauma) or with allergies
   3. Mastoiditis
   4. Furuncle
   5. Temporomandibular joint dysfunction
   6. Mumps
   7. Dental abscess
   8. Tonsillitis
   9. Foreign body
   10. Trauma

D. Diagnostic Tests
   1. Usually no diagnostic tests are ordered
   2. Tympanocentesis for culture and sensitivity of middle ear effusion is the gold standard for diagnosis of AOM and is recommended to guide choice of therapy in persistent and recurrent AOM
   3. Tympanometry is useful, particularly in recurrent cases and when there is suspicion of fluid behind the TM without clinical signs
   4. Acoustic reflectometry helps diagnose AOM by analyzing sound pressure and reflected sound in the eardrum
   5. Consider ordering sinus films in patients with recurrent otitis media
   6. Order CBC with differential and blood cultures in patients who appear toxic, have a high fever, are not drinking and voiding, or are immunocompromised
   7. Consider audiometry post treatment

V.   Plan/Management

A.   General management concepts (see following table)

GENERAL CONCEPTS OF MANAGEMENT	
1. Be cautious	Remember favorable natural history of AOM (80% of cases resolve spontaneously)
2. Prescribe antibiotics sparingly	Antibiotics improve resolution by only about 15% Antibiotics increase risk of bacterial resistance

3. Modify risk factors	Improve odds of resolution:
	    Avoid passive smoking
	    Control food and inhalant allergies
	    Treat sinusitis

4. Avoid unproven therapies	Antihistamines/decongestants Homeopathy and naturopathy Folk remedies such as "sweet oil"

B.   Treatment with antibiotics
1.   Antibiotics for correctly diagnosed AOM provide a small benefit (reduce pain and the risk of developing contralateral AOM and mastoiditis); the following outcomes are not affected by antibiotic use: Tympanic membrane perforation, pain and fever resolution at 4-7 days, recurrent AOM
2.   Some experts recommend that patients who have AOM without bulging tympanic membranes should be managed with a delayed antibiotic-prescribing strategy; provide patient with prescription for antibiotic to be used only if otalgia or fever persist or there is no clinical improvement after 48-72 hours
3.   Amoxicillin is the first line antibiotic (see following table)
    a.   In patients with low risk for drug-resistant *S. pneumoniae* (DRSP) prescribe 500 mg BID
    b.   In patients at high risk for DRSP, increase dose to 80-90 mg/kg/day
4.   For patients allergic to penicillins and cephalosporins, prescribe azithromycin or clarithromycin (for dosing, see table THIRD-LINE ANTIBIOTICS V.B.6.); increasing resistance to trimethoprim/ sulfamethoxazole and erythromycin/sulfisoxazole has been found, but in some areas these antibiotics may also be effective

RECOMMENDED FIRST-LINE ANTIBIOTIC FOR MEDICAL MANAGEMENT*		
Generic (Trade) Name *Duration of treatment*	**Dosing**	**Comment**
Amoxicillin (Amoxil) *10 day treatment* OR	500 mg tabs BID	Use this lower dose in uncomplicated AOM and in patients at low risk for DRSP Inexpensive, few adverse effects Disadvantage: Ineffective against beta-lactamase producing organisms
Amoxicillin (Amoxil) 10 day treatment*	80-90 mg/kg/day in 2 or 3 divided doses	Use this increased dose in patients with high risk of DRSP

* Shortened courses of antibiotics may be acceptable for patients who have mild, uncomplicated AOM, no underlying medical condition, no history of chronic or recurrent otitis media, and whose symptoms improve within 72 hours

5.   Use second-line antibiotics (see following table) for patients with following clinical features:
    a.   Received antibiotics within one month of course of treatment (consider high dose amoxicillin or one of the second-line antibiotics)
    b.   Failed to respond by third day of treatment with amoxicillin
    c.   Have complicated infections
    d.   Have ipsilateral conjunctivitis suggesting *H. influenzae* infection

RECOMMENDED SECOND-LINE ANTIBIOTICS FOR MEDICAL MANAGEMENT

Generic (Trade) Name *Duration of treatment*	Dosing	Comment
Amoxicillin-clavulanate (Augmentin) *10 day treatment** -OR- (Augmentin ES-600) *10 day treatment**	250-500 mg tab TID -OR- 80-90 mg/kg/day in 2 divided doses (available 600 mg/5 mL)	- Broad spectrum - 15-20% patients have gastrointestinal upset
Cefuroxime (Ceftin) *10 day treatment**	250-500 mg cap BID	- Broad spectrum
Ceftriaxone (Rocephin) *1-5 day treatment*	50-75mg/kg/day IM injection QD	- Good choice if patient is vomiting, has diarrhea, refuses oral medications, or is toxic

* Shortened courses of antibiotics may be acceptable for patients who have mild, uncomplicated AOM, no underlying medical condition, no history of chronic or recurrent otitis media, and whose symptoms improve with 72 hours

> 6. Use third-line antibiotics for special cases; see following table

RECOMMENDED THIRD-LINE ANTIBIOTICS FOR MEDICAL MANAGEMENT

Generic (Trade) Name *Duration of treatment*	Dosing	Comment
Azithromycin (Zithromax) *5 day treatment*	500 mg tab QD Day 1; 250 mg Days 2-5	- Broad spectrum
Cefprozil (Cefzil) *10 day treatment**	500 mg tab BID	- Broad spectrum
Cefpodoxime (Vantin) *10 day treatment**	200 mg tab BID	- Broad spectrum - Take tabs with food
Ceftibuten (Cedax) *10 day treatment**	400 mg cap QD	- Broad spectrum; convenient dosing - Take suspension on empty stomach; caps may be taken without regard for meals
Clarithromycin (Biaxin) *10 day treatment**	250-500 mg cap BID	- Broad spectrum - Well tolerated
Loracarbef (Lorabid) *10 day treatment**	200-400 mg caps BID	- Broad spectrum - Must take on an empty stomach

*Shortened courses of antibiotics may be acceptable for patients who have mild, uncomplicated AOM, no underlying medical condition, no history of chronic or recurrent otitis media, and whose symptoms improve with 72 hours

C. Management of pain
1. Usually, an analgesic such as acetaminophen or ibuprofen is all that is needed
2. Topical pain relievers such as Auralgan Otic solution (fill ear canal and insert moistened cotton plug) every 1-2 hours may be beneficial; **do not use if TM is ruptured**

D. Treatment of persistent and recurrent AOM
1. If no response in 2-3 days and patient is not toxic switch to a second-line or third-line antibiotic
2. Tympanocentesis with culture of middle ear fluid can guide antibiotic selection and can be beneficial in draining the effusion and breaking the cycle of persistent and recurrent AOM
3. Clindamycin is another possible choice, but is ineffective against *H. influenzae* and *M. catarrhalis*; consider if tympanocentesis confirms that pathogen is *S. pneumoniae*
4. Consider consultation with specialist if 2-3 courses of recommended treatments fail

5.   If middle ear fluid cultures are not available, previous treatment and current symptoms may provide clues to likely pathogen (see following table)

CLUES TO ETIOLOGY OF PERSISTENT AND RECURRENT AOM	
Clinical feature	**Pathogen**
Increased otalgia & fever Spontaneous perforation	More likely to be *S. pneumoniae*
Therapy in preceding month with amoxicillin, erythromycin-sulfisoxazole, azithromycin, antibiotic prophylaxis Epidemiological features: History of recurrent AOM, contact with individuals treated with antibiotics	More likely to be resistant *S. pneumoniae*
Mild symptoms Preceding therapy was with high-dose amoxicillin	Less likely to be *S. pneumoniae*
Otitis-conjunctivitis syndrome	More likely to be *H. influenzae*
Preceding therapy was with amoxicillin	More likely to be β-lactamase-positive *H. influenzae*
Preceding therapy was with third-generation cephalosporin	Less likely to be *H. influenzae*

Adapted from Pichichero, M.E., Reiner, S.A., Brook, I., Gooch, W.M. III, Yamauchi, T., Jenkins, S.G., et al. (2000). Controversies in the medical management of persistent and recurrent acute otitis media: Recommendations of a clinical advisory committee. *Annals of Otology, Rhinology, and Laryngology, 109*, 2-12.

E.   Nasal and oral decongestants are usually ineffective in preventing or treating AOM, but may provide symptomatic relief of associated symptoms that often accompany AOM

F.   Antihistamines are not recommended unless the predisposing factor for developing AOM is an allergy; antihistamines may thicken the secretions and aggravate the problem

G.   Treatment of tympanic membrane perforation involves prescription of oral antibiotic supplemented with topical antibiotic for maximum of 10 days; select one of the following topical antibiotics:
1.   Ofloxacin otic solution 3% (Floxin Otic): Instill 5-10 drops BID
2.   Combination of neomycin sulfate, polymyxin-B and hydrocortisone (Cortisporin Otic suspension) 3-4 drops in each ear, 3-4 times a day

H.   Consult specialist in following cases:
1.   Hearing loss bilaterally of 20 dB or more
2.   Chronic or persistent infection with evidence of mastoid involvement
3.   Cholesteatoma formation or chronic perforation
4.   Recurrent infections in healthy adults because of remote possibility of nasopharyngeal cancer

I.   Follow Up
1.   Assess patient in 48-72 hours for symptom improvement
2.   Typically, return visits are scheduled several days after completion of drug therapy or recheck in 2-3 weeks from initial visit; some authorities recommend delaying follow-up for 4-6 weeks if the patient is asymptomatic and reports that the infection has resolved
3.   For patients treated with prophylactic antibiotics, evaluate every 4 weeks

OTITIS MEDIA WITH EFFUSION

I.   Definition: Accumulation of serous fluid in the middle ear **without signs and symptoms of acute infection** (previously referred to as serous otitis media [OM], nonsuppurative OM, or secretory OM)

II.   Pathogenesis

A.   Loss of patency of the eustachian tube with subsequent negative pressure and effusion behind the tympanic membrane (TM)

B.   Risk factors are similar to those of acute otitis media (see section ACUTE OTITIS MEDIA)

III. Clinical Presentation

    A.   Effusion may occur in adults but is less common than in children

    B.   Patient are often asymptomatic, but may have mild pain, sensation of stuffiness or fullness in ear, or popping and crackling sounds in ear with chewing, yawning, or blowing nose

    C.   A small number of patients may experience vertigo or ataxia

    D.   Tympanic membrane is often retracted, opaque, and has a diffuse light reflex
        1.   Bubbles or a fluid level may be present behind the tympanic membrane
        2.   Decreased tympanic membrane movement with insufflation (pneumatic otoscopy) is usually present

    E.   Chronic effusion may result in chronic hearing loss

    F.   Complications are rare, but may include chronic drainage and perforation, cholesteatoma, and facial nerve paralysis

IV. Diagnosis/Evaluation

    A.   History
        1.   Determine onset, duration, character of symptoms
        2.   Inquire about rhinitis, cough, and fever
        3.   Question about pain and decreased hearing acuity level
        4.   Inquire about recent upper respiratory infection and allergies
        5.   Inquire about past episodes of otitis media and treatments received
        6.   Ask about family history of allergies

    B.   Physical Examination
        1.   Measure vital signs
        2.   Examine nasal passages and pharynx
        3.   Examine tympanic membranes (TM) for fluid level, retraction, diffuse light reflex and/or bubbles
        4.   Assess TM mobility with pneumatic otoscopy (removal of cerumen is mandatory)
            a.   Recommended for primary diagnosis
            b.   Accuracy of diagnosis with pneumatic otoscopy is 70-79%
        5.   Perform Rinne and Weber tests (see section on HEARING LOSS)
        6.   Palpate neck and jaw for adenopathy
        7.   Examine neck and head for anatomical abnormalities

    C.   Differential Diagnosis
        1.   Nasopharyngeal carcinoma
        2.   Anatomic abnormalities

    D.   Diagnostic Tests
        1.   Tympanometry (indirect measure of tympanic membrane compliance and estimate of middle ear pressure)
            a.   Often falsely positive due to impacted cerumen, foreign body, TM perforation, or improper placement of instrument tip on the ear canal wall
            b.   Pneumatic otoscopy recommended for primary diagnosis, followed by tympanometry as confirmatory test
            c.   Tympanogram is flat with an effusion
        2.   Audiometry
            a.   Patients with fluid in both ears for three months should undergo hearing evaluation; prior to three months, audiometry is an option
            b.   Hearing impairment is defined as equal to or worse than 20 decibels (dB) hearing threshold level in the better-hearing ear
        3.   Acoustic reflectometry; experts disagree about the value of this test

V. Plan/Management

A. For asymptomatic patients (normal hearing, speech) watchful waiting with vigilant monitoring is usually recommended, but patients who do not have resolution of effusion within 2 months may be candidates for antibiotic therapy
   1. Watchful waiting is becoming the preferred approach due to accumulating evidence that antibiotic use increases the risk for both colonization and invasive disease with penicillin-resistant *Streptococcus pneumoniae*; additional rationale for this recommendation:
      a. The majority of cases spontaneously resolve without antibiotic treatment
      b. Effect of antibiotics is marginal and often short-lived; antibiotics increase short-term resolution by approximately 15%
      c. Incidence of delayed suppurative complications from effusion is small
   2. If antibiotic therapy is chosen, prescribe a beta-lactamase stable antibiotic such as the following:
      a. Amoxicillin-clavulanate (Augmentin) 250-500 mg TID
      b. Clarithromycin (Biaxin) 250-500 mg BID

B. Assess hearing status and structural integrity of TM with audiometry and pneumatic otoscopy every 3-4 months

C. Patients with bilateral OME for greater than 3 months and hearing loss (defined as 20 dB hearing threshold level or worse in the better-hearing ear) should be referred to an ENT specialist for possible placement of tympanostomy tubes

D. Oral corticosteroids are sometimes recommended as a last-resort alternative to surgery: Dangers of this approach are chickenpox exacerbation, immunosuppression and adverse effects such as insomnia, changes in behavior, and weight gain

E. Consider autoinflation of eustachian tube with plastic nasal cannula attached to balloon

F. Patient education, modification of risk factors, and controlling concurrent illnesses are important
   1. Limit passive smoke exposure
   2. Treat concurrent illnesses such as sinusitis and allergic rhinitis
   3. Emphasize importance of follow up
   4. Discuss the possibility of hearing loss due to this condition

G. Most studies indicate that decongestants and antihistamines are ineffective; the role of allergies in patients with effusions is still uncertain

H. Referral to speech therapist may be needed for language delay or a speech problem

I. Nasopharyngeal cancer is a remote possibility in a healthy adult and consultation with an otolaryngologist is necessary if there is suspicion of this condition

J. Follow Up
   1. Assess every 4-6 weeks or sooner if ear pain or other bothersome symptoms occur
   2. If effusion persists at 3-month follow-up visit, hearing evaluation is indicated

ALLERGIC AND NONALLERGIC RHINITIS

I. Definition: Inflammation of mucous membranes of the nose, usually accompanied by edema of mucosa and a nasal discharge. Rhinitis may be allergic or nonallergic

II. Pathogenesis

A. Allergic rhinitis: An IgE-mediated inflammatory disease involving the nasal mucosa membranes
   1. When a person with a genetic predisposition to allergy is exposed to a strong allergic stimulus, antigen IgE-antibody molecules are produced and bind to mast cells in the respiratory epithelium
   2. Re-exposure to offending allergen causes a hypersensitivity to offending allergen and triggers the release of histamines and other mediators

3. Histamine release results in immediate local vasodilation, mucosal edema, and increased mucous production
4. A late-phase reaction sometimes occurs 4-8 hours after the original reaction in persons with severe disease; results in hyper-responsiveness to antigenic and nonantigenic stimuli and is linked to development of chronic disease
5. Most common form is the seasonal pattern due to inhalant pollen allergens
6. Year-round perennial type is difficult to diagnose and treat; usually related to house dust mites, mold, cockroaches, and animal dander; in adults, food allergies are a rare cause

B. Nonallergic Rhinitis
1. Vasomotor rhinitis or idiopathic perennial nonallergic rhinitis: Unknown etiology but possibly due to abnormal autonomic responsiveness or vascular dysfunction; unrelated to allergy, infection, structural lesions, systemic diseases, or drug use
2. Atrophic or geriatric rhinitis: Perennial nonallergic rhinitis resulting from progressive degeneration and atrophy of nasal mucous membranes and bones of nose
3. Chronic inflammatory diseases such as midline granuloma, Wegener's granuloma, and sarcoidosis present with chronic nasal congestion and rhinitis
4. Rhinitis medicamentosus or rebound rhinitis is due to overuse of topical decongestant
5. Rhinitis of pregnancy is due to hormonal increase (will not be discussed further)
6. NARES syndrome (non-allergic rhinitis with eosinophilia syndrome) occurs infrequently in adults who have nasal eosinophils but negative skin and *in vitro* tests
7. Gustatory rhinitis may be due to an overly sensitive cholinergic reflex that can be triggered by eating or cold air
8. Other causes: infections (chronic rhinosinusitis), anatomic problems (adenoidal hypertrophy, nasal polyps, deviated nasal septum), trauma, foreign bodies, neoplasm, cocaine abuse, and rhinitis associated with systemic diseases such as hypothyroidism

III. Clinical Presentation of allergic rhinitis and vasomotor rhinitis

A. Allergic rhinitis
1. Prevalence is increasing worldwide
2. Onset of symptoms is most common between ages 10-20; rarely begins before age 4 or after age 40
3. Usually involves the triad of nasal congestion, sneezing, and clear rhinorrhea
4. Nasal itching, nasal obstruction, nasal pain, post-nasal drip, coughing, sore throat, and itching and puffiness of eyes may occur
5. Individuals with allergic rhinitis are more likely to develop asthma over time than other individuals
6. There is an increased prevalence of acute and chronic bacterial sinusitis among patients with allergic rhinitis
7. Signs include the following:
   a. Pale, boggy nasal mucosa with clear thin secretions
   b. Enlarged nasal turbinates which may obstruct airway flow
   c. "Allergic shiners" or a dark discoloration beneath both eyes
   d. Cobblestone appearance of the conjunctiva
   e. "Dennie's lines" or extra wrinkles below the lower eyelids
   f. Transverse nasal crease due to chronic upward wiping of the nose
   g. Nasal salute
   h. Mouth-breathing
   i. Short upper lip
   j. Enlarged tonsils and adenoids
8. Associated with significant comorbidities and complications such as asthma, sinusitis, nasal polyposis, and otitis media with effusion (OME)

B. Vasomotor rhinitis
1. Onset is usually in adult life
2. Rapid onset of nasal congestion and a pronounced and noticeable postnasal drip are typical; unlike allergic rhinitis, pruritus is absent
3. Triggers of attacks are the following: abrupt changes in temperature and barometric pressure, odors, smoke, and emotional stress
4. Negative family history of allergy
5. Nasal smear and skin tests are negative
6. Patients are usually unresponsive to environmental controls and medications

IV. Diagnosis/Evaluation

    A. History
        1. Question about onset, duration, and progression of symptoms
        2. Explore relationship of symptoms to season, place, time of day, and activity
        3. Question about contact with offending allergens and other triggers such as exposure to cold air, ingestion of spicy foods, odors, and changes in temperature and barometric pressure
        4. Determine occupational exposure and obtain a detailed environmental history to identify precipitating factors
        5. Question about nasal stuffiness or obstruction, sensation of pressure over and under the eyes, itching of the eyes, nose and pharynx, sneezing, color, consistency, amount of nasal and postnasal discharges, and sensation of needing to constantly clear throat
        6. Ask about mouth breathing, changes in hearing and smell acuity, snoring during sleep, and fatigue
        7. Inquire about self-treatment, particularly duration and use of nasal sprays
        8. Inquire about family history and past history of allergies
        9. Assess impact on patient's quality of life

    B. Physical Examination
        1. Check pulse and blood pressure as sympathomimetic decongestants may increase both
        2. Measure temperature which should be normal
        3. Inspect eyes for allergic "shiners," tearing, conjunctival injection, lid swelling, and periorbital edema
        4. Palpate for sinus tenderness
        5. Examine ears to rule out otitis media and to check for serous otitis media
        6. Assess for nasal obstruction and polyps
        7. Inspect nasal mucosa noting color, edema, and type and color of nasal discharge
        8. Assess pharynx for tonsillar enlargement and inflammation
        9. Palpate lymph nodes
        10. Always check breath sounds to rule out concurrent asthma

    C. Differential Diagnosis; see pathogenesis (II.A.B.) for causes
        1. Patients with persistent sinusitis, asthma, or OME need evaluation for presence of allergies
        2. Suspect upper respiratory infections with a history of contagion, presence of fever, purulent nasal discharge, inflamed nasal mucosa, and absence of eosinophils on nasal smear
        3. Suspect foreign body or an anatomical problem if rhinitis is unilateral

    D. Diagnostic tests (diagnosis is usually made from the history and physical and no tests are required)
        1. Skin testing for allergies is the gold standard test; compare results with the clinical history
            a. Two types are available: epicutaneous (prick or scratch test) and intradermal (antigen is injected between skin layers)
            b. Warn patients to avoid use of antihistamines, decongestants, and corticosteroids before testing as these may interfere with results
        2. Nasal smear is often helpful; eosinophils are elevated with allergic rhinitis whereas an infection is likely if neutrophils predominate; peripheral eosinophil count is not useful
        3. Nasal cytology helps in differentiating allergic rhinitis from other forms (e.g., vasomotor, infectious rhinitis)
        4. Because serum IgE levels are elevated in 30-40% of patients with allergic rhinitis and increased levels occur in nonallergies, this testing has limited value
        5. *In vitro* serum allergy tests (radioallergosorbent, fluoroallergosorbent, and multiple allergosorbent tests) are expensive and not as specific nor as sensitive as skin testing
        6. If there is any question of an infectious process obtain a CBC
        7. Fiberoptic nasal endoscopy and/or rhinomanometry may be needed to rule out associated diseases such as sinusitis and anatomical problems; consult specialist

V. Plan/Management

    A. Allergic rhinitis
        1. Effective long-term management may prevent or reduce general respiratory tract inflammation and lower airway hyper-reactivity, thereby decreasing incidence and worsening of asthma and other diseases (e.g., otitis media, sinusitis)
        2. Patient Education: Allergen avoidance is the most effective form of treatment.
            a. The bedroom is considered the room that must be the most allergen-free
            b. Try to eliminate dust and allergen exposure in the household (see table that follows)

MEASURES OF ENVIRONMENTAL CONTROL IN THE HOME

→ Vacuum weekly (some vacuums spread dust and mites, so the vacuum should be cleaned regularly) or perform damp mopping

→ Dust furniture and all horizontal surfaces weekly with a damp cloth

→ Encase mattress and pillow in allergen-impermeable cover; wash sheets and blankets in hot water weekly

→ Remove carpets from bedroom; avoid lying on upholstered furniture; remove carpets laid on concrete

→ Avoid rubber mattress

→ Recommend keeping windows and doors closed to decrease influx of mold and pollen; may necessitate air conditioning in the summer (have AC unit professionally cleaned to clear mold/mildew off coils)

→ Reduce indoor humidity to less than 50%

→ Eliminate or restrict exposure to pets; use high efficiency particulate air (HEPA) filter or electrostatic air purifier if pets remain in house; wash pets weekly

→ To control cockroaches, use poison traps or bait; do not leave food or garbage exposed

→ Use clothes dryer rather than hanging clothes outside to air dry

→ Wear high-efficiency mask and long-sleeved shirt when gardening; bathe and change clothes immediately after coming inside

3. Inform patients that they may access information such as pollen counts on TV weather stations as well as on the internet (see following table for Websites)

WEBSITES FOR PATIENT INFORMATION

Organization	Website
American Academy of Allergy, Asthma and Immunology	www.aaaai.org
American College of Asthma, Allergy and Immunology	www.acaai.org
Asthma and Allergy Foundation of America	www.aafa.org

4. Drug therapy is indicated when allergen avoidance is ineffective or impractical
    a. No recommended first-line drug of choice; choice of medication depends on the patient's symptoms, adverse drug reactions, adherence factors, risk of drug interactions, and cost (see table COMPARATIVE EFFICACY)
    b. Because of potentially dangerous side effects (sedation and performance impairment) of first generation antihistamines, second generation antihistamines or nasal corticosteroids for severe cases are often considered the first-line drugs

COMPARATIVE EFFICACY OF MEDICATIONS

	Pruritus	Rhinorrhea	Nasal Blockage	Eye Symptoms
Oral antihistamines	+++	++	±	+++
Oral decongestants	---	±	+++	---
Antihistamine/decongestant combinations	+++	++	+++	+++
Intranasal decongestants	---	---	+++	---
Intranasal corticosteroids	+++	+++	++(+)	+
Intranasal cromolyn	+	+	±	---
Intranasal ipratropium	---	+++	---	---

5. Second generation antihistamines (see table that follows)
    a. Advantages: Fewer adverse drug effects and simpler dosing schedule than first-generation antihistamines
    b. Disadvantages: No relief for rhinorrhea and nasal congestion; do not control underlying inflammatory response

COMPARISON OF SECOND GENERATION ANTIHISTAMINES

	Cetirizine (Zyrtec)	Desloratadine (Clarinex)	Fexofenadine (Allegra)	Loratadine (Claritin and Claritin Reditabs*)
Formulation	Tablets: 5 mg, 10 mg Syrup: 1 mg/mL	Tablets: 5 mg	Tablets: 30 mg, 60 mg, 180 mg Capsules: 60 mg	Tablets: 10 mg Syrup: 1 mg/mL
Dosage	5 or 10 mg QD	5 mg QD (Initially 5 mg EOD**)	60 mg BID or 180 mg QD (Initially 60 mg QD)	10 mg QD (Initially 10 mg EOD**)
Sedation	Yes	No	No	No
Dry mouth and urinary retention	Yes	No	No	No
Interactions	Potentiates CNS depression with alcohol and other CNS depressants	None known	Avoid aluminum or magnesium-containing antacids	None known

*Rapidly disintegrating tablets; dissolve on tongue; swallow with or without water
** EOD - every other day

6. First generation antihistamines (see table that follows)
   a. Advantages: Inexpensive; anticholinergic properties may reduce rhinorrhea; early onset of action is useful for intermittent symptoms
   b. Disadvantages: Numerous adverse effects such as drowsiness, impaired performance, anticholinergic effects such as dry mouth, urinary retention, and constipation; do not relieve nasal congestion; must be cautious when used in the elderly; may worsen asthma symptoms; do not control underlying inflammatory response
   c. Warn patients to avoid driving cars or operating heavy machinery when beginning therapy
   d. Avoid or use cautiously in patients with prostate hypertrophy and angle-closure glaucoma
   e. Rule of thumb is to use the smallest dose that is effective
   f. Slowly titrate drugs beginning with one dose at bedtime for several days, then add a small morning dose; tolerance to sedative effects occurs after 1-2 weeks of dosing

FIRST GENERATION ANTIHISTAMINES

	Dose (mg)
Ethanolamine	
Diphenhydramine (Benadryl)*†	25-50 TID/QID
Clemastine (Tavist)†	1 BID
Alkylamine	
Chlorpheniramine (Chlor-Trimeton)†	4 QID or 8 BID
Piperazine	
Hydroxyzine (Atarax, Vistaril)	10-25 TID/QID
Piperidine	
Cyproheptadine (Periactin)	4 TID

*Benadryl may decrease cognitive function in elderly patients
†Over-the-counter medication

7. Azelastine HCl nasal spray (Astelin) is the first topical antihistamine
   a. Advantages: Effective in reducing allergic symptoms, has good safely profile, and is more beneficial in relieving nasal obstruction than oral antihistamines
   b. Disadvantages: Causes sedation and has a bitter taste
   c. Prescribe 2 sprays per nostril BID
8. Oral decongestants are often combined with antihistamines to enhance effectiveness and/or counterbalance sedative side effects (see table that follows); products containing phenylpropanolamine are banned because of increased risk of stroke in young women

COMMON COMBINATION ANTIHISTAMINE/DECONGESTANT PRODUCTS

Antihistamine/Decongestant	Brand Name	Dose
Chlorpheniramine 4 mg/ pseudoephedrine 60 mg	Deconamine	1 tab TID/QID
Fexofenadine 60 mg/pseudoephedrine 120 mg	Allegra-D	1 tab BID
Loratadine 10 mg/pseudoephedrine 240 mg	Claritin-D 24 Hour	1 tab QD

9. For patients with significant nasal congestion, a topical decongestant may be needed first
   a. Minimal side effects but ineffective for pulmonary and ocular allergic symptoms
   b. Never use beyond 3-4 days
   c. Prescribe oxymetazoline (Neo-Synephrine 12-Hour Spray) 2-3 sprays in each nostril up to every 10-12 hours
10. Steroid sprays are often drug of choice, particularly for severe cases, because they are the most effective and potent agents available for treatment (see table that follows)
    a. Advantages: Control nasal congestion and rhinorrhea; few adverse effects; control underlying anti-inflammatory response; greater efficacy of steroid sprays than antihistamines were found in several studies
    b. Disadvantages: Expensive; slow onset of activity; do not relieve ocular symptoms; adverse effects are epistaxis, nasal irritation, and, very rarely, septal perforation
    c. May be combined with antihistamines for enhanced effectiveness
    d. Steroid sprays have a slow onset of activity; warn patients they might <u>not</u> see effects for 2 weeks after initiating therapy
    e. Use on a regular basis and reduce dose when benefit is obtained

INTRANASAL CORTICOSTEROIDS

Medication	Dosing
Beclomethasone (Beconase AQ)	1-2 sprays in each nostril BID
Fluticasone propionate (Flonase)	1 spray in each nostril QD
Mometasone furoate (Nasonex)	2 sprays in each nostril QD
Triamcinolone (Nasacort AQ)	2 sprays in each nostril QD; reduce dose as condition improves

11. Oral corticosteroids are reserved for short-term therapy for patients with severe disease
12. Mast cell stabilizers are usually reserved for patients with chronic or severe symptoms
    a. Advantages: Good safety profile, control underlying inflammatory response
    b. Disadvantages: Less effective than other therapies in relieving nasal obstruction; frequent dosing makes it difficult for patients to adhere; expensive
    c. Prevent symptoms from starting and are generally not beneficial once an attack has started; can use prophylactically (e.g., just before visiting a home with a cat)
    d. Recommend over-the-counter, intranasal cromolyn sodium (NasalCrom) 1 spray in each nostril every 4 to 6 hours
    e. Concomitant use of decongestants may be useful to relieve congestion
13. Intranasal ipratropium
    a. Advantages: Excellent safety profile and few adverse reactions
    b. Disadvantage: Effective for only rhinorrhea; minimal effect on other symptoms
    c. Prescribe ipratropium bromide 0.03% aqueous solution (Atrovent nasal spray) 2 sprays in each nostril 2-3 times daily
14. Application of saline to nasal mucosa acts as a mild decongestant and can liquify mucus and prevent crusting; administer 2-4 times a day
15. Allergic conjunctivitis which often accompanies allergic rhinitis may require flushing eyes with artificial liquid tears or use of one of the following ophthalmic solutions:
    a. Naphazoline HCl 0.025% and pheniramine maleate 0.3% (Naphcon A) 1-2 drops in each eye up to 4 times daily
    b. Cromolyn sodium 4% (Crolom) 1-2 drops in each eye 4-6 times daily
16. Leukotriene modifiers: Some research studies have found these drugs effective in relieving symptoms; use montelukast (Singulair) for patients who don't benefit from or tolerate nasal steroids and/or antihistamines

17. For patients with nasal polyps, refer to specialist
18. Patient education
    a. Remind patients with perennial allergic rhinitis to take medications regularly rather than sporadically when symptoms occur
    b. Teach patients to read drug labels before taking over-the-counter medication as many cold products and sleep aids contain antihistamines
    c. Teach patient proper administration of intranasal medications (see following table)

INSTRUCTIONS FOR USE OF INTRANASAL MEDICATION
✓ Clear nasal passages or blow nose before administering medication
✓ Keep head upright and tilted slightly forward; breathe out slowly
✓ Squeeze the pump or press down the canister as you slowly breathe through nose
✓ Spray medication away from nasal septum
✓ Spray each nostril separately and wait at least 1 minute before second spray
✓ If possible, avoid sneezing or blowing nose for 5-10 minutes after spraying
✓ Cleanse medicine canister device after each use

19. Allergen immunotherapy (also see table that follows)
    a. Consider this therapy for patients who have demonstrable evidence of specific IgE antibodies to clinical relevant allergens after skin testing and who wish to avoid or reduce the long-term use of medications
    b. Immunotherapy is effective for pollen, fungi (molds), animal dander, dust mites, and cockroaches
    c. Decision to begin therapy should depend on degree to which symptoms can be reduced by avoidance and medication, amount and type of medications needed for symptom control, and the adverse effects of medications

GUIDELINES FOR THE SAFE AND EFFECTIVE USE OF ALLERGEN IMMUNOTHERAPY
• Contraindications: Severe asthma uncontrolled by pharmacotherapy, significant cardiovascular disease, and use of beta-adrenergic blocking agents
• Use very cautiously in older adults with comorbid conditions
• Whenever possible, use standardized extracts to prepare vaccine treatment
• Efficacy of immunotherapy depends on achieving an optimal therapeutic dose of each of the clinically relevant constituents in the vaccine
• Routine periodic skin testing or *in vitro* IgE antibody testing of patients receiving immunotherapy is not recommended
• Only administer the vaccine in settings where prompt recognition and treatment of anaphylaxis are assured
• Inject agent subcutaneously into triceps muscle with a 26- or 27-gauge syringe with a 3/8- or ½-inch nonremovable needle
• Patients should remain in clinician's office at least 20-30 minutes after injections
• The usual frequency of vaccine administration is 1-2 injections per week, at least 2 days apart
• When the maintenance dose is reached, the interval between injections can be progressively increased as tolerated to 4-6 weeks
• Clinical improvement is usually seen within 1 year after a patient reaches maintenance dose
• Evaluate patients every 6-12 months during immunotherapy
• Carefully consider stopping immunotherapy after 3-5 years

Adapted from Li, J.T., Lockey, R.F., Bernstein, I.L, Portnoy, J.M, & Nicklas, R.A. (2003). Allergen immunotherapy: A practice parameter. *Annals of Allergy, Asthma, and Immunology, 90*, 1-40.

B. Nonallergic rhinitis; difficult to relieve symptoms
    1. Nonspecific broad-based therapy includes topical azelastine or topical corticosteroids
    2. Symptomatic-specific therapy
        a. Decongestants for patients whose symptoms are primarily obstructive
        b. Topical ipratropium bromide for patients whose symptom is primarily rhinorrhea
        c. A nasal spray of physiological saline solution or a more thorough cleansing of nose with powered irrigators such as the Grossan irrigator may be helpful for postnasal drainage, sneezing, and congestion
    3. Patient education: increase water intake, decrease caffeine and alcohol intake (both have a diuretic effect), and consider adding humidity to bedroom

C. Follow up of all types of rhinitis
    1. Schedule visits in 2-3 weeks to review patient education topics and check therapy results
    2. Schedule quarterly or biannual rechecks depending on patient's level of comfort and health

EPISTAXIS

I. Definition: Nasal bleeding from any cause

II. Pathogenesis

    A. The nose acts as a conduit to allow air into the lungs and has a very well vascularized mucosa with a complex interior surface composed of folds and irregularities

    B. The blood supply of the nose comes from both the internal and external carotid systems

    C. More than 90% of bleeds are related to local irritation and most occur in the absence of a specific underlying anatomic lesion

    D. Bleeding is typically due to disruption of the nasal mucosa: dry nasal mucosa, infection, allergy, trauma (nose picking, forceful blowing, injury), foreign body, neoplasm, cocaine use

    E. Epistaxis is infrequently due to systemic diseases: liver disease, hypertension (hypertension does not cause nasal bleeding but may exacerbate the problem), bleeding disorders (such as thrombocytopenia and problems related to chemotherapy for cancer), hereditary hemorrhagic telangiectasia (Rendu-Osler-Weber disease), granulomatous disease (Wegener's, sarcoidosis)

    F. The following medications may be associated with bleeds: aspirin, warfarin, dipyridamole, antihistamines, nasal steroids, diuretics

    G. Site of the bleeding helps to determine the cause
        1. Anterior bleeds usually involve the Kiesselbach's plexus (triangle of the anterior portion of the septum) and result from local irritation, cracks in dry nasal mucosa, or trauma
        2. Posterior bleeds are usually just superior or inferior to the posterior tip of inferior turbinate and are associated with systemic causes or facial trauma

III. Clinical Presentation

    A. Approximately 10% of the population experiences at least one significant nosebleed

    B. Over 90% of nosebleeds are anterior
        1. Generally less severe and easier to control than posterior nosebleeds
        2. Usually are unilateral, continuous, and have moderate bleeding

    C. Posterior bleeds are often intermittent, severe, and difficult to treat
        1. Tend to occur in older persons
        2. Blood may flow into pharynx and lungs

IV. Diagnosis/Evaluation

    A. History; quickly assess patient and, if stable, begin history
        1. Question about onset, duration, pattern, and severity (quantity) of bleeding
        2. Ask about an increase in nasal mucus; if yes, determine color, character, and quantity
        3. Ask if nasal obstruction is present, and if so, is it an acute or chronic occurrence
        4. Ask about bleeding into pharynx which commonly indicates a posterior bleed
        5. Ask about occupational exposure to irritating chemicals or dust; ask about dry, indoor environment
        6. Inquire about medication usage; ask about cocaine use if appropriate
        7. Inquire about previous episodes and treatments
        8. Ask about trauma (injury, nose picking, forceful blowing)

9. Question about other medical conditions (infections, allergies, bleeding disorders, hypertension)
10. Inquire about history of clotting problems (easy bruising, hematuria, melena, heavy menstrual flow)

B. Physical Examination; patient is best examined sitting and leaning forward
1. Assess blood pressure and pulse
2. Use gentle suction with a bulb syringe removing blood and secretions to make visualization of the involved vessels possible
3. Locate bleeding site if possible; 90% are in the anterior septum; posterior site is indicated by persistent drainage of blood down the pharynx
4. If systemic illnesses are likely assess the following:
    a. Skin for pallor, rash, purpura, petechiae, telangiectasias
    b. Lymph nodes for enlargement due to malignancy or other illnesses
    c. Percuss sinuses to assess for sinusitis

C. Differential Diagnosis (see Pathogenesis II.C.-G.)

D. Diagnostic Tests; history and physical examination should guide selection of tests
1. Extensive evaluation should be reserved for cases that are recurrent or particularly severe
2. Hemoglobin or hematocrit if significant blood loss has occurred
3. CBC with differential, platelets, PT, and PTT if bleeding disorders are suspected

V. Plan/Management

A. Use the approaches outlined in the table below for anterior nose bleeds

---

MANAGEMENT OF ANTERIOR NOSE BLEEDS

- First, apply pressure to anterior nasal septum while head is tilted forward; continue pressure for 10-15 minutes (patient should be sitting and leaning forward)
- Then, if clot formation and bleeding cessation do not occur, do the following
    ✓ Place a small piece of cotton soaked in 1:1000 epinephrine or a vasoconstricting nosedrop such as phenylephrine (Neo-Synephrine) or oxymetazoline (Afrin) into the vestibule of the nose
    ✓ Press against the bleeding site for 10 to 15 minutes to promote vasoconstriction
    ✓ Remove to observe for bleeding (almost all venous types of anterior nosebleeds are stopped with this treatment)
- If bleeding continues, but has slowed considerably
    ✓ Repeat treatment
    ✓ Apply ice pack over the nose as an additional therapy
- If these remedies fail,
    ✓ Anesthetize the mucous membrane with 4% lidocaine or 4% cocaine (apply to cotton ball and hold in place for several minutes)
    ✓ Apply a silver nitrate stick to the bleeding site
- Finally, if bleeding persists consider the following (consider consultation with a specialist)
    ✓ Use adherent materials such as oxidized cellulose (Oxycel, Surgicel), microfibrillar collagen (Avitene), or absorbable gelatin sponge (Gelfoam) placed at the bleeding site; these agents dissolve in a few days
    ✓ A compressed nasal tampon (Merocel) can also be placed in nares and left in place for 1-3 days; usually tampon is impregnated with antibiotic ointment and patient is treated with antistaphylococcal antibiotics

---

B. Patients with anterior bleeds who do not respond to above treatments should be referred to emergency department for cautery and/or packing; refer recurrent and severe cases to specialist

C. Patients with posterior bleeds should be immediately referred to otolaryngologic specialist; while awaiting consult, efforts to control bleeding should be limited to spraying nose with topical anesthetic or vasoconstricting substance such as 5% oxymetazoline or 4% cocaine

D. Patient education
1. Instruct patient regarding management of simple nose bleeds at home
    a. Sit up, lean forward, spray nose with over-the-counter nasal sprays (Afrin, Neo-Synephrine), then apply and press cotton soaked with nasal spray against bleeding area
    b. Apply petrolatum-based ointment to septum to prevent further drying
    c. Limit heavy lifting, straining, bending over, intake of spicy or hot foods, hot showers, and medications that might affect hemostasis

2. Teach about prevention of nosebleeds
   a. Increase humidity in home through use of humidifier, especially during winter months
   b. Advise liberal use of lubricant such a petrolatum in nares to promote hydration
   c. Recommend trial of nasal saline drops, particularly at night
   d. Teach to avoid traumatizing nose

E. Follow Up: None indicated for cases due to local trauma or inflammation

FOREIGN BODY IN THE NOSE

I. Definition: Presence of object(s) in the nasal cavity

II. Pathogenesis: Intentional placement of an object in nose, or occasionally accidental placement of a foreign body while patient is attempting to sniff or smell the object

III. Clinical Presentation

A. The key feature is unilateral symptoms
   1. Symptoms include unilateral obstruction, mild discomfort, sneezing, and occasionally epistaxis
   2. Unilateral purulent, foul-smelling, nasal discharge can also occur over time
   3. When an alkaline disk battery is lodged, the symptoms are more acute and may include electrical burns and necrosis

B. Complications include local infection, inflammation, chronic sinusitis, and rhinolith (occurs when foreign body remains in nose for long time and becomes calcified); aspiration can be avoided by prompt and skilled removal

IV. Diagnosis/Evaluation

A. History
   1. Inquire about onset and duration of symptoms
   2. Determine type of foreign body

B. Physical Examination
   1. Test both nares for patency
   2. Examine both nares with nasal speculum; powerful illumination and adequate visualization is mandatory (see Plan/Management V.A. for strategies to improve visualization)

C. Differential Diagnosis
   1. Suppurative rhinitis
   2. Sinusitis
   3. Adenoiditis
   4. Nasal or nasopharyngeal tumors
   5. Nasal polyps

D. Diagnostic Tests: X-rays may be helpful if the object is radiopaque or has become calcified, but usually no tests are needed

V. Plan/Management

A. Use topical decongestant such as Neo-Synephrine to reduce mucosal edema, remove secretions with a small suction tip, and then, visualize object with an endoscope

B. Method of removal depends on location and type of foreign body; consider the following:
   1. For shallow objects, occlude the uninvolved nostril and have the patient blow forcefully out or remove with a Frazier tip suction
   2. For hard objects, a right-angle hook can be placed behind the object and pulled out slowly; insert instruments perpendicular to the plane of the face and avoid instrumenting the medial wall to prevent damage to the turbines

3. Soft objects can be grasped with alligator forceps if the patient is cooperative; instruments introduced into the nasal passage require a steady hand resting on the patient's head
4. Some experts recommend removal with a Fogarty or small Foley catheter
   a. Catheter is placed beyond the foreign body and then inflated with 2-3 ml of saline solution
   b. Then gently draw catheter out, expelling the object
   c. Aspiration is a risk because foreign body may be pushed posteriorly into the nasopharynx

C. After removal of object if local irritation is present, use saline drops 2-3 times/day for 2-3 days or antibacterial ointment such as bacitracin or mupirocin; use sterile water if the foreign object was an alkaline battery

D. For uncooperative patients, or when the nasal passage is completely occluded by an expanding foreign object such as plant materials, beans, or other seeds, or when there is marked edema and inflammation, referral to a specialist is indicated

E. Always refer to a specialist if the foreign body appears to be going deeper

F. Follow Up
   1. Advise to return if signs of retained foreign body develop (purulent discharge or epistaxis)
   2. Evaluate healing of mucosa in 2 days

RHINOSINUSITIS

I. Definition: Acute, subacute, or chronic inflammation of the mucous membranes that line the paranasal sinuses and concomitant inflammation of nasal mucosa

A. Acute rhinosinusitis: Abrupt onset of infection with duration of symptoms of less than 4 weeks

B. Subacute rhinosinusitis: Persistent occurrence of purulent nasal discharge despite therapy; epithelial damage is usually reversible; minimal to moderate symptoms last 4-12 weeks

C. Chronic rhinosinusitis: Prolonged inflammation and/or repeated or inadequately treated acute infection; irreversible damage to the mucosa is present, symptoms last >12 weeks

D. Recurrent acute rhinosinusitis: Four or more episodes per year with each episode of at least seven days' duration; absence of intervening signs and symptoms

II. Pathogenesis

A. Etiological factors
   1. Main factor is obstruction of the sinus ostia (small opening in which the maxillary, frontal, ethmoid, and sphenoid sinuses all drain into nasal cavity) that leads to lower levels of oxygen within sinuses, decreased clearance of foreign material, and mucus stasis which creates a good environment for pathogens to grow; the following are predisposing factors:
      a. Recent upper respiratory infection
      b. Allergic rhinitis
      c. Environmental pollutants (smoke)
      d. Anatomic abnormalities such as a deviated septum or adenoidal hypertrophy
      e. "Aspirin triad" of aspirin sensitivity, asthma, and nasal polyps
      f. Medication side effects (antiosteoporosis agents, hormone replacement sprays, or rhinitis medicamentosa from abuse of topical decongestants and cocaine)
      g. Diving and swimming
      h. Extension of dental abscess
      i. Neoplasms
      j. Hormone-based turbinate edema as occurs during pregnancy
      k. Trauma
      l. Foreign body
   2. Other patients have problems with mucus stasis due to immune deficiency, immotile cilia syndrome, or cystic fibrosis

B.   Pathogens in acute sinusitis
1.   Common
a.   Viruses (viral rhinosinusitis occurs more often than bacterial rhinosinusitis)
b.   *Streptococcus pneumoniae*; penicillin-resistant *S. pneumoniae* is becoming common
c.   *Haemophilus influenzae* (may be ß-lactamase producing)
d.   *Moraxella catarrhalis* ([may be ß-lactamase producing]; prevalence greater among children than adults)
e.   *Streptococcus pyogenes*
2.   Less common
a.   Streptococcus species
b.   *Chlamydia pneumoniae*
c.   *Staphylococcus aureus*
d.   Fungi (e.g., *Aspergillus fumigatus*) (more common in patients who are immunosuppressed or have diabetes mellitus)

C.   Pathogens in chronic or subacute sinusitis are usually polymicrobial but commonly include the following:
1.   Anaerobic bacteria
2.   *Staphylococcus aureus*

D.   Anaerobes are common in sinusitis resulting from dental infections

III.   Clinical Presentation

A.   Most sinus disease involves the maxillary and anterior ethmoidal sinuses

B.   Acute bacterial rhinosinusitis has the following characteristics (see following table):

DIAGNOSTIC PREDICTORS OF BACTERIAL RHINOSINUSITIS*	
Major factors	Facial pain or pressure (requires another major factor for diagnosis)
	Facial congestion or fullness
	Nasal obstruction
	Nasal purulence or discolored postnasal discharge
	Hyposmia or anosmia
	Fever (acute sinusitis only)
Minor factors	Headache
	Halitosis
	Fatigue
	Dental pain
	Cough
	Ear pain, pressure, or fullness
	Fever (nonacute sinusitis)

*Diagnosis of bacterial rhinosinusitis depends on the presence of at least 2 major factors or 1 major factor and 2 minor factors
Adapted from Lanza, D.C., & Kennedy, D.W. (1997). Adult rhinosinusitis defined. In J.B. Anon (Ed.). Report of the Rhinosinusitis Task Force Committee Meeting. *Otolaryngology–Head and Neck Surgery, 111*(Suppl), S1-S7.

1.   Other clinical features include sore throat, early morning periorbital swelling, toothache, malaise, increased pain with coughing, bending over, or sudden head movement, and lack of response to decongestants
2.   Signs and symptoms are prolonged for at least for 10 days

C.   Subacute or chronic sinusitis has the following characteristics:
1.   Nasal discharge, nasal congestion, or cough lasting >30 days
2.   Hallmark is dull ache or pressure across midface or headache
3.   Other symptoms include thick postnatal drip, "popping" ears, eye pain, halitosis, chronic cough, and fatigue

D.   Thick, tenacious, brown secretions are characteristic of fungal sinusitis

E.   All types of sinusitis may exacerbate asthma

F.   Diabetics and immunosuppressed patients often experience severe, invasive sinus disease

G.   Complications include contiguous spread or hematogenous dissemination of infection and can result in life-threatening intraorbital (cellulitis, abscess) and intracranial suppuration (cavernous sinus thrombosis, meningitis, subdural empyema, brain abscess); patients with frontal headaches and associated frontal sinusitis are at greatest risk for intracranial complications

IV.   Diagnosis/Evaluation

A.   History
       1.   Question regarding onset, duration, and seasonality of symptoms
       2.   Ask whether symptoms are improving or worsening
       3.   Inquire about the laterality and quality (mucoid, purulent, serous) of nasal discharge; change in color or consistency is not a specific sign of bacterial infection
       4.   Ask about fever and systemic symptoms such as fatigue
       5.   Question about character (dry, productive) and timing (day, night, continual) of cough
       6.   Ask patient to describe pain and what aggravates it
       7.   Ask about timing and quality of headaches and morning puffiness about the eyes
       8.   Ask about past episodes and treatments
       9.   Inquire about past medical history such as allergies, diabetes mellitus, immunodeficiency, asthma
       10.   Question about smoking, recent trauma to the nose, recent upper respiratory infections
       11.   Inquire about family history of allergies, immunodeficiency, chronic respiratory complaints

B.   Physical Examination
       1.   Determine vital signs
       2.   Examine eyes, noting peri-orbital swelling and presence of allergic shiners; if proptosis, impaired visual acuity, or impaired extraocular mobility are present, computerized tomography is needed to rule out suppurative complications
       3.   Examine nasal mucosa for erythema, edema, and discharge
       4.   Determine patency of both nasal nares
       5.   Anterior rhinoscopy (use of nasal speculum and otoscope) is important; use of topical decongestant before examination may facilitate inspection
             a.   Does not allow visualization of middle meatus, but can view inferior turbinate and can evaluate quality of mucus within anterior nose
             b.   Determine presence of polyps, septal deviation, and other anatomical deformities
       6.   Examine ears, throat, and mouth for signs of inflammation
       7.   Transilluminate and percuss frontal and maxillary sinuses
       8.   Examine teeth and gingivae for caries and inflammation; tap maxillary teeth with tongue blade because 5% to 10% of maxillary sinusitis is due to dental root infection
       9.   Palpate neck and jaw for lymphadenopathy
       10.   Auscultate heart and lungs
       11.   Perform a neurological examination to rule out complications

C.   Differential Diagnosis
       1.   Any condition that results in rhinitis (see Pathogenesis II.A.)
       2.   Differentiating viral from bacterial rhinosinusitis is difficult because viral infection frequently precedes bacterial infection
             a.   Typically, in bacterial rhinosinusitis symptoms worsen after 5 days and persist for at least 10 days; persistence of respiratory symptoms without evidence that they are beginning to resolve suggests bacterial infection
             b.   Symptoms are more severe and patients with bacterial infections often have purulent nasal discharge for 3-4 days and fever >102°F (39°C) (see table DIAGNOSTIC PREDICTORS OF BACTERIAL RHINOSINUSITIS, III.B.)

D.   Diagnostic Tests
       1.   None indicated for typical presentation and for first episode of acute rhinosinusitis
       2.   Sinus aspiration with culture is the "gold standard" test (impractical in most primary care settings)
       3.   Radiologic studies are not routinely ordered and must be interpreted cautiously
             a.   The common cold often includes radiologic evidence of sinus involvement (abnormal images only reflect inflammation, they do not pinpoint whether the inflammation is viral, bacterial or allergic in origin)
             b.   Order radiographs to confirm clinical impression and in the following: patients with frontal headaches, refractory cases, when complications are suspected, and when diagnosis is unclear

(1) Sinus x-rays
    (a) Need antero-posterior, lateral, and occipitomental (Waters view) views
    (b) An air-fluid level or complete opacification of the sinuses and thickening of the mucosal lining are most diagnostic
    (c) Accuracy of diagnosing ethmoid disease is questionable with x-rays
(2) Computerized tomography (CT scan) is gold standard of radiographic study, but is reserved for recalcitrant cases and patients in need of surgery

4. Flexible fiberoptic rhinoscopy, after the topical application of a vasoconstrictor and anesthetic, may be indicated
5. CBC with differential indicated for severely ill patients
6. Allergy testing when the history suggests an allergic disease
7. Consider ordering nasal cytology (diagnosis of allergic rhinitis, eosinophilia syndrome), a sweat chloride test (diagnosis of cystic fibrosis), and tests for immunodeficiency in recurrent cases

V. Plan/Management

A. Treatment of acute and subacute rhinosinusitis
  1. Antibiotics
    a. Although 40% of cases recover spontaneously without drugs, antibiotics are indicated for correctly diagnosed bacterial infections because they arrest progression to chronic sinusitis and concomitant permanent mucosal damage and also prevent complications
    b. Duration of treatment is controversial; 10-14 days is usually recommended; some experts suggest that antibiotics be continued until patient is free of symptoms and then for an additional 7 days
    c. First line drug is amoxicillin (Amoxil) 500 mg TID; but should not be drug of choice in certain patients (see table RISK FACTORS PROMPTING USE OF SECOND-LINE DRUGS); in areas with high resistance to *S. pneumoniae* double the dosage
    d. Trimethoprim-sulfamethoxazole and erythromycin-sulfisoxazole are sometimes recommended as first line drugs, however, because they have substantial resistance to *S. pneumoniae*, other antibiotics should be used

RISK FACTORS PROMPTING USE OF SECOND-LINE DRUGS
Antibiotic use in previous 4-6 weeks
Resistance common in community
Active or passive smoking
Allergy to penicillin or amoxicillin
Frontal or sphenoidal sinusitis
Complicated ethmoidal sinusitis
Possibly severe and protracted symptoms

Adapted from Brook, I., Gooch, W.M., III, Jenkins, S.G., et al. (2000). Medical management of acute bacterial sinusitis: Recommendations of a Clinical Advisory Committee on Pediatric and Adult Sinusitis. *Annals of Otology, Rhinology, and Laryngology, 109,* 2-20.

    e. Second line drugs
      (1) Amoxicillin/clavulanate (Augmentin) 500-875 mg BID or Augmentin XR, 2 tabs every 12 hours
      (2) Cefdinir (Omnicef) 300 mg BID
      (3) Cefuroxime axetil (Ceftin) 250-500 mg BID
      (4) Cefpodoxime proxetil (Vantin) 200-400 mg BID
    f. Third line drugs (useful for patients who are penicillin and cephalosporin sensitive): Gatifloxacin, levofloxacin, or moxifloxacin
    g. Switch to another drug if there is lack of response at ≥72 hours; a good choice is high-dose amoxicillin/clavulanate; use a total of 3-3.5 g/day
    h. A single dose of ceftriaxone (50 mg/kg/day) IM or IV can be given if patient has difficulty taking oral antibiotics (e.g., vomiting)

2. Decongestants or saline nasal spray at the time of diagnosis of acute sinusitis and in acute episodes of subacute and chronic sinusitis can improve patency of ostiomeatal unit
   a. Topical decongestants should be used no longer than 3-4 days. Use oxymetazoline (Neo-Synephrine 12 hour spray 0.05%) 2-3 sprays in each nostril up to every 10-12 hours
   b. Alternatively, use saline nasal drops, 2-3 drops in each nostril BID-QID (1/4 tsp of salt in 8 oz of boiled water)
   c. Oral decongestants are not as effective as topical agents but can be used for a longer time period
      (1) Use cautiously in patients with hypertension
      (2) Pseudoephedrine hydrochloride (Sudafed) 60 mg every 4-6 hours
3. Nasal corticosteroids are not recommended for the treatment of acute rhinosinusitis

B. Treatment of chronic sinusitis
   1. Antibiotics: prescribe a β-lactamase stable antibiotic such as amoxicillin/clavulanate (Augmentin) or clarithromycin (Biaxin) and extend treatment for 2-4 weeks
   2. Topical nasal steroid sprays may be effective, but should not be used during acute episodes or exacerbations; prescribe one of the following:
      a. Beclomethasone (Beconase AQ) 1-2 sprays in each nostril BID
      b. Fluticasone propionate (Flonase), 1 spray in each nostril QD
      c. Decrease dosages as symptoms improve

C. For acute sinusitis due to dental infection prescribe amoxicillin/clavulanate (Augmentin)

D. Treatment of fungal infections involves surgery and broad-spectrum antibiotics for intercurrent bacterial infections

E. Oral antihistamines should not be used unless patient has allergies as they tend to slow the movement of secretions out of the sinuses

F. Referral to a specialist is needed for the following:
   1. Recurrent, recalcitrant symptoms
   2. Exquisite pain with palpation or percussion of the face
   3. Possibility of cellulitis or other severe complications
   4. Periorbital swelling
   5. Uncontrolled asthma, nasal polyposis, or severe allergies

G. Functional endoscopic sinus surgery which removes only affected tissue has improved the surgical treatment of sinus disease

H. Patient Education
   1. Instruct patient to return for further evaluation if symptoms are not improved within 48 hours
   2. Teach patient about the complications of sinusitis, particularly the need to return if there is swelling in the periorbital area
   3. Humidify the air
   4. Increase fluid intake
   5. Steam inhalation and warm compresses often help relieve pressure
   6. Sleep with head of bed elevated
   7. Avoid allergens and excessively dry heat
   8. Avoid swimming/diving and air travel during acute period
   9. Avoid use of antihistamines unless there is an allergic basis to disease
   10. Encourage cessation of smoking
   11. Teach proper application of nasal sprays (see table on instructions for use of intranasal medications in ALLERGIC RHINITIS section)
   12. Patients who have recurrent sinusitis should be instructed to begin decongestants at the first sign of sinusitis to facilitate sinus drainage and decrease development of infection

I. Follow Up
   1. If no decrease in symptoms in 48-72 hours, patient should be re-evaluated; refer to specialist if symptoms are actually worsening
   2. Schedule return visit for 10-14 days
   3. Patients with chronic sinusitis who do not have marked improvement in four weeks with continuous medical therapy may require needle aspiration of a maxillary sinus or surgery

PHARYNGITIS

I.   Definition: Inflammation of the pharynx and surrounding lymph tissue (tonsils)

II.   Pathogenesis

    A.   Viruses are the most common pathogens; the following are common viral infections:
        1.   Infections due to rhinovirus, adenovirus, influenza, parainfluenza, coronavirus, echovirus, respiratory syncytial virus
        2.   Herpangina due to Coxsackie virus and echovirus
        3.   Hand, foot, and mouth syndrome due to Coxsackie virus
        4.   Infectious mononucleosis caused by Epstein-Barr virus
        5.   Human immunodeficiency virus (HIV) infection

    B.   Bacteria (listed common to rare)
        1.   Group A β-hemolytic streptococcus
        2.   *Neisseria gonorrhoeae*
        3.   *Corynebacterium diphtheriae*
        4.   Streptococci of serogroups *C* and *G* (often associated with contaminated food or water)

    C.   Other atypical agents that occur primarily in adults include *Mycoplasma pneumoniae* (uncommon) and *Chlamydia trachomatis* (rare)

    D.   Fungus: *Candida albicans*

    E.   Peritonsillar abscess: Often due to anaerobic bacteria, but may be due to Group A streptococci, *Haemophilus influenzae*, or *Staphylococcus aureus*

    F.   Noninfectious causes
        1.   Allergic rhinitis or post-nasal drip
        2.   Mouth breathing
        3.   Trauma from heat, alcohol, irritants such as marijuana or sharp objects
        4.   Subacute thyroiditis in females

III.   Clinical presentation of common causes of pharyngitis

    A.   Pharyngitis due to respiratory viruses such as adenovirus, influenza, parainfluenza, respiratory syncytial virus
        1.   Sore throat is often accompanied by conjunctivitis, coryza, cough, diarrhea
        2.   Typically patient is afebrile and has gradual onset of symptoms

    B.   Herpangina
        1.   Small oral vesicles or ulcers may be on tonsils, pharynx, or posterior buccal mucosa
        2.   Fever, headache, and malaise often accompany sore throat

    C.   Hand, foot, and mouth syndrome: usually oral lesions and sore throat are accompanied by lesions on hands and feet; may have lesions on arms, legs, buttocks as well

    D.   Infectious mononucleosis: Exudative tonsillitis with fever, fatigue, lymphadenopathy, and palatal petechiae (see section on INFECTIOUS MONONUCLEOSIS)

    E.   Primary HIV infection resembles signs and symptoms of mononucleosis with sore throat, fever, malaise, myalgia, photophobia, lymphadenopathy, and rash; duration is few days to 2 weeks

F. Pharyngitis due to Group A β-hemolytic streptococci; referred to as strep throat or GAS pharyngitis
    1. Epidemiology
        a. Mode of transmission is usually via direct projection of large droplets or physical transfer of respiratory secretions; rarely due to contaminated articles or ingestion of contaminated milk or other food
        b. Prolonged carriage of streptococci may occur in the throat or upper respiratory tract for weeks to months
        c. Incubation period usually ranges from 2-5 days
        d. Period of communicability: During incubation period and clinical illness or approximately 10 days; after 24 hours of antibiotic therapy, person is no longer infectious
        e. Predominantly a disease of children 5-15 years, but can occur in all age groups
        f. Commonly seen in 5-10% of adults with pharyngitis
        g. Occurs in winter or early spring
    2. Symptoms include sudden onset of fever >101°F, headaches, and sore throat with dysphagia and without cold-type symptoms such as nasal congestion
    3. Erythema of tonsils and pharynx with white or yellow exudate occur
    4. "Strawberry" tongue presents as a thick white coat with hypertrophied red papillae
    5. Tender and enlarged anterior cervical lymph nodes are often present
    6. Abdominal pain, vomiting, and headache may occur, whereas upper respiratory symptoms suggest viral pharyngitis
    7. Without proper antimicrobial treatment, streptococcal pharyngitis can lead to serious suppurative (direct extension from pharyngeal infection) and nonsuppurative complications (arise from immune responses to acute infection)
        a. Suppurative adenitis involving tender, enlarged nodes (see section CERVICAL ADENITIS)
        b. Scarlet fever or scarlatina (suppurative)
            (1) "Sandpaper" rash due to a vascular response to bacterial exotoxin occurs
            (2) Exanthem appears 24-48 hours after infection and lasts 4-10 days
            (3) Presents as fine, pin-head sized eruptions, often confluent, on an erythematous base which blanches on pressure
            (4) Rash rapidly becomes generalized but is typically absent on the face which usually has a flushed appearance with circumoral pallor
            (5) Petechiae may be present in a linear pattern along the major skin folds in the axillae and antecubital fossa (Pastia's sign)
            (6) Rash fades 3-4 days after onset
            (7) Desquamation of the skin usually occurs at the end of first week and disappears by end of 3 weeks
        c. Peritonsillar abscess (suppurative) (see III.K.)
        d. Glomerulonephritis (nonsuppurative) appears 1-3 weeks after pharyngeal infection (proper treatment with antimicrobials does not prevent)
        e. Rheumatic fever (nonsuppurative); criteria for diagnosis is seen in table that follows
            (1) Leading cause of cardiac death in individuals between 5 and 24 years; chronic cardiac valve disease and mitral regurgitation are the major complications
            (2) Carditis is a new or changed murmur, a pericardial friction rub or effusion, and a recent or worsening heart enlargement with or without heart failure
            (3) Polyarthritis, the most common major manifestation, is a benign condition involving the larger joints such as the knees, ankles, elbows, and wrists
            (4) Sydenham's chorea, a benign sign, presents as purposeless, involuntary, rapid movements of the trunk and/or extremities
            (5) Subcutaneous nodules are painless and freely movable; located under the skin over the extensor surfaces of joints (e.g., elbows, knees, and wrists)
            (6) Rheumatic fever lasts an average of less than 3 months; fewer than 5% of the cases persist for more than 6 months

```
┌─────────────────────────────────────────────────────────────────────────────┐
│ ╔═══════════════════════════════════════════════════════════════════════╗ │
│ ║  CHARACTERISTICS OF ACUTE RHEUMATIC FEVER (JONES CRITERIA, UPDATED 1992) ║ │
│ ╟───────────────────────────────────────────────────────────────────────╢ │
│ ║  Two major manifestations or one major and 2 minor manifestations are   ║ │
│ ║  required to make the diagnosis:                                        ║ │
└─────────────────────────────────────────────────────────────────────────────┘
```

Two major manifestations or one major and 2 minor manifestations are required to make the diagnosis:

Major manifestations	Minor manifestations
Carditis	Clinical
Polyarthritis	Fever
Chorea	Arthralgias
Erythema marginatum (rare)	Previous acute rheumatic fever or evidence of pre-existing rheumatic heart disease
Subcutaneous nodules	Laboratory
	Acute phase reaction
	Leukocytosis
	Elevated erythrocyte sedimentation rate
	Abnormal C-reactive protein
	Prolonged PR interval or other electrocardiographic changes

Plus Evidence of a preceding streptococcal infection such as elevated or increasing antistreptolysin-O or other streptococcal antibodies, positive throat culture for group A streptococcus, recent scarlet fever

Adapted from Dajani, A.S., et al. (1993). Guidelines for the diagnosis of rheumatic fever: Jones criteria, updated 1992. *Circulation, 87,* 302-307.

G. Pharyngitis due to *Corynebacterium diphtheriae* (rare in US)
   1. Grayish brown, adherent membrane on the nasal mucosa, tonsils, uvula, or pharynx
   2. Bleeding occurs when membrane is removed

H. Pharyngitis due to *Neisseria gonorrhoeae* and *Chlamydia trachomatis*
   1. Seen in those patients who practice orogenital sex
   2. Commonly presents as a chronic sore throat

I. Pharyngitis due to *Mycoplasma pneumoniae*
   1. Uncommon in children <5 years of age, but seen in adolescents and adults
   2. Signs and symptoms indistinguishable from streptococcal disease

J. Pharyngitis due to *Candida albicans*
   1. Thin diffuse or patchy exudate on mucous membranes
   2. Patients typically have history of antibiotic use or are immunosuppressed

K. Peritonsillar abscess
   1. Most common in older children and adults following an episode of tonsillitis
   2. Often presents with gradually increasing unilateral ear and throat pain
   3. Dysphagia, dysphonia, drooling, and trismus (difficulty opening mouth) are common
   4. Muffled "hot potato" voice may be present
   5. The affected tonsil is usually grossly swollen medially and erythematous and may displace uvula and soft palate to contralateral side
   6. Swelling and erythema of the soft palate are characteristic
   7. Fluctuance may be felt with palpation of affected side
   8. Enlarged and very tender lymph nodes are usually present

IV. Diagnosis/Evaluation

A. History
   1. Determine onset and duration of symptoms
   2. Question about rhinorrhea and coughing (suggestive of viral agent)
   3. Inquire about trismus, drooling and dysphagia (suggestive of peritonsillar abscess)
   4. Ask about mouth lesions (suggestive of herpangina, hand, foot, and mouth syndrome, and thrush)
   5. Inquire about skin changes and exanthems
   6. Determine other associated symptoms such as abdominal pain, headache, and fatigue
   7. Ascertain that sore throat is not significantly reducing intake of fluids
   8. Inquire about possible streptococcal exposure
   9. Inquire about immunization status
   10. If applicable, inquire about sexual practices

B. Physical Examination
   1. Do not attempt to examine the pharynx of a patient who has drooling, stridor, or trouble breathing (may have epiglottitis)
   2. Measure vital signs
   3. Observe appearance for signs of toxicity and distress
   4. Inspect skin for color and exanthems
   5. Palpate skin for texture and turgor, noting whether the skin has a "sandpaper" rash
   6. Inspect mouth for lesions and thrush
   7. Examine ears for concurrent otitis media or effusion
   8. Visualize throat and pharynx for exudate and swelling (unilateral swelling occurs with peritonsillar abscess)
   9. Palpate jaw and neck for adenopathy and nuchal rigidity
   10. Perform complete heart and lung examinations
   11. Depending on history of sexual activity, may need to perform genitourinary examination
   12. Palpate abdomen

C. Differential Diagnosis
   1. Stomatitis
   2. Rhinitis or sinusitis with post nasal drip
   3. Epiglottitis
   4. Thyroiditis
   5. Oropharyngeal anthrax (typically accompanied by ulcers at base of tongue and may have neck swelling and difficulty breathing)

D. Diagnostic Tests
   1. Diagnosis of GAS should be suspected on clinical presentation and epidemiological grounds (patient's age, the season, and family and community epidemiology) and then supported by results of a laboratory test
      a. Patients with acute onset of sore throat, fever, headache, pain on swallowing, anterior cervical node enlargement, and abdominal pain who do not have features suggestive of a viral syndrome (cold-type symptoms, conjunctivitis, diarrhea) should be tested
      b. A positive throat culture (sensitivity of 90-95%) or rapid antigen detection testing (RADT) (sensitivity 60-95%) provides confirmation of diagnosis
      c. A negative RADT should be confirmed with throat culture results; in adults, the clinician may forgo culture testing, as the incidence of GAS and risk for rheumatic fever is low in the adult population
      d. Follow-up cultures are not routinely indicated for asymptomatic patients who complete their courses of antibiotics; patients with history of rheumatic fever or who develop pharyngitis during outbreaks of rheumatic fever or glomerulonephritis should have follow-up testing
      e. Testing of asymptomatic household contacts for GAS is not recommended except during outbreaks or when contacts have increased risk of developing complications; also test contacts who have rheumatic fever, glomerulonephritis, or symptoms suggestive of GAS
   2. Consider heterophil agglutination, or mono spot test
   3. Consider CBC with differential; expect WBC elevation with bacterial infection and WBC decrease with viral agent
   4. Obtain culture on Thayer-Martin medium if gonococcal pharyngitis is suspected
   5. If acute HIV infection is suspected, measure HIV RNA levels or obtain p24 antigen
   6. Consider viral cultures of throat and mouth lesions
   7. Tests for diagnosing peritonsillar abscess
      a. Consider ultrasonography or computed tomographic scanning
      b. Needle aspiration of abscess and culture; performed by trained clinician
   8. To diagnose diphtheria, order culture of pseudomembrane in Loeffler's or tellurite selective medium

V. Plan/Management

A. For viral pharyngitis (i.e., herpangina, hand, foot, and mouth syndrome, and infectious mononucleosis), treatment is symptomatic, such as pain medication and use of hard candy, lozenges, or warm saline gargles to soothe throat

B. Streptococcal pharyngitis
   1. Therapy is aimed at preventing suppurative complications such as rheumatic fever and decreasing infectivity
   2. A delay of treatment as long as 9 days after acute onset does not increase risk of rheumatic fever

3. Treatment of choice is oral or intramuscular penicillin
   a. Penicillin V (Veetids) 500 mg BID or TID PO for 10 days (take on empty stomach)
   b. Benzathine penicillin G (IM) 1,200,000 units
      (1) Be familiar with signs, symptoms, and treatment of anaphylaxis and observe patient for 30 minutes after injection.
      (2) Bring medication to room temperature before injecting to reduce discomfort
4. Antibiotics for patients allergic to penicillin
   a. Because of the increase in macrolide-resistant group A streptococcus, always prescribe penicillin unless patient has a penicillin allergy
   b. Prescribe erythromycin stearate: 1 g per day, divided into 2 or 4 doses
   c. First- and second-generation cephalosporins and azithromycin are acceptable alternatives to erythromycin; however, remember that 15% of penicillin-allergic persons also are allergic to cephalosporins
5. Treatment of patient who has recurrence of streptococcal pharyngitis shortly after completing recommended antibiotic therapy includes one of following:
   a. Retreat with same antibiotic
   b. Prescribe an alternative oral antibiotic such as amoxicillin-clavulanic acid (Augmentin) 500 mg BID or clindamycin (Cleocin) 150-300 mg every six hours; take with full glass of water
   c. Administer IM dose of benzathine penicillin G
   d. Administer benzathine penicillin G with rifampin PO (20 mg/kg/day in 2 divided doses for 4 days; maximum daily dose is 600 mg); addition of rifampin to benzathine penicillin may be helpful in eradicating streptococci from pharynx
   e. Also, rifampin 20 mg/kg/day PO once daily added during the final 4 days of a 10-day course of oral penicillin V might increase rate of eradication
6. Treatment of asymptomatic contacts is not recommended except in cases at increased risk of frequent infections or nonsuppurative streptococcal sequelae
7. Treatment of streptococcal pharyngeal carriers;
   a. Antibiotics are not indicated except for the following:
      (1) During outbreaks of acute rheumatic fever or poststreptococcal glomerulonephritis
      (2) During an outbreak of GAS pharyngitis in a closed or semi-closed community
      (3) Family history of rheumatic fever exists
      (4) Multiple episodes of documented, symptomatic GAS pharyngitis continue to occur within a family over weeks despite appropriate antibiotic therapy
      (5) Family has excessive anxiety of GAS pharyngitis
      (6) When tonsillectomy is considered due to chronic strep carriage
      (7) When a case of GAS toxic shock syndrome or necrotizing fasciitis has occurred in a household contact
   b. To eliminate carriage, prescribe clindamycin (Cleocin) 600 mg/day in 2-4 divided doses

C. Acute rheumatic fever (ARF)
   1. Treatment of first attack of ARF depends on severity; consult with specialist
   2. Prevention of recurrent attacks of ARF or secondary prevention
      a. Continuous prophylaxis is recommended for patients with a well-documented history of ARF
      b. Begin prophylaxis, after full course or antibiotics to eradicate residual Group A β-hemolytic streptococci even if throat culture is negative; promptly treat family members who have current or previous rheumatic fever
      c. Prescribe one of the following medication regimens (see following table)

SECONDARY PROPHYLAXIS OF ACUTE RHEUMATIC FEVER		
Drug	Dose	Frequency
Benzathine penicillin G IM	1,200,000 units	Every 3-4 weeks
Penicillin V PO	250 mg	BID
Sulfadiazine PO	>60 pounds (27 kg): 1 gm	QD
	≤60 pounds (27 kg): 500mg	QD
Erythromycin PO*	250 mg	BID

*For patients allergic to penicillin and sulfadiazine

Adapted from Dajani, A., et al., 1995. Treatment of acute streptococcal pharyngitis and prevention of rheumatic fever: A statement for health professionals. *Pediatrics, 96*, 758-764.

        d.   Duration of continuous prophylaxis is controversial. Duration of treatment is dependent on risk of recurrence. Risk increases with multiple, previous attacks and in persons who have increased risk of exposure to streptococcal infections such as school teachers, health professionals, or military recruits; additional recommendations for therapy duration are as follows:

           (1)   ARF without carditis: 5 years or until age 21 years, whichever is longer

           (2)   ARF with carditis but without residual heart disease (no valvular disease): 10 years or well into adulthood, whichever is longer

           (3)   ARF with carditis and residual heart disease: at least 10 years since last episode and at least until age 40 years

    3.   Short-term antibiotic prophylaxis for bacterial endocarditis prior to certain procedures (including dental and surgical procedures) is needed for patients with rheumatic valvular heart disease (see pages 736-740 in *Red Book 2002, Report on the Committee on Infectious Diseases* for recommended regimens)

D.   Pharyngeal gonorrhea is usually treated with ceftriaxone (Rocephin) 250 mg IM or a single dose of oral quinolone (ciprofloxacin, 500 mg, or ofloxacin, 400 mg) plus either a single dose of azithromycin (1 g) or doxycycline (100 mg) BID for 7 days

E.   Diphtheria needs immediate consultation with a specialist and is usually treated with equine antitoxin and penicillin or erythromycin; notify public health department

F.   For pharyngitis due to *Mycoplasma pneumoniae* and *Chlamydia trachomatis*, treat with erythromycin (Ery-Tab) 500 mg BID for 10 days

G.   *Candida albicans* (see section on CANDIDIASIS)

H.   Peritonsillar abscess needs an immediate referral to a specialist

    1.   Initially, in outpatient setting, prescribe drug of choice, penicillin, and a pain medication

    2.   Needle aspiration, incision and drainage, or abscess tonsillectomy are current surgical approaches to management

I.   Patient Education

    1.   Teach parents and patients to immediately call office if the pain becomes more severe or if dyspnea, drooling, difficulty swallowing, and inability to fully open mouth develop

    2.   Advise increased fluid intake

    3.   Patients with streptococcal pharyngitis should not return to school or work until they have been on antibiotic therapy for a full 24 hours

    4.   Reinforce that patients will usually feel well in 24-48 hours, but that it is important to take full 10-day course of antibiotic to prevent complications, particularly rheumatic fever

    5.   Assure family that rheumatic fever does not occur with appropriate antibiotic therapy

J.   Follow Up

    1.   If no significant improvement in 3-4 days patient should return for re-evaluation

    2.   Patients with streptococcal pharyngitis: Post-treatment throat cultures are indicated only for patients who have high risk for rheumatic fever or who are still symptomatic after treatment

APHTHOUS STOMATITIS

I.   Definition: Chronic Inflammation of the oral mucosal tissue with ulcers often called canker sores

II.   Pathogenesis

A.   Etiology is uncertain, but heightened immunologic response to oral mucosal antigens probably plays a role

    1.   Common in persons with leukemia, neutropenia, and HIV infection

    2.   Increased prevalence in patients with autoimmune diseases such as Crohn's disease, Behçet's syndrome, Reiter's syndrome, and ulcerative colitis

B. Contributing factors include the following:
1. Allergies to coffee, chocolate, potatoes, cheese, figs, nuts, citrus fruits, and gluten
2. Stress
3. Generalized physical debility
4. Viral and bacterial pathogens
5. Trauma
6. Nutritional deficiencies such as vitamin B_{12}, folate, and iron
7. Hormones
8. Medications such as antihypertensives, antineoplastics, gold salts, and nonsteroidal anti-inflammatory drugs

C. Regardless of cause, when mucosal breakdown occurs, the lesions are invaded by mouth flora and become secondarily infected

III. Clinical Presentation

A. Less prevalent in men and in chronic smokers

B. In approximately 1/3 of patients, recurrences continue for numerous years

C. Lesions divided into 3 categories
1. Minor
a. Most common type; often present initially in childhood or adolescence
b. Lesions are usually singular (but may be multiple), shallow, small (<1 cm), and painful
c. Lesions appear on labial or buccal mucosa, tongue, soft palate, and floor of mouth; rarely do lesions appear on attached gingiva and hard palate as occurs in herpes simplex
d. Prodromal burning or tingling may precede ulcers
e. Typically lesions heal in 7-14 days and tend to recur
2. Major
a. This severe form presents with lesions that are deep and large (>1 cm)
b. Lesions take 6 weeks or longer to heal with possible scarring
3. Herpetiform
a. Typically present as crops of small (1-5 mm) painful ulcers from 3 to >12
b. Lesions are initially round or oval and later coalesce to form large ulcers with irregular margins

IV. Diagnosis/Evaluation

A. History
1. Ask about onset and duration of symptoms
2. Inquire about fever, rashes on other parts of body, and systemic symptoms
3. Question regarding nutritional deficiencies, stressors, allergies, recent mouth trauma, infections, and risk factors for sexually transmitted diseases
4. Obtain medication history
5. Inquire about systemic diseases
6. Ask about past episodes and previous treatments

B. Physical Examination
1. Determine vital signs
2. Assess hydration status; patients may not be drinking fluids due to mouth pain
3. Assess skin for lesions on other parts of body
4. Perform complete head, ears, eyes, nose, mouth, and throat examinations; note location, number and distribution of lesions
5. Palpate neck and jaw for adenopathy
6. Auscultate chest
7. May need complete physical examination if systemic disease is suspected

C. Differential Diagnosis
1. Oral cancer (consider if lesions are present for more than 6 weeks, are unresponsive to therapy, and have unusual presentations such as indurated or rolled borders)
2. Oral candidiasis (white patches in mouth) (see CANDIDIASIS section)
3. Hand-foot-and-mouth disease (papulovesicular lesions with erythematous halo on hands and feet as well as mouth)

4. Herpes simplex virus (see HERPES SIMPLEX section)
   a. Vesicles form before ulcers develop and are confined to pharynx, tonsils and soft palate in primary herpes and are on the vermilion borders of lip in secondary herpes
   b. Tzanck smear is positive for inclusion-bearing giant cells
5. Syphilis (risk factors, skin lesions on hands and feet, and positive RPR/FTA tests are present)
6. Vincent's stomatitis (ulcers appear on gingivae and are covered by purulent, gray exudate)
7. Herpangina
   a. More common in children than adults
   b. Multiple distinctive papular, vesicular, and ulcerative lesions on anterior tonsillar pillars, soft palate, tonsils, pharynx, and posterior buccal mucosa
8. Behçet's syndrome (lesions are similar to aphthous stomatitis, but with this syndrome genital ulceration, uveitis, and retinitis are also present)
9. Reiter's syndrome (uveitis, conjunctivitis, and arthritis are present)
10. Acute necrotizing ulcerative gingivitis (history of periodontal disease is present)
11. Trauma due to dental appliances or rough surfaced teeth
12. Varicella (chickenpox)
13. Pemphigus (presence of bullous lesions in mouth and other parts of body and Tzanck smear from lesions reveals acantholytic cells)
14. Oropharyngeal anthrax (ulcers at base of tongue; initially edematous and hyperemic)

D. Diagnostic Tests
   1. Usually none indicated
   2. Order vitamin B_{12}, folate, and iron levels if nutritional deficiencies are suspected
   3. Consider CBC with differential to assist in ruling out anemias
   4. Consider Tzanck smear for distinguishing herpetic stomatitis from other causes
   5. Consider HIV testing when ulcers are large and slow to heal
   6. Biopsy is needed if cancer is suspected

V. Plan/Management

A. Pharmacologic treatment includes one of following:
   1. Liquid antacids or 3% hydrogen peroxide/water solution, 1:1 as a gargle
   2. Xylocaine (Lidocaine 2%) viscous solution; may apply to lesions every 3 hours or use 15 mL as a gargle or mouthwash and swallow every 3 hours (maximum 8 doses/day)
   3. Diphenhydramine 5 mg/mL (Benadryl) elixir mixed 1:1 with attapulgite (Kaopectate) or aluminum hydroxide, magnesium hydroxide (Maalox). May be used as mouth rinse QID
   4. Corticosteroid creams can provide pain relief and promote healing, but be cautious as they worsen viral infections; apply thin layer of triamcinolone acetonide 0.1% (Kenalog) in paste vehicle, Orabase, after meals and HS (moderate potency)
   5. Tetracycline syrup (Sumycin) 250 mg/10 mL syrup QID for 7-14 days; rinse for 2 minutes and then expectorate; contraindicated in pregnant women and children <8 years old
   6. Dexamethasone elixir (Decadron) 0.5 mg/5 mL; rinse with 5 mL every 12 hours and then expectorate
   7. Remind patient not to eat or drink for 20 minutes after this treatment

B. Treat severe, recurrent aphthous ulcers with one of following:
   1. May require oral corticosteroids: Initially, in adults, prescribe prednisone 30-60 mg/day with tetracycline syrup QID for 5 days, then, decrease to 5-20 mg every other day for 10 days
   2. Ask pharmacist to mix clobetasol propionate 0.05% (Temovate) ointment with an equal amount of Orabase; dry ulcer site lightly and apply sufficient paste to cover lesion three to six times daily

C. Alternative agents include zinc gluconate lozenges; oral vitamins (vitamin B, vitamin B complex, lysine), sage and chamomile mouthwash, and juices (carrot, celery, cantaloupe); limited research is available on the efficacy of these agents

D. Thalidomide (Thalomid) 200 mg once or twice a day for 3-8 weeks is used in HIV-infected patients who have severe, nonhealing ulcers; contraindicated in other patients because of risk of adverse effects and teratogenicity

E. Patient Education
   1. Warn that using steroid pastes or elixirs could result in secondary fungal infection
   2. Encourage good nutrition and increased fluid intake
   3. Stress the importance of good oral hygiene

4. Avoid spicy, salty, and acidic foods and drinks
5. Use soft-bristled toothbrush and avoid foods with sharp surfaces and talking while chewing
6. Aphthous ulcers are not contagious, so there is no danger in spreading

F. Follow Up
1. Immediately in elderly persons not taking fluids
2. In severe cases, reschedule in 2-3 days
3. Consult specialist if not healed in 2-3 weeks

GINGIVITIS AND PERIODONTITIS

I. Definitions:

A. Gingivitis: Inflammation of the gingiva

B. Periodontitis: Oral inflammation that results in loss of supporting bony structure of the teeth

II. Pathogenesis

A. Poor dental hygiene which allows plaque to accumulate on the teeth is the major causative factor

B. Initiating factors in the development of periodontal disease include bacterial plaque and calculus
1. The initial changes in healthy gingiva after only a few days of plaque accumulation include an acute inflammation of the junctional epithelium (attachment of the gingiva to the enamel surface of the tooth)
2. Within 2-4 weeks after the beginning of plaque (transparent deposit of primarily bacteria and their byproducts) formation, the gingivitis becomes established
3. At some point, chronic gingivitis may progress to periodontitis, which is characterized by bone loss, loss of attachment, pocket formation, tooth mobility, and loss of teeth

C. Systemic factors that alter inflammatory and immune responses so that the host's defenses against bacteria or their metabolites are compromised include the following:
1. Hormonal: Pregnancy gingivitis is an exaggerated inflammatory response that may be caused by hormonal changes, especially in the third trimester
2. Nutritional: Vitamin C deficiency is well established
3. Drug therapy: Hyperplasia is associated with the use of phenytoin (Dilantin), cyclosporine, and calcium channel blockers
4. Systemic diseases such as diabetes mellitus
5. Immunosuppression such as HIV infection
6. Hematologic disorders such as leukemia

D. Local factors that modify the immunoinflammatory response and contribute of the progress of plaque-induced periodontal disease include the following:
1. Trauma from occlusion (bruxism) which tends to accelerate pocket formation and bone loss
2. Food impaction which occurs most frequently due to an impinging overbite
3. Mouth breathing and exposure and drying of the facial gingiva of the maxillary anterior teeth
4. Cigarette smoking

III. Clinical Presentation

A. Approximately two-thirds of young adults and 80% of middle-aged and older adults suffer from periodontal disease

B. Most common cause of tooth loss in adults; occurs at all ages, but increases in prevalence and severity with age

C. Whereas dental caries damage the tooth itself, the supporting structures for the tooth, the gingiva, cementum, alveolar bone, and periodontal membrane are damaged by gingivitis and periodontitis

D. Gingivitis may be acute, subacute, recurrent, and chronic and includes any of the following signs:
   1. Redness (normal gingiva is coral-pink) and edema of gingival tissue
   2. Bleeding upon provocation
   3. Changes in consistency and contour, presence of calculus and/or plaque
   4. Lack of radiographic evidence of crestal bone loss
   5. In chronic forms, gingiva has a fibrous appearance that pits with pressure

E. Major complication of untreated gingivitis is periodontitis
   1. Patients present with red, bleeding gums, unpleasant taste in mouth, but usually pain is absent (unless acute infection superimposed on chronic process)
   2. Signs of gingivitis as described above are present and there are also periodontal pockets around the teeth containing purulent matter
   3. As periodontitis progresses, teeth loosen, spread apart, causing difficulty chewing, pain, and acute abscess formation
   4. Eventually, the alveolar bone is destroyed and teeth are deprived of support and lost

IV. Diagnosis/Evaluation

   A. History
      1. Ask about onset and duration of symptoms
      2. Ask about bleeding from gums after brushing
      3. Inquire regarding dental hygiene habits
      4. Question about bruxism, mouth breathing, and problems with occlusion
      5. Obtain medication history

   B. Physical Examination
      1. Examine teeth and gingiva for presence of plaque, and for hyperplasia or recession of gums
      2. Examine gums for areas of erosion
      3. Determine if gingival hyperplasia is generalized or localized

   C. Differential Diagnosis
      1. Dental abscess
      2. Stomatitis

   D. Diagnostic Tests: None indicated.

V. Plan/Management

   A. Treatment of gingivitis usually requires 1-3 dental visits and is aimed at elimination of local etiologic factors (plaque and calculus) which will result in a reversal of the gingival inflammation
      1. Plaque and calculus are removed using appropriate instruments
      2. Patient education in proper plaque control measures (use of soft-bristled toothbrush that facilitates cleaning of teeth and gingiva; use of dental floss)
      3. Patients are scheduled for return visits for professional cleaning every 6 months
      4. Mouthwashes such as chlorhexidine gluconate 0.12% (Peridex) used BID are beneficial
      5. Correction of plaque-retentive factors (caries, tooth malposition, overhanging margins) is important

   B. Patients with phenytoin-induced gingival hyperplasia usually require periodontal surgery

   C. Mouth-breathing associated gingivitis usually is difficult to correct, but good plaque control can control the process in most cases

   D. Periodontitis can be effectively treated provided early diagnosis and referral are instituted
      1. The first phase of treatment is similar to that for gingivitis described above
      2. Phase 2 of treatment involves surgery to improve the gingival architecture that remains

   E. Follow up should be by the dentist to whom patient was referred

TOOTHACHE (PULPITIS)

I. Definition: A suppurative process that usually results from pulpal infection

II. Pathogenesis

    A. Inflammation involving pulp tissue, the central portion of the tooth containing vital soft tissue, occurs due to injury of some type

    B. Dental caries, a bacterial disease characterized by demineralization of tooth enamel and dentine, is the most frequent type of injury that causes pulpitis; pain does not occur until decay impinges on the pulp and an inflammatory response develops

    C. Diverse flora, including gram-positive anaerobes and bacteroides are the organisms most often involved in the infectious process

III. Clinical Presentation

    A. Constant, throbbing pain is the most frequent presenting complaint

    B. Affected tooth is extremely sensitive to touch and pain is intensified with the application of heat or cold (thermal sensitivity)

    C. Tooth may be slightly extruded so that occlusal contact gives rise to exquisite pain

    D. The affected area of the jaw is tender to palpation

    E. Systemic manifestations may or may not be present and are usually limited to regional lymphadenopathy, malaise, and fever

    F. Complications include periapical abscess and cellulitis

IV. Diagnosis/Evaluation

    A. History
        1. Inquire about recent toothache
        2. Inquire about occurrence of fever and chills
        3. Inquire about heart murmur or defect
        4. Determine type of medication taken for pain relief and when it was last taken

    B. Physical Examination
        1. Determine if febrile
        2. Inspect and gently percuss teeth to determine location of affected tooth
        3. Examine adjacent tissue for signs of inflammation
        4. Observe for facial symmetry and examine jaw in area for signs of cellulitis
        5. Examine for regional lymphadenopathy
        6. Auscultate heart (risk of sepsis and complications increase with valvular disease)

    C. Differential Diagnosis
        1. Mumps
        2. Cellulitis
        3. Pericoronitis (painful wisdom teeth)
        4. Sinusitis
        5. Myofascial inflammation
        6. Migraine headache
        7. Neuralgias

    D. Diagnostic Tests: Should be done by dentist who will see patient

V.   Plan/Management

A.   Patients with toothaches generally fall into one of three categories ranging from least to most serious (see following table for treatment)

TREATMENT OF TOOTHACHE

Category 1:   Patients who are afebrile, with no extraoral swelling (no facial asymmetry present) or intraoral swelling
- ✓ Prescribe analgesics: A nonsteroidal anti-inflammatory drug (NSAID) or acetaminophen (300 mg) with codeine (30 mg) (Tylenol #3), 1-2 tabs, every 4 hours
- ✓ Recommend warm salt water rinses (swish and spit) every 3-4 hours
- ✓ Refer to dentist within 24 hours

Category 2:   Patients who have either slight extraoral or intraoral swelling, or who have a low-grade fever
- ✓ Prescribe analgesics (as above) and
- ✓ Prescribe antibiotics: Treatment of choice is Penicillin V (Pen-Vee-K) 250-500 mg Q 6-8 hours x 5-7 days
- ✓ Patients allergic to penicillin should be treated with erythromycin
- ✓ Recommend warm salt water rinses (swish and spit) every 3-4 hours
- ✓ Refer to dentist within 12-24 hours

Category 3:   Patients who have fever ≥101°F (38.5°C) with intraoral and/or extraoral swelling (causing facial asymmetry)
- ✓ Emergency consultation and treatment by dentist is needed
- ✓ Management must be immediate because the consequences of delayed treatment can be serious and occasionally life threatening!

B.   Treatment by the dentist for these toothache categories varies from extraction to root canal to incision and drainage, and to hospitalization for IV antibiotic therapy for patients with cellulitis

C.   Patient education includes prevention of dental caries such as decreasing ingestion of sugar-containing foods, performing regular toothbrushing and flossing, appropriate use of fluoride, and regular visits to dentist

D.   Follow up should be done by dentist

CERVICAL ADENITIS

I.   Definition: Acute pyogenic infection of a cervical lymph node

II.   Pathogenesis

A.   Usually reactive or secondary to an upper respiratory tract infection or dental infection; less frequently due to trauma

B.   Pathogens:
1.   *Staphylococcus aureus* and *Streptococcus pyogenes* account for 80% of unilateral cervical adenitis
2.   Increasingly, anaerobic pathogens are being identified
3.   Less common pathogens: viruses and group B streptococci, *Mycobacterium avium* complex, and *M. scrofulaceum*

III.   Clinical Presentation

A.   Typically, patient is afebrile or has a low-grade fever, malaise, and an upper respiratory infection or dental infection

B.   Usually presents as tender, soft, warm, rapidly enlarging lymph node with erythema of the overlying skin and possibly with fistulas to the skin; node ranges from 2-6 cm

C.   Most common sites are the submandibular and anterior cervical areas

IV.   Diagnosis/Evaluation

A.   History
1.   Ascertain duration and onset of node enlargement
2.   Ask if node is increasing in size and whether overlying skin has changed in color
3.   Ask about pain during eating which suggests parotid gland involvement
4.   Question about dysphagia, odynophagia, stridor, speech disorders, or a sensation of a lump in the throat
5.   Inquire about associated constitutional symptoms
6.   Question about recent infections, trauma, insect bites, pet scratches, tuberculosis contact, drug usage, and foreign travel

B.   Physical Examination
1.   Measure vital signs
2.   Observe for general state of health
3.   Carefully examine scalp and face for skin lesions
4.   Assess for facial-nerve weakness that can be caused by a parotid gland tumor
5.   Thoroughly examine ears, eyes, nose, throat, and mouth
6.   Carefully examine neck for other masses and nuchal rigidity
7.   Carefully palpate cervical mass to determine exact anatomic location, presence of tenderness, mobility, and consistency; examine skin overlying node for color
8.   Thoroughly examine areas of lymph nodes
9.   Inspect skin for lesions and rashes
10.   Assess respiratory status
11.   Palpate abdomen for organomegaly

C.   Differential Diagnosis (see Figure 9.1 for common location of masses of the neck)
1.   Congenital cysts (these conditions need referral and usually surgery)
      a.   Thyroglossal duct cyst (located at midline and typically moves with swallowing or tongue protrusion)
      b.   Brachial cleft cysts (small dimple or opening anterior to middle portion of the sternocleidomastoid muscle)
      c.   Cystic hygromas (fluid-filled, compressible mass in the posterior triangle just behind the sternocleidomastoid muscle and in the supraclavicular fossa)
2.   Salivary gland disorders; salivary glands are located in area of lymph nodes and enlarged glands may be confused as cervical adenitis; care must be taken to distinguish glands from nodes; for example, enlargement of the parotid gland obliterates the angle of the mandible
3.   Cervical lymphadenopathy (see section on LYMPHADENOPATHY)
      a.   Viral infections (most common)
            (1)   Often due to herpesviruses, adenoviruses, enteroviruses, and Epstein-Barr virus
            (2)   Nodes are typically bilateral, discrete, oval, soft, and minimally tender
      b.   Bacterial infections of the upper respiratory tract and mouth
      c.   Cat scratch disease (see CAT SCRATCH DISEASE section)
      d.   Kawasaki disease (see KAWASAKI DISEASE section)
      e.   Atypical mycobacterium
      f.   Toxoplasmosis
      g.   Systemic disorders such as lupus, rheumatoid arthritis, sarcoidosis, histoplasmosis

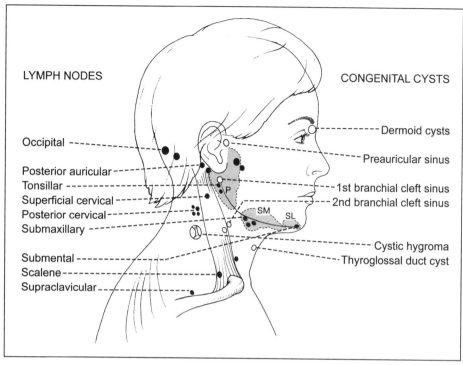

Figure 9.1. Common Location of Masses of the Face and Neck
P = Parotid gland; SM = Submandibular gland; SL = Sublingual gland

4. Abscesses, furuncles, and soft tissue tumors (arise from cutaneous or subcutaneous tissue)
5. Lipoma is a benign, subcutaneous tumor composed of fat cells and may be located in back of neck (other common sites are trunk and extremities); consistency is soft and rubbery
6. Malignancy
   a. Neck mass is usually persistent and enlarging
   b. Node is often supraclavicular, firm and fixated to skin and underlying tissue
   c. Patient often has persistent fever, weight loss, voice change, and hearing loss
   d. Patient may have lesion in oral cavity or pharynx or unilateral nasal obstruction
   e. Smokers, alcoholics, African Americans, and older individuals are at most risk
7. Generalized lymphadenopathy is usually caused by systemic disease (see LYMPHADENOPATHY section)
8. Thyroid nodules or goiters may be confused with enlarged nodes

D. Diagnostic Tests; often no tests are needed
   1. Ultrasound is helpful in establishing whether mass is solid, cystic, or fluctuant
   2. In moderately or severely ill patients, consider CBC, sedimentation rate, throat culture, and blood culture
   3. PPD should be considered if tuberculosis is suspected
   4. Heterophil tests or titers for Epstein-Barr virus, cytomegalovirus, and toxoplasma may be indicated to rule-out specific viral infections
   5. Consider aspiration and culture in patients who have large, fluctuant nodes which do not respond to initial therapy
   6. Biopsy of node is needed when malignancy is suspected

V. Plan/Management

A. For patient who appears well with minimal pain, close observation for 2-3 days and symptomatic treatment may be all that is needed
   1. Prescribe analgesic such as Tylenol or nonsteroidal anti-inflammatory agent
   2. Warm compresses every 4 hours

B. For the patient with moderate to severe adenitis prescribe one of following antibiotics:
   1. Amoxicillin/clavulanic acid (Augmentin) 500 mg TID or 875 mg BID
   2. Cephalexin (Keflex) 500 mg BID

C. Patient education
   1. Emphasize that patient should immediately return if difficulty swallowing or breathing occurs
   2. Reinforce that follow-up is important if symptoms persist

D. Patients with lymph node enlargement persisting more than 2 weeks without regression with antibiotic therapy need further evaluation and possible referral to a specialist

E. Follow Up
   1. Return to clinic if symptoms not resolved in 2-3 days
   2. For the patient who appears well and is treated only symptomatically, re-evaluate symptoms at 3-5 day intervals; some nodes take many weeks to regress but other nodes regress spontaneously within 2-3 weeks without pharmacological treatment
   3. Re-evaluate patients who are treated with antibiotics after completion of therapy
   4. Individualize follow-up for patients who are at risk for systemic or serious disorders

REFERENCES

Agency for Health Care Policy & Research. (1999). *Diagnosis and treatment of acute bacterial rhinosinusitis. Summary, evidence report/technology assessment.* (AHCPR Publ. No. 99-E016). Rockville, MD.

Agency for Healthcare Research & Quality. (2000). *Management of acute otitis media. Summary, evidence report/technology assessment.* (AHRQ Publ. No. 15). Rockville, MD. http://www.ahrq.gov/clinic/epcsums/otitisum.htm

Agency for Healthcare Research and Quality. (2002). *Management of allergic and nonallergic rhinitis. Summary, evidence report/technology assessment.* (AHRQ Publ. No. 54). Rockville MD. http://www.ahrq.gov/clinic/epcsums/rhinsum.htm

Agency for Healthcare Research and Quality. (2003). Management of allergic rhinitis in the working-age population. Summary, evidence report/technology assessment. Number 67. AHRQ Publication No. 03-E013. Agency for Healthcare Research and Quality, Rockville MD. http://www.ahrq.gov/clinic/epcsums/rhinworksum.htm

American Pharmaceutical Association Pediatric Disorders Protocol Panel. (2000). American Pharmaceutical Association drug treatment protocols: Management of pediatric acute otitis media. *Journal of American Pharmacy Association, 40,* 599-608.

Bachur, R. (2001). Minor trauma. In C. Green-Hernandez, J.K. Singleton, & D.Z. Aronzon (Eds.). *Primary care pediatrics.* Philadelphia: Lippincott.

Balk, E.M., Zucker, D.R., Engels, E.A., Wong, J.B., Williams, J.W., & Lau, J. (2001). Strategies for diagnosing and treating suspected acute bacterial sinusitis. *Journal of General Internal Medicine, 16,* 701.

Bartnik, G., Fabijanska, A., & Rogowski, M. (2001). Effects of tinnitus retraining therapy (TRT) for patients with tinnitus and subjective hearing loss versus tinnitus only. *Scandinavian Audiology Supplement, 52,* 206-208.

Bisno, A.L. (2001). Acute pharyngitis. *New England Journal of Medicine, 344,* 205-211.

Bisno, A.L., Gerber, M.A., Gwaltney, J.M. Jr., Kaplan, E.L., & Schwartz, R.H. (2002). Practice guidelines for diagnosis and management of group A streptococcal pharyngitis. *Clinical Infectious Diseases, 35,* 113-125.

Bisno, A.L., Peter, G.S., & Kaplan, E.L. (2002). Diagnosis of strep throat in adults. Are clinical criteria really good enough? *Clinical Infectious Diseases, 35,* 126-129.

Bluestone, C.D., Gates, G.A., Klein, J.O., Lim, D.J., Mogi, G., Ogra, P.L., et al. (2002). Panel reports: 1. Definitions, terminology, and classification of otitis media. *Annals of Otology, Rhinology, and Laryngology, 111,* 8-18.

Bluestone, C.D., Klein, J.O., Rosenfeld, R.M., Berman, S., Casselbrant, M.L., Chonmaitree, T., et al. (2002). Panel reports: 9. Treatment, complications, and sequelae. *Annals of Otology, Rhinology, and Laryngology, 111,* 102-119.

Braunwald, E., Fauci, A.S., Kasper, D.L., Hauser, S.L., Longo, D.L., & Jameson, J.L. (2002). Hearing disorders. *Harrison's principles of internal medicine (15th ed.).* New York: McGraw-Hill.

Brook, I., Gooch, W.M., III, Jenkins, S.G., Pichichero, M.E., Reiner, S.A., Shar, L., et al. (2000). Medical management of acute bacterial sinusitis: Recommendations of a Clinical Advisory Committee on Pediatric and Adult Sinusitis. *Annals of Otology, Rhinology, and Laryngology, 109,* 2-20.

Buchman, C.A., & Wamback, B.A.,. (2002) Otitis externa. In R.E. Rakel & E.T. Bope (Eds.). *Conn's current therapy 2002.* Philadelphia: Saunders.

Casselbrant, M.L., Gravel, J.S., Margolis, R. H., Bellussi, L., Dhooge, I., Downs, M.P., et al. (2002). Panel reports: 8. Diagnosis and screening. *Annals of Otology, Rhinology, and Laryngology, 111,* 95-99.

Consensus Panel, Hannley, M.T., Denneny, J.C., III, & Holzer, S.S. (2000). Consensus Panel Report: Use of ototopical antibiotics in treating common ear diseases. *Otolaryngology–Head and Neck Surgery, 122,* 934-940.

Culpepper, L., & Froom, J. (1997). Routine antimicrobial treatment of acute otitis media: Is it necessary? *JAMA, 278,* 1643-1645.

Dajani, A.S., et al. (1993). Guidelines for the diagnosis of rheumatic fever: Jones criteria, updated 1992. *Circulation, 87,* 302-307.

Dajani, A., Taubert, K., Ferrieri, P., Peter, G., Shulman, S., and other committee members. (1995). Treatment of acute streptococcal pharyngitis and prevention of rheumatic fever: A statement for health professionals. *Pediatrics, 96,* 758-764.

Dajani, A.S., Taubert, K.A., Wilson, W., Bolger, A.F., Bayer, A., Ferrieri, P., et al. (1997). Prevention of bacterial endocarditis: Recommendations by the American Heart Association. *JAMA, 277,* 1794-1801.

Dolitsky, J.N., & Ward, R.F. (2001). Foreign bodies of the ear, nose, airway, and esophagus. In R.A. Hoekelman. *Primary pediatric care.* St. Louis: Mosby.

Douglass, A.B., & Douglass, JM. (2003). Common dental emergencies. *American Family Physician, 67,* 511-516.

Ebell, M.H., Smith, M.A., Barry, H.C., Ives, K., & Carey, M. (2000). Does this patient have strep throat? *JAMA, 284,* 2912-2918.

Forzley, G.J. (1994). Cerumen impaction removal. In J.L. Pfenninger, & G.C. Fowler (Eds.), *Procedures for primary care physicians.* St. Louis: Mosby.

Goroll, A.H., & Mulley, A.G., Jr. (2000). Approach to the patient with chronic nasal congestion and discharge. In A.H. Goroll, & A.G. Mulley, Jr. (Eds.), *Primary care medicine.* Philadelphia: Lippincott, Williams & Wilkins.

Goroll, A.H., & Mulley, A.G., Jr. (2000). Management of aphthous stomatitis. In A.H. Goroll, & A.G. Mulley, Jr. (Eds.), *Primary care medicine.* Philadelphia: Lippincott, Williams & Wilkins.

Gulya, A.J. (2000). Evaluation of hearing loss. In A.H. Goroll & A.G. Mulley, Jr. (Eds.), *Primary care medicine.* Philadelphia: Lippincott.

Hayden, M.L. (2001). Allergic rhinitis: A growing primary care challenge. *Journal of the American Academy of Nurse Practitioners, 13,* 545-551.

Haynes, J.H., & Newkirk, G.R. (1994). Removal of foreign bodies from the ear and nose. In J.L. Pfenninger, & G.C. Fowler (Eds.), *Procedures for primary care physicians.* St. Louis: Mosby.

Hayes, C.S., & Williamson, H., Jr. (2001). Management of group A beta-hemolytic streptococcal pharyngitis. *American Family Physician, 63,* 1557-1565.

Hendley, J.O. (2002). Otitis media. *New England Journal of Medicine, 347,* 1169-1174.

Herendeen, N.E., & Szilagyi, P.G. (2001). Cystic and solid masses of the face and neck. In R.A. Hoekelman et al., (Ed.). *Primary pediatric care,* St. Louis: Mosby.

Huovinen, P. (2002). Macrolide-resistant group A streptococcus–Now in the United States. *New England Journal of Medicine, 346,* 1243-1245.

Kleinegger, C.L. (2002). Diseases of the mouth. In R.E. Rakel & E.T. Bope, (Eds.). *Conn's current therapy 2002.* Philadelphia: Saunders.

Krouse, J.H., Mirante, J.P., & Christmas, D.A., Jr. (1999). *Office-based pediatric otolaryngology and audiology.* Philadelphia: Saunders.

Lanza, D.C., & Kennedy, D.W. (1997). Adult rhinosinusitis defined. In J.B. Anon (Ed.). Report of the Rhinosinusitis Task Force Committee Meeting. *Otolaryngology–Head and Neck Surgery, 111*(Suppl), S1-S7.

Leberman, P. (2002). Nonallergic rhinitis. In R.E. Rakel, & E.T. Bope (Eds.). *2002 Conn's current therapy.* Philadelphia: Saunders.

Leibovitz, E., & Dagan, R. (2001). Otitis media therapy and drug resistance–Part 1: Management principles. *Infectious Medicine, 18,* 212-216.

Li, J.T., Lockey, R.F., Bernstein, I.L, Portnoy, J.M, & Nicklas, R.A. (2003). Allergen immunotherapy: A practice parameter. *Annals of Allergy, Asthma, and Immunology, 90,* 1-40.

MacLeod, D.K. (1999). Chronic dental and oral problems. In L.R. Barker, J.R. Burton, & P.D. Zieve (Eds.), *Principles of ambulatory medicine.* Baltimore: Williams & Wilkins.

McBride, D.R. (2000). Management of aphthous ulcers. *American Family Physician, 62,* 149-154, 160.

McKenna, M.W. (2002). Epistaxis. In R.B. Taylor (Ed.). *Manual of family practice.* Philadelphia: Lippincott Williams & Wilkins.

Nudelman, J. (2001). How should we treat acute maxillary sinusitis? *American Family Physician, 63,* 837-838.

Osguthorpe, J.D. (2001). Adult rhinosinusitis: Diagnosis and management. *American Family Physician, 63,* 69-76.

Owens, T.P., Jr. (2000). Removal of impacted cerumen. In R.E. Rakel (Ed.). *Saunders manual of medical practice (2nd ed.)*. Philadelphia: Saunders.

Piccirillo, J.F., Mager, D.E., Frisse, M.E., Brophy, R.H., & Goggin, A. (2001). Impact of first-line vs second-line antibiotics for the treatment of acute uncomplicated sinusitis. *JAMA, 286,*1849-1856.

Pichichero, M.E. (2000). Acute otitis media: Part 1. Improving diagnostic accuracy. *American Family Physician, 61,* 2051-2056.

Pichichero, M.E. (2000). Acute otitis media: Part II. Treatment in an era of increasing antibiotic resistance. *American Family Physician, 61,* 2410-2416.

Pichichero, M.E., Reiner, S.A., Brook, I., Gooch, W.M. III, Yamauchi, T., Jenkins, S.G., et al. (2000). Controversies in the medical management of persistent and recurrent acute otitis media: Recommendations of a clinical advisory committee. *Annals of Otology, Rhinology, and Laryngology, 109, 2-12.*

Rabinowitz, P.M. (2000). Noise-induced hearing loss. *American Family Physician, 61,* 2749-2756, 2759-2760.

Rosenfeld, R.M., Casselbrant, M.L., & Hannley, M.T. (2001). Implications of the AHRQ evidence report on acute otitis media. *Otolaryngology–Head and Neck Surgery, 125,* 440-448.

Sander, R. (2001). Otitis externa: A practical guide to treatment and prevention. *American Family Physician, 63,* 927-936, 941-942.

Schantz, N.V. (1994). Management of epistaxis. In J.L. Pfenninger, & G.C. Fowler (Eds.), *Procedures for primary care physicians.* St. Louis: Mosby.

Sheeler, R.D., Houston, M.S., Radke, S., Dale, J.C., & Adamson, S.C. (2002). Accuracy of rapid strep testing in patients who have had recent streptococcal pharyngitis. *Journal of the American Board of Family Practitioners, 15,* 261-265.

Sinus and Allergy Health Partnership. (2000). Antimicrobial treatment guidelines for acute bacterial rhinosinusitis. *Otolaryngology–Head and Neck Surgery, 123,* S1-S29.

Snow, V., Mottur-Pilson, C., Cooper, R.J., Hoffman, J.R. for the American Academy of Physicians–American Society of Internal Medicine. (2001). Principles of appropriate antibiotic use for acute pharyngitis in adults. *Annals of Internal Medicine, 134,* 506-508.

Snow, V., Mottur-Pilson, C., Cooper, R.J., Hickner, J.M. for the American Academy of Physicians–American Society of Internal Medicine. (2001). Principles of appropriate antibiotic use for acute sinusitis in adults. *Annals of Internal Medicine, 134,* 495-497.

Steyer, T.E. (2002). Peritonsillar abscess: Diagnosis and treatment. *American Family Physician, 65,* 93-96.

Takata, G.S., Chan, L.S., Shekelle, P., Morton, S.C., Mason, W., & Marcy, S.M. (2001). Evidence assessment of management of acute otitis media: I. The role of antibiotics in treatment of uncomplicated acute otitis media. *Pediatrics, 108,* 239-247.

Williams, J.W., Aguilar, C., Makela, M., Cornell, J., Hollman, D.R., Chiquette, E., & Simel, D.L. (2002). Antibiotics for acute maxillary sinusitis (Cochrane review). In *The Cochrane library.* Oxford: Update Software Ltd.

Windom, H.H. (2002). Allergic rhinitis caused by inhalant factors. In R.E. Rakel, & E.T. Bope (Eds.). *2002 Conn's current therapy.* Philadelphia: Saunders.

Wirtschafter, A., Cherukuri, S., & Benninger, M.S. (2002). Anthrax: ENT manifestations and current concepts. *Otolaryngology–Head and Neck Surgery, 126,* 8-13.

Yueh, B., Shapiro, N., MacLean, C.H., & Shekelle, P.G. (2003). Screening and management of adult hearing loss in primary care: Scientific review. *JAMA, 289,* 1976-1985.

Problems of the Upper Airways, Lower Respiratory System

BETSY HERNANDEZ WARREN & CONSTANCE R. UPHOLD

ASTHMA

I.   Definition: Chronic inflammatory disorder of the airways which causes bronchial hyper-responsiveness to stimuli and recurrent episodes of respiratory symptoms which are usually associated with reversible airflow obstruction

II.   Pathogenesis

    A.   Inflammation plays a central role
        1.   Results from complex interactions among many cells and cellular elements (mast cells, eosinophils, T lymphocytes, macrophages, neutrophils, and epithelial cells)
        2.   Inflammation is associated with airway obstruction, airway hyperresponsiveness, respiratory symptoms, and disease chronicity

    B.   Airway obstruction leads to airflow limitation and is usually widespread, recurrent, variable, and reversible either with treatment or spontaneously; obstruction is due to the following:
        1.   Acute bronchoconstriction results from airway hyperresponsiveness after exposure to a variety of stimuli such as allergens, drugs (aspirin, nonsteroidal anti-inflammatory drugs), stimuli (exercise, cold air, irritants) and possibly stress
        2.   Airway wall edema and mucosal thickening are caused by increased microvascular permeability and leakage
        3.   Chronic mucus plug formation sometimes occurs in severe, intractable cases
        4.   Airway wall remodeling may develop in severe cases, causing persistent abnormalities in lung function which are unresponsive to treatment

    C.   Factors contributing to asthma severity:
        1.   Inhaled allergens such as animal allergens, house-dust mites, outdoor allergens, indoor fungi, and cockroaches
        2.   Occupational exposures
        3.   Irritants such as tobacco smoke and pollution
        4.   Rhinitis/sinusitis
        5.   Gastroesophageal reflux
        6.   Sensitivity to aspirin, other nonsteroidal anti-inflammatory drugs, and sulfites
        7.   Topical and systemic beta-blockers
        8.   Viral respiratory infection

    D.   Adult-onset asthma may be related to allergies, but some adults have coexisting sinusitis, nasal polyps, and sensitivity to aspirin or nonsteroidal anti-inflammatory drugs; occupational exposure to workplace materials may also be a factor

III.   Clinical Presentation

    A.   Underdiagnosis and inappropriate therapy are major factors in morbidity and mortality

    B.   Symptoms typically begin in childhood or adolescence, but can develop in adulthood

    C.   Exercise-induced bronchospasm occurs with loss of heat and/or water from lungs during exercise; cough, shortness of breath, chest pain or tightness, wheezing or endurance problems may develop during exercise

    D.   Spectrum ranges from few mild episodes in a lifetime to daily debilitating symptoms; classification of asthma severity is based on symptoms and lung function before treatment (see table CLASSIFICATION OF THE SEVERITY OF ASTHMA)

CLASSIFICATION OF THE SEVERITY OF ASTHMA*

Step/ Category	Symptoms**	Nighttime Symptoms	Lung Functions***
STEP 4 Severe Persistent	• Continual symptoms • Limited physical activity • Frequent exacerbations	Frequent	• FEV$_1$ or PEF ≤60% predicted • PEF variability >30%
STEP 3 Moderate Persistent	• Daily symptoms • Daily use of inhaled short-acting beta$_2$-agonist • Exacerbations affect activity • Exacerbations are ≥2 times a week	>1 time a week	• FEV$_1$ or PEF >60%-<80% predicted • PEF variability >30%
STEP 2 Mild Persistent	• Symptoms >2 times a week but <1 time a day • Exacerbations may affect activity	>2 times a month	• FEV$_1$ or PEF ≥80% predicted • PEF variability 20-30%
STEP 1 Mild Intermittent	• Symptoms ≤2 times/week • Asymptomatic & normal PEF between exacerbations • Exacerbations brief (from a few hours to few days) • Intensity may vary	≤2 times a month	• FEV$_1$ or PEF ≥80% predicted • PEF variability <20%

*The presence of one of the features of severity is sufficient to classify patient in that category. A patient should be assigned to the most severe grade in which any feature occurs

**Patients at any level of severity can have mild, moderate, or severe exacerbations

*** FEV$_1$ = Forced expiratory volume in one second; PEF = Peak expiratory flow

Adapted from National Institutes of Health. National Heart, Lung, and Blood Institute. (1997). *The Expert Panel Report 2: Guidelines for the diagnosis and management of asthma*. National Asthma Education Program. NIH Publ. #97-4051. Bethesda, MD.

IV.   Diagnosis/Evaluation

    A.   History

        1.   Identify the symptoms likely to be due to asthma (see table KEY INDICATORS)

KEY INDICATORS OF ASTHMA

✓   Wheezing
✓   History of any of the following:
- Cough worse at night or in early morning
- Recurrent difficulty breathing
- Recurrent tightness in chest

✓   Reversible airflow limitation and diurnal variation as measured by peak flow meter
✓   Symptoms occur or are worsened by any of the following:
- Exercise, viral infection, animals, house-dust mites, mold, smoke, pollen, changes in weather, laughing, hard crying, airborne chemicals or dusts, menses

✓   Symptoms occur or worsen at night, awakening the patient

Adapted from National Institutes of Health. National Heart, Lung, and Blood Institute. (1997). *The Expert Panel Report 2: Guidelines for the diagnosis and management of asthma*. National Asthma Education Program. NIH Publ. #97-4051. Bethesda, MD.

        2.   Assess onset and duration of symptoms (number of days/nights per week/month)

        3.   Determine whether symptoms are seasonal, continuous, episodic, or diurnal

        4.   Determine profile of asthma attacks or exacerbations

        5.   Assess past and present management strategies and responses

        6.   Inquire about factors known to be related to asthma

        7.   Determine family history of asthma, allergy, sinusitis, rhinitis, or nasal polyps

        8.   Assess impact of disease on family, finances, school, work, activity, sleep, and behavior

        9.   Assess patient's and family's knowledge level, understanding of treatments, sociocultural beliefs

      10.   For persons with occupational asthma, inquire about number of sick days taken from work per month

      11.   At each follow-up visit assess whether the goals of therapy are being met

B. Physical Examination
  1. Determine pulse rate and respiratory rate
  2. Assess for signs of dehydration such as delayed capillary refill, poor skin turgor, and dry mucous membranes
  3. Observe for use of accessory respiratory muscles, retractions, nasal flaring, diaphoresis, and cyanosis
  4. Observe for hyperexpansion of thorax (hunched shoulders or chest deformity)
  5. Observe for flexural eczema or other manifestations of allergic skin conditions
  6. Assess for nasal discharge, mucosal swelling, frontal tenderness, postnasal discharge, nasal polyps, and allergic shiners (dark discoloration beneath both eyes)
  7. Auscultate and percuss lungs
     a. Wheezing during forced exhalation is no longer believed to be a reliable indicator
     b. In mild, intermittent asthma, wheezing may be absent between attacks; in severe asthma, wheezing may be absent due to diminished breath sounds
  8. Perform a complete cardiac examination

C. Differential Diagnosis
  1. Underdiagnosis of asthma is common
  2. Remember that recurrent episodes of coughing and wheezing are usually due to asthma
  3. The following should be included in the differential diagnosis:
     a. Vocal cord dysfunction can cause recurrent wheezing
     b. Enlarged lymph nodes, tumors
     c. Pulmonary infections such as pneumonia, tuberculosis, mycoplasma and respiratory syncytial virus
     d. Gastroesophageal reflux
     e. Chronic obstructive pulmonary disease
     f. Congestive heart failure
     g. Pulmonary embolism
     h. Cough secondary to drugs such as ACE inhibitors

D. Diagnostic Tests: regular monitoring of pulmonary function is essential, particularly for patients who do not perceive their symptoms until airways are severely obstructed
  1. Spirometry tests
     a. Recommended at following intervals:
        (1) Time of diagnosis
        (2) After treatment when symptoms and peak flow reading are stabilized to document attainment of normal airway function
        (3) Every 1-2 years to monitor maintenance of airway function
     b. More frequent testing is needed in the following cases: to check accuracy of peak flow, when precision is needed to determine treatment response, and when peak flow readings may be unreliable such as when patients are young, elderly, or have neuromuscular problems
  2. Order an exercise challenge test to confirm exercised-induced bronchospasm
  3. Other tests to consider: chest x-ray or CBC if infection is suspected; skin testing or *in vitro* testing for patients with persistent asthma exposed to perennial indoor allergens
  4. Peak expiratory flow (PEF) meters
     a. **Should be used to monitor lung function not to confirm diagnosis**
     b. Daily monitoring is not mandatory for all patients, but is important for patients after an exacerbation and for patients with moderate-to-severe persistent asthma
     c. Teach patients to determine their best PEF (see table PATIENT EDUCATION OF PEAK FLOW METER)

PATIENT EDUCATION OF THE PEAK FLOW METER

1. Demonstrate and have return demonstration of use of peak flow meter
   - Stand, do not sit
   - Place indicator at bottom of numbered scale
   - Take deep breath
   - Close lips around mouthpiece
   - Blow out as hard and fast as possible in a single blow
2. Teach patient to repeat #1 two more times and record the best of the three blows
3. Instruct patients how to determine their personal best peak flow number
   - Take readings twice a day for 2-3 weeks: upon awakening or between 12 noon & 2:00 PM
   - Take readings before and after inhaling beta$_2$-agonist
4. Explain that personal best peak flow numbers are categorized into zones to help patients self-manage their illnesses and to assess progression of disease and need for additional therapy
   - Green Zone: 80% of patient's personal best and denotes good control
   - Yellow Zone: 50-<80% of patient's personal best and denotes caution and the need to take a short-acting inhaled beta$_2$-agonist
   - Red Zone: <50% of patient's personal best and denotes severe asthma exacerbation and the need to take short-acting inhaled beta$_2$-agonist and call health care provider or emergency room or go directly to hospital
5. Explain to patient that once their personal best peak flow is documented they may decrease peak flow readings to once a day in the morning. If morning reading is <80% of personal best, instruct patient to monitor more frequently

Adapted from National Institutes of Health. National Heart, Lung, and Blood Institute. (1997). *The Expert Panel Report 2: Guidelines for the diagnosis and management of asthma.* National Asthma Education Program. NIH Publ. #97-4051. Bethesda, MD.

V.   Plan/Management

   A.   Referral to an asthma specialist is recommended in the following situations:
      1. Life-threatening or severe persistent asthma (step 4) is present
      2. Goals of asthma therapy are not fulfilled after 3 to 6 months of treatment
      3. Signs and symptoms are atypical or diagnosis is uncertain
      4. Other illnesses such as sinusitis, gastroesophageal reflux, or chronic obstructive pulmonary disease complicate the airway disease
      5. Immunotherapy is a treatment consideration
      6. Continuous oral corticosteroids or high-dose inhaled corticosteroids or two bursts of oral steroids in 1 year are needed

   B.   Control of the factors contributing to asthma severity is important
      1. Instruct patient to avoid the following:
         a. Allergens (see table MEASURES OF ENVIRONMENTAL CONTROL in ALLERGIC AND NONALLERGIC RHINITIS section)
         b. Environmental tobacco smoke
         c. Exercise when levels of pollution are high
         d. Beta-blockers
         e. Foods containing sulfite and other foods to which they are sensitive
      2. Caution patients with severe persistent asthma, nasal polyps, or a history of sensitivity to aspirin or nonsteroidal anti-inflammatory drugs that there is risk of severe and possibly fatal exacerbations when using these drugs
      3. Treat patients for rhinitis, sinusitis, and gastroesophageal reflux if present
      4. Recommend annual influenza vaccination

   C.   General pharmacological principles: a stepwise pharmacological approach is recommended (see table STEPWISE APROACH IN ADULTS)

STEPWISE APPROACH FOR MANAGING ASTHMA IN ADULTS

Preferred treatments are in bold print

Medications Needed to Maintain Long-Term Control

Daily Medications

STEP 4
Severe
Persistent

Preferred treatment:
- **High-dose inhaled corticosteroids AND Long-acting inhaled beta₂-agonists**

AND, if needed:
- Corticosteroid tablets or syrup long-term (2 mg/kg/day, generally do not exceed 60 mg/day). (Make repeat attempts to reduce systemic corticosteroids and maintain control with high-dose inhaled corticosteroids)

STEP 3
Moderate
Persistent

Preferred Treatment: (Listed alphabetically)
- **Low-to-medium dose inhaled corticosteroids and long-acting inhaled beta₂-agonists**

Alternative Treatment:
- Increase inhaled corticosteroids within medium-dose range

OR
- Low-to-medium dose inhaled corticosteroids and either leukotriene modifier or theophylline

If needed (particularly in patients with recurring severe exacerbations)

Preferred treatment:
- **Increase inhaled corticosteroids within medium-dose range and add long-acting inhaled beta₂-agonists**

Alternative Treatment: (Listed alphabetically)
- Increase inhaled corticosteroids within medium-dose range and add either leukotriene modifier of theophylline

STEP 2
Mild
Persistent

Preferred Treatment:
- **Low-dose inhaled corticosteroids**

Alternative Treatment: (Listed alphabetically)
- Cromolyn, leukotriene modifier, nedocromil, OR sustained release theophylline to serum concentration of 5-15 mcg/mL

STEP 1
Mild
Intermittent

- **No daily medication needed**
- Severe exacerbations may occur, separated by long periods of normal lung function and no symptoms. A course of systemic corticosteroids is recommended

QUICK RELIEF
All patients

- Short-acting bronchodilator: 2-4 puffs **short-acting inhaled beta₂-agonists** as needed for symptoms
- Intensity of treatment will depend on severity of exacerbation; up to 3 treatments at 20-minute intervals or a single nebulizer treatment as needed. Course of systemic corticosteroids may be needed
- Use of short-acting beta₂-agonists >2 times/week in intermittent asthma (daily, or increasing use in persistent asthma) may indicate the need to initiate (increase) long-term control therapy

Step down
Review treatment every 1 to 6 months; a gradual stepwise reduction in treatment may be possible

Step up
If control is not maintained, consider step up. First: review patient medication technique, adherence, and environmental control

Adapted from National Institute of Health. National Heart, Lung and Blood Institute (2002). *NAEPP Expert Panel Report guidelines for diagnosis and management of asthma – update on selected topics 2002.* National Asthma Education and Prevention Program. NIH Publ. #02-5075, Bethesda, MD.

1. The dose and dosing interval are dictated by the asthma severity with the goal of suppressing airway inflammation and preventing exacerbations
2. As needed, begin therapy at a high level (short course of systemic corticosteroids plus inhaled corticosteroids or use of medium-to-high dose of inhaled corticosteroids) to promptly control symptoms and then lower level
3. Cautiously and very gradually step down therapy after control is achieved and sustained for several weeks or months
   a. Generally, the last medication added should be the first medication reduced
   b. Inhaled corticosteroids may be reduced 25% every 2-3 months to the lowest dose possible to maintain control

4. Continual monitoring is imperative; control is indicated by the following:
   a. Peak expiratory flow (PEF) less than 10-20% variability
   b. PEF consistently greater than 80% patient's personal best
   c. Minimal symptoms
   d. Minimal need for short-acting inhaled beta$_2$-agonist
   e. Absence of nighttime awakenings
   f. No activity limitations
5. Other actions needed if control is not achieved and sustained at any step
   a. Assess patient adherence and technique in using medication
   b. Step up to next higher step of care or temporarily increase anti-inflammatory therapy such as with a burst of prednisone
   c. Reassess for factors that diminish control
   d. Consult a specialist
6. Long-term control drugs are used daily to maintain control of persistent asthma; quick-relief drugs treat acute symptoms and exacerbations
7. See next three tables for information and dosing of long-term control medications
8. Quick relief medications can be used at all steps to rapidly control symptoms (see table)

LONG-TERM CONTROL MEDICATIONS

1. Corticosteroids are the most potent and effective agents
   ✓ Oral/systemic form used for prompt control when initiating long-term therapy
   ✓ Inhaled form is preferred for long-term control
   ✓ Benefits outweigh risk of adverse effects; to reduce adverse effects, the following are recommended:
   - Use with spacers/holding chambers
   - Rinse mouth after use
   - Use lowest possible dose to maintain control
   - Consider a long-acting beta$_2$-agonist rather than a higher dose inhaled corticosteroid
   - Do not give varicella vaccine to patients receiving ≥2 mg/kg or 20 mg/day of oral prednisone
   ✓ In postmenopausal women, consider supplements of calcium, vitamin D, estrogen, and bisphosphonate therapy

2. Cromolyn sodium and nedocromil are mild to moderate anti-inflammatory medications
   ✓ Comparison of nedocromil and cromolyn
   - Nedocromil is more potent in inhibiting bronchospasm due to exercise, cold dry air, and bradykinin aerosol; more effective in nonallergic patients using inhaled corticosteroids
   - Nedocromil may help reduce dose requirements of corticosteroids

3. Long-acting beta$_2$-agonists are used with anti-inflammatory medications; helpful for nocturnal symptoms
   ✓ Salmeterol and Formoterol are **not used for treatment of acute symptoms or exacerbations**
   ✓ Daily use of these drugs should not exceed recommended amounts
   ✓ Even if symptoms improve, patients should **not** stop anti-inflammatory medication

4. Methylxanthines (mainly sustained-release theophylline) are used as adjuvant to inhaled corticosteroids for prevention of nocturnal symptoms
   ✓ Although not preferred, sustained-release theophylline may be alternative for long-term preventive therapy when cost or adherence in using inhaled medications is problematic
   ✓ Essential to monitor serum concentration levels
   ✓ Smoking increases metabolism of theophylline

5. Leukotriene modifiers are alternatives to low doses of inhaled corticosteroids or cromolyn or nedocromil for persons with mild persistent asthma (need more research and experience)
   ✓ Zafirlukast (Accolate) has an interaction effect with warfarin; essential to closely monitor prothrombin times and adjust appropriately
   ✓ Zileuton (Zyflo)
   - May infrequently cause liver toxicity; essential to monitor liver enzymes
   - May inhibit metabolism of terfenadine, warfarin, and theophylline
   ✓ Montelukast sodium (Singulair)

USUAL DOSAGES FOR LONG-TERM-CONTROL MEDICATIONS

Medication	Dosage Form	Dose
Inhaled Corticosteroids *(See table: Estimated Comparative Daily Dosages for Inhaled Corticosteroids)*		
Systemic Corticosteroids *(applies to all three corticosteroids)*		
Methylprednisolone Prednisolone Prednisone	2, 4, 8, 16, 32 mg tablets 5 mg tablets, 5 mg/5cc, 15 mg/5 cc 1, 2.5, 5, 10, 20, 50 mg tablets; 5 mg/cc, 5 mg/5cc	▪ 7.5-60 mg daily in a single dose in AM or QOD as needed for control ▪ Short-course "burst" to achieve control: 40-60 mg/day as single or 2 divided doses for 3-10 days
Long-Acting Inhaled Beta$_2$-Agonists *(Should not be used for symptom relief or for exacerbations. Use with inhaled corticosteroids)*		
Salmeterol Formoterol	MDI 21 mcg/puff DPI 50 mcg/blister DPI 12 mcg/single-use capsule	2 puffs q 12 hours 1 blister q 12 hours 1 capsule q 12 hours
Combined Medication		
Fluticasone/Salmeterol	DPI 100, 250, or 500 mcg/50 mcg	1 inh BID; dose depends on severity of asthma
Cromolyn and Nedocromil		
Cromolyn Nedocromil	MDI 1 mg/puff Nebulizer 20 mg/ampule MDI 1.75 mg/puff	2-4 puffs TID-QID 1 ampule TID-QID 2-4 puffs BID-QID
Leukotriene Modifiers		
Montelukast	4 or 5 mg chewable tablet 10 mg tablet	10 mg QHS
Zafirlukast	10 or 20 mg tablet	40 mg daily (20 mg tablet BID)
Zileuton	300 or 600 mg tablet	2,400 mg daily (give tablets QID)

ESTIMATED COMPARATIVE DAILY DOSAGES FOR INHALED CORTICOSTEROIDS

Drug	Low Daily Dose	Medium Daily Dose	High Daily Dose
Beclomethasone CFC 42 or 84 mcg/puff	168-504 mcg	504-840 mcg	>840 mcg
Beclomethasone HFA 40 of 80 mcg/puff	80-240 mcg	240-480 mcg	>480 mcg
Budesonide DPI 200 mcg/inh	200-600 mcg	600-1,200 mcg	>1,200 mcg
Flunisolide 250 mcg/puff	500-1,000 mcg	1,000-2,000 mcg	>2,000 mcg
Fluticasone MDI: 44, 110, or 220 mcg/puff DPI: 50, 100, or 250 mcg/inh	88-264 mcg 100-300 mcg	264-660 mcg 300-600 mcg	>660 mcg >600 mcg
Triamcinolone acetonide 100 mcg/puff	400-1,000 mcg	1,000-2,000 mcg	>2,000 mcg

QUICK-RELIEF MEDICATIONS

1. Therapy of choice is a short-acting beta$_2$-agonist
   - ✓ Use of >1 canister in 1 month signifies poor control & need to begin or increase anti-inflammatory drug
   - ✓ Regularly scheduled, daily use of these drugs is **not** recommended

2. Anticholinergics (ipratropium bromide) may provide additive benefit to inhaled beta$_2$-agonist or may be alternative quick-relief drug for patients unable to tolerate inhaled beta$_2$-agonist

3. Oral/systemic corticosteroids are used for moderate-to-severe exacerbations and can speed resolution of airflow obstruction and reduce rate of relapse

Adapted from National Institutes of Health. National Heart, Lung, and Blood Institute. (1997). *The Expert Panel Report 2: Guidelines for the diagnosis and management of asthma.* National Asthma Education Program. NIH Publ. #97-4051. Bethesda, MD.

D.   Treatment of **Step 1: Mild Intermittent Asthma in Adults**
1.   No daily medicine needed; prescribe short-acting inhaled beta$_2$-agonist on an as-needed basis (see table)

DOSAGES FOR INHALED SHORT-ACTING BETA$_2$-AGONISTS

Medication	Dosage Form	Adult Dose	Comments
	Metered-Dose Inhaler		
Albuterol (Ventolin) Albuterol HFA (Proventil HFA) Pirbuterol (Maxair Autohaler)	90 mcg/puff, 200 puffs 200 mcg/puff, 400 puffs	2 puffs TID-QID prn	Increasing or regular use on a daily basis indicates the need for additional long-term-control therapy
	Dry Powder Inhaler		
Albuterol Rotacaps (Ventolin)	200 mcg/capsule	1-2 capsules Q 4-6 hours prn	
	Nebulizer solution		
Albuterol (Ventolin)	5 mg/mL (0.5%)	1.25-5 mg (0.25-1 cc) in 2-3 cc of saline Q 4-8 hours	May mix with cromolyn or ipratropium nebulizer solutions
Levalbuterol (Xopenex)	0.63 mg/3 mL 1.25 mg/3 mL	0.63 mg-1.25 mg in 3 cc TID Q 6-8 hours	Advantage for patients who have significant side effects to albuterol
Bitolterol (Tornalate)	2 mg/mL (0.2%)	0.5-3.5 mg (0.25-1 cc) in 2-3 cc of saline Q 4-8 hours	May not mix with other nebulizer solutions

Adapted from National Institutes of Health. National Heart, Lung, and Blood Institute. (1997). *The Expert Panel Report 2: Guidelines for the diagnosis and management of asthma.* National Asthma Education Program, Office of Prevention, Education and Control. NIH Publication #97-4051. Bethesda, MD.

2.   Treatment of **exercise-induced bronchospasm**; use one of following:
a.   Short-acting inhaled beta$_2$-agonist 1-2 puffs 5 minutes prior to exercise
b.   Inhaled cromolyn sodium (Intal) or nedocromil (Tilade) 2 puffs 10 minutes prior to exercise
c.   Formoterol (Foradil Aerolizer) is indicated when administered on an occasional as needed basis for the acute prevention of exercise-induced bronchospasm (dose one capsule [one 12 microgram inhalation] inhaled at least 15 minutes prior to exercise; additional doses should not be used for 12 hours)
d.   Inhaled corticosteroids are recommended for long-term control
3.   Treatment of **mild exacerbations** due to viral respiratory infections: prescribe short-acting beta$_2$-agonist every 4-6 hours for approximately 24 hours
4.   Treatment of **moderate-to-severe exacerbations:**
a.   Use both of the following:
(1)   Give short-acting beta$_2$-agonist by nebulizer or MDI (with close supervision can give 3 treatments spaced every 20-30 minutes)
(2)   Also, prescribe systemic corticosteroid; patients with history of severe exacerbations should start corticosteroids at first sign of infection (see table USUAL DOSAGES FOR LONG-TERM CONTROL MEDICATIONS)
b.   Oxygen is recommended for most patients
c.   Careful, vigilant monitoring of patient's condition is paramount

E.   Treatment of **Step 2: Mild Persistent Asthma:** Use inhaled short-acting beta$_2$-agonist on an as-needed basis
1.   Prescribe inhaled corticosteroids at a low dose (see table DAILY DOSAGES OF INHALED CORTICOSTEROIDS); when taking several inhaled medications simultaneously, always use beta$_2$-agonist first to open airway and then use steroid inhaler for greater penetration of medication

2. Alternative treatment (select one)
   a. Cromolyn (Intal) or Nedocromil (Tilade)
   b. Sustained-release theophylline is an alternative, but is not preferred because of modest effectiveness and potential for toxicity; prescribe drug to achieve a serum concentration of between 5 and 15 mcg/mL (periodic monitoring is necessary to maintain a therapeutic level)
   c. Leukotriene receptor antagonists (zafirlukast, zileuton, or montelukast sodium) are alternative drugs
3. For exacerbations, see V.D.3.4. and V.L.

F. Treatment of **Step 3: Moderate Persistent Asthma:** Consultation with an asthma specialist is advised
   1. Preferred treatment is low-to-medium dose of inhaled corticosteroids and long-acting beta$_2$-agonists such as formoterol (Foradil) or salmeterol (Serevent); for patients on fluticasone (Flovent) when salmeterol is being added to regimen, fluticasone/salmeterol (Advair Diskcus) is an option
   2. Alternative treatment: Increase inhaled corticosteroid within medium-dose range – OR – low-to-medium dose inhaled corticosteroid and either leukotriene modifier or theophylline
   3. Additional plan: If symptoms are not optimally controlled with initial plan, either of the following two strategies is recommended
      a. Increase inhaled corticosteroid within medium-dose range and add long-acting inhaled beta$_2$-agonist
      b. Increase inhaled corticosteroid within medium-dose range and add either leukotriene modifier or theophylline (alternative)

G. Treatment of **Step 4: Severe Persistent Asthma:** Consult specialist
   1. Preferred treatment: High-dose inhaled corticosteroids AND long-acting inhaled beta$_2$-agonists
   2. Additionally, if needed, prescribe an oral systemic corticosteroid
      a. Prescribe lowest possible dose (single daily dose on alternate days)
      b. Do not exceed 60 mg/day
      c. Carefully monitor for adverse side effects such as secondary infections, electrolyte imbalances, hypertension, peptic ulcers, dermal atrophy, carbohydrate intolerance, osteoporosis, cataracts, glaucoma, and psychological effects (euphoria, depression)
      d. Conscientiously try to reduce systemic corticosteroids once symptoms are controlled and maintain control with high-dose inhaled corticosteroids that have less adverse effects
      e. For exacerbations see V.D.3.4. and V.L.

H. Special considerations in older adults
   1. Chronic obstructive pulmonary disease may coexist with asthma; trial of systemic corticosteroids will determine whether the airflow obstruction is reversible; if reversible, long-term asthma medication may be beneficial
   2. Adjustments in medication may be needed due to increased adverse effects in the elderly and the effects of co-morbid conditions (heart disease, COPD, diabetes)

I. Treatment of exercise-induced bronchospasm (EIB) (see V.D.2.)

J. Home management of exacerbations
   1. Increase inhaled beta$_2$-agonist (up to three treatments of 2-4 puffs by MDI at 20 minute intervals or a single nebulizer treatment)
      a. If good response: continue beta$_2$-agonist every 3-4 hours for 24-48 hours; patients on inhaled corticosteroids should double dose for 7-10 days; contact clinician for followup instructions
      b. If response is incomplete: Add oral corticosteroid and continue beta$_2$-agonist and contact clinician within the day
      c. If poor response: Add oral corticosteroid, repeat beta$_2$-agonist immediately; if distress is severe go to emergency department or call 911
   2. Continue more intensive treatment for several days as recovery from exacerbations is often slow

K. Route of administration: inhaled route more effectively delivers medication to lung, has reduced side effects, and the onset of action is shorter than oral medications (see following tables on descriptions and how to use various delivery devices)

AEROSOL DELIVERY DEVICES

Device/Drugs*	Therapeutic Issues
Metered-dose inhaler (MDI) Beta$_2$-agonists Corticosteroids Cromolyn sodium and Nedocromil Anticholinergics	Takes coordination to actuate and inhale. Mouth washing is effective in reducing systemic absorption
Breath-actuated MDI Beta$_2$-agonists	Best for patients unable to coordinate inhalation and actuation (may be particularly useful in elderly). Cannot be used with currently available spacer/ holding chamber devices
Dry powder inhaler (DPI) Beta$_2$-agonists Corticosteroids	Delivery may be ≥MDI depending on device and technique. Mouth washing is effective in reducing systemic absorption
Space/holding chamber	Easier to use than MDI alone
	Decrease oropharyngeal deposition. Reduce potential systemic absorption of inhaled corticosteroid preparations that have higher oral bioavailability; recommended for all patients on medium-to-high doses of inhaled corticosteroids
	May be as effective as nebulizer in delivering high doses of beta$_2$-agonists during severe exacerbations
Nebulizer Beta$_2$-agonists Cromolyn Anticholinergics Corticosteroids	Use for high-dose beta$_2$-agonists and anticholinergics in moderate-to-severe exacerbations in all patients
	Less dependent on patient coordination or cooperation

*See additional tables for directions on how to use metered-dose inhaler, dry powder capsules, nebulizers, and Diskcus

Adapted from National Institutes of Health. National Heart, Lung, and Blood Institute. (1997). *The Expert Panel Report 2: Guidelines for the diagnosis and management of asthma*. National Asthma Education Program. NIH Publ. #97-4051. Bethesda, MD.

DIRECTIONS ON HOW TO USE AN INHALER*

- Remove the cap, hold the inhaler upright and shake it

- Tilt your head back slightly and slowly exhale

- Put the inhaler 1-2 inches from your mouth (open mouth technique) -- OR -- Enclose mouthpiece with your lips (closed mouth technique); do **not** use closed mouth technique for corticosteroids -- OR -- Use spacer/holding chamber** (slowly inhale or tidal breathe immediately after actuation; actuate only once into chamber per inhalation or if face mask is used, allow 3-5 inhalations per actuation)

- Press down on the plunger and take a full, deep, slow, even breath (breathe in through mouth, not through nose)

- Hold your breath for 10 seconds, then exhale slowly through your nose

- Wait one minute before taking next puff

- Rinse your mouth afterward to prevent possible fungal infection

- Keep mouthpiece clean

*Counsel regarding danger of overuse of inhaler. Patients should be using <u>no</u> more than 1 canister (200 metered dose inhalations of a beta$_2$-agonist) in a month
**Spacers/holding chambers are particularly recommended for older adults and for patients using inhaled corticosteroids

Adapted from National Institutes of Health. National Heart, Lung, and Blood Institute. (1997). *The Expert Panel Report 2: Guidelines for the diagnosis and management of asthma*. National Asthma Education Program. NIH Publ. #97-4051. Bethesda, MD.

DIRECTIONS ON HOW TO USE DRY POWDER CAPSULES

- Close mouth tightly around mouthpiece
- Inhale deeply and rapidly
- Minimally effective inspiratory flow is device dependent

DIRECTIONS ON HOW TO USE A NEBULIZER

- Measure correct amount of normal saline solution and place into cup (if medicine is premixed, go to step 3)
- Measure correct amount of medicine and put into cup with saline solution
- Fasten mouthpiece to the T-shaped part and then fasten this unit to the cup
- Put mouthpiece in mouth and seal lips tightly around
- Turn on the air compressor machine
- Take slow, deep breaths through mouth
- Hold breath 1-2 seconds before exhaling
- Continue until medicine is depleted from cup (approximately 10 minutes)
- Do not forget to clean nebulizer; cleaning removes germs and prevents infection as well as keeps nebulizer from clogging

Adapted from National Institutes of Health. (1992). *Teach your patients about asthma: A clinician's guide.* National Asthma Education Program, Office of Prevention, Education and Control. Publication #92-2737. Bethesda, MD.

DIRECTIONS ON HOW TO USE DISKCUS

- Hold device level with one hand
- With thumb of the other hand on the thumbgrip, push thumb away from you until you hear the mouthpiece snap into position
- With mouthpiece towards you, slide the lever away from you until you hear a click (each time the lever is pushed back a dose is available for inhalation)
- Breathe out as far as comfortable while holding device level and away from your mouth
- With the mouthpiece to your lips, breathe in deeply and steadily through the device
- Hold your breath for around 10 seconds, then breathe out slowly
- To close the device, slide the thumbgrip back towards you and click the device shut (the device will be reset and ready for next scheduled dose)
- Remember to never exhale into device
- Keep the device dry; never wash any part of the device

Adapted from GlaxoWellcome. (1995) Patient instructions for use of Serevent Diskcus (salmeterol xinafoate) inhalation powder. Research Triangle Park, NC.

L. Patient Education: establish a partnership with patient and include patient in developing goals and plan; important components of patient education include the following:
1. Basic facts about asthma
2. Roles of medications
3. Discuss asthma triggers and ways to avoid or control them (see V.B.)
4. Review techniques and ask patient to demonstrate use of inhaler, spacer, nebulizer, or Diskcus (many drug failures are due to improper use of equipment)
5. Counsel regarding overuse of inhalers which could result in tachyarrhythmias and death
6. Teach how to recognize symptom patterns that indicate poor asthma control; may need to keep a daily diary of symptoms, peak flow readings, and medications
7. Develop a written action plan based on peak flow readings (see Expert Panel Report 2, 1997)
8. Extensive teaching on exacerbation management is needed
   a. Discuss indicators of worsening asthma, specific recommendations for using beta$_2$-agonist rescue therapy, early administration of systemic corticosteroids, and directions on seeking medical care
   b. Patients at high risk of asthma-related death include those using >2 canisters per month of beta$_2$-agonists, difficulty perceiving airflow obstruction, co-morbidity, severe psychiatric or psychosocial problems, low socioeconomic status, illicit drug use, and prior history of severe exacerbations, intubation, hospitalizations, frequent ER visits
9. Good web site resources (see following table)

WEBSITE RESOURCES

Organization	Website
Allergy and Asthma Network/Mothers of Asthmatics, Inc.	http://www.aanma.org
Asthma and Allergy Foundation of America	http://www.aafa.org
National Asthma Education and Prevention Program, National Heart, Lung, and Blood Information Center	http://www.nhlbi.nih.gov
Asthma in America	http://www.asthmainamerica.com

M.   Follow Up
1.   For acute exacerbations with incomplete or poor responses see patient within 24 hours and then re-evaluate in 3-5 days
2.   After exacerbation has resolved completely, schedule follow up visits every 1-3 months
3.   For patients on theophylline, check serum drug levels after 2 weeks from initiation of therapy; then every 4 months
4.   Follow up for other patients depends on symptom severity, symptom control, knowledge level, social support and other resources; for new asthmatics, frequent visits are important to monitor disease as well as for patient education

BRONCHITIS, ACUTE

I.   Definition: Infection of the tracheobronchial tree that causes reversible bronchial inflammation

II.   Pathogenesis

A.   Mucous membrane of tracheobronchial tree becomes hyperemic, edematous, with increased bronchial secretions and destruction of epithelium and impaired mucociliary activity

B.   Pathogens
1.   In >90% of cases, the infection has a nonbacterial cause; the viruses most frequently associated with lower respiratory tract disease include influenza B, influenza A, parainfluenza, respiratory syncytial virus
2.   *Bordetella pertussis, Mycoplasma pneumoniae, Chlamydia pneumoniae* as a group are associated as the nonviral causes in 5-10% of cases
3.   Secondary bacterial invasion by *Streptococcus pneumoniae, Moraxella catarrhalis* and *Haemophilus influenzae* type B usually occur in patients with underlying lung disease

III.   Clinical Presentation

A.   Cough, with or without sputum, particularly at night, is hallmark symptom; sputum may be clear or purulent

B.   Most patients are afebrile with mild symptoms

C.   Symptoms such as fever, substernal pain, and possibly mucoid sputum production, dyspnea, or bronchospasm with wheezing occur occasionally (fever is a common sign especially the first 48 hours but often resolves over a few days)

D.   Symptoms typically last 7-14 days but may continue for 3 weeks (cough lasting longer than 3 weeks exceeds case definition for acute bronchitis)

E.   Smokers have more frequent, longer, and more severe episodes than nonsmokers

F.   Some patients with acute bronchitis have an underlying predisposition to bronchial reactivity which may turn into more chronic bronchial inflammation which characterizes asthma

G.   Adults with acute bronchitis due to pertussis typically have a chronic cough which is often paroxysmal and may or may not have the typical "whooping"; adults with unrecognized pertussis may transmit pathogen to nonimmune children (limit suspicion and treatment unless there are documented outbreaks)

IV.   Diagnosis/Evaluation

A.   History
1.   Determine onset, duration and characteristics of cough, particularly ask about night coughing
2.   Inquire about frequency and pattern of previous episodes of coughing
3.   Ask about associated symptoms such as fever, pharyngitis, dyspnea, chest pain

4. Questions about the appearance of the sputum are not considered helpful as purulent sputum occurs when inflammatory cells are present and neither the character nor production of sputum is predictive of a bacterial etiology
5. Inquire about infectious illnesses of other household members
6. Always ask if patient or household members smoke
7. Inquire about past medical history, particularly respiratory diseases
8. Determine immunization history of patient and household members

B. Physical Examination
1. Assess eyes, ears, nose, and throat for signs of inflammation
2. Palpate and transilluminate sinuses
3. Perform a heart examination
4. Perform a complete lung examination; inspect, palpate, percuss, and auscultate
5. Palpate for lymph nodes

C. Differential Diagnosis
1. Pneumonia and acute bronchitis are extremely difficult to differentiate. The following characteristics are more consistent with <u>pneumonia</u> than bronchitis in adults:
   a. Fever >100.4°F oral body temperature (>38°C)
   b. Increased respiratory rate (>24 breaths/minute)
   c. Increased heart rate (>100 beats/minute)
   d. Rigors and constitutional symptoms
   e. Pleuritic chest pain
   f. Rusty/bloody sputum
   g. Focal consolidation with rales, egophony, fremitus
   h. X-ray abnormalities
2. Upper respiratory infection and sinusitis
3. Tuberculosis
4. Asthma should be considered in patients who have repetitive episodes of acute bronchitis
5. Allergies
6. Cystic fibrosis
7. Nonpulmonary causes of cough such as congestive heart failure, reflux esophagitis, and bronchogenic tumors

D. Diagnostic Tests: Acute bronchitis is a diagnosis of exclusion
1. Order a chest x-ray if the patient has severe symptoms to confirm or rule out the diagnosis of pneumonia
2. Consider PPD if patient is at risk for tuberculosis
3. Consider diagnostic pulmonary function testing or provocative testing with a methacholine challenge test when asthma is suspected; to diagnose asthma, abnormalities in tests must persist after the acute phase
4. If a diagnosis of pertussis is suspected, consult local public health officials concerning appropriate diagnostic tests (culture or polymerase chain reaction)
5. CBC and sputum cultures are not necessary unless diagnosis is uncertain

V. Plan/Management

A. Antibiotic treatment is NOT recommended in uncomplicated acute bronchitis, as most cases of acute bronchitis are viral; even patients who have a persistent cough (>10 days) usually do not need antibiotics

B. Only symptomatic treatment is needed in most cases

C. Consider a trial of inhaled albuterol (Ventolin) 2 puffs every 6 hours for 7 days for patients with troublesome cough and evidence of bronchial hyperresponsiveness; the effect of anticholinergic bronchodilator treatment in acute bronchitis is unknown

D. Consider prescribing erythromycin for 14 days for patients in frequent contact with nonimmunized infants due to risk of pertussis infection; however, careful surveillance of infant is probably more beneficial than treating contagious patient

E. Patient Education
1. Antihistamines should be avoided because they dry out secretions; expectorants have not been found to relieve symptoms
2. Cough suppressants should be avoided except if patient is unable to sleep due to irritating cough
3. Encourage smoking cessation
4. Website resources
   a. American Thoracic Society (http://www.thoracic.org)
   b. National Heart, Lung, and Blood Information Center (http://www.nhlbi.nih.gov)

F. Follow Up
1. Return to clinic if symptoms persist longer than 7-14 days or if condition worsens; although previously patients with symptoms lasting over one week were treated with antibiotics for a bacterial etiology, today it is recognized that even viral infections may persist for 3 weeks
2. Patients who do not improve after 4 to 6 weeks need further evaluation (see section on COUGH)

CHRONIC OBSTRUCTIVE PULMONARY DISEASE

I. Definition: A complex syndrome of chronic airway obstruction or airflow limitation which is generally progressive and may be accompanied by airway hyperactivity; patients with nonremitting asthma are classified as suffering from COPD, but most frequently COPD is caused by the following two conditions:

A. Emphysema is a pathologic diagnosis based on a permanent abnormal dilation and destruction of the alveolar ducts and air spaces distal to the terminal bronchioles

B. Chronic bronchitis is a clinical diagnosis based on the presence of a cough and sputum production occurring on most days for at least a 3-month period during 2 consecutive years without another explanation; cough is not necessarily accompanied by airflow limitation

II. Pathogenesis

A. Emphysema is characterized by airway obstruction, hyperinflation, loss of lung elastic recoil, and destruction of the alveolar-capillary interface which decreases gas exchange

B. Chronic bronchitis is characterized by thickened bronchial walls, hyperplasia and hypertrophied mucous glands, and mucosal inflammation in the bronchial walls, large central airways, and later, in the small airways

C. COPD has predominantly neutrophilic inflammation versus asthma which has predominantly eosinophilic inflammation

D. Predisposing Factors
1. Tobacco smoke (primary cause in 80-90% of cases)
2. Recurrent or chronic respiratory infections and hyper-responsive airways such as from asthma or atopy
3. Occupational and environmental exposure to atmospheres polluted with dust, chemical fumes, and "second hand" tobacco smoke
4. α_1-antitrypsin deficiency (suspect this in patients under 45 years who have significant COPD symptoms whether or not they smoke)

III. Clinical Presentation

A. Fourth leading cause of death in U.S.; World Health Organization anticipates by 2020 will be third common cause of death

B. In COPD, both elements of emphysema and chronic bronchitis are present but usually one condition predominates

C. Begins early in adult life, but significant symptoms do not become apparent until the middle years; most patients have been smoking at least 20 cigarettes per day for 20 or more years before symptoms develop (however 10% of nonsmokers will develop the disease)

D. Most common symptom is gradually progressing exertional dyspnea

E. Other symptoms include chronic cough, wheezing, recurrent respiratory infections, fatigue, weight loss, and decreased libido

F. Signs include tachypnea, increased use of accessory muscles, increased anterior-posterior chest diameter, hyper-resonance on percussion, decreased heart and breath sounds, prolonged expiration during quiet breathing, wheezes and rhonchi

G. Once COPD is established, the patient's condition tends to gradually worsen; however, early detection of the disease with treatment and modifications in risk factors can significantly alter the disease course

H. Characterized by episodes of acute exacerbations
    1. Three clinical findings occur during an exacerbation: worsening dyspnea, increase in sputum purulence, and increase in sputum volume
    2. Triggered by environmental exposures and tracheobronchial infections that can lead to acute respiratory decompensation; infection is most common cause of death in these patients

I. Pulmonary hypertension and cor pulmonale are caused by chronic hypoxemia that may result in symptoms and signs of right-sided heart failure:
    1. Dyspnea at rest
    2. Fatigue and possibly syncope and angina during exertion
    3. Impaired cognitive function
    4. Peripheral edema, weight gain
    5. Cyanosis and neck vein distension
    6. Holosystolic murmur and S_3 gallop
    7. Hepatomegaly
    8. Erythrocytosis
    9. Renal function abnormalities

J. Left ventricular heart failure can also develop in patients with severe COPD

IV. Diagnosis/Evaluation

    A. History
        1. Ask patient to specifically describe how far he/she can walk before becoming dyspneic; determine number of stairs patient can climb before stopping to rest
        2. Explore symptoms and limitations experienced in daily living both at rest and with exercise
        3. If cough is present, ask patient to describe onset, characteristics, and amount and color of sputum production
        4. Question about signs and symptoms of infection such as chills and fever
        5. Inquire about associated symptoms such as fatigue, angina, insomnia, edema, weight gain, changes in voiding, weight loss
        6. Determine number of pillows patient sleeps on at night
        7. Essential to explicitly ask about patterns of cigarette smoking (age at initiation, quantity smoked per day, and whether or not still smoking); inquire about passive smoking
        8. Inquire about occupational and environmental exposure to irritants
        9. Thoroughly explore past medical history to include previous hospitalizations for respiratory disorders
        10. Consider questioning patients with severe symptoms about their wishes concerning intubation and resuscitation
        11. Consider asking patient to complete a health-related quality of life tool

    B. Physical Examination
        1. Observe general appearance, noting color, posture, gait, affect, and degree of respiratory distress when walking
        2. Closely monitor weight
        3. Assess vital signs, being alert for fever, tachycardia, and tachypnea
        4. Observe for clubbing

5. Observe chest for increased anterior-posterior diameter, retractions, accessory muscle use, and pursed-lip breathing
6. Percuss, palpate, and auscultate lungs (note wheezes, decreased breath sounds, and prolonged forced expiratory time)
7. Auscultate heart
8. Palpate for organomegaly
9. Palpate extremities, assessing for peripheral edema and presence and quality of pulses

C. Differential Diagnosis
    1. Consider asthma in younger persons, particularly smokers
    2. Congestive heart failure
    3. Acute bronchitis
    4. Bronchiectasis
    5. Obliterative bronchiolitis
    6. Diffuse panbronchiolitis

D. Diagnostic Tests
    1. All persons with altered lung function as well as persons at risk for COPD should be evaluated with spirometry; assess airflow obstruction with FEV_1 (forced expiratory volume in one second), FVC (total volume forcibly exhaled), and FEV_1/FVC ratio; spirometry defines severity, helps in determining prognosis, and measures response to therapy and disease progression
        a. Early screening for at risk individuals is important; patients have a large reserve of pulmonary function and usually do not develop COPD symptoms until quite severe airflow obstruction is present
            (1) When the ratio of FEV_1 to FVC (FEV_1/FVC) is one second lower than normally expected, airflow limitation is present
            (2) A decline in the FEV_1 greater than expected (normally there is less than a 30 mL decrease per year) helps identify patients at risk for COPD
        b. Diagnosis of COPD is established when FEV_1/FVC ratio is ≤70%
        c. Staging of COPD is based on FEV_1 (see table CLASSIFICATION OF COPD BY SEVERITY)

CLASSIFICATION OF COPD BY SEVERITY	
Stage	**Characteristics**
0: At Risk	• Normal spirometry • Chronic symptoms (cough, sputum production)
I: Mild COPD	• FEV_1/FVC <70% • FEV_1 ≥80% predicted • With or without chronic symptoms (cough, sputum production)
II: Moderate COPD	• FEV_1/FVC <70% • 30% ≤ FEV_1 <80% predicted (IIA: 50% ≤ FEV_1 80% predicted) (IIB: 30% ≤ FEV_1 50% predicted) • With or without chronic symptoms (cough, sputum production, dyspnea)
III: Severe COPD	• FEV_1/FVC <70% • FEV_1 <30% predicted or FEV_1 <50% predicted plus respiratory failure or clinical signs of right heart failure

FEV_1: forced expiratory volume in one second; FVC: forced vital capacity; respiratory failure: arterial partial pressure of oxygen (PaO_2) less than 8.0 kPa (60 mm Hg) with or without arterial partial pressure of CO_2 ($PaCO_2$) greater than 6.7 kPa (50 mm Hg)

Adapted from National Institutes of Health, National Heart, Lung, and Blood Institute (2001). *Executive Summary. Global strategy for the diagnosis, management, and prevention of chronic obstructive pulmonary disease.* NIH Publ. #2701A, Bethesda, MD.

        d. Spirometry 10 minutes after administration of a short-acting beta₂-agonist confirms presence and reversibility of airflow obstruction; an increase of ≥15% in FEV_1 indicates the presence of a substantial reversible component
    2. For newly diagnosed patients, obtain chest x-ray which is diagnostic only of severe emphysema but is essential to rule out other abnormalities; lung hyperinflation, flattening of diaphragms, and increased retrosternal airspace occur in severe emphysema
    3. For patients 45 years old or younger who have a familial history of emphysema or roentgenographic evidence of panlobular emphysema consider testing for $α_1$-protease inhibitor deficiency

4. Arterial blood gases (ABGs) are not necessary in Stage 1 but are important to monitor disease progression in Stages II and III; ABGs determine need for oxygen therapy and facilitate diagnosis of respiratory failure
5. Other testing is usually not needed except in special situations:
    a. Consider ordering carbon monoxide diffusing capacity when the patient has dyspnea out of proportion to severity of airflow limitation
    b. Order CBC with differential, Gram's stain, and culture of sputum, and administer tuberculin skin test (PPD) if infection is suspected
    c. For patients with severe airflow obstruction, order electrocardiogram to assess for cardiac dysfunction and presence of cor pulmonale

V. Plan/Management

A. Prevention of further damage is essential; treatment is also aimed at increasing airflow, decreasing respiratory symptoms and exacerbations
    1. Cessation of smoking is the single most important intervention especially in early stage of disease as lung function improves initially and annual decline of FEV_1 is slowed (see section TOBACCO USE AND SMOKING CESSATION)
    2. Prevention of infection is important
        a. Pneumococcal vaccination is not recommended for general use in COPD population
        b. Yearly prophylactic vaccination against influenza is recommended
        c. Consider prescribing amantadine (Symmetrel) or oseltamivir (Tamiflu) following exposure to influenza A virus for unimmunized persons who are at high risk for influenza or persons who have acute influenza infection
            (1) Amantadine (Symmetrel): Over 65 years of age prescribe 100 mg/day; under 65 years prescribe 100 mg BID for 2-7 days depending on patient characteristics or clinical improvement (treatment and prophylaxis have similar dosages)
            (2) Oseltamivir (Tamiflu): Start within 2 days of symptom onset or exposure; Treatment: ≥13 years, 75 mg BID for 5 days; reduce to 75 mg QD if decreased creatinine clearance; Prophylaxis: ≥13 years, after close contact with infected individual prescribe 75 mg QD for at least 7 days
    3. Elimination of environmental irritants may be beneficial
        a. In areas of high ozone environments (e.g., industrialized cities) counsel patients to limit or avoid outdoor activities when the air quality is poor
        b. Advise patients that extremes in temperature, humidity, high altitudes, and air travel can trigger hyper-reactivity in irritated airways
    4. Avoid potentially harmful drugs such as antihistamines, cough suppressants, sedatives, tranquilizers, beta-blockers, and narcotics
    5. Early treatment of recurrent and chronic infections is important; however, many exacerbations may be due to viral infections of upper respiratory tract and antibiotics may not be indicated
        a. Indicators of infection are change in color, consistency, and amount of sputum, increased dyspnea, and possibly fever; may also have increased malaise, fatigue, insomnia
        b. Approximately one-half of exacerbations are due to bacterial infections; major pathogen is *Haemophilus influenzae* (20-40% of strains are resistant to beta-lactam antibiotics); other bacterial pathogens include *Streptococcus pneumoniae* and *Moraxella catarrhalis*
        c. Antibiotic therapy is warranted in some patients but not in younger patients who are in stage 1 with mild symptoms and infrequent exacerbations
            (1) For patients ≤60 years with mild-to-moderate impairment of lung function (FEV_1 ≥50% predicted) and who have <4 exacerbations per year prescribe one of the following antibiotics:
                (a) Doxycycline (Vibramycin) 100 mg capsule BID for 5-10 days
                (b) Sulfamethoxazole-trimethoprim (Septra DS) 1 tab BID for 5-10 days
                (c) Amoxicillin-clavulanate (Augmentin) 500 mg tab TID or 875 mg tab BID for 5-10 days
            (2) For older patients with moderate or severe impairments and frequent exacerbations (4 or more per year) prescribe one of the following:
                (a) Clarithromycin (Biaxin) 500 mg tab BID for 7-14 days
                (b) Azithromycin (Zithromax) 500 mg tab day 1, 250 mg tab daily days 2-5
                (c) Moxifloxacin (Avelox) 400 mg tab daily for 5-10 days

B. Pharmacological therapy: use a stepwise approach based on stage of COPD, patient's symptoms, and patient's tolerance to specific drugs
1. **For patients in Stage I or with mild COPD** prescribe short-acting beta$_2$-agonist as needed; prescribe albuterol (Ventolin) or metaproterenol (Alupent), both metered dose inhalers (MDI) with or without spacers, 1-2 puffs TID or QID as needed (prn or rescue therapy) or as prophylaxis before exercise (not to exceed 8-12 puffs in 24 hours)
    a. There is no evidence that early, regular use of these medications alters progression of COPD
    b. Carefully dose these drugs to patients with cardiac disease because of the potential of arrhythmias
2. **For patients in Stage II or with moderate COPD**, prescribe a regular treatment with one or more bronchodilators and possibly an inhaled corticosteroid (see V.B.3.a.b.) (prescribe corticosteroid ONLY if the patient has a documented spirometric response to this drug or for patients in Stage IIB)
    a. Inhaled therapy is preferred
    b. The choice of which bronchodilator to prescribe depends on the patient's response in terms of symptom relief and adverse effects as well as availability
        (1) Anticholinergic agent, ipratropium bromide (Atrovent), has the advantage of low incidence of side effects and absence of tachyphylaxis; prescribe MDI, 2-6 puffs every 6-8 hours (because of slow onset and long duration of action use only on a regular basis)
        (2) Short-acting beta$_2$-agonists are another choice; there is recent concern that these agents might increase risk of myocardial infarction (MI)
            (a) Prescribe albuterol (Ventolin) or metaproterenol (Alupent), (MDI), 1-4 puffs every 4-6 hours daily as needed or on a regular basis
            (b) Nebulized beta$_2$-agonists are usually no more effective than MDIs, but are helpful in patients who have trouble using inhalers
        (3) Long-acting beta$_2$-agonists are more convenient; they may reduce the adhesion of bacteria such as *Haemophilus influenzae* to airway epithelial cells; also, they are particularly beneficial in patients who have reversible disease with nocturnal attacks of wheezing; prescribe one of the following:
            (a) Salmeterol (Serevent) MDI 21 mcg/inh, 2 puffs every 12 hours (Serevent Diskcus is not indicated for maintenance in COPD)
            (b) Formoterol (Foradil Aerolizer) 12 mcg/inh, 1 inhalation every 12 hours (Aerolizer Inhaler should never be washed and should be kept dry; capsules should be handled with dry hands)
        (4) Theophylline is effective, but inhaled bronchodilators are preferred because they have less potential toxicity; prescribe sustained release theophylline (Theo-24 or Uniphyl) 400 mg preferably at HS for nocturnal bronchospasm
            (a) Additional benefits of theophylline include increase in cardiac output, improved contraction and delayed fatigue of diaphragm, stimulation of respiratory center, and diuresis
            (b) Has a narrow therapeutic window; titrate dosage to achieve safe levels in range of 8-12 µg/ml
            (c) In a smoker, theophylline dosage is approximately 50% higher than that required by nonsmoker
            (d) In a patient with hypoxia, congestive heart failure, or liver disease the dosage is 25%-50% lower than dose required of nonsmoker
            (e) Theophylline interacts with several drugs; prescribe cautiously
    c. Consider combining drugs with different mechanisms and durations of action
        (1) Combinations may increase degree of bronchodilation for equivalent or lesser adverse effects
        (2) Albuterol and ipratropium are available in the same MDI; Combivent 2 puffs QID with maximum of 12 puffs per day
3. **For patients in Stage III or severe COPD**, prescribe regular treatment with one or more bronchodilators (see V.B.2.b.) and an inhaled corticosteroid if patient has significant symptoms and lung response to this therapy or if patient has recurrence of exacerbations
    a. Prescribe a trial of 6 weeks to 3 months of one of the following inhaled corticosteroids to identify patients who may benefit from this therapy:
        (1) Beclomethasone (Beclovent) MDI 2 puffs BID
        (2) Triamcinolone (Azmacort) MDI 2 puffs BID
    b. Long-term treatment with oral corticosteroids is not recommended and may cause steroid myopathy which may lead to muscle weakness, decreased functionality, and respiratory failure in patients in Stage III

351

C.   Treatment of exacerbations; consider the following:
1.   Evaluate patient for cause and severity such as airway infection, pneumonia, cardiac failure, pulmonary embolism, or spontaneous pneumothorax
2.   Increase the dose and/or frequency of the existing bronchodilator therapy
3.   Add an anticholinergic until symptoms improve, if patient is not already taking one
4.   Oral corticosteroids shorten recovery time and should be considered as an additional drug if the patient's baseline FEV_1 is <50%; prescribe prednisolone 40 mg per day for 10 days
5.   For more severe cases, high-dose nebulizer therapy on a prn basis for the acute episode may be helpful
6.   Noninvasive intermittent positive pressure ventilation (NIPPV) improves blood gases and pH, and reduces mortality
7.   Prescribe an antibiotic only if patient has worsening dyspnea and cough as well as increased sputum volume and purulence (see V.A.5.)

D.   Considerations when prescribing medications
1.   Frequent errors in medication management are inadequate teaching about how to use inhalers, suboptimal dosing, inadequate monitoring, and failure to advise patient to take medicine before exercising.
2.   Teach patient correct method of using inhaler (see table DIRECTIONS ON HOW TO USE AN INHALER in ASTHMA section)

E.   Formal or individualized patient education and pulmonary rehabilitation programs are beneficial
1.   Components of successful programs include individual and family education: information about disease process, smoking cessation, medication administration, maintenance of home oxygen equipment, strategies to attain and maintain normal weight, avoidance of infection, sexual counseling, discussion of extraordinary life-support measures, and exercise training
2.   Encourage exercise
     a.   Exercise training has been shown to increase exercise tolerance whereby the patient is able to perform a given level of exercise at a lower oxygen consumption and a lower minute ventilation
     b.   Upper extremity training can help lessen diaphragmatic work and concomitant fatigue
     c.   Lower-extremity exercise is sometimes beneficial
     d.   Pursed-lip breathing and diaphragmatic exercises may be helpful
3.   Nutritional therapy
     a.   Small frequent feedings may reduce gastric distention, thereby improving diaphragmatic breathing
     b.   High fat, reduced carbohydrate (CHO) diet is suggested; increased CHO intake may lead to dyspnea and increased ventilation as a result of a high CO_2 production

F.   Supplemental oxygen therapy has been shown to prolong life and improve quality of life in hypoxemic patients
1.   Indications for supplemental oxygen:
     a.   Pa O_2 ≤55 mm Hg or SaO_2 ≤88% breathing ambient air
     b.   Pa O_2 56 to 59 mm Hg or SaO_2 89% with concurrent cor pulmonale or polycythemia
     c.   Pa O_2 ≥60 mm Hg or SaO_2 ≥90% with significant exercise- or sleep-induced hypoxemia which reverses with supplemental oxygen or other compelling medical justification
2.   Prescribe oxygen at a flow rate sufficient to produce a PaO_2 ≥65 mm Hg or a SaO_2 ≥90% at rest and with activity
     a.   Oxygen prescription should include the oxygen dose (L/min), number of hours per day that oxygen is needed, and the type of delivery device (nasal cannula, demand-flow device, reservoir cannula, or transtracheal oxygen catheter); typically given by nasal cannula at flow rates of 0.5 to 4 liters per minute
          (1)   Ambulatory oxygen sources that enable patients to exercise are recommended
          (2)   Instillation of oxygen directly into the trachea (transtracheal oxygen) using a catheter has both cosmetic and physiologic advantages; almost any patient with chronic, stable hypoxemia can be considered a candidate for this technology
     b.   May need to increase flow rate by 1 L/min at night or during exercise
     c.   May need to increase flow rate when patient travels by air
3.   Re-evaluate patients 1-3 months after initiation of oxygen therapy, because many patients (30-45%) do not need long-term therapy

G. Therapies that are **NOT** effective:
1. Increased fluid intake is not helpful unless patient is dehydrated
2. Oral expectorants and nebulized water and salt are not beneficial
3. Although coughing may be an annoying symptom, regular use of antitussives is contraindicated in stable COPD patients.
4. Postural drainage and chest percussion are only helpful for patients who have excessive secretions or a non-productive cough
5. Use of iodinated glycerol (Organidin) has not been shown to be effective in previous research, but some clinicians suggest a short-term-trial period for patients with increased amounts of tenacious sputum; discontinue drug if there is no therapeutic benefit; may affect thyroid function with long-term use
6. Narcotics and vasodilators are contraindicated in COPD

H. Consult specialist concerning patient who has cor pulmonale; recommended treatment is oxygen therapy, diuretics and possibly digoxin (in left-sided congestive heart failure only)

I. α_1-antitrypsin augmentation is expensive but is approved for use in patients with this deficiency

J. Hospitalization is usually required for patients who continue to deteriorate with acute exacerbations despite therapy, patients with serious comorbid conditions, patients without home support, patients with altered mentation, and patients with worsening hypoxemia and/or hypercapnia

K. Surgical options are available
1. Lung volume reduction surgery
2. Lung transplantation; selection criteria include the following: Limited life expectancy (<3 years), age <60 years, failure of maximal medical therapy, and no extra-pulmonary organ failure

L. Follow Up
1. For acute attack contact patient by phone in 24-48 hours
2. If patient is on theophylline, measure drug levels 2 weeks after initiation of therapy and at regular intervals thereafter
3. Schedule follow up visits every 3-6 months for stable, chronic disease
4. Teach patient to immediately consult health care provider when signs and symptoms of respiratory infection or respiratory distress develop

COMMON COLD

I. Definition: An acute, mild and self-limiting syndrome caused by a viral infection of the upper respiratory tract mucosa

II. Pathogenesis

A. Inflammation of all or part of the mucosal membranes from the nasal mucosa to the bronchi

B. Etiology is usually rhinoviruses, coronaviruses, or other viruses

C. Incubation period averages 48 hours with a range of 12 hours to 5 days; maximum viral shedding occurs in first 2-4 days

D. Transmission occurs through direct contact with infectious secretions on skin and environmental surfaces and air-borne droplets

III. Clinical Presentation

A. Adults average 2-4 colds per year

B. Characterized by one or more of the following symptoms:
1. General malaise with low grade or no fever
2. Nasal discharge, obstruction or congestion
3. Sneezing, coughing, sore throat and hoarseness
4. Conjunctivae may be watery and inflamed

C. Usually self-limited (lasting approximately 5-7 days), but can predispose patient to bacterial infections such as otitis media, sinusitis, pneumonia and exacerbation of chronic conditions such as asthma

IV. Diagnosis/Evaluation

A. History – Question about the following:
1. Respiratory distress (wheezing, dyspnea, stridor), inability to swallow, drooling and severe headaches which indicate the need for immediate evaluation
2. Fever, chills, anorexia, nausea, vomiting, and diarrhea
3. Duration, character, and timing (day and/or night) of cough
4. Facial, head, ear, throat, or chest pain
5. Number and seasonal pattern of previous colds within 1 year
6. Exposure to others with similar symptoms
7. Medication use
8. Past medical and family history; particularly history of allergies, asthma, or other respiratory problems
9. History of tobacco use and passive tobacco exposure

B. Physical Examination
1. Measure temperature, pulse and blood pressure
2. Examine conjunctivae, ears, nose and throat
3. Sinus percussion and transillumination
4. Palpate cervical lymph nodes for enlargement and tenderness
5. Perform a complete lung examination

C. Differential Diagnosis
1. Allergic rhinitis (nasal mucosa may be pale and boggy rather than erythematous and swollen as in common cold)
2. Foreign body (especially if nasal discharge is unilateral, purulent and malodorous)
3. Sinusitis
   a. Thick, opaque, and discolored nasal discharge are typical of the common cold and do not indicate a more severe, sinus infection
   b. Symptoms persisting or worsening for >10-14 days with facial swelling and tenderness and mucopurulent sputum are suggestive of sinusitis
4. Influenza (arthralgias are usually present)
5. Streptococcal pharyngitis
6. Otitis media
7. Pneumonia

D. Diagnostic Tests
1. Usually none are indicated
2. Throat culture or quick strep test if symptomatic or history of streptococcal exposure

V. Plan/Management

A. Decongestants cause vasoconstriction and reduce nasal secretions and congestion; topical decongestants are effective for short-term therapy and provide rapid decrease in airway resistance whereas oral decongestants are best when treatment is needed for more than 3-4 days
1. Topical decongestants should be used no longer than 3-4 days because of potential for rebound congestion; suggest one of the following:
   a. Oxymetazoline hydrochloride 0.05% (Afrin 12-Hour Nasal Spray) 2-3 sprays each nostril BID
   b. Phenylephrine hydrochloride 1% (Neo-Synephrine Spray) 1 spray each nostril every 3-4 hours as needed

2. Oral decongestants (not as effective); suggest one of the following:
   a. Pseudoephedrine hydrochloride (Sudafed) 60 mg, 1 tablet every 4-6 hours
   b. Pseudoephedrine sulfate (Afrin 12-Hour Tablets) 120 mg, 1 tablet every 12 hours

B. Intranasal ipratropium bromide 0.06% (Atrovent) 2 sprays per nostril TID or QID reduces nasal discharge, severity of rhinorrhea and sneezing; not recommended as first-line agent for these symptoms but may prove useful in patients with disease-state contraindications to oral decongestants such as severe hypertension or angle-closure glaucoma

C. Equivocal research is available on the benefits of zinc acetate or zinc gluconate lozenges
   1. Therapy should be initiated within 24 hours of symptom onset
   2. Adverse effects of bad taste and nausea limit use of lozenges
   3. Zinc is not safe in pregnancy
   4. Dosages of zinc
      a. Zinc acetate lozenges (12.8 mg elemental zinc) 1 every 2 to 3 hours while awake
      b. Zinc gluconate lozenges (Hall's Zinc Defense) 1 every 2 hours for 4 days while awake

D. Although controversial, some researchers found a decrease in the duration and severity of cold symptoms with the use of Vitamin C 1 gram daily

E. Symptomatic treatment of cough (choose one of the following options)
   1. Dexbrompheniramine 6 mg/pseudoephedrine sulfate 120 mg (Drixoral Cold & Allergy) one tab BID for 1 week
   2. Naproxen (Naprosyn) 500 mg loading dose then 500 mg TID for 5
   3. Ipratropium (Atrovent) 0.06% nasal spray (42 μg per spray) 2 sprays per nostril TID for 4 days

F. Acetaminophen or nonsteroidal anti-inflammatory agents (NSAIDs) such as ibuprofen are effective in relieving fever and headaches

G. Nonpharmacologic approaches to relieve symptoms
   1. Saline nose drops or sprays: 2-3 drops in each nostril BID to QID of commercial products (Ocean, Salinex) or homemade solution (1/4 tsp salt in 8 oz boiled water)
   2. Steamy showers or inhalation of steam
   3. Fluids or hydration help loosen secretions and prevent upper airway obstruction; warm fluids such as tea and chicken soup can increase the rate of mucus flow
   4. Salt-water gargle for sore throat
   5. Hard candy or throat lozenge for sore throat and cough

H. Treatments that are not recommended
   1. Antihistamines are ineffective because nasal congestion in colds is not mediated by histamine receptors; antihistamines may increase upper airway obstruction by impairing flow of mucus
   2. With exception of increased water intake, expectorants such as guaifenesin provide no benefit in cold management

I. Patient Education
   1. Review the etiology, course, and proper treatment of the common cold
      a. Explain that colds are caused by viruses which are not eradicated with antibiotics
      b. Reinforce that the indiscriminate use of antibiotics can cause adverse effects such as diarrhea, yeast infection, and drug resistance
   2. Emphasize that cold remedies are to relieve symptoms and prevent complications rather than cure infection
   3. Advise rest and increased oral fluid intake
   4. Increase humidity of the air at home
   5. Discuss ways to prevent the spread of colds; all household members should frequently wash hands

J. Follow Up: none indicated unless symptoms worsen after 3-5 days, new symptoms develop, or symptoms do not improve or resolve after 10-14 days

COUGH, PERSISTENT

I. Definition: Host defense mechanism to clear airway of secretions and inhaled particles which lasts at least 3 weeks or longer

II. Pathogenesis

   A. The most common causes are from postnasal drip or clearing of the throat due to rhinitis or tracheobronchitis, bacterial sinusitis, asthma, gastroesophageal reflux, chronic bronchitis due to cigarette smoking or environmental irritants

   B. Other causes include physical irritants, foreign body aspiration, tuberculosis, and psychogenic factors

   C. Worrisome causes of coughing include mediastinal or pulmonary masses such as tumors or nodes

   D. Greater than 90% of patients with chronic cough have postnasal drip syndrome, asthma, gastroesophageal reflux or a combination of these conditions

III. Clinical presentation of important causes of persistent cough

   A. Tuberculosis
       1. Initially cough is minimally productive of yellow or green mucus which is worse upon arising in morning
       2. As disease progresses, cough becomes more productive
       3. Associated symptoms include fatigue, night sweats, dyspnea, and hemoptysis

   B. Gastroesophageal reflux
       1. May have history of heartburn, dysphagia, sour or bitter taste in mouth, and frequent use of antacids
       2. Symptoms are often aggravated by meals and relieved by sitting up

   C. Asthma
       1. Often occurs at night or after exercise, laughing, or exposure to cold air
       2. May be seasonal in occurrence and have a strong family history
       3. Cough may be nonproductive or productive but not purulent
       4. Associated symptoms include wheezing and intercostal retractions

   D. Aspirated foreign body
       1. Cough may persist for weeks or even months
       2. Fixed, localized wheezing audible when chest is auscultated

   E. Viral infections
       1. Infrequently last beyond 2 weeks
       2. Often occur during the winter
       3. Cough is often nonproductive
       4. Usually accompanying symptoms are mild and include rhinitis and nasal congestion

   F. Bacterial infections such as pneumonia
       1. Cough may be productive and purulent but this is not always the case
       2. Associated symptoms may include fever and respiratory distress

   G. Postnasal drip syndrome
       1. Usually related to chronic sinusitis or allergic rhinitis
       2. Patient often complains of clear nasal discharge, nasal congestion, tickle in throat, and frequent throat clearing

   H. Chronic bronchitis
       1. Often dry, hacking cough
       2. Worse in the morning

I. Carcinoma of the lung
   1. Cigarette smoking accounts for the majority of cases
   2. Characteristic of the cough depends on location of the primary tumor

J. Cough related to psychogenic factors (rare)
   1. Disappears during sleep; worsens when attention is drawn to it and during times of emotional stress
   2. Lacks other associated physical symptoms

K. Pertussis is a diagnosis of exclusion
   1. Characteristic but infrequently heard whoop with coughing and vomiting; fever is absent or minimal
   2. History of contact with known case
   3. Striking more teenagers and young adults; speculation is that pertussis vaccination given during infancy may lose its effectiveness as one ages
   4. Duration of symptoms is 6-10 weeks
   5. Complications include seizures, encephalopathy and death; infants have most severe disease

L. Diseases associated with intentional release of biologic agents
   1. Inhalation anthrax caused by inhalation of infectious spores
      a. Incubation period of 1-6 days
      b. First phase is a nonspecific illness characterized by nonproductive cough, mild fever, malaise, myalgias, and mild chest or abdominal pain
      c. Within 2-3 days, the second phase abruptly begins and involves fever, acute dyspnea, diaphoresis, and cyanosis
         (1) Stridor may be present due to obstruction of trachea by enlarged lymph nodes, mediastinal widening, and subcutaneous edema of chest and neck
         (2) In about half of patients meningitis develops with obtundation and nuchal rigidity
         (3) Within 24-36 hours of the second stage, shock, associated hypothermia, and death occurs
   2. Pneumonic plague occurs when *Yersinia pestis* infects lungs
      a. Cough with mucopurulent sputum, hemoptysis, and chest pain are clinical features along with nonspecific symptoms such as fever, headache, and weakness
      b. Chest radiograph shows evidence of bronchopneumonia
      c. Pneumonia progresses for 2-4 days and without treatment, patients may have respiratory failure, shock, and eventual death
   3. Inhalational tularemia can occur alone from exposure via aerosol or can be spread hematogenously from other forms of tularemia
      a. Three to five days after exposure, patient has abrupt onset of nonspecific febrile illness such as dry cough, headaches, myalgias, and weakness
      b. In subsequent 7 days, pleuropneumonitis develops in many cases

IV. Diagnosis/Evaluation

A. History
   1. Determine duration of cough
   2. Determine characteristics of cough
      a. Productive (white, purulent, bloody) or nonproductive; productive cough may suggest infection
      b. Quality (raspy, barking, harsh, wet); paroxysms of cough occur in pertussis and foreign body aspiration
      c. Temporal occurrence (night, morning, or seasonal)
         (1) Nighttime cough suggests asthma, sinusitis with postnasal drip
         (2) Cough associated with exercise may indicate asthma, cardiac disease (rare), and bronchiectasis
   3. Ask about associated symptoms such as fatigue, rhinitis, epistaxis, tickle in throat, pharyngitis, night sweats, dyspnea, fever, heartburn, hemoptysis, weight loss
      a. Hemoptysis signals concern for tuberculosis, cancer, or foreign body (see section on HEMOPTYSIS)
      b. Weight loss and fever suggest tuberculosis or HIV infection
   4. Ask if the cough is preceded by feeding or choking episodes
   5. Inquire about precipitating factors such as exercise, cold air, laughing
   6. Explore environmental and occupational exposure
   7. Inquire about infectious illness of other household members
   8. Always ask about smoking or the exposure to passive smoking
   9. Ask about medications, particularly angiotensin-converting enzyme (ACE) inhibitors

10. Explore family history of cystic fibrosis, malabsorption, asthma, and allergies
11. Inquire about past medical history such as allergies, frequent infectious diseases, obstructive airway disease, cardiac disease
12. Ask about pertussis immunization status

B. Physical Examination
1. Observe patient for signs of respiratory distress such as cyanosis, shortness of breath on ambulating, intercostal retractions, accessory muscle use
2. Observe general appearance, noting whether patient appears robust or fatigued and wasted
3. Listen for the quality of spontaneous coughing during the interview
4. Assess eyes, ears, nose, and throat
   a. Conjunctivitis, rhinitis, and pharyngitis suggest infection
   b. Cobblestoning in oropharynx suggests allergies or chronic sinusitis but may not always be present in postnasal drip syndrome
5. Check for tenderness of sinuses
6. Palpate lymph nodes
7. Observe for tracheal deviation which suggests mediastinal mass or foreign body aspiration
8. Perform a complete lung exam including inspection, palpation, percussion, and auscultation
9. Perform a complete cardiac exam as chronic cardiovascular problems may present with persistent cough

C. Differential Diagnosis: see pathogenesis section

D. Diagnostic Tests
1. Order tuberculin skin test (PPD) and chest x-ray for unexplained persistent cough
2. If diagnosis is unclear after PPD and chest x-ray, order spirometry to detect airway obstruction as in asthma
3. Consider a CBC with differential if infection, anemia, carcinoma are likely possibilities
4. Cough that is productive should have Gram's stain of sputum as well as cultures
5. If asthma is suspected, a methacholine challenge should be considered
6. To determine pertussis, culture nasopharyngeal mucus (obtained by aspiration or with a Dacron or calcium alginate swab)
7. To detect pathologic gastroesophageal reflux, 24-hour pH probe monitoring may be needed
8. Oximetry may be helpful to quickly evaluate the patient's respiratory status and later may be used to assess response to treatment
9. Other possible tests to order depend on characteristics of patient and include sinus x-rays, immunologic testing, allergy testing, or a barium swallow for detecting structural lesions
10. More invasive tests such as bronchoscopy may be needed
11. At first suspicion of patients exposed to intentional release of biologic agents, notify local or state health department, local hospital epidemiologist, and local or state laboratory; definitive tests can be arranged through a reference laboratory

V. Plan/Management

A. Treat all known causes: antibiotic therapy for bacterial infections, bronchodilators for asthma, and antihistamines for allergies

B. Treatment of pertussis; drug of choice is erythromycin 40-50 mg/kg per day orally in 4 divided doses for 14 days

C. Treatment for diseases associated with intentional release of biologic agents: consult infectious disease specialist immediately and obtain information from national sources (see table WEBSITES: RESPONDING TO BIOTERRORISM); usual treatment is the following:
1. Inhalation anthrax
   a. Ciprofloxacin 400 mg every 12 hours (begin with IV treatment and switch to oral therapy);
   b. Alternatively use doxycycline 100 mg every 12 hours and one or two additional drugs such as rifampin, vancomycin, penicillin, ampicillin, chloramphenicol, imipenem, clindamycin, and clarithromycin

2. Pneumonic plague
   a. Antibiotics must be given within 24 hours of first symptoms
   b. Streptomycin, gentamicin, the tetracyclines, and chloramphenicol are effective agents
3. Inhalational tularemia: drugs of choice are doxycycline and ciprofloxacin

WEBSITES: RESPONDING TO BIOTERRORISM	
Agency	**Website**
Centers for Disease Control and Prevention	http://www.bt.cdc.gov
US Army Medical Research; Research Institute of Infectious Diseases	http://www.usamriid.army.mil/education/bluebook.html
Association for Infection Control Practitioners	http://www.apic.org
The Johns Hopkins Center for Civilian Biodefense	http://www.hopkins-biodefense.org

D. Discuss need to stop cigarette smoking and avoid environmental irritants

E. Air humidification and keeping the throat moist are simple suggestions that may be beneficial; adequate hydration with at least 1500 mL of fluid daily

F. Cough suppressants such as dextromethorphan or codeine may be beneficial in improving sleep and rest (use only at bedtime)

G. Expectorants and mucolytic agents are ineffective

H. A stepwise approach may be beneficial by progressing from simple to more aggressive diagnostic tests and treatments in patients with persistent, mild-to-moderate coughing of unknown etiology
   1. Initial screen: Eliminate environment irritants (smoking, cough-producing medications, etc.)
   2. Step 1: Treat empirically for postnasal drip with first generation antihistamine-decongestant combination (post nasal drip syndrome is non-histamine mediated and second generation antihistamines do not appear to be effective); add nasal steroids or order CT of sinuses if symptoms persist
   3. Step 2: Evaluate and treat possible asthma with inhaled cromolyn, steroids, and bronchodilators
   4. Step 3: Order chest radiographs and CT of sinuses if asthma is not confirmed; treat specific, identified disease
   5. Step 4:
      a. Treat for GERD if no abnormalities found in Step 3: Antireflux measures and high-dose proton-pump inhibitor (may take 2 to 3 months of intensive therapy before cough starts to improve)
      b. Order endoscopy or 24-hour esophageal pH monitoring
   6. Step 5:
      a. Perform bronchoscopic examination if no abnormalities are found and previous treatments are unsuccessful
      b. Repeat course of antihistamine-decongestant combination
      c. Consider less common diagnoses such as cancer, tuberculosis, congestive heart failure, sarcoidosis, bronchiectasis, etc.

I. In undiagnosed patients with risk factors for cancer such as smoking or occupational exposure, consider referral to specialist

J. Follow Up
   1. Frequency of return visits will depend on patient's condition
   2. Patients who have a complete work-up with no abnormalities should be seen at least every 1-3 months if their coughing persists

EPIGLOTTITIS (SUPRAGLOTTITIS)

I. Definition: Inflammation of the soft tissues above the glottis

II. Pathogenesis

    A. Caused primarily by *Haemophilus influenzae* type B

    B. Involves rapid and pronounced inflammation of the epiglottis and surrounding areas which results in edema and subsequent mechanical obstruction to the flow of air

    C. The swollen epiglottis may be pulled down into the larynx during inspiration and create complete airway obstruction

    D. The inflammation may also result in increased secretions and exudate which can compound the airway obstruction

III. Clinical Presentation

    A. Previous to current vaccine era, primarily a disease in ages 2 to 4 years, but because most adults have not been vaccinated against *Haemophilus influenzae* type b (HIB), acute epiglottitis has become primarily a disease of adults

    B. Symptoms are an abrupt onset of severe sore throat, fever, hoarseness, and painful swallowing

    C. Usual appearance is an individual in sitting position, leaning forward with head extended, jaw thrust forward, mouth open, tongue protruding, and drooling

    D. As the condition progresses may have dysphagia, stridor, respiratory distress, anxiety and later exhaustion and limpness with diminished breath sounds; adults typically do not have as much stridor and dyspnea as children

    E. Signs include cervical adenopathy and a "beefy red" pharynx with copious secretions

IV. Diagnosis/Evaluation

    A. History: Quickly question patient and family members about onset and characteristics of symptoms and level of alertness

    B. Physical Examination
        1. Quickly assess vital signs and respiratory status such as respiratory rate, cyanosis, retractions, use of accessory muscles, nasal flaring
        2. Quickly auscultate lungs; may have inspiratory stridor and expiratory rhonchi
        3. If epiglottitis is suspected, do **NOT** attempt to examine pharynx with a tongue depressor because occlusion of airway may result

    C. Differential Diagnosis
        1. Croup
        2. Bacterial tracheitis
        3. Aspiration of foreign body
        4. Diphtheria
        5. Peritonsillar abscess
        6. Angioneurotic edema

D. Diagnostic Tests
    1. Tentative diagnosis must be made quickly on the basis of the history and clinical presentation
    2. After admission to hospital the following are performed:
        a. Laryngoscopy to visualize epiglottis; performed in operating room in case of airway obstruction and need for intubation
        b. Lateral neck radiography is important when expert direct laryngoscopy is unavailable; "thumb sign" or swelling of epiglottis and the vallecular sign (decrease in the vallecular air space) confirm the diagnosis
        c. Computed tomography of the neck is recommended when diagnosis cannot be confirmed and when complications are suspected.
        d. Blood and surface cultures are obtained after intubation to confirm the presence of *H. influenzae*

V. Plan/Management

A. Immediate transport to the hospital as this is a medical emergency; airway must be established by endotracheal tube or tracheostomy

B. Attempt to keep patient calm

C. Initial in-hospital treatment is cefotaxime sodium (Claforan), ceftizoxime sodium (Cefizox), or ceftriaxone sodium (Rocephin)

D. Chemoprophylaxis of index case and household contacts is recommended with rifampin (Rifadin) when there is invasive *H. influenzae* type B infection and there is a child <4 years old in the household who is unimmunized, incompletely immunized, or immunocompromised
    1. Infant 0-1 month: 10 mg/kg/day QD for 4 days
    2. Child >1 month to adult: 20 mg/kg/day QD for 4 days (maximum of 600 mg/day QD for 4 days)

E. Follow up after discharge from the hospital will depend on the patient's condition

HEMOPTYSIS

I. Definition: Expectoration of both blood-tinged and grossly bloody sputum

II. Pathogenesis

A. Inflammation of the tracheobronchial mucosa is the causative factor in many cases
    1. Minor mucosal erosions can occur from upper respiratory infections and bronchitis
    2. Bronchiectasis
    3. Tuberculosis (TB)
    4. Endobronchial inflammation due to sarcoidosis

B. Bronchogenic carcinoma may injure the mucosa whereas metastatic lung cancer rarely results in hemoptysis

C. Injury to the pulmonary vasculature is an important cause
    1. Lung abscess
    2. Necrotizing pneumonias such as those caused by *Klebsiella*
    3. Aspergillomas
    4. Pulmonary infarction secondary to embolization

D. Elevations in pulmonary capillary pressure can result in hemoptysis
    1. Pulmonary edema
    2. Mitral stenosis
    3. Wegener's granulomatosis
    4. Goodpasture's syndrome
    5. Arteriovenous malformations

E. Bleeding disorders and excessive anticoagulant therapy are additional causes

F. Chest trauma is a less common cause

G. Patients with cryptogenic hemoptysis (indeterminate etiology) have a normal or nonlocalizing chest radiograph and nondiagnostic fiberoptic bronchoscopies; 90% of patients experience resolution of hemoptysis by 6 months

H. Acute and chronic bronchitis followed by bronchogenic carcinoma, TB, pneumonia, and bronchiectasis are the most common causes in adults

I. Pneumonic plague due to intentional release of biologic agents is a rare cause

III. Clinical presentation of important causes of hemoptysis

A. Blood that is coughed is bright red, frothy, has an alkaline pH, and is mixed with sputum rather than hematemesis that is darker brown, has an acid pH, and may be mixed with food particles

B. Blood-streaked sputum is common, usually occurs with nonthreatening conditions, and often arises from the nasal mucosa and oropharynx rather than the lower respiratory tract

C. Bronchiectasis
   1. Occasional, foul-smelling, blood-tinged sputum is characteristic
   2. Patient usually has chronic, productive cough which may be worse when lying down
   3. Dyspnea, fever, pleurisy may be present

D. Lung tumors account for about 20% of the cases of hemoptysis in adults but hemoptysis is an uncommon symptom in children with malignancies
   1. Occur most frequently in persons over age 40 and in smokers
   2. Patient often has a change in cough pattern
   3. Chest ache may be an accompanying symptom

E. Pneumonia
   1. Sputum appears red-brown or red-green and is mixed with pus
   2. May have fever, pleuritic chest pain, and malaise

F. Pulmonary infarction secondary to pulmonary emboli
   1. Characterized by a sudden onset of pleuritic pain in conjunction with hemoptysis
   2. Diaphoresis and syncope often are present
   3. Signs include tachypnea, tachycardia, rales, fever, shock, fourth heart sound, pleural rub, or cyanosis
   4. Frequently patient has a history of phlebitis, calf pain, or immobilization of the legs

G. Pulmonary edema
   1. Characteristically has pink, frothy sputum
   2. Diaphoresis, tachypnea, tachycardia are present
   3. Jugular venous distention, hepatomegaly, and ankle edema may be present

IV. Diagnosis/Evaluation

A. History
   1. Inquire about onset and whether hemoptysis is a recurrent problem
   2. Explicitly determine that the bleeding is originating from the lungs rather than from vomiting blood or expectorating blood from nasopharyngeal bleeding
   3. Ask patient to describe the color, consistency, and characteristics of sputum
      a. Pink sputum is suggestive of pulmonary edema fluid
      b. Putrid sputum suggests a lung abscess
      c. Currant-jelly-like sputum may indicate necrotizing pneumonia
      d. Copious amounts of purulent sputum mixed with blood points toward bronchiectasis
   4. Ask patient to quantify amount of bleeding or if possible collect the sputum
   5. Inquire about associated symptoms such as recent weight loss, fatigue, persistent cough, dyspnea, wheezing, fever, night sweats, excessive bruising, hematuria

6. Determine whether patient has had recent respiratory inflammation or infection
7. Inquire about past medical history; particularly ask about previous lung, cardiac, hematological, and immunological problems
8. Inquire about exposure to tuberculosis
9. Ask about patterns of cigarette smoking
10. Inquire about history of chest trauma
11. Ask about use of anticoagulant drugs
12. Explore environmental exposure to such things as asbestos
13. Ask about family history of hemoptysis, respiratory, cardiac, and hematological problems
14. Inquire about date of last chest x-ray and tuberculin skin test

B. Physical Examination
1. Assess vital signs, particularly noting fever and tachypnea
2. Observe skin for ecchymosis, telangiectasis, and nails for clubbing; clubbing is consistent with neoplasm, bronchiectasis, lung abscess and other severe respiratory problems
3. Examine nose, sinuses and pharynx for source of bleeding
4. Inspect neck for jugular venous distention which is suggestive of heart failure
5. Palpate for lymph nodes; lymphadenopathy is associated with TB, sarcoidosis, and malignancy
6. Perform a complete lung and cardiovascular exam
7. Check for ankle edema

C. Differential Diagnosis: hemoptysis is a symptom; see pathogenesis for possible causes
1. Most cases of blood-tinged sputum are upper-respiratory in nature and do not need extensive workup
2. Differentiate hemoptysis from epistaxis, hematemesis and bleeding from nasopharyngeal sources

D. Diagnostic Tests
1. Order chest x-ray; inspiratory and expiratory films may demonstrate local air trapping if foreign body aspiration is suspected
2. Computed tomography and magnetic resonance imaging may detect additional abnormalities unrecognized on chest x-ray
3. Administer tuberculin skin test (PPD) unless there has been a positive PPD in the past
4. Consider Gram's stain of sputum for suspected infections, an acid-fast stain for suspected tuberculosis, and cytologic examination of three sputum samples for malignant cells
5. Consider bronchoscopy for patients who smoke, who are over 40 years of age, and who have normal chest x-rays; also consider for patients with persistent, recurrent hemoptysis or massive bleeding
6. Consider ventilation-perfusion scanning or angiography when pulmonary embolization is suspected
7. PT, PTT, platelet count, and bleeding time are necessary when more than one site of bleeding is present

V. Plan/Management

A. Consider consultation with a specialist for patients who are at increased risk for malignancy and those cases in which bronchoscopy is indicated

B. Patients expectorating more than 25-50 mL of blood in 24 hours require hospitalization

C. Treat any underlying illness or infection

D. Because blood is irritating to the tracheobronchial tree and triggers a cough response, consider prescribing a mild cough suppressant. However, instruct patient to continue expectorating as mucus and blood can accumulate and cause additional problems

E. Patient Education
1. Instruct patient to record episodes of hemoptysis and collect all blood that is expectorated
2. Instruct patient to return to clinic or emergency room if bleeding increases, has clots, or if patient has respiratory distress, diaphoresis, chest pain, or tachypnea

F. Follow Up
1. For mild blood-streaking of sputum with respiratory infection, all blood streaking should resolve in 2-3 days. If blood-streaking of sputum persists, patient needs a reevaluation
2. Patients with hemoptysis which involves expectoration of blood, not just minimal amounts of blood-streaked sputum, should have follow up visit within 12-48 hours

PNEUMONIA, COMMUNITY-ACQUIRED

I. Definition: "Acute infection of the pulmonary parenchyma that is associated with at least some symptoms of acute infection and is accompanied by the presence of an acute infiltrate on a chest radiograph or auscultatory findings consistent with pneumonia (altered breath sounds and/or localized rales) and occurs in a patient who is not hospitalized or residing in a long-term care facility for ≥14 days before onset of symptoms" (Barlett, et al., 1998)

II. Pathogenesis

A. Mainly results from aspiration of pathogens into the lower respiratory tract from oropharyngeal contents

B. Less commonly, pathogens spread to lungs hematogenously from distant foci such as bacterial endocarditis or from aerosolized particles

C. Aspirated pathogens are usually cleared before infection develops unless there are alterations in the normal protective mechanisms such as depressed mucociliary transport by ethanol and narcotics or by obstruction of bronchus by mucus or tumors

D. Pathogens
1. *Streptococcus pneumoniae* is the most common cause of morbidity and mortality from community-acquired pneumonia (CAP); accounts for 30%-50% of bacteremic pneumonia
2. *Haemophilus influenzae* is becoming a more common pathogen
3. *Legionella* species is an important pathogen in up to 30% of severe pneumonias
4. Gram-negative pathogens account for 20-40% of causative agents in the elderly
5. Pathogens according to the 2001 American Thoracic Society (ATS) categories:
   a. Outpatient pneumonia without cardiopulmonary disease or modifying factors (following does not include patients at risk for HIV): *Streptococcus pneumoniae* (pneumococcus), *Mycoplasma pneumoniae, Chlamydia pneumoniae, Haemophilus influenzae,* respiratory viruses
   b. Outpatient pneumonia with cardiopulmonary disease (CHF or COPD) and/or other modifying factors (following does not include patients at risk for HIV): *Streptococcus pneumoniae* (including drug-resistant *S. pneumoniae* - DRSP), *Mycoplasma pneumoniae, Chlamydia pneumoniae,* mixed infection (bacteria plus atypical pathogen or virus), *Haemophilus influenzae,* enteric gram-negatives, respiratory viruses
   c. Hospitalized patients with community-acquired pneumonia, not in ICU (excluding patients at risk for HIV): *Streptococcus pneumoniae* (including DRSP), *Haemophilus influenzae, Mycoplasma pneumoniae, Chlamydia pneumoniae,* mixed infection (bacteria plus atypical pathogen), viruses; in addition, for those patients with cardiopulmonary disease and/or modifying factors consider enteric gram-negatives (such as the Enterobacteriaceae), aspiration (anaerobes), *Legionella* species, *Mycobacterium tuberculosis,* endemic fungi
   d. Hospitalized patients with severe community-acquired pneumonia, in ICU (excluding patients at risk for HIV): *Streptococcus pneumoniae* (including DRSP), *Legionella* species, *Haemophilus influenzae,* enteric gram-negative bacilli (predominantly Enterobacteriaceae), *Staphylococcus aureus, Mycoplasma pneumoniae,* respiratory viruses; *Pseudomonas aeruginosa* (consider this organism for patients who have had prolonged broad-spectrum antibiotic therapy, bronchiectasis, malnutrition, or diseases and therapies associated with neutrophil dysfunction)

E. Bacterial pneumonia is often associated with concurrent viral infection which may suppress the immune system and disrupt the respiratory tract mucosa

III. Clinical Presentation

A. In US, pneumonia is the sixth leading cause of death and the number one cause of death from infectious disease

B. The epidemiology of pneumonia has undergone changes in recent years; pneumonia is increasingly common among elderly patients and those with coexisting illness; in the elderly the clinical expression of various types of pneumonia is atypical, obscured, and may even be absent

C. Symptoms suggestive of pneumonia include the following:
   1. Fever or hypothermia, chills, sweats
   2. New cough with or without sputum production; in patient with chronic cough, change in color of respiratory secretions
   3. Chest discomfort and/or dyspnea
   4. Nonspecific symptoms such as fatigue, myalgias, abdominal pain, headaches, anorexia, and worsening of an underlying chronic illness

D. Signs include respiratory rate >20/minute, tachycardia, crackles heard on auscultation and signs of consolidation

E. Complications of pneumonia include the following:
   1. Metastatic infection (meningitis, arthritis, endocarditis, pericarditis, peritonitis and empyema) occurs in as many as 10% of patients with bacteremic pneumonia
   2. Bacteremia, renal failure, heart failure, pulmonary embolus with infarction, and acute myocardial infarction

F. The following are risk factors for mortality: increased age, alcoholism, active malignancies, immunosuppression, neurological disease, congestive heart failure, and diabetes

G. Increasingly, research has found considerable overlap in the symptoms, signs, and radiographic findings of the various types of pneumonia; even though it is usually not prudent to base empiric treatment on clinical findings, this section summarizes literature on the clinical presentation of pneumonia due to specific pathogens
   1. Pneumococcal pneumonia (due to *S. pneumoniae*)
      a. May occur in previously healthy adults after an upper respiratory infection; but occurs predominantly in elderly and patients with other co-morbid medical conditions
      b. Often presents with abrupt onset of high fever, shaking chills, productive cough of purulent or rusty sputum, headache, prostration, and pleuritic chest pain
      c. Bacteremia occurs in 15-30% of cases
   2. *Haemophilus influenzae*
      a. Predilection for the elderly, cigarette smokers, and patients with chronic obstructive pulmonary disease or pre-existing illnesses but may affect healthy persons
      b. Symptoms similar to other bacterial pneumonias
      c. Often occurs after an episode of influenza
   3. *Staphylococcus* species occur in patients with specific risk factors such as residence in nursing home, alcohol abuse, chronic disease, or during influenza epidemics
   4. *Moraxella catarrhalis*
      a. Occurs in patients with chronic obstructive pulmonary disease or other underlying chronic illness
      b. Symptoms are usually mild and patients do not usually have myalgias, chills, pleuritic chest pain, or extreme prostration
   5. Pneumonia due to gram-negative bacilli rarely occurs in previously healthy adults
      a. Risk factors include old age, residence in chronic care facility, alcohol abuse, malnutrition, and chronic illness
      b. High risk for complications and high (20-30%) mortality rate
   6. Pneumonia due to *M. pneumoniae*
      a. Only 3-10% of all community-acquired pneumonia in adults between ages 35-60 is due to *M. pneumoniae*, but common in adults <35 years
      b. Close contact is necessary for transmission and epidemics have occurred in military housing, schools, etc.
      c. Usually symptoms are mild and course is self-limited
      d. Hacking cough, fever, malaise, and headache are common symptoms
      e. Symptoms may last up to 6 weeks despite treatment
      f. Erythema multiforme is associated with *M. pneumoniae*

7. Pneumonia due to *Chlamydia pneumoniae* has presentation and course similar to pneumonia due to *M. pneumoniae*
8. Pneumonia due to *Legionella pneumophila*
    a. *Legionella* is an opportunistic pathogen; rarely occurs in healthy young adults
    b. Symptoms are more severe with a fatality rate of 10-30% of all cases
    c. Unique characteristics are hyponatremia, neurologic symptoms (confusion, headache), gastrointestinal symptoms (nausea, diarrhea), hematuria, and elevated serum transaminase
9. Viral pneumonia
    a. Uncommon in adults except in the immunosuppressed patient
    b. Influenza viruses most common cause of viral pneumonia with fever, chills, dry hacking cough, and pharyngitis
    c. Respiratory syncytial virus is increasingly being recognized as cause of pneumonia in adults
    d. Cytomegalovirus and herpes simplex viruses cause treatable pneumonia in immunosuppressed patients
    e. Viral pneumonias have more prolonged prodromal illness, milder symptoms, less elevated white count than bacterial pneumonias
    f. Chest x-rays do not usually reveal lobar distribution of infiltrate and pleural effusions as in bacterial pneumonias
10. *Pneumocystis carinii* presents with insidious onset of fever, cough, and dyspnea in the immunocompromised person
11. Pneumonia due to anaerobes is most common in patients with poor dental hygiene; putrid sputum is associated with anaerobic infections

IV. Diagnosis/Evaluation

A. History
    1. Determine whether onset was gradual, involving mild upper respiratory symptoms or abrupt with rapid onset of fever and cough
    2. Inquire about associated symptoms such as rhinorrhea, fever, chills, myalgias, pharyngitis, chest pain, and neurological symptoms
    3. Ask patient to describe cough and sputum
    4. Inquire about recent infectious illnesses in the patient's household
    5. Inquire about past medical history such as acquired immunodeficiency, asthma, chronic obstructive pulmonary disease, smoking history, tuberculosis, alcohol and drug abuse

B. Physical Examination
    1. Assess vital signs
    2. Observe for respiratory disease such as cyanosis, tachypnea, intercostal retractions, accessory muscle use, nasal flaring, and grunting
    3. Assess for signs of dehydration, particularly in the elderly
    4. Auscultate lungs; typical findings are the following:
        a. Localized diminished breath sounds
        b. Rales and tubular breath sounds
        c. Egophony (changes patient's "ee" to what sounds like "ay")
        d. Bronchophony (voice sounds are louder and clearer than usual)
        e. Whispered pectoriloquy (whispered sounds are louder and clearer than normal)
    5. Palpate chest for tactile fremitus (palpate for increased areas of vibration as patient says "ninety-nine")
    6. Percuss chest for dullness which is typical over consolidated lung tissue
    7. Perform a cardiac examination
    8. Assess mental status

C. Differential Diagnosis: There is no combination of clinical findings that can rule in a diagnosis of pneumonia; however, some researchers found that absence of vital sign abnormalities or any abnormalities on chest auscultation substantially lessened the likelihood of pneumonia
    1. Chronic pulmonary diseases such as asthma, chronic bronchitis, or emphysema
    2. Atelectasis
    3. Lung abscess
    4. Pulmonary embolism
    5. Damage from physical agents such as near drowning and smoke inhalation
    6. Congestive heart failure
    7. Neoplasms
    8. Sarcoidosis

9. Intrapulmonary hemorrhage
10. Consider illnesses associated with intentional release of biological agents: inhalational anthrax, pneumonic plague, inhalational tularemia

D. Diagnostic Tests
   1. Chest radiograph is recommended as respiratory complaints alone are poorly predictive of finding an acute infiltrate on x-ray; order PA and lateral chest x-ray to aid in the following:
      a. To differentiate pneumonia from other conditions that mimic it
      b. To uncover specific etiologies or conditions such as lung abscess or pneumonia caused by *Pneumocystis carinii*
      c. To identify co-existing conditions such as pleural effusion or bronchial obstruction
      d. To evaluate the severity of disease by identifying multilobar pneumonia or pleural effusion which indicates a severe illness
      e. As a baseline measure and to assess response to treatment
   2. Sputum Gram's stain is desirable (if properly collected and examined) as it may be helpful for focusing initial empiric therapy; culture of expectorated sputum especially if drug-resistant bacteria are suspected (both tests lack sensitivity and specificity)
   3. Routine laboratory tests such as CBC, glucose, serum electrolytes, hepatic enzymes, and tests of renal function are helpful in deciding which patients should be hospitalized, especially in patients >65 years of age or patients with coexisting illness
   4. Consider pulse oximetry in patients with underlying chronic heart or lung disease (may help define need for hospitalization)
   5. Patients who are admitted should, in addition to the above, have the following: arterial-blood gas analysis, two sets of blood cultures, serologic test for HIV infection (any patients with risk factors and those aged 15-54), deep cough sputum for Gram's stain and culture, test for *Mycobacterium tuberculosis* with acid-fast stain and culture for selected patients (cough >1 month); urinary antigen assay for *Legionella* in selected patients (seriously ill, immunosuppressed, >40 years, or patients nonresponsive to β-lactam antibiotics)
   6. Patients with pleural effusion should have a diagnostic thoracentesis
   7. Consider tuberculin skin test (PPD)
   8. Patients over 40 and all smokers should have chest x-ray at 4-8 weeks post-treatment to rule out bronchogenic carcinoma which has a similar presentation as pneumonia; patients who were hospitalized should also have one to establish a new radiographic baseline

V. Plan/Management

A. Consider consultation with a specialist for a patient who appears toxic, has hemoptysis, severe dyspnea, a history of a serious, chronic disease

B. The Pneumonia Severity Index (Fine, et. al. 1997) indicates that the following factors predict high risk outcomes and should be considered in clinical decision making for hospitalization (see versions of the index on the Internet at http://www.emedhomon.com/dbase.cfm)
   1. Age >50 years
   2. Comorbid condition (neoplastic disease, CHF, cerebrovascular disease, renal disease, liver disease)
   3. Physical examination findings (altered mental status, respiratory rate >30/minute, systolic blood pressure <90 mm Hg, temperature <35°C or >40°C, pulse ≥125/minute)
   4. Laboratory findings (pH <7.35, BUN ≥30 mg/dL, sodium <130 mEq/L, glucose ≥250 mg/dL, hematocrit <30%, PO_2 <60 mm Hg, pleural effusion on x-ray)

C. Empiric treatment of pneumonia is often necessary because available diagnostic tests fail to reveal the pathogen in 40-50% of all cases and most test results (sputum, blood cultures, serologies) are not available at the time of initial presentation
   1. Research has found that patients treated in the early stage of their disease progress better than patients in whom treatment is delayed
   2. The patient stratification approach recommended by the 2001 American Thoracic Society is a valuable aid; it is based on an assessment of the place of therapy, the presence of cardiopulmonary disease (COPD, CHF), and the presence of modifying factors (risk factors for DRSP, enteric gram-negatives, *Pseudomonas aeruginosa*)
      a. Risk factors for DRSP: age >65, β-lactam therapy within the past 3 months, alcoholism, immunosuppressive illness or therapy, and exposure to a child in a day care center

b. Risk factors for enteric gram-negatives: residence in a nursing home, underlying cardiopulmonary disease, multiple medical comorbidities, recent antibiotic therapy

c. Risk factors for *P. aeruginosa:* structural lung disease such as bronchiectasis, broad-spectrum antibiotic therapy for >7 days within the past month, malnutrition, and chronic corticosteroid therapy with >10 mg/day

D. The goal is to avoid excessively broad antibiotic therapy. Select as narrow a spectrum of therapy as possible based on the ATS patient stratification guidelines (see table PATIENT STRATIFICATION/THERAPY OPTIONS to direct therapy of choice to specific subsets of patients; see table OUTPATIENT TREATMENT ANTIMICROBIAL OPTIONS to prescribe correct dosages and scheduling)

PATIENT STRATIFICATION AND THERAPY OPTIONS

PATIENT GROUP (Excludes patients at risk for HIV)	THERAPY
Group I: Outpatients, no cardiopulmonary disease, no modifying factors (in roughly 50-90% of cases no etiology was identified)	Advanced generation macrolide: azithromycin or clarithromycin (erythromycin is not active against *H. influenzae* and the advanced generation macrolides are better tolerated) OR Doxycycline (tetracycline should be used only if the patient is allergic to or intolerant of macrolides as many isolates of *S. pneumoniae* are resistant)
Group II: Outpatients, with cardiopulmonary disease, and/or other modifying factors (in 50-90% of cases no etiology was identified)	Beta–lactam (oral cefpodoxime, cefuroxime, amoxicillin/clavulanate; or parenteral ceftriaxone followed by oral cefpodoxime) PLUS Macrolide or doxycycline OR Antipneumococcal fluoroquinolone alone
Group III: Hospitalized patients, not in ICU a. Cardiopulmonary disease and/or modifying factors including being from a nursing home	Intravenous beta-lactam (cefotaxime, ceftriaxone, ampicillin/sulbactam, high-dose ampicillin) PLUS Intravenous or oral macrolide or doxycycline OR Intravenous antipneumococcal fluoroquinolone alone
b. No cardiopulmonary disease, no modifying factors	Intravenous azithromycin alone (If macrolide allergic or intolerant: doxycycline and a beta-lactam) OR Monotherapy with an antipneumococcal fluoroquinolone
Group IV: Hospitalized patients, in ICU a. No risks for *Pseudomonas aeruginosa*	Intravenous beta-lactam (cefotaxime, ceftriaxone) PLUS EITHER Intravenous macrolide (azithromycin) OR Intravenous fluoroquinolone
b. Risks for *Pseudomonas aeruginosa*	Selected intravenous antipseudomonal beta-lactam (cefepime, imipenem, meropenem, piperacillin/tazobactam) *plus* intravenous antipseudomonal quinolone (ciprofloxacin) OR Selected intravenous antipseudomonal beta-lactam (cefepime, imipenem, meropenem, piperacillin/tazobactam) *plus* intravenous aminoglycoside PLUS EITHER macrolide (azithromycin) OR intravenous nonpseudomonal fluoroquinolone

Adapted from American Thoracic Society (2001). Guidelines for the management of adults with community-acquired pneumonia. *American Journal of Respiratory and Critical Care Medicine, 163,* 1730-1754.

OUTPATIENT TREATMENT ANTIMICROBIAL OPTIONS*

Consideration of potential pathogen should direct therapy choice (antimicrobials are listed in no specific order)

✓ Macrolides

- Clarithromycin extended release (Biaxin XL) available 500 mg tablets; 2 tablets QD (with food) for 7-14 days (1 Pac has 7 days)
- Clarithromycin (Biaxin) 250-500 mg every 12 hours for 7-14 days
- Azithromycin (Zithromax) 500 mg day 1, then 250 mg daily for 4 days (take 1 hour before meals or 2 hours after meals)

✓ Fluoroquinolones

- Levofloxacin (Levaquin) 500 mg QD for 7-14 days (take with full glass of water)
- Moxifloxacin (Avelox) 400 mg QD for 10 days
- Gatifloxacin (Tequin) 400 mg QD for 7-14 days

✓ Doxycycline (Vibramycin) 100 mg BID

Beta-lactam Options

✓ Amoxicillin/Clavulanate (Augmentin) 500 mg tab TID or 875 mg every 12 hours or Augmentin XR (amoxicillin 1000 mg, clavulanic acid 62.5 mg) two XR tabs every 12 hours

✓ Some second-generation cephalosporins

- Cefuroxime axetil (Ceftin) 250-500 mg every 12 hours
- Cefpodoxime (Vantin) 200 mg tab every 12 hours for 14 days (take with food)
- Ceftriaxone (Rocephin) 1-2 gram IM or IV once daily or in 2 divided doses followed by oral cefpodoxime

*Duration of treatment varies. Most bacterial infections can be treated until a patient is afebrile for 72 hours. *C. pneumoniae, M. pneumoniae,* and Legionnaires' disease should be treated for 10-14 days. Immunocompromised patients require longer treatments (21 days).

Adapted from American Thoracic Society (2001). Guidelines for the management of adults with community-acquired pneumonia. *American Journal of Respiratory and Critical Care Medicine, 163,* 1730-1754.

E.   Patient Education
1.   Increase oral fluids
2.   Avoid cough suppressants and cigarettes

F.   Prevention: more emphasis is being placed on the role of vaccination in preventing pneumonia than in the past
1.   Pneumococcal vaccination is a strategy to control the expansion of drug-resistant pneumococci; approximately 90% of penicillin-resistant pneumococci are serotypes covered by the vaccine (see table RECOMMENDATIONS FOR ADULT IMMUNIZATIONS in section PERIODIC HEALTH EVALUATION FOR ADULTS)
2.   Yearly influenza immunization is recommended for at-risk populations and health care workers

G.   Follow Up
1.   Contact patient with moderate-to-severe symptoms within 24 hours by phone or in office
2.   With effective antimicrobial therapy, some improvement in the clinical manifestations of pneumonia should be seen within 48-72 hours; however, antimicrobial therapy should not be changed within first 72 hours unless there is a marked clinical deterioration
a.   Consult specialist if there is little improvement or deterioration after 48-72 hours of therapy
b.   Sampling of lower respiratory tract secretions with bronchoscopy and other diagnostic tests such as computerized tomography are often needed if there is no improvement; however, there may be a high false-negative rate when performed while the patient is on antibiotics
3.   For patients with moderate and severe symptoms who are improving, schedule return visit in 3-4 days after treatment is initiated to assess response; then, evaluate patients in 2-3 weeks
4.   For patients >40 years and all smokers, another return visit should be scheduled in 4-8 weeks to obtain second chest x-ray to rule out bronchogenic carcinoma, which has a similar presentation as pneumonia

TUBERCULOSIS

I. Definition: Necrotizing bacterial infection most commonly infecting the lungs; other important definitions include the following:

   A. Positive tuberculin skin test: applies to a person who has likely infection with *Mycobacterium tuberculosis*, an acid-fast bacillus

   B. Exposure: applies to a person who has recent contact with an individual with suspected or confirmed, contagious pulmonary tuberculosis (TB) and whose tuberculin skin test is non-reactive, physical examination is normal, and chest x-ray is normal; some exposed persons have infection (and eventually develop a positive tuberculin skin test) whereas some do not

   C. Latent TB infection: applies to a person who has a positive tuberculin skin test, absent physical findings of disease, and a chest x-ray which is either normal or has only granulomas or calcifications in lung and/or regional lymph nodes

   D. TB disease: applies to a person with infection who has signs, symptoms, and x-ray manifestations that appear to be caused by *M. tuberculosis*; disease may be pulmonary or extrapulmonary

II. Pathogenesis

   A. Primary or initial infection occurs by inhalation of the etiologic agent, *Mycobacterium tuberculosis*; it is dispersed as droplet nuclei (small airborne particles) from persons who have infectious pulmonary or laryngeal TB when they cough, sneeze, speak, or sing

   B. The duration of infectivity is variable, but the majority of adult and adolescent patients are noncontagious within a few weeks of starting appropriate therapy; children <12 years are usually not contagious because their lesions are small and cough is minimal

   C. Incubation period from infection to development of a positive reaction to tuberculin skin test is 2-10 weeks

   D. Close contacts of persons who have infectious TB are at the highest risk of becoming infected; infection rates range from 21%-23% for the contacts of infectious TB patients

   E. Approximately 90% of primary TB infections remain in a latent or dormant infection stage:
      1. Persons in this stage are not infectious
      2. Persons with latent TB infection may develop active clinical disease after periods of stress or at times when the body is undergoing change or fighting an infection

   F. The most common site for clinical TB (73% of cases) is the lungs; however, TB is a systemic disease which can result in disseminated TB (miliary TB) or infections in the bones and joints as well as in the lymphatic, genitourinary, and central nervous systems

   G. Current classification system (see table CLASSIFICATION SYSTEM) is based on pathogenesis

Class	Type	Description
CLASSIFICATION SYSTEM FOR TB*		
0	No TB exposure Not infected	No history of exposure Negative reaction to tuberculin skin test
1	TB exposure No evidence of infection	History of exposure Negative reaction to tuberculin skin test
2	TB infection No disease	Positive reaction to tuberculin skin test Negative bacteriologic studies (if done) No clinical, bacteriological, or radiographic evidence of TB
3	TB, clinically active	*M. tuberculosis* cultured (if done) Clinical, bacteriological, or radiographic evidence of current disease
4	TB Not clinically active	History of episode(s) of TB **or** Abnormal but stable radiographic findings Positive reaction to the tuberculin skin test Negative bacteriologic studies (if done) **and** No clinical or radiographic evidence of current disease
5	TB suspected	Diagnosis pending

*All persons with class 3 or class 5 TB should be reported promptly to state and local health departments

Source: US Department of Health and Human Services, Centers for Disease Control and Prevention. (2000). *Core curriculum on tuberculosis* (4th ed.). Atlanta, GA.

III.   Clinical Presentation

A.   Of the estimated 10-15 million persons in the U.S. who are infected with *M. tuberculosis*, about 10% of those with normal immune systems will develop TB disease if there is no intervention

B.   Although the number of TB cases has declined since 1993, the incidence of drug-resistant tuberculosis is increasing

C.   Outbreaks of multidrug-resistant TB (MDR-TB) -- resistant to both isoniazid (INH) and rifampin (RIF) -- are a serious concern; these outbreaks have been associated with a high prevalence of HIV infection among the outbreak cases, a high mortality rate, and a high transmission rate of MDR-TB to heath-care and correctional facility workers
    1.   Transmission of drug-resistant TB is the same as drug-susceptible TB
    2.   Two types of drug resistance
        a.   Primary resistance occurs in persons who are initially infected with resistant organisms
        b.   Secondary resistance or acquired resistance occurs during TB therapy because the regimen was inadequate or the regimen was not taken appropriately

D.   Presenting symptoms of TB in adults are often vague
    1.   Productive, prolonged cough over 3 weeks' duration
    2.   Chest pain
    3.   Hemoptysis
    4.   Increased fatigue, malaise, anorexia, weight decrease
    5.   Periodic fever, night sweats

E.   Symptoms of extrapulmonary TB depend on the site affected; hematuria may occur in TB of the kidney, and back pain may occur in TB of the spine

F.   Certain persons are at higher risk for exposure to or infection with *M. tuberculosis*
    1.   Close contacts of person known or suspected to have TB
    2.   Foreign-born persons from areas where TB is common
    3.   Residents and employees of high-risk congregate settings
    4.   Health care workers who serve high-risk patients
    5.   Medically underserved, low-income populations

6.   High-risk racial or ethnic minority populations
7.   Children exposed to adults in high-risk categories
8.   Persons who inject illicit drugs

G.   Certain persons are at higher risk of developing TB disease once infected (see table INDIVIDUALS AT RISK FOR TB DISEASE)

INDIVIDUALS AT RISK FOR DEVELOPING TB DISEASE ONCE INFECTED

- HIV infection

- Anyone with associated diabetes, silicosis, prolonged corticosteroid therapy, other immunosuppressive therapy, cancer of the head and neck, hematologic and reticuloendothelial disease, end-stage renal disease, intestinal bypass or gastrectomy, chronic malabsorption syndromes, low body weight (10% or more below the ideal)

- Recent infection with *M. tuberculosis* (within the past 2 years), chest radiograph findings suggestive of previous TB (in a person who received inadequate or no treatment)

- Substance abuse (especially drug injection)

Source: U.S. Department of Health & Human Services, Centers for Disease Control and Prevention. (2000). *Core curriculum on tuberculosis* (4th ed.). Atlanta, GA.

IV.   Diagnosis/Evaluation

A.   History
1.   Inquire about onset and duration of weight loss, fatigue, fever, night sweats, anorexia, cough, hemoptysis, chest pain, as well as localized symptoms in other body organs such as hematuria, enlarged lymph nodes
2.   Consider risk factors (country of origin, age, occupation, ethnic or racial group, HIV, substance use)
3.   Ask about history of TB exposure, infection, or disease
4.   Ask about results and dates of TB skin tests and chest x-rays
5.   Determine whether patient has had previous TB treatment; may need to contact the local health department to confirm
6.   Assess medical conditions that increase risk for TB disease (see III.G., table INDIVIDUALS AT RISK FOR TB DISEASE)
7.   Inquire about travel to developing countries where TB is common

B.   Physical Examination
1.   Observe for skin pallor
2.   Palpate for lymphadenopathy
3.   Inspect, palpate, percuss, and auscultate chest (rales in upper posterior chest, bronchovesicular breathing, and whispered pectoriloquy are often positive findings in patients with TB)
4.   Complete physical exam is needed if disseminated TB is suspected

C.   Differential Diagnosis
1.   Malignancy
2.   Silicosis
3.   Chronic obstructive pulmonary disease
4.   Asthma
5.   Bronchiectasis
6.   Pneumonia

D.   Diagnostic Tests
1.   Testing is performed to identify infected individuals at higher risk for TB exposure or infection and to identify individuals at higher risk for TB disease once infected; regular tuberculin testing of high risk groups is recommended (no need to repeat PPD on person with a known positive tuberculin skin test)

a. Preferred method of testing is the Mantoux tuberculin skin test 5 TU-PPD

    (1) The skin test is the only way to diagnose TB infection before the infection has progressed to TB disease; generally, takes 2 to 10 weeks after infection for person to react positively to skin test (persons who recently had contact with someone with TB and have a negative tuberculin skin test should be re-tested 10-12 weeks after last exposed to infectious TB)

    (2) Administer intradermal injection of 0.1 mL of purified protein derivative (PPD) tuberculin containing 5 tuberculin units (TU) into inner surface of forearm; should produce a discrete pale wheal 6-10 mm in diameter

        (a) Monitor for reactions 48-72 hours after application

        (b) Measure only the area of induration and record in millimeters

    (3) Interpretation of PPD (see table POSITIVE PPD)

POSITIVE PPDs

- ≥5 mm if patient is one of the following: known HIV+, recent contacts of infectious TB case, chest x-ray with fibrotic changes or findings suggestive of previous TB, organ transplant and other immunosuppressed patients (receiving the equivalent of >15 mg/day of prednisone for >1month)

- ≥10 mm if patient is one of the following: recent arrival (<5 years) from high-prevalence country, injection drug users, residents and employees of high-risk congregate settings, mycobacteriology laboratory personnel, person with medical risk factors, children <4 years of age, or children and adolescents exposed to adults in high-risk categories

- ≥15 mm: all persons with no known risk factor for TB

Source: U.S. Department of Health and Human Services, Centers for Disease Control and Prevention. (2000). *Core curriculum on tuberculosis* (4th ed.). Atlanta, GA.

    (4) Anergy testing

        (a) Does **not** rule out diagnosis of TB based on a negative skin test; persons may have a condition known as anergy in which the tuberculin reactions are decreased or disappear

        (b) Although routine anergy testing is no longer routinely recommended, consider anergy on an individual basis in persons with negative skin tests who have the following: HIV infection, severe or febrile illness, immunosuppressive therapy, live-virus vaccinations, viral infections or overwhelming TB infection

        (c) Determine anergy by administering two delayed-type hypersensitivity antigens such as mumps or *Candida* by the Mantoux technique; persons with a reaction ≥3 mm are not anergic

        (d) If anergy is present, probability of infection should be evaluated and persons judged at high risk of exposure should be considered for preventive therapy

    (5) Two-step testing is used to differentiate boosted reactions from reactions due to new infection; should be performed in adults who will be retested periodically, such as health care workers

        (a) Some individuals with TB infection may have a negative skin test when tested several years after an infection; however, the skin test may stimulate their ability to react to tuberculin and cause positive reactions to subsequent tests (boost) which may be misinterpreted as new infections

        (b) To distinguish a boosted reaction from a new infection when the first test is negative, administer a second skin test 1-3 weeks after first test

            (i) If second test is negative: person is uninfected and any subsequent positive test should be classified as a new infection

            (ii) If second test is positive: person is infected and should be treated accordingly

b. Chest radiograph or sputum smears may be the recommended first screening test in populations where risk of transmission is high and difficulties in administering and reading tests exist, such as jails or homeless shelter

c. The QuantiFERON-TB test (QFT) was approved by the Food and Drug Administration (FDA) in 2001 as an aid for detecting latent *M. tuberculosis* infection (LTBI)

    (1) QFT can be considered for LTBI screening in the following:

        (a) Initial and serial testing of persons with an increased risk (recent immigrants, injection-drug users, and residents and employees of prisons and jails)

        (b) Initial and serial testing of persons whose future activity might place them at increased risk for exposure (healthcare workers and military personnel)

        (c)   Testing of persons who undergo screening but who are not considered to have an increased probability of infection (entrance requirements for certain schools and workplaces)

     (2)   QFT is not recommended in the following:

        (a)   Evaluation of persons with suspected tuberculosis

        (b)   Assessment of contacts of persons with infectious tuberculosis

        (c)   Screening of children aged <17 years, pregnant women, or for persons with clinical conditions that increase the risk for progression of LTBI to active TB

        (d)   Detection of LTBI after skin test results

        (e)   Confirmation of tuberculin skin test results

        (f)   Diagnosis of *M. avium* complex disease

     (3)   QFT results may be confirmed with tuberculin skin testing; the probability of LTBI is greatest when both are positive

     (4)   QFT testing should be through a qualified laboratory; collection and transport of blood is required within 12 hours

  2.   Diagnosis of active disease

    a.   Order three sputum specimens for **both** smear examination and culture in patients suspected of pulmonary or laryngeal TB

     (1)   A presumptive diagnosis of TB can be made with detection of acid-fast bacilli (AFB); results can usually be obtained in 24 hours

     (2)   A positive sputum culture for *M. tuberculosis* is essential to confirm diagnosis but often takes several weeks for results to be obtained

     (3)   Drug susceptibility testing should be done on the initial *M. tuberculosis* isolate; testing should also be performed on additional isolates from patients whose cultures fail to convert to negative within 2 months of beginning therapy or if there is clinical evidence of failure to respond to therapy

     (4)   Aerosol induction to stimulate sputum production, bronchoscopy, or gastric aspiration should be done if the patient cannot produce a sputum specimen and there is suspicion of TB

    b.   A tuberculin skin test is helpful in making diagnosis and should be applied, but absence of a reaction to the test does not exclude diagnosis; see anergy testing IV.D.1.a.(4)

    c.   Order posterior-anterior chest x-ray

     (1)   Abnormalities are suggestive but are not diagnostic of TB; x-rays may rule out possibility of pulmonary TB in an asymptomatic person with a positive skin test

     (2)   In pulmonary TB, abnormalities are often present in apical or posterior segments of upper lobes or superior segments of lower lobes; in HIV infected persons, other abnormalities are often present

  3.   Baseline laboratory testing is ordered after TB is diagnosed (also see V.C. for specific baseline laboratory tests that should be ordered when patients are prescribed specific medications)

    a.   For latent TB infection, baseline testing is not routinely recommended for all patients at the start of treatment; obtain baseline hepatic measurements for the person whose initial evaluation suggests liver disease, patients with HIV infection, women who are pregnant or within 3 months postpartum, and persons with a history of chronic liver disease

    b.   For TB disease, baseline testing includes measurements of hepatic enzymes, bilirubin, serum creatinine, blood urea nitrogen (BUN), CBC, and platelet count; measure serum uric acid if pyrazinamide is used; test visual acuity if ethambutol is used; test hearing function if streptomycin is used

V.   Plan/Management

    A.   Latent TB infection (LTBI) therapy reduces the risk that TB infection will progress to actual disease

      1.   LTBI therapy is indicated for persons who would benefit from treatment (see table CANDIDATES FOR TREATMENT OF LTBI)

CANDIDATES FOR TREATMENT OF LTBI

❖ Positive skin test result ≥5 mm:
- ✓ HIV-positive persons
- ✓ Recent contacts of a TB case
- ✓ Persons with fibrotic changes on chest radiograph consistent with old TB
- ✓ Patients with organ transplants and other immunosuppressed patients

❖ Positive skin test result ≥10 mm:
- ✓ Recent arrivals (<5 years) from high-prevalence countries
- ✓ Injection drug users
- ✓ Residents and employees of high-risk congregate settings
- ✓ Mycobacteriology laboratory personnel
- ✓ Persons with high-risk clinical conditions

❖ Positive skin test result ≥15 mm:
- ✓ Persons with no known risk factors for TB may be considered

❖ Other candidates:
- ✓ Persons who are close contacts with infectious cases and have a negative TB skin test reaction (<5 mm) should be considered for LTBI treatment (after TB disease has been ruled out); children <4 years, immunosuppressed persons, and others who may develop TB disease quickly after infection; close contacts with negative initial reaction should be retested 10-12 weeks after last exposure to TB

❖ Consult specialist for pregnant women

Source: U.S. Department of Health and Human Services, Centers for Disease Control and Prevention. (2000). *Core curriculum on tuberculosis* (4th ed.). Atlanta, GA.

2. Before initiating treatment for LTBI:
   a. Exclude possibility of TB disease as this would require multiple drug therapy
   b. Question history of previous treatment for LTBI or disease
   c. Explore characteristics of person (preventive therapy might **not** be indicated in the following persons: persons at high risk for adverse reactions to isoniazid (INH) such as those with acute or active liver disease, persons who cannot tolerate INH, persons likely to be infected with drug-resistant *M. tuberculosis*, persons who are highly unlikely to complete course of preventive therapy)
   d. Recommend HIV testing if there are risk factors

3. There are several drug treatment regimens available for the treatment of LTBI (see table REGIMEN OPTIONS FOR LTBI)
   a. Dispense only a 1-month supply of drug at a time (2 weeks only if taking rifampin and pyrazinamide)
   b. Monthly question for the following: compliance, symptoms of neurotoxicity (paresthesias of hands and feet), signs of hepatitis, signs and symptoms of active TB disease (if taking rifampin and pyrazinamide must be reassessed every 2 weeks)
   c. In patients prone to developing neuropathy, pregnant women, and persons with seizure disorders prescribe pyridoxine (vitamin B_6) 10-50 mg/day
   d. New, short-course preventive treatment regimens are currently being investigated; however 9-month Isoniazid is considered optimal

REGIMEN OPTIONS FOR TREATMENT OF LTBI	
Type of Patient	**Dosage***
⚹ Adults (without HIV infection)	INH 300 mg QD for 6 months or 9 months** (minimum of 180 doses within 9 months for the 6 month regimen; minimum 270 doses within 12 months for 9 month regimen); four months of daily rifampin is an acceptable alternative; because of the risks of liver injury, the two-month rifampin and pyrazinamide combination should be used with caution, especially if the patient is taking other medications associated with liver injury or those with alcoholism
⚹ Adults with HIV infection	INH 300 mg QD for 9 months *OR* Rifampin 10 mg/kg/day QD (Maximum dose of 600 mg) and pyrazinamide 15-30 mg/kg/day QD (Maximum dose of 2 grams) for 2 months*** (minimum of 60 doses in 3 months); available data do not show excessive risk for severe hepatitis associated with this RIF-PZA treatment in HIV-infected adults
⚹ Adults with positive skin test, chest x-ray demonstrating old fibrotic lesions, no evidence of active disease, no history of treatment for TB	INH 300 mg QD for 9 months *OR* 4 months of rifampin (with or without isoniazid) *OR* 2 months of rifampin plus pyrazinamide cautiously
⚹ Adults with close contacts of infectious patients who have INH-resistant TB	<u>HIV negative persons</u>: 4 month regimen of daily rifampin *OR* 2 months with a rifamycin and pyrazinamide cautiously <u>HIV positive persons</u>: 2 month regimen with a rifamycin and PZA
⚹ Pregnancy and Breast-feeding	INH daily or twice weekly (dosages as above) Pyridoxine supplementation Breast-feeding not contraindicated

*INH can also be given 2 times weekly in dose of 15 mg/kg when compliance is doubtful and direct observation is needed (minimum of 76 doses administered within 12 months)

9-month regimen is considered optimal; twice-weekly 6 month regimen should have a minimum of 52 doses within 9 months; 2-month RIF-PZA treatment regimen should be used with **caution due to risk of severe liver injury

***Twice-weekly regimens should consist of at least 16 doses in 2 months or 24 doses in 3 months; PZA dose for twice weekly regimen 4 grams (50-70 mg/kg/day)

Source: US Department of Health and Human Services, Centers for Disease Control and Prevention. (2000). *Core curriculum on tuberculosis* (4th ed.). Atlanta, GA.

    B.   Treatment of active disease (uncomplicated, intrathoracic TB): initial treatment should include four drugs: isoniazid (INH), rifampin (RIF), pyrazinamide (PZA), and either ethambutol (EMB) or streptomycin (SM)

          1.   See tables that follow for regimens and dosages of initial drug therapy in adults and in patients with special considerations; when drug susceptibility results are available, the regimen should be altered as appropriate

REGIMEN OPTIONS FOR INITIAL TREATMENT OF PULMONARY AND EXTRAPULMONARY TB

TB without HIV Infection

Option 1	Option 2	Option 3
Administer daily INH, RIF, PZA, and EMB or SM for 8 wks, followed by 16 weeks* of INH and RIF daily for 2-3 times/ week;** EMB or SM should be continued until susceptibility to INH and RIF is demonstrated. In areas where the INH resistance rate is <4%, EMB or SM may not be necessary for patients with no individual risk factors for drug resistance. Consult a TB medical expert if the patient is symptomatic or smear or culture positive after 3 months.	Administer daily INH, RIF, PZA, and SM or EMB for 2 weeks followed by 2 times/week** administration of the same drugs for 6 weeks (by DOT#), and subsequently, with 2 times/week** administration of INH and RIF for 16 weeks (by DOT).** After the 8-week induction phase, continue EMB or SM until susceptibility to INH and RIF is demonstrated, unless drug resistance is unlikely. Consult a TB medical expert if the patient is symptomatic or smear or culture positive after 3 months.	Treat by DOT, 3 times/week** with INH, RIF, PZA, and EMB or SM for 6 months.*** Consult a TB medical expert if the patient is symptomatic or smear or culture positive after 3 months. This regimen has been shown to be effective for INH-resistant TB.

*For adults with forms of extrapulmonary TB (miliary TB, bone and joint TB, or TB meningitis), response to therapy should be closely monitored and treatment should be altered accordingly

**All regimens administered 2 times/week or 3 times/week should be monitored by DOT for the duration of therapy

***The strongest evidence from clinical trials is the effectiveness of all 4 drugs given for the full 6 months. There is weaker evidence that SM can be stopped after 4 months if the isolate is susceptible to all drugs. The evidence for stopping PZA before the end of 6 months is equivocal for the 3 times/week regimen, and there is no evidence on the benefit of this regimen with EMB for less than the full 6 months

#DOT = Directly observed therapy

OPTIONS FOR INITIAL TREATMENT OF PULMONARY AND EXTRAPULMONARY TB IN SPECIAL CIRCUMSTANCES

Smear-and culture negative pulmonary TB	Pulmonary and extrapulmonary TB when PZA is contraindicated
Administer INH, RIF, PZA, and EMB or SM following option 1, 2, or 3 for initial therapy in table above for 8 weeks followed by INH, RIF, PZA, and EMB or SM daily or 2-3 times per week (DOT) for 8 weeks. If drug resistance is unlikely, EMB or SM may be unnecessary and PZA may be discontinued after 2 months	Administer INH, RIF, and EMB or SM daily for 4-8 weeks followed by INH and RIF daily or 2 times per week (DOT) for 28-32 weeks. EMB or SM should be continued until susceptibility to INH and RIF is demonstrated. If drug resistance is unlikely, EMB or SM may be unnecessary

DOSAGE RECOMMENDATIONS FOR FIRST-LINE DRUGS IN INITIAL TREATMENT OF TB

Drugs	Dosage		
	Daily	2 times/week	3 times/week
Isoniazid	5 mg/kg Max 300 mg	15 mg/kg Max 900 mg	15 mg/kg Max 900 mg
Rifampin*	10 mg/kg Max 600 mg	10 mg/kg Max 600 mg	10 mg/kg Max 600 mg
Pyrazinamide*	15-30 mg/kg Max 2 gm	50-70 mg/kg Max 4 gm	50-70 mg/kg Max 3 gm
Ethambutol**	15-25 mg/kg	50 mg/kg	25-30 mg/kg
Streptomycin	15 mg/kg Max 1 gm	25-30 mg/kg Max 1.5 gm	25-30 mg/kg Max 1.5 gm

* Dispense no more than a 2-week supply of RIF-PZA at a time to facilitate periodic clinical assessments due to the risk of severe liver injury
** No maximum doses. Calculate dosage on lean body weight in obese patients

Source: US Department of Health and Human Services, Centers for Disease Control and Prevention. (2000). *Core curriculum on tuberculosis* (4th ed.). Atlanta, GA.

2. Second-line TB drugs may be prescribed after consulting a specialist: capreomycin, kanamycin, ethionamide, para-aminosalicylic acid, cycloserine, ciprofloxacin, levofloxacin, ofloxacin, amikacin, clofazimine

3. Treatment of persons with additional medical conditions must be individualized
   a. For patients with impaired renal function avoid streptomycin, kanamycin and capreomycin
   b. In patients with HIV infection, duration of treatment is the same as HIV-negative adults; HIV positive adults should be aggressively assessed for response to treatment and treatment should be prolonged if response is slow or suboptimal
4. Treatment of drug-resistant TB
   a. In patients with documented INH resistance during initial four-drug therapy, discontinue INH and continue RIF, PZA, and EMB or SM for entire 6 months *OR* treat with RIF and EMB for 12 months
   b. Consult specialist for multidrug-resistant TB
5. Directly observed therapy (DOT) is one method to ensure adherence
   a. DOT requires that a health-care provider or other designated person observe patient while ingesting anti-TB medications
   b. All patients with TB caused by organisms resistant to either INH or RIF and all patients receiving intermittent therapy should receive DOT

C. Monitoring drug therapy includes the following:
1. Patients treated for TB should have baseline measurements of hepatic enzymes, bilirubin, serum creatinine or BUN, CBC, and platelet count; measure serum uric acid if pyrazinamide is used; test visual acuity if EMB is used; test hearing function if SM is used
2. At minimum, assess patients monthly and evaluate for adverse drug reactions
3. Drug interactions: current literature and package inserts should be consulted
   a. INH and phenytoin interact; monitor serum level of phenytoin
   b. Rifampin may increase the clearance of drugs metabolized by the liver: methadone, Coumadin, glucocorticoids, estrogens, oral hypoglycemic agents, digitalis, anticonvulsants, ketoconazole, fluconazole, cyclosporine and protease inhibitors; women should use birth control method other than oral contraceptives, such as barrier methods
4. Specific guidelines for drug monitoring
   a. INH: Baseline hepatic enzymes; repeat tests if abnormal or risks for adverse reactions
   b. Rifampin: baseline CBC, platelets, hepatic enzymes; repeat as needed
   c. PZA: Baseline uric acid and hepatic enzymes; repeat as needed (asymptomatic hyperuricemia is not an indication for discontinuing the drug)
   d. RIF-PZA combination therapy: Serum aminotransferase (AT) and bilirubin at baseline and at 2, 4, and 6 weeks of treatment; stop treatment if AT >5 times the upper limit of normal in an asymptomatic person, AT greater than normal range when accompanied by symptoms of hepatitis, or a serum bilirubin greater than normal range
   e. Ethambutol: Baseline and monthly visual acuity and color vision tests
   f. Streptomycin: Baseline hearing test and kidney function; repeat as needed
5. Monitoring response to therapy includes the following:
   a. Sputum exam at least monthly until conversion to negative; then, at least one sputum at completion of therapy; most important response to treatment is culture conversion
   b. For patients with multi-drug resistant TB, monthly sputum evaluation should continue for entire course of treatment
   c. Chest radiographs are less important than sputums but chest film at completion of treatment provides a baseline for future comparisons
   d. Patients with sputum that remains culture positive beyond 3 months should be evaluated for disease due to drug-resistant organisms
   e. When waiting for drug susceptibility results, continue the original drug regimen or augment regimen with at least three new drugs; **never** add one drug to a failing regimen

D. BCG vaccination should be undertaken only after consultation with health department; vaccination is used in many countries but is not generally recommended in US

E. Patient Education: teach about possible reactions to medicines
1. INH
   a. Hepatic toxicity is the most common adverse reaction
   b. Instruct patient to immediately report nausea, loss of appetite, vomiting, unexplained fever over 3 days, abdominal tenderness (all hepatitis-suggesting symptoms)
   c. Peripheral neuropathy may be prevented by taking daily 10-50 mg of pyridoxine (vitamin B_6)

2. Rifampin
   a. GI upset, hepatitis, bleeding problems, flu-like symptoms, and rash
   b. Warn patient that tears, urine, saliva, etc., may turn orange-red; may permanently stain contact lenses
3. Pyrazinamide: hyperuricemia, gout (rare), hepatitis, joint aches, rash, and GI upset
4. Ethambutol: Optic neuritis and rash
5. Streptomycin: Hearing and balance changes and renal toxicity

F. Additional patient education also includes discussion of mode of transmission and need to cover nose and mouth when coughing or sneezing; no sharing of eating utensils

G. A good website resource is the CDC National Center for HIV, STD, and TB Prevention, Division of Tuberculosis Elimination (http://www.cdc.gov/nchstp/tb/default.htm)

H. Follow Up (see V.C.4.-5. for follow-up guidelines for drug and response monitoring)
   1. Patient must have sputum examination at least monthly until conversion to negative, most important objective measure of response to treatment is culture conversion; patients whose sputum no longer has *M. tuberculosis* after two months should have at least one additional sputum smear and culture at the completion of therapy
   2. Patients with multi-drug resistant TB need monthly sputum evaluations for entire course of therapy
   3. Monitor adverse drug reactions and response to treatment monthly while on drug therapy
   4. Order chest films at end of therapy as they provide baseline comparison with future films

REFERENCES

American Academy of Pediatrics. (2000). In L.K. Pickering (Ed.). *Red Book: Report of the Committee on Infectious Disease.* (25th ed.). Elk Grove Village, IL: Author.

American Thoracic Society. (2001). Guidelines for the management of adults with community-acquired pneumonia: Diagnosis, assessment of severity, antimicrobial therapy, and prevention. *American Journal of Respiratory and Critical Care Medicine, 163,* 1730-1754.

Bach, P.B., Brown, C., Gelfand, S.E., & McCrory, D.C. (2001). Management of acute exacerbations of chronic obstructive pulmonary disease: A summary and appraisal of published evidence. *Annals of Internal Medicine, 134,* 600-620.

Barnes, P.J. (2000). Chronic obstructive pulmonary disease. *New England Journal of Medicine, 343,* 269-280.

Bartlett, J.G., Breiman, R.F., Mandell, L.A., & File, T.M., Jr. (1998). Guidelines from the Infectious Disease Society of America. Community-acquired pneumonia in adults: Guidelines for management. *Clinical Infectious Diseases, 26,* 811-836.

Busse, W.W., & Lemanske, R.F., Jr. (2001). Asthma. *New England Journal of Medicine, 344,* 350-362.

Cain, W.A. (2002). Tularemia. *American Journal for Nurse Practitioners, 5,* 24-26.

Centers for Disease Control and Prevention. (2002). Guidelines for using the QuantiFERON-TB test for diagnosing latent *Mycobacterium tuberculosis* infection. *MMWR, 51,* 1-5.

Centers for Disease Control and Prevention. (2001). Recognition of illness associated with the intentional release of a biologic agent. *MMWR, 50(41),* 893-897.

Centers for Disease Control and Prevention. (2001). Update: Fatal and severe liver injuries associated with rifampin and pyrazinamide for latent tuberculosis infection, and revisions in American Thoracic Society/CDC recommendations-United States, 2001. *MMWR, 50(34),* 733-735.

Celi, B.R. (1998). Standards for the optimal management of COPD: A summary. *Chest, 113,* 283S-287S.

Dewan, N.A. (2002). COPD exacerbations: To x-ray or not to x-ray. *Chest, 122,* 1118-1121.

Drazen, J M., Israel, E., & O'Byrne, P.M. (1999). Treatment of asthma with drugs modifying the leukotriene pathway. *New England Journal of Medicine, 340,* 197-206.

Fine, M.J., Auble, T.E., Yealy, D.M., Hanusa, B.H., Weissfeld, L.A., Singer, D.E., Coley, C.M., Marrie, T.J., & Kapoor, W.N. (1997). A prediction rule to identify low-risk patients with community-acquired pneumonia. *New England Journal of Medicine, 336,* 243-250.

German, J.A., & Harper, M.B. (2002). Environmental control of allergic diseases. *American Family Physician, 66,* 421-426.

GlaxoWellcome. (1995). Patient instructions for use of Serevent Diskcus® (salmeterol xinafoate) inhalation powder. Research Triangle Park, NC.

Gonzales, R., Bartlett, J.G., Besser, R.E., Cooper, R.J., Hickner, J.M., Hoffman, J.R., & Sande, M.A. (2001). Principles of appropriate antibiotic use for treatment of uncomplicated acute bronchitis: Background. *Annals of Internal Medicine, 134,* 521-529.

Gonzales, R., & Sande, M.A. (2000). Uncomplicated acute bronchitis. *Annals of Internal Medicine, 133,* 981-991.

Guthrie, R. (2001). Community-acquired lower respiratory tract infections: Etiology and treatment. *Chest, 120,* 2021-2034.

Hall, C.B. (2001). Respiratory syncytial virus and parainfluenza virus. *New England Journal of Medicine, 344,* 1917-1928.

Halm, E.A., & Teirstein, A.S. (2002). Management of community-acquired pneumonia. *New England Journal of Medicine, 347,* 2039-2045.

Hueston, W.J., & Mainous, A.G. (1998). Acute bronchitis. *American Family Physician, 57,* 1270-1276.

Hunter, M.H., & King, D.E. (2001). COPD: Management of acute exacerbations and chronic stable disease. *American Family Physician, 64,* 603-612, 621-622.

Inglesby, T.V., O'Toole, T., Henderson, D.A., et al. (2002). Anthrax as a biological weapon 2002: Updated recommendations for management. *JAMA, 287,* 2236-2252.

Irwin, R.S., & Madison, J.M. (2000). The diagnosis and treatment of cough. *New England Journal of Medicine, 343,* 1715-1721.

Irwin, R.S., & Madison, J.M. (2001). Symptom research on chronic cough: A historical perspective. *Annals of Internal Medicine, 134,* 809-814.

Jasmer, R.M., Saukkonen, J.J., Blumberg, H.M., Daley, C.L., Bernardo, J., Vittinghoff, E., King, M.D., Kawamura, M., & Hopewell, P.C. (2002). Short-course rifampin and pyrazinamide compared with isoniazid for latent tuberculosis infection: A multicenter clinical trail. *Annals of Internal Medicine, 137,* 640-647.

Kormos, W. A. (2000). Approach to the patient with acute bronchitis or pneumonia in the ambulatory setting. In A.H. Goroll & A.G. Mulley, Jr. (Eds.), *Primary care medicine: Office evaluation and management of the adult patient* (4th ed.). Philadelphia: Lippincott, Williams and Wilkins.

Kormos, W.A. (2000). Management of the common cold. In A.H. Goroll & A.G. Mulley, Jr. (Eds.), *Primary care medicine: Office evaluation and management of the adult patient* (4th ed.). Philadelphia: Lippincott, Williams and Wilkins.

Knutson, D., & Braun, C. (2002). Diagnosis and management of acute bronchitis. *American Family Physician, 65,* 2039-2044

Miyashita, N., Fukano, H., Okimoto, N., Hara, H, Yoshida, K., Niki, Y., & Matsushima, T. (2002). Clinical presentation of community-acquired *Chlamydia pneumoniae* pneumonia in adults. *Chest, 121,* 1776-1781.

Mysliwiec, V., & Pina, J.S. (1999). Bronchiectasis: The 'other' obstructive lung disease. *Postgraduate Medicine, 106*(1), 123-31.

National Institutes of Health. National Heart, Lung, and Blood Institute. (1997). *The Expert Panel Report 2: Guidelines for the diagnosis and management of asthma.* National Asthma Education Program, Office of Prevention, Education and Control. NIH Publication #97-4051. Bethesda, MD.

National Institutes of Health. National Heart, Lung, and Blood Institute. (2002). N*AEPP Expert Panel Report Guidelines for the diagnosis and management of asthma.* Update on selected topics 2002. National Asthma Education and Prevention Program. NIH Publ. #02-5075, Bethesda, MD.

National Lung Health Education Program Executive Committee. (1998). Strategies in preserving lung health and preventing COPD and associated diseases: The National Lung Health Education Program. *Chest, 113,* 123S-S154S.

Naureckas, E.T., & Solway, J. (2001). Mild asthma. *New England Journal of Medicine, 345,* 1257-1262.

Niederman, M.S. (1998). Community-acquired pneumonia: A North American perspective. *Chest, 113,* 179S-182S.

Nightingale, J.A., Rogers, D.F., & Barnes, P.J. (2002). Comparison of the effects of salmeterol and formoterol in patients with severe asthma. *Chest, 121,* 1401-1406.

Novartis Pharmaceuticals Corporation. (2001). Foradil® Aerolizer (formoterol fumarate inhalation powder) package insert. East Hanover, NJ.

Prasad, A.S., Fitzgerald, J.T., Bao, B., Beck, F.W.J., & Chandrasekar, P.H. (2000). Duration of symptoms and plasma cytokine levels in patients with the common cold treated with zinc acetate. *Annals of Internal Medicine, 2000,* 245-252.

Petty, T.L. (1998) Supportive therapy in COPD. *Chest, 113,* 256S-262S.

Philip E.B. (1997). Chronic cough. *American Family Physician, 56,* 1395-1402.

Rodriguez-Roisin, R. (2000). Toward a consensus definition for COPD exacerbations. *Chest, 117,* 398S-401S.

Rosenstein, N., Phillips, W.R., Gerber, M.A., Marcy, M., Schwartz, B., & Dowell, S.F. (1998). The common cold--principles of judicious use of antimicrobial agents. *Pediatrics, 101,* 181-184.

Sack, J.L. & Brock, C.D. (2002). Identifying acute epiglottitis in adults. *Postgraduate Medicine, 112,* 81-86.

Scott, J., & Orzano, A.J. (2001). Evaluation and treatment of the patient with acute undifferentiated respiratory tract infection. *Journal of Family Practice, 50,* 1070-1077.

Senior, R.M., & Anthonisen, N.R. (1998). Chronic obstructive pulmonary disease. *American Journal of Respiratory and Critical Care Medicine, 157,* S139-S147.

Singh, D., Sutton, C., & Woodcock, A. (2002). Tuberculin test measurement variability due to the time of reading. *Chest, 122,* 1299-1301.

Slovis, B.S., Plitman, J.D., & Haas, D.W. (2000). The case against anergy testing as a routine adjunct to tuberculin skin testing. *JAMA, 283,* 2003-2007.

Small, P.M., & Fujiwara, P.I. (2001). Management of tuberculosis in the United States. *New England Journal of Medicine, 345,* 189-200.

Snow, V., Mottur-Pilson, C., & Gonzales, R. (2001). Principles of appropriate antibiotic use for treatment of acute bronchitis in adults. *Annals of Internal Medicine, 134,* 518-520.

Snow, V., Lascher, S., & Mottur-Pilson, C. for the Joint Expert Panel on Chronic Obstructive Pulmonary Disease of the American College of Chest Physicians and the American College of Physicians-American Society of Internal Medicine. (2001). Evidence base for management of acute exacerbations of chronic obstructive pulmonary disease. *Annals of Internal Medicine, 134,* 595-599.

Swartz, M.N. (2001). Recognition and management of anthrax – An update. *New England Journal of Medicine, 345,* 1621-1626.

US Department of Health and Human Services, Centers for Disease Control and Prevention. (2000). *Core curriculum on tuberculosis* (4th ed.). Atlanta, GA.

US Department of Health and Human Services, National Institutes of Health, National Heart, Lung, and Blood Institute. (2001). *Executive summary: Global strategy for the diagnosis, management, and prevention of chronic obstructive pulmonary disease* (NIH Publication No. 2701A). Bethesda, MD.

Voelkel, N. F. (2000). Raising awareness of COPD in primary care. *Chest, 117,* 372S-375S.

Weg, J.G., & Haas, C.F. (1998). Long-term oxygen therapy for COPD: Improving longevity and quality of life in hypoxemic patients. *Postgraduate Medicine, 103,* 143-155.

ZuWallack, R.L., Mahler, D.A., Reilly, D., Church, N., Emmett, A., Rickard, K., & Knobil, K. (2001). Salmeterol plus theophylline combination therapy in the treatment of COPD. *Chest, 119,* 1661-1670.

Cardiovascular Problems

JEAN E. DEMARTINIS, CONSTANCE R. UPHOLD & MARY VIRGINIA GRAHAM

Peripheral Vascular Disorders
Deep Venous Thrombosis

Leg Ulcers

Peripheral Arterial Disease: Chronic Lower Extremity Arterial Occlusive Disease

Varicose Veins

ATRIAL FIBRILLATION

I. Definition: Supraventricular tachyarrhythmia characterized by uncoordinated atrial activation with deterioration of atrial mechanical function and usually associated with an irregular ventricular response; see table that follows

CLASSIFICATION SCHEME FOR ATRIAL FIBRILLATION*	
Category	**Definition**
First detected episode of AF**	New onset of AF whether or not symptomatic or self-limited (50% of patients revert to sinus rhythm within 24 hours without treatment)
Recurrent AF	Two or more episodes
Paroxysmal AF	Attacks terminate spontaneously, are limited in duration, *recurrent*, and occur at variable time intervals
Persistent AF	Attacks are not self-terminating, but rather terminate with pharmacological or electrical cardioversion; sustained AF that usually leads to permanent status
Permanent AF	AF that is resistant to pharmacological or electrical cardioversion
Lone AF	AF occurring in young individuals (<60 years of age) without clinical or echocardiographic evidence of identifiable cardiopulmonary disease or known precipitating factors
Alcohol-related AF	AF associated with alcoholism; binge drinking episodes precipitate AF (called "holiday heart syndrome")

*Applies to episodes of AF that last more than 30 seconds and are unrelated to a reversible cause
**Acute AF is onset within 48 hours

Adapted from Fuster, V., Ryden, L.E., Asinger, R.W., Cannon, D.S., Crijns, H.J., Frye, R.L., et al. (2001). ACC/AHA/ESC guidelines for the management of patients with atrial fibrillation: A report of the American College of Cardiology/American Heart Association Task Force on Practice Guidelines and the European Society of Cardiology Committee for Practice Guidelines and Policy Conferences (Committee to Develop Guidelines for the Management of Patients With Atrial Fibrillation). *Journal of the American College of Cardiology 38*, 1266i-1266lxx and available at: www.acc.org.

II. Pathogenesis

  A. Atrial fibrillation (AF) is frequently triggered by alterations in autonomic tone, acute or chronic changes in atrial wall tension, or atrial ectopic foci called premature atrial contractions (PAC)
   1. Once initiated, the multifocal, reentrant impulses occur at a truly rapid rate (350-600/minute) entering the atrioventricular (AV) node at random
   2. Fortunately, normal conduction through the AV junction is slowed and not all of the atrial impulses reach the ventricles; the resulting ventricular rate is slower than the atrial rate, typically between 120-180 complexes/minute, in the absence of drug therapy or AV node disease, and is irregular
   3. However, with hemodynamic decline, the ventricular rate may become overly accelerated or the response may be inadequate, leading to severe bradycardia, or even sudden cardiac death

  B. The rapid reentrant impulses result in incomplete contractions and ineffective emptying of the atria causing a decline in cardiac output and stasis of blood within the atria, which may result in thrombus formation and complications such as peripheral embolization and stroke

  C. Hemodynamic compromise in AF is often worse in patients with disorders reliant on the atrial component of ventricular filling, such as dilated and hypertrophic cardiomyopathies and aortic stenosis

  D. Factors which predispose patients to develop AF include the following:
   1. Organic heart disease that causes atrial distention such as ischemia or infarction, hypertension, valvular disorders, obstructive cardiomyopathy, rheumatic heart disease, or Wolff-Parkinson-White syndrome (Although AF may complicate a myocardial infarction because of the left ventricular dysfunction and volume overload of the left atrium, ischemia itself is a rare cause of AF)
   2. Metabolic diseases such as hyperthyroidism, hypothyroidism, and diabetes mellitus
   3. Right atrial stretch due to pulmonary embolus and acute or chronic lung disease
   4. High adrenergic tone secondary to stress, alcohol withdrawal, sepsis, excessive physical exertion, or caffeine intake
   5. Inflammatory conditions causing myocarditis such as pericarditis or endocarditis
   6. Vagally mediated AF episodes may occur during sleep, after a large meal, or during a period of rest after exercise or activity
   7. The most common predisposing factors are acute respiratory illnesses, such as pneumonia or acute asthma, cardiothoracic surgery, hyperthyroidism, and coronary artery disease

III. Clinical Presentation

A. Some patients are asymptomatic, some feel palpitations or irregular pulse, others have life-threatening symptoms from pulmonary edema; fatigue and nonspecific symptoms are most common

B. Patients with rapid ventricular responses often complain of shortness of breath, fatigue, dizziness, chest pain, palpitations, fullness in neck, or near syncope or syncope secondary to decreased blood pressure

C. Complications:
1. A major complication is arterial embolization that may lead to stroke
2. AF can precipitate angina in patients with CAD and worsen symptoms of heart failure
3. AF can cause congestive heart failure (CHF) and severe cardiomyopathy in patients with otherwise normal hearts and restoration of sinus rhythm can reverse both conditions
4. AF increases myocardial vulnerability and decreases the fibrillation threshold which can enhance development of ventricular tachyarrhythmias and sudden death

D. In the past, patients with AF and preexisting left ventricular failure or coronary obstruction had a poor prognosis; today, prognosis is fair if patients are closely followed and participate in cardiac rehabilitation

IV. Diagnosis/Evaluation; important to characterize the pattern of the arrhythmia (paroxysmal or persistent), determine the cause, and define associated cardiac and extra-cardiac factors

A. History
1. Inquire about onset, pattern, and duration of symptoms
2. Ask patient to describe all symptoms such as palpitations, dyspnea, fatigue, dizziness, near syncope or syncope, leg edema, or calf pain
3. Ask about chest pain to determine if it is related to ischemic heart disease, pulmonary embolism, or other disorders
4. Explore whether patient has weight change, mood change, hair loss, heat or cold intolerance, or tremors that are often associated with thyroid disorders, particularly thyrotoxicosis
5. Determine the number of previous episodes, what relieved symptoms, and previous treatments
6. Explore precipitating factors such as stress, sleep deprivation, unusual activity, bath in hot tub, excessive caffeine or alcohol ingestion, ingestion of large meals, or drug use
7. Carefully explore previous medical history; focus on cardiovascular, respiratory, and neurological systems
8. Ask about family medical history, including heart disease, hypertension, diabetes, thyroid disorders, lung problems, or conduction abnormalities (genetic transmission is gaining recognition as an important component of AF)
9. Obtain medication history
10. Ask about quality of life issues

B. Physical Examination
1. Observe general appearance and signs of respiratory distress and altered levels of consciousness; note apathetic appearance which may be related to thyroid problems
2. Assess postural blood pressure in supine, sitting, and standing positions
3. Assess pulse; in patients with AF pulse is irregularly irregular; intensity of the peripheral pulse and the first heart sound varies with each beat, depending on the allowed ventricular filling time
4. Observe skin for pallor or flushing
5. Perform an eye exam, noting lid lag that is associated with thyroid disease
6. Assess neck for thyromegaly, jugular venous distention, irregular jugular venous pulsations, and carotid artery bruits
7. Auscultate lungs
8. Perform a complete cardiovascular (CV) examination, assessing for murmurs indicative of valvular disease, a pericardial friction rub, or signs of hypertrophy
9. Perform a neurological examination; assess reflexes and observe for resting tremors
10. Perform a mental status examination; particularly in the elderly, AF can lead to cognitive changes

C. Differential Diagnosis: see factors under pathogenesis

D. Diagnostic Tests (baseline studies); see V.K. for additional tests required at follow up visits
1. Order an electrocardiogram (ECG) to identify rhythm, left ventricular hypertrophy, p-wave duration and morphology, bundle-branch block (BBB), prior myocardial infarction, other atrial arrhythmias

a. Diagnosis requires ECG documentation of at least a single lead
b. AF is characterized by rapid, irregular, fibrillatory waves that vary in size, shape, and timing; ventricular rate is irregularly irregular
c. 12-lead recording is helpful in identifying other potential problems such as a re-entry focus, BBB, and left or right atrial or ventricular hypertrophy
2. Order chest x-ray to evaluate for pulmonary status and pulmonary vascular status, and to assess for cardiomegaly
3. Order thyroid function tests
4. Order a complete resting transthoracic echocardiogram with 2-D Doppler flow imaging to identify valvular heart disease, sizes of atria, left ventricle (LV) size and function, peak right ventricle pressure, LV hypertrophy, left atrial thrombus (low sensitivity), and pericardial disease
a. Measures cardiac wall motion, and contractility of the left ventricle and resulting ejection fraction (EF) rate (normal EF >50%)
b. Most important indicator of heart failure
c. Helpful in predicting the success of cardioversion (a dilated left atrium or severe left ventricular failure has a low success rate)
5. Consider the following additional tests:
a. Metabolic panel (electrolytes, blood sugar, BUN, creatinine, liver enzymes)
b. Complete blood count
c. Ambulatory ECG readings with or without exercise testing may be helpful in establishing diagnosis and, later, may be used to evaluate the adequacy of rate control therapy over time; use a 24-48 hour Holter monitor or Event monitor that can be used for days to weeks
d. Transesophageal echocardiograms (TEE) are the most *sensitive* for identifying left atrial thrombi, but are expensive
e. If pulmonary embolus is suspected order D-dimer
f. If congestive heart failure is suspected order brain natriuretic peptide (BNP)

V. Plan/Management:

A. General Principles
1. Goals are to control symptoms, control ventricular rate, prevent thromboembolism and stroke, and prevent recurrences
2. Emphasis now is placed on long-term control of heart rate with calcium channel blockers, beta-blockers, and digoxin
3. Less focus is placed on controlling heart rhythm with antiarrhythmic medications; however, if patients have symptoms despite adequate rate control, these patients may need an antiarrhythmic drug
4. The following mnemonic is helpful: **'RCC'–Rate control, Clot control, Cardioversion (rhythm control)**
5. Individualize plan based on clinical presentation, hemodynamic tolerance, time of onset of AF, and any underlying comorbid condition
6. Immediate **symptom relief should be first priority**

B. Hospitalization is usually required for treatment of acute AF, particularly if ventricular rate is >170 per minute or <40 per minute and patient has underlying cardiac disease (consult cardiologist)
1. Patients often revert to sinus rhythm when predisposing factors are removed
2. Intravenous drug therapy with beta-blockers or calcium channel blockers is indicated if symptoms persist (collaborate with cardiologist in drug selection and dosage)
3. If patient is hemodynamically compromised, immediate electrical or direct-current-cardioversion (DC/CV) is performed

C. **Rate Control:** (see following table for drug options)
1. Increased importance is now placed on rate control than in the past
2. For patients who have mild stable symptoms with no cardiovascular compromise, oral therapy to control ventricular rate with an AV nodal blocking agent may be the only therapy needed; may be used for immediate control and sometimes long-term control
3. Drugs to control ventricular rate do not convert an acute episode back to sinus rhythm and they do not prevent recurrences of AF
4. These drugs may result in an inappropriately low ventricular response rate; rate is considered controlled when the ventricular response ranges between 60 and 80 beats per minute (bpm) at rest and 90-115 bpm during moderate exercise

DRUGS TO CONTROL VENTRICULAR RATE

Drug	Usual Maintenance Dose	Major Adverse Effects
Calcium Channel Blockers (CCB)*		
Diltiazem (Cardizem)	120-360 mg PO daily in divided doses, slow release available	Hypotension, heart block, heart failure
Verapamil (Calan)	120-360 mg PO daily in divided doses, slow release available	
β-blockers (BB)*		
Metoprolol (Lopressor)	25-100 mg PO in divided doses	Hypotension, heart block, bradycardia, asthma, heart failure
Metoprolol CR (Toprol XL)	25-200 mg PO daily; replace short-acting Lopressor with long-acting form prior to discharge	
Atenolol (Tenormin)	25-100 mg PO in one or two divided doses	
Digoxin (Lanoxin)**	0.125-0.375 PO daily	Digitalis toxicity, heart block, bradycardia

*Start at the lower doses and titrate slowly in elderly patients
**Digoxin should be reserved for the elderly and those with left ventricular dysfunction

5. Calcium channel blockers (CCB) reduce both the resting and exercise heart rates and may improve exercise tolerance
   a. Best given in a slow release, once daily preparations
   b. Diltiazem and verapamil are equally effective (the dihydropyridines such as nifedipine are ineffective)
   c. Generally, CCBs should **not** be used in patients with heart failure (HF) due to systolic dysfunction and should be used cautiously in all patients with HF
6. Beta-blockers (BB) block AV nodal conduction and counteract increased sympathetic activity
   a. Particularly beneficial when AF is associated with activity, stress, hyperthyroidism, or other hyperadrenergic states such as acute myocardial infarction or sepsis; probably drug of choice for patients with coronary artery disease and systolic dysfunction
   b. Control ventricular response at rest and during exercise, but exercise tolerance is reduced
   c. Use with caution in patients with reactive airway disease (RAD), chronic obstructive pulmonary disease, and systolic heart failure
   d. May cause sinus bradycardia or AV block
   e. Initiate BBs gradually in patients with HF
7. Digoxin slows the ventricular rate by blocking conduction through the AV node
   a. Because of slow onset, cannot be used for acute rate control
   b. No longer considered as a first line drug for ventricular rate control in patients with preserved performance of the left ventricle (ejection fraction [EF] >40%); little positive effect in otherwise healthy patients under 65 years of age
   c. May be used as monotherapy in controlling ventricular response when patient has left ventricular dysfunction (EF <40%)
   d. Cannot be used as sole agent to control rate with exercise
   e. Digoxin's main role may be in combination with CCBs and BBs
   f. Major disadvantages: Limited effect on exercise heart rate; toxicity can occur relatively rapidly; slow onset of action
   g. Reduce dosage of digoxin if patient is also receiving quinidine
8. Clonidine may also be effective in controlling ventricular response, but further studies are needed
9. Combination therapy may be required to achieve rate control
   a. Use cautiously and avoid excessive slowing of rate
   b. Combination of digoxin with BBs is most effective

D. **Clot Control:**
   1. Anticoagulant therapy is recommended for the prevention of stroke and other embolic complications; involves a balance between stroke prevention and avoidance of hemorrhagic complications
      a. All patients over 75 years with persistent or permanent AF should be given warfarin if no contraindications exist (stroke risk increases 30% in patients over 75 years of age)
      b. Prescribe warfarin to patients with persistent or permanent AF who are under 75 years of age, and who have one of the following 5 features:
         (1) History of HF, mitral stenosis, prosthetic heart valves, coronary artery disease
         (2) Hypertension
         (3) Diabetes

        (4)   Thyrotoxicosis

        (5)   History of transient ischemic attack or minor non-hemorrhagic cerebrovascular accident

    c.   In patients 65-75 years without any of the five preceding factors use either warfarin or aspirin; if aspirin is used, prescribe buffered (Ascriptin) or enteric coated (Ecotrin) aspirin 325 mg PO daily

    d.   Recommend aspirin or nothing in patients under 60-65 years who have none of the five preceding features

2.   Anticoagulation with oral dosing of warfarin (Coumadin) is totally individualized

    a.   Titrate dosage to maintain International Normalized Ratio (INR) within 2.0-3.0 range; persons at high risk for embolism (mechanical valves, recurrent thromboembolism) should be maintained at INR of 2.5-3.5 range

    b.   Initially, INR should be monitored daily as loading doses of warfarin are initiated until therapeutic level is attained or every 2-3 days if outpatient until therapeutic level is attained

    c.   After therapeutic level is achieved, monitor INR every 1-2 weeks for several weeks to ensure maintenance of therapeutic level, then every 1-2 months

3.   Hospitalized patients are started on continuous low-dose heparin intravenously immediately or given low-molecular-weight heparin (LMWH) subcutaneously; oral dosing of warfarin can also begin at the same time or be withheld until closer to discharge (ideally patient will have reached therapeutic INR with warfarin, and heparin will be discontinued prior to discharge)

4.   Prescribe warfarin pre and post cardioversion (see V.F.2., V.G.2.b., and V.H.2.b.)

5.   Patient education in relation to warfarin

    a.   Teach patient to report any signs of bleeding

    b.   Numerous medications such as acetaminophen, some antiarrhythmics, some antibiotics, phenytoin, nonsteroidal antiinflammatory agents, and selective serotonin reuptake inhibitors increase INR; other drugs such a rifampin, carbamazepine, antihistamines, antianxiety agents, and antacids decrease INR

    c.   Foods and beverages such as green tea, alcohol, broccoli, and tomatoes may affect warfarin levels

E.   **Cardioversion (pharmacological and electrical) to restore sinus rhythm:**

1.   Clinicians can either try to restore sinus rhythm (cardioversion) or allow persistent AF and just control ventricular rate; the following factors should guide the clinician's decision about whether to attempt restoration of sinus rhythm or not:

    a.   Benefits of cardioversion in patients with rate control are reduced symptoms, prevention of embolism, and improved ejection fraction

    b.   Risk of cardioversion is proarrhythmia

    c.   Patients with urgent, acute AF or patients who are symptomatic during rate control are typically considered for cardioversion

    d.   Younger patients with structurally normal hearts appear to benefit from attempts to restore rate control more than older patients with comorbid conditions

    e.   In elderly patients with other comorbidities who can tolerate persistent AF, cardioversion with drugs or electrical cardioversion is often **not** attempted

2.   In about half the cases, AF spontaneously converts to normal sinus rhythm so it may be prudent to delay the decision of cardioversion for 24 hours if the patient is hemodynamically stable

3.   Either pharmacological or electrical cardioversion can be initially attempted as there is no evidence that risk of stroke differs between the two therapies

4.   Pharmacological cardioversion is usually tried first as it is less invasive, even though it is less effective than electrical cardioversion

F.   **Cardioversion: Pharmacological** (also see table V.H. for drugs effective for maintenance of sinus rhythm)

1.   Drug selection is based on potential for adverse effects; because of dangers of proarrhythmia, drugs are usually initiated in the hospital with continuous cardiac monitoring (collaborate with cardiologist in selecting drug and in deciding dose and route of administration)

2.   Before initiating pharmacological cardioversion, several decisions about anticoagulation must be made

    a.   If the patient's condition is stable, a transthoracic echocardiogram or transesophageal echocardiogram can be obtained for evaluation of thrombus formation, and if no evidence of thrombus, drug therapy can be initiated immediately without long-term anticoagulation

    b.   In other cases, anticoagulation is recommended for 3-4 weeks prior to pharmacological cardioversion, but based on individual assessment, pharmacological cardioversion may begin any time after drug therapy for rate control and anticoagulation has been initiated

3. Successful in 10-30% of cases, depending on drug used and duration of the arrhythmia; less effective than electrical cardioversion, but the latter requires conscious sedation or anesthesia
4. Most recurrences happen within three months after cardioversion of the first episode AF, regardless of antiarrhythmic drug used, indicating either failure of drug, too low a dose or both, and suggests need to reevaluate drug therapy
5. If a single agent fails, consider combination of antiarrhythmic drugs
6. Pharmacological cardioversion is most effective when initiated within 7 days of onset of AF
7. The following are drugs with proven efficacies: Dofetilide, flecainide, propafenone, amiodarone, quinidine
8. Procainamide, sotalol, and digoxin are less effective or have been inadequately studied

G. **Electrical cardioversion (DC/CV)** is the most effective means of restoring sinus rhythm (SR) but can result in embolisms, hypotension, pulmonary edema, and major arrhythmias
  1. DC/CV involves delivery of an electrical shock synchronized with R wave of ECG
  2. Elective DC/CV is undertaken when the restoration of sinus rhythm is not deemed urgent
    a. Treatment of choice when the duration of the AF is greater than 48 hours and less than 12 months and when the atria are of normal size (not enlarged and boggy)
    b. Prescribe anticoagulant therapy warfarin for 3-4 weeks prior to cardioversion; some providers prefer 4-6 weeks of therapeutic anticoagulation
  3. For acute episodes deemed urgent, DC/CV can be attempted within 24-48 hours (the sooner the better) after first episode AF when patient is otherwise asymptomatic
  4. For patients with minimal symptoms, it may be sufficient to perform DC/CV after appropriate anticoagulation therapy without the pre-administration of an antiarrhythmic drug; if AF recurs, the DC/CV can be repeated in combination with the use of an antiarrhythmic drug, such as propafenone or amiodarone
  5. Unfortunately, the majority of patients with long-standing AF revert back to AF after cardioversion; each successive attempt is less successful in long-term maintenance of SR and at some point one must weigh the risk of aggressive re-attempt vs. mainstay with anticoagulation and rate control

H. **Long-term maintenance of sinus rhythm** (SR) after initial cardioversion (see tables that follow for dosing/adverse effects and selection of drug with selected disorders)
  1. After pharmacological cardioversion, consider the following agents (see table that follows for suggested antiarrhythmic drug for selected patients):
    a. Class III drugs are used less for acute conversion and more for maintenance
      (1) Amiodarone is a first-line drug and has the lowest incidence of proarrhythmia but in high doses can cause pulmonary fibrosis, hepatitis and thyroid conditions
      (2) Class III drugs such as sotalol and dofetilide are newer agents and are probably as effective as other antiarrhythmic drugs, but may cause torsades de pointes
        (a) Sotalol possesses nonselective β-blocker activities, making it a good choice for patients with CAD who have normal left ventricular function
        (b) Dofetilide appears to be more effective for cardioversion of atrial flutter than of AF; also safe in patients with HF
    b. Alternatively, Class IC agents such as flecainide and propafenone which lengthen the PR interval and width of QRS interval may be prescribed
      (1) May be first-line drugs in patients with true lone AF, those with LV hypertrophy, and those without coronary artery disease; effective for acute conversion of AF
      (2) Do not use in patients with structural heart disease because of high risk of potentially fatal proarrhythmia
    c. Class IA drugs
      (1) Quinidine was the traditional drug of choice, but is used less today because of its adverse effects
      (2) Disopyramide and procainamide have anticholinergic properties in addition to the proarrhythmias and thus, are no longer in favor as first or second line choices
  2. After electrical cardioversion (DC/CV) the following are recommended:
    a. Continue rate and clot control (for at least 4-6 weeks) and reassess for reversion to AF
    b. If reversion to AF, continue or reinitiate anticoagulation therapy and DC/CV once again after 3-6 weeks therapeutic INRs and concurrently prescribe a drug to control rate and an antiarrhythmic drug to maintain sinus rhythm
    c. If episode free for greater than 6 months to one year, try discontinuing the antiarrhythmic drug and maintain heart rate control with one or a combination of AV nodal blocking drugs

Drugs Used to Maintain Sinus Rhythm in Patients with Atrial Fibrillation*

Type[§]	Drug	Daily Dosage	Potential Adverse Effects
IA	Quinidine (Quinidex)	600-1500 mg	Torsade de pointes, GI upset, enhanced AV nodal conduction
	Disopyramide (Norpace)	400-750 mg	Torsade de pointes, HF, glaucoma, urinary retention, dry mouth
	Procainamide (Procanbid)	1000-4000 mg	Torsade de pointes, lupus-like syndrome, GI symptoms
IC	Flecainide (Tambocor)	200-300 mg	Ventricular tachycardia, congestive HF, enhanced AV nodal conduction (conversion to atrial flutter)
	Propafenone (Rythmol)	450-900 mg	Ventricular tachycardia, congestive HF, enhanced AV nodal conduction (conversion to atrial flutter)
III	Sotalol HCl (Betapace)	240-320 mg	Torsade de pointes, congestive HF, bradycardia, exacerbation of chronic obstructive or bronchospastic lung disease
	Amiodarone (Cordarone)**	100-400 mg	Photosensitivity, pulmonary toxicity, polyneuropathy, GI upset, bradycardia, torsade de pointes (rare), hepatic toxicity, thyroid dysfunction
	Dofetilide (Tikosyn)[†]	500-1000 mcg	Torsade de pointes

*Prescribe lower doses in the elderly
[§]Vaughn Williams class
** A loading dose of 600 mg per day is usually given for one month or 1000 mg per day over 1 week
[†] Dose should be adjusted for renal function and QT-interval response during inhospital initiation phase

Adapted from Fuster, V., Ryden, L.E., Asinger, R.W., Cannon, D.S., Crijns, H.J., Frye, R.L., et al. (2001).

Suggested Approach to Selection of Antiarrhythmic Therapy to Maintain Sinus Rhythm in Patients with Selected Disorders

Disorder	Suggested Antiarrhythmic Therapy
Lone atrial fibrillation or hypertension	Propafenone, flecainide, sotalol, disopyramide, dofetilide, amiodarone, and possibly quinidine
Coronary artery disease **without** congestive heart failure	Sotalol, dofetilide, amiodarone, disopyramide
Congestive heart failure or ejection fraction <35%	Dofetilide, amiodarone

Adapted from Falk, R.H. (2001). Atrial fibrillation. *New England Journal of Medicine, 344,* 1067-1078.

I. Patient Education
   1. Remind patients to quit smoking, avoid sleep deprivation, and limit their use of stimulants (i.e., caffeine, sodas, chocolate) and alcohol
   2. Teach relaxation techniques to reduce stress
   3. Teach patients and family members to watch for signs of complications such as extremely rapid heart rate, edema and weight gain, increasing dyspnea on exertion, and chest pain
   4. Teach signs and symptoms of digitalis toxicity (arrhythmias, anorexia, nausea, vomiting, diarrhea, lethargy, confusion, and visual disturbances such as scotomas and color perception changes) and/or adverse effects of other drugs
   5. Intensive teaching is needed for patients on warfarin (see V.D.5.)

J. For patients with permanent AF and disabling symptoms the following are sometimes successful: Ablation of atrioventricular node and pacemaker implantation, focal ablation, the maze procedure, pacemaker therapy, and implantable atrial defibrillators

K. Follow Up: Close follow up is essential
   1. Patients who have their first episodes of AF that terminate spontaneously should return to clinic within 24-48 hours for reevaluation, and then in one week
   2. Patients who are on rate control and anticoagulation prior to elective electrical conversion should return at regular intervals for bloodwork for INRs and in week 4 to assess and schedule DC/CV if INRs have remained therapeutic; after DC/CV they should return in one week
   3. Patients who were directly cardioverted should return in one week; they should be followed with periodic electrocardiograms to assess for rhythm changes
   4. Follow up monitoring for patients on selected medications:
      a. Warfarin: Order INRs every 1-2 months
      b. Amiodarone

(1) At baseline order chest x-ray; pulmonary function testing (PFT); complete metabolic panel including liver function tests; and thyroid tests

(2) Repeat lab testing in 3 then 6 month intervals

(3) Repeat chest x-ray yearly and PFT if respiratory symptoms occur

c. Other antiarrhythmic drugs

(1) Measure liver enzymes the first 4-8 weeks of therapy

(2) Patients with risk factors for developing cardiac complications to therapy should have electrocardiograms ordered the first weeks of drug therapy and then in 3-6 months

(3) Monitoring of serum levels of drugs every 6 months may reduce risk of toxicity

d. Patients on digoxin should be carefully monitored for digitalis toxicity (serum drug levels are not routinely ordered); electrolytes, BUN, creatinine and ECG are often ordered 1-2 weeks after therapy is initiated, and then every 6 month to one year

CHEST PAIN

I. Definition: Chest discomfort or a sensory response to noxious stimuli associated with actual or potential tissue damage involving the chest wall, thoracic organs, and adjacent structures

II. Pathogenesis

A. Chest wall pain may be caused by irritation, trauma, and/or compression of the muscles, cartilaginous structures, nerves, or bones comprising the chest wall area

B. Pain originating from the lungs or adjacent structures may be caused by irritation/inflammation of the lung tissue, pleura (called pleurisy), or diaphragm secondary to inflammation, infection, chronic disease, and/or neoplasm; or reactive airway/bronchospasm due to irritation or inflammation of the bronchi

C. Cardiac pain is often secondary to a low-flow state to the myocardium through coronary arteries blocked or partially blocked by atherosclerotic plaques causing spasm, tissue hypoxia, anaerobic metabolism, lactic acidosis, and increased prostaglandin secretion; other causes of cardiac pain involve the irritation of structures of the mediastinum near the heart, such as in pericarditis

D. Pain due to gastrointestinal problems results from structural defects (luminal laxity, obstruction, or distention) and/or mucosal or organ tissue irritation, inflammation, or infection involving the esophagus and abdominal organs

E. Pain related to psychogenic disorders may be secondary to anxiety, depression, anxiety-tension syndromes, illicit drug use, or neuroses or other psychiatric disorders

III. Clinical Presentation

A. Chest pain resulting from musculoskeletal or nerve origins is variable and may last from a few seconds to several days or even a month or more and may be sharp, dull, or aching and may be aggravated by deep inspiration and cough; the chest is tender on palpation (called point-tenderness) or along the dermatome

1. Musculoskeletal pain tends to occur with movement, stretching, or palpation of the inflamed muscle/tendon and involved body part

2. Bone pain is usually well localized and described as intensely tender

3. Costochondritis is characterized by sharp, usually well localized pain (but may radiate across anterior chest and down the arms) and is most intense at the costochondral junction (junction of the anterior ribs and sternum); may have warmth, erythema, and swelling at junction worsening with deep breath or cough

4. Nerve irritation or compression has characteristic types of chest pain

a. Herpes zoster (see section on HERPES ZOSTER) causes pain along dermatomes and typically precedes a persistent vesicular rash; commonly affects elderly and immunosuppressed patients; patients may have pain along the dermatomes long after the rash has healed

b. Nerve root compression results in pain and motor and sensory deficits (numbness or tingling) in the neck, chest, and upper arm

B. Pleural causes of chest pain typically present as pain worsened by deep inspiration and coughing or spasm secondary to cold weather and increased activity
    1. Bacterial pneumonia is one of the most common causes of pleuritic pain and is characterized by abrupt onset of fever, chills, leukocytosis, and purulent sputum
    2. Pulmonary embolus (PE) is another common cause of pleuritic pain; patients present with sudden onset of dyspnea, tachypnea, tachycardia, hypotension, and possibly hemoptysis; remember, however, that many patients with PE may be asymptomatic
        a. Rales and a pleural friction rub may be present; may exhibit decreased or absent breath sounds distal to PE
        b. May progress to pulmonary hypertension, acute right heart failure, or respiratory arrest
        c. Typically associated with risk factors such as immobility, surgery, pregnancy, oral contraceptives, pelvis or lower extremity trauma (fat embolus)
        d. Patients with history of large bone fracture, malignancy, deep venous thrombosis, previous pulmonary embolus, congestive heart failure, chronic obstructive pulmonary disease, obesity, and hypercoagulability conditions are more prone to developing a PE
    3. Spontaneous pneumothorax or hemothorax secondary to trauma or disease can cause acute, unilateral, stabbing pain with dyspnea
        a. Typically, auscultation reveals decreased breath and voice sounds
        b. Incidence is highest in young men or in older patients with chronic obstructive pulmonary disease; other risk factors include cigarette smoking, lung cancer, and Valsalva maneuver
        c. Be on the alert for mediastinal shift and cardiopulmonary compromise

C. Chest pain due to cardiac diseases may be mild to severe, transient (generally exertional and relieved by rest) or constant (often radiating to neck, jaw, or arms; sometimes the back)
    1. Pericarditis presents with one of two types of pain: Pleuritic pain resulting from spread of the inflammation from the relatively insensitive pericardium to the pain-sensitive parietal pleura or with steady substernal or left precordial pain that resembles angina (aggravated by swallowing and deep breathing with radiation to the left shoulder, upper back and neck)
        a. Pain is paroxysmal and decreases upon sitting and leaning forward
        b. Characterized by a friction rub
        c. Associated signs are fever, tachycardia, pulsus paradoxus, tamponade, elevated sedimentation rate, and leukocytosis
        d. Classic sign if accompanied by tamponade is narrowed pulse pressure
        e. Risk factors include infection, autoimmune disease, recent myocardial infarction, cardiac surgery, malignancy, uremia, and drugs such as procainamide, hydralazine, isoniazid
    2. Pain with angina pectoris is often located in the shoulder, mid-back, or midsternal; radiates to the neck, jaw, epigastrium, shoulder, or arm, and is aggravated by exertion or stress; pain usually lasts less than 10 minutes and is relieved with rest or nitroglycerin (see section on ISCHEMIC HEART DISEASE)
    3. Patients with myocardial infarction (MI) commonly complain of sudden onset of substernal pain which may radiate and is associated with weakness, dyspnea, diaphoresis, nausea, vomiting, palpitations, and anxiety; pain usually lasts 20-30 minutes or longer and is unrelieved or only partially relieved by nitroglycerin or morphine (see section on ISCHEMIC HEART DISEASE)
    4. Patients with mitral valve prolapse (MVP) are often asymptomatic, but chest pain, fatigue, palpitations (especially when lying supine on left side), lightheadedness, dizziness, shortness of breath, headaches, and mood swings may be present; only 15% of patients experience moderate to severe symptoms
        a. Pain is sharp, fleeting, localized over mid or left chest wall; rarely radiates
        b. Pain is not relieved by nitroglycerin; usually pain is unrelated to exertion
        c. Pain may be brief or last for several days
        d. MVP can progress to mitral insufficiency with enlargement of left atrium and left ventricle, and congestive heart failure
        e. Hallmark diagnostic sign is a mid-systolic click and late systolic murmur
        f. Echocardiogram will reveal extent of regurgitation and may reveal abnormally thickened, billowing mitral valve leaflets
    5. Dissecting aortic aneurysm (AA) often presents with excruciating, tearing, or knifelike pain, sudden in onset and lasting for hours; pain can also be nagging and constant
        a. Usually pain is located in the anterior chest but may be in the abdomen or back and move as the dissection progresses; often radiates to thoracic area of back
        b. Signs include lowered or elevated blood pressure (classically, a widening pulse pressure develops), dissociation of arm blood pressures, absent pulses, paralysis, pulsus paradoxus, and murmur of aortic insufficiency
        c. Risk factors include hypertension, connective tissue disease, pregnancy, arterio-atherosclerosis, and cigarette use

6. Cocaine-induced chest pain may present with severe, sharp, pressure-like or squeezing substernal pain
   a. Associated symptoms include euphoria, mydriasis, hyperstimulation, paranoia, delusions, followed by depression, nausea, and muscle twitching
   b. Complications include myocardial ischemia and infarction, arrhythmias, respiratory failure, and circulatory collapse

D. Pain from disorders of the gastrointestinal system can mimic cardiovascular symptoms
   1. Gastroesophageal reflux presents with burning and substernal pain that starts in the epigastrium and radiates upward toward the throat, and is related to consuming a large meal, lying down, or bending over; pain is usually relieved by ingestion of antacid or food (see section on GASTROESOPHAGEAL REFLUX DISEASE)
   2. Esophageal spasm presents as an intense, substernal, sharp pain radiating to interscapular region; unfortunately, also relieved by nitroglycerin as with true angina; but unlike angina it may persist as a dull ache long after the acute attack
   3. Other gastrointestinal problems such as cholecystitis, peptic ulcer disease, and pancreatitis resemble cardiac pain, but they can be distinguished by their association with eating and their relief with antacids; however, remember: 10% of patients with acute MIs relate that their chest pain is relieved by antacids

E. Chest pain may be due to psychiatric or mental health disorders
   1. Patients with psychogenic problems often describe pain as generalized, constantly present, and aggravated by any effort, particularly at times of stress
      a. Associated symptoms include dyspnea, fatigue, headache, hyperventilation, and other somatic symptoms
      b. Pain absent on weekends and at non-stress times indicates an anxiety-tension syndrome
   2. Patients with panic disorders often have chest pain that is accompanied by intense fear, tachypnea, palpitations, diaphoresis, trembling, nausea, dizziness, syncope or near syncope, and chills or hot flashes

F. Chest pain not associated with any abnormal finding in the history or physical examination is often termed idiopathic; symptoms are usually self-limited and resolve within two years; rule out psychogenic causes before making this diagnosis

IV. Diagnosis/Evaluation

A. History (length of history will depend on patient's clinical presentation); perform a rapid history for any patient with a suspected emergent condition such as MI or dissecting AA
   1. Determine the pattern and whether onset was sudden, gradual, recurrent, or new
   2. Ask patient to describe the pain's location, regions of radiation, quality, intensity, duration, time of onset, and whether paroxysmal or constant
   3. Determine the quantity of pain, use the visual analog scale from 0 to 10 (10 is the worst pain ever experienced and 0 indicates no pain); cardiac chest pain should never be allowed to persist greater than 0, as is allowable for skeletal muscle pain
   4. Inquire about aggravating factors such as exercise or activity, stress, food intake, movement, coughing, emotional experiences, or cold temperatures
   5. Inquire about relieving factors -- rest, use of nitroglycerin, antacids, food intake
   6. Ask about associated symptoms such as fatigue, dyspnea, hemoptysis, fever, chills, cough, sputum production, exanthem, diaphoresis, dizziness, syncope or near syncope, nausea, diarrhea, cyanosis, pallor, leg pain, or edema
   7. Ask if a coexistent illness is present or if other members of the household are sick
   8. Explore stress-related factors in school, work, or home environments
   9. Ask about risk factors for ischemic heart disease
   10. Explore past medical history; get family history related to cardiovascular disease

B. Physical Examination
   1. Observe general appearance of patient, assessing for level of distress and anxiety
   2. Measure vital signs
      a. Take blood pressure in both arms (dissecting AA presents with discrepancy in readings between arms)
      b. If unable to detect, use Doppler and/or take thigh pressure to assess presence and compare with arm pressures
      c. Obtain postural pressures; lying, sitting, and standing measurements are best
   3. Inspect skin for pallor, cyanosis, jaundice, or herpetic rash

4. Examine eyes, including funduscopy
5. Assess neck for lymphadenopathy, thyromegaly, tracheal shift, or jugular venous distention
6. Auscultate carotid arteries for bruits
7. Examine chest wall for herpes lesions and signs of trauma, lifts, or heaves
8. Palpate chest wall, noting tenderness and swelling or the presence of thrills
9. Perform a complete examination of the heart, noting extra heart sounds, murmurs, clicks, hums, rubs, S_3 or S_4 sounds, or irregular irregularities
10. Auscultate lungs for equal breath sounds, a pleural rub, crackles, or wheezes
11. Auscultate abdomen for bowel sounds and bruits
12. Palpate abdomen for tenderness and masses (particularly in the right upper quadrant and epigastrium), organomegaly, bounding pulses, and ascites
13. Palpate for femoral pulses
14. Assess lower extremities for cyanosis, diminished pulses, unilateral swelling, and other signs of phlebitis
15. Patients who present with pain that changes with movement should have a musculoskeletal and neurological exam performed, focusing on focal tenderness, muscular weakness, and motor and sensory deficits

C. Differential Diagnosis: Generally, pain should be considered cardiovascular and life threatening until proven otherwise (see following table)

CHEST PAIN: DIFFERENTIAL DIAGNOSIS		
Cardiac Ischemic Syndromes • Acute myocardial infarction • Stable angina • Variant angina Myocarditis Pericarditis Valvular Disease • Aortic stenosis • Mitral valve prolapse • Hypertrophic obstructive cardiomyopathy **Musculoskeletal** Cervical radiculopathy Costochondritis Muscle strain/spasm	**Gastrointestinal** Biliary colic Esophageal spasm Esophagitis/gastritis Gastric/duodenal ulcer Gastroesophageal reflux disorder **Neurologic** Herpes zoster Nerve root compression **Vascular** Aortic dissection Pulmonary embolism Pulmonary hypertension	**Pulmonary** Bronchitis/bronchospasm Empyema Pleural effusion Pleuritis Pneumonia Pneumothorax Pulmonary edema Pulmonary embolism Pulmonary hypertension

1. A detailed history (if condition allows) is extremely important in assisting the clinician in ruling in and ruling out potential diagnoses
2. Age and sex of the patient can also help narrow the differential diagnosis: Women <40 years of age without risk factors for coronary disease rarely have a cardiac problem; conversely, always first consider a cardiac problem in men >40 years with significant family history or risk factors
3. Risk factors provide important information to arrive at a diagnosis
4. Quality, location, radiation, and intensity of pain are nonspecific symptoms and are usually not helpful in arriving at a diagnosis

D. Diagnostic tests are based on data collected in the history and physical examination
   1. For suspected cardiac or cardiopulmonary problems consider ordering the following:
      a. Pulse oximetry to assess for oxygen desaturation
      b. Creatinine phosphokinase (CPK) with isoenzymes, troponin T and I, high-sensitivity C-reactive protein (hsCRP), and brain natriuretic peptide (BNP) when myocardial ischemia is suspected
      c. Electrocardiogram (ECG) when a cardiac diagnosis cannot be ruled out immediately, or when significant risk factors exist
      d. Echocardiography is helpful in diagnosing mitral valve prolapse or other valvular abnormalities, pericarditis, and to assess for wall motion and ejection fraction
      e. Immediate cardiac catheterization for patients with suspected acute MI

      f.   Consider exercise stress echocardiogram for ruling in or ruling out a cardiac diagnosis in light of a negative ECG and negative cardiac enzymes

      g.   Radionuclide scans using thallium or cardiolyte with treadmill, or with dobutamine or adenosine infusions may be helpful in further differentiating cause or extent of injury if cardiac in origin

2. The Erlanger Chest Pain Evaluation Protocol is helpful in identifying and excluding acute coronary syndromes (see following table)

3. Computed tomography with contrast, transesophageal echocardiography, and aortic angiography are diagnostic tests for aortic dissection

4. Consider ordering a chest x-ray when there is suspicion of following: Chest trauma (rib fractures), pulmonary diseases (pneumonia or tuberculosis, pneumothorax, pulmonary embolus), or a widened mediastinum (dissecting abdominal aneurysm)

5. Consider a lung CT scan or ventilation/perfusion scan for suspected PE

6. Consider Gram's stain of sputum for suspected pulmonary infections

7. Order a complete metabolic profile including liver enzymes and a CBC for all patients; include amylase and lipase if pancreatitis is suspected

8. An acid perfusion (Bernstein) test or more invasive tests such as esophageal manometry, barium x-ray studies, and endoscopy may be helpful in diagnosing specific gastrointestinal problems

---

THE ERLANGER CHEST PAIN EVALUATION PROTOCOL

A positive result in one or more of the following is considered a positive protocol

- Initial ECG reflecting acute or reciprocal injury
- Baseline CK-MB level ≥10 ng/mL and index of ≥5% **or** cTn-I level ≥2 ng/mL
- Serial 12-lead ECG monitoring indicating new or evolving injury or ischemia
- Minimum 1.5-ng/mL increase in CK/MB level **or** minimum 0.2-ng/mL increase in cTn-I level in 2 hours
- Clinical diagnosis of ACS (despite a negative evaluation at 2 hours)
- Reversible perfusion defect on nuclear stress scan vs resting scan

ECG, electrocardiogram; CK-MB, creatine kinase MB band; cTn-I, cardiac troponin I; ACS, acute coronary syndrome

---

Adapted from Fesmire, F.M., Hughes, A.D., Fody, E.P., Jackson, A.P., Fesmire, C.E., Gilbert, M.A., et al. (2002). The Erlanger Chest Pain Evaluation Protocol: A one-year experience with serial 12-lead ECG monitoring, two-hour delta serum marker measurements, and selective nuclear stress testing to identify and exclude acute coronary syndromes. *Annals of Emergency Medicine, 40*, 584-594.

V.   Plan/Management

    A.   Relief of pain is based on the etiology; remember cardiac pain must be relieved to level 0

    B.   Treatment of musculoskeletal problems such as costochondritis is usually symptomatic with pain medications such as nonsteroid anti-inflammatory drugs or acetaminophen and local ice and heat applications (see chapter on MUSCULOSKELETAL PROBLEMS)

    C.   Treatment of pulmonary problems

1. Pneumonia, bronchitis, asthma, bronchospasm (see RESPIRATORY chapter)

2. Pulmonary embolus requires hospitalization and intravenous anticoagulation; typically patient is then placed on long-term oral anticoagulation

3. Carefully assess vital signs and watch for mediastinal shift in patients with a pneumothorax

      a.   A small, stable pneumothorax without evidence of respiratory compromise requires only observation for several days until stabilization and resolution

      b.   Hospitalization and insertion of chest tubes is needed for a large, expanding pneumothorax or tension pneumothorax

    D.   Treatment of cardiac pain (also see section on ISCHEMIC HEART DISEASE)

1. Hospitalization and immediate referral to cardiologist is required for myocardial infarction and AA

2. Pericarditis is treated with aspirin, non-steroidal anti-inflammatory drugs, or, for severe cases, corticosteroids; hospitalization is required for patients with signs of cardiac tamponade

3. Mitral valve prolapse

      a.   No specific treatment is indicated for most patients, except for reassurance about a good prognosis

      b.   The major therapeutic dilemma is whether to recommend antibiotic prophylaxis against infective endocarditis when certain invasive procedures are performed; prophylaxis is often recommended for patients who have the following:

<blockquote>
(1) Moderate to severe mitral regurgitation and/or thickened leaflets
(2) Murmur of mitral regurgitation, but not in those who have only a click
(3) If there is uncertainty about the diagnosis of mitral regurgitation refer to cardiologist
</blockquote>

    c. Patients with severe mitral regurgitation may require valve surgery
    d. Patients with annoying arrhythmias may benefit from a beta-blocker such as atenolol or metoprolol XL

E. Treatment of abdominal problems (see chapter on GASTROINTESTINAL PROBLEMS)

F. Treatment of psychogenic problems
    1. Reassure patient that pain does not have a cardiac etiology
    2. Counseling and psychotherapy may be helpful

G. Patient Education
    1. Refer to specialist if acute cardiac or serious conditions are identified; otherwise, educate patient and family about the diagnosis and treatment and how best to comply with the prescribed regimen
    2. To avoid panic, carefully explain to the patient or parents that the history, physical exam, and diagnostic results revealed no cardiac abnormality
    3. Educate patients and families about problems other than cardiac that can cause "chest pain," how to recognize them, and when to seek medical attention
    4. Allow time for the patient to express concerns and questions
    5. Teach about risk factors for cardiac disease and strategies to reduce risks

H. Follow up is variable depending on diagnosis and patient's condition

CHRONIC HEART FAILURE

I. Definition: A multifaceted clinical syndrome that results from any structural or functional cardiac factor that diminishes the ability of the ventricle to fill with or eject blood; because not all patients have volume overload at initial or subsequent evaluations, the term "heart failure" is preferred over the older term "congestive heart failure"

A. Heart failure (HF) is not equivalent to cardiomyopathy or to left ventricular dysfunction which are terms that describe potential structural reasons for the development of HF; rather, HF is a clinical syndrome characterized by specific symptoms (dyspnea and fatigue) and signs (fluid retention)

B. Chronic heart failure has been defined as the state in which there is an inability of the heart to pump blood in a relative amount sufficient to meet the metabolic needs of the peripheral tissues, or to do so only when filling pressure is increased; may result from disorders of the pericardium, myocardium, endocardium, or great vessels, but most often is secondary to impaired left ventricular function (systolic and/or diastolic)

II. Pathophysiology: Injuries to the heart predispose the individual to HF; exhaustion of the compensatory hemodynamic and neurohormonal mechanisms causes the signs and symptoms of the syndrome

A. As the heart's ability to pump is reduced, several cardiac compensatory mechanisms occur as follows:
    1. The heart compensates by dilating to increase cardiac output via the Frank-Starling mechanism
    2. Ventricular hypertrophy develops to handle the greater preload (end-diastolic volume) and hyperplasia develops to maintain cardiac output by increasing contractility or contractile mass
    3. Initially, these two mechanisms provide improvement in symptoms but over time the heart decompensates and functioning is compromised

B. Neurohormonal systems are also triggered secondary to the stress response with the decreased efficiency of the heart's pumping:
    1. Plasma renin activity, ACTH, aldosterone, and plasma arginine vasopressin (ADH) levels are increased resulting in systemic vasoconstriction and sodium and water retention which, if excessive, lead to increased atrial pressure and/or pulmonary congestion
    2. Increased sympathetic tone occurs with increased levels of epinephrine and norepinephrine which initially improves cardiac output and blood pressure, but eventually increases oxygen demand, accelerates myocardial cell death, and causes excessive increases in ventricular preload and afterload (dynamic resistance against which the heart contracts)

C. The underlying injury to the heart may be due to left ventricular systolic dysfunction (LVSD), diastolic dysfunction, or both
  1. Left-ventricular systolic dysfunction (most common) has preserved filling but impaired emptying due to decreased myocardial contractility, chamber dilation, and hypertrophy, resulting in decreased cardiac output and left ejection fraction <35-40% (called cardiac or left ventricular remodeling); common causes are the following:
     a. Dilated cardiomyopathies, viral cardiomyopathies, cor pulmonale
     b. Reduction in contractile muscle mass (e.g., myocardial infarction)
  2. Ventricular diastolic dysfunction has normal emptying with preserved performance of the left ventricles and normal or near normal systolic function, but restriction in ventricular filling or disturbances in the relaxation properties of the heart; underlying pathologic processes include myocardial ischemia, some left ventricular hypertrophy (LVH), left atrial enlargement, hyperplasia, and fibrosis; common causes are the following:
     a. Most patients with isolated diastolic dysfunction have hypertension or coronary artery disease (CAD) or both (especially in the presence of renal dysfunction, diabetes, aortic stenosis, or atrial fibrillation)
     b. Elderly, hypertensive persons may develop hypertrophic-like features, with small ventricular cavity dimensions, and increased intraventricular gradients leading to diastolic dysfunction and possibly pulmonary edema, but do not have impaired systolic function
     c. Pericardial disease (pericarditis, pericardial tamponade) and increased ventricular stiffness (restrictive or hypertrophic cardiomyopathy, amyloidosis, sarcoidosis) are uncommon
  3. Several conditions are associated with both systolic and diastolic dysfunction such as ventricular hypertrophy, hyperplasia, and myocardial ischemia; myocardial infarction (MI) is the most common, potentially reversible cause of heart failure

D. Major causes of HF
  1. Ischemic heart disease/coronary artery disease (approximately two-thirds of patients with LVSD)
  2. Remainder have a nonischemic cardiomyopathy, which may have an identifiable cause (e.g., hypertension, thyroid disease, valvular disease, alcohol use or myocarditis) or may have no known cause (e.g., idiopathic dilated cardiomyopathy)
  3. Myocarditis (bacterial, viral, toxic) is an uncommon cause but may occur in young patients with acute onset of symptoms and unexplained heart failure

E. Patients with previously compensated HF may decompensate as a result of any of the following factors:
  1. Inadequate therapy or lack of compliance with drugs or treatment regimens
  2. Uncontrolled hypertension
  3. Cardiac arrhythmias
  4. Endocrine disorders (thyrotoxicosis, uncontrolled diabetes)
  5. Pulmonary infection/pneumonia
  6. Pulmonary embolism
  7. Excessive intake of fluids and/or dietary sodium
  8. Stress/emotional turmoil
  9. Anemia
  10. Liver and renal disease
  11. Sleep apnea or general sleep disturbances
  12. Alcoholism and cocaine use
  13. Over-aggressive diuresis and afterload reduction in patients with marked diastolic dysfunction

III. Clinical Presentation

A. HF is the most common Medicare diagnosis-related group (DRG); hospitalizations and deaths due to HF have steadily increased despite advances in treatment

B. Majority of patients are women; common in elderly patients and in the African-American population

C. Signs and symptoms develop gradually or abruptly as occurs with acute HF; acute HF can be grouped clinically into acute pulmonary edema, cardiogenic shock, and/or acute decompensation of chronic HF

D. In left-ventricular systolic dysfunction, signs and symptoms are not reliable indicators of cardiac functioning; patients with severely impaired ventricular performance may be completely asymptomatic until they overexert themselves; common signs and symptoms are presented in the following table

SIGNS AND SYMPTOMS OF VENTRICULAR SYSTOLIC DYSFUNCTION

Symptoms

Dyspnea on exertion	Frothy white to pinkish sputum	Bloating	Weakness
Orthopnea	Abdominal pain	Constipation	CNS symptoms
Paroxysmal nocturnal dyspnea	Anorexia	Exercise intolerance	Nocturia
Cough	Nausea	Fatigue	Presyncope/syncope

Signs

Fine or course crackles, generally bibasilar	Peripheral edema, generally symmetric	Tachycardia
	Jugular venous distention	Pallor
S$_3$ gallop	Hepatomegaly	Cyanosis
Erratic respiratory patterns	Hepatojugular reflex	

E. Diastolic dysfunction occurs in about 20-40% of all cases; presentation ranges from no symptoms to dyspnea, pulmonary edema, signs of right HF (abdominal complaints, peripheral edema), and exercise intolerance; since patients with predominantly diastolic dysfunction have different natural histories and require different treatment strategies this category will be discussed separately (see section V.K.)

F. A new staging system of HF was developed by American College of Cardiology/American Heart Association (see following table)
   1. The staging system helps to classify patients reliably and objectively in the course of their disease; appropriate treatments can be targeted at each stage to reduce morbidity and mortality
   2. Intended to complement but not to replace the New York Heart Association (NYHA) functional classification (see III.G.)
   3. Only stages C & D qualify for the traditional clinical diagnosis of HF for diagnostic and coding purposes
   4. System recognizes that HF has established risk factors and structural prerequisites and that the evolution of HF has asymptomatic and symptomatic phases
   5. Patients are expected to advance from one stage to the next unless the disease is slowed or stopped by treatment

STAGING SYSTEM FOR HEART FAILURE

Stage	Description
A	Patients that are at high risk for developing HF, but have no structural disorder of the heart
B	Designates patients with a structural disorder of the heart but who have never developed symptoms
C	Classifies patients with past or current symptoms of HF associated with underlying structural heart disease
D	Identifies patients with end-stage disease who require extra specialized treatments to survive

Adapted from Hunt, S.A., Baker, D.W., Chin, M.H., Cinquegrani, G., Feldman, A.M., Francis, C.G., et al. (2001). ACC/AHA guidelines: Evaluation and management of chronic heart failure in the adult: A report of the American College of Cardiology/ American Heart Association Task Force on Practice Guidelines. Available at: http://www.acc.org/clinical/guidelines/failure/hf_index.htm

G. The NYHA functional classification system primarily gauges *the severity of symptoms* in patients who are in evolutionary Stages C or D above (see following table)
   1. Reflects a subjective assessment by a clinician and changes frequently over short periods of time
   2. Recommended treatments do not typically vary across the classes

NEW YORK HEART ASSOCIATION FUNCTIONAL CLASSIFICATION

Functional Class	Descriptive Findings in Patients with Cardiac Disease
I	No physical limitation in activity
II	Slight limitation in ordinary physical activity, resulting in fatigue, palpitations, dyspnea or angina
III	Marked limitation in activity; patients are comfortable at rest, but ordinary activity leads to symptoms
IV	Symptoms are present at rest; any activity leads to increased discomfort

IV.   Diagnosis/Evaluation

    A.   History
1. Specifically ask about previous heart disease such as CAD, atherosclerosis, MI, hypertension, valvular disease, and myopathies
2. Ask about difficulty with breathing and increased fatigue
    a. Ask how far patient can walk without SOB
    b. Determine how many pillows are needed to sleep comfortably
    c. Ask about waking at night with SOB
    d. Ask about reductions in activities of daily living and social or recreational activities
3. Inquire about type, frequency, duration, and self-treatment of chest pain
4. Inquire about amount of weight gain; ask whether gain was rapid or more gradual over weeks
5. Question about other associated symptoms such as edema, abdominal complaints, palpitations, frequent colds with congestion, awakening with a cough
6. Inquire about risk factors for coronary heart disease
7. Ask about personal and family history of sudden unexplained death; cardiovascular/peripheral vascular, thyroid, hepatic, endocrine (diabetes), and renal diseases; hypercholesterolemia
8. Explore possibility of patient having sleep apnea (e.g., snoring in sleep)
9. Obtain medication history (prescription, over the counter, herbal)
10. Explore sexual function, cognitive function, social support, illicit drug use, and alcohol consumption
11. At initial and follow-up visits, ask about type, severity, and duration of symptoms and the degree to which symptoms impair activities of daily living

    B.   Physical Examination; elevated jugular venous pressure and a third heart sound have the most prognostic significance
1. Observe overall appearance, noting whether patient is in any distress when sitting or walking
2. Inspect skin for color, moisture, and turgor
3. Carefully measure vital signs, noting changes in blood pressure, tachycardia, or tachypnea
4. Measure weight at every visit; changes in weight may be signs of fluid status, but are less reliable during long periods of follow-up as patients often lose skeletal mass and body fat as HF progresses
5. Perform a complete eye examination with funduscopy
6. Palpate thyroid
7. Observe neck for venous distention and hepatojugular reflux, auscultate carotid arteries for bruits
8. Perform a complete heart examination; HF patients often have extra heart sounds (S_3 sound/ventricular gallop), murmurs, increased second pulmonic heart sounds, and a point of maximal impulse (PMI) that has shifted to the left and downward
9. Perform a complete lung examination, listening for rales/crackles
10. Perform an abdominal examination, noting hepatomegaly and ascites
11. Assess for peripheral edema in the presacral area, scrotum in men, and extremities (grade extremity edema on scale of 1+-4+ pitting or non-pitting)
12. Assess peripheral pulses; check capillary refill
13. Perform a mental status examination as confusion may occur, especially in elderly patients

    C.   Differential Diagnosis: Since HF is a syndrome it is important to determine the underlying causes of the HF; however, the following conditions mimic the presentation of HF or may occur concomitantly with HF
1. Dyspnea
    a. Chronic obstructive pulmonary disease
    b. Asthma
    c. Ischemic nephropathy caused by bilateral renal artery stenosis
    d. Pulmonary emboli
2. Chest pain (see section on CHEST PAIN)
    a. Pulmonary emboli
    b. Bacterial endocarditis
    c. Pericarditis
    d. MI
3. Edema
    a. Renal disease
    b. Liver disease
    c. Peripheral vascular disease: peripheral edema is often due to venous insufficiency
    d. Endocrine disorders
    e. Untoward effect of medications, particularly some calcium channel blockers such as amlodipine

D. Diagnostic Testing: Goals are to evaluate for alternative diagnoses, to get baseline data, to determine the type of cardiac dysfunction, and to determine degree of ventricular impairment, and prognosis
  1. A complete resting transthoracic echocardiogram, coupled with 2-D Doppler flow studies, is the single most useful test to order initially
      a. Measures chamber size, wall thickness, wall mobility, valvular function and flow gradients, and left-ventricular ejection fraction (EF)
      b. Determines if primary abnormality is pericardial, myocardial, or valvular; and, if myocardial, differentiates diastolic from systolic dysfunction
      c. EF <35-40% denotes heart failure, but patients with EF >40% may still have HF due to valvular disease or diastolic dysfunction
  2. Initially, order a 12-lead electrocardiogram to uncover the following:
      a. Myocardial infarction (ST-T wave changes and Q waves)
      b. Arrhythmias due to thyroid disease, HF caused by either rapid or slow ventricular rate, or tachy-brady syndrome
      c. Low voltage that accompanies pericardial effusion
      d. Left-ventricular hypertrophy that may cause diastolic dysfunction
  3. Initially, order a chest x-ray to determine heart size and assess pulmonary congestion and to detect pulmonary diseases or infection; serial chest x-rays are not recommended
  4. The following laboratory tests are recommended to detect disorders that lead to or exacerbate HF:
      a. Blood glucose to detect if diabetes is a contributing factor
      b. Complete blood count (detects anemia, infection)
      c. Electrolytes (including calcium and magnesium); serial monitoring of potassium levels is also recommended
          (1) Hypokalemia is an adverse effect of diuretics and increases risk of digitalis toxicity
          (2) Hyperkalemia may complicate treatment with angiotensin converting enzyme (ACE) inhibitors and spironolactone
      d. Urinalysis to determine proteinuria which may be a result of nephrotic syndrome or to determine presence of red blood cells or cellular casts which suggests glomerulonephritis
      e. Blood urea nitrogen and serum creatinine; if creatinine is elevated this denotes volume overload due to renal failure; if BUN is elevated disproportionately to creatinine this may indicate marked reduction in cardiac output; serial monitoring is also recommended
      f. TSH to detect hypo/hyperthyroidism
      g. Liver function tests to determine if liver disease is a contributing factor
  5. The following tests should be considered in special cases:
      a. Brain natriuretic peptide (BNP) (some authorities suggest serial measurements of BNP); high values are associated with greater left ventricular dysfunction
      b. High sensitivity C-reactive protein (hsCRP)
      c. Cardiac enzymes to rule out myocardial infarction
      d. Serum iron and ferritin to rule out anemia and hemochromatosis
      e. Serum albumin which, if decreased, may be related to increased extravascular volume
      f. Screening tests for HIV infection in high-risk patients
      g. Serum antinuclear antibody, rheumatoid factor, urinary vanillylmandelic acid, and metanephrines to detect autoimmune conditions
      h. Noninvasive stress testing with echocardiogram to detect ischemia, particularly for patients who are possible candidates for revascularization or radionuclide stress testing to detect stress-induced ischemia
      i. Six minute walk test to assess functional capacity for those patients that cannot complete a regular treadmill stress test
  6. Additional studies (usually ordered in consultation with a cardiologist)
      a. Radionuclide angiography provides good images in obese patients and those with severe chronic lung disease; detects segmental wall motion abnormalities and determines left and right ventricular EFs
      b. Cardiac catheterization for patients with coronary artery disease and angina, when diagnosis of HF is uncertain after noninvasive techniques, in young patients to exclude congenital coronary anomalies, or in patients whose HF is refractory to medical therapy and an ischemic etiology is suspected
      c. Myocardial biopsy may be useful in young patients with sudden onset of heart failure in whom cardiomyopathy or myocarditis is suspected
      d. Routine Holter monitoring or signal-averaged electrocardiography for patients with arrhythmias and syncope
      e. If positive emission tomography (PET) is available, it is an excellent test to assess cardiac muscle viability in relation to EF and wall motion problems, but it is quite expensive
  7. Follow-up diagnostic testing is important (see V.M. for recommendations)

V.   Plan/Management: Goals are to improve patient's quality of life by reducing symptoms, increase patient's ability to perform activities of daily living (ADLs), decrease morbidity, and prolong survival as long as possible

    A.   Hospitalize patients with any of the following:
        1.   Pulmonary edema with marked pulmonary rales and signs/symptoms of hypoxia
        2.   Cardiogenic shock with severe hypotension, oliguria, and/or mental status changes
        3.   Clinical or ECG evidence of myocardial ischemia or infarction
        4.   Oxygen saturation <90% which is not due to pulmonary diseases
        5.   Anasarca (generalized infiltration of edema fluid into subcutaneous connective tissue)
        6.   Severe, complicating medical illnesses such as pneumonia
        7.   Symptomatic hypotension or syncope
        8.   Heart failure that is nonresponsive to outpatient therapy
        9.   Inadequate social support for safe outpatient management; particularly if patient is nonadherent to therapy

    B.   Patients should only be discharged from hospital when symptoms are controlled, all reversible causes of morbidity have been treated or stabilized, and patients and caregivers have understanding of the disease

    C.   General principles of management for all stages of HF
        1.   Individualize treatments based on HF stage (see figure 11.1)

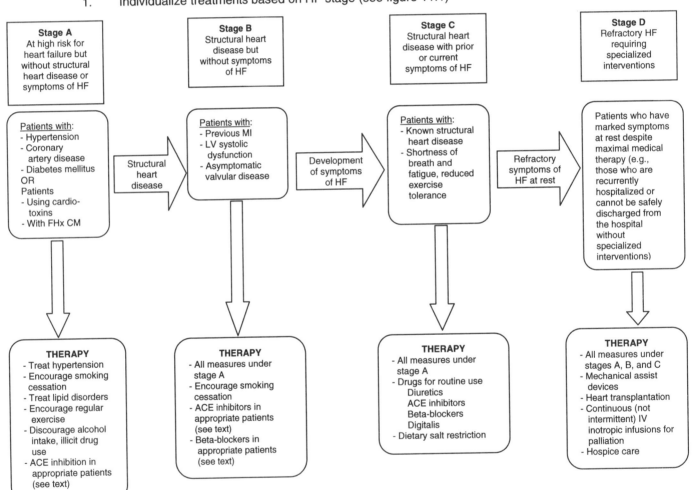

Figure 11.1. Stages in the Evolution of Heart Failure and Recommended Therapy by Stage
FHx CM indicates family history of cardiomyopathy; MI, myocardial infarction; LV, left ventricular; and IV, intravenous

Adapted from Hunt, S.A., Baker, D.W., Chin, M.H., Cinquegrani, M.P., Feldman, A.M., Francis, G.S., et al. (2001). Evaluation and management of chronic heart failure in the adult (2001). Available at http://www.add.org/clinical.guidelines/failure/hf_index.html

2.   Certain drugs are commonly used to treat HF (see following table)

DRUGS COMMONLY USED FOR TREATMENT OF CHRONIC HEART FAILURE		
Drug	Initial Dose	Maximum Dose
*Loop diuretics**		
Bumetanide	0.5-1.0 mg QD or BID	Titrate to achieve dry weight (up to 10 mg daily)
Furosemide	20-40 mg QD or BID	Titrate to achieve dry weight (up to 400 mg daily)
Torsemide	10-20 mg QD or BID	Titrate to achieve dry weight (up to 200 mg daily)
ACE Inhibitors		
Captopril	6.25 mg TID	50 mg TID
Enalapril	2.5 mg BID	10-20 mg BID
Fosinopril	5-10 mg QD	40 mg QD
Lisinopril	2.5-5.0 mg QD	20-40 mg QD
Quinapril	10 mg BID	40 mg BID
Ramipril	1.25-2.5 mg QD	10 mg QD
Beta-receptor blockers		
Bisoprolol	1.25 mg QD	10 mg QD
Carvedilol	3.125 mg BID	25 mg BID; 50 mg BID for patients >85 kg
Metoprolol tartrate	6.25 mg BID	75 mg BID
Metoprolol succinate extended release**	12.5-25 mg QD	200 mg QD
Digitalis glycosides		
Digoxin	0.125-0.25 mg QD	0.125-0.25 mg QD

ACE indicates angiotensin converting enzyme
*   Thiazide diuretics are not listed in this table but may be appropriate for patients with mild heart failure or associated hypertension or as a second diuretic in patients refractory to loop diuretics above
** Referred to in some publications as Metoprolol CR/XL

Adapted from Hunt, S.A., Baker, D.W., Chin, M.H., Cinquegrani, M.P., Feldman, A.M., Francis, G.S., et al. (2001). Evaluation and management of chronic heart failure in the adult (2001). Available at http://www.acc.org/clinical/guidelines/failure/hf_index.html

3.   Initially prescribe low doses and slowly titrate to maximum dosage recommendations; the larger doses are those shown to be effective in reducing mortality

D.   Therapy for **patients at high risk for developing left ventricular dysfunction (Stage A)**; identification and early modification of certain factors can reduce risk of HF (see preceding Figure in V.C.1.)
   1.   Treat hypertension: Lower both systolic and diastolic blood pressures; select drugs that are useful for treatment of both hypertension and HF (see section on HYPERTENSION)
   2.   Treat lipid disorders (see section on HYPERLIPIDEMIA)
   3.   Treat diabetes: Control hyperglycemia (see section on DIABETES)
   4.   Manage atherosclerotic disease (see section on ISCHEMIC HEART DISEASE)
   5.   Prescribe ACE inhibitor to patients with diabetes, hypertension, atherosclerotic disease, and who have associated cardiovascular risk factors
   6.   Control conditions that may cause cardiac injury
      a.   Advise about dangers of tobacco, alcohol, cocaine, and illicit drug use
      b.   Carefully weigh the benefits and risks of using certain cancer treatments such as ionizing radiation and certain chemotherapeutic agents (anthracyclines or trastuzumab)
      c.   Treat other diseases that may adversely affect heart, especially thyroid disorders and supraventricular tachyarrhythmias
   7.   Other measures, such as control of dietary sodium, nutritional supplements, and regular exercise, enhance general health, but do not prevent dysfunction to the heart

E.   Therapy for **patients with asymptomatic left ventricular dysfunction (Stage B)**:
   1.   All the measures used in Stage A (V.D.) are recommended in Stage B
   2.   For patients with history of recent or remote myocardial infarction (MI) **and/or** reduced EF prescribe an ACE inhibitor and a beta-blocker
   3.   For patients with hemodynamically significant valvular stenosis or regurgitation, referral for valve replacement or repair is recommended
   4.   Teach patients to monitor for signs of limitations of exercise tolerance or unexplained fatigue so that their clinicians can intensify efforts to detect HF

F.   General management of **patients with symptomatic left ventricular dysfunction (Stage C)**
   1.   All the measures used in Stage A (V.D.) are recommended in Stage C
   2.   Patient education is important: Moderately restrict sodium intake (<3 g daily), perform daily weight measurements, participate in physical activity except during periods of acute decompensation, and obtain immunizations for influenza and pneumonia

3. Avoid the use of the following three classes of drugs that can exacerbate HF
   a. Antiarrhythmic agents may have cardiodepressant and proarrhythmic effects; only amiodarone does not adversely affect survival
   b. Calcium channel blockers are associated with increased risk of cardiovascular events; only amlodipine does not adversely affect survival
   c. Nonsteroidal anti-inflammatory agents can cause sodium retention, peripheral vasoconstriction, and can lessen efficacy and increase toxicity of diuretics and ACE inhibitors
4. Closely monitor patients for hypokalemia and hyperkalemia which can both affect cardiac excitability and conduction and lead to sudden death; avoid serum potassium concentrations in the range of 3.5 to 3.8 mmol/L or 5.2 to 5.5 mmol/L

G. Pharmacological treatment of **patients with symptomatic left ventricular dysfunction (Stage C):** In most cases, patients are routinely managed with a combination of 4 types of drugs: A diuretic, an ACE inhibitor, a beta-adrenergic blocker, and (usually) digitalis
   1. **Diuretics:** Appropriate use of this class of drugs is often key to success of other drugs and is the cornerstone of HF treatment; prescribe for patients who have evidence of fluid retention
      a. Produce symptomatic benefits quicker than any other drugs and only drugs used in HF that can adequately control fluid retention
      b. Diuretics should not be used alone nor should ACE inhibitors be substituted for diuretics
      c. Loop diuretics are the preferred diuretic agent for most patients
         (1) Furosemide is most commonly prescribed
         (2) Newer agents such as torsemide have better absorption and may be more effective
      d. Thiazide diuretics may be effective for patients with mild HF or as a second diuretic for patients refractory to loop diuretics alone
      e. Initiate with low dose of diuretic and increase dose until urine output increases and weight decreases (about 0.5 to 1.0 kg daily)
      f. Once fluid retention has resolved, continue diuretics to prevent recurrence of volume overload; periodically adjust dose
         (1) Patient can be taught to make changes in dose if weight increases or decreases beyond a specified range
         (2) As HF progresses, the dose of the diuretic will often need to be increased
      g. Diuretic resistance can be overcome by intravenous administration of diuretics, use of two or more diuretics (e.g., furosemide and metolazone), or use of diuretics with drugs that increase renal blood flow (positive inotropic agents)
      h. Potassium deficits are adverse effects of diuretics
         (1) To correct, prescribe short-term use of potassium supplements, or if severe, add magnesium
         (2) Using ACE inhibitors alone or in combination with potassium-retaining agent, spironolactone, often prevents deficit and potassium supplementation may not be needed
      i. Excessive diuresis (overdiuresis), reduction in blood pressure, and activation of the neurohormonal system may occur when diuretics are used concurrently with other drugs
         (1) Hypotension, tachycardia, reduced jugular venous distention, prerenal azotemia, hyponatremia, hypokalemia, hypomagnesemia, near syncope/syncope, and dehydration occur with overdiuresis
         (2) Withhold diuretic for 24-72 hours if overdiuresis occurs
   2. **ACE inhibitors** prevent further development of HF, alleviate symptoms, reduce hospitalizations, and improve patient survival
      a. An ACE inhibitor should be prescribed to all patients with HF due to left ventricular systolic dysfunction unless patient has a known contraindication or cannot tolerate
         (1) Contraindication is significant hyperkalemia
         (2) Do not prescribe to patients who have experienced life-threatening adverse effects (angioedema or anuric renal function) during previous drug exposure or to pregnant patients
         (3) Do not give to hypotensive patients who are at immediate risk of cardiogenic shock
         (4) Use cautiously in patients with low systemic blood pressure (BP) (systolic BP <80 mm Hg), markedly increased serum creatinine (>3 mg/dL), bilateral renal artery stenosis, or elevated serum potassium (>5.5 mmol/L)
      b. Select drug from preceding table (V.C.2.) and titrate slowly, aiming for highest maintenance dose as this dose has been shown to reduce risk of cardiovascular (CV) events; ramipril, captopril, enalapril, and lisinopril should be given preference for selection as these drugs were found to reduce mortality in clinical trials
      c. Symptom improvement may require several weeks or months to become apparent

    d.   Even if symptoms do not improve, long-term use of ACE inhibitor should be continued to reduce the risk of death or hospitalizations

    e.   Abrupt withdrawal can lead to clinical deterioration and should be avoided except if life-threatening complications such as angioedema occur

    f.   Important to minimize the occurrence of sodium retention or depletion because changes in salt and water balance can attenuate or exaggerate the CV and renal effects of treatment

        (1)   Ensure that patients are given appropriate doses of diuretics

        (2)   Assess renal function and serum potassium within 1-2 weeks of drug initiation and periodically thereafter

    g.   Adverse effects include hypotension, worsening renal function, potassium retention, cough, and angioedema

    h.   Effects of specific drugs

        (1)   Captopril (Capoten) and enalapril (Vasotec) work quickly to reduce acute symptoms; prescribed for early treatment but are not practical for extended home use

        (2)   Lisinopril (Zestril), fosinopril (Monopril), quinapril (Accupril), and ramipril (Altace) have advantage of once-daily dosing

3.   **Beta-blockers** lessen symptoms, improve clinical status, improve systolic function, and reduce morbidity and mortality

    a.   Prescribe to all patients with **stable** HF due to left ventricular dysfunction unless they have contraindications to use or cannot tolerate; even patients with mild symptoms should use a beta-blocker as these drugs reduce disease progression

        (1)   Do not prescribe until patient is in stable condition (e.g., when she/he is discharged from ICU, has no or minimal evidence of fluid overload or volume depletion, has not required recent treatment with an intravenous positive inotropic agent)

        (2)   Do not prescribe to patients with reactive airway disease, symptomatic bradycardia, or advanced heart block (unless treated with a pacemaker)

    b.   In general, beta-blockers are used with an ACE inhibitor, a diuretic (particularly if patient had current or recent history of fluid retention), and usually with digitalis; beta-blockers often cause fluid retention and thus a diuretic is needed to maintain sodium balance

    c.   Initiate at very low doses and gradually increase; every effort should be made to reach target doses shown to be effective in clinical trials

    d.   Closely monitor for changes in vital signs and symptoms during initiation and titration; patients should weigh themselves daily and dosage of diuretic should be adjusted as needed to restore pretreatment weight levels

    e.   Symptoms may take 2-3 months to improve

    f.   Even if symptoms do not improve, long-term therapy should be continued to prevent cardiac deterioration

    g.   Adverse reactions include fluid retention, worsening HF, fatigue, bradycardia, hypotension

    h.   Metoprolol extended release (Toprol XL) and carvedilol (Coreg) are the most commonly used and have best research results; also used for patients with dilated cardiomyopathies

        (1)   Metoprolol is selective for beta-1 receptors and is less likely to cause bronchoconstriction than nonselective beta-blockers

        (2)   Carvedilol is a nonselective beta-blocker and is preferred for patients with hypertension

4.   **Digitalis**

    a.   Treatment with digoxin for 1-3 months was found to improve symptoms, quality of life, and exercise tolerance; long-term therapy had little effect on mortality

    b.   Use in conjunction with diuretics, an ACE inhibitor, and a beta-blocker

    c.   Do not prescribe to patients with significant sinus or atrioventricular block (unless treated with a pacemaker); use cautiously in patients taking other drugs that depress sinus or atrioventricular nodal function (e.g., amiodarone or beta-blocker)

    d.   Consider adding digitalis to patients who have the following:

        (1)   Dilated heart and in whom the symptoms of HF appear to be due to a decreased inotropic state of heart muscle (EF <40-45% or the presence of an S_3 gallop)

        (2)   Atrial fibrillation and rapid ventricular rates

        (3)   Severe HF and patients in whom symptoms persist despite optimal doses of other medications

    e.   Prescribe digoxin (the recommended digitalis agent): Initiate and maintain at dose of 0.125 to 0.25 mg QD; use low dose for patients who are >70 years, have impaired renal function, low lean body mass, or who are on the following medications: Verapamil, quinidine, amiodarone, clarithromycin; St. John's wort can decrease digoxin levels by 25%

    f.   In approximately 5-7 days full digitalization will be achieved

g.   Drug is well tolerated by most patients; digitalis toxicity typically is associated with levels >2 ng/mL, but may occur with lower levels, especially if patient has hypokalemia, hypomagnesemia, or hypothyroidism; clinical manifestations include the following:
   (1)   Slowing of heart rate
   (2)   Anorexia, nausea, vomiting, and diarrhea
   (3)   Neurologic symptoms such as fatigue, confusion, muscle weakness, and visual disturbances (halos around light or red-green vision)
h.   If patient is digitalis-toxic, often withdrawal of digoxin is all that is needed
i.   Concomitant use of quinidine, verapamil, spironolactone, flecainide, propafenone, or amiodarone increases likelihood of digitalis toxicity

5.   **Pharmacological interventions to be considered for <u>selected</u> patients with symptomatic left ventricular dysfunction (Stage C)**
   a.   Consider addition of spironolactone in patients who have symptoms at rest despite use of diuretics, ACE inhibitor, digoxin, and (usually) a beta-blocker; not recommended for patients with mild to moderate HF
      (1)   Prescribe only to patients who have serum potassium <5.0 mmol/L and a serum creatinine <2.5 mg/dL; monitor potassium and creatinine closely
      (2)   Prudent to stop potassium supplements as hyperkalemia may occur
   b.   Angiotensin II-receptor antagonists promote physiologic responses similar to those of ACE inhibitors but should be used only if patient is intolerant of ACE inhibitor (cough, angioedema); valsartan (Diovan) initiated at 40 mg BID and titrated to 160 mg BID as tolerated is an approved drug for HF
   c.   Combination use of hydralazine and isosorbide dinitrate is a therapeutic option for patients who cannot take ACE inhibitor; because of adherence problems (large number of pills) and high incidence of adverse reactions, angiotensin II-receptor antagonists are usually preferred in patients who cannot tolerate ACE inhibitors
      (1)   Prescribe isosorbide dinitrate (Isordil) 5 -10 mg TID and hydralazine (Apresoline) 10 mg QID as initial doses; particularly helpful in patients with hypertension or severe mitral regurgitation
      (2)   If patient tolerates initial doses, gradually increase isosorbide dinitrate to 40 mg TID and hydralazine to 75 mg QID as far as patient's hemodynamic parameters will tolerate
      (3)   To avoid nitrate tolerance, prescribe a minimal 10-hours of nitrate-free period at night

H.   Treatment of **patients with refractory end-stage HF (Stage D)**
   1.   All the measures used in Stages A, B, C are recommended in Stage D, except that great caution should be exercised in using both ACE inhibitors and beta-blockers in patients with refractory HF
      a.   Do not administer ACE inhibitor or beta blocker if patient has systolic BP <80 mm Hg or signs of peripheral hypoperfusion; do not use beta-blocker if fluid retention is present or patient had recently required treatment with intravenous positive inotropic agent
      b.   Consider combination use of hydralazine and isosorbide dinitrate (see V.G.5.c.) or spironolactone (see V.G.5.a.) if patients cannot tolerate ACE inhibitor and beta-blocker
   2.   Meticulously identify and control fluid retention
      a.   As HF advances, declines in renal perfusion can limit kidneys' abilities to respond to diuretic therapy
      b.   When patients become resistant to therapy either because there is significant renal failure (serum creatinine >2-4 mg/dL) or when there is severe heart failure, add metolazone (Zaroxolyn) 2.5-10 mg QD
      c.   Restriction of dietary sodium to <2 g daily is beneficial
      d.   Hospitalization is required for patients whose fluid overload does not resolve with above therapies; intravenous diuretics and/or use of mechanical methods to remove fluids are often prescribed
   3.   Patients are also often hospitalized and given intravenous (IV) infusions of peripheral vasodilators (nitroglycerin or nitroprusside) and positive inotropic agents (dobutamine, dopamine, or milrinone)
      a.   Positive inotropic agents result in dramatic improvement in symptoms and positive changes in the way patients feel during short-term continuous IV infusions when used with IV diuresis
      b.   Therapies may be accompanied by worsening azotemia and may actually increase mortality

    c.   For patients who cannot be weaned from IV or oral therapy, an indwelling line may be placed for continuous infusion of dobutamine or milrinone

        (1)   IV infusions at home should be used only as last resort to provide palliative care and to allow the patient to die comfortably at home

        (2)   Long-term use of regularly scheduled intermittent infusions at home, in an out-patient clinic setting, or short-stay unit is strongly discouraged, even in advanced HF

    d.   Nesiritide (Natrecor), a B-type natriuretic peptide, works similarly to the body's own hormone BNP and was found to produce hemodynamic improvements without the dangerous sequelae of the inotropes; may be the future first-line drug for treatment of refractory HF

    4.   Mechanical and surgical strategies: Cardiac transplantation is only established surgical approach for refractory HF, but alternate surgical and mechanical approaches are under development

I.   Management recommendations for **patients with HF and concomitant diseases**

    1.   For patients with hypertension, use drugs that control both conditions (diuretics, ACE inhibitors, beta-blockers); avoid calcium channel blockers

    2.   For patients with diabetes, use typical therapy of diuretics, ACE-inhibitors, and beta-blockers; do **not** avoid beta-blockers for fears of masking symptoms of hypoglycemia or exacerbating glucose intolerance or insulin resistance

    3.   For patients with angina

        a.   Consider coronary revascularization

        b.   Consider adding nitrates to relieve symptoms

        c.   Generally, avoid calcium channel blockers (CCB); amlodipine is the only CCB that should be considered; this drug was found to improve survival but experience with this drug exists mainly in patients not taking beta-blockers

    4.   For patients with supraventricular arrhythmias

        a.   Generally avoid CCBs

        b.   Beta blockers are drugs of choice to slow ventricular response; if beta blockers are ineffective or contraindicated, amiodarone may be a useful alternative (other antiarrhythmics should **not** be used in patients with HF)

        c.   Prescribe warfarin to achieve a target range of international normalized ration of 2.0 to 3.0

    5.   For patients with history of sudden death, ventricular fibrillation, or destabilizing ventricular tachycardia consider implantable cardioverter-defibrillator (alone or combined with amiodarone)

J.   Promising Interventions under active investigation include synchronized biventricular pacing and enhanced external counterpulsation (EECP)

K.   Treatment of **diastolic dysfunction** (recommendations do not include therapy for hypertrophic cardiomyopathy because the pathophysiologic features and therapy significantly differ from other causes of diastolic dysfunction)

    1.   Goals are to lower elevated filling pressures without significantly reducing cardiac output by controlling physiologic factors (blood pressure, heart rate, blood volume, and myocardial ischemia)

    2.   Try to achieve BP goals lower than those recommended for patients with uncomplicated hypertension (e.g., <130 mm Hg systolic and <80 mm Hg diastolic)

        a.   Calcium channel blockers are not contraindicated in this subgroup, but carefully monitor for reduction in left ventricular performance and development of LVSD; discontinue CCB at that time

        b.   ACE inhibitors can also be prescribed; they directly improve ventricular relaxation and cause regression of hypertrophy/cardiac remodeling

    3.   Initially prescribe small doses of diuretics with careful monitoring to control pulmonary congestion and peripheral edema; however, beware of excessive diuresis, as this can reduce stroke volume and cardiac output causing SOB, hypotension, tachycardia, and subsequent chest pain

    4.   Control ventricular rate; beta-blockers are a good choice as they enhance ventricular relaxation and improve compliance

    5.   In general, do <u>not</u> use digoxin as this drug will further increase the contractility and deplete cardiac muscle reserves

    6.   Heart transplantation is an option in patients whose symptoms are refractory to optimal medical/surgical management

L.   Patient Education

    1.   Provide information on nature of heart failure, drugs, and dietary restrictions

    2.   Encourage regular exercise such as walking or cycling for stable patients according to cardiac rehabilitation guidelines; start with a supervised exercise program, advancing to home program

    3.   Teach patients to restrict dietary sodium to as close to 2 grams per day as possible; patients with poorly compensated heart failure may require further reductions in salt intake to 500 mg or 1 gram

4. Advise patient to avoid excessive fluid intake; fluid restriction is not recommended unless patient is hyponatremic; 32-48 ounces of water per day is standard suggestion
5. Teach patients to monitor weight as an indirect measure of fluid retention
   a. Advise patient to weigh daily at the same time of day with no shoes and similar clothing
   b. Advise patient to call clinician if weight increases by 2-3 pounds in <4 days
6. Teach a weight-based diuresing protocol to patients that can understand instructions and who are usually compliant with treatments
   a. Obtain baseline dry weight
   b. If weight increases by 4-5 pounds (usually with edema and increased shortness of breath) and the normal food intake has not increased, instruct patient to increase dosage of her/his regularly prescribed diuretic (taken in divided doses throughout the day – not in evening) until weight returns to baseline (amount of increase in dosage is individually determined)
7. Advise patients to consume no more than one drink per day (one drink equals a glass of beer or wine, or drink with no more than 1 ounce of alcohol)
8. Emphasize that patient should not smoke or chew tobacco
9. Teach patient to recognize symptoms of worsening heart failure and what to do if symptoms occur
10. Inform patient and family of the prognosis so decisions and plans for the future can be made
11. Recommend weight reduction in obese patients and elimination of undue stress
12. Instruct patient to eliminate or cautiously use drugs that precipitate exacerbation of HF: Nonsteroidal anti-inflammatory drugs, anti-arrhythmic agents (disopyramide and flecainide), glucocorticoids, androgens, estrogens
13. Discuss sexual practices, sexual difficulties, and coping strategies
14. Remind patient to obtain vaccinations against influenza and pneumococcal disease
15. Teach **PACE** to help patients *pace* themselves through their activities of daily living (ADL)
    a. **P**: Plan ahead – plan activities for the time of day when energy is greatest and symptoms are at lowest level; wait one hour after eating or bathing
    b. **A**: Assign activities – decide what activities can be done and what should be assigned to others
    c. **C**: Choose what is important – list activities in order of importance, do what has to be done
    d. **E**: Energy saving – use movements that conserve energy, teach to relax, and use rest breaks; sit to work or play when possible
16. Teach patients to slow down or stop activities if the following symptoms develop: Chest pain (angina), rapid heart rate, unusual shortness of breath, palpitations, excessive sweating, weakness, faintness, dizziness, leg pain, or cramping

M. Follow Up
1. All patients who have been hospitalized should be evaluated by phone or office visit within one week of discharge to determine if they are stable and to check their understanding of and adherence with the treatment plan
2. Patients treated as outpatients:
   a. Contact within 24 hours
   b. Then, schedule return visit for every 1-2 weeks until patient is symptom-free and dry weight is maintained
3. When patient is symptom-free, schedule visits for every 3-6 months
   a. Consider referring patient to heart failure/heart improvement program
   b. Monitor lipids, anticoagulants, blood pressure measurements, and patient's journals on a regular basis
4. Order certain laboratory tests after initiating certain drug therapies:
   a. Order blood urea nitrogen, serum creatinine, and electrolyte levels initially, at 2 weeks, at 8 weeks, and then every 6 months if patient is stable
   b. If patient is taking diuretics, order uric acid at 3 months and then annually
   c. If patient is taking an ACE inhibitor, monitor urinalysis for protein monthly for 2-4 months and then annually; monitor creatinine and liver enzymes every 3-6 months depending on patient's baseline data
   d. Although not routinely done, consider checking serum digoxin level in 2 weeks after beginning drug treatment or if suspicion of nonadherence or digitalis toxicity

HYPERTENSION IN ADULTS

I.   Definition: Persistent elevation of the systolic blood pressure (SBP) at 140 mm Hg or higher and the diastolic blood pressure (DBP) at 90 mm Hg or higher, or taking antihypertensive medications; for patients with diabetes or progressive renal disease, treatment goal is lowered to 130/85 (or to 125/75 in patients with renal disease and severe proteinuria)

II. Pathogenesis

    A.   Any factor producing an alteration in peripheral vascular resistance, heart rate, or stroke volume affects systemic arterial blood pressure through four control mechanisms:
        1.   The arterial baroreceptor and chemoreceptor systems
        2.   Regulation of body fluid volume
        3.   The renin-angiotensin system
        4.   Vascular autoregulation

    B.   Approximately 90-95% of hypertensive individuals have essential hypertension (HTN) with no identifiable etiology; likely due to multiple factors in some or all of the above four control mechanisms

    C.   Blood pressure (BP) remains elevated, if not treated, because of an overall net increase in peripheral arterial resistance secondary to the inappropriate renal retention of salt and water and/or the increased endogenous pressure activity because of malfunctions in the four control mechanisms (II.A.1-4.)

    D.   Secondary hypertension is defined as BP elevation from an identifiable cause; primary mechanisms in all causes of HTN include the following: (also see table SECONDARY HYPTERTENSION, IV.C.2.)
        1.   Increased secretion of catecholamines causing vasoconstriction (e.g., pheochromocytoma)
        2.   Increased release of renin that starts the renin-angiotensin cascade (e.g., renal artery stenosis)
        3.   Increased sodium and water retention, expanding blood volume (e.g., Cushing's syndrome)

III. Clinical Presentation

    A.   About 1 in 4 persons have HTN in US
        1.   Typically appears between ages 30-55
        2.   More common in elderly and nonwhite races
        3.   Only about 25% of hypertensive persons have BPs controlled at or below target levels
        4.   Persons who are normotensive at 55 years of age have a 90% lifetime risk of developing hypertension

    B.   Fewer than 5-8% of adult hypertensive patients have secondary HTN

    C.   Environmental factors such as obesity, psychogenic stress, high fat and sodium intake, oral contraceptives, and large alcohol intake may increase BP levels

    D.   BP fluctuations have a reasonably predictive circadian pattern; in untreated hypertensive patients, BP rises in morning when awakening and declines by approximately 10-20% during sleep

    E.   Most patients are asymptomatic but some have varying degrees of target organ disease (TOD) that may not appear until after 10-20 years of disease progression
        1.   For persons 40-70 years, each increment of 20 mm Hg in systolic BP or 10 mm Hg in diastolic BP doubles risk of cardiovascular disease (CVD) across the entire BP range (115/75 mm Hg to 185/155 mm Hg)
        2.   Higher levels of both SBP and DBP are related to increased risks of morbidity, disability, and mortality due to cardiac, renal, and cerebral diseases
        3.   Systolic pressure of more than 140 mm Hg is a stronger predictor of cardiovascular events than is diastolic pressure in persons >50 years

    F.   "White coat" hypertension is BP that is intermittently elevated and increases only in the clinician's office
        1.   An intermittent vaso-vagal response is accountable for the transient elevation in BP
        2.   Treating this 'false' hypertension can produce significant hypotension, but essential or secondary hypertension disguised as "white coat" hypertension left untreated will have deleterious sequelae

3. Chronic, frequent intermittent vaso-vagal responses, particularly if BP responses are quite high, should be treated to prevent possibility of stroke (e.g. low-dose beta-blocker or antianxiety drugs)

G. Classification of adult BP is based on the impact of risk; classification is for persons who are not taking antihypertensive medications and who have no acute disease (see following table)
   1. Classification is based on average of 2 or more properly measured seated BP readings taken at each of 2 or more visits following an initial screening
   2. When systolic and diastolic pressures fall into different categories, the higher category should be selected to classify the individual's blood pressure stage

CLASSIFICATION OF BLOOD PRESSURE FOR ADULTS AGE 18 AND OLDER*

Category	Systolic (mm Hg)		Diastolic (mm Hg)
Normal	<120	and	<80
Prehypertension	120-139	or	80-89
Stage 1 hypertension	140-159	or	90-99
Stage 2 hypertension	≥160	or	≥100

Adapted from The JNC 7 Report. (2003). The Seventh Report of the Joint National Committee on Prevention, Detection, Evaluation, and Treatment of High Blood Pressure. *JAMA, 289*, 2560-2572.

H. Malignant hypertension, now referred to as *persistent severe hypertension*, results from hypertension left untreated or that which is refractory to treatment and BP continues to rise unchecked
   1. Characterized by chronically elevated systolic blood pressure (SBP) and a diastolic blood pressure (DBP) >110 to 120 mm Hg
   2. Symptoms include severe headaches, visual impairment (double vision, blurring), papilledema, and retinal hemorrhages or exudates

I. Prevalence of isolated systolic hypertension (ISH) increases after the age of 60 years
   1. Hypothesized to be a result of increased cardiac output or atherosclerosis-induced changes in blood vessel compliance or both in elderly persons
   2. ISH is SBP of 140 mm Hg or greater with a DBP <90 mm Hg
   3. ISH is now considered " true" hypertension and treatment is indicated to reduce the SBP
   4. Among the elderly, SBP is a better predictor of events such as coronary heart disease (CHD), stroke, heart failure, renal disease than is DBP

J. Widened pulse pressure (high SBP paired with low DBP) indicates large artery stiffness and is a major mechanism determining CHD risk in older adults

IV. Diagnosis/Evaluation: Goals are to identify type of hypertension (primary or secondary), ascertain the presence of other cardiovascular risk factors, and determine the extent of target organ involvement

A. History
   1. Ask about the duration and levels of elevated blood pressure as well as successes/failures or adverse effects of previous treatment regimens
   2. Inquire about symptoms that suggest secondary hypertension such as palpitations, sweating, dizziness, and abdominal and back pain (also see IV.C.)
   3. Question about symptoms of stress, cardiovascular disease, cerebrovascular disease, peripheral vascular disease, renal disease, diabetes, dyslipidemia, gout, sexual dysfunction
   4. Inquire about weight control, physical activities, tobacco use, or sedentary lifestyle
   5. Explore dietary intake of sodium, alcohol, caffeine, cholesterol, saturated fats, or appetite suppressants
   6. Ask about patient and family histories of hypertension, premature coronary heart disease (CHD), stroke, cardiovascular disease (CVD), diabetes, dyslipidemia, and renal disease
   7. Obtain a medication history including illicit drugs and drugs that may elevate BP (oral contraceptives, steroids, nonsteroidal anti-inflammatory drugs, decongestants, appetite suppressants, cyclosporine, tricyclic antidepressants, monoamine oxidase inhibitors)
   8. Explore psychosocial and environmental factors that may impact on blood pressure control

B. Physical Examination
1. Obtain two or more blood pressure measurements with patient in chair (not on examination table) and feet on floor and arm supported at heart level; measurement in standing position is needed periodically, especially in those at risk for postural hypotension
   a. Measurements should begin after at least 5 minutes of rest; patients should refrain from smoking and caffeine ingestion for at least 30 minutes prior to measurement
   b. Bladder of cuff should encircle at least 80% of arm
   c. Systolic BP is point at which first of 2 or more sounds is heard (phase 1) and diastolic BP is point before disappearance of sounds (phase 5)
2. Ambulatory BP monitoring
   a. Consider using an automated noninvasive ambulatory blood pressure monitoring device for patients with the following
      (1) "White-coat" hypertension
      (2) Drug resistance
      (3) Nocturnal pressure changes
      (4) Episodic HTN
      (5) Hypotensive symptoms associated with antihypertensive medications or autonomic dysfunction
      (6) Carotid sinus syncope and pacemaker syndrome (ECG monitoring also needed)
   b. Awake hypertensive individuals have BP of more than 135/85 mm Hg and during sleep 120/75 mm Hg
   c. Provides measure of percentage of elevated BP readings, overall BP load, and extent of BP reduction during sleep
3. Self-measurement of BP is informative and can be recorded in a journal; validated electronic devices or aneroid sphygmomanometers are recommended; finger monitors are inaccurate; BP of more than 135/85 mm Hg at home is considered hypertension
4. Measure height, weight, waist circumference, and determine body mass index (BMI)
   a. BMI of ≥27 kg/m^2 correlates closely with elevated BP
   b. Excess body fat accumulated in the torso with a waist circumference of ≥34 inches for women and ≥39 inches for men indicates increased risk for cardiovascular disease
5. Perform a funduscopic exam, noting arteriolar narrowing, arteriovenous nicking, hemorrhages, exudates, or papilledema
6. Assess neck for distended veins, carotid bruits, and thyromegaly
7. Perform a complete heart exam, noting tachycardia, shift in point of maximal impulse (PMI), precordial heave, clicks, murmurs, arrhythmias, and third and fourth heart sounds
8. Perform complete lung exam, noting rales and evidence of bronchospasm
9. Perform abdominal exam, noting bruits, enlarged kidneys, masses, and abnormal aortic pulsation
10. Assess extremities for abnormal peripheral arterial pulsations, bruits, and edema
11. Perform a complete neurologic exam

C. Differential Diagnosis
1. Important to correctly identify patients who are truly hypertensive from those who appear to be hypertensive because of faulty or incorrect B/P measurements
2. Important to eliminate secondary causes of hypertension (see following table); clues to presence of secondary cause are the following:
   a. Hypertension presenting for first time in individuals <25 years of age in the absence of family history or in older adults >60 years of age
   b. Acute onset of severe HTN at any age that is not due to antihypertensive drug withdrawal
   c. Adherent patients whose BPs do not lower with antihypertensive medications or whose BPs are normalized and then become refractory to treatment
   d. Patients with certain clinical manifestations:
      (1) Central obesity, hirsutism, purple stria, and ecchymosis (e.g., Cushing's syndrome)
      (2) Widening pulse pressure, acute anterior chest and mid-back pain, impending feeling of doom (e.g., dissecting abdominal aneurysm)
      (3) Weight loss, nervousness, exophthalmos, tremors, fatigue, palpitations (e.g., hyperthyroidism)
      (4) Paroxysmal complaints of headache, perspiration, palpitations, and dizziness (e.g., pheochromocytoma)

CAUSES OF SECONDARY HYPERTENSION

Acute Stress
Alcoholism
Acute alcohol withdrawal
Burns
Chronic intermittent vaso-vagal response
Hyperventilation
Hypoglycemia
Psychogenic

Vascular Disorders
Arteriosclerosis
Coarctation of the aorta
Increased intravascular volume
Sickle cell crisis

Dissecting Aortic Aneurysm

Endocrine Disorders
Acromegaly
Adrenal disorders
   Cortical
      Cushing's syndrome
      Primary aldosteronism
   Medullary
      Pancreatitis
      Pheochromocytoma
Hypothyroidism
Hyperthyroidism

Neurologic Disorders
Autonomic dysreflexia
Increased intracranial pressure
   Brain tumor
   Encephalitis
   Respiratory acidosis
Sleep apnea

Medications
Abrupt medication withdrawal
Amphetamine use
Anabolic and adrenogenic steroids
Antihistamine/decongestants
Cocaine use
Cyclosporine
Ergot Alkaloids
Erythropoietin
Glucocorticoids
Heavy metal poisons (lead, arsenic)
Mineralocorticoids
Monoamine oxidase inhibitors
NSAIDs
Oral contraceptives
Sympathomimetics
   Ephedrine
   Phenylephrine
Tricyclic antidepressants

Problems with Pregnancy
Pregnancy induced HTN
Eclampsia

Renal Disorders
Renal artery stenosis
Renal parenchymal disease
   Acute glomerulonephritis
   Chronic pyelonephritis
   Connective tissue diseases
   Diabetic nephropathy
   Hydronephrosis
   Polycystic disease
Renin-producing tumors
Renovascular diseases
   Atherosclerosis
   Vasculitis

Severe Anemia

Tyramine-Containing Foods
Aged cheeses (esp. cheddar)
Beer, wine
Chicken liver
Yeast extract

D. Diagnostic Tests
   1. Before beginning therapy order the following: Urinalysis; complete blood count; blood glucose (fasting, if possible); potassium, creatinine, calcium; fasting lipid panel; electrocardiogram
   2. Optional tests include measurement of urinary albumin excretion or albumin/creatinine ratio
   3. Consider additional tests for persons with suspected secondary cause/s: Creatinine clearance, urinary microalbumin determination, 24-hour urinary protein, uric acid, glycosylated hemoglobin (HgA1c), thyroid-stimulating hormone (TSH), drug levels, erythrocyte sedimentation rate (ESR), cortisol level, C-reactive protein (hsCRP), brain natriuretic peptide (BNP) level, vascular angiogram, CT scan or ultrasound of suspected organs, graded exercise test (exercise treadmill test [ETT] with or without accompanying "limited view" echocardiogram), and/or complete resting echocardiogram with 2-D Doppler flow imaging

V. Plan/Management

  A. Goals of management
     1. Maintain arterial pressure below 140 mm Hg SBP and 90 mm Hg DBP and lower if tolerated while controlling the modifiable risk factors; for patients with diabetes or progressive renal disease, goal is 130/80 mm Hg (or to 125/75 mm Hg for patients with renal disease and proteinuria >1 g/24 hours) (see V.L.4.5)
     2. The primary focus of treatment should be on achieving systolic BP goal

  B. Treatment regimens are based on stage of blood pressure and risk stratification (see following tables)

CARDIOVASCULAR RISK STRATIFICATION

Major Risk Factors

Hypertension*
Smoking
Age (>55 for men; >65 for women)
Diabetes mellitus*

Physical inactivity
Dyslipidemia*
Sex (men and postmenopausal women)

Obesity (BMI ≥30)*
Family history of cardiovascular disease: women under age 65 or men under age 55
Microalbuminuria or estimated GFR <60 mL/min

Target Organ Damage/Clinical Cardiovascular Disease (TOD/CCD)

Heart Diseases
  Left ventricular hypertrophy
  Angina/prior myocardial infarction
  Prior coronary revascularization
  Heart failure

Stroke or transient ischemic attack
Nephropathy
Peripheral arterial disease
Retinopathy

* Components of metabolic syndrome
Adapted from The JNC 7 Report. (2003). The Seventh Report of the Joint National Committee on Prevention, Detection, Evaluation, and Treatment of High Blood Pressure. *JAMA, 289*, 2560-2572.

CLASSIFICATION AND MANAGEMENT OF BLOOD PRESSURE FOR ADULTS

BP Classification	Systolic BP, mm Hg*		Diastolic BP, mm Hg*	Lifestyle Modification	Management — Initial Drug Therapy: Without Compelling Indication	Management — Initial Drug Therapy: With Compelling Indication
Normal	<120	and	<80	Encourage		
Prehypertension	120-139	or	80-89	Yes	No antihypertensive drug indicated	Drug(s) for the compelling indications**
Stage 1 hypertension	140-159	or	90-99	Yes	Thiazide-type diuretics for most; may consider ACE inhibitor, ARB, β-blocker, CCB, or combination	Drug(s) for the compelling indications. Other antihypertensive drugs (diuretics, ACE inhibitor, ARB, β-blocker, CCB) as needed
Stage 2 hypertension	≥160	or	≥100	Yes	2-Drug combination for most (usually thiazide-type diuretic and ACE inhibitor or ARB or β-blocker or CCB)⁺	Drug(s) for the compelling indications. Other antihypertensive drugs (diuretics, ACE inhibitor, ARB, β-blocker, CCB) as needed

* Treatment determined by highest BP category
** Treat patients with chronic kidney disease or diabetes to BP goal of <130/80 mm Hg
⁺ Initial combined therapy should be used cautiously in those at risk for orthostatic hypotension
Adapted from The JNC 7 Report. (2003). The Seventh Report of the Joint National Committee on Prevention, Detection, Evaluation, and Treatment of High Blood Pressure. *JAMA, 289*, 2560-2572.

C. Lifestyle modifications are helpful in lowering blood pressure and can reduce other risk factors for premature cardiovascular disease (see table that follows); adoption of healthy lifestyles by all individuals is critical for prevention of high BP and mandatory for those with hypertension
   1. Considered as **first line measures** for those at risk, who are borderline, or who have a confirmed diagnosis (see risk stratification table above)
   2. Lifestyle modifications should be addressed from a multifactorial, multidisciplinary perspective

LIFESTYLE MODIFICATIONS FOR PRIMARY PREVENTION OF HYPERTENSION

- Maintain normal body weight for adults (body mass index, 18.5-24.9 kg/m^2)
- Reduce dietary sodium intake to no more than 100 mmol/day (approximately 6 g of sodium chloride or 2.4 g of sodium per day)[*†]
- Limit daily alcohol consumption to no more than 1 oz (30 mL) of ethanol (e.g., 24 oz of beer, 10 oz wine, or 2 oz of 100-proof whisky); women and lighter weight people should limit daily consumption to 0.5 oz (15 mL) of ethanol
- Engage in regular aerobic physical activity such as a brisk walk (at least 30 minutes per day, most days of week)[§]
- Maintain an adequate intake of dietary potassium (>90 mmol [3500 mg] per day)
- Consume a diet that is rich in fruits and vegetables and in low-fat dairy produces with a reduced content of saturated and total fat (see table on DASH diet that follows)

* Remember 2.4 gm of sodium equals approximately 1 teaspoon of salt
† African-Americans and elderly persons are particularly sensitive to changes in dietary sodium chloride
§ Weight bearing exercises with light weights are a positive adjunct to any exercise regime, however, lifting heavy weights may be harmful because BP rises; advise patients to initiate exercise programs gradually and to receive ongoing professional surveillance of their conditions

Adapted from Whelton, P.K., He, J., Appel, L.J., Cutler, J.A., Havas, S., & Kotchen, T.A. (2002). Primary prevention of hypertension: Clinical and Public Health Advisory from the National High Blood Pressure Education Program. *JAMA, 288,* 1882-1888.

DASH DIET*	
Food/Servings	**Food Examples**
Grains & grain products--7 to 8 daily	Whole wheat breads, English muffins, pita bread, bagels, cereals, oatmeal, grits
Fruits & vegetables--4 to 5 fruit servings daily; 4 to 5 vegetable servings daily	Apricots, bananas, grapes, oranges, grapefruit, melons, strawberries, tomatoes, peas, carrots, potatoes, broccoli, squash, leafy greens
Dairy foods (low-fat or nonfat)--2 to 3 daily	Skim or 1% milk, nonfat or low-fat yogurt, nonfat or part-skim cheese
Meats, poultry & fish--2 or fewer daily	Lean meats only; trim visible fat, remove skin from poultry; broil, roast or boil
Nuts, seeds & legumes--4 to 5 a week	Almonds, peanuts, mixed nuts, sunflower seeds, kidney beans, lentils

*For DASH diet details visit the following website: nhlbi.nih.gov/health/public/heart/hbp/dash/
Adapted from Joint National Committee on Detection, Evaluation, and Treatment of High Blood Pressure. (1997). The sixth report of the Joint National Committee on Detection, Evaluation, and Treatment of High Blood Pressure (JNV VI). *Archives of Internal Medicine, 157,* 24-14-2446.

3. Other lifestyle approaches have uncertain or unproven efficacy
    a. Calcium supplementation results in only a small reduction in BP, but it is prudent to have an adequate calcium intake in any diet (1000-1200 mg/day for adults)
    b. Fish oil supplementation with relatively high doses of omega-3 polyunsaturated fatty acids has modest effects on BP but increased intake may reduce the risk of CHD and stroke
    c. Smoking cessation is important in reducing risk of CHD and may decrease spikes in BP
    d. Relaxation therapies, transcendental meditation, yoga, biofeedback, and psychotherapy reduce BP at least transiently, but there is no evidence of their long-term efficacies

D. Begin pharmacological therapy and continue lifestyle modifications if lifestyle changes fail to achieve goal BP (see specific timeline in table in V.B. RISK STRATIFICATION AND TREATMENT)
    1. Goal of pharmacological therapy is to achieve target BP level with a minimum of side effects
    2. See table that follows for available antihypertensive medications

ORAL ANTIHYPERTENSIVE DRUGS*

Drug	Trade Name	Usual Dose Range, Total mg/day* (Frequency per Day)	Selected Side Effects and Comments*
Diuretics (partial list)			Short-term: Increase cholesterol and glucose levels; biochemical abnormalities: Decrease potassium, sodium, and magnesium levels, increase uric acid and calcium levels; rare: Blood dyscrasias, photosensitivity, pancreatitis, hyponatremia
Thiazide diuretics			
Chlorthalidone (G)H	Hygroton	12.5-25 (1)	
Hydrochlorothiazide (G)	Hydrodiuril	12.5-50 (1)	
Indapamide	Lozol	1.25-5 (1)	(Less or no hypercholesterolemia)
Metolazone	Mykrox	0.5-1.0 (1)	
	Zaroxolyn	2.5-5 (1)	
Loop diuretics			
Bumetanide (G)	Bumex	0.5-2 (2)	(Short duration of action, no hypercalcemia)
Furosemide (G)	Lasix	20-80 (2)	(Short duration of action, no hypercalcemia)
Torsemide	Demadex	2.5-10 (1)	
Potassium-sparing agents			Hyperkalemia
Amiloride hydrochloride (G)	Midamor	5-10 (1)	
Triamterene (G)	Dyrenium	50-100 (1)	
Adrenergic inhibitors			
Central alpha-agonists			Sedation, dry mouth, bradycardia, withdrawal hypertension
Clonidine hydrochloride (G)	Catapres	0.1-0.8 (2)	(More withdrawal)
Guanfacine hydrochloride (G)	Tenex	0.5-2 (1)	(Less withdrawal)
Methyldopa (G)	Aldomet	250-1,000 (2)	(Hepatic and "autoimmune" disorders)
Reserpine	Serpasil	0.05-0.25 (1)	(Nasal congestion, sedation, depression, activation of peptic ulcer)
Alpha-blockers			Postural hypotension
Doxazosin mesylate	Cardura	1-16 (1)	Not for use as monotherapy, increased risk for heart failure
Prazosin hydrochloride (G)	Minipress	2-20 (2-3)	
Terazosin hydrochloride	Hytrin	1-20 (1)	
Beta-blockers			Bronchospasm, bradycardia, heart failure, may mask insulin-induced hypoglycemia; less serious: impaired peripheral circulation, insomnia, fatigue, decreased exercise tolerance, hypertriglyceridemia (except agents with intrinsic sympathomimetic activity)
Acebutolol ' I	Sectral	200-800 (1)	
Atenolol (G) '	Tenormin	25-100 (1)	
Betaxolol '	Kerlone	5-20 (1)	
Bisoprolol fumarate '	Zebeta	2.5-10 (1)	
Metoprolol tartrate (G) '	Lopressor	50-100 (1-2)	
Metoprolol succinate '	Toprol-XL	50-100 (1-2)	
Nadolol (G)	Corgard	40-120 (1)	
Penbutolol sulfateI	Levatol	10-40 (1)	
Pindolol (G)I	Visken	10-40 (2)	
Propranolol hydrochloride (G)	Inderal	40-160 (2)	
	Inderal LA	60-180 (1)	
Timolol maleate (G)	Blocadren	20-40 (2)	
Combined alpha- and beta-blockers			Postural hypotension, bronchospasm
Carvedilol	Coreg	12.5-50 (2)	
Labetalol hydrochloride (G)	Normodyne, Trandate	200-800 (2)	
Direct vasodilators			Headaches, fluid retention, tachycardia
Hydralazine hydrochloride (G)	Apresoline	25-100 (2)	(Lupus syndrome) headaches, peripheral edema
Minoxidil (G)	Loniten	2.5-80 (1-2)	(hirsutism)

(Continued)

415

ORAL ANTIHYPERTENSIVE DRUGS* *(CONTINUED)*

Drug	Trade Name	Usual Dose Range, Total mg/day* (Frequency per Day)	Selected Side Effects and Comments*
Calcium channel blockers (CCB)			
Nondihydropyridines			Conduction defects, worsening of systolic dysfunction, gingival hyperplasia (Nausea, headache)
Diltiazem hydrochloride	Cardizem SR	60-180 (2)	
	Cardizem CD, Dilacor XR, Tiazac	180-420 (1)	
Verapamil hydrochloride	Isoptin SR, Calan SR	120-360 (1-2)	Higher dosing goes to BID in this case (constipation)
	Verelan, Covera HS	120-360 (1)	
Dihydropyridines			Edema of the ankle, flushing, headache, gingival hypertrophy
Amlodipine besylate	Norvasc	2.5-10 (1)	
Felodipine	Plendil	2.5-20 (1)	
Isradipine	DynaCirc CR	2.5-10 (2)	
Nicardipine	Cardene SR	30-120 (2)	
Nifedipine	Procardia XL, Adalat CC	30-60 (1)	
Nisoldipine	Sular	10-40 (1)	
Aldosterone-receptor blockers			
Eplerenone	Inspra	50-100 (1-2)	
Spironolactone	Aldactone	25-50 (1-2)	(Gynecomastia)
			(Continued)
ACE inhibitors (ACE I)			Common: cough; rare: angioedema, hyperkalemia, rash, loss of taste, leukopenia
Benazepril hydrochloride	Lotensin	10-40 (1-2)	
Captopril (G)	Capoten	25-100 (2)	
Enalapril maleate	Vasotec	2.5-40 (1-2)	
Fosinopril sodium	Monopril	10-40 (1)	
Lisinopril	Prinivil, Zestril	10-40 (1)	
Moexipril	Univasc	7.5-30 (1)	
Quinapril hydrochloride	Accupril	10-40 (1)	
Ramipril	Altace	2.5-20 (1)	
Trandolapril	Mavik	1-4 (1)	
Angiotensin II receptor blockers (ARB)			Angioedema (very rare), hyperkalemia
Candesartan	Atacand	8-32 (1)	
Eprosartan	Teveten	400-800 (1-2)	
Irbesartan	Avapro	150-300 (1)	
Losartan	Cozaar	25-100 (1-2)	
Olmesartan	Benicar	20-40 (1)	
Telmisartan	Micardis	20-80 (1)	
Valsartan	Diovan	80-320 (1)	

*These dosages may vary from those listed in the *Physicians' Desk Reference* which may be consulted for additional information. The listing of side effects is not all-inclusive, and side effects are for the class of drugs except where noted for individual drugs (in parentheses); clinicians are urged to refer to the package insert for a more detailed listing

H(G) indicates generic available

I Has intrinsic sympathomimetic activity

' Cardioselective

**Also acts centrally

Adapted from The JNC 7 Report. (2003). The Seventh Report of the Joint National Committee on Prevention, Detection, Evaluation, and Treatment of High Blood Pressure. *JAMA, 289*, 2560-2572.

E. Recent trends in pharmacological therapy
1. Most patients will require two or more antihypertensive drugs; multiple drugs or combination drug treatment is increasingly recommended as first line therapy in high risk patients such as those with diabetes or those with higher BP levels
   a. Multiple drug therapy provides faster BP control and, thus, may enhance medication adherence
   b. Diuretics should be included in multidrug regimens unless patient is unable to take
2. Even slight elevations in BP above normal levels are associated with increased risk of CV disease; renewed interest is being placed on strictly meeting target BP levels

3. Increased focus on monitoring and treatment of elevated SBP and pulse pressure is recommended
4. Patient education, patient participation, and medication adherence strategies are emphasized

F. Selecting the initial drug (see table that follows and V.K. for overview of classes of drugs)
  1. Choice of therapy is based on combined assessment of the following: Co-morbidities, age, race/ethnicity, response to previously used drugs, including the presence or absence of adverse reactions
  2. Thiazide diuretics are first-line choice if there are no indications for another type of drug; they have excellent efficacy in lowering BP and reducing clinical events and they have good tolerability and are inexpensive; may consider ACE inhibitor, ARB, beta blockers, CCB, or combination
  3. See table CONSIDERATIONS FOR SELECTING THE INITIAL ANTIHYPERTENSIVE DRUGS; most patients should use thiazide diuretic either alone or in combination with one of the other classes but there are compelling reasons to use other drugs as first-line
  4. To improve adherence ask the following questions and collaborate with the patient in the decision of which drug to initially prescribe
    a. How much money can the patient afford to pay for drug(s)?
    b. What are the patient's risk factors and co-morbidities?
    c. What clinical adverse reactions does the patient perceive as most troublesome?
  5. Certain drugs are preferred for patients with coexisting conditions (see following table)

CONSIDERATIONS FOR SELECTING THE INITIAL ANTIHYPERTENSIVE DRUG*	
Indication	**Drug Therapy**
Compelling Indications Unless Contraindicated	
Diabetes mellitus	Thiazide diuretics, ACE I, ARB, beta blocker, CCB
Heart failure (asymptomatic with ventricular dysfunction)	ACE I, beta blocker
Heart failure (symptomatic ventricular dysfunction or end-stage heart disease)	ACE I, beta blocker, ARB, aldosterone blocker along with loop diuretic
Chronic kidney disease	ACE I, ARB
Post-myocardial infarction	ACE I, beta blocker, aldosterone blocker
Stable angina	Beta blocker
Acute coronary syndrome	Beta blocker, ACE I
Recurrent stroke prevention	ACE I and thiazide diuretic
May Have Favorable Effects on Comorbid Conditions	
Atrial tachycardia and fibrillation	Beta-blockers, CCB (non-DHP)
Cyclosporine-induced hypertension (caution with the dose of cyclosporine)	CCB
Dyslipidemia	Alpha-blockers
Essential tremor	Beta-blockers (non-CS)
Hyperthyroidism	Beta-blockers
Migraine	Beta-blockers (non-CS), CCB (non-DHP)
Osteoporosis	Thiazides
Preoperative hypertension	Beta-blockers
Prostatism (BPH)	Alpha-blockers
Raynaud syndrome	CCB
May Have Unfavorable Effects on Comorbid Conditions*	
Bronchospastic disease	Beta-blockers[†]
Depression	Beta-blockers, central alpha-agonists, reserpine[†]
Dyslipidemia	Beta-blockers (non-ISA), diuretics (high-dose)
Gout	Diuretics
2° or 3° heart block	Beta-blockers,[†] CCB (non-DHP)[†]
Heart failure due to left ventricular dysfunction	CCB (except amlodipine besylate, felodipine), Cardura
Hyperkalemia	Aldosterone antagonists and potassium sparing diuretics
Liver disease	Labetalol hydrochloride, methyldopa[†]
Peripheral vascular disease	Beta-blockers
Pregnancy	ACE I,[†] ARB
Renal insufficiency	Potassium-sparing agents
Renovascular disease	ACE I if creatinine significantly increased

(Continued)

Demographic Factors and Effects	
African Americans	Diuretics and calcium channel blockers may have most favorable effects
Elderly	Thiazides or beta-blockers plus thiazides are recommended; also consider long-acting dihydropyridine calcium antagonists

*ACE I indicates angiotensin-converting enzyme inhibitors; ARB indicates angiotensin receptor blocker, BPH, benign prostatic hyperplasia; CCB, calcium channel blocker; DHP, dihydropyridine; ISA, intrinsic sympathomimetic activity; MI, myocardial infarction; and non-CS, noncardioselective.

**Trial-based evidence supports use of ACE I to reduce proteinuria and BP, both of which improve renal function. ARBs have similar action. These drug classes may move up to "compelling indications" category in the next Joint National Committee report.

***These drugs may be used with special monitoring unless contraindicated.

†Contraindicated.

Adapted from National High Blood Pressure Education Program, National Institutes of Health, National Heart, Lung, and Blood Institute. (1997). *The Sixth Report of the Joint National Committee on Detection, Evaluation, and Treatment of High Blood Pressure* (NIH Publication No. 98-4080). Bethesda, MD: US Government Printing Office.

G. Recommended drug regimen
1. For most patients, start with a low to moderate dose of a single drug and titrate upward as directed
2. In **patients with Stage 2** begin one of the following modifications:
   a. Give drug therapy with minimal delay and possibly start with higher doses
   b. Give a 2-drug combination for most patients (usually a thiazide diuretic and ACE I or ARB or beta blocker or CCB)
3. **Patients with SBP ≥200 mm Hg and ≥DBP 120 mm Hg** require more aggressive initial therapy and may need to be hospitalized for IV drug therapy if symptoms or target organ damage are present (see V. N. for details regarding hypertensive urgency versus emergency)
4. For low and medium-risk patients, monotherapy may be sufficient to reach target BP goal; if BP is still uncontrolled after 2 weeks to 2 months of drug therapy, consider these options:
   a. Increase dose of the initial drug until target BP goal or maximum recommended dosage is reached; do not increase the dose prematurely (allow sufficient time for drug to be effective)
   b. Reconsider drug choice
      (1) Substitute an agent from another class if the patient is having no response or significant adverse effects
      (2) If diuretic was not selected initially, choose it as second-step drug; a diuretic should be included in most regimens as its addition potentiates the effects of other drugs
   c. Consider a multiple drug regimen (see V.H. below)

H. Multiple drug therapy or combination drugs (see table below)
1. Combinations of low doses of agents from different classes may provide additional efficacy and reduce likelihood of dose-dependent adverse effects
2. Single drugs used concomitantly or one combination drug may be prescribed; combination drugs may be most cost-effective and promote best patient adherence
3. Combined use of ACE inhibitor and calcium channel blocker reduces proteinuria and results in less pedal edema than with use of a calcium channel blocker alone; examples include Lexxel 5-2.5 (enalapril, felodipine) and Lotrel 2.5 mg/10 mg (amlodipine, benazepril)
4. Beta blocker/diuretic combinations such as Tenoretic 50 (atenolol, chlorthalidone) may be beneficial
5. Metolazone and a loop diuretic provide additive effects when used in patients with renal failure (there is no single combination drug for these two choices as yet)
6. Spironolactone with a thiazide diuretic as one pill (Aldactazide) is effective for heart failure
7. Many ACE and ARB drugs have been combined with a thiazide diuretic in one pill (Zestoretic, Prinzide, Atacand/HCT, Diovan/HCT); these drugs work well to reduce edema and fluid overload in patients with HTN/ heart failure or chronic renal insufficiency
8. Refer to a *PDR* or *Pharmacopoeia* for specific choices as number of combination drugs is increasing
9. Initiate and titrate each drug separately, and then, if needed substitute a combination drug

COMBINATION DRUGS

Drug	Trade Name
Beta-adrenergic blockers and diuretics	
Atenolol, 50 or 100 mg/chlorthalidone, 25 mg	Tenoretic
Bisoprolol fumarate, 2.5, 5, 0r 10 mg/hydrochlorothiazide, 6.25 mg	Ziac*
Metoprolol tartrate, 50 or 100 mg/hydrochlorothiazide, 25 or 50 mg	Lopressor HCT
Nadolol, 40 or 80 mg/bendroflumethiazide, 5 mg	Corzide
Propranolol hydrochloride, 40 or 80 mg/hydrochlorothiazide, 25 mg	Inderide
Propranolol hydrochloride (extended release), 80, 120, or 160 mg/hydrochlorothiazide, 50 mg	Inderide LA
Timolol maleate, 10 mg/hydrochlorothiazide, 25 mg	Timolide
ACE inhibitors and diuretics	
Benazepril hydrochloride, 5, 10, or 20 mg/hydrochlorothiazide, 6.25, 12.5, or 25 mg	Lotensin HCT
Captopril, 25 or 50 mg/hydrochlorothiazide, 15 or 25 mg	Capozide*
Enalapril maleate, 5 or 10 mg/hydrochlorothiazide, 12.5 or 25 mg	Vaseretic
Moexipril HCl 7.5 or 15 mg/hydrochlorothiazide 12.5 or 25 mg	Univasc
Quinapril HCl 10 or 20 mg/hydrochlorothiazide 12.5 or 25 mg	Accupril
Lisinopril, 10 or 20 mg/hydrochlorothiazide, 12.5 or 25 mg	Prinzide, Zestoretic
Angiotensin II receptor antagonists and diuretics	
Candesartan cilexetil 16 or 32 mg/hydrochlorothiazide 12.5 mg	Atacand HCT
Eprosartan mesylate 600 mg/hydrochlorothiazide 12.5 or 25 mg	Teveten HCT
Irbesartan 75, 150, or 300 mg/hydrochlorothiazide 12.5 mg	Avalide
Losartan potassium, 50 or 100 mg/hydrochlorothiazide, 12.5 mg	Hyzaar
Telmisartan 40 or 80 mg/hydrochlorothiazide 12.5 mg	Micardis HCT
Valsartan 80 or 160 mg/hydrochlorothiazide 12.5 mg	Diovan HCT
Calcium antagonists and ACE inhibitors	
Amlodipine besylate, 2.5 or 5 mg/benazepril hydrochloride, 10 or 20 mg	Lotrel
Verapamil hydrochloride (extended release), 180 or 240 mg/trandolapril, 1, 2, or 4 mg	Tarka
Felodipine, 5 mg/enalapril maleate, 5 mg	Lexxel
Diuretic and diuretic	
Triamterene, 37.5, 50, or 75 mg/hydrochlorothiazide, 25 or 50 mg	Dyazide, Maxzide
Spironolactone, 25 or 50 mg/hydrochlorothiazide, 25 or 50 mg	Aldactazide
Amiloride hydrochloride, 5 mg/hydrochlorothiazide, 50 mg	Moduretic
Central acting drug and diuretic	
Methyldopa, 250 or 500 mg/hydrochlorothiazide, 15, 25, 30, or 50 mg	Aldoril
Reserpine, 0.125 mg/hydrochlorothiazide, 25 or 50 mg	Hydropres
Reserpine, 0.125 or 0.25 mg/chlorothiazide, 250 or 500 mg	Diupres

*Approved for initial therapy.

Adapted from The JNC 7 Report. (2003). The Seventh Report of the Joint National Committee on Prevention, Detection, Evaluation, and Treatment of High Blood Pressure. *JAMA, 289*, 2560-2572.

I.   Drug interactions may be helpful or harmful (see Table DRUG INTERACTIONS)

DRUG INTERACTIONS

Class of Agent	Increase Efficacy	Decrease Efficacy	Effect on Other Drugs
Diuretics	• Diuretics that act at different sites in the nephron (e.g., furosemide + thiazides)	• Resin-binding agents • NSAIDs • Steroids	• Diuretics raise serum lithium levels • Potassium-sparing agents may exacerbate hyperkalemia due to ACE inhibitors
Beta-blockers	• Cimetidine • Quinidine • Food	• NSAIDs • Withdrawal of clonidine • Agents that induce hepatic enzymes, including rifampin and phenobarbital	• Beta-blockers may mask and prolong insulin-induced hypoglycemia • Heart block may occur with nondihydropyridine calcium channel blockers • Beta-blockers increase angina-inducing potential of cocaine
ACE inhibitors	• Chlorpromazine or clozapine	• NSAIDs • Antacids • Food decreases absorption (moexipril)	• ACE inhibitors may raise serum lithium levels • ACE inhibitors may exacerbate hyperkalemic effect of potassium-sparing diuretics

(Continued)

DRUG INTERACTIONS *(CONTINUED)*

Class of Agent	Increase Efficacy	Decrease Efficacy	Effect on Other Drugs
Calcium channel blockers	• Grapefruit juice (some dihydropyridines) • Cimetidine or ranitidine (hepatically metabolized calcium channel blockers)	• Agents that induce hepatic enzymes, including rifampin and phenobarbital	• Cyclosporine levels increase[H] with diltiazem hydrochloride, verapamil hydrochloride, mibefradil dihydrochloride, or nicardipine hydrochloride (but not felodipine, isradipine, or nifedipine) • Nondihydropyridines increase levels of other drugs metabolized by the same hepatic enzyme system, including digoxin, quinidine, sulfonylureas, and theophylline • Verapamil hydrochloride may lower serum lithium levels
Alpha-blockers			• Prazosin may decrease clearance of verapamil hydrochloride
Central alpha₂-agonists and peripheral neuronal blockers		• Tricyclic antidepressants • Monoamine oxidase inhibitors • Sympathomimetics or phenothiazines antagonize guanethidine monosulfate or guanadrel sulfate • Iron salts may reduce methyldopa absorption	• Methyldopa may increase serum lithium levels • Severity of clonidine hydrochloride withdrawal may be increased by beta-blockers • Many agents used in anesthesia are potentiated by clonidine hydrochloride

[H]This is a clinically and economically beneficial drug-drug interaction because it both retards progression of accelerated atherosclerosis in heart transplant recipients and reduces the required daily dose of cyclosporine.

Adapted from National High Blood Pressure Education Program, National Institutes of Health, National Heart, Lung, and Blood Institute. (1997). *The Sixth Report of the Joint National Committee on Detection, Evaluation, and Treatment of High Blood Pressure* (NIH Publication No. 98-4080). Bethesda, MD: US Government Printing Office.

J. Long-term therapy
    1. For chronic maintenance, use 24-hour formulations whenever possible to cover morning surge in B/P, for smooth persistent control, and to enhance compliance
    2. After BP is controlled for 1 year, consider decreasing dosages and/or number of drugs
    3. Recommend a baby aspirin (81-160mg/day) or one ASA 325 mg/day to improve cardiovascular outcomes over that expected with effective BP control alone

K. Overview of classes of antihypertensive agents
    1. Diuretics:
        a. Advantages: Inexpensive, effective, have additive and synergistic effects with other drugs, and in small doses have few adverse effects
        b. Disadvantages: In higher doses have adverse effects such as impaired glucose tolerance, increased lipids, electrolyte imbalance; approximately 15-30% of patients become hypokalemic on hydrochlorothiazide; consider the following for patients with hypokalemia:
            (1) Monitor magnesium (magnesium deficiency is often associated with hypokalemia)
            (2) Prescribe K+ supplement such as K-Dur 20 mEq tablets (take one tablet at breakfast and one at dinner) or a K+ sparing diuretic
        c. Types:
            (1) Thiazides: More effective than loop diuretics except in patients with serum creatinine >221 mmol/L (2.5 mg/dL)
            (2) Loop diuretic: Use in patients with renal impairment
            (3) Potassium sparing agents
                (a) Avoid or reverse hypokalemia from other diuretics; may cause hyperkalemia, particularly when combined with an ACE inhibitor or potassium supplement
                (b) Avoid when serum creatinine is >221 mmol/L (2.5 mg/dL)
    2. Beta-blockers
        a. Beta-blockers are classified as either with intrinsic sympathomimetic activity (ISA) or without ISA; both types are equally effective, but those without ISA were found to reduce nonfatal myocardial infarctions (MI), sudden death, and all-cause mortality
        b. Beta-blockers are somewhat less effective in treating African American and elderly patients
        c. May cause depression and fatigue in some patients
        d. Use cautiously with calcium channel blockers as this combination, although quite effective, increases risk for bradycardia and/or heart block

3. Alpha-blockers
   a. An alpha blocker is **absolutely contraindicated as first line drug for monotherapy** as researchers found a 25% higher risk for major CV events associated with doxazosin and a doubling of the risk for development of heart failure
   b. May be used cautiously as second or third drug in regimen; causes postural effects so titrate based on standing blood pressure; start first dose at bedtime; start low and titrate slowly
   c. Beneficial in patients with benign prostatic hypertrophy
4. Central alpha agonists
   a. No longer widely used because they depress central nervous system, cause fatigue, lethargy, and cognitive impairment
   b. Helpful in patients with panic attacks; methyldopa is drug of choice for HTN in pregnancy
5. Peripheral acting adrenergic antagonists: Rarely used; adverse reactions include postural hypotension, impotence, diarrhea, weight gain, and depression (reserpine)
6. Calcium channel blockers (CCB)
   a. Mechanism of action
      (1) The non-dihydropyridines, verapamil and diltiazem, reduce heart rate, slow ventricular conduction, and depress contractility (may reduce sinus rate and produce heart block), therefore more effective in rate control than BP control
      (2) Dihydropyridines have little effect on contractility and conduction but are good peripheral vasodilators (may cause dizziness, headache, edema, and tachycardia)
   b. Short acting dihydropyridines, particularly nifedipine, should no longer be used because of increased risk of MI and mortality after MI
   c. Extended release forms of the dihydropyridines are still used effectively in BP management and are better agents at reducing BP than the non-dihydropyridine derivatives
   d. In those with isolated systolic hypertension, who remain at increased risk of stroke, the initial use of CCB therapy continues to be supported by trial-based evidence
7. ACE Inhibitors
   a. ACE inhibitors are good initial selections, particularly if the patient has concomitant disease
   b. Effective as monotherapy in patients with left ventricular dysfunction, after MI, in diabetes; not as effective as monotherapy in African American patients unless used with a diuretic
   c. Few side effects except ticklish dry cough, particularly in older, female, white or Asian patients, and patients with chronic heart failure; one alarming side effect is angioedema
   d. Avoid or use with caution in combination with potassium supplements, salt substitutes, or potassium-sparing diuretics; may need to adjust doses if used with hypoglycemic agents
   e. A short-acting agent such as captopril (Capoten) may be useful as initial drug to determine effectiveness and patient's reactions; for chronic maintenance switch to long-acting agent
   f. ACE inhibitors in low doses are protective of the kidneys in patients with concomitant HTN and chronic renal insufficiency (CRI) with creatinine <2.3, with or without heart failure; contraindicated in advancing renal failure
8. Angiotensin II receptor blockers (ARB)
   a. Main advantage over ACE inhibitors is the lack of undesirable side effects, specifically cough and angioedema
   b. Only modestly increases potassium levels
   c. Similar to ACE inhibitors in reducing proteinuria and may have an even better positive effect on creatinine levels in patients with CRI
9. Aldosterone blocker, eplerenone (Inspra), recently approved for treatment of hypertension

L. Special situations
1. Frequently monitor BP in **women on oral contraceptives and estrogen replacement therapy**
2. **Older persons** have orthostatic falls in BP; measure BP standing and in seated or supine position
   a. Cautiously use drugs that increase postural changes in BP (peripheral adrenergic blockers, alpha-blockers, and high dose diuretics) or drugs that cause cognitive dysfunction (central alpha$_2$-agonist)
   b. Lower initial doses may be needed but standard doses and multiple drugs are needed by majority
3. **Isolated systolic hypertension** (ISH): In older persons with stage 2 or 3 ISH, diuretics and dihydropyridine CCB have been found to reduce morbidity and mortality
4. Patients with **chronic renal insufficiency** with greater than 1 gram per day of proteinuria should be treated toward a goal BP of 125/75 mm Hg or less; those with less proteinuria should have goal BP of 130/80 mm Hg; ACE inhibitors or ARBs are recommended
5. Patients with **diabetes** should have target BP goal of 130/80 mm Hg or less; ACE inhibitors or ARBs are recommended; thiazide diuretics, beta-blockers, and CCBs are also good choices
6. Aim for a goal BP of less than 120/75 mmHg in patients with **heart failure**; in fact, a SBP closer to 100 mm Hg, <u>without producing symptoms of hypotension</u>, is optimal

7. In **African Americans**, prevalence, severity and impact of hypertension are increased; may have reduced response to monotherapy with beta blocker, ACE inhibitors, or ARBs

8. **Low dose aspirin therapy** should be considered when BP is controlled because risk of hemorrhagic stroke is increased in patients with uncontrolled hypertension

M. **Resistant or refractory hypertension**: BP that cannot be reduced below 140/90 mm Hg in patients adhering to adequate and appropriate triple-drug regimen which includes diuretic and drugs prescribed at maximum dosage or SBP which cannot be reduced below 160 mm Hg in older patients with ISH
   1. Consider the following:
      a. White coat hypertension
      b. Incorrect measurement techniques
      c. Inadequate doses or inappropriate drug combinations
      d. Volume overload (renal damage, excess salt intake, inadequate diuretic therapy)
      e. Drug-related causes (drug interactions, drug actions [NSAIDs, both nonselective and COX-2 inhibitors, may cause refractory HTN])
      f. Associated conditions (renal artery stenosis; dissecting aortic aneurysm, sleep apnea, chronic pain, increased alcohol intake, insulin resistance)
   2. Always consider nonadherence with therapeutic regimen if BP is not controlled
   3. Refer to specialist if goal BP cannot be achieved, especially if multiple comorbid diseases coexist

N. **Hypertensive crises**: Urgency versus emergency (see table that follows)
   1. Severe elevated BP alone, in the absence of clinical manifestations or new or progressive target organ damage, rarely requires *emergency* therapy, but rather requires *urgent* attention
   2. **Urgencies**: Situations in which it is desirable to reduce BP within a few hours to 24 hours (upper levels of stage 3 hypertension, without significant TOD, but may have significant headaches or vision disturbances)
   3. **Emergencies**:
      a. Situations that require immediate BP reduction to prevent or limit TOD (hypertensive encephalopathy, intracranial hemorrhage, papilledema, unstable angina, MI, heart failure, pulmonary edema, aneurysm, eclampsia)
      b. The initial goal of therapy is to reduce the mean arterial pressure by no more than 25% (within minutes to 2 hours) then toward 160/100 mm Hg in 2 to 6 hours
   4. Parenteral drugs should be used for emergencies; oral doses of ACE inhibitors, alpha$_2$-agonists, beta-blockers, or calcium channel blockers can be used for urgencies
   5. Do **NOT** administer sublingual fast-acting nifedipine because of potential serious adverse effects

PHARMACOLOGIC TREATMENT FOR HYPERTENSIVE URGENCIES AND EMERGENCIES

Drug Class with Example(s) and Dosage	Monitoring	Comments
HYPERTENSIVE URGENCIES		
ACE Inhibitors -Captopril (Capoten)—first-line agent 25 mg PO; may repeat in 30 min -Enalapril (Vasotec)—second-line agent 5 mg PO, may repeat in 30 min	BP should be checked at 15-min intervals over first hour, at 30-min intervals over second hour, then hourly	Very effective first-line therapy in hypertensive *urgency* with diastolic BP >110 mm Hg when patient has no end-organ problems and oral treatment over several hours is indicated
Centrally Acting Alpha$_2$ Agonist Clonidine (Catapres) 0.1-0.2 mg loading dose, followed by 0.1 mg every 20 min to 1 hr up to 0.7-0.8 mg total	Monitor level of consciousness BP should be checked at 15-min intervals over first hour, at 30-min intervals over second hour, and then hourly	• Effective second-line treatment of hypertensive urgency • Sedation is a common side effect • After 8 hrs, clonidine dosing may begin again if necessary
Adrenergic Inhibitor -Labetalol is the most commonly used agent in this group—see under Hypertensive Emergencies for discussion -Oral dose determined per patient situation	BP should be checked at 15-min intervals over first hour, at 30-min intervals over second hour, and then hourly	• Effective second-line treatment of hypertensive urgency • Be particularly watchful for the development of heart block—adrenergic blockade of normal cardiac conduction

(Continued)

Calcium Channel Blockers

Diltiazem (Cardizem) and verapamil (Calan) are drugs of choice in this category but are currently used cautiously; therapy must be completely individualized	• Monitor pulse closely • BP should be checked at 15-min intervals over first hour, at 30-min intervals over second hour, and then hourly	• May be effective and efficient choice if BP elevation is secondary to a tachyarrhythmia • Be particularly watchful for the development of heart block—adrenergic blockage of normal cardiac conduction • Sublingual nifedipine or a fast-acting form of nifedipine is now **contraindicated** in the treatment of hypertensive emergency

HYPERTENSIVE EMERGENCIES (Drugs listed in order of rapidity of action, with most rapid listed first)

Vasodilators

-Sodium nitroprusside (Nipride) 0.25-10 µg/kg/min as IV infusion (maximal dose for 10 min only) -Fenoldopam mesylate 0.1-0.3 µg/kg/min as IV infusion -Nitroglycerine 5-200 µg/kg/min as IV infusion -Nicardipine hydrochloride 5-15 mg/h IV -Hydralazine hydrochloride 10-20 mg IV 10-50 mg IM -Enalaprilat 1.25-5 mg q 6 h IV	• For all of these drugs, careful and continuous monitoring of IV lines and blood pressure is essential • Monitor for too rapid a fall in BP or increase in pulse • Monitor for side effects; most cause GI disturbance in varying degrees such as nausea/vomiting, tachycardia, headache, flushing, sweating—all secondary to increased vasodilation • IV use of these drugs restricted to hospital emergency room and intensive care settings; drug titration continued until normotensive status prevails and persists	• Nipride, fenoldopam, and nicardipine are most commonly used in hypertensive emergencies, with certain precautions to indicate which drug to use in a given situation • Nitroglycerine is drug of choice when coronary ischemia is also present (may use with extreme caution in combination with sodium nitroprusside) • Enalaprilat may be most effective with acute left ventricular failure; however, it must be avoided in acute myocardial infarction

Adrenergic Inhibitors

-Esmolol hydrochloride 250-500 µg/kg/min IV for 1 min, then 50-100 µg/kg/min for 4 min; may repeat sequence -Phentolamine 5-15 mg IV -Labetalol hydrochloride 20-80 mg IV bolus q 10 min 0.5-2.0 mg/min IV infusion	In addition to foregoing outcome and monitoring considerations, be particularly watchful for development of heart block—adrenergic blockade of normal cardiac conduction	• Labetalol is the only one of this group that is commonly used for most hypertensive emergencies, except in acute heart failure • All of these drugs may be used in combination with vasodilators to increase effectiveness • Esmolol and phentolamine are reserved for specific underlying causes of increased blood pressure (i.e., aortic dissection and catecholamine excess, respectively)

O. Follow Up
1. Patients treated with lifestyle modifications should be seen after 3-6 months; when their blood pressures are stabilized, they should be seen every 6-12 months
2. Patients who begin or change drug therapy should be seen every 1-2 weeks to 1 month until their BPs are stable (remember that many ACE Inhibitors, ARBs, and CCBs do not peak until 3-4 weeks); patients in Stage 2 or with complicating comorbid conditions should be seen more frequently
3. Once patients achieve target BP goals and BPs are stable, schedule visits for every 3-6 months
4. Patients with emergent and urgent hypertension should be seen within 24 hours
5. Elderly patients, patients with TOD, patients with co-morbidities, and patients with a history of emergent or urgent hypertensive episodes should be followed more closely

ISCHEMIC HEART DISEASE: CORONARY ARTERY DISEASE, STABLE ANGINA PECTORIS, AND THE ACUTE CORONARY SYNDROMES

I.   Definition: Ischemic heart disease (IHD) is the broad umbrella term used to describe heart diseases that occur as a result of inadequate oxygen and blood supply to the myocardium secondary to decreased blood flow through atherosclerotic coronary arteries; its clinical expressions range from the asymptomatic preclinical phase through stable angina pectoris (AP) to the acute coronary syndromes (ACS) and sudden cardiac death

   A.   Coronary artery disease (CAD): Primarily refers to atherosclerotic narrowing of the major epicardial coronary arteries

   B.   Angina pectoris (AP): Syndrome characterized by deep, poorly localized chest pain or arm discomfort
        1.   Stable AP: Chest discomfort is associated with physical exertion or emotional stress and relieved with rest or sublingual nitroglycerin
        2.   Unstable AP (UAP): Considered part of the acute coronary syndrome (see I.D.)
             a.   Involves chest or arm discomfort in which episodes are severe and prolonged and may occur at rest
             b.   Resultant acute myocardial ischemia is not of sufficient severity and duration to result in myocardial necrosis, but is often associated with unstable plaque disease and patients are at increased risk for myocardial infarction (MI)
        3.   Variant angina (Prinzmetal's angina): Syndrome of rest pain and reversible ST segment elevation without subsequent enzyme evidence of acute myocardial infarction

   C.   Acute myocardial infraction (AMI): Considered part of the acute coronary syndrome; an acute process of myocardial ischemia with sufficient severity and duration to result in permanent myocardial damage

   D.   Acute coronary syndrome (ACS): Any constellation of clinical signs and symptoms suggestive of unstable angina pectoris or acute myocardial infarction; ACS is used as a clinical classification because both unstable angina pectoris and acute MI initially present with similar signs and symptoms and, thus are initially managed in a similar fashion
        1.   All disorders falling within this syndrome involve an acute process of myocardial ischemia that is of sufficient severity and duration to cause damage/necrosis of cardiac musculature that can lead to permanent irreversible myocardial damage
        2.   ACS is classified into three categories:
             a.   Unstable angina pectoris (UAP)
             b.   Non–ST-segment elevation MI (NSTEMI)
             c.   ST-segment elevation MI (STEMI): Immediate reperfusion therapy should be considered

II. Pathogenesis

   A.   Coronary artery disease (CAD) is due to blockages consisting of fats, platelets and other debris that form fatty streaks, fibrous plaques, and complicated lesions in the large and medium-sized arteries of the heart
        1.   Fatty streaks (earliest lesions of atherosclerosis) are accumulation of lipid-filled smooth-muscle cells as well as tissue macrophages and fibrous tissue in focal areas of the intima; fatty streaks appear in all children by age 10
        2.   Fibrous plaques are elevated areas of intimal thickening and represent the most characteristic lesion of advancing atherosclerosis; appear in men before women and in the aorta before the coronary arteries
        3.   Complicated lesions are calcified fibrous plaques containing various degrees of necrosis, thrombosis, and ulceration; these are the lesions usually associated with symptoms

   B.   Angina pectoris (AP) is due to myocardial ischemia that occurs when the cardiac workload and myocardial oxygen demand exceed the ability of the coronary arteries to supply oxygenated blood; involves reversible myocardial ischemia resulting from significant underlying CAD

C. Acute Coronary Syndromes (ACS)
   1. In unstable angina pectoris, artery blockages may be large, ruptured or involve a lesion; a blood clot or thrombus may form around the damage which can be so large that blood flow is impeded or completely blocked; still reversible at this point
   2. In acute myocardial infarction, irreversible necrosis and cellular death occur when an atherosclerotic plaque completely blocks a major coronary artery or branch or a plaque ruptures with an associated thrombus that occludes the coronary lumen; immediate intervention can limit the amount of irreversible damage that will ultimately persist and scar

D. Risk factors for development of coronary artery disease:
   1. Age (men over age 40 years and postmenopausal women)
   2. Hypertension
   3. Hyperlipidemia
   4. Diabetes mellitus
   5. Cigarette smoking
   6. Family history of premature CAD (individual whose father died of CAD before the age of 60)

E. Possible risk factors include oral contraceptives, personality type, sedentary living, obesity (particularly with a truncal distribution), stress, and high stored iron levels

F. Other conditions may exacerbate symptoms secondary to myocardial ischemia:
   1. Aortic stenosis
   2. Hypertrophic cardiomyopathy
   3. Anemia
   4. Gastrointestinal bleeding
   5. Chronic obstructive pulmonary disease
   6. Arteriovenous (AV) fistula in dialysis patients

G. Other factors may play a role in the development of CAD:
   1. Destabilization of atherosclerotic plaques may result from inflammatory processes and infection; highly sensitive C-reactive protein (hsCRP) rises in presence of inflammation and may be a good marker of cardiac injury or a predictor of future cardiac events
      a. Infection with *Chlamydia pneumoniae* has been linked with CAD; reinfection with this pathogen may trigger an AMI
      b. Infection with *Helicobacter pylori* has a role in development of IHD
   2. Homocysteine, an amino acid, has been linked with increased risks of IHD
   3. Elevated fasting triglyceride levels have been associated with coronary risk
   4. Cardiovascular disease has been associated with pathogenic low-density lipoprotein modification due to oxidation damage by free radicals

III. Clinical Presentation

A. Ischemic heart disease (IHD)
   1. Leading non-traumatic cause of disability and death in US, but the incidence in IHD has declined by 20% over the last 20 years (rate of decline is slower among women then men)
   2. Men die earlier from IHD than women, but after age 60, one in 4 women as well as men die of IHD
   3. IHD is characteristically silent until critical stenosis, thrombosis, aneurysm, or embolus develop
   4. Signs and symptoms develop gradually as the atheroma extends in the vessels; fatigue, intermittent claudication, and mild angina on exertion are often the initial complaints

B. Stable angina pectoris (AP)
   1. Stable AP is often hard for the patient to describe, but typically involves poorly localized tightness, pressure, or aching in the chest or arm that lasts 5 minutes or less
   2. Associated symptoms include dyspnea, nausea or vomiting, gas, sweating, dizziness, weakness, lightheadedness, presyncope/syncope, and palpitations
   3. Chronic stable AP is controlled or relieved by rest and/or medications and there is no change in the frequency or pattern of 'break-through' ischemic pain within the preceding 6 weeks
   4. Patients have a good prognosis with an annual mortality rate of <4%; these patients are excellent candidates for reversal of IHD through risk reduction and lifestyle modifications

C. Variant angina (Prinzmetal's angina): Some patients have coronary vasospasms alone, but most patients have angiographically significant CAD

D. Acute Coronary Syndrome (ACS)
1. Unstable angina pectoris (UAP) has three principal presentations:
   a. Angina that is no longer relieved by rest or medications; angina is usually >20 minutes
   b. New-onset severe angina
   c. Acceleration of angina: Increase in frequency, severity, and/or duration of occurrence; marked limitations of ordinary physical activity (walking 1-2 blocks on level ground and climbing one flight of stairs) or inability to carry on any physical activity without discomfort
   d. **Note**: Ischemia confirmed by ST-segment changes in association with recurrent rest pain, by a positive or unequivocal stress test, or by presence of small elevations in troponin that do not meet the criteria for MI is consistent with UAP
2. AMI: Classified as non-ST-segment elevation MI or ST-segment elevation MI
   a. Diagnosed by a typical rise and gradual fall of troponins or more rapid rise and fall of creatine kinase (CK-MB); often accompanied by Q waves and dynamic ST-segment change ≥1 mm on the electrocardiogram (ECG) (see section IV. D. for further details)
   b. Signs include S_3 gallop, rales, new or worsening mitral regurgitation murmur, and hypotension
   c. Typical symptoms: Severe ischemic discomfort that lasts more than 20-30 minutes and is not relieved by rest or sublingual nitroglycerin; substernal compression or crushing chest pain, pressure/heaviness in chest, and radiating pain in neck, jaw, shoulder, back or arms
   d. In US, about 25% of all MIs are "silent" or go undetected because of atypical presentations such as discomfort in arm, neck, back, or jaw without chest pain or pain radiation
   e. Women, diabetic patients, and elderly patients often have atypical chest pain and symptoms; elderly patients may have generalized weakness, stroke, syncope, or change in mental status
   f. Postinfarction angina pectoris, congestive heart failure, arrhythmias, and arterial embolus are common complications

IV. Diagnosis/Evaluation: Patients with chest pain >20 minutes need a rapid, focused evaluation to identify a potential AMI which may require immediate reperfusion therapy or other catastrophic conditions such aortic dissection; see V.K. for care of patient while awaiting transport to emergency room

A. History should be done at intervals with urgent and emergent needs addressed first
1. Ask patient to describe pain or discomfort: Ask about onset, location, radiation, quality, severity (use 0 –10 scale), duration, precipitating/aggravating factors, alleviating/relieving factors
2. Ask about associated symptoms such as arm and neck discomfort, shortness of breath, nausea or vomiting, gas, sweating, dizziness, weakness, presyncope/syncope, and palpitations
3. Carefully explore presence of symptoms suggestive of diseases other than myocardial ischemia or AMI (see differential diagnosis and section on CHEST PAIN); focus on the cardiovascular, pulmonary, musculoskeletal, gastrointestinal, and neurological/psychological systems
4. Inquire about past history or cardiac disease, particularly coronary artery bypass graft (CABG), CAD, angina, and AMI
5. Obtain a thorough personal and family medical history including congenital heart defects, diabetes, hyperlipidemia, hypertension, and sudden cardiac death, particularly in younger relatives
6. Inquire about personal or family history of risk factors for CAD
7. Explore medication history including nitroglycerin, prescription, over-the-counter, and herbal use; explore compliance with prescribed regimen
8. Ask about illicit drug use; particularly, ask about cocaine use in patients <40 years with suspected ACS (cocaine causes coronary vasospasm, thrombosis, increased heart rate and arterial pressure)
9. Ask about risk reduction strategies and lifestyle changes
10. Ask patient to describe support network, life and job stressors, use of alcohol, and exposure to certain environments such as cold or windy weather

B. Physical Examination
1. Observe general appearance, noting signs of distress such as dyspnea, pallor, diaphoresis, weakness, confusion
2. Frequently measure vital signs including blood pressure in both arms, heart rate, temperature
3. In certain patients, as time and severity of symptoms allows, measure fat distribution, obtain a waist to hip ratio, and use charts readily available to assess body mass index (BMI)
4. Perform a complete eye examination, including funduscopy
5. Examine neck for jugular venous distention, thyromegaly, and bruits
6. Perform a complete heart exam
7. Perform a complete exam of the lungs

8. Examine abdomen for organomegaly, pain on palpation of right or left upper quadrant and pain that radiates to back may indicate cholecystitis or pancreatitis, respectively; mid-epigastric pain radiating upward is suggestive of reflux disease, gastritis, or ulcers
9. Assess peripheral pulses; presence of bruits or pulse deficits identifies patients with higher likelihood of significant CAD
10. Assess extremities for edema, cyanosis, and clubbing
11. Perform musculoskeletal exam of the thorax, assessing for point tenderness in area of chest pain

C. Differential Diagnosis (also see section on CHEST PAIN for other conditions)
　1. Four main conditions mimic acute MI and need to be diagnosed, evaluated, and immediately treated (see table that follows)
　2. Any of these following problems can co-exist with evolving myocardial ischemia as precipitating etiologies and thus, concomitant myocardial ischemia/infarction should always be ruled out

FOUR SERIOUS CONDITIONS THAT MIMIC ACUTE MYOCARDIAL INFARCTION	
Condition	**Clinical Findings**
Acute pericarditis with or without tamponade	Pericardial friction rub Tamponade is associated with pulsus paradoxus and narrowed pulse pressure
Aortic dissection	Pain in back, asymmetry of pulses and blood pressures in both arms, murmur or aortic regurgitation, widening pulse pressure
Spontaneous pneumothorax	Acute dyspnea, pleuritic chest pain, absent breath sounds
Pulmonary emboli	Pleuritic chest pain, tachypnea, wheezing, hemoptysis

　3. The following features are **not** characteristic of myocardial ischemia and point to a noncardiac source of chest pain but do **not** exclude the possibility of a cardiac cause (see table that follows)

CLINICAL FEATURES THAT ARE NOT CHARACTERISTIC OF MYOCARDIAL ISCHEMIA
➡ Pleuritic pain
➡ Pain or discomfort that is located primarily or only in the middle or lower abdominal region
➡ Pain that may be localized at the tip of one finger, particularly over the left ventricular apex
➡ Pain reproduced with movement or palpation of the chest wall or arms
➡ Very brief episodes of pain, lasting a few seconds or less
➡ Constant pain, lasting many hours
➡ Pain radiating into the lower extremities

D. Diagnostic Tests: Provide critical information for risk stratification of patients with IHD versus information on symptoms that are not clearly of a cardiac nature
　1. Patients with suspected AMI or unstable angina (resting chest pain >20 minutes or recent syncope or presyncope) should be immediately transferred to emergency department or chest pain specialty unit where the following diagnostic tests are recommended (also see section on CHEST PAIN for the description of the Erlanger Chest Pain Evaluation Protocol that is used to identify and exclude acute coronary syndromes [ACS])
　　a. 12-lead electrocardiogram (ECG); normal in approximately 25% of patients with angina (see table that follows for findings indicative of myocardial ischemia)

FINDINGS ON ELECTROCARDIOGRAM THAT INDICATE MYOCARDIAL ISCHEMIA OR DAMAGE
➡ Q waves (≥0.03 seconds in width & ≥1 mm in depth)
➡ ST-T wave elevation >1 mm in 2 or more contiguous leads
➡ ST-T wave depression of at least 0.5 mm in 2 or more contiguous leads
➡ Deep symmetrical T-wave inversion of at least 1 mm in two or more contiguous leads
➡ Location of myocardial stress, injury or infarction

　　b. Biochemical markers (see table for advantages and disadvantages of each): Order cardiac-specific troponin; creatine kinase (CK-MB) by mass assay is also acceptable
　　　(1) If patient has negative cardiac markers within 6 hours of onset of pain, another sample should be drawn in the 6- to 12-hour frame

(2) Serial enzymes may be discontinued provided patient's signs and symptoms have resolved; if enzymes are negative but significant symptoms persist, further evaluation is indicated

   c. Consider ordering the following:
  (1) Myoglobin or CK-MB subforms in addition to troponin for patients who present within 6 hours of symptom onset (tests are early markers of cardiac injury)
  (2) Highly sensitive C-reactive protein (hsCRP) and other markers of inflammation
  (3) Total CK (without MB), aspartate aminotransferase (AST, SGOT), beta-hydroxybutyric dehydrogenase and/or lactate dehydrogenase (LDH) have been replaced by troponins and CK-MB in most settings

BIOCHEMICAL MARKERS FOR EVALUATION OF PATIENTS WITH SUSPECTED MYOCARDIAL ISCHEMIA

Marker	Advantage	Disadvantage	Comment
Cardiac troponins	• Detection of recent MI up to 2 weeks after onset • Greater sensitivity and specificity than CK-MB	• Low sensitivity in very early phase of MI (<6 hrs after symptom onset) and requires repeat measurement at 8-12 hrs if negative • Limited ability to detect late minor reinfarction • May be released with myocardial injury of diverse origins (myocarditis, trauma)	Best biomarker of cardiac damage
CK-MB	• Rapid, cost-efficient, accurate assays • Ability to detect early reinfarction	• Present in low levels in healthy individuals • Elevated with severe skeletal muscle injury • Low sensitivity during early MI (<6 hrs after symptom onset) or later after symptom onset (>36 hrs) • Low sensitivity for minor myocardial damage (detectable with troponins)	Acceptable in most clinical circumstances
CK-MB Isoforms	• Early detection of MI (3-6 hrs)	• Specificity profiles similar to that of CK-MB • Current assays require special expertise	Useful for early detection of MI
Myoglobin	• Useful in early detection of MI • Useful in ruling out MI • High sensitivity	• Very low specificity in settings of skeletal muscle damage • Rapid return to normal range limits detection of later presentations of myocardial damage	Useful for early detection of MI

Adapted from Braunwald, E., Antman, E.M., Beasley, J.W., Califf, R.M., Cheitlin, M.D., Hochman, J.S., et al. (2002). ACC/AHA guideline update for the management of patients with unstable angina and non-ST-segment elevation myocardial infarction: A report of the American College of Cardiology/American Heart Association Task Force on Practice Guidelines (Committee on the Management of Patients With Unstable Angina). Available at: http://www.acc.org/clinical/guidelines/unstable/unstable.pdf.

  2. A variety of tests are available to establish a diagnosis of CAD and to quantify the severity of ischemic heart disease; order these tests for patients who are asymptomatic or whose clinical manifestations are consistent with stable angina or CAD and who are not in acute distress
  a. 12-lead electrocardiogram and cardiac biomarkers (see above table) to detect myocardial damage
  b. Chest x-ray provides information about heart size and heart failure and is helpful in ruling out pulmonary edema, pleural effusions, dilated aortic root, pneumonia or other lower respiratory tract diseases that may exacerbate ischemic symptoms
  c. Recommendations for noninvasive testing (see table that follows)

RECOMMENDATIONS OF ACC/AHA FOR NONINVASIVE TESTING FOR THE DIAGNOSIS OF OBSTRUCTIVE CAD AND RISK STRATIFICATION IN ASYMPTOMATIC PATIENTS

- Exercise ECG testing without an imaging modality in asymptomatic patients with possible myocardial ischemia on ambulatory ECG (AECG) monitoring or with severe coronary calcification on electron-beam computed tomography (EBCT) in the absence of one of the following ECG abnormalities:
  - ✓ Pre-excitation (Wolff-Parkinson-White) syndrome
  - ✓ Electronically paced ventricular rhythm
  - ✓ More than 1 mm of ST depression at rest
  - ✓ Complete left bundle-branch block
- Exercise perfusion imaging or exercise echocardiography in asymptomatic patients with possible myocardial ischemia on AECG monitoring or with severe coronary calcification on EBCT who are able to exercise and have one of the following baseline ECG abnormalities:
  - ✓ Pre-excitation (Wolff-Parkinson-White) syndrome
  - ✓ More than 1 mm of ST depression at rest
- Adenosine or dipyridamole myocardial perfusion imaging in patients with severe coronary calcification on EBCT but with one of the following baseline ECG abnormalities:
  - ✓ Electronically paced ventricular rhythm
  - ✓ Left bundle-branch block
- Adenosine or dipyridamole myocardial perfusion imaging or dobutamine echocardiography in patients with possible myocardial ischemia on AECG monitoring or with coronary calcification on EBCT who are unable to exercise
- Exercise myocardial perfusion imaging or exercise echocardiography should be performed if exercise treadmill ECG testing in asymptomatic patients results in intermediate-risk or high-risk Duke treadmill score
- Adenosine or dipyridamole myocardial perfusion imaging or dobutamine echocardiography should be performed if exercise treadmill ECG testing in asymptomatic patients results in inadequate exercise ECG

Adapted from Gibbons, R.J., Abrams, J., Chatteerjee, K., Daley, J., Deedwania, P.C., Douglas, J.S., et al. (2003). ACC/AHA 2002 guideline update for the management of patients with chronic stable angina—summary article: A report of the American College of Cardiology/American Heart Association Task Force on Practice Guidelines (Committee on the Management of Patients with Chronic Stable Angina). *Journal of American College of Cardiology, 42,* 159-168.

(1) Exercise ECG testing is contraindicated in patients with UAP, uncontrolled hypertension, suspected severe valvular disease, decompensated heart failure (HF), neurological or orthopedic disease that may make it hazardous to walk on treadmill

(2) Exercise echocardiogram images assess cardiac architecture, wall motion, valves, performance of left ventricle at rest and during peak exercise (achievement of target heart rate)

    (a) Negative result: No evidence of ischemic symptoms or echocardiogram changes and the patient reaches target heart rate

    (b) Positive result: Ischemic symptoms (discomfort), ST changes, or new ST shift develops

    (c) Unequivocal result: Submaximal test (stopped for other non-cardiac reasons before target heart rate reached) with minimal or no change on echocardiogram

(3) Adenosine or dipyridamole myocardial perfusion imaging may be helpful if stress echocardiogram alone is insufficient for diagnosing condition

    (a) Augments information from regular stress echocardiogram by pinpointing existing areas of ischemia, identifying affected artery(ies), detecting old versus new MI, and revealing if stress induces changes in echocardiogram

    (b) If patient is high risk for bronchospasm use of adenosine is contraindicated in most cases

    (c) Dipyridamole thallium test is infrequently used because adenosine produces better results with less adverse effects

d. A complete resting echocardiogram with 2-dimensional color Doppler to immediately assess cardiac architecture, wall motion, valve performance and flow gradients, and performance of left ventricle (ejection fraction) may also be of benefit in patients with unknown CAD status or for an update on a patient with known disease whose status has changed

e. PET scan is best test to differentiate the viability and extent of ischemia versus infarction; usually not needed and is expensive

f.   Cardiac catheterization is recommended for patients with high-risk criteria that suggest ischemia on noninvasive testing (i.e., persistent symptoms of UAP, confirmed elevations in cardiac enzymes, ECG changes, and/or positive or unequivocal stress test results). **Note**: If patient has significant symptoms upon admission with acute ST changes (particularly ST-elevation), immediate heart catheterization is warranted

    (1)   Gold standard for diagnosis of CAD

    (2)   Allows direct visualization of coronary arteries via fluoroscopic arteriography

    (3)   Provides evidence of wall motion and ejection fraction as well as other hemodynamic parameters

    (4)   Delineates lesions and assists in determining whether percutaneous transluminal coronary angioplasty (PTCA) with or without other intervention (e.g. cutting balloon, stent) is indicated or if coronary artery bypass graft (CABG) would be best option

g.   Research indicates that high sensitivity C-reactive protein (hs-CRP) is a good indicator of severity of injury or predictor of future cardiac events

    (1)   Not recommended for widespread use to screen the entire adult population; in patients with stable coronary disease or ACS, hs-CRP measurement may be useful as an independent marker of prognosis for recurrent events, including death, MI, and restenosis after percutaneous coronary intervention

    (2)   First assess traditional cardiovascular disease risk factors and calculate an absolute Framingham risk score before considering hs-CRP testing

    (3)   Consider test for moderate-risk patients (10% to 20% risk of developing coronary heart disease in the next 10 years) to tip the scale for more aggressive treatment to prevent heart disease

    (4)   hs-CRP results should be expressed as mg/L only

    (5)   Measure hs-CRP twice (about 2 weeks apart) and then use the average

    (6)   Do not test patients with obvious inflammatory or infectious conditions such as rheumatoid arthritis or gingivitis because these conditions elevate hs-CRP levels

    (7)   If hs-CRP level is >10 mg/L, test should be repeated and patient examined for infection or inflammation

    (8)   Serum hs-CRP level of <1.0 mg/L is considered low risk; 1.0-3.0 mg/L is considered average risk; and >3.0 mg/L is considered high risk

h.   Homocysteine concentrations may be useful in patients with a strong family history of CAD

i.   Additional tests include CBC with differential, complete metabolic panel including liver enzymes, fasting blood sugar analysis, fasting lipid panel, thyroid function tests, lipase, amylase, bilirubin, and brain natriuretic peptide (BNP) may be beneficial

3.   New diagnostic methods:

a.   Intravascular ultrasound (IVUS) is a promising new technique used during a heart catheterization to view the vessel and plaque dimensions from within the artery; direct comparison with traditional angiography shows IVUS to be a better predictor of percentage of luminal blockage and indicator of exact lesion proportions

b.   Electron-beam computed tomography (EBCT) is a new noninvasive method of detecting atherosclerosis of the coronary arteries through visualization of calcium deposits in the vessel wall; further research is needed regarding efficacy of method and value of the results

c.   Transthoracic coronary Doppler flow echocardiography is a simple, inexpensive, and validated technique for noninvasively measuring coronary flow reserve, detecting lesions in the left anterior descending artery, but is ineffective in visualizing other arteries; insufficient research is available to determine its role

V.   Plan/Management (see websites of the American College of Cardiology [www.acc.org] and the American Heart Association [www.americanheart.org] for updates of management guidelines)

A.   Primary prevention of the major modifiable risk factors for CAD:

1.   Complete cessation of smoking is strongly recommended (see section on SMOKING CESSATION)

2.   Lipid management with primary goal of low density lipids (LDL) <100 mg/dL and secondary goals of non-HDL cholesterol (<130 mg/dL), high density lipids (HDL) >40 mg/dL, and triglycerides (TG) <150 (see section on DYSLIPIDEMIA)

3.   Three dietary strategies are effective in CAD prevention:

a.   Substitution of nonhydrogenated unsaturated fats for saturated hydrogenated, and *trans*-fats

b.   Increased consumption of fruits, vegetables, nuts, and whole grains and decreased consumption of refined grain products

c.   Increased consumption of omega-3 fatty acids from fish, fish oil supplements, or plant sources; for example, at least 2 servings per week of fish is recommended (see table that follows)

RECOMMENDATIONS FOR OMEGA-3 FATTY ACID INTAKE	
Population	**Recommendation**
Patients without documented CHD	Eat a variety of (preferable oily) fish at least twice a week. Include oils and foods rich in α-linolenic acid (flaxseed, canola, and soybean oils; flaxseed and walnuts)
Patients with documented CHD	Consume about 1 g of EPA* + DHA* per day, preferable from oily fish. EPA + DHA supplements could be considered in consultation with the clinician
Patients needing triglyceride lowering	2-4 g of EPA + DHA per day provided as capsules under a clinician's care

*EPA = eicosapentaenoic acid   DHA = docosahexaenoic acid

Adapted from Kris-Etherton, P.M., Harris, W.S., Appel, L.J. for Nutrition Committee. (2002). Fish consumption, fish oil, omega-3 fatty acids, and cardiovascular disease. *Circulation, 106*, 2747-2757.

4. Maintenance of ideal body weight: Start intensive diet and appropriate physical activity intervention in patients >120% of ideal weight for height, particularly emphasize need for weight loss in patients with metabolic syndrome (waist circumference >102 cm (40 inches) in men or >88 cm (35 inches) in women; triglycerides >150 mg/dL; HDL cholesterol <40 mg/dL in men and <50 mg/dL in women; fasting serum glucose >110 mg/dL; blood pressure ≥130/85 mm Hg) (see section on OBESITY)

5. Therapy to lower non-HDL cholesterol in patients with documented or suspected CAD and triglyceride levels >200 mg/dL, with a target non-HDL cholesterol <130 mg/dL

6. Encourage regular exercise with the minimum goal of 30 minutes 3-4 times per week of moderate-intensity activity supplemented by an increase in daily lifestyle activities

7. Antiplatelet agents/anticoagulation: The US Preventive Services Task Force strongly recommends that clinicians discuss aspirin chemoprevention with adults who are at increased risk of CAD
   a. See II.D. through E. for risk factors or to calculate risk, use the "CV Risk Tool" at www.med-decisions.com or other tools at www.intmed.mcw.edu/clincalc/heartrisk.html
   b. Initiate aspirin 75-325 mg/d if not contraindicated
   c. For post-MI patients not able to take aspirin or when clinically indicated, consider clopidogrel (Plavix) 75 mg per day or warfarin (Coumadin) to reach International Normalized Ratio (INR) of 2.0-3.0

8. Control blood pressure with goal of 140/90 mm Hg; or <130/85 mm Hg if patient has heart failure, renal insufficiency, or diabetes (see section on HYPERTENSION)

9. Hormone replacement therapy (HRT) is no longer recommended for primary prevention
   a. Women taking HRT for established indications and who have vascular disease may continue to take HRT provided there are not better alternative therapies
   b. Discontinue HRT if a woman develops an acute CAD event
   c. Women who are immobilized should discontinue HRT or venous thromboembolism prophylaxis should be initiated

10. Other preventive therapies are still under investigation and cannot be recommended at present for expressed purpose of preventing CAD:
    a. Antioxidant therapy from diet or dietary supplementation of vitamin E (400 IU/day) or vitamin C (1,000-1,500 mg/day)
    b. Supplementation of folic acid 0.4 mg per day to reduce homocysteine levels
    c. Because of increased risk of negative sequelae and potential for cancer development, beta carotene is now contraindicated as a supplement

B. Treatment **in patients with stable angina who have infrequent anginal attacks**
   1. Correct treatable disorders: Hypertension, anemia, valvular disease, hyperthyroidism, and HF
   2. Treat risk factors (see V.A.)
   3. Initiate beta blocker (BB) or calcium channel blocker (CCB) therapy if patient is not already on secondary to coexisting conditions
   4. Angiotensin converting enzyme (ACE) inhibitors are recommended for routine secondary prevention for most patients with known CAD, particularly diabetics without severe renal disease
   5. Prescribe nitroglycerin (Nitrostat), 1 tablet (0.4 mg) sublingually or nitroglycerin spray (Nitrolingual) 1 spray onto or under tongue (do not inhale) on a prn basis (see table that follows)
   6. Sublingual nitroglycerin or lingual aerosol nitroglycerin may be prescribed for prophylactic use; instruct patient to take tablet or spray, wait 5-10 minutes, and then proceed with activity such as exercise or sexual intercourse

PATIENT EDUCATION FOR TREATMENT OF ANGINAL DISCOMFORT WITH NITROGLYCERIN

- ✓ Discontinue activity or remove self from stressful event when anginal discomfort lasts >2-3 minutes
- ✓ If pain does not subside immediately, sit down and take nitroglycerin
- ✓ Tell patient to wait 5 minutes before taking another dose (watch for signs and symptoms of hypotension—if these occur, stop taking NTG tabs and call 911)
- ✓ Instruct patient to **call 911** if pain is not relieved after 3 doses or if pain persists for >15-20 minutes
- ✓ Remind patient to keep tablets no longer than 3-4 months after opening the bottle and to keep in same brown bottle from which supplied
- ✓ Teach patients to not carry nitroglycerin bottle in pockets, especially on hot days (potency will be greatly reduced)
- ✓ Instruct patient that nitroglycerin is not an analgesic and that repeated use is not harmful or addictive
- ✓ Instruct patients to take the nitroglycerin at onset of pain
- ✓ Remind patient to call provider to make an office visit if taking NTG more frequently or if pain is more frequent or severe or is precipitated by less effort or now occurs at rest; keep journal recording pattern of anginal pain

C. **When the anginal attacks become more regular and predictable in patients with stable angina pectoris,** nitrates, beta-blocking (BB) agents or calcium channel blockers (CCB), and ACE inhibitors (particularly for diabetes without severe renal disease) are the mainstays of treatment and can be prescribed on a chronic basis (each of the drug classes will be described in further detail in sections D, E, F, and G that follow)
    1. Initially patients should be prescribed a BB as first line agent
    2. It is also now conventional to start with two drugs; BB and nitrates work well in combination
    3. CCBs are second line agents for patients whose symptoms persist despite treatment with nitrates and beta-blockers and to select patients in whom BBs are contraindicated as noted below
    4. If initial therapy fails, cautiously try triple drug therapy or substitute a drug
        a. Be careful in combining a BB with a negative inotropic calcium channel blocker such as verapamil or diltiazem; this combination can induce severe bradycardia or AV block
        b. BBs work well with amlodipine (Norvasc)
    5. In addition, prescribe an ACE inhibitor to reduce incidence of cardiovascular disease, myocardial infarction, and stoke in patients at high risk for, or have, vascular disease
    6. Selection of medication(s) depends on specific patient comorbid conditions (see section on HYPERTENSION IN ADULTS for details regarding BB, CCB and comorbid conditions)

D. Beta-blocking (BBs) agents decrease heart rate and contractility
    1. Advantages: Efficacy in angina prophylaxis and cardioprotective effects after AMI
    2. Disadvantages: May cause serious side effects, cannot be prescribed in certain patients (e.g., sinus bradycardia, sick sinus syndrome, vasospastic angina, and those prone to bronchospasm)
    3. Patients who have constant, effort-induced angina or chest pain, which develops consistently with walking a certain distance, are ideal candidates for BB
    4. The following BBs are possible agents, but other BBs are equally effective
        a. Metoprolol (Lopressor) 25-50 mg bid or Metoprolol CR (Toprol XL) 25-100mg per day
        b. Atenolol (Tenormin): Initially 50 mg once daily, may increase after one week to 100 daily which can be given in one or two divided doses
        c. Nadolol (Corgard): Initially 40 mg daily; increase if needed at 3-7 day intervals with usual maintenance dose of 40-80 mg daily and maximum dose of 240 mg daily

E. Long-acting nitrates are vasodilators and are widely used
    1. Advantages: Efficacy, multiple delivery routes, reasonably well tolerated, have modest antiplatelet effects, some products are inexpensive
    2. Two relative contraindications to long-acting nitrates are a history of migraine or cluster headaches and demonstrated orthostatic hypotension
    3. Isosorbide dinitrate (Isordil Titradose) is a good choice: Start with 5-20 mg every 4-6 hours orally; maintenance dose is 10-40 mg every 6 hours; allow a daily dose free interval of at least 14 hours
    4. Alternatively, use isosorbide mononitrate (Imdur) long-acting preparation; 20 mg bid or 30-60 mg daily initially, up to 120-240 mg depending on patient tolerance of dose level; headache or hypotension may occur with high doses
    5. Nitroglycerin 2% ointment (Nitro-Bid ointment) may be preferable: Apply ointment with an applicator, usually to chest and occlude; initially apply 1/2 inch BID; maximum dose is 2 inches BID
    6. Nitroglycerin patch (Transderm-Nitro patch) is convenient but expensive: Initially one 0.2 mg/hr or 0.4 mg/hr patch for 12-14 hrs/day; remove for 10-12 hours/day

7. The absorption of the drug when using either the patch or the ointment is dependent on the site used (i.e., epidermal thickness, vascularity and amount of hair); instruct patient to use on upper body and alternate sites
8. Although most patients experience headaches initially, the headaches can usually be relieved with acetaminophen and usually abate after 1-2 weeks

F. Calcium channel blockers (CCB) are another option; these agents dilate coronary arteries, prevent coronary vasospasm, and produce vasodilation
   1. Advantages: Prevent attacks, effectively treat attacks, useful in patients with coronary artery spasm, usually well tolerated, and may have a possible antiatherogenic effect
   2. Disadvantages: Serious adverse effects and nuisance adverse effects such as constipation and peripheral edema; do not have cardioprotective effects after a myocardial infarction
   3. Prescribe one of the following:
      a. Amlodipine (Norvasc): Initially 5 mg QD; may increase to 10 mg QD; few side effects, but is notorious for causing lower leg and ankle edema
      b. Nifedipine (Procardia XL) is the most potent vasodilator of this group of agents: initially 30-60 mg daily (take HS to reduce side effects). Titrate over 7-14 days with a maximum dose of 90 mg/day (use this drug cautiously in patients taking digitalis)
      c. Diltiazem HCl (Cardizem CD): Initially 120-180 mg once daily; titrate at 7-14 day intervals with maximum 480 mg daily (do not prescribe in patients who have an abnormal atrioventricular conducting system)
      d. Verapamil HCl (Calan): Initially 80 mg every 6-8 hours, increase daily or weekly with maximum daily dose of 480 mg (do not use in patients with left ventricular failure, sinus bradycardia or heart block)

G. ACE inhibitors improve outcomes, particularly in diabetics who do not have severe renal disease; one acceptable therapy is ramipril (Altace) 10 mg/day

H. Percutaneous transluminal coronary angioplasty (PTCA) with or without stent placement and CABG are options for patients with stable angina who cannot be controlled with medications

I. Alternative therapies for patients with stable angina refractory to medical therapies who are not candidates for percutaneous intervention or revascularization
   1. Spinal cord stimulation
   2. Enhanced external counterpulsation
   3. Surgical laser transmyocardial revascularization

J. Patients with **variant angina (Prinzmetal's angina)**
   1. Coronary spasms are usually relieved with nitroglycerin, long-acting nitrates, and CCBs
   2. Smoking cessation is important

K. Patients who present with signs and symptoms of **acute coronary syndrome (AMI or unstable angina)** need immediate transport to the hospital; call 911
   1. While awaiting transport to hospital, patients should be quickly assessed and kept quiet on bedrest
   2. Administer oxygen 2-4 liters by nasal prongs
   3. Give aspirin 160-325 mg; if an enteric-coated aspirin is the only preparation available, the tablet should be chewed or crushed
      a. There are no longer any absolute contraindications to use aspirin except allergy; there are relative contraindications such as those who have risk of hemorrhagic stroke
      b. Continue aspirin therapy 75-325 mg/d at least for 30 days; indefinitely is better
   4. Give nitroglycerin SL or spray every 5 minutes times three doses or until chest pain is perceived as '0' on scale of 0-10; monitor for hypotension and hold dose if blood pressure excessively drops
   5. Morphine is recommended when symptoms are not immediately relieved with nitroglycerin or when acute pulmonary congestion and/or severe agitation is present

L. **Initial, urgent care of patients with unstable angina (UAP), NON-ST-segment MI (NSTEMI), and ST-segment MI (STEMI)**; usually treated by a cardiology in hospital
   1. Antiplatelet therapy is the cornerstone of treatment; three classes of drugs are beneficial:
      a. Aspirin (ASA) should be initiated as soon as possible after symptom presentation and should be continued indefinitely

b. Clopidogrel (Plavix)
   (1) Administered if patient is unable to take ASA
   (2) Administered if patient is not planning to have catheterization and percutaneous transluminal coronary angioplasty (PTCA) or CABG or in patients planning to have PTCA or CABG and who are NOT at high risk for bleeding; add to ASA at admission and continue for up to 9 months
c. Platelet glycoprotein IIb/IIIa antagonists (abciximab [ReoPro], eptifibatide [Integrilin]); typically, administered in addition to ASA and heparin if cardiac catheterization and percutaneous transluminal coronary angioplasty (PTCA) are planned and may also be administered just prior to PTCA
2. Parenteral anticoagulant therapy with unfractionated heparin or subcutaneous low-molecular-weight heparin should be added to antiplatelet therapy
3. Management of pain is critical; patient should never have pain above a level of above "0"
4. In addition, one of the following treatment strategies are recommended:
   a. Early conservative strategy in which coronary angiography is reserved for patients with evidence of recurrent ischemia or a strongly positive stress test despite vigorous medical therapy
   b. Early invasive strategy in which patients without obvious contraindication to coronary revascularization are recommended for coronary angiography and if possible, angiographically directed revascularization with either PTCA with stenting or CABG

M. Care of **hospitalized patient with ST-segment MI (STEMI)**
   1. Antiplatelet and anticoagulant therapies should be given (see V.L.1.2.)
   2. Intravenous thrombolytic therapy or alternatively, PTCA, should be administered within the first 4-6 hours (or longer) after AMI; these therapies substantially reduce mortality if given within appropriate time frame but each has advantages and disadvantages
      a. Thrombolytic therapy with commonly used fibrinolytic agents streptokinase (Streptase), alteplase (TPA), tenecteplase (TNKase), or reteplase (Retavase) has adverse effects of bleeding and numerous contraindications for use (previous hemorrhagic stroke, known intracranial neoplasm, active or recent internal bleeding, suspected aortic dissection, severe uncontrolled hypertension, current use of anticoagulants in therapeutic doses, recent trauma, pregnancy)
      b. PTCA is gaining favor as preferred option, but must be performed in a facility with an effective primary PTCA team

N. **Post acute coronary syndrome (UAP/NSTEMI or STEMI) care** is based on the condition of the patient; initial plan is usually done in conjunction with a cardiologist
   1. A thorough patient education program is usually started in the hospital and followed after discharge; program should include nature of disease, cardiac drugs, modification of risk factors, and guidelines for resumption of employment, sexual activities, and physical exertion; patients should be encouraged to join a formalized cardiac rehabilitation program
   2. Selection of appropriate regimen is highly individualized and the mnemonic **ABCDE** (**A**spirin and antianginals; **B**eta-blockers and blood pressure; **C**holesterol and cigarettes; **D**iet and diabetes; **E**ducation and exercise) is useful in guiding treatment

O. **Pharmacological therapy** for patients with **acute coronary syndrome (UAP/NSTEMI or STEMI) following an acute event and/or for long-term management**
   1. Antiplatelet therapy (see V. A. 7.) (ASA and/or clopidogrel) is recommended
   2. Prescribe sublingual nitroglycerin as needed; prescribe long-acting nitrate therapy for patients with residual ischemia or break-through angina
   3. β-blockers reduce the risk of mortality, infarction, or reinfarction; particularly beneficial in higher-risk patients with electrical or mechanical complications, prior MIs, and compensated heart failure
      a. See V. D. 4 and section HYPERTENSION IN ADULTS for possible good choices
      b. Increase β-blockers to amount required to produce significant attenuation of heart rate and blood pressure response to exercise without causing significant side effects
      c. β-blockers should be administered within hours post-MI and therapy should continue for at least 2-5 years, preferably for life
   4. Consider prescribing an angiotensin converting enzyme (ACE) inhibitor (reduces mortality risks after acute MI, particularly in patients with anterior MI, left ventricular dysfunction [ejection fraction <40], heart failure, or diabetes); may prescribe one of following since they are all good choices:
      a. Captopril (Capoten) 3 days post-MI start with 6.25 mg, gradually increase to 12.5 mg TID, then increase to 25-50 mg TID; less attractive for long-term use because of TID dosing schedule
      b. Enalapril (Vasotec) initially 2.5 daily and slowly increase to maintenance dose of 10 mg BID

      c.   Ramipril (Altace) initially 2.5 mg BID and increase to usual maintenance dose of 5 mg BID
- (1)   Frequently used drug with documented efficacy
- (2)   Once a day dosing schedule enhances adherence
- (3)   Prescribe for 4-6 weeks; if <40% left ventricular ejection fraction or patient has symptoms of heart failure, ACE inhibitor should be continued for at least 3 years

5.   Routine use of CCBs is not usually recommended; amlodipine (Norvasc) 5-10 mg daily may be beneficial in patients with severe chronic heart failure and an ejection fraction <30%

6.   For patients with acute coronary syndrome, pre-discharge initiation of cholesterol-lowering agents has become the standard of care for those with hypercholesterolemia diagnosed on admission; post-discharge continuation of aggressive therapy is recommended
- a.   A fibrate or niacin is recommended if high-density lipoprotein cholesterol is <40 mg/dL, occurring as an isolated finding or in combination with other lipid abnormalities
- b.   HMG-CoA reductase inhibitor (statin) and diet for LDL cholesterol >100 mg/dL are recommended
- c.   The benefits of statins extend beyond their lipid-lowering effects; statins may improve clinical outcomes by improving endothelial and platelet function and reducing vascular inflammation

P.   Follow Up varies depending on the severity of the disease
1.   Encourage patients to enroll in a formal or home cardiac rehabilitation program
2.   Re-evaluate patients with stable angina every 2-6 months and have a repeat ECG and stress testing every 1-2 years; emphasize that patient should immediately call clinician if symptoms increase or pattern changes as additional testing and evaluation will be needed
3.   Low risk medically treated patients and revascularized patients who are stable should be seen in 2-6 weeks; thereafter, schedule return visits periodically
4.   High risk patients should return in 1-2 weeks and then need frequent visits depending on condition

PRESYNCOPE/SYNCOPE

I.   Definitions:

A.   Presyncope or Near Syncope: Sensation of dizziness, lightheadedness, and an impending loss of consciousness

B.   Syncope: Sudden transient loss of consciousness and loss of postural tone and motor control with spontaneous recovery

II.   Pathogenesis

A.   Usually due to any mechanism that decreases cerebral blood flow; results in decreased delivery of oxygen and nutrients to brain

B.   Pathophysiologic abnormalities underlying presyncope/syncope
1.   Neurocardiogenic types of syncope are associated with a reflex-mediated, vasomotor instability resulting from a decrease in vascular resistance and/or venous return causing peripheral venous and arterial pooling and subsequent decreased cerebral perfusion.
- a.   Conditions are usually benign and include vasovagal episodes, situational crises, orthostatic hypotension, drugs, and carotid sinus disorders
- b.   Vasodepressor syncope or the 'simple faint' occurs in response to stress and is the most common cause of presyncope/syncope, accounting for 20-40% of all syncopal episodes
2.   Cardiac causes associated with decreased cardiac output or obstruction of blood flow within heart or pulmonary circulation
- a.   Electrical etiology such as arrhythmias and heart block
- b.   Mechanical etiology such as idiopathic hypertrophic subaortic stenosis (IHSS) now referred to as hypertrophic obstructive cardiomyopathy (HOCM), valvular diseases, myxoma, myocardial infarction, and aortic dissection (due to rupture into the pericardial space causing a cardiac tamponade)
3.   Neurologic, vascular, or psychogenic causes include cerebrovascular diseases (due to hypoperfusion of the vertebrobasilar vascular system), subclavian steal syndrome, seizures, migraines, and psychiatric illnesses

4. Metabolic causes such as hypoglycemia, hypoxia, and hyperventilation; these disorders usually lead to somnolence and coma rather than syncope

C. Most common causes are vasovagal/vasodepressive episodes, heart disease, arrhythmias, orthostatic hypotension, and seizures

D. Approximately 48% of all patients who have syncope have an unexplained cause

III. Clinical Presentation of important causes of presyncope/syncope (elderly are at the greatest risk for most causes of presyncope/syncope)

A. Vasovagal, vasodepressor syncope (psychological activation of the stress-mediated autonomic system causes an intense vagal drive and transient decrease in cardiac output)
1. Often precipitated by trigger events that include noxious stimuli, unpleasant sights or smells, fear, anxiety, anticipated pain, alcohol, a large meal, micturition, defecation, cough, sneezing, or swallowing
2. Symptoms occur in the standing or seated position
3. Typically patient has prodromal symptoms such as nausea, warmth, lightheadedness, weakness, diaphoresis, constriction of visual fields, epigastric discomfort, and a sensation of impending faint
4. At first, patient has increased heart rate, but then becomes bradycardic
5. Unconsciousness is usually brief (seconds to minutes once the patient reaches the supine position) and in the recovery stage the patient may have weakness, lightheadedness, or fatigue, but no confusion or signs of injury; usually after the episode, the patient remembers the event and does not have loss of bowel and bladder control
6. Occasionally, hypotension and hypoperfusion are so profound that cerebral hypoxia and seizure activity occur, but there is no loss of consciousness or only a brief loss of consciousness

B. Orthostatic hypotension is common, particularly in the elderly
1. Reflex vasoconstriction and increase in heart rate fail to occur when the patient stands, leading to inadequate cerebral perfusion
2. Defined as systolic blood pressure fall of 20 mm Hg or more on standing
3. Possible etiologic factors
a. Condition may be idiopathic; often this type occurs after patient has been exposed to a warm environment
b. Medications such as diuretics and autonomic blocking agents
c. Blood loss often due to a gastrointestinal bleed
d. Dehydration

C. Drug-induced syncope is most likely when patients are taking nitrates, vasodilators, β-blockers, anti-Parkinson drugs, antidepressants, analgesics, and central nervous system antidepressants

D. Carotid sinus hypersensitivity
1. Occurs primarily in elderly patients who have underlying atherosclerotic disease
2. Condition is associated with pressure on carotid sinus which can occur with tumors and tissue scars in neck causing marked reflex bradycardia

E. Typical presentation of syncope due to cardiac disease
1. Symptoms often worsen on standing and improve with lying down; although patients with arrhythmias may have symptoms when supine
2. May have generalized weakness, fatigue, and pallor; some patients are asymptomatic
3. Syncope may be the presenting symptom in older patients with acute myocardial infarction
4. Sudden onset without warning, sensation of rapid heart action without aura, or seizure suggests cardiac origin
5. Exertional or effort syncope are common manifestations with advancing valvular aortic stenosis; patients with HOCM may also experience effort syncope
6. Patients who experience syncope due to underlying cardiac disease appear to be at increased risk of disease from all causes

F. Arrhythmias often present with brief loss of consciousness, lack of prodrome, and palpitations

G. Subclavian steal syndrome
   1. Occlusion of proximal subclavian artery leading to reversal of flow in the adjacent vertebral artery during arm exercise
   2. Blood flow is redirected from brain and ischemic symptoms develop
   3. Syncope occurs with arm exercise

H. Cerebrovascular disease; patients usually have visual, auditory, or vestibular symptoms

I. Seizures
   1. May have signs and symptoms of blue face, frothing at mouth, myoclonic jerks, tongue biting, tonic spasms, staring, or repetitive facial grimacing which are not common with other types of syncope
   2. Commonly associated with warning symptoms (auras) such as certain smells, sounds or visual cues; these warning *symptoms* differ from the *triggers* that can initiate a sudden vasovagal/vasodepressive syncopal episode
   3. After seizure, postictal symptoms such as disorientation and headache are common

J. Psychological distress often involves circumoral numbness and digital paresthesia
   1. History of generalized anxiety disorder, panic disorder, somatization, or depression is common
   2. Estimated that up to 20% of patients presenting with syncope have psychiatric illness
   3. Hysteria, a form of conversion reaction, may result in apparent loss of consciousness, especially if an audience is present, and is characterized by a graceful fainting to the floor while exhibiting otherwise normal vital signs and physical findings

IV. Diagnosis/Evaluation (see also section on DIZZINESS)

A. History; important to determine whether patient has serious disorder (e.g., cardiac disease, stroke, gastrointestinal bleeding, intracranial tumor) or a benign condition
   1. Ask patient to briefly describe in own words the sensation he/she experiences
   2. If possible obtain a description of the episode and events preceding the episode from a witness
   3. Differentiate feelings of fainting from vertigo, imbalance, fatigue, weakness, or anxiety; specifically ask the following types of questions:
      a. Is there a sensation of movement or rotation? (vertigo)
      b. Is the sensation similar to when you get out of bed too quickly? (orthostatic hypotension)
      c. Does it feel like you can't keep your balance? (disequilibrium)
   4. Ascertain that patient did not actually lose consciousness which may indicate an emergent problem
   5. Ask about frequency of syncopal or near syncopal episodes, even though frequency does not correlate well with specific causes
   6. Ask about duration of episode; brief duration is more common with vestibular disorders
   7. Inquire about associated symptoms such as hearing loss, heart palpitations, neurological problems
   8. Determine if sensation occurs after exertion or when one arises to sitting or standing position
      a. Disequilibrium occurs primarily when one is standing or walking
      b. Benign positional vertigo often occurs with a change of position or when lying down
   9. Determine precipitants such as cough with loss of consciousness (post-tussive syncope), emptying of distended bladder (postmicturition syncope), warm, crowded environment (simple faint), or shaving or tight collar (carotid sinus hypersensitivity)
   10. Ask about symptoms occurring after episode; disorientation after an event is most common in patients who have seizures
   11. Inquire about past medical history including history of cardiac disease or risk factors, trauma, infection, seizures, thyroid disease, metabolic problems, anxiety, and medication/drug use

B. Physical Examination
   1. Vital signs should include check for orthostatic hypotension (see following table)

DETERMINING ORTHOSTATIC HYPOTENSION

➡ Measure in lying (ideally) or sitting position first

➡ Measure immediately after standing and then, after patient stands for 2-5 minutes, measure again

➡ Normally, systolic pressure falls no more than 10 mm Hg, diastolic pressure rises 2-5 mm Hg, and heart rate increases 5-20 beats (if there is no increase in heart rate, consider a cardiac problem). A drop in systolic pressure of 20 mm Hg or more indicates orthostasis

---

2. Measure blood pressure in both arms; differences in pulse intensity and blood pressure (more than 20 mm Hg) in two arms suggests aortic dissection and subclavian steal syndrome
3. Perform cardiac examination noting forceful left ventricular impulse, murmurs, or arrhythmias
4. Auscultate neck for carotid bruits
5. Perform a thorough neurological examination
6. Perform dizziness simulation tests such as following:
   a. Valsalva maneuver
   b. Carotid sinus massages help to determine autonomic impairment; tests should be done cautiously in facilities where cardiac monitoring and emergency equipment are available; if patient has bruits or history of cardiac or cardiovascular disease, massage should be performed by a specialist
7. Determine if hyperventilation evokes symptomatology by asking patient to breathe rapidly for 1-3 minutes
8. Other special tests:
   a. Ask patient to flex and extend arm at least 10 times to reproduce symptoms of subclavian steal syndrome
   b. Ask patient to flex and extend neck to reproduce symptoms of vertebrobasilar insufficiency
9. Complete psychological examination may be helpful

C. Differential Diagnosis: One way to sort out the many causes of dizziness is to differentiate the sensations the patient experiences into 3 categories:
   1. Presyncope/syncope: Feeling of lightheadedness or feeling that one is about to faint
   2. Vertigo: Sensation of abnormal movements of the body or surroundings (see section on DIZZINESS)
   3. Disequilibrium or imbalance due to multiple sensory deficits: Sensation of feeling drunk, seasick, or unsteady on one's feet; subtle, enduring symptom that one cannot keep balance and might fall
      a. Patient often has frequent falling, near-falling, or bumping into things
      b. Typically, the patient is elderly with peripheral neuropathy from alcohol or diabetes or has a combination of visual, hearing, sensory, and motor impairments

D. Diagnostic Tests; routine laboratory testing is not recommended; instead, laboratory testing should be done based on results of history and physical examination
   1. Electrocardiogram (ECG) should be core of the workup for most patients
   2. Consider pregnancy testing in women of child-bearing age, especially those for whom tilt table or electrophysiologic testing is being considered
   3. Tilt-testing may be frightening to the patient, and some patients, especially the elderly, may not be able to tolerate
      a. Upright tilt testing at 60-80° for at least a 15 minute baseline tilt or for 45 minutes is ordered in patients in whom cardiac causes of syncope have been excluded and who have infrequent syncopal episodes
      b. Tilt-table testing with isoproterenol is recommended for patients with negative results on passive tilt-table test who have a high pretest probability of neurally mediated syncope; it is not clear whether prolonged tilt procedures of 45-60 minutes offer better specificity or sensitivity compared with shorter tilt periods and the addition of isoproterenol or adenosine
   4. Order 24-hour Holter monitor or prolonged ambulatory continuous-loop ECG recordings using an Event monitor (patient activates system when a syncopal episode occurs) in patients who have the following:
      a. Normal heart and frequent episodes of syncope
      b. Heart disease or an abnormal ECG or symptoms suggestive of arrhythmias
   5. Echocardiogram is useful for detecting suspected heart disease such as valve dysfunction
   6. Exercise stress testing is important in patients experiencing exertional syncope
   7. Intracardiac electrophysiologic studies are needed when symptoms are suggestive of cardiac syncope, but no abnormality is uncovered with noninvasive tests
   8. Computerized tomography (CT) scan or magnetic resonance imaging (MRI) is warranted if intracranial abnormalities (patient has focal neurologic signs) are suspected
   9. Electroencephalogram (EEG) may be indicated to detect seizure disorders
   10. Order carotid and transcranial Doppler ultrasonography for patients with bruits and who experience drop attacks (sudden loss of postural tone without a clear-cut loss of consciousness)
   11. Lung ventilation-perfusion is reserved for patients with suspected pulmonary embolism
   12. Consider other tests such as fasting blood glucose, hematocrit/hemoglobin, electrolytes, toxicology screens, thyroid function tests, and stool for occult blood based on patient symptomatology

V. Plan/Management

A. Admit to hospital the patients with known serious cardiovascular disease or new findings of cardiovascular disease, significant ECG changes, and patients who have chest pain; consider hospitalization for patients with disabling episodes of syncope, patients who have symptoms suggestive of coronary disease or pulmonary embolus, patients who have sudden loss of consciousness with injury, rapid pulses, or exertional syncope, and patients >70 years of age

B. Depending on etiological factors, consultation with a specialist is often needed; surgical procedures are considered for some conditions such as valvular and cerebrovascular diseases

C. Simple faint may resolve rapidly by elevating patient's feet and legs

D. Patients with recurrent, disabling episodes of vasovagal syncope may benefit from the following:
1. Medications such as β-blockers (metoprolol [Lopressor 25-50 mg bid or Toprol XL 25 –50 mg/day], atenolol [Tenormin] 25-50 mg/day, or anticholinergic agents [transdermal scopolamine, one patch every 2-3 days])
2. If symptoms are not relieved by first-line drugs, consider the following:
a. Fludrocortisone acetate (Florinef) 0.1 to maximum of 0.3 mg/day; contraindicated in patients with congestive heart failure
b. Midodrine 2.5 mg TID titrating up to 10 mg TID per patient tolerance, specific for orthostatic hypotension, may use in combination therapy with Florinef
c. Fluoxetine (Prozac) 10-20 mg/day
3. Measures to expand volume include increased salt intake and custom-fitted counter pressure support garments from ankle to waist
4. Atrioventricular pacing can be considered in patients with clinically important bradycardia in response to upright tilt testing or in variable tachy-brady syndromes

E. Orthostatic hypotension
1. Prevention
a. Wear elastic stockings, only if patient feels they help; there are no randomized control trials to date that indicate compression stockings add a statistically significant beneficial effect
b. Change positions slowly
c. Sleep with head of bed elevated
d. Exercise legs before standing
e. Eat multiple small meals
f. Avoid alcohol
g. Avoid hot environments and hot showers or baths
h. Stay well hydrated, which can be beneficial even within the fluid restrictions that often accompany HF
2. Treatment: Medications in section V.D. may be prescribed if symptoms are more disabling

F. Advise patient not to drive automobiles until symptoms are resolved; refer to laws in each state for clinician's responsibilities in reporting condition

G. Follow up is variable depending on diagnosis

DEEP VENOUS THROMBOSIS

I. Definition: Acute formation of blood clots in the deep venous system of the lower extremities

II. Pathogenesis

A. Etiology of deep venous thrombosis is unknown, but the triad of stasis, injury to the vascular intima, and altered blood coagulability are central to the process

B. Current theory indicates that procoagulant enzymes, factor Xa and thrombin, are able to proliferate unchecked because of a single point mutation of the coagulation factor V (FV) gene that regulates both coagulation and anticoagulation; the mutation renders FVa less susceptible to proteolytic inactivation by activated protein C (APC) and impairs the anticoagulation aspect of FV, thus allowing a thrombus to form

C.   Deep venous thrombosis (DVT) occurs as blood clots in the tibial veins and can progress proximally to involve the popliteal, femoral, and even the iliac veins

D.   Venous thromboembolism (VTE) occurs as microscopic particles, larger pieces, or the entire venous thrombus breaks free becoming mobile and following the venous return pathway through the heart to the lungs, where they can lodge in the vessels infarcting lung tissue distal to the occlusion/s, called pulmonary emboli (PE)

III.   Clinical Presentation

A.   Major risk factors for DVT include cancer, orthopedic surgery, femoral fracture, major surgery of all types, acute myocardial infarction, prolonged bed rest, and pregnancy/childbirth

B.   Individuals status post stroke can develop DVT secondary to immobility of affected extremities and prolonged bedrest; (**Note**: DVT does not cause stokes; arterial thrombi, as discussed in a previous section or this chapter, cause strokes)

C.   Old age is also a significant risk factor for DVT with the underlying cause probably related to inactivity

D.   Use of oral contraceptives is also associated with DVT, although the current oral contraceptives contain considerably less estrogen than in previous years

E.   Most patients present with pain, tenderness, swelling, erythema, and warmth of the affected extremity; however, swelling alone may be the only presenting symptom. Some patients may be totally asymptomatic initially

F.   The incidence of thrombi in the calves is higher than that in the thighs with thrombi in the thighs alone being least common

G.   Pulmonary embolism occurs in almost 40% of patients when the thigh veins are involved; the risk of a large PE when only the calf veins are involved is minimal, but small or microemboli to the lungs commonly originate in the calf veins

H.   Pulmonary embolism can kill quickly if the embolus is large enough, with up to 90% of those affected dying within the first few hours; the presence of a small or microembolus or emboli is much more common and is successfully treated in the majority of cases

I.   The prevention of VTE is the primary reason why diagnosis and treatment of venous thrombosis is urgent

IV.   Diagnosis/Evaluation

A.   History
       1.   Inquire about onset and duration of symptoms (usually pain, tenderness, erythema, warmth and swelling of the involved extremity)
       2.   Inquire about risk factors for DVT such as recent surgery, pregnancy, previous phlebitis, prolonged inactivity, use of oral contraceptives or hormone replacement therapy
       3.   Inquire regarding recent trauma to the affected leg

B.   Physical Examination
       1.   Examine the affected extremity for tenderness on palpation, warmth, firmness, and swelling or presence of palpable cord (**Note**: In superficial thrombophlebitis, but not in DVT, thrombosed vein is often palpable)
       2.   Observe for a positive Homan's sign
       3.   Palpate femoral, popliteal, post-tibial, and pedal pulses, comparing sides
       4.   **Note:** It is virtually impossible to distinguish DVT from other processes on the basis of history and physical examination alone

C.   Differential Diagnosis
       1.   Cellulitis
       2.   Trauma
       3.   Popliteal (Baker's) cyst

4. Heart failure; renal failure (bilateral edema would be present)
5. Superficial thrombophlebitis
6. Muscle/tendon strain

D. Diagnostic Tests
1. Should be ordered by the specialist to whom patient is referred
2. Most commonly ordered test is real-time B-mode compression ultrasonography (US) in which the lack of compressibility of a venous segment documents thrombosis; the gold standard test for diagnosis of venous thromboembolism is contrast venography, but this test is not often performed
3. Invasive vascular angiography with contrast is indicated if surgical intervention is being considered
4. The D-dimer assay and spiral CT of chest or ventilation/perfusion (VQ) scan are appropriate tests to rule-in-or rule-out PE; angiography is the gold standard for testing for PE

V. Plan/Treatment

A. Patients with acute DVT require hospitalization for anticoagulation therapy initially with subcutaneous low molecular weight heparin (LMWH) (enoxaparin, dalteparin), or intravenous unfractionated heparin (UFH); the primary role of these agents is to "bridge" the patient to warfarin and not to replace it

B. Once patient has been fully transitioned from heparin to warfarin, monitoring the INR can be done by the primary care clinician
1. Guidelines suggest continuing anticoagulation with warfarin in most patients with simple DVT for about 3 months, unless contraindicated (LMWH can be used as sole agent if warfarin contraindicated)
2. For DVT with first episode VTE about 6 months
3. Recurrent DVT with FTE about 12 months
4. If symptoms isolated to a calf thrombosis, treat for about 6-12 weeks

C. Follow Up: By specialist to whom patient was referred
1. Weekly follow-up as required for bloodwork—can extend lab draws to 3-4 weeks once INR stabilized
2. Optimal duration of oral anticoagulation treatment after initial episode of DVT or in recurrent disease is currently under intense investigation—preliminary data appear to indicate need for longer treatment intervals than previously recommended

LEG ULCERS

I. Definition: Chronic slow-to-heal, circumscribed, crater-like lesions of the lower extremity between knee and ankle and/or involving foot due to vascular disease

II. Pathogenesis

A. Many possible causes, but 80% to 90% are caused by venous insufficiency; the next two most common etiologies are arterial insufficiency and neuropathy

B. The leg is uniquely vulnerable to nonhealing wounds due to its anatomy and hemodynamics
1. The heart pumps blood to the lower extremities, but it is the calf muscle pump that moves blood from the foot and leg back to the heart during upright posture
   a. Effective calf muscle pumping requires full range of motion of the ankle and sufficient calf muscle to empty the deep system during muscle contraction
   b. Additional requirements are patent veins in both the deep and superficial systems with well-functioning one-way valves that ensure forward and prevent backward flow
2. Damage to any of the components of the calf muscle pump can cause dysfunction of the pump; however, the venous valves (that direct blood from the superficial, relatively low-pressure veins of the saphenous system through the perforating veins that then drain into the deep veins) are most prone to early failure
   a. If high-pressure regurgitation into the saphenous system occurs because of one-way valve failures in the perforators, varicosities, edema, and soft tissue injury in the superficial system will follow

b. Ulceration may develop spontaneously, but in many cases, some minor trauma leads to the wound formation

III. Clinical Presentation

A. Chronic venous insufficiency is the most common cause of leg ulcers between knee and ankle, accounting for 80% to 90% of ulcers
   1. Virtually all patients with venous ulcers have a history of ankle edema and discomfort preceding the development of ulceration
      a. Unlike the pitting edema associated with salt-retaining conditions such as heart failure and nephrotic syndrome, the edema that precedes venous ulcer formation accumulates under high pressure, creating tissue damage and is thus exquisitely tender
      b. Soft tissue tenderness noted when checking patient for edema may be the earliest physical finding of venous disease
   2. Fine, petechial hemorrhage on the edematous skin indicates leakage of red blood cells from damaged vessels
      a. Hemoglobin deposited in the tissues is digested, but the iron remains in the dermis as hemosiderin and produces a brown or brown-red pigmentation in skin surrounding ulcer
      b. Eczematous changes may be present; the dermatitis is often pruritic, excoriated, and prone to colonization with *Staphylococcus aureus*
   3. Ulcer is usually superficial with shaggy borders and with heavy exudate covering the base of the ulcer
   4. Patient usually complains of aching discomfort when the leg is dependent with pain relief when the leg is elevated

B. Arterial insufficiency: Along with neuropathic ulcers, is the second most common cause of leg ulcers (much less common than venous ulcers)
   1. Ulcers usually begin with trauma and thus are located in areas where trauma is most likely to occur (pressure sites, bony prominences, toes)
   2. Ulcers are usually quite painful and have a "punched out" defect with a sharply demarcated border
   3. Surrounding skin is likely to have hair loss and be pale and atrophic with a shiny, fragile, and transparent appearance
   4. Patient usually complains of severe pain exacerbated by elevation or exertion and relieved by dangling the affected leg (dependency) and rest

C. Neuropathic/diabetic ulcers
   1. Characteristic location is an area of pressure (arches, plantar surface, heels, toes)
   2. Ulcers have appearance similar to those of arterial insufficiency ulcer ("punched out" appearance)
   3. Ulcer is fairly insensitive, although there may be tingling, burning sensation that increases at night and decreases with exercise

D. The following table compares physical findings in leg ulcers

COMPARISON OF THREE COMMON TYPES OF LEG ULCERS			
	Venous	**Arterial**	**Neuropathic/Diabetic**
Location	Gaiter area of leg*/medial leg	Pressure sites/ toes, heels, foot	Pressure sites/ plantar, arches, heels, toes
Lesion features	Shallow, partial thickness with irregular borders/shaggy	Punched-out, eschar (blackened if necrotic)	Punched-out
Surrounding skin	Hyperpigmented, thickened, with dermatitis—stasis changes	Hair loss, not hyperpigmented, atrophic	Hair loss, not hyperpigmented, callus
Palpation findings	Non-pitting, tender, tight edema; peripheral pulses may be normal	Peripheral pulses decreased, capillary refill time increased	Altered sensation of touch, vibration, peripheral pulses decreased

*An area between the foot and upper calf, that extends from about 2.5 cm below malleoli to the point at which calf muscles become prominent posteriorly

IV. Diagnosis/Evaluation

A. History
   1. Ask about onset, location, duration, and progress of lesion (slow or rapid development)
   2. Ask if the ulcer is painful, and whether elevating or dangling the affected leg makes the pain better or worse

442

3. Ask if leg edema is prominent at the end of the day
4. Ask about exercise: Does it make the pain better or worse?
5. Obtain past medical history including medication history; ask about previous surgeries, trauma, history of previous ulcers or prior episodes of deep venous thrombosis (DVT)
6. Ask about treatments tried (topical antiseptics and topical corticosteroids can impair normal wound healing)
7. Inquire about tobacco use and interest in smoking cessation
8. Ask about lifestyle, employment, and how the wound has affected quality of life

B. Physical Examination
1. Examine leg when patient is standing or dangling leg; evaluate for edema in skin surrounding ulcer and determine if edema is painful
2. Evaluate for femoral, popliteal, dorsalis pedis, and posterior tibial pulses; test for light touch and vibratory sensation; check capillary refilling time; observe for dependent rubor (arterial insufficiency and neuropathy as cause of the ulcer can be excluded by evaluating the peripheral pulses and sensation)
3. Examine the ulcer looking for characteristics of location, size, lesion features (color, drainage, odor), appearance of surrounding skin, and findings on palpation
4. To measure both the vertical (depth) and horizontal areas of the wound in millimeters, place plastic sandwich bag over ulcer, trace with magic marker, discard side of bag that came in contact with ulcer; use tracing for future comparison (area is a better measure of wound size than diameter because it accommodates for irregularity)

C. Differential Diagnosis
1. Neoplasms (e.g., Kaposi's sarcoma, metastatic tumor)
2. Trauma
3. Infection (bacterial, fungal)
4. Cellulitis

D. Diagnostic Tests
1. Extensive diagnostic evaluation is not needed for most patients with intact sensation and normal arterial blood flow; the likelihood that the ulcer is due to venous disease is >90%
2. Order Doppler studies to assess vascular status if normal arterial blood flow cannot be conclusively established via physical examination
3. Ankle brachial index (ABI) is a useful approach to rule out significant arterial occlusive disease (see PERIPHERAL ARTERIAL DISEASE section for technique of performing ABI)
4. Order radiographs of ulcer site whenever osteomyelitis is suspected
5. Wound cultures are not routinely recommended since most wounds are heavily contaminated with a variety of bacteria; wounds that do not rapidly respond to conservative treatment outlined below require histopathology of the ulcer and adjacent tissue

V. Plan/Management

A. Patients with arterial ulcers and neuropathic/diabetic ulcers must be referred for expert evaluation and management

B. Guidelines for hospital admission of patients with chronic venous leg ulcers are contained in the following table; patients should be immediately referred for treatment

CRITERIA FOR HOSPITALIZATION	
• Suspected systemic infection	• Acute deep venous thrombosis
• Extensive regional infection	• Extensive leg edema
• Metabolic derangement	• Multiple ulcers
• Severe anemia/malnutrition	• Large (2-3 cm) or deep ulcers
• Acute arterial occlusion, pain, absent pulses	• Poor social support or neglect/ poor hygiene

C. Management of small, shallow venous ulcer that meet the following criteria can be accomplished in outpatient setting with compliant patient with good support
1. There is no evidence of infection at the site and the patient is afebrile
2. At least 50% of the ulcer base contains pale pink to beefy red tissue, "proud flesh"
3. Patient's nutritional status is adequate
4. Edema is minimal
5. None of the conditions identified in the table above are present

D.   The following approaches to management of venous ulcers are usually effective
1.   Wound debridement may need to be accomplished using mechanical, enzymatic, or autolytic methods
2.   Wound cleansing should be done with saline or water. Avoid soaps and antiseptics
3.   Moist wound-healing techniques are widely available in a variety of materials that have subtle differences; however, they all have in common that they provide a moist healing environment for the ulcer and they are compatible with compression bandages
4.   Choice of dressing is determined by the condition of the wound and surrounding skin

Minimum drainage	Hydrocolloid dressing
Highly exudative	Calcium alginate
Dry wound base	Hydrogel dressing

a.   If periwound skin is particularly fragile or if patient has dermatitis, a foam dressing or hydrogel is indicated
b.   Whenever the amount of wound drainage overcomes the ability of the dressing to contain it, the dressing should be changed; in general, patients are seen once or twice a week for dressing changes
5.   Edema control during wound healing may require application of compression wraps
a.   Unna boots (zinc oxide-impregnated bandage) and/or flexible cohesive bandages
b.   Various types of fitted compression stockings have been shown to assist in acceleration of healing of venous stasis ulcers and have been found to reduce rates of recurrence if used over the long term
c.   Intermittent pneumatic compression (IPC) has implications in treating swelling in venous leg ulcers but effectiveness and appropriate duration and frequency are still unknown, as are the differences between various types of IPC; further trials are required before widespread use is encouraged
6.   The role of nutritional and vitamin supplementation and various biological growth factors (GF) in managing chronic ulcers needs further study; however, an appropriate nutritional plan is recommended if undernourishment is suspected and leg ulcers are not healing
7.   Recent research results indicate that treatment with pentoxifylline in venous stasis ulcers improves healing and microcirculation and should be considered in slow-to-heal venous ulcers; pentoxifylline in combination with compression therapy may prove to have added benefits for healing
8.   Wounds that do not demonstrate improvement after 4-6 weeks of treatment require biopsy for histology and quantitative bacteriology and patient should be referred to a wound care specialist for management

E.   Follow Up: Weekly until healing is assured

PERIPHERAL ARTERIAL DISEASE: CHRONIC LOWER EXTREMITY ARTERIAL OCCLUSIVE DISEASE

I.   Definition: Narrowing or obstruction of the lumen of peripheral arteries that eventually compromises the normal metabolic processes in the lower extremities producing symptoms of arterial insufficiency (other common peripheral arterial diseases encountered in primary care—abdominal aortic aneurysm and carotid artery disease are not considered here)

II.   Pathogenesis

A.   Atherosclerosis is the cause of peripheral arterial disease; it is a systemic disease process that usually spares the upper extremities

B.   Atherosclerotic lesions contain fatty streaks, fibrous plaques, and complicated lesions that affect all arteries system-wide; there is, however, a segmental distribution of the lesions
1.   Lesions are prone to develop at major arterial bifurcations, in areas of arterial fixation, and at points of arterial angulation

444

2. With gradual development of these lesions, collateral vessels form and can compensate for the segmental obstructive processes
3. Over time, as further main arterial involvement occurs, collateral channels may lose their effectiveness or become occluded, and symptoms of claudication may develop; rest pain and tissue necrosis are not inevitable but can occur with disease progression

III. Clinical Presentation

A. Peripheral arterial disease (PAD) affects approximately 8-10 million persons (men and women equally) in the US and is an important manifestation of systemic atherosclerosis; the age-adjusted prevalence of the disorder is 12% but reaches 20% if only persons >70 years of age are considered

B. Major risk factors for PAD are older age (>40 years), cigarette smoking, and diabetes mellitus; other important risk factors are hyperlipidemia, hypertension, and hyperhomocysteinemia

C. The relative risk of death from cardiovascular causes is approximately the same in persons with PAD—even those with **no history** of MI or ischemic stroke—as it is in persons **with a history** of coronary or cerebrovascular disease

D. Up to 40% of patients with PAD experience typical claudication, defined as walking-induced pain in one or both legs, primarily affecting the calves, that fails to cease with continued walking and is relieved only by rest; muscle pain in the buttocks, thighs, or hips is also experienced by some patients, but calf pain is most common
1. Tends to occur in the same muscle groups each time the patient walks the same distance with the same degree of exertion; symptoms occur sooner if pattern varies (walks uphill or at a faster pace); does not occur with standing
2. Patient describes the pain as muscle cramps or fatigue
3. If the walking distance required to induce pain varies substantially from day to day or if the person must sit or lie down for more than a few minutes to obtain relief, a nonvascular cause for the pain (such as spinal stenosis) should be suspected

E. The severity of claudication increases slowly over time; approximately 25% experience worsening symptoms, and 5% require an amputation within 5 years

F. Complaints of pain at rest suggest critical leg ischemia—defined as ischemic pain in the distal foot, ischemic ulceration, or gangrene
1. Occurs in approximately 5-10% of patients with PAD; risk of limb loss is substantial and the annual mortality rate is 25%
2. Patients complain of rest pain when supine and some pain relief by dangling the involved leg over the side of bed or standing up, indicating that blood flow is marginal and that gravity can increase flow slightly

IV. Diagnosis/Evaluation

A. History
1. Inquire about onset and duration of symptoms
2. Ask if leg pain occurs with exercise or if it is present with rest
3. Ask patient how far he/she can walk before developing cramping pain; determine which muscle groups are involved (calf, thigh, hips, buttock)
4. In males, ask if erectile dysfunction is present
5. Ask patient if dangling legs over the side of the bed or getting up and walking a short distance relieves pain (in arterial disease, the response should be "yes")
6. Ask if hair on toes, lower legs has been lost
7. Obtain tobacco use history and interest in smoking cessation
8. Obtain past medical history; ask patient if he/she has been diagnosed with diabetes mellitus, high blood pressure, hyperlipidemia
9. Inquire regarding present medications

B. Physical Examination
1. Examine skin, hair, and nails, observing for brittle nails, absence of hair on toes and anterior tibial areas; note skin color and texture (poor perfusion results in thin, parchment-like atrophic skin that is generally pale in color when elevated)
2. Assess for *dependent* rubor or 'mottled' appearance to skin (a sign of severe ischemia), ischemic lesions (always examine areas between toes), and gangrenous areas

445

3. Perform a detailed vascular exam including blood pressure in both upper extremities, palpation of peripheral pulses and abdominal aorta; auscultate aortic and groin regions for bruits
   a. Decreased, absent, or asymmetrical pulses help pinpoint exact site of partial or complete occlusion
   b. The "five P's"—pallor, pain, pulselessness, paresthesia, and paralysis are classic signs of acute arterial occlusion
   c. Bruits are present over narrowed arteries
4. Perform a neurosensory exam of the legs

C. Differential Diagnosis
   1. Diabetic neuropathy
   2. Arterial embolism
   3. Spinal Stenosis
   4. Lumbar disk disease

D. Diagnostic Tests
   1. A useful tool for the evaluation of PAD—the ankle-to-arm ratio of systolic blood pressure (or ankle-brachial ratio)—is easily measured with standard blood pressure cuffs and a Doppler device
   2. Other vascular testing should be done by specialist to whom patient is referred
   3. In patients with premature disease (age <50 years), obtain serum homocysteine level

---

PROCEDURE FOR DETERMINING ANKLE BRACHIAL INDEX (ABI)

- Position the patient supine with the extremities at the level of the heart
- The first step is to measure the systolic brachial pressure in **both** the left and the right arms by placing the Doppler probe (transducer) on the long axis of the brachial artery angled at 45-60 degrees; inflate the cuff 20 to 30 mm Hg beyond the last audible Doppler arterial signal; the systolic pressure is defined as the pressure at which the first audible Doppler signal returns once cuff deflation has begun
- Select the higher of these two values as the brachial artery pressure measurement (**Note:** There should be a difference of less than 10 mm Hg between the two arm measurements)
- The next step is to measure the systolic blood pressure in the dorsalis pedis (DP) and posterior tibial (PT) arteries in each ankle
- Select the higher of the two pressures in each ankle
- The right and left ankle-brachial index values are determined by dividing the higher ankle pressure in each leg by the higher arm pressure

$$\text{Right ABI} \quad \frac{\text{Higher right-ankle pressure}}{\text{Higher arm pressure}} \qquad \text{Left ABI} \quad \frac{\text{Higher left-ankle pressure}}{\text{Higher arm pressure}}$$

INTERPRETATION OF ABI

ABI	Interpretation
1.0-1.1	Normal with no evidence of arterial occlusive disease
0.9	Indicative of minimal disease
0.5 - <0.9	Significant arterial occlusive disease; patients often have exercise claudication
<0.5	Severe disease; patients often have pain at rest

V. Plan/Management

A. Management of PAD includes risk-factor modification, antiplatelet therapy, and strategies for effective treatment for claudication

RISK FACTOR MODIFICATION

Smoking Cessation
- ✓ Reduces the risk of death from vascular causes and slows the progression to critical leg ischemia (see section on TOBACCO USE AND SMOKING CESSATION for details on strategies to assist patients to quit smoking)

Hyperlipidemia
- ✓ Several large clinical trials have documented the benefits of lower cholesterol levels in patients with coronary artery disease; in patients with PAD, therapy with a statin not only lowers serum cholesterol concentrations, but also improves endothelial function and other markers of atherosclerotic risk
- ✓ Current recommendation for patients with PAD is to achieve a serum LDL cholesterol concentration of <100 mg/dL and a serum triglyceride concentration of <150 mg/dL (see section on DYSLIPIDEMIA for management recommendations)

Diabetes Mellitus
- ✓ As a major risk factor for PAD, glucose control in persons with either type 1 or type 2 disease should be monitored closely (intensive control of blood glucose prevents the microvascular complications of diabetes but its effects on macrovascular complications are less clear)
- ✓ Recommendation for glycosylated hemoglobin is <7.0 percent (see section on DIABETES MELLITUS for additional information relating to management)

Hypertension
- ✓ The JNC-VI recommends that patients with PAD receive aggressive management of hypertension
- ✓ *Use of angiotensin-converting-enzyme inhibitors in patients with PAD may confer protection against cardiovascular events independent of that expected from blood-pressure reduction (see section on HYPERTENSION for additional management considerations)*

Elevated Homocysteine Concentration
- ✓ Increases risk of death from cardiovascular causes; also an independent risk factor for PAD
- ✓ Causes of high serum concentrations include genetic defects in homocysteine metabolism, alterations in vitamin B_{12} metabolism, and folate deficiency
- ✓ *Supplementing the diet with B vitamins and folic acid can lower serum homocysteine concentrations; however, no clinical trials have demonstrated that reducing homocysteine concentration benefits patients with PAD*

ANTIPLATELET-DRUG THERAPY

Patients with PAD are at high risk for cardiovascular disease and death because atherosclerosis is a systemic disease; antiplatelet drugs reduce the risks of nonfatal myocardial infarction, ischemic stroke, and death from vascular causes

Aspirin is considered to be the primary antiplatelet drug for preventing ischemic events in patients with PAD
- ✓ The American College of Chest Physicians recommends aspirin at doses of 81 to 325 mg once daily for patients with PAD

An alternative is *clopidogrel (Plavix)* which has FDA approval for the prevention of atherosclerotic events in patients with atherosclerosis, including those with PAD
- ✓ Dosing is 75 mg once daily (see PDR for precautions, contraindications, interactions, and adverse reactions)

Note: Ticlopidine (Ticlid) has been used in the past, but concern about its life-threatening hematological adverse reactions severely limits its use to very select circumstances

THERAPY FOR CLAUDICATION: NONPHARMACOLOGIC AND PHARMACOLOGIC

- Patients with PAD have substantial limitations in exercise performance and overall functional capacity
- Impairment in the ability to walk has a very detrimental impact on quality of life, disrupting both work and leisure activities
- The primary nonpharmacologic therapy for claudication is a formal exercise-training program, described in more detail below
- Drugs that improve functional status are also described below

B. All patients with claudication as the major symptom limiting exercise should be referred to an exercise-training program for rehabilitation with treadmill or track walking 3 to 5 times per week
   1. Such programs carry little risk and the likelihood of substantial benefits associated with exercise are great
   2. Emphasize to patient that spontaneous improvement in walking capacity without structured intervention of some type does not occur; supervised walking on a regular basis is essential for relief of disability **(Note:** Clinician provided advice to patients with claudication to "go home and walk," has little data to support its efficacy even though it continues to be commonly given)
   3. A rigorous exercise-training program may be at as beneficial as angioplasty and perhaps more beneficial than bypass surgery

C.   Limitations of exercise-training therapy are that the patient must be motivated and best results are in a supervised setting modeled after cardiac rehabilitation
    1.   Recently, a growing recognition of the benefits of exercise training for patients with claudication symptoms has led to the establishment of a Current Procedural Terminology code (93668) for exercise rehabilitation for claudication
    2.   Emphasize to patient that exercise training must also be maintained or the benefits are lost

D.   Prior to the initiation of an exercise program, the patient should undergo treadmill exercise testing with 12-lead electrocardiographic monitoring. Essential components of an exercise training program for patients with claudication are summarized in the table below

---

ESSENTIAL COMPONENTS OF A WALKING PROGRAM

- Patients should begin each session with a five-minute warm-up period to increase the heart rate slowly, promote flexibility, and allow for stretching of the large muscle groups used for walking
- Initially, the patient should aim to walk for about 5 to 10 minutes before stopping to rest for a few minutes
- Gradually, the length of time spent in walking should be increased so that the patient is walking for about 35 minutes out of a 50-minute period (35 minutes spent in walking and 15 minutes spent in resting) [**Note:** The warm-up and cool-down periods are not included in the 50-minute period]
- Patient should be instructed to continue walking for as long as possible (even though leg pain is experienced) before stopping to rest with the goal of walking more and resting less
- A five-minute cool-down period should be included at the end of the session to allow the heart rate to return to baseline values and to continue stretching the large muscle groups
- The program should last for a lifetime; exercise must be maintained for the benefit to be maintained

---

E.   Drug therapies for claudication that improve functional status are the following
    1.   Cilostazol (Pletal) improves the ability to exercise; dosing is 100 mg BID
    2.   Pentoxifylline (Trental) provides a more modest benefit; usual dosing is 400 mg extended release tab TID with meals
    3.   Consult PDR for dosing, precautions, contraindications, drug interactions, and adverse effects before prescribing these and any other medications

---

COUNSELING RELATED TO PROPER FOOT CARE

Assessment of Feet: Demonstrate to patient
- How to inspect feet for changes in color and temperature, and for signs of skin irritation and injury (scratches, cuts, fissures, blisters, erosions)
- On subsequent visits, **ask** patient to demonstrate to you how he/she assesses feet to determine if this important self-care activity is being properly performed

Foot Care: Instruct patient as follows
- Keep feet clean by bathing at least once daily in lukewarm water
- Gently apply a moisturizer to feet after carefully patting feet dry
- Wear clean, cotton socks that are changed daily (if patient's feet tend to sweat, recommend synthetic socks which wick moisture away from the feet)
- Use strand of lamb's wool (Dr. Scholl's Lamb's Wool) between overriding toes
- Nails should be cut with extreme care, in good light, and only if vision is normal (if any doubt about patient's ability to do this, refer to podiatrist)

Protect Feet from Injury: Instruct patient as follows
- Wear properly fitting shoes to prevent calluses, corns, and blisters
- Use a night light after going to bed to avoid hitting toes or shins on furniture when getting out of bed during the night; house slippers should be worn—advise patient never to go barefoot
- Do not expose feet to extremes of temperature—no hot water soaks or use of heating pads on feet and legs and wear socks to bed in winter to protect from cold

If Symptoms Become Worse: Advise patient as follows
- Call at first sign of difficulty (sudden change in symptoms such as prolonged pain, numbness, or decline in mobility); a delay can lead to limb loss if gangrene or osteomyelitis ensues
- Seek urgent/emergent care if there are sudden changes in symptoms such as prolonged pain, numbness, or tingling or if there is a limitation in movement of affected leg

---

F.   Refer patients with moderate to significant arterial occlusive disease to an expert for management
    1.   Extensive disease may be treated with bypass with either prosthetic or autogenous vein grafts (depending on the vessels involved)

2. Short focal lesions, particularly involving the common iliac artery, are effectively treated with percutaneous transluminal angioplasty (PTCA), with or without a stent
3. **Note:** Recent studies have shown promising results for the use of endovascular brachytherapy (radiation within angioplastied area) to prevent restenosis after angioplasty in improvement of long-term arterial patency)

G. Follow Up
1. In patients with minimal disease, frequent follow up may be needed to evaluate response to risk modification strategies (particularly smoking cessation), to assess adherence to the exercise (walking) program, and to determine efficacy of any medications that have been prescribed
   a. Approximately 75% of patients will improve on such a regimen
   b. Patients who fail to improve or whose condition worsens with a 3 to 6 month trial of conservative therapy should be referred to an expert for management
2. In patients with more than minimal disease, follow up should be with specialist to whom patient was referred

VARICOSE VEINS

I. Definition: Prominent, dilated, tortuous, superficial blood vessels of the lower extremities

II. Pathogenesis

A. Either incompetence of the valves or weakness of the venous wall itself causes dilatation of the vein lumen and subsequent valve inadequacy

B. A self-perpetuating cycle ensues of venous reflux leading to further dilation and valve failure

C. Eventually, the superficial veins widen, elongate, and become tortuous

D. Factors that increase and prolong intraluminal vein pressure such as pregnancy, obesity, and wearing of constricting garments may also play a role in varicose vein development

III. Clinical Presentation

A. Varicosities most often involve the veins of the greater saphenous system and its tributaries; thus, occurrence is usually in the medial and anterior thigh, calf, and ankle regions

B. The presenting symptoms of varicose veins are variable and often bear little relationship to the severity of the varicosities

C. Occur twice as frequently in women as in men and occurs most often in the 20-40 year age group

D. Typically, patients complain of local aching, a feeling of heaviness, or burning pain in the area of the varicosities; worse at the end of the day and after prolonged standing

E. Mild edema of the ankles that is worse in summer and at the end of the day may also be present

F. Infrequently, pruritus due to stasis dermatitis may occur in the region of a severe and chronically dilated vein, but this is unusual with uncomplicated varicose veins

G Ulceration due solely to varicose veins is extremely rare; ulceration almost always implies problems with the deep venous system

H. Large varices may be subject to trauma and bleeding; much more commonly, however, the distended vein will thrombose, leading to superficial phlebitis

I. Subcutaneous varicose veins (sunburst varices) are not truly varicose veins, but are dilations of subcutaneous venous plexuses that are spider-like in arrangement and appear purplish in color

IV.   Diagnosis/Evaluation

    A.   History
        1.   Inquire about onset, location, and presence of any symptoms such as pain, feeling of heaviness, and edema after standing for several hours
        2.   Inquire about what makes condition better or worse
        3.   Determine if cosmetic concerns are a high priority

    B.   Physical Examination
        1.   Note the extent and location of the varicosities
        2.   Observe for signs of pathology of the deep venous system (thrombophlebitis, stasis changes, ulceration, edema

    C.   Differential Diagnosis
        1.   Arterial insufficiency
        2.   Orthopedic problems (bones and joints)
        3.   Neurologic problems

    D.   Diagnostic Tests: None indicated with typical presentation of uncomplicated varicose veins
        1.   May want to try Trendelenburg test; a simple test to evaluate venous incompetency
            a.   With patient supine, lift the leg above the level of the heart until veins empty
            b.   Then quickly lower the leg, observing how fast varicosities fill; the more rapid the filling time, the more incompetent the system
        2.   For more accurate diagnosis of venous architecture, ultrasonic duplex scanning using a B-mode imager with a pulsed Doppler instrument can provide better imaging and flow patterns

V.   Plan/Management

    A.   All patients can benefit from proper elastic support stockings of medium weight and periodic elevation of the extremity during the day
        1.   Stockings can be below the knee, but should be obtained from a surgical company such as Jobst, or TED; department and drugstore stockings are usually unsatisfactory
        2.   Ace wraps are not recommended because they are difficult to apply correctly, cumbersome, cosmetically unattractive, and patient compliance is usually poor

    B.   Obese patients need to be encouraged to lose weight (see section on OBESITY)

    C.   Prolonged standing should be avoided as much as possible

    D.   Women should be advised to avoid constricting panty girdles, tight garters or other garments that may constrict superficial venous return at the thigh level

    E.   Patients may be referred for sclerotherapy, a simple, cost-effective office procedure; several treatments are often necessary

    F.   Indications for referral for surgery include persistent symptomatic varicose veins after conservative treatment (above) has been tried; patient desire for removal because of cosmetic reasons, or episodes of superficial thrombophlebitis
        1.   Conventional vein stripping has been surgical method of choice
        2.   However, endovenous saphenous vein obliteration, an innovative operative procedure for primary greater saphenous vein tributaries, may offer advantages over a stripping operation based on reduced postoperative pain, shorter sick leaves, and faster return to normal activities; further research is needed

    G.   Follow Up: In 3-6 months to determine if conservative treatment has relieved symptoms and to assess need for referral for additional treatment

REFERENCES

Ades, P.A. (2001). Cardiac rehabilitation and secondary prevention of coronary heart disease. *New England Journal of Medicine, 345*, 892-902.

Agodoa, L.Y., Appel, L., Bakris, G.L., Beck, G., Bourgoignie, J., Briggs, J.P., et al. (2001). Effect of ramipril vs amlodipine on renal outcomes in hypertensive nephrosclerosis: A randomized control trial (AASK). *JAMA, 285*, 2719-2728.

Albers, G.W., Dalen, J.E., Laupacis, A., Manning, W., Petersen, P., & Singer, D.E. (2001). Antithrombotic therapy in atrial fibrillation. *Chest, 119*(Suppl.), 194S-206S.

Alderman, M.H., Furberg, C.D., Kostis, J.B., Laragh, J.H., Psaty, B.M., Ruilope, L.M., et al. (2002). Hypertension guidelines: Criteria that might make them more clinically useful. *American Journal of Hypertension, 15,* 917-923.

ALLHAT Officers and Coordinators for the ALLHAT Collaborative Research Group. (2002). Major outcomes in high-risk hypertensive patients randomized to angiotensin-converting enzyme inhibitor or calcium channel blocker vs. diuretic: The antihypertensive and lipid-lowering treatment to prevent heart attack trial (ALLHAT). *JAMA, 288*, 2981-2997.

Alpert, J.S., Antman, E., Apple, F., Armstrong, P.W., Bassand, J.P., de Luna, A.B., et al. (2000). Myocardial infarction redefined. A consensus document of The Joint European Society of Cardiology/American College of Cardiology Committee for the Redefinition of Myocardial Infarction. *Journal of the American College of Cardiology, 36*, 959-969.

Atrial Fibrillation Follow-up Investigation of Rhythm Management (AFFIRM) Investigators. (2002). A comparison of rate control and rhythm control in patients with atrial fibrillation. *New England Journal of Medicine, 347,* 1825-1833.

August, P. (2003). Initial treatment of hypertension. *New England Journal of Medicine, 348,* 610-617.

Basile, J. N. (2001). Hypertension 2001: How will JNC VII be different from JNC VI? *Southern Medical Journal, 94*, 889-890.

Becker, R.C., & Pechet, L. (2001). Fibrinolytics, anticoagulants, and platelet antagonists in clinical practice. In R. Becker & J. Alpert (Eds.), *Cardiovascular medicine: Practice and management* (Chapter 18). New York: Arnold.

Braunwald, E., Antman, E.M., Beasley, J.W., Califf, R.M., Cheitlin, M.D., Hochman, J.S., et al. (2002). ACC/AHA guideline update for the management of patients with unstable angina and non-ST-segment elevation myocardial infarction: A report of the American College of Cardiology/American Heart Association Task Force on Practice Guidelines (Committee on the Management of Patients With Unstable Angina). Available at: http://www.acc.org/clinical/guidelines/unstable/unstable.pdf.

Brenner, B.M., Cooper, M.E., Zeeuw, D., Keane, W.F., Mitch, W.E., Parving, H.H., et al. (2001). Effects of losartan on renal and cardiovascular outcomes in patients with type 2 diabetes and nephropathy. *New England Journal of Medicine, 345*, 861-869.

Brewster, D.C. (2000). Evaluation of arterial insufficiency of the lower extremities. In A.H. Goroll & A.G. Mulley, Jr. (Eds) *Primary care medicine.* Philadelphia: Lippincott/Williams & Wilkins.

Brewster, D.C. (2000). Evaluation of peripheral venous disease. In A.H. Goroll & A.G. Mulley, Jr. (Eds.). *Primary care medicine.* Philadelphia: Lippincott/Williams & Wilkins.

Buffon, A., Biasucci, L.M., Liuzzo, G., D'Onofrio, G., Crea, F., & Maseri, A. (2002). Widespread coronary inflammation in unstable angina. *New England Journal of Medicine, 347,* 5-12.

Burton, C.S. (2002). Leg ulcers. In R.E. Rakel & E.T. Bope (Eds.), *Conn's current therapy.* Philadelphia: Saunders.

Cannon, C.P., Battler, A., Brindis, R.G., Cox, J.L., Ellis, S.G., Every, N.R., et al. (2001). American College of Cardiology key elements and data definitions for measuring the clinical management and outcomes of patients with acute coronary syndromes: A report of the American College of Cardiology Task Force on Clinical Data Standards (Acute Coronary Syndromes Writing Committee). *Journal of the American College of Cardiology, 38,* 2114-2130. Available at www.acc.org.

Carman, T.L., & Fernandez, B.B. (2000). A primary care approach to the patient with claudication. *American Family Physician, 61,* 1027-1034.

Chombanian, A.V., Bakris, G.L., Black, H.R., Cushman, W.C., Green, L.A., Izzo, J.L. Jr., et al. (2003). The Seventh Report of the Joint National Committee on Prevention, Detection, Evaluation, and Treatment of High Blood Pressure. The JNC 7 Report. *JAMA, 289*, 2560-2572.

Committee on Health and Science Policy, The American College of Chest Physicians, Consensus Panel on Antithrombotic Therapy. (2001). *Sixth ACCP Consensus Conference on Antithrombotic Therapy, Quick Reference Guide.* Northbrook, IL: DuPont Pharmaceuticals Company.

Cosmi, B., Conti, E., & Coccheri, S. (2001). Anticoagulants (heparin, low molecular weight heparin, and oral anticoagulants) for intermittent claudication. *Cochrane Database of Systematic Reviews, 3*, CD001999.

Davidson, M.H. (2002). Strategies to improve Adult Treatment Panel III Guideline adherence and patient compliance. *The American Journal of Cardiology, 89*(Suppl.), 8C-22C.

Dawson, D.L., Hiatt, W.R., Creager, M.A., & Hirsch, A.T. (2002). Peripheral arterial disease: Medical care and prevention of complications. *Preventive Cardiology, 5*, 119-130.

DeMartinis, J. (2001). Relaxation and stress management. In Denise Robinson, & C.P. Kish (Eds.), *Core concepts in advanced practice nursing* (Chapter 44). St. Louis, MS: Mosby.

DeMartinis, J. (2003). Clients with hypertensive disorders: Promoting positive outcomes. In J. Black & J. Hawks (Eds.), *Medical-surgical nursing: Clinical management for positive outcomes* (7th ed.). Philadelphia: W.B. Saunders.

DeMartinis, J. (2003). Principles and methods of the basic physical examination. In R. Jones and R. Rospond (Eds.), *Patient assessment in pharmacy practice* (Chapter 4). Baltimore, MD: Lippincott/Williams & Wilkins.

Diercks, D.B., Gibler, W.B., Liu, T., Sayre, M.R., & Storrow, A.B. (2000). Identification of patients at risk by graded exercise testing in an emergency department chest pain center. *American Journal of Cardiology, 86*, 289-292.

Donnelly, R., & Yeung, J. M. (2001). Assessment and management of intermittent claudication: importance of secondary prevention. *International Journal of Clinical Practice* (Suppl. 119), 2-9.

Epperly, T.D., & Fogarty, J.P. (2001). Syncope. In M.B. Mengel & L.P. Schwiebert (Eds.). *Ambulatory medicine: The primary care of families* (3rd ed.). New York: Lange Medical Books/McGraw-Hill.

Falk, R.H. (2001). Atrial fibrillation. *New England Journal of Medicine, 344,* 1067-1078.

Falk, R.H. (2002). Management of atrial fibrillation—Radical reform or modest modification. *New England Journal of Medicine, 347,* 1883-1884.

Farrell, M.H., Foody, J.M., & Krumholz, H.M. (2002). ß-blockers in heart failure: Clinical applications. *Journal of the American Medical Association, 287,* 890-897.

Feinstein, S.B., Voci, P., & Pizzuto, F. (2002). Noninvasive surrogate markers of atherosclerosis. *The American Journal of Cardiology 89*(Suppl.), 31C-44C.

Fesmire, F.M., Hughes, A.D., Fody, E.P., Jackson, A.P., Fesmire, C.E., Gilbert, M.A., et al. (2002). The Erlanger Chest Pain Evaluation protocol: A one-year experience with serial 12-lead ECG monitoring, two-hour delta serum marker measurements, and selective nuclear stress testing to identify and exclude acute coronary syndromes. *Annals of Emergency Medicine, 40*, 584-594.

Foody, J.M., Farrell, M.H., & Krumholz, H.M. (2002). ß-blocker therapy in heart failure. *Journal of the American Medical Association, 287*, 883-889.

Furberg, C.D., Psaty, B.M., Pahor, M., & Alderman, M.H. (2001). Clinical implications of recent findings from the Antihypertensive and Lipid-Lowering Treatment to Prevent Heart Attack Trial (ALLHAT) and other studies of hypertension. *Annals of Internal Medicine, 135*, 1074-1078.

Fuster, V., Ryden, L.E., Asinger, R.W., Cannon, D.S., Crijns, H.J., Frye, R.L., et al. (2001). ACC/AHA/ESC guidelines for the management of patients with atrial fibrillation: A report of the American College of Cardiology/American Heart Association Task Force on Practice Guidelines and the European Society of Cardiology Committee for Practice Guidelines and Policy Conferences (Committee to Develop Guidelines for the Management of Patients With Atrial Fibrillation). *Journal of the American College of Cardiology 38*, 1266i-1266lxx. Available at: www.acc.org.

Gerstenfeld, E.P., & Mittleman, R.S. (2001). Atrial fibrillation: Current management. In R. Becker & J. Alpert (Eds.), *Cardiovascular medicine: Practice and management* (Chapter 20). New York: Arnold.

Gibbons, R.J., Abrams, J., Chatteerjee, K., Daley, J., Deedwania, P.C., Douglas, J.S., et al. (2003). ACC/AHA 2002 guideline update for the management of patients with chronic stable angina—summary article: A report of the American College of Cardiology/American Heart Association Task Force on Practice Guidelines (Committee on the Management of Patients with Chronic Stable Angina). *Journal of American College of Cardiology, 42,* 159-168.

Goroll, A.H., May, L.A., & Mulley, A.G. (2000). Evaluation of chest pain. In A.H. Goroll & A.G. Mulley, Jr. (Eds). *Primary care medicine.* Philadelphia: Lippincott/Williams & Wilkins.

Haider, A.W., Larson, M.G., Franklin, S.S., & Levy, D. (2003). Systolic blood pressure, diastolic blood pressure, and pulse pressure as predictors of risk for congestive heart failure in the Framingham Heart Study. *Annals of Internal Medicine, 138,* 10-16.

Hansson, L. (2002). Hypertension management in 2002: Where have we been? Where might we be going? *American Journal of Hypertension, 15*(Suppl.), S101-S107.

Hargett, F. (2001). Peripheral vascular disease. In M.B. Mengel & L.P. Schwiebert (Eds.). *Ambulatory medicine: The primary care of families* (3rd ed., Chapter 87), New York: Lange Medical Books/McGraw-Hill.

Heart Protection Study Collaborative Group. (2002). MRC/BHF Heart Protection Study of cholesterol lowering with simvastatin in 20536 high-risk individuals: A randomized placebo-controlled trial. *Lancet, 360,* 7-22.

Hiatt, W.R. (2001). Medical treatment of peripheral arterial disease and claudication. *New England Journal of Medicine, 344*, 1608-1621.

Hirsch, J., & Lee, A.Y. (2002). How we diagnose and treat deep vein thrombosis. *Blood, 99*, 3102-3110.

Hobbs, J. (2001). Chest pain. In M.B. Mengel & L.P. Schwiebert, (Eds.), *Ambulatory medicine: The primary care of families* (3rd ed.), New York: Lange Medical Books/McGraw-Hill.

Homocysteine Studies Collaboration. (2002). Homocysteine and risk of ischemic heart disease and stroke. *JAMA, 288,* 2015-2022.

Hu, F.B., & Willett, W.C. (2002). Optimal diets for prevention of coronary heart disease. *JAMA, 288,* 2569-2578.

Humphrey, L.L., Chan, B.K.S., & Sox, H.C. (2002). Postmenopausal hormone replacement therapy and the primary prevention of cardiovascular disease. *Annals of Internal Medicine, 137,* 273-284.

Hunt, S.A., Baker, D.W., Chin, M.H., Cinquegrani, M.P., Feldman, A.M., Francis, G.S., et al. (2001). ACC/AHA guidelines for the evaluation and management of chronic heart failure in the adult: A report of the American College of Cardiology/American Heart Association Task force on Practice Guidelines (Committee to Revise the 1995 Guidelines for the Evaluation and Management of Heart Failure). American College of Cardiology Web site. Available at: http//www.acc.org/clinical/guidelines/failure/hf_index.htm.

Isaacsohn, J., Black, D., Troendle, A. & Orloff, D. (2002). The impact of the National Cholesterol Education Program Adult Treatment Panel III guidelines on drug development. *The American Journal of Cardiology, 89*(Suppl.), 45C-49C.

Jackson, M.R., & Clagett, G.P. (2001). Antithrombotic therapy in peripheral occlusive disease. *Chest, 119*(Suppl.) 45C-49C.

Johnson, S. (2002). Compression hosiery in the prevention and treatment of venous leg ulcers. *Journal of Tissue Viability 12,* 67, 70, 72-74.

Joint European Society of Cardiology/American College of Cardiology Committee. (2002). Myocardial infarction redefined—A consensus document of the Joint European Society of Cardiology/American College of Cardiology Committee for the redefinition of myocardial infarction, *Journal of the American College of Cardiology, 36,* 959- 969.

Joint European Society of Cardiology/American College of Cardiology Committee. (2002). Myocardial infarction redefined—A consensus document of the Joint European Society of Cardiology/American College of Cardiology Committee for the redefinition of myocardial infarction, *Journal of the American College of Cardiology, 36,* 959-969.

Kalayoglu, M.V., Libby, P., & Byrne, G.I. (2002). *Chlamydia pneumoniae* as an emerging risk factor in cardiovascular disease. *JAMA, 288,* 2724-2731.

Kershaw, G.R. (2001). Comprehensive management of hypertension and its complications. In R. Becker & J. Alpert (Eds.), *Cardiovascular medicine: Practice and management.* New York: Arnold.

Kris-Etherton, P.M., Harris, W.S., Appel, L.J. for Nutrition Committee. (2002). Fish consumption, fish oil, omega-3 fatty acids, and cardiovascular disease. *Circulation, 106,* 2747-2757.

Krum, H., Roecker, E.B., Mohacsi, P., Rouleau, J.L., Tendera, M., Coats, A.J.S., et al. (2003). Effects of initiating carvedilol in patients with severe chronic heart failure. *JAMA, 289,* 712-718.

Kushner, I., & Sehgal, A.R. (2002). Is high-sensitivity C-reactive protein and effective screening test for cardiovascular risk? *Archives of Internal Medicine, 162,* 867-869.

Lee, A.Y., & Hirsch, J. (2002). Diagnosis and treatment of venous thromboembolism. *Annual Review of Medicine, 53,* 15-33.

Meyer, T.E., Chung, E.S., & Gaasch, W.H. (2001). Evaluation and management of patients with heart failure in clinical practice. In R. Becker & J. Alpert (Eds.), *Cardiovascular medicine: Practice and management.* New York: Arnold.

Moser, M. (2002). Update on the management of hypertension: Do recent clinical trial results indicate a change in national recommendations for therapy? *Journal of Clinical Hypertension, 4*(Suppl.), 20-31.

National Cholesterol Education Program (NCEP), National Institutes of Health, National Heart, Lung, and Blood Institute. (2001). *Executive summary of the third report of the National Cholesterol Education Program (NCEP) Expert Panel on Detection, Evaluation, and Treatment of High Blood Cholesterol in Adults (Adult Treatment Panel III).* NIH Publication No. 01-3305. Bethesda, MD: US Government Printing Office.

National High Blood Pressure Education Program Working Group on Hypertension Control in Children and Adolescents. (1996). Update on the 1987 task force report on high blood pressure in children and adolescents: A working group report from the National High Blood Pressure Education Program. *Pediatrics, 98,* 649-658.

National High Blood Pressure Education Program, National Institutes of Health, National Heart, Lung, and Blood Institute. (1997). *The Sixth Report of the Joint National Committee on Detection, Evaluation, and Treatment of High Blood Pressure* NIH Publication No. 98-4080. Bethesda, MD: US Government Printing Office.

Nutrition Committee of the AHA. (2000). AHA dietary guidelines: Revision 2000: A statement for healthcare professionals from the nutrition committee of the American Heart Association. *Circulation, 102,* 2284-2299.

Ockene, J.K., & Ockene, I.S. (2001). Primary prevention of cardiovascular disease: Helping patients change lifestyle behaviors. In R. Becker & J. Alpert (Eds.), *Cardiovascular medicine: Practice and management.* New York: Arnold.

Opie, L. (2001). *Drugs for the heart* (3rd ed.). Philadelphia, WB Saunders.

Paquette, D., & Falanga, V. (2002). Leg ulcers. *Clinics of Geriatric Medicine, 18* (1), 77-88.

Pasternak, R. (2002). Adult Treatment Panel II versus Adult Treatment Panel III: What has changed and why? *The American Journal of Cardiology 89*(Suppl.), 3C-7C.

Pearson, T.A., Mensah, G.A., Alexander, R.W., Anderson, J.L., Cannon R.O., Criqui, M., et al. (2003). Markers of inflammation and cardiovascular disease. Application to clinical and public health practice. A statement for healthcare professionals from the Centers for Disease Control and Prevention and the American Heart Association. *Circulation, 107*, 499-511.

Pineo, G.F. & Hull, R.D. (2001). Outpatient management of thrombotic disorders. In R. Becker & J. Alpert (Eds.). *Cardiovascular medicine: Practice and management.* New York, Arnold.

Regensteiner, J.G., & Hiatt, W.R. (2002). Current medical therapy for patients with peripheral arterial disease: A critical review. *American Journal of Medicine, 112*, 49-57.

Ridker, P.M., Rifai, N., Rose, L., Buring, J.E., & Cook, N.R. (2002). Comparison of C-reactive protein and low-density lipoprotein cholesterol: Levels in the prediction of first cardiovascular events. *New England Journal of Medicine, 347*, 1557-1565.

Ryan, T.J., Antman, E.M., Brooks, N.H., Califf, R.M., Hillis, L.D., Hiratzka, L.F., et al. (1999). ACC/AHA guidelines for the management of patients with acute myocardial infarction: 1999 update: A report of the American College of Cardiology/American Heart Association Task Force on Practice Guidelines (Committee on Management of Acute Myocardial Infarction). Available at www.acc.org.

Sacks, F.M., Svetkey, L.P., & Vollmer, W.M. (2001). Effects on blood pressure of reduced dietary sodium and the dietary approaches to stop hypertension (DASH) diet. *New England Journal of Medicine, 344*, 3-10.

Schroeder, S.A. (2001) . Chest pain. In R.A. Hoekelman (Ed.). *Primary pediatric care* (4th ed.), St. Louis: Mosby.

Sheldon, R., Rose, S., Ritchie, D., Connolly, S.J., Koshman, M., & Lee, M.A. (2002). Historical criteria that distinguish syncope from seizures. *Journal of the American College of Cardiology, 40,* 142-143.

Sloane, P.D., Coeytaux, R.R., Beck, R.S., & Dallara, J. (2001). Dizziness: State of the science. *Annals of Internal Medicine, 134,* 823-832.

Smith, S.C., Blair, S. N., Bonow, R. O., Brass, L. M., Cerqueira, M.D., Dracup, K., et al. (2001). AHA/ACC guidelines for preventing heart attack and death in patients with atherosclerotic cardiovascular disease: 2001 update: A Statement for Healthcare Professionals From the American Heart Association and the American College of Cardiology. *Circulation, 104*, 1577-1579. Available at: www.acc.org or www.circulationaha.org.

Stevenson, L.W. (2002). Beta-blockers for stable heart failure. *New England Journal of Medicine, 346,* 1346-1347.

Stewart, K.J., Hiatt, W.R., Regensteiner, J.G., & Hirsch, A.T. (2002). Exercise training for claudication. *New England Journal of Medicine, 347*, 1941-1951.

Talner, N.S., & Carboni, M.P. (2000). Chest pain in the adolescent and young adult. *Cardiology in Review, 8*, 49-56.

Topol, E.J., Califf, R.M., Van de Werf, F., Willerson, J.T., Booth, J., White, H., et al. (Gusto V Investigators). (2001). Reperfusion therapy for acute myocardial infarction with fibrinolytic therapy or combination reduced fibrinolytic therapy and platelet glycoprotein IIb/IIIa inhibition: The Gusto V randomized trial. *The Lancet, 357*, 1905-1914.

US Preventive Services Task Force. (2002). Aspirin for the primary prevention of cardiovascular events: Recommendation and rationale. *Annals of Internal Medicine, 136,* 157-160.

Weitz, J.I., & Bates, S.M. (2000). Beyond heparin and aspirin: New treatments for unstable angina and non-Q-wave myocardial infarction. *Archives of Internal Medicine, 160,* 749-758.

Wells, T.G. (2002). Antihypertensive therapy: Basic pharmacokinetic and pharmacodynamic principles as applied to infants and children. *American Journal of Hypertension*, 15(Suppl.), 34S-37S.

Whelton, P.K., He, J., Appel, L.J., Cutler, J.A., Havas, S., Kotchen, T.A., et al. (2002). Primary prevention of hypertension: Clinical and public health advisory from the National High Blood Pressure Education Program. *JAMA, 288*, 1882-1888.

Wing, L.M.H., Reid, C.M., Ryan, P., Beilin, L.J., Brown, M.A., Jennings, G.L.R., et al. (2003). A comparison of outcomes with angiotensin-converting-enzyme inhibitors and diuretics for hypertension in the elderly. *New England Journal of Medicine, 348,* 583-592.

Wissing, UE., Wengstrom, A.C., Skold, G., & Unosson, M. (2002). Can individualized nutritional support improve healing in therapy-resistant leg ulcers? *Journal of Wound Care, 11,* 15-29.

Writing Group for the Women's Health Initiative Investigators. (2002). Risks and benefits of estrogen plus progestin in healthy postmenopausal women. Principle results from the Women's Health Initiative (WHI) randomized controlled trial. *Journal of the American Medical Association, 288*, 321-333.

Wyse, D.G., Waldo, A.L., DiMarco, J.P., Domanski, M.J., Rosenberg, Y., Schron, E.B. et al. (2002). A comparison of rate control and rhythm control in patients with atrial fibrillation. The Atrial Fibrillation Follow-up Investigation of Rhythm Management Investigators (AFF/RM). *New England Journal of Medicine, 347,* 1825-1833.

Young, J.B., Abraham, W.T., Stevenson, L.W., Horton, D., Elkayam, U., & Bourge, R.C. (2002). Intravenous nesiritide vs nitroglycerin for treatment of decompensated congestive heart failure: A randomized controlled trial. *Journal of the American Medical Association, 287,* 1531-1540.

Gastrointestinal Problems

Mary Virginia Graham

ACUTE ABDOMINAL PAIN

I.   Definition: Recent onset of severe abdominal pain

II.   Pathogenesis

    A.   Major mechanisms of acute abdominal pain include obstruction of a hollow viscus, capsular distention, peritoneal irritation, mucosal ulceration, vascular compromise, traumatic wall injury, and referral from an extra-abdominal site

    B.   Types of abdominal pain can be helpful in determining the cause
        1.   Visceral pain is deep, dull, crampy, poorly localized, and originates from a solid or hollow viscus; this pain occurs when noxious stimuli trigger visceral nociceptors
        2.   Somatoparietal pain is sharp, well localized, and originates from noxious stimulation of the parietal peritoneum and generally is more intense and more precisely located than is visceral pain
        3.   Referred pain is pain that is experienced at a distance from the disease process and is explained by the embryologic origins of the structures involved

III. Clinical Presentation

    A.   Location of pain may provide clues to common causes of abdominal pain from both intra-abdominal and extra-abdominal sources

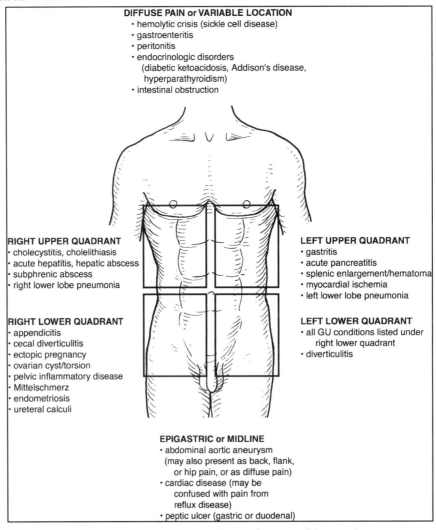

DIFFUSE PAIN or VARIABLE LOCATION
- hemolytic crisis (sickle cell disease)
- gastroenteritis
- peritonitis
- endocrinologic disorders
  (diabetic ketoacidosis, Addison's disease, hyperparathyroidism)
- intestinal obstruction

RIGHT UPPER QUADRANT
- cholecystitis, cholelithiasis
- acute hepatitis, hepatic abscess
- subphrenic abscess
- right lower lobe pneumonia

LEFT UPPER QUADRANT
- gastritis
- acute pancreatitis
- splenic enlargement/hematoma
- myocardial ischemia
- left lower lobe pneumonia

RIGHT LOWER QUADRANT
- appendicitis
- cecal diverticulitis
- ectopic pregnancy
- ovarian cyst/torsion
- pelvic inflammatory disease
- Mittelschmerz
- endometriosis
- ureteral calculi

LEFT LOWER QUADRANT
- all GU conditions listed under right lower quadrant
- diverticulitis

EPIGASTRIC or MIDLINE
- abdominal aortic aneurysm
  (may also present as back, flank, or hip pain, or as diffuse pain)
- cardiac disease (may be confused with pain from reflux disease)
- peptic ulcer (gastric or duodenal)

Figure 12.1. Location of Pain: Clues to Diagnosis

B. Obstruction may occur in the bowel, biliary tree, and ureters with the severity of the pain dependent on both the speed of onset and the degree of distention
   1. Pain due to an acute obstruction is usually colicky and wavelike in nature; patients are restless, frequently shifting positions, and lack peritoneal signs
   2. Obstruction of the small bowel is greatest when the obstruction is jejunal and the patient may be comfortable between bouts of pain; obstruction of the large bowel may result in constipation; large bowel obstruction is generally less painful and distention is usually greater than is seen with small bowel obstruction
   3. Obstruction of the cystic duct by a stone produces acute pain, which is fairly steady and unremitting; in acute cholecystitis, the pain is typically in the right upper quadrant or epigastrium, radiating to the scapular region, and associated with nausea and vomiting (see CHOLECYSTITIS)
   4. Obstruction within the urinary tract can present as abdominal pain; the pain usually begins in the back and flank and radiates into the lower abdomen and groin; hematuria is frequently present

C. Peritoneal irritation can cause severe pain due to the rich innervation of the parietal peritoneum; suggests that a condition requiring surgical intervention is present
   1. An inflamed appendix is a common cause of peritoneal pain
   2. With peritoneal irritation, rebound tenderness is prominent on physical examination because pain is accentuated by pressure changes in the peritoneum

D. Vascular compromise including acute arterial insufficiency or dissection or rupture of an abdominal aortic aneurysm can present with severe abdominal pain; with an abdominal aneurysm, a pulsating mass may be palpated in the epigastrium

E. Mucosal ulceration or inflammation of the gastrointestinal tract is usually accompanied by pain; with duodenal ulcer disease, the pain is usually burning or aching and is not usually severe unless there is perforation or penetration into the pancreas

F. Gastroenteritis is characterized by the onset of crampy, diffuse abdominal pain
   1. Fever, nausea, vomiting, and diarrhea are often associated symptoms and bowel sounds are frequently hyperactive
   2. Abdominal exam does not elicit rebound tenderness

G. Capsular distention of the well-innervated capsule surrounding organs such as the liver causes a constant, aching abdominal pain; pain due to splenic capsular distention as may occur with blunt trauma is located in the left upper quadrant and with subdiaphragmatic peritoneal irritation, pain may radiate to the ipsilateral shoulder

H. Traumatic injury to the abdominal muscle wall can produce pain that is constant, aching, and made worse with movement or pressure on the abdomen

I. Referral of pain from an extra-abdominal source such as the chest, particularly with conditions such as lower lobe pneumonia, may present as abdominal pain; an acute inferior myocardial infarction may present as upper abdominal pain, with nausea and vomiting

J. Lower abdominal pain may occur in women with sexually transmitted diseases, ectopic pregnancies, disorders of the ovaries, or other pelvic pathology; depending on the cause of the pain, patient may also experience vaginal discharge, bleeding, or irregular menses

IV. Diagnosis/Evaluation: Determine if patient has an emergent problem BEFORE proceeding with the complete evaluation (patient should be examined promptly for evidence of obstruction, peritoneal irritation, vascular compromise, or cardiopulmonary disease)

   A. History
      1. Determine onset, location, and quality of pain
      2. Ask patient to rate pain on scale of 0 to 10; ask if pain interferes with sleep
      3. Ask if pain has changed since onset (progression of pain)
      4. Determine if pain is referred to or radiates to other sites
      5. Ask about aggravating and relieving factors
      6. Ask about associated symptoms of vomiting, marked change in bowel habits (either diarrhea or constipation), melena, or urogenital symptoms (see Clinical Presentation on previous pages for clues to possible causes). Ask regarding associated fever or chills

7.   In women of childbearing age, ask about symptoms indicating pelvic pathology–dyspareunia, abnormal vaginal discharge, and irregular menstrual bleeding; inquire regarding chance of being pregnant
8.   Obtain past medical history, surgical history, and medication history
9.   Obtain social history including alcohol and tobacco use

B.   Physical Examination
   1.   Determine if patient is febrile; assess for orthostatic hypotension
   2.   Observe general appearance for pallor, perspiration, restlessness, signs of peritonitis, toxicity
   3.   Perform a complete exam focusing on possible extra-abdominal sources of the abdominal pain
   4.   To examine the abdomen, position patient with hips flexed; observe for surgical scars and distension; auscultate for bowel sounds; palpate abdomen, beginning in non-painful region
      a.   Determine areas of localized tenderness, masses, liver and spleen size
      b.   Assess for rigid abdomen, guarding, rebound tenderness, presence of abdominal bruits, CVA tenderness (see following table ASSESSING FOR REBOUND TENDERNESS)
      c.   Assess for positive Murphy's sign (pain and "inspiratory arrest" when patient takes a deep breath while examiner applies pressure in area of gallbladder, a sign that suggests cholecystitis)
      d.   Assess for positive obturator and psoas signs (see techniques in Figures 12.2. and 12.3.)

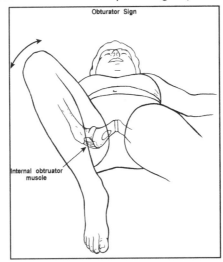

Figure 12.2. Obturator Sign.
Passively flex the right hip and knee and internally rotate the leg at the hip, stretching the obturator muscle. Right-sided abdominal pain is a positive sign, indicating irritation of the obturator muscle by an inflamed appendix

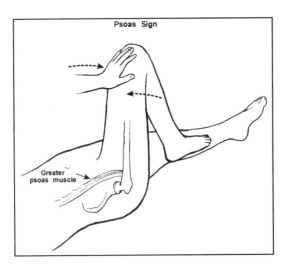

Figure 12.3. Psoas Sign.
With the patient in the supine position, instruct him/her to lift the right thigh against the resistance of the examiner's hand, which is placed just above the patient's knee. Increased pain with the maneuver is a positive test, indicating irritation of the psoas by a possibly inflamed appendix

e. Assess for hernias
5. Percuss the liver span and assess for fluid wave (**Note:** Percussion tenderness is a very sensitive sign of peritoneal irritation)
6. Percuss the back for costovertebral angle tenderness
7. Perform pelvic exam on women to evaluate cervix, assess for cervical motion tenderness (CMT), adnexal tenderness, or abnormal masses
8. Perform digital rectal exam to assess for occult bleeding, to obtain stool for occult blood, and to evaluate for fecal impaction, prostate enlargement, tenderness and hemorrhoids
9. In elderly patients, be aware that signs of acute peritoneal irritation may be absent, especially initially when the only manifestation may be unexplained low-grade fever, tachycardia, diminished bowel sounds, and vague abdominal discomfort without frank rebound tenderness or guarding

---

ASSESSING FOR REBOUND TENDERNESS

After thorough exam of the abdomen, evaluate for peritoneal irritation as follows

➡ Using the flat of your hand, press on the area identified by the patient as most painful
➡ Press sufficiently to depress the peritoneum. The patient will experience pain with this maneuver
➡ Keep pressing with a constant pressure and, as the patient adjusts to the constant pressure over a 30 to 60 second period, the pain lessens in intensity and may even subside
➡ Then, without warning, remove your hand suddenly to just above skin level
➡ Observation of the patient's face may be the best index of a complaint of pain and peritoneal irritation

---

10. When psychogenic pain is suspected
    a. First, rule out serious pathology by history and physical exam
    b. After establishing that abdominal exam is negative, use deep palpation while patient is distracted; lack of tenderness is characteristic
    c. Push down slowly, firmly, and deeply on abdomen with stethoscope, distracting patient by appearing to auscultate

C. Differential Diagnosis
   1. Many causes of acute abdominal pain
   2. Need to rule out all emergent conditions

D. Diagnostic Tests
   1. Initial basic testing in office setting includes the following
      a. CBC with differential and urinalysis are routinely done
      b. Electrolytes, BUN, creatinine should be measured if there is vomiting or diarrhea
   2. If pregnancy is possible, obtain serum hCG β-subunit determination
   3. Consider testing for gonorrhea and chlamydia, based on patient history
   4. Consider obtaining abdominal flat plate and upright for bowel obstruction, free air, ileus, or abnormal calcification
   5. Other laboratory tests such as ultrasonography may be ordered based on history and physical examination
   6. Immediately refer patients with evidence of acute obstruction, peritonitis, or bowel ischemia for emergent evaluation and treatment
      a. Ultrasound or computed tomography are the usual tests
      b. If conditions such as ovarian torsion, ectopic pregnancy, or pelvic abscess are suspected, transvaginal ultrasonography is more sensitive than transabdominal

V. Plan/Management

A. Consultation with a specialist is necessary if diagnosis is unclear and/or patient is unstable

B. Management depends on findings from H&P, diagnostic tests, and specialist recommendations

C. Recent research suggests that judicious use of pain medication may enable a more accurate evaluation of acute abdominal pain

D. Follow up is variable depending on diagnosis

ACUTE DIARRHEA

I. Definition: Abrupt onset of increased fluid content of the stool above the normal value of approximately 10 mL/kg/day, that resolves in less that 14 days; implies an increased frequency of bowel movements also which can range from 4 to 5 to more than 20 per day

II. Pathogenesis

A. Increased water content of the stools results from an imbalance in the function of the small and large intestinal processes involved in the absorption of organic substrates and water

B. Imbalance in the intestinal handling of water and electrolytes involves one or a combination of four basic mechanisms
1. Osmotic: Occurs when poorly absorbed, osmotically active substances are ingested, creating an osmotic gradient that encourages movement of water into the lumen and subsequently into the stool–examples are ingestion of lactose in a lactase-deficient person, sorbitol, mannitol, magnesium-containing antacids in excess
2. Secretory: There is increased small intestinal secretion or reduced absorption–cholera has been the prototype of secretory diarrhea; in recent years, however, a growing number of infectious agents such as enterotoxigenic *Escherichia coli* have been associated with this mechanism; a number of noninfectious causes exist as well
3. Exudative: Intestinal mucosa becomes inflamed, causing mucus, blood, and pus to leak into the lumen; examples are invasive infections of small and/or large intestine by bacterial agents as well as non-infectious conditions such as inflammatory bowel disease
4. Motility disturbances: Contact time with bowel mucosa is limited which interferes with reabsorption of fluids–examples are irritable bowel disease and medications such as erythromycin

III. Clinical Presentation

A. Most diarrheal illnesses are self-limited or viral, and nearly half last less than one day
1. In the US, diarrheal illnesses are most likely to occur during the winter months
2. These illnesses are commonly associated with noroviruses—in families and in outbreaks including those in nursing homes—or rotaviruses in infants and children

B. In infectious diarrhea, the clinical presentation and the course of the illness are greatly influenced by the host and by the infecting organism
1. Age and nutritional status appear to be the most important host factors–elderly patients can become volume depleted very rapidly
2. Characteristics of the infecting organism also result in a variable pattern of clinical features–for example, patients with **viral** diarrhea tend to have dehydration, vomiting, and watery stools. On the other hand, fever, cramping abdominal pain, and blood mixed with stools are more common in patients with invasive **bacterial** pathogens such as *Salmonella, Shigella*, and *Campylobacter*

C. Relative frequency of occurrence of diarrheal illnesses by specific infectious agents is outlined below
1. Viral pathogens—noroviruses (i.e., Norwalk-like viruses)—cause a watery diarrhea without leukocytes or blood in the stools (rotaviruses and astroviruses are common viral agents in children, but not in adults)

Noroviruses
✓ Members of the family *Calciviridae*
✓ Well-recognized etiologic agents of nonbacterial acute gastroenteritis (AGE)
✓ By far the leading cause of outbreaks of AGE among adults
✓ Self-limited
✓ At risk for complications are elderly persons and those with severe underlying medical conditions—because of volume depletion and electrolyte disturbances
✓ Hospitalization of adults with norovirus who are otherwise healthy is rare

2. Diarrhea caused by *Shigella*, *Salmonella*, and *Campylobacter* share certain inflammatory features (an inflammatory etiology can be suspected on the basis of fever, tenesmus, or bloody stools). All three agents are common causes of diarrhea

3. *Clostridium perfringens* and *Staphylococcus aureus* also are common causes of diarrhea; enterotoxigenic *Escherichia coli* (ETEC) is also common, but only among travelers to developing countries

4. *Giardia lamblia* is a relatively uncommon cause of diarrhea

D. Distinguishing features as well as clinical presentation of commonly occurring infectious causes of acute diarrhea are summarized in the table on pages 462-463

E. In addition to infectious causes of acute diarrhea, medications such as laxatives, antibiotics, antihypertensive agents, cardiovascular agents, and magnesium containing antacids as well as substances such as alcohol can cause diarrhea

F. Dietary causes of acute diarrhea include nonabsorbable sugar substitutes such as sorbitol, food intolerance or allergy, and excessive caffeine

G. Extra-intestinal infections–for example, middle ear, lung, and urinary tract infections can result in acute diarrhea via an unknown mechanism; the diarrhea is usually mild and self-limited

H. Chronic diarrhea (lasting at least 2 weeks or frequent recurrences after initial attack) also often presents in primary care settings

I. Some of the more common causes of chronic diarrhea along with their associated signs and symptoms are listed here:
1. Irritable bowel syndrome: recurrent abdominal pain, diarrhea alternates with constipation; the most common of the motility disorders causing chronic diarrhea (see IRRITABLE BOWEL SYNDROME section for a discussion of this condition)
2. Inflammatory bowel diseases: destruction of the bowel wall compromises absorption of electrolytes; characterized by bloody stools, abdominal pain, fever, and extraintestinal manifestations involving skin, joints, liver, and heart
3. Malabsorption of fat or carbohydrate
   a. With fat malabsorption, there are foul, bulky, greasy stools and the signs and symptoms are those associated with the resultant caloric and vitamin deficiencies (weight loss, ecchymosis, glossitis, peripheral neuropathy)
   b. With carbohydrate malabsorption, patients report bloating, abdominal cramps and diarrhea after intake of dairy products
4. Chronic laxative abuse can also cause diarrhea; occurs often in patients with bulimia; substances appear in the stool and the stool can be tested if laxative abuse is suspected

COMMONLY OCCURRING INFECTIOUS CAUSES OF ACUTE GASTROENTERITIS (AGE): DISTINGUISHING FEATURES

Infectious Agent	Mode of Transmission	Incubation Period	Associated Signs and Symptoms	Character-istics of Stool	Laboratory Examination of Stool	Important to Remember
Viral Norovirus (i.e., Norwalk-like virus)	By hands contaminated through the fecal-oral route directly from person-to-person, through contaminated food or water, or by contact with contaminated surfaces or fomites	12-48 hrs	Sudden onset of nausea, vomiting, abdominal cramps Fever	Watery No occult or gross blood	No WBCs in stool	By far the leading cause of outbreaks of gastroenteritis, causing approximately 23 million cases each year Infection lasts 12-60 hours Because of high infectivity and persistence in the environment, transmission of noroviruses is difficult to control through routine sanitary measures Cruise-ship outbreaks of noroviruses were common in 2002
Bacterial *Staphylococcus aureus*	Ingestion of food containing a preformed toxin produced by enterotoxicogenic staphylococci Food products most commonly involved are ham, poultry, filled pastries, egg/potato salads Contamination is via food handlers Not transmissible from person-to-person	Very short--30 minutes to 6 hours	Nausea, vomiting, abdominal cramps Fever is uncommon	Soft, but not watery No occult or gross blood	No WBCs in stool	Onset is abrupt Look for a common source pattern
Clostridium perfringens	Ingestion of food contaminated by the organism Once ingested, an enterotoxin is produced in the lower intestine of the host, producing symptoms Beef, poultry, Mexican-style foods are common sources Not transmissible from person-to-person	8-12 hours	Nausea, vomiting, moderate-to-severe mid-epigastric pain Fever is uncommon	Watery No occult or gross blood	No WBCs in stool	Onset is not as abrupt as in staphylococcal food poisoning because enterotoxin is not preformed, but is produced in host's intestine Look for a common source pattern Look for recent ingestion of foods served from steam tables
Campylobacter jejuni	Ingestion of contaminated food, including unpasteurized milk and untreated water OR by direct contact with fecal material from infected persons/animals Main vehicles of transmission: Improperly cooked poultry, un-treated water, unpasteurized milk Person-to-person spread is not common	1-7 days	Nausea, vomiting, abdominal pain, malaise Fever	Watery Occult and gross blood	WBCs in stool Positive culture	Abdominal pain can mimic that produced by appendicitis Mild infection lasts 1-2 days with most patients recovering in <7 days Outbreaks in child care centers are uncommon

(continued)

462

COMMONLY OCCURRING INFECTIOUS CAUSES OF ACUTE GASTROENTERITIS (AGE): DISTINGUISHING FEATURES (*CONTINUED*)

Infectious Agent	Mode of Transmission	Incubation Period	Associated Signs and Symptoms	Character-istics of Stool	Laboratory Examination of Stool	Important to Remember
Salmonella	Major modes: Ingestion of food of animal origin, including poultry, red meat, eggs, and unpasteurized milk Other modes: Ingestion of contaminated water, contact with infected animals such as pet turtles/reptiles Direct person-to-person transmission (fecal-oral) are less common than other modes	6-72 hours; usually <24 hours	Nausea, vomiting, abdominal cramping Fever	Watery Occult and gross blood	WBCs in stool Positive culture	Most likely to occur in children <5 (peaks in first year of life) and adults >70 Outbreaks of this infection are rare in day care centers Report all confirmed cases to local public health department
Shigella	Ingestion of contaminated food or water and homosexual transmis-sion most common routes in adults Fecal-oral transmission is most common route in children Feces of infected humans are source of infection No animal reservoir known	1-7 days; usually 2-4 days	Abdominal pain Fever	Watery Occult and gross blood	WBCs in stool Positive culture	Most common in children 1-4 years of age Important problem in child care centers in US Report all confirmed cases to the local health department
Enterotoxigenic *Escherichia coli* (ETEC)	One of at least 5 different groups of diarrhea-producing strains of *E. coli* Most commonly from food or water contaminated with human or animal feces Most common cause of "travelers' diarrhea," acquired by travelers to developing countries	10 hours to 6 days	Abdominal cramps Usually no fever	Watery No occult or gross blood	No WBCs (usually); can be present Positive culture	The enterotoxin that is produced by the organism promotes fluid secretion in the small bowel which results in a watery diarrhea History of recent travel to a developing country is important epidemiologic information Causes travelers' diarrhea in all ages
Protozoal *Giardia*	Main route of spread is fecal-oral transfer of cysts from feces of an infected person Many common source outbreaks are traced to contaminated drinking water Humans are principle reservoir but organism can infect animals such as dogs, cats, beavers	1-4 weeks	Abdominal pain associated with flatulence, disten-tion, and anorexia Passage of foul-smelling stools No fever	Soft, watery No occult or gross blood	Positive stool for O & P	Most often represents an acute presentation of chronic or recurrent diarrhea

IV. Diagnosis/Evaluation: Focus of initial clinical evaluation is to assess severity of the illness, determine need for rehydration, and identify likely causes based on history and clinical findings

    A. History: Important to assess both clinical and epidemiological features

Relevant Clinical Features: Determine the Following
• When (duration) and how the illness began (e.g., was onset abrupt or gradual)
• Stool characteristics–whether watery, bloody, mucous-containing, purulent, greasy
• Frequency of bowel movements and relative quantity of stool produced
• If dysenteric symptoms are present–fever, tenesmus, blood and/or pus in stool
• If symptoms of volume depletion are present–thirst, tachycardia, orthostasis, decreased urine output, lethargy, decreased skin turgor
• If associated symptoms are present–nausea, vomiting, abdominal pain, cramps, headache, myalgias, altered sensorium–and gauge their severity

Relevant Epidemiological Risk Factors for Particular Diarrheal Illnesses and Their Spread: Determine the Following
• Recent travel to developing countries
• Day-care employment
• Consumption of unsafe foods (e.g., raw meats, eggs, shellfish, unpasteurized milk)
• Swimming in or drinking untreated surface water from a lake or stream
• Recent visit to a petting zoo or recent contact with reptiles or pets with diarrhea
• Knowledge of other ill persons (such as in households, dormitories, at social functions, or on cruise ships)
• Recent or regular medications (antibiotics, antacids)
• Underlying medical conditions predisposing to infectious diarrhea (AIDS, prior gastrectomy)
• Sexual practices that include receptive anal intercourse or oral-anal sexual contact
• Occupation as a food handler

    B. Physical Examination
       1. Determine if patient is febrile and assess for dehydration

Assess for Dehydration
• Note general appearance, level of alertness
• Measure pulse, blood pressure, presence or absence of postural hypotension
• Assess mucous membranes
• Observe for tears and sunken eyes
• Measure skin turgor and capillary refill

       2. Weigh patient and determine if there has been a weight loss (more of an issue in chronic diarrhea)
       3. Examine abdomen for tenderness, rigidity, abnormal tympany, bowel sounds, liver/spleen enlargement
       4. Perform rectal exam for tenderness, masses; obtain stool for occult blood

    C. Differential Diagnosis: Diarrhea is a symptom. Refer to common causes of acute and chronic diarrhea under section III. above

D. Diagnostic Tests
1. Microbiologic investigation is usually not necessary for patients presenting within 24 hours after onset of diarrhea
2. Any diarrheal illness lasting >24 hours, especially if accompanied by fever, blood/pus in stools, systemic illness, dehydration, or recent use of antibiotics should prompt evaluation of a fecal specimen

Stool Testing
• Patients with systemic illness, fever, or blood/pus in stools require stool testing for salmonella, shigella, and Campylobacter (microscopic examination for fecal polymorphonuclear leukocytes or immunoassay for the neutrophil marker lactoferrin [Leukotest by TechLab])
• Patients presenting with an acute onset of bloody diarrhea (especially *without* fever) should have fecal testing for Shiga toxin along with cultures for E. coli 0157:H7
• Bloody diarrhea in recent travelers to regions where E. histolytica is endemic (e.g., Asia, tropical Africa, South America) indicates need for fecal testing for that pathogen
• Recent ingestion of shellfish requires special cultures for vibrio species
• Exposure to untreated water (e.g., hikers and travelers to developing countries) and illnesses that last more than 7 days should prompt evaluation for the protozoal pathogens—Giardia and cryptosporidium
• If recent antibiotics, chemotherapy, or hospitalization, test for *C. difficile* toxins A and B

3. Additional diagnostic testing such as complete blood cell count and serum chemistries may also be indicated in selected cases, depending on the clinical findings

V. Plan/Management

A. Acute diarrhea is almost invariably a benign, self-limited condition, subsiding within one or two days–age and the nutritional status of the patient are important factors in determining risk for severe dehydration with patients at the extremes of the age range (very young and very old) being the most vulnerable

B. Appropriate management of acute dehydration, electrolyte status, and nutrition remains the cornerstones of therapy; whether or not the cause of the diarrhea is determined, supportive therapy must be instituted immediately to rehydrate (if necessary) and maintain hydration status and to maintain adequate nutrition through refeeding as soon as possible

C. Supportive therapy should focus on attaining and maintaining adequate hydration status through appropriate fluid intake. Water or sports drinks may be used for hydration as well as the commercial rehydration products such as Pedialyte and Rehydralyte

D. The decision to treat patients with suspected bacterial or parasitic enteritis must be based on stool culture or testing for specific organisms
1. Keep in mind that any consideration of antimicrobial therapy must be carefully weighed against unintended and potentially harmful consequences
2. Unintended consequences include development of antimicrobial-resistant infections, side effects of treatment, and suprainfections when normal flora are eradicated
3. Situations in which empirical antibiotics are commonly recommended without obtaining a fecal specimen are the following
   a. Travelers' diarrhea, in which enterotoxigenic E. coli or other bacterial pathogens are likely causes and prompt therapy can reduce duration from 3-5 days to <1-2 days
   b. When giardiasis is suspected, based on patient's history of travel or water exposure, consider empirical treatment of diarrhea that has lasted longer than 10-14 days
4. In addition, patients with febrile diarrheal illnesses, particularly when moderate to severe invasive disease is suspected, should be considered for empirical treatment (prior to treatment, a fecal specimen should be obtained for testing)

E. Counseling and control measures for patients with identified infectious agents as the cause of acute diarrheal illness as well as recommended pharmacologic management are contained in the following table

TREATMENT OF AGE CAUSED BY COMMONLY OCCURRING INFECTIOUS AGENTS

Infectious Agent	Pharmacologic Management	Counseling and Control Measures
Viral Norovirus (i.e., Norwalk-like virus)	✓ No specific antiviral therapy is available	✓ Emphasize importance of frequent, vigorous handwashing with soap and water ✓ Contaminated food and water can spread virus from person-to-person; sharing of utensils and dishes should be avoided ✓ **Infected persons should be excluded from handling food** ✓ Disinfecting of possibly contaminated surfaces (e.g., sinks and commode seats) should be with freshly prepared chlorine solutions at concentrations of ≥1,000 ppm
Bacterial Staphylococcus aureus	✓ Antibiotics are not recommended	✓ Proper cooking and refrigeration of food helps prevent the disease ✓ Persons with staphylococcal infections should be excluded from handling food
Clostridium perfringens	✓ Antibiotics are not recommended	✓ C. perfringens should not be allowed to proliferate in food (beef, poultry, gravies, and Mexican-style foods are common sources) ✓ Foods should never be held at room temperature to cool, but should be refrigerated promptly, and reheated thoroughly before serving ✓ Foods should not be kept in warming devices or serving tables for long periods of time
Campylobacter infections	✓ Erythromycin (Ery-Tab), given early in the course of infection, shortens duration of illness and prevents relapse • Dosing: 250 mg PO QID x 5-7 days	✓ Persons who prepare food should practice frequent handwashing, wash surfaces that have been exposed to raw poultry, and thoroughly cook poultry ✓ Pasteurization of milk and chlorination of water supplies are essential ✓ Infected food handlers who are asymptomatic need not be excluded from work if proper personal hygiene measures are maintained ✓ Outbreaks are uncommon in child care centers
Salmonella infections (non-typhi species)	✓ Antimicrobial therapy is not routinely recommended for uncomplicated gastroenteritis caused by non-typhi species of Salmonella because it can prolong excretion of the organism ✓ Treatment is recommended for patients at an increased risk of invasive disease such as persons with valvular heart disease, uremia, or HIV infection. Consult specialists for treatment recommendations	✓ Emphasis should be on good hand-washing and personal hygiene ✓ There must be proper sanitation in food processing and preparation; **infected persons should be excluded from handling food** ✓ Eggs and other foods of animal origin should be cooked thoroughly before ingestion ✓ Raw eggs as well as food containing raw eggs should not be eaten ✓ Handwashing when handling pet turtles and other reptiles is important ✓ Outbreaks of Salmonella infection are rare in child care centers ✓ Vaccination for typhoid is recommended only for international travelers ✓ Report all cases of Salmonella infection to local public health department so that proper investigation of outbreak can be conducted

(Continued)

TREATMENT OF AGE CAUSED BY COMMONLY OCCURRING INFECTIOUS AGENTS *(CONTINUED)*

Infectious Agent	Pharmacologic Management	Counseling and Control Measures
Shigella	✓ To shorten course and prevent further spread, may treat with trimethoprim-sulfamethoxazole • Dosing: 1 DS tab BID x 3-5 days ✓ Intestinal motility patterns are considered important in recovery from infection, therefore anti-diarrhea drugs should not be given	✓ Emphasis should be on good hand-washing and personal hygiene, particularly among workers in group care settings such as child care and group living facilities ✓ There must be proper sanitation in food processing and preparation; **infected persons should be excluded from handling food** ✓ Prevention of contamination of food by flies during preparation and serving is required ✓ Insuring that water supply is not contaminated is important ✓ Outbreak of Shigella infection must be reported to the local health department for investigation
Escherichia coli infection (enterotoxigenic) [ETEC], major cause of **Travelers' Diarrhea**	✓ May treat with trimethoprim-sulfamethoxazole • Dosing: 1 DS tab, BID x 3 days ✓ Ciprofloxacin is an alternative agent for adults • Dosing: 500 mg BID x 3 days	✓ When traveling in developing countries or in any area where water supply is questionable, drink only bottled water ✓ Avoid all raw fruits and vegetables that may not have been properly washed (unless can peel and eat)
Protozoal *Giardia*	✓ Drug of choice is metronidazole • Dosing: 250 mg TID x 5 days ✓ Alternative drug is furazolidone • Dosing: 100 mg QID x 7-10 days ✓ In pregnant women, paromomycin is recommended for treatment of symptomatic infections. Consult PDR for dosing recommendations	✓ Emphasize sanitation and personal hygiene, especially in group care settings ✓ Hand washing after diaper changes and after personal toilet use by workers cannot be overemphasized; persons with diarrhea (both workers and children) should be excluded from day care until problem resolves ✓ Adequate filtration of municipal water supply prevents water-borne outbreaks in metropolitan areas ✓ Boiling of water by campers, backpackers will eliminate cysts; drinking from streams is risky ✓ Treatment of asymptomatic carriers is not recommended except for prevention of household transmission to pregnant women ✓ Outbreaks in day care centers require reporting to local public health department for epidemiological investigation

F. Several products are available to provide some symptomatic relief to patients during a diarrheal illness; these agents do not alter the course of the illness or reduce fluid loss
   1. The following anti-diarrheal agents are available and may be used in selected cases of diarrheal illnesses for no longer than 3 days where there are no contraindications
   2. Use of these agents have not been shown to be beneficial in the management of acute diarrhea and patients should be advised of this
   3. Loperamide (Imodium) is the antimotility agent of choice—it inhibits intestinal peristalsis and has antisecretory properties. Unlike other opiates (codeine, diphenoxylate, paregoric) it does not penetrate the nervous system and has no substantial addiction potential

ANTI-DIARRHEAL AGENTS FOR ACUTE DIARRHEA

Agents	Medication	Dosage
Antimotility agents	Imodium A-D (OTC), available as 1 mg/5mL syrup and 2 mg caplets	4 mg initially, then 2 mg after each unformed stool. Maximum 8 mg/day; use for 2 days
	Lomotil, available as 2.5 mg tabs and liquid, 2.5 mg/5 mL	2 tabs QID (maximum 20 mg/day) for 2-3 days only
Adsorbents	Kaolin-pectin mixture (Kaopectate) liquid	30-120 mL after each loose stool
Antisecretory agents	Bismuth subsalicylate (Pepto-Bismol) available as 262 mg chewable tabs and 262 mg/15 mL liquid	2 tabs or 30 mL Q 30-60 minutes (Maximum 8 doses/day)

G. Patients with chronic diarrhea require treatment of the underlying cause
   1. Refer to sections on HIV/AIDS and IRRITABLE BOWEL SYNDROME for management of patients with these conditions
   2. If *Giardia* is suspected, obtain diagnostic tests and treat as described in the table above
   3. If a medication that the patient is taking is producing the diarrhea, change medication if possible
   4. If inflammatory bowel disease or a malabsorption syndrome such as sprue or lactase deficiency is suspected, refer to a specialist for management

H. Public health considerations
   1. Food handlers in food service establishments should be tested for viral and bacterial pathogens if they have diarrhea because of their potential to transmit infection to large numbers of persons
   2. Workers in day-care centers and residents in institutional facilities such as nursing homes and prisons who have a diarrheal illness should be evaluated for bacterial or parasitic infection because gastrointestinal illnesses in such settings may indicate that a disease outbreak is occurring
   3. When a disease outbreak is suspected due to an observed increased incidence of diarrheal illness among a particular group, diagnostic testing to facilitate identification of the etiologic agent and to define the extent of the outbreak should be undertaken; the suspected outbreak should be reported to public health authorities
   4. Rapid implementation of control measures at the first sign of a suspected acute gastroenteritis outbreak is critical in preventing additional cases

> Disease reporting to appropriate public health officials is the cornerstone of public-health surveillance, outbreak detection, and control and prevention efforts
> ✓ Reporting requirements and procedures differ by jurisdictions
> ✓ Requirements for the reporting of disease can be obtained from the state or local health department or from the CDC http://www.cdc.gov/epo/dphsi/phs/infdis.htm
> ✓ Can also be obtained at the Web site of the Council of State and Territorial Epidemiologists at http://www.cste.org

I. General counseling and patient education (in addition to counseling and control measures in the table above) include the following
   1. Hand-washing with soap after toileting and before food preparation is very effective
   2. Human feces must always be considered potentially hazardous and should be handled as hazardous waste
   3. Select populations (such as food handlers and day-care attendants) require additional education about food safety and these persons should be referred to appropriate resources for education
   4. Immunocompromised persons (e.g., HIV-infected, cancer chemotherapy recipients, persons receiving long term oral steroids or immunosuppressive agents) are more susceptible to infection from a variety of enteric pathogens and can reduce their risk through safe food-handling and preparation practices
   5. General educational information on food safety is available from the following Web sites

Websites
http://www.cdc.gov/ncidod/dbmd/diseaseinfo/foodborneinfections_g.htm
http://www.fightbac.org
http://www.foodsafety.gov
http://www.healthfinder.gov
http://www.nal.usda.gov/fnic/foodborne/foodborn.htm

   6. CDC encourages local and state health departments to test for noroviruses when investigating outbreaks of suspected viral AGE; contact CDC's Viral Gastroenteritis Section, telephone 404-639-3577 for assistance

J. Follow Up
   1. In 48 hours if diarrhea has not resolved
   2. In certain situations such as those involving food-handlers, daycare workers, and healthcare workers with laboratory-confirmed bacterial or parasitic diarrheal disease, confirmation that the disease has been cured or that the person is no longer a fecal carrier must be obtained; consult local public health officer to find out more about regulations pertaining to persons in these categories before the patient is allowed to return to work

NAUSEA AND VOMITING

I. Definition

    A.   Nausea: An unpleasant sensation of the throat or epigastric region alerting one that vomiting is imminent

    B.   Vomiting: The forceful oral expulsion of gastric contents

II. Pathogenesis

    A.   Three consecutive phases of emesis include nausea, retching, and vomiting
        1.   Nausea is entirely subjective and is commonly described as a sensation immediately preceding vomiting; may or may not lead to the act of vomiting
        2.   When vomiting does occur, it is preceded by retching which is repetitive active contractions of the abdominal musculature which generate the pressure gradient that leads to evacuation of the stomach
        3.   Vomiting is a highly specific physical event that results in the rapid, forceful evacuation of gastric contents in a retrograde way from the stomach and up to and out of the mouth

    B.   Vomiting is triggered by afferent impulses received in the vomiting center (VC) believed to be located in the medulla

    C.   Sensory centers such as the cerebral cortex, visceral afferents from the pharynx and gastrointestinal tract, and the chemoreceptor trigger zone (CTZ) are responsible for sending the impulses to the vomiting center

    D.   Once the VC is stimulated, efferent pathways to the salivation center, respiratory center, and the pharyngeal, gastrointestinal, and abdominal musculature work in concert to produce vomiting

III. Clinical Presentation

    A.   Nausea and vomiting are among the most common symptoms that children and adults experience and may be associated with a variety of clinical presentations

    B.   A broad range of both pathologic and physiologic conditions may evoke these symptoms; only the most common causes are listed in the box below

---

Toxic etiologies and medications
- Acute gastroenteritis, both viral and bacterial
- Nongastrointestinal infections including urinary tract infection
- Numerous medications including cardiovascular medications (e.g., digoxin, calcium channel blockers); hormonal preparations (e.g., oral contraceptives); antibiotics/antivirals, (e.g., erythromycin, acyclovir); analgesics (e.g., aspirin, NSAIDs); cancer chemotherapy (e.g., methotrexate)

Disorders of the gut and peritoneum
- Mechanical obstruction, e.g., small bowel obstruction, gastric outlet obstruction
- Functional disorders, e.g., gastroparesis, irritable bowel syndrome
- Organic disorders, e.g., peptic ulcer disease, cholecystitis, pancreatitis, hepatitis

CNS causes
- Migraine
- Increased intracranial pressure from malignancy, hemorrhage, infarction, abscess, other etiologies
- Labyrinthine disorders, e.g., motion sickness, labyrinthitis, tumors, Ménière's disease

Endocrinologic and metabolic causes
- Pregnancy
- Uremia, diabetic ketoacidosis, hyperthyroidism

Postoperative nausea and vomiting

Iatrogenic, as occurs in bulimia

IV. Diagnosis/Evaluation

   A.   History
        1.   Question about onset, duration, quantity and quality of vomitus (undigested food, yellow-green bilious material, blood)
        2.   Determine if this is an acute (few days) or chronic (> 4 weeks) problem
             a.   Acute onset of nausea and vomiting suggests gastroenteritis, pancreatitis, cholecystitis, or a medication-related side effect
             b.   A more insidious onset of nausea, without vomiting, should raise suspicion of gastroparesis, a drug-related side effect, or metabolic disorders
        3.   Ask about timing of vomiting and relation to meals
             a.   Vomiting that occurs in the morning before meals is typical of that related to pregnancy, uremia, alcohol ingestion, and increased intracranial pressure
             b.   Vomiting that occurs more than 1 hour after meal ingestion suggests gastroparesis or gastric outlet obstruction
        4.   Ask about associated symptoms such as abdominal pain, diarrhea, dizziness, headache
             a.   Abdominal pain preceding vomiting usually indicates an organic lesion such as an obstruction
             b.   With small bowel obstruction, pain is typically prominent, severe, and colicky; may temporarily improve after a vomiting episode
        5.   Ask if systemic symptoms of fever and malaise are present
        6.   Ask about past medical history and medication history
        7.   Ask if others in household are ill to identify a common source cause

   B.   Physical Examination
        1.   Observe general appearance for pallor, perspiration, restlessness, signs of peritonitis, toxicity; determine if febrile
        2.   Assess hydration status: Check for dry mucous membranes, decreased skin turgor, tachycardia, and oliguria
        3.   Assess cardiovascular status (pulse, blood pressure; check for postural hypotension)
        4.   Examine abdomen for tenderness, rigidity, abnormal tympany, bowel sounds, liver and spleen size
        5.   Perform rectal exam for tenderness, masses; stool for occult blood

   C.   Differential Diagnosis: Vomiting is a symptom; see Pathogenesis for possible causes

   D.   Laboratory Tests: Selection of laboratory studies should be directed by findings from history and physical examination
        1.   Goals of testing are twofold: To assist in identifying cause and to evaluate the consequences of vomiting
        2.   Basic laboratory tests include the following
             a.   Complete blood count and erythrocyte sedimentation rate
             b.   Serum chemistries to document acid-base, electrolyte status
             c.   Pregnancy test in women
             d.   Drug levels, if indicated

V. Plan/Management

   A.   Patients suspected of having an emergent condition involving the gastrointestinal tract, such as mechanical obstruction, perforation, or peritonitis should be immediately transported to the emergency department for evaluation and management

   B.   If central nervous system symptoms are present (headache, vertigo, neck stiffness, and focal neurologic deficits), refer the patient for emergent evaluation and management

   C.   If medications are believed to be the cause and can safely be switched, consider this option (nausea frequently subsides with many medications over time)

   D.   All underlying causes detected in history, physical examination, and laboratory testing should be either treated or referred for management

   E.   Most acute episodes of nausea and vomiting are caused by viral gastroenteritis or (less commonly) motion sickness, and are self-limiting; supportive therapy is all that is indicated

   F.   Nonpharmacologic interventions to promote hydration

470

- Discontinue solid foods
- Encourage clear liquids only (not milk) until at least 4 hours have passed without vomiting
- Start with 1 tbsp (15 cc) every 10 minutes
- If vomiting does not occur, double the amount each hour
- If vomiting does occur, allow stomach to rest briefly and then start again
- Key is to gradually increase amount of fluid until taking 8 oz every hour
- May use glucose-electrolyte solutions developed for infants/small children such as Pedialyte or Rehydralyte (may combine with flavored gelatin to make more palatable) or sports drinks such as Gatorade which contain salt and sugar in addition to water
- Goal is to ingest 1000 to 1500 mL/day
- Resume normal diet as soon as tolerated (usually, 4 hours after vomiting ceases)

G. Pharmacologic therapy is usually not indicated; however, for selected patients (for example, those with electrolyte disturbances, severe anorexia/weight loss, motion sickness, pregnancy, or with chemotherapy-induced nausea and vomiting) antiemetic therapy may be indicated

---

Emetrol (OTC): Do not dilute or take fluids 15 minutes before or after. Can be used in pregnancy
  ✓ 15-30 mL at 15 minute intervals as needed
Promethazine (Phenergan) is the agent of choice for n/v from gastroenteritis: Available as 12.5, 25, 50 mg tabs and rectal supp
  ✓ 25 mg Q 8-12 hrs
Prochlorperazine (Compazine): Available 5, 10 mg tabs; 10, 15, 30 mg spansules; 25 mg rectal supp
  ✓ Tabs/5-10 mg 3-4 times day; spansules/10 mg Q 12 hrs; rectal supp/25 mg BID
Trimethobenzamide (Tigan) works well for gastroenteritis and motion sickness: Available as 100, 250 mg caps and rectal supp--100, 200 mg
  ✓ 250 mg caps OR 200 mg rectal supp 3-4 x day
Scopolamine (Transderm Scop) works well for prevention and treatment of motion sickness: Available as 0.33 mg patch
  ✓ Apply one patch in hairless area behind ear 4 hours prior to when antiemetic effect is needed
  ✓ Replace after 3 days

H. The 5-HT$_3$ antagonist drugs have dramatically reduced vomiting associated with chemotherapy treatment (these drugs have been unsuccessful in controlling chemotherapy-induced nausea, however); examples of these drugs are Ondansetron (Zofran) and Dolasetron (Anzemet) [patients receiving chemotherapy will have these medications prescribed by the oncologist]

I. Follow Up: None needed unless failure to respond to nonpharmacologic or pharmacologic therapy

CONSTIPATION

I. Definition: Diminished frequency of defecation, incomplete evacuation, or stools that are too hard or too small

II. Pathogenesis

A. Fecal continence is defined as the ability to control defecation voluntarily and requires normal contractions of the anal sphincters, normal sensory receptors in the rectum and anus (to identify the rectal contents as liquid, solid, or gaseous), and a normal rectal reservoir

B. Movement of a fecal bolus into the rectum stimulates several automatic, coordinated reflexes
  1. The lower colon, including the rectum, contracts and the internal sphincter relaxes
  2. The external sphincter initially contracts, but the initial contraction is followed by a total inhibition of both the external and internal sphincters
  3. Intra-abdominal pressure is voluntarily increased (Valsalva maneuver), the pelvic floor descends and stool is expelled

C. The distal colon and rectum provide storage for feces until defecation is convenient; defecation can be postponed by contracting the external anal sphincter and the gluteal muscles

D. Constipation is a major feature of two disorders of colorectal motility: Slow transit constipation and pelvic floor dysfunction
   1. **Slow-transit constipation** or "colonic inertia," is believed to be the most common mechanism of constipation. It is characterized by slower than normal movement of contents from the proximal to the distal colon and rectum (basis of this disorder may be dietary or even cultural); two subtypes of slow-transit constipation are believed to exist
      a. Colonic inertia is thought to result from reduced numbers of high-amplitude peristaltic sequences–a reduction that causes impaired mass movement of colonic contents
      b. Increased, uncoordinated motor activity in the distal colon is the second subtype–a functional barrier or resistance to normal transit is created by this dysfunction in motor activity
      c. Distinction between the two subtypes requires colonic manometry and is most often made in research settings
   2. **Pelvic floor dysfunction** is characterized by normal or slightly slowed colonic transit overall and a failure to evacuate contents adequately from the rectum where residue is stored for prolonged periods of time
   3. **Combination syndromes** are frequently observed in patients who present with elements of both slow transit and disorders of evacuation (pelvic floor dysfunction)
      a. Often present in conjunction with other features of the irritable bowel syndrome (IBS)
      b. Presence of pain as a major presenting complaint would evoke the strong possibility of IBS

E. Constipation may also arise secondary to other conditions (or medications used to treat medical conditions) including the following
   1. Primary diseases of the colon including stricture, tumor, anal fissure, proctitis
   2. Endocrine and metabolic disorders such as hypothyroidism and diabetes mellitus
   3. Neurologic disturbances such as parkinsonism and spinal cord lesions
   4. Medications such as anticholinergics, antiparkinsonian agents, calcium channel blockers, diuretics, and antacids

III. Clinical Presentation

A. Prevalence of constipation has been reported to be as high as 20% among the general adult population in the US; prevalence is highest among African-Americans, women, and older persons

B. Constipation accounts for 2.5 million healthcare visits per year, the majority of which are in primary care settings; more than $800 million is spent on laxatives in the US each year

C. Constipation is associated with inactivity, low calorie intake, the number of medications being taken, low income, and low educational level (association does not equate to causality)
   1. Interestingly, constipation has not been reported to be associated with a low intake of fiber in research studies to date (study design is believed to account for this failure)
   2. Although inactivity is associated with constipation, exercise has not clearly been shown to be an effective treatment

D. Rome II criteria for defining chronic functional constipation in adults are contained in the box below

> To meet criteria, two or more of the following signs/symptoms must have been present for at least 12 weeks during the previous 12 month period
> ➡ For more than 25% of defecations, person must
>   • Strain to defecate
>   • Produce lumpy or hard stools
>   • Experience sensation of incomplete evacuation
>   • Experience sensation of anorectal obstruction
>   • Use manual maneuvers (e.g., digital evacuation) to facilitate evacuation of stool
> ➡ Have fewer than 3 defecations per week
> ➡ Loose stools are not present
> ➡ There are insufficient criteria for diagnosis of irritable bowel syndrome

Adapted from Thompson, W.G., Longstreth, G.F., Drossman, D.A., Heaton, K.W., Irvine, K.J., Muller-Lissner, S.A. (1999). Functional bowel disorders and functional abdominal pain. *Gut, 45* (suppl 2), 1143-1147.

E. Constipation is a symptom, not a disease; therefore patients presenting with a complaint of constipation should be evaluated for underlying causes and treated appropriately based on the following priority
    1. First, life-threatening or treatable conditions must be excluded as the cause (see *Important Red Flags* in box below)
    2. Second, patients who may benefit from referral to an expert for specialized testing must be identified
    3. Finally, effective therapy must be provided for the majority of patients who have neither a life-threatening nor disabling disorder, but whose primary need is for control of symptoms

IV. Diagnosis/Evaluation

A. History
    1. Determine what the patient means by constipation (Is it small stools, infrequent stools, a feeling of fullness, or difficulty/pain with passing stools?); [for most patients, frequency is usually the issue, as frequency is the characteristic that is easiest to set standards for]
    2. Determine how long the problem has been present (acute constipation is more often associated with organic disease than is long-standing constipation)
    3. Ask about the current regimen and bowel pattern ("How often does a 'call to stool' occur?" "Is the call always answered, usually answered, or almost always ignored or put off?")
    4. To determine if patient meets Rome II criteria for constipation–ask about straining to defecate, consistency and size of stools, sensation of incomplete evacuation, sensation of anorectal obstruction; ask patient if manual maneuvers are necessary to facilitate defecation; ask if loose stools are present (see section on IRRITABLE BOWEL SYNDROME to determine if patient meets criteria for that condition)
    5. Ask about associated symptoms and signs that are considered "red flags" suggesting the presence of an underlying gastrointestinal organic disorder

---

Important Red Flags
- Abdominal pain
- Nausea, vomiting
- Melena, rectal bleeding, rectal pain
- Fever
- Weight loss

---

    6. Determine if patient has a history of signs and symptoms of a neurologic, endocrine, or metabolic disorder
    7. Ask about dietary intake and activity level (fiber-poor diet, inadequate fluid intake, and sedentary lifestyle may contribute to problem)
    8. Determine if there have been any recent changes in patient's life that could be producing stress (e.g., travel, change in job, family problems)
    9. Inquire about current medications (including over-the-counter products) and laxative use; ask if suppositories or enemas are used in addition to oral agents
    10. Obtain past medical and surgical history; determine if there is a family history of colon cancer

B. Physical Examination
    1. Weigh patient and determine if there has been a weight loss
    2. Assess abdomen for tenderness, masses, distension, and high-pitched or absent bowel sounds
    3. Perineal/rectal exam should focus on the following

With patient in the left lateral position, with buttocks separated
- ✓ Examine perianal skin for evidence of fecal soiling and for fissures
- ✓ Test anal reflex by light pinprick or scratch
- ✓ Perform digital examination to evaluate resting tone of the sphincter segment, ask patient to tighten sphincter by squeezing down on examining finger to determine tone with augmentation by a squeezing effort
- ✓ Check for fecal impaction, especially in elderly patients with a history of chronic constipation
- ✓ Obtain stool for testing for occult blood

---

    4. Perform a focused neurologic examination

C. Differential Diagnosis
1. Functional causes such as diet, motility disturbance, and irritable bowel syndrome
2. Structural abnormalities such as anorectal disorders, tumors, or strictures
3. Endocrine and metabolic conditions such as diabetes mellitus, hypothyroidism, and electrolyte disturbances
4. Neurologic conditions such as spinal cord lesions and parkinsonism
5. Smooth muscle and connective tissue disorders such as scleroderma
6. Psychogenic conditions such as anxiety, depression, and somatization
7. Drugs such as antacids, anticholinergics, antidepressants, calcium channel blockers, narcotics, and nonsteroidal anti-inflammatory agents

D. Diagnostic Tests: Purpose is to exclude conditions that are either treatable or important to diagnose early
1. Complete blood cell count; TSH, serum glucose, creatinine, calcium
2. Evaluation of the colon is appropriate, particularly in patients >50 years of age, or in those patients who have not had previous screenings for colorectal cancer and colitis; colonoscopy or flexible sigmoidoscopy and barium enema are effective in excluding lesions that could cause constipation

V. Plan/Management

A. Patients who are found to have a life-threatening condition should be referred immediately for emergent care by an expert

B. Patients who are found to have underlying disorders that are treatable (such as hypothyroidism) should be treated appropriately; if medications are suspected of causing the constipation, the medications should be adjusted when possible to avoid those with constipating effects

C. Patients who meet the diagnostic criteria for irritable bowel syndrome should be treated according to the recommendations in the section IRRITABLE BOWEL SYNDROME

D. Patients who are not in the above three categories (i.e., absence of a life-threatening condition or treatable underlying condition, and who fail to meet diagnostic criteria for irritable bowel syndrome) should be managed with a treatment regimen emphasizing dietary fiber, adequate fluid intake, increased physical activity, and long-term laxative use

E. Recommend a **gradual** increase in fiber intake; this can be done via adding high-fiber containing foods to the diet or through use of a fiber supplement
1. Refer to section on NUTRITION for foods to recommend to increase fiber intake to the recommended dietary allowance or simply recommend bran, 1 cup/day
2. If the patient prefers to use a fiber supplement, prescribe products such as psyllium (Perdiem, Metamucil), methylcellulose (Citrucel), or polycarbophil (FiberCon)
3. Advise patients that high fiber diets and fiber supplements usually increase gaseousness, but this symptom often decreases over the first week or two
4. Counsel patients to drink plenty of fluids for fiber supplement to work (**Note:** 8 oz water with each dose)
5. Immediate response should not be expected but should result in softer stools within 7-10 days or so; patient can then increase or decrease daily dose of fiber based on quantity and quality of stools
6. Patients who gradually increase fiber intake will be able to tolerate fiber better than those who attempt a rapid increase

F. Encourage patient to consume adequate amounts of water each day; recently the dictum to drink eight, 8 ounce glasses of water each day has been called into question because of its lack of a scientific basis (most experts still agree that 6 glasses [8 ounces each] is certainly reasonable)

G. Whereas physical activity has not clearly been shown to be an effective treatment for constipation, current recommendations from the Institute of Medicine are for adults to engage in 60 minutes of moderate intensity physical activity each day
1. Counseling the patient to increase activity levels (if presently below the current standard) is important for a healthy lifestyle in general, and thus should be recommended without hesitation
2. Emphasize the total amount of activity can be accomplished in 10-15 minute segments throughout the day

H. Most patients also require a laxative, and an inexpensive saline agent such as milk of magnesia should be recommended as first-line therapy: Start with 15-30 mL/day and advise patients to titrate dose until soft, but not liquid stools are achieved
    1. If this agent is not satisfactory after an adequate trial, more expensive agents such as lactulose and polyethylene glycol (PEG) without electrolytes can be considered
        a. Lactulose (Kristalose), 10-20 g/day QD, available as 10 g/packet, 20 g/packet [advise patient that lactulose is a nonabsorbable carbohydrate, and as such is limited by its extreme potential to produce gas]
        b. Polyethylene glycol (PEG) [MiraLax], 17 g in 8 ounces of water QD
    2. Use of a stimulant agent such as bisacodyl (Dulcolax), two 5 mg tabs PO at bedtime 2 or 3 times a week may also be considered as a "rescue" medication for occasional use
    3. Long-term use of laxatives such as milk of magnesia, lactulose, and PEG without electrolytes is generally considered safe although no laxative is approved for chronic use; stimulant laxatives are best used short-term and no more often than 2 or 3 times a week to allow the colon to fill properly

I. Most patients with simple or slow transit constipation are controlled by the above regime
    1. Patients who fail to respond to an adequate trial of increased fiber, adequate fluids, increased physical activity and use of a laxative should be referred for expert evaluation and management
    2. Patients with pelvic floor dysfunction (see above description) frequently fail to respond well to standard laxative programs and often require referral

J. Follow Up
    1. In 2-4 weeks to determine initial efficacy of treatment program
    2. Then in 3-6 months to evaluate for continued efficacy

IRRITABLE BOWEL SYNDROME

I. Definition: Chronic, benign gastrointestinal disorder characterized by abdominal pain, bloating, and disturbed defecation that cannot be explained by structural or biochemical abnormalities

II. Pathogenesis:

A. A number of pathophysiologic features have been proposed as playing a role in the development of the irritable bowel syndrome (IBS)
    1. **Altered bowel motility**: Changes in the contractility of the colon and small bowel. Such factors as psychological or physical stress, ingestion of food, ingestion of a high fat meal, and fasting have all been implicated in altering bowel motility in patients with IBS
    2. **Visceral hypersensitivity**: Differences in the way that the brain of affected persons modulates afferent signals from the dorsal-horn neurons through the ascending pathways suggest a primary central defect of visceral pain processing (an alternative hypothesis is that rather than true visceral hypersensitivity, hypervigilance may be responsible for the low pain threshold of IBS patients)
    3. **Psychosocial factors**: Psychological stress including a history of abuse in childhood can alter motor function in the small bowel and colon; one theory is that experiences early in life may affect the central nervous system in such a way as to confer a predisposition to a state of hypervigilance
    4. **Neurotransmitter imbalance**: Serotonin and a number of other neurotransmitters are known to influence bowel contractility and visceral sensitivity and may well provide links between the enteric and central nervous systems
    5. **Infection and inflammation**: Much evidence points to a role for infection in the initiation of (or a contribution to) activation of peripheral sensitization or hypermotility in affected persons

B. Presently, no single conceptual model can explain all cases of the irritable bowel syndrome

III. Clinical Presentation

A. Irritable Bowel Syndrome (IBS) is a common malady affecting approximately 15% of the adult population in the US and accounts for 28% of referrals to gastroenterologists from primary care clinicians; it is uncommon for IBS to present de novo in patients after the age of 50

B. Women are affected more often than men (3:1); IBS accounts for 12% of all visits to primary care settings
   1. Whether this female to male distribution represents a true predominance of the disorder among women or merely reflects the fact that women are more likely than men to seek medical care is unclear
   2. Estimates are that only about 25% of persons with this condition actually seek medical care and that those who do seek care are more likely to have behavioral and psychiatric problems than those who fail to seek care
   3. Healthcare costs for IBS are very high with ABS patients incurring an average of 1.6-fold more medical expense than an asymptomatic individual
   4. IBS patients undergo appendectomies, cholecystectomies, and hysterectomies at higher rates than the general population
   5. IBS patients miss three times as many days of work each year than persons without IBS

C. Most cases present before age 45, and most common presentation is that of abdominal pain and bloating along with altered bowel habits with either diarrhea or constipation predominating
   1. Constipation-predominant patients pass hard, pellet-like stools
   2. Diarrhea-prone patients report frequent loose stools often occurring after meals with urgency

D. Location and intensity of abdominal pain is highly variable
   1. Pain is hypogastric in 25%, right-sided in 20%, left-sided in 20%, and epigastric in 10% of patients
   2. Pain is usually crampy or achy and can be precipitated by meal ingestion, stress, or emotional turmoil
   3. Pain that is progressive, interferes with sleep, is associated with anorexia or weight loss is not part of the syndrome—an organic cause needs to be identified

E. Symptoms are most often intermittent, though some patients have daily problems and a small percentage of patients are refractory to treatment, with pain that is disabling

F. The symptom-based diagnostic classification system below can be helpful in evaluating patients

G. The syndrome can be divided into four subcategories according to the predominance of the symptom experienced by the patient: abdominal pain, diarrhea, constipation, or constipation alternating with diarrhea

---

ROME II CRITERIA FOR DIAGNOSIS OF IRRITABLE BOWEL SYNDROME

Presence for at least 12 weeks (not necessarily consecutive) in the preceding 12 months of abdominal discomfort or pain that cannot be explained by structural or biochemical abnormalities and that has at least 2 of the following 3 features:
- Pain relieved with defecation; and/or
- Onset is associated with a change in frequency of stooling (diarrhea or constipation); and/or
- Onset is associated with a change in consistency or form of stool (loose, watery, or pellet-like)

Adapted from Thompson, W.G., Longstreth, C.F., Drossman, D.A., Heaton, K.W., Irvine, K.J., Muller-Lissner, S.A. (1999). Functional bowel disorders and functional abdominal pain. *Gut, 45* (Suppl2), 1143-1147.

IV. Diagnosis/Evaluation

A. History
   1. Ask about onset, duration, location, and severity of abdominal pain and changes over time
   2. Ask questions relating to Rome II diagnostic criteria outlined above

> - Has the abdominal pain/discomfort been present for at least 12 weeks during the last 12 months?
>   ✓ Is pain relieved with defecation?
>   ✓ Is pain associated with a change in frequency of stool?
>   ✓ Is pain associated with change in consistency of stool?
> - Determine which of 4 symptoms is predominant–abdominal pain, diarrhea, constipation, or constipation alternating with diarrhea

3. If diarrhea is present, question about blood in diarrhea, awakening in night because of diarrhea (if positive response to either question, points to inflammatory bowel disease rather than IBS)
4. If constipation is present, determine if slow transit constipation or pelvic floor dysfunction constipation or a combination of the two is present (see section on CONSTIPATION)
5. Determine if alarm markers are present

Alarm Markers in Patients Being Evaluated for IBS

- Evidence of gastrointestinal bleeding such as occult blood in the stool, rectal bleeding, or anemia
- Anorexia or weight loss
- Fever
- Persistent diarrhea causing dehydration
- Severe constipation or fecal impaction
- Family history of gastrointestinal cancer, inflammatory bowel disease, or celiac sprue
- Onset of symptoms at ≥50 years of age

---

6. Inquire if psychological stress occurred at about time the disorder appeared or intensified
7. Obtain diet history to determine usual diet and eating patterns
8. Ask about drug/alcohol use/present medications used
9. Ask detailed questions about previous diagnostic evaluations by other healthcare providers; determine outcomes of previous treatments
10. In women, take menstrual history

B. Physical Examination
1. Determine if weight loss has occurred by weighing patient and comparing with previous weight
2. Perform abdominal exam for tenderness, guarding, rigidity, abnormal bowel sounds, masses, liver or spleen enlargement (abdominal compression may elicit tenderness which is vague and poorly localized)
3. Perform rectal exam for tenderness, masses; stool for occult blood
4. **Note:** There should be no abnormalities on physical examination and no findings suggestive of a structural disorder; the physical exam serves mainly to exclude other diagnoses and to reassure the patient

C. Differential Diagnosis
1. Lactase deficiency
2. Cancer of the colon
3. Inflammatory bowel disease
4. Diverticulitis
5. Enteric infection
6. Malabsorption
7. Endometriosis

D. Diagnostic Tests
1. Complete blood count, blood-chemistry tests, liver-function tests, and erythrocyte sedimentation rate
2. Measurement of thyrotropin
3. Patients who are <50 years of age should have a flexible sigmoidoscopy
4. Patients who are ≥50 years of age should have a colonoscopy; barium enema and flexible sigmoidoscopy are often substituted for colonoscopy
5. In patients with diarrhea, a biopsy specimen should be obtained from the mucosa of the descending colon to rule out microscopic colitis

V. Plan/Management

A. For patients with typical presentation who meet the Rome II criteria and who demonstrate no abnormalities on physical examination or laboratory testing (and if alarm markers are not present), diagnosis of irritable bowel syndrome, a diagnosis of exclusion, can be made

B. Establishment of an effective patient-clinician relationship based on education and reassurance is important in order to maximize the efficacy of treatment and is fundamental to any treatment plan

C. The most reasonable approach to treating IBS is to use the patient's predominant symptom as a guide
1. Based on the history, determine which subcategory best describes the patient: Is the predominant symptom abdominal pain, diarrhea, constipation, or constipation alternating with diarrhea?
2. Implement a treatment plan based on the predominant symptom as a beginning point

D. For patients in all subcategories–abdominal pain, diarrhea, constipation, or alternating constipation and diarrhea–use of a food intake and symptom diary can be helpful. This approach serves the purpose of helping the patient take responsibility for his/her own care and also helps to identify whether exacerbation of symptoms occurs after consuming certain foods, or if certain events (exercise, menses, stressful situations) make condition worse
1. For a two-week period, ask patient to record symptom, date/time of occurrence, description of severity (scale of 0-10), factors associated with symptom (diet, activity, menses, stressful event, etc.); emotional responses (what person feels); thoughts and cognition (what person thinks)
2. Review the symptom diary with the patient on return visit as a way of evaluating his/her progress in "gaining control" of the condition; decide with the patient if the symptom diary approach is helpful and worthwhile to continue on subsequent visits

E. **For patients in whom the predominant symptom is abdominal pain**, the following approach can be used
1. Elimination of gas-forming foods may be helpful (lactose, legumes, broccoli, cauliflower, cabbage, onions, cucumbers); if symptoms improve, these foods can be gradually reintroduced
2. Prescribe an antispasmodic agent—dicyclomine hydrochloride or hyoscyamine sulfate—refer to table below for dosage guidelines; these drugs reduce abdominal pain or bloating through anticholinergic pathways
3. Consider prescribing a secondary tricyclic amine such as nortriptyline or desipramine (refer to table below for dosage guidelines) which delays intestinal transit and may blunt perception of visceral distention

F. **For patients in whom the predominant symptom is diarrhea**, the following approach can be used
1. Use of fiber supplements to add bulk to the stool may occasionally improve diarrhea (Note: Insoluble fiber such as methylcellulose [Citrucel] works well for persons with IBD because, unlike soluble fiber such as psyllium husk [e.g., Metamucil products], it is non gas-producing)
   a. Unfortunately, insoluble fiber—unlike soluble fiber—has no role in lowering cholesterol or normalizing blood sugar in persons who could benefit from such effects
   b. Dietary fiber may also be recommended (see fiber recommendations in section on NUTRITION)
2. Advise patient to avoid foods that exacerbate symptoms (based on food diary experience); common foods that increase symptoms are those that contain sorbitol such as sugarless gum and dietetic candy
3. Use of antidiarrheal agents such as loperamide or bismuth subsalicylate may help decrease the frequency of bowel movements and improve consistency of stool (refer to table below for dosage guidelines)

G. **For patients in whom the predominant symptom is constipation**, the following approaches can be used
1. Increase dietary fiber as above under V.F.1.
2. Prescribe use of a laxative such as milk of magnesia, lactulose, or polyethylene glycol solution (PEG); these medications are generally considered safe for long-term use although no laxative is approved for chronic use
   a. Milk of magnesia may be the best choice for many patients because it is inexpensive and effective—dosing is 15-45 mL PO once daily at bedtime
   b. Hyperosmolar agents such as polyethylene glycol (PEG) without electrolytes (MiraLax) and nonabsorbable sugars such as lactulose (Kristalose) are generally well-tolerated but may have side effects of bloating and flatulence (refer to table below for dosage guidelines)
   c. Patients should be advised to titrate dose of laxative until stool is soft, but not liquid
3. Tegaserod maleate (Zelnorm) has been approved by the FDA for short-term treatment of women with irritable bowel syndrome with constipation as the predominant symptom
   a. Activates 5-HT$_4$ receptors on neurons in GI tract thereby promoting motility and also decreasing visceral sensation
   b. Recommended duration of treatment is 4-6 weeks with an additional 4-6 weeks as an option for responders; cost of 60 2-mg or 6-mg tabs is approximately $150

c. Dose at 6 mg orally BID before meals; consult PDR for contraindications, interactions, and precautions

d. IBS is a chronic disease–long term efficacy and safety of this drug have not been established and is best reserved for use in a specialty setting

H. **For patients in whom there is constipation alternating with diarrhea**, the patient should be advised to self-monitor condition and to respond appropriately (based on recommendations in V.F. and G. above for management of diarrhea and constipation), depending on whether the symptom at the time is diarrhea or constipation

DOSAGE GUIDELINES FOR DRUGS COMMONLY USED TO TREAT IRRITABLE BOWEL SYNDROME

Drug	Dose
Anticholinergic agents	
Dicyclomine hydrochloride	20 mg q 6 h; can be increased to 40 mg q 6 h if tolerated
Hyoscyamine sulfate	0.125-0.25 mg sublingually q 4 h (0.375 mg extended-relief tablets: 1-2 tablets q 12 h)
Antidiarrheal agents	
Loperamide	4 mg/day initially, with a maintenance dose of 4-8 mg/day, in a single or divided dose
Bismuth subsalicylate	30 mL/dose; can repeat dose up to 4 times/day
Osmotic laxatives	
Lactulose	10-20 g dissolved in 120 mL (4 oz) of water, taken daily
Polyethylene glycol solution	17 g dissolved in 240 mL (8 oz) of water, taken daily
Tricyclic compounds	
Amitriptyline	25-75 mg/day
Nortriptyline	25-75 mg/day
Desipramine	25-75 mg/day

Adapted from Horwitz, G.J. & Fisher, R.S. (2001). The irritable bowel syndrome. *New England Journal of Medicine, 344*, 1849.

I. Discuss with all patients–whether their predominant symptom is abdominal pain, diarrhea, constipation, or diarrhea alternating with constipation–that modifications in lifestyle are well recognized for their potential benefit on symptom management

1. Stress reduction is important, and can be accomplished via the use of relaxation audiotapes, books, or meditation taught by behavioral therapists or others in group settings

2. Biofeedback can sometimes help decrease stress and reduce gut hypersensitivity

3. Regular exercise can reduce stress and increase feelings of well-being; current recommendations are for adults to engage in 60 minutes of moderate intensity physical activity each day

J. Follow Up

1. Frequent follow up is important; first follow up visit should be in 2 weeks, then monthly, then every 3-6 months

2. Patients who fail to respond to therapy after an adequate trial should be referred to an expert in the diagnosis and management of functional bowel disorders for evaluation and management

PEPTIC ULCER DISEASE

I. Definition: A circumscribed ulceration of the gastrointestinal mucosa occurring in areas exposed to acid and pepsin and most often caused by *Helicobacter pylori* infection

II. Pathogenesis

A. In the majority of cases of both duodenal and gastric ulcer, infection with *Helicobacter pylori* produces damage to the mucosa and thus is causally related to ulcer development

1. The gastric mucosa is well protected against bacterial infections, but *H. pylori* is highly adapted to overcome resistant factors

2. After being ingested, *H. pylori* bacteria must evade the bactericidal activity of the gastric luminal contents and enter the mucous layer, a process that is aided by (1) urease production by the bacteria which converts urea into carbon dioxide and ammonia, thereby enabling its survival in an acidic milieu; and, (2) motility of the organism which is essential for colonization and attachment to epithelial cells

3. *H. pylori* causes continuous gastric inflammation in virtually all infected persons
4. Once the defect in the mucosa occurs, the presence of both acid and pepsin contribute to ulcer formation

B. Infection with *H. pylori* occurs worldwide and the prevalence is higher in developing countries (over 80%) compared with industrialized countries (ranges from 20% to 50%)
1. Infection is acquired by oral ingestion of the bacterium and is mainly transmitted within families in early childhood
2. In industrialized countries, direct transmission from person to person is believed to occur via saliva, vomitus, or feces; water may be important in the transmission in developing countries
3. Overall prevalence of *H. pylori* infection is strongly correlated with socioeconomic conditions

C. A less common cause of peptic ulcer formation is damage to the mucosa caused by use of nonsteroidal anti-inflammatory drugs (NSAIDs); most experts believe that *H. pylori* also plays a role in ulcers that are commonly referred to as "NSAID-induced"
1. NSAIDs damage the mucosa through a direct action
2. A systemic effect also occurs whereby endogenous prostaglandin synthesis is inhibited

D. Cigarette smoking increases gastric acid secretion thereby increasing the risk of occurrence and recurrence of ulcers

E. Cause and effect relationship between psychological stress and ulcer development has not been demonstrated

F. Diet has no role in causing ulcers, but certain foods exacerbate symptoms in some people; alcohol ingestion can cause acute gastritis and may interfere with healing

G. Uncommon etiologies such as gastrinoma, mastocytosis, and annular pancreas account for some ulcer formation; some ulcer formation remains in the idiopathic category

III. Clinical Presentation

A. *H. pylori* is responsible for the majority of duodenal (up to 95%) and gastric (about 80%) ulcers; the lifetime risk of peptic ulcer in persons infected with *H. pylori* is approximately 3% in the US
1. *H. pylori* infection is usually chronic in adults and will not resolve without specific therapy
2. The clinical course of the infection is highly variable and is influenced by both microbial and host factors

B. There is no symptom complex that can adequately differentiate gastric from duodenal ulcers; however, the following characteristics may provide some helpful but not conclusive data
1. Duodenal ulcers (DU) have the following characteristics
   a. Classically, distress of duodenal ulcer occurs 1-3 hours after meal and may awaken patient from sleep in early morning. Pain is relieved by food, antacids, or vomiting (distress-food-relief pattern)
   b. Much more common than gastric ulcers
   c. Rarely harbor malignancy
2. Gastric ulcers (GU) have the following characteristics
   a. A similar distress-food-relief pattern may exist, but food may also exacerbate the pain
   b. Nausea, vomiting, anorexia, and weight loss may be more common in GU than in DU
   c. About 2-4% of gastric ulcers harbor malignancy
   d. NSAID related ulcers are more likely to be gastric than duodenal

C. Epigastric distress is the classic and most common symptom for both duodenal and gastric ulcers; if actual pain occurs, it is typically aching or burning

D. Other dyspeptic symptoms such as nausea, vomiting, belching, and bloating also occur

E. The elderly and patients with NSAID-related ulcers are often symptom-free until bleeding or perforation occurs

IV.   Diagnosis/Evaluation

   A.   History
      1.   Question about presence, location of distress/pain
      2.   If distress/pain are present, determine onset, duration, character of pain, and effect of food/antacids on pain
      3.   Ask about associated symptoms of nausea, vomiting, and heartburn
      4.   Question about presence of alarm markers: anemia, weight loss, or gastrointestinal bleeding
      5.   Obtain past medical history and medication history
      6.   Obtain social history, specifically, smoking, alcohol use, stress in family and at work
      7.   Ask about regular use of NSAIDs, oral corticosteroids
      8.   Inquire about PUD in first-degree relatives

   B.   Physical Examination
      1.   Perform abdominal exam for tenderness (specifically in epigastric area), rigidity, abnormal bowel sounds, masses, liver/spleen enlargement
      2.   Perform digital rectal exam for tenderness, masses; obtain stool for occult blood

   C.   Differential Diagnosis
      1.   Neoplasm of the stomach
      2.   Pancreatitis
      3.   Diverticulitis
      4.   Nonulcer dyspepsia

   D.   Diagnostic Tests
      1.   All patients should receive the following tests to detect bleeding
         a.   Stool for fecal occult blood
         b.   Complete blood count (CBC) to rule out bleeding
      2.   Patients over the age of 50 with new onset of dyspeptic/ulcer symptoms **or** those with alarm markers including anemia, weight loss, or gastrointestinal bleeding, should be referred for endoscopy
      3.   *H. pylori* infection can be diagnosed by noninvasive methods or via endoscopic biopsy of the gastric mucosa
         a.   Noninvasive methods include the urea breath test, serologic tests, and stool antigen assays; both urea breath tests and stool antigen assays have very good sensitivity and specificity (>90%) and can be used for the initial diagnosis as well as for follow-up of eradication therapy (serologic tests are cheap and widely used for the diagnosis of *H. pylori* infection prior to treatment, but are of limited usefulness in determining the success of therapy)
         b.   Patients who are referred for endoscopy because of age or presence of alarm markers can be diagnosed for the presence of *H. pylori* infection via a urease test on an antral-biopsy specimen

V.   Plan/Management

   A.   Patients who are diagnosed with *H. pylori* infection can be treated with any of the FDA-approved treatment options for *H. pylori* eradication listed in the table below; empiric antibiotic therapy without *H. pylori* testing is discouraged

FDA-APPROVED TREATMENT OPTIONS FOR *H. PYLORI* ERADICATION

- Omeprazole (40 mg daily) plus clarithromycin (500 mg TID) for 2 weeks, then omeprazole (20 mg daily) for 2 weeks
- Omeprazole (20 mg BID) plus clarithromycin (500 mg BID) plus amoxicillin (1 g BID) for 10 days
- Lansoprazole (30 mg BID) plus clarithromycin (500 mg BID) plus amoxicillin (1 g BID) for 10 days
- Lansoprazole (30 mg BID) plus amoxicillin (1 g BID) plus clarithromycin (500 mg TID) for 10 days
- Lansoprazole (30 mg TID) plus amoxicillin (1 g TID) for 2 weeks*
- Esomeprazole (40 mg daily) plus clarithromycin (500 mg BID) plus amoxicillin (1 g BID) for 10 days
- Ranitidine bismuth citrate (400 mg BID) plus clarithromycin (500 mg TID) for 2 weeks, then ranitidine bismuth citrate (400 mg BID) for 2 weeks
- Ranitidine bismuth citrate (400 mg BID) plus clarithromycin (500 mg BID) for 2 weeks, then ranitidine bismuth citrate (400 mg BID) for 2 weeks

*This dual-therapy regimen has restrictive labeling. It is indicated for patients who are either allergic to or intolerant of clarithromycin or for infections with known or suspected resistance to clarithromycin

Adapted from Suerbaum, S. & Michetti, P. (2002). *Helicobacter pylori* infection. *New England Journal of Medicine, 347*, 1181.

B. The goal of *H. pylori* treatment is the complete elimination of the organism; once achieved, reinfection rates are low
   1. The use of two or more antimicrobial agents increases rates of cure and reduces the risk of selecting for resistant *H. pylori*
      a. Frequency of clarithromycin resistance is presently about 10%
      b. Resistance to amoxicillin remains uncommon
   2. The benefit of treatment is durable

C. For follow-up of eradication therapy, use of either the urea breath test or stool antigen tests is recommended
   1. Urea breath test should not be performed before an interval of four weeks have elapsed in order to avoid false negative results
   2. For stool antigen tests, an eight-week interval must be allowed after therapy

D. Eradication is more difficult when there is a treatment failure with the first attempt which most often fails due to poor patient compliance or development of antibiotic resistance; optimal strategy for retreatment has not been established, but the following options are available
   1. Retreat with a regimen using a proton pump inhibitor with a different antibiotic for at least 14 days
   2. Consider referral to an expert when there is treatment failure for additional diagnostic testing

E. Patients who are *H. pylori* negative can be treated with proton pump inhibitors or H_2 receptor-antagonists to assist ulcer healing

TREATMENT WITH ANTISECRETORY DRUGS

Treatment With H_2 Receptor Antagonists

Four agents presently available	Cimetidine (Tagamet) 800 mg daily at bedtime or 400 mg BID for up to 8 weeks
Equally effective when prescribed in equipotent doses	Famotidine (Pepcid) 40 mg daily at bedtime or 20 mg BID for up to 8 weeks
All 4 agents are relatively expensive	Nizatidine (Axid) 300 mg daily at bedtime or 150 mg BID for up to 8 weeks
Can be given in split-dose, evening, or nighttime doses	Ranitidine (Zantac) 300 mg daily at bedtime or 150 mg BID for up to 8 weeks
Fewer drug interactions with famotidine and nizatidine	

Proton-Pump Inhibitors

Five agents presently available	Omeprazole (Prilosec), 20 mg/day
Omeprazole is now off patent	Lansoprazole (Prevacid), 30 mg/day
Require activation in the acidic compartments of the stimulated parietal cell	Esomeprazole (Nexium), 20-40 mg/day
	Pantoprazole (Protonix), 40 mg/day
Thus, should not be given in fasting state or at bedtime	Rabeprazole (Aciphex), 20 mg/day
Most effective when given 30 to 60 minutes **before meals** (consult PDR for specific drug)	Treatment should be given for 4 to 8 weeks

F. Patients who continue to have symptoms after 4 weeks on any of the above regimens should be referred for further diagnostic workup

G. Counsel all patients regarding the following lifestyle changes
1. Patient should discontinue use of NSAIDs, and use acetaminophen for pain control if possible; if use of an NSAID is deemed necessary, refer to H. below
2. All patients who smoke should be counseled to stop (see section on TOBACCO USE AND SMOKING CESSATION for recommendations relating how to assist patients to quit smoking)
3. No dietary restrictions are necessary unless certain foods are associated with problems
4. Alcohol, if patient drinks, should be used in moderate amounts only (no more than 2 drinks/day for men <65; no more than 1 drink/day for women and for both men and women >65); alcohol should be consumed with food
5. Consider using stress reduction techniques that may improve the quality of life for some patients

H. Prevention of NSAID ulcers in patients without active *H. pylori* infection
1. Consider preventive therapy for patients taking NSAIDs based on risk factors
2. Patients with a prior history of ulcer disease, those who are using NSAIDs with steroids or anticoagulants, and those who have coexisting conditions that would seriously limit ability to cope with ulcer complications are appropriate candidates for preventive therapy
   a. Proton pump inhibitors (PPIs) have been shown to prevent both duodenal and gastric ulcers
   b. Generally, lansoprazole is preferred because of fewer drug interactions; consult PDR for dosing
   c. Use of Cox-2 inhibitors such as Celebrex is not indicated, as this class of drugs was recently found to be no more effective than older NSAIDs (e.g., diclofenac) in terms of preventing ulcers and other gastrointestinal complications in susceptible patients
   d. Another option is to prescribe low-dose misoprostol plus an H_2-receptor antagonist to prevent ulcers in patients taking NSAIDs

I. Follow Up
1. Patients who have been prescribed therapy for eradication of *H. pylori* infection should be scheduled for retesting for treatment efficacy based on whether urea breath test or stool antigen tests are used (see V.C. above)
2. Patients who remain symptomatic after treatment outlined above should be managed according to the recommendations in V.D. above
3. Patients who have been prescribed acid suppression therapy should be evaluated for treatment efficacy after one month; patients whose symptoms are controlled should be continued another 2 to 4 weeks on therapy; patients who remain symptomatic should be referred for additional diagnostic evaluation

GASTROESOPHAGEAL REFLUX DISEASE (GERD)

I. Definition: Reflux of gastric contents into the esophagus resulting in a symptomatic condition

II. Pathogenesis

A. The lower esophageal sphincter allows for the flow of solids and liquids between the esophagus and the stomach and several structures at the gastroesophageal junction operate to maintain an antireflux barrier

B. The sphincter mechanism at the lower end of the esophagus is composed of both the intrinsic smooth muscle of the distal esophagus and the skeletal muscle of the crural diaphragm

C. Transient relaxation of this sphincter mechanism (involving the simultaneous relaxation of the lower esophageal sphincter and crural diaphragm) is the major mechanism of gastric reflux
1. A neural reflex mediated through the brain stem is responsible for transient relaxation of the smooth muscle of the distal esophagus
2. Mechanism of relaxation of the crural diaphragm has not been established

D.   Recently, hiatal hernia has once again emerged as an important factor in the pathogenesis of GERD
     1.   Most patients with moderate-to-severe reflux disease have hiatal hernia
     2.   This condition may promote reflux in a number of ways

E.   Pathologic reflux differs from physiologic reflux in both frequency and volume of refluxed material

F.   Excessive reflux overwhelms the intrinsic mucosal defense mechanisms producing symptoms and signs of esophageal inflammation; potentially serious complications include strictures, erosive esophagitis, and the development of Barrett esophagus

III. Clinical Presentation

A.   The most commonly recognized manifestation of GERD is heartburn or a substernal sensation in the chest; the frequency of other reflux-related symptoms, such as regurgitation, is also common, but less well described
     1.   Heartburn, regurgitation, or both, most often occur within 60 minutes after eating, especially after consuming a large or fatty meal
     2.   Symptoms are made worse by recumbency or bending—maneuvers that increase intra-abdominal pressure

B.   Numerous studies have indicated that cessation of smoking, decreasing fat intake, attaining a healthy weight (for overweight persons), avoiding recumbency for 3 hours postprandially, and elevation of the head of the bed decrease distal esophageal acid exposure; in addition, avoidance of certain foods including chocolate, tomato-based foods, alcohol, peppermint, caffeinated products, citrus fruits and drinks, and onions and garlic can reduce symptom occurrence in some people

C.   Signs and symptoms that are more likely to be associated with underlying esophageal pathology than others are the following: Difficulty swallowing (dysphagia), pain on swallowing (odynophagia), anemia, weight loss, and hematemesis

IV. Diagnosis/Evaluation

A.   History
     1.   Inquire about onset, duration, and progression of symptoms(s) [usually heartburn, regurgitation, or both] (patients with symptoms that are present for >5 years are at increased risk for Barrett esophagus and esophageal cancer compared with the general population and with those with symptoms of shorter duration)
     2.   Determine if heartburn is aggravated by meals and relieved by sitting up or antacids
     3.   Determine if patient smokes
     4.   Diagnosis can be made on basis of history alone if patient presents with typical symptoms and has none of the alarm features suggesting complicated disease (see III.C. above)

B.   Physical Examination
     1.   Determine if patient is overweight
     2.   Perform abdominal exam for masses, tenderness; check for occult blood in stool

C.   Differential Diagnosis
     1.   Cardiac chest pain
     2.   Esophagitis/esophageal motility/structural disorders
     3.   Esophageal tumor
     4.   Dyspepsia, peptic ulcer disease, biliary tract disease

D.   Diagnostic Tests
     1.   The presence of one or more alarm features (see III.C. above) in patients with reflux indicates need for further diagnostic testing; upper endoscopy is usually the preferred test, but a barium swallow is a reasonable alternative if dysphagia is present
     2.   Upper endoscopy is also indicated in any patient with long-standing GERD symptoms, particularly those aged 50 years or older
     3.   Diagnostic testing is usually not indicated in patients who are not in the above categories (no alarm features, no long-standing symptoms, and age <50 years)

V.   Plan/Management

A.   Patients <50 years of age with typical symptoms of mild, episodic GERD that is not long-standing, and with no alarm features suggesting complicated disease can be treated empirically with lifestyle modifications and patient-directed therapy with antacids and over-the-counter acid suppressants; these interventions (described below) are designed to decrease distal esophageal acid exposure and are effective in up to 20% of patients with GERD

Lifestyle Modification

Advise patient as follows:
➡ Weight loss (for overweight and obese patients), even as little as 10 pounds, may decrease symptoms (see section on OBESITY for strategies to assist patients to lose weight)
➡ Quitting smoking is a crucial change since tobacco use reduces esophageal sphincter tone (see section on TOBACCO USE AND SMOKING CESSATION for strategies to assist patients to quit smoking)
➡ Elevate head of bed on 15 cm blocks or sleep on wedge-shaped bolster
➡ Eat smaller meals, and do not eat for 3 hours prior to lying recumbent
➡ Avoid large, high fat meals and avoid foods that may aggravate the problem (see III.B. above)

Patient-Directed Therapy

➡ Antacids and antirefluxants such as alginic acid are useful in the milder forms of GERD (compared with H_2 receptor antagonists (H_2RAs), these products have a more rapid response but a shorter duration of action)
➡ H_2RAs available in an over-the-counter form are usually ½ of the standard prescription dose; these doses have been shown to reduce gastric acid, particularly after a meal and generally may be used interchangeably
➡ H_2RAs are especially useful when taken before an activity that may result in reflux symptoms (heavy meal or exercise)

B.   Patients who have an incomplete symptomatic response to lifestyle modifications and patient-directed therapy may be managed with **one** of the following approaches

---

Step-down approach: Empirical trial of a proton pump inhibitor (PPI) at standard dosing and then decreasing to least potent acid suppression dose at which the patient is symptom free—with either a PPI or, preferably, a H_2RA

  Rationale: PPIs provide rapid symptomatic relief and healing of erosive esophagitis in the highest percentage of patients and at a higher cost

Step-up approach: Start therapy with H_2RAs and intensify therapy as necessary with PPIs (this approach should only be used in patients who have not tried therapeutic doses of H_2RAs before evaluation)

  Rationale: H_2RAs given in divided doses are effective treatment in many patients with less severe GERD and are often used in a cost-restrictive environment

Whether using the step-down or the step-up approach, close monitoring to ensure response of symptoms to therapy, and to allow for the tapering of the medication to the lowest dose at which the patient is symptom-free is important

---

Dosing of Proton Pump Inhibitors	**Dosing of H_2 receptor antagonists**
Omeprazole, 20 mg/day	Cimetidine, 400 mg BID
Lansoprazole, 30 mg/day	Ranitidine, 150 mg BID
Rabeprazole, 20 mg/day	Nizatidine, 150 mg BID
Pantoprazole, 40 mg/day	Famotidine, 20 mg BID
Esomeprazole, 20-40 mg/day	

C.   For most patients, GERD is a chronic condition, and maintenance therapy has become the rule rather than the exception; this is especially true for patients who develop erosive esophagitis (diagnosed via upper endoscopy) who often need maintenance therapy after healing in order to avoid recurrences; many patients requiring PPIs to heal mucosal disease can continue taking H_2RAs for maintenance; in reflux patients who again become symptomatic while receiving H_2RAs, long-term maintenance therapy with PPIs may be needed

1.   Drug safety is an important concern with the long-term use of PPIs because of the profound decrease in gastric acid secretion; consult PDR for length of time a specific PPI is approved for use as maintenance therapy

2.   Length of time that the different H_2RAs are approved for use as maintenance therapy also varies; consult PDR

D.   Educational materials for patients and clinicians are contained in the box below

For Patients	
American College of Gastroenterology	http://www.acg.gi.org/acg-dev/patientinfo/frame_gerd.html
National Institutes of Health	http://www.niddk.nih.gov/health/digest/pubs/heartbrn/heartbrn.htm
Mayo Clinic's heartburn information site	http://www.mayohealth.org/home?id=5.1.1.8.7
National Library of Medicine's online tutorial	http://www.nlm.nih.gov.medlineplus/tutorials/gerd/id159101.html
For Clinicians	
American College of Gastroenterology's forum on GERD	http://www.acg.gi.org/phyforum/gifocus/2evi.html
American College of Gastroenterology's guidelines for the diagnosis and treatment of GERD	http://www-east.elsevier.com/ajg/issues/9406/ajg1123fla.htm

Education Resources

Adapted from Shaheen, D., & Ransohoff, D.F. (2002). Gastroesophageal reflux, Barrett esophagus, and esophageal cancer: Clinical applications. *JAMA, 287*, p. 1985

E. Antireflux surgery is a maintenance option for patients with well-documented GERD but its place in management remains controversial

F. Follow Up
1. Patients who respond to lifestyle modifications and patient-directed therapy do not require follow-up unless symptoms persist or alarm features develop
2. Patients who are managed with either a step-down or step-up approach to pharmacological therapy should be evaluated every 2-4 weeks x 2 months in order to evaluate response of symptoms to therapy and to taper the dose to the lowest one at which the patient is symptom-free
3. Patients who do not respond as expected to therapy should be immediately referred to a gastroenterologist for further evaluation

ABDOMINAL HERNIAS

I. Definition: Protrusion of an abdominal viscus or part of a viscus through the abdominal wall

A. Incarcerated hernias are hernias that cannot be reduced and the contents of the hernial sac cannot be returned to the peritoneal cavity

B. Strangulated hernias are hernias that occur when the blood supply to the viscera lying within the hernial sac is obliterated or cut off

II. Pathogenesis

A. A hernia is a defect in the normal musculofascial continuity of the abdominal wall and is either congenital or acquired

B. Acquired hernias may occur from any condition that increases intra-abdominal pressure such as obesity, chronic cough, ascites, chronic constipation with straining, and lifting heavy objects

C. Distinction between congenital and acquired hernias is often unclear as hernias can be acquired because of a congenital predisposition
1. Distinction has little implication for management
2. Distinction may be very important when work-related injury is claimed

III. Clinical Presentation

A. The symptoms of reducible hernias are related to the degree of pressure of contents rather than to size

B. Most patients with reducible hernias are asymptomatic or complain of only mild pain, whereas patients with strangulated hernias have colicky abdominal pain, nausea, vomiting, abdominal distention, and hyperperistalsis

C.   Inguinal hernias are classified as direct (portions of the bowel and/or omentum protrude directly through the floor of the inguinal canal and emerge at the external inguinal ring) or indirect (pass through the internal abdominal ring, traverse the spermatic cord through the inguinal canal and emerge at the external inguinal ring) [see Figure 12.4]

1.   Approximately 75% of abdominal hernias are inguinal; most common type of hernia in both genders but occurs more frequently in men
2.   Indirect hernias are more common in younger persons since they are due to a congenital defect in which the processus vaginalis remains patent
    a.   However, the incidence of inguinal hernias increases with advancing age and is approximately four times more common after age 50 years than before
    b.   Indirect hernias often enter the scrotum
3.   Direct hernias occur mainly in the middle and later years of life and are due to a weakness in the abdominal structures. Direct hernias usually reduce and rarely enter the scrotum
4.   Symptoms of both direct and indirect hernias include a dull ache in the groin and a bulge localized in the groin or extended into the scrotum (referred to as a complete hernia); in women a complete hernia may enter the labia majora as a labial hernia

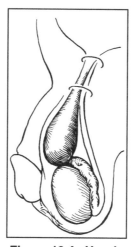

Figure 12.4. Hernia

D.   Femoral hernias: Protrusion of omentum through the femoral canal
1.   Second most common abdominal hernia in both women and men; rare in children
2.   Occurs 3-5 times more commonly in females than males
3.   Incidence increases with age and with increased pressure produced by pregnancy and straining
4.   Risk of strangulation is high
5.   In women, may have signs of intestinal obstruction

E.   Incisional hernias: Protrusion of bowel and/or omentum through a surgical incision
1.   Risk factors are post-operative wound infection, dehiscence, malnutrition, obesity, and smoking
2.   Bulge can usually be seen through incision
3.   If not repaired immediately, an intestinal obstruction can develop

F.   Umbilical hernias: Protrusion of bowel and/or omentum through the umbilical ring
1.   So common in infants and young children that it can be considered a normal variation
    a.   Incidence varies widely with race, affecting African-American children much more often
    b.   Low birth weight infants are more often affected; males and females are affected equally
2.   Also occurs in middle-aged multiparous women, patients with cirrhosis and ascites, chronically ill patients, and elderly patients
3.   Infrequently, patient may have vague, intermittent pain and tenderness
4.   Most umbilical hernias in infants close spontaneously (many close within the first year of life and the majority are closed by the fifth year); infrequently, these hernias may become incarcerated and/or strangulated

G.   Epigastric hernias: Protrusion of fat or omentum through the linea alba between the umbilicus and the xiphoid
1.   Most common in men between the ages of 20-50
2.   Presents as small, painless, subcutaneous mass

IV.   Diagnosis/Evaluation

A.   History
    1.   Inquire about circumstances and time of onset of hernia
    2.   Ask about presence of **alarm markers**: acute onset of colicky abdominal pain, nausea, vomiting (suggests entrapment/strangulation in person with known hernia)
    3.   Inquire about groin pain and swelling
    4.   Determine whether patient can reduce hernia
    5.   Ask about aggravating and alleviating factors (worse with standing, straining, coughing?)

B.   Physical examination is directed at determining type of hernia, distinguishing hernias from other causes of inguinal swelling/pain, and identification of hernias that require no therapy, those that should be referred for elective surgery, and those for which emergency surgery is indicated
    1.   Patients with reducible hernias should be examined in both standing and supine positions
    2.   Carefully inspect abdomen and groin, with and without patients performing Valsalva maneuver
    3.   With hernias that are not reducible, assess for discoloration, edema, elevated temperature, tenderness, and signs of bowel obstruction
    4.   Do not try to reduce strangulated hernias, because reduction can cause gangrenous bowel to enter the peritoneal cavity
    5.   Examination for inguinal hernias involves the following:
        a.   In men, if a suspected hernia is not visible the examiner's finger should gently invaginate the scrotum and advance toward the head and laterally into the inguinal canal to the external inguinal ring; then the patient should cough or strain and the examiner should feel for a bulge at the examining finger (see Figure 12.5)
        b.   With a direct hernia, when the finger is inserted through the external canal a bulge will be felt striking the side of the finger
        c.   With an indirect hernia, when the finger is inserted through the external canal, the bulge will be felt at the fingertip when the patient coughs
        d.   In females, it is more difficult to establish the diagnosis of inguinal hernia; locate the external inguinal ring by identifying the inguinal ligament and os pubis; place hand over inguinal ring and palpate for bulge when patient coughs
    6.   Femoral hernias are more difficult to diagnose
        a.   The external opening of the femoral canal can be located just medial to the femoral artery and deep to the inguinal ligament
        b.   Ask patient to cough and palpate for swelling and impulse within the femoral canal
    7.   To detect umbilical and incisional hernias, inspect abdomen while patient lifts head from a supine position while bearing down to tense abdominal wall
    8.   Check the groin area for lymphadenopathy and other masses that are unchanged with position or Valsalva; groin pain but no mass suggests a musculoskeletal etiology

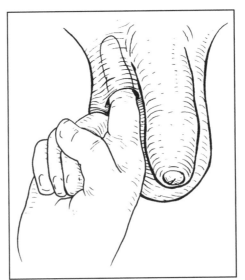

Figure 12.5. Technique of Examination for Inguinal Hernia.

C. Differential Diagnosis
    1. Inguinal hernias (see sections on HYDROCELE and VARICOCELE)
        a. Hydrocele
        b. Varicocele
        c. Spermatocele
        d. Epididymal cysts
        e. Testicular tumor
        f. In children, undescended testes
    2. Femoral hernias
        a. Enlarged lymph node
        b. Lipoma
        c. Direct inguinal hernia
        d. Saphenous varix
        e. Psoas abscess
    3. Other causes of groin pain/swelling include muscle strain, inguinal adenopathy, and hip arthritis
    4. Incisional, umbilical, and, to a lesser extent, epigastric hernias are usually not confused with other conditions

D. Diagnostic Tests: Often none needed, may order ultrasound if uncertain about abdominal mass

V. Plan/Management

A. Patients with asymptomatic, easily reducible inguinal hernia can be managed with watchful waiting
    1. Elective surgery should be considered in younger patients
    2. Obviously, should signs of incarceration develop, the patient should be referred for surgery

B. Patients with symptomatic, reducible inguinal hernia should be referred for elective repair

C. Patients with nontender incarcerated inguinal hernia of recent onset, with no signs of inflammation/ obstruction, can be referred to a specialist for an attempt at reduction before referral to surgeon

D. Patients with reducible femoral hernias should be referred for immediate elective repair because of high rate of strangulation

E. Umbilical hernias in adults should be managed as follows
    1. Umbilical hernia presenting as small, asymptomatic fascial defect without protrusion may be followed expectantly
    2. If PE reveals herniation, refer for repair because there is a high risk of incarceration and strangulation

F. Patients with small-neck incisional hernias should undergo immediate repair

G. Factors associated with hernia formation should be corrected, if possible

H. Patients who are managed conservatively should receive detailed instruction about symptoms of incarceration and strangulation

I. Follow Up: Return visits will usually occur after surgery; for patients who do not undergo immediate surgery follow up is only needed for problems

HEMORRHOIDS

I.   Definition: Vascular cushions located in the distal rectum and anal canal whose exact function is unknown; contrary to popular misconceptions, hemorrhoids are normal anatomic structures

II. Pathogenesis

   A.   The anal canal extends from the opening of the anus to the internal anal sphincter with a total length in adults of about 4 cm
      1.   The lowest 2 cm is cutaneous tissue and the upper 2 cm is covered by mucosa
      2.   The junction of these two areas is marked by a saw-tooth, or dentate, line known as the pectinate line

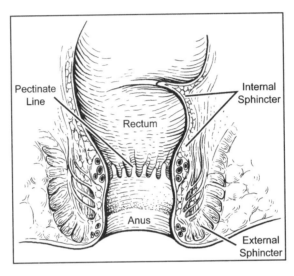

Figure 12.6. Normal Anatomy–the Anal Canal.

   B.   Anal cushions, part of the normal anatomy of the anal canal, become displaced through an unknown mechanism

   C.   Prolapse of a vascular anal cushion through the anal canal results in entrapment by the internal anal sphincter and the result is hemorrhoid formation

   D.   Prolapse may be initiated by any of the following:
      1.   Shearing force from passage of large firm stool
      2.   Increase in venous pressure from heart failure or pregnancy
      3.   Straining that occurs with lifting or defecation

   E.   In most cases of hemorrhoids, however, no definite cause can be identified

III. Clinical Presentation

   A.   Classic sign is bleeding, which is usually painless, and bright red (because it is produced by presinusoidal arterioles), and anal discomfort

   B.   Occurs most often in persons over age 50; uncommon in persons under 25 except women who have been pregnant

   C.   Rectal itching, pain, or burning may be present

D. Hemorrhoids are usually classified as either internal, external, or mixed
1. External hemorrhoids are below the pectinate line (see illustration) and covered by cutaneous tissue; pain from this type is caused by thrombosis that provokes swelling of the overlying skin
2. Internal hemorrhoids are above the pectinate line and covered by the mucosa of the anal canal; this type will be noticed when they protrude or produce bleeding or soiling

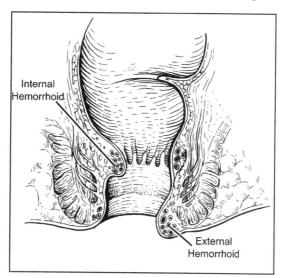

Internal Hemorrhoid

External Hemorrhoid

Figure 12.7. Hemorrhoids by Type

IV. Diagnosis/Evaluation

A. History
1. Inquire about onset, duration of symptoms--pain, itching, burning; occurrence of bleeding
2. Ask about past medical history of hemorrhoids, recent pregnancy, liver disease, anorectal surgery, or chronic constipation

B. Physical Examination
1. Inspect anal area and perform digital rectal exam (unless patient is experiencing a great deal of pain)
2. Anoscopy is recommended in moderate to severe cases

C. Differential Diagnosis
1. Hypertrophic anal papilla, seen with anal fissure, Crohn's disease
2. Anal tags
3. Prolapse of rectal mucosa (much more common in elderly)
4. Anorectal abscess
5. Perianal tumors
6. Perianal thrombosis

D. Diagnostic Tests: None indicated; consider hemoglobin

V. Plan/Management

A. For mild hemorrhoidal symptoms from either internal or external hemorrhoids, advise
1. High fiber diet and bulk-forming agents (see section on CONSTIPATION)
2. Use of witch-hazel pads (Tucks) or gel (Tucks Gel) both over-the-counter products that are applied up to 6 x day
3. Sitz baths 1-2 x day

B. For moderate hemorrhoidal symptoms, recommend the nonpharmacologic measures listed above
1. Use of the following can also be recommended
   a. Anusol HC-1 ointment (OTC); apply 3-4 x/day for 7 days
   b. Preparation H ointment (OTC); apply up to 4 x/day
   c. Topical ointments are most effective applied with a finger cot inside the anus
2. Note that ointments applied correctly are much more effective than suppositories

C. For severe external hemorrhoidal symptoms, refer patient for excision of the clot and overlying skin under local anesthesia
    1. Most patients are seen several days after the onset of symptoms when severe pain is subsiding and are best managed with the above described therapies
    2. The thrombosis will resolve within 4-6 weeks; some patients will have a residual skin tag at the site of the thrombosed external hemorrhoid, but most are asymptomatic

D. Internal hemorrhoids that remain symptomatic after the conservative therapy described above can be effectively treated using such therapies as elastic ligation (banding), sclerotherapy, and infrared photocoagulation with elastic ligation being the most effective and least expensive of these methods

E. Follow Up: None needed unless persistence, recurrence of symptoms

DYSPHAGIA

I. Definition: Abnormalities of deglutition that may be related to initiation of the swallowing reflex in the oropharynx or propulsion of the food bolus through the esophagus

II. Pathogenesis

A. Dysphagia is often classified by location: oropharyngeal versus esophageal
    1. Oropharyngeal dysphagia refers to dysfunctional transfer of a food bolus in the pharynx past the upper esophageal sphincter into the esophagus
    2. Esophageal dysphagia results from disordered peristaltic motility or conditions that obstruct the flow of a food bolus through the esophagus into the stomach

B. A second way that dysphagia is classified is by mechanism: motility versus structural disorders
    1. Motility disorders are caused by neuromuscular or neurologic diseases
    2. Structural disorders include strictures, webs and rings, tumors, and extrinsic masses, all of which can result in luminal stenosis

C. Motility disorders and structural disorders can cause both oropharyngeal dysphagia and esophageal dysphagia

III. Clinical Presentation

A. Swallowing problems are most common among adults >50, particularly among hospitalized or nursing home patients

B. Patients with oropharyngeal dysphagia present with difficulty initiating swallowing that is often associated with coughing, choking, or nasal regurgitation
    1. Frequently presents as part of a broader complex of signs and symptoms of the underlying central nervous system or neuromuscular disorder or structural disorder
    2. Most often associated with stroke, Parkinson's disease, or other degenerative disorders; local structural lesions such as head and neck malignancy, radiation changes, and pharyngeal or hyopharyngeal webs are less common

C. Patients with esophageal dysphagia present with the sensation of food sticking in their throat or chest; patients with esophageal dysphagia are virtually always able to accurately localize symptoms to the level of the obstruction (unlike patients with oropharyngeal dysphagia)
    1. Esophageal motor disorders such as achalasia, scleroderma, and diffuse esophageal spasm are the most common causes of motor or motility disorders, with achalasia being the most common cause
    2. Benign esophageal stricture and esophageal cancer are among the structural causes

D. Achalasia is a slowly progressive motor disorder characterized by loss of peristaltic activity in distal esophagus
   1. Lower esophageal sphincter also fails to relax properly causing an obstruction at the esophagogastric junction
   2. Substernal chest pain often is present (reported in up to 50% of patients)
   3. Difficulty with swallowing both solids and liquids is reported with very cold liquids often provoking symptoms
   4. Repeated swallowing and performing the Valsalva maneuver may help propel food and fluids into stomach

E. Scleroderma can cause both a decrease in lower esophageal tone and a lack of propulsive motor activity in the esophagus
   1. Approximately 75% of these patients have esophageal involvement of some type
   2. Reflux is more common in these patients than is dysphagia which can be helpful in distinguishing it from other motor disorders

F. Structural lesions causing mechanical obstruction via luminal stenosis produce characteristic signs and symptoms in both classifications of dysphagia–oropharyngeal and esophageal
   1. More difficulty swallowing solids than liquids; with time, difficulty for liquids may also be present (dysphagia is a late sign of mechanical obstruction, and lumen must be reduced by approximately 40% before the person is symptomatic)
   2. Duration of symptoms before causing obstruction is relatively short (less than 1 year) for malignancy as compared with benign causes of obstruction
   3. Most persons with tumor are over age 50 and report marked weight loss
   4. Patients with stricture due to severe esophagitis usually have a long-standing history of reflux

G. Numerous commonly prescribed medications can cause dysphagia in either the oropharyngeal or esophageal stages of swallowing through (1) direct esophageal mucosal injury, (2) reduction of lower esophageal sphincter tone, or (3) by causing abnormal dryness of the mouth or xerostomia
   1. Examples of drugs causing mucosal injury to esophagus: antibiotics (doxycycline, tetracycline, clindamycin, trimethoprim-sulfamethoxazole), alendronate, and nonsteroidal anti-inflammatory drugs
   2. Examples of drugs causing reduced sphincter tone and xerostomia: atropine, scopolamine, ACE inhibitors, antihistamines, diuretics, opiates, antipsychotics
   3. Consult PDR for more complete information

IV. Diagnosis/Evaluation

A. History: Focus on (1) differentiating a motility disorder from a mechanical obstruction, and (2) determining if the dysphagia is oropharyngeal or esophageal in location
   1. Determine duration and progression of symptoms
      a. Is dysphagia new?
      b. Is it chronic and recurrent with some intervening periods of swallowing that are relatively normal?
      c. Was the onset fairly abrupt and is the condition progressing?
      d. **Note:** Gradual onset, slow progression, and chronic course suggest a motor disorder whereas a more rapid onset and progressive course suggest an obstruction
   2. Question regarding swallowing difficulty–is it for solids, liquids, or both; ask if there is temperature sensitivity, especially to cold substances
      a. With motility disorders, there is equal difficulty with solids and liquids, symptoms are aggravated by cold substances (liquid or solid) and passage of bolus is assisted with repeated swallowing and Valsalva maneuver
      b. With mechanical obstruction, there is more difficulty with solids than liquids, cold substances have no effect, and swallowing a bolus is not helped by Valsalva maneuver or repeated swallowing
   3. Ask if there is choking, regurgitation of fluid into the nose and if the difficulty with swallowing seems to be localized in the suprasternal area or if it is lower in the chest
   4. Ask if there is pain on swallowing (odynophagia)
   5. Determine if reflux is a problem
   6. Ask if there has been weight loss
   7. Obtain past medical history related to neurological disease, chronic reflux disease, esophagitis
   8. Obtain a good medication history to determine if medications are playing a role in the condition

B. Physical Examination
1. Examine the skin for pallor, signs of scleroderma (sclerodactyly, telangiectasia, calcinosis) and hyperkeratotic palms and soles (rarely found, but suggest esophageal carcinoma)
2. Examine mouth for adequate saliva production (if adequate, mucosa should appear pink and well-hydrated); examine floor of mouth, tongue and lips with a gloved hand to detect masses and abnormal motor function; view the soft palate
3. Palpate for enlarged lymph nodes in neck; palpate for thyroid enlargement
4. Perform abdominal exam for masses, tenderness, enlargement of liver/spleen
5. Perform rectal exam to obtain stool for occult blood (presence of occult blood in stool may be a sign of neoplasm or esophagitis)
6. Neurological examination should include testing of patient's mental status, motor and sensory functioning, deep tendon reflexes, and cranial nerves (gag reflex, palatal movement, and tongue protrusion), as well as a cerebellar examination
7. Observing the patient swallowing a variety of liquids and solids can be helpful

C. Differential Diagnosis: Many causes can be divided into motor and obstructive categories
1. Motor diseases include the following: Stroke, myasthenia gravis, multiple sclerosis, Parkinson's disease, amyotrophic lateral sclerosis, achalasia, scleroderma, diffuse esophageal spasm
2. Obstructing diseases/lesions include the following: tumor, radiation changes, prior head and neck surgeries, stricture, webs and rings, extrinsic masses

D. Diagnostic Tests
1. Radiographic contrast study (barium study) is often the initial test employed in evaluating patients with dysphagia and provides the best balance between detecting both structural and motor disorders; the type of barium study ordered varies depending on whether the swallowing problem is localized to the oropharyngeal or esophageal area
   a. The standard barium esophagogram, performed as part of an upper gastrointestinal series, is satisfactory when the location of the swallowing problem is known to be the esophagus
   b. If pharyngeal function needs to be assessed, a videoradiographic barium study is required
2. Endoscopy is a poor test for detecting motility disorders, but a good test for detecting strictures and permits dilatation in a single session; also an excellent test for detecting mucosal inflammation and mass lesions
3. Additional tests such as manometric studies and pH probe studies may be indicated based on results of the barium studies and endoscopy
4. Consultation with a specialist is recommended prior to and after any diagnostic testing is undertaken in order to help determine the most cost-effective approach in diagnostic testing based on findings from the history and physical examination

V. Plan/Management

A. Regardless of etiology and pending definitive diagnosis, an adequate caloric intake that can be swallowed with a minimum of difficulty should be advised
1. Liquid or soft diets work best if mechanical obstruction is suspected
2. If motor disturbances are suspected, small amounts that are eaten slowly work best

B. Patient should be referred to a specialist for management

C. Follow up should be done by specialist

CHOLECYSTITIS

I.   Definition: Acute or chronic inflammation of the gallbladder

II.   Pathogenesis

    A.   Pathogenesis of cholesterol gallstones (most common type in US) is multifactorial

    B.   High bile cholesterol levels (supersaturation with constituents in bile exceeding their maximum solubilities) initiate a cascade of events resulting in development of a crystal nucleus, stone growth, delayed gallbladder emptying, and resultant stasis of gallbladder contents
        1.   Delayed or incomplete emptying of bile from gallbladder can promote sludge formation
        2.   Gallstone formation is usually preceded by formation of biliary sludge (viscous gel-like substance composed of mucin, precipitates of cholesterol, and calcium bilirubinate)
        3.   Synthesis and secretion of bile mucin (a necessary component in sludge formation) is stimulated by prostaglandins; thus, inflammation and other stimuli known to enhance prostaglandin secretion increase risk for gallstone formation

    C.   Symptoms develop from mechanical obstruction, local inflammation, or a combination of these factors

    D.   Cholecystokinin is the most potent physiologic stimulator of gallbladder contraction; pain occurs when gallbladder contracts against an obstructing stone

III.   Clinical Presentation

    A.   Acute cholecystitis accounts for 3%-9% of hospital admissions for acute abdominal pain

    B.   Gallstones are more common in women, obese persons, and persons with a rapid weight loss; gallstones frequently develop during pregnancy but usually do not become symptomatic until after delivery

    C.   Pain is often colicky, located in the right upper quadrant with radiation to the flanks and occasionally the right shoulder; biliary colic localizes to the mid epigastrium as often as to the right upper quadrant

    D.   Pain of classic acute cholecystitis occurs within one hour after eating a large meal, lasts for several hours, and is followed by a residual aching that can last for days

    E.   Abdominal discomfort most often follows consumption of a fatty meal; may be associated with anorexia, nausea, vomiting, and fever

    F.   Most patients report a prior episode

    G.   Symptoms may be minimal in the elderly

IV.   Diagnosis/Evaluation

    A.   History
        1.   Question about onset, duration, location, radiation of pain; determine if pain is severe and persistent
        2.   Ask about presence of associated symptoms and provocative and palliative factors; specifically ask if pain is precipitated by a heavy meal or aggravated by deep inspiration, and if there is fat intolerance
        3.   Question regarding prior episodes of similar symptoms
        4.   If female of childbearing age, ask if pregnant during past year
        5.   Obtain past surgical and medical history
        6.   Obtain medication history

B. Physical Examination
   1. Determine if febrile
   2. Examine abdomen for right upper quadrant abdominal tenderness and involuntary guarding, indicative of early peritoneal inflammation
   3. Check for Murphy's sign—pain and arrested inspiration occurring when examiner's fingers are hooked underneath the right costal margin during deep inspiration
   4. An enlarged gallbladder may be palpable in right upper quadrant

C. Differential Diagnosis
   1. Peptic ulcer disease
   2. Pancreatitis
   3. Viral hepatitis
   4. Appendicitis

D. Diagnostic Tests
   1. Obtain CBC with differential and chemistry profile to determine if liver enzymes are elevated
   2. Order right upper quadrant ultrasound for the confirmation or exclusion of gallstone disease; patient needs to fast at least 8 hours prior to ultrasonography as gallstones are better visualized in a distended, bile-filled gallbladder
   3. **(Note: Test has a sensitivity >95% in detecting stones in the gallbladder)**

V. Plan/Management: Consultation with a specialist is indicated for additional evaluation, possible hospitalization

A. Previously, the diagnosis of acute cholecystitis was followed by a several week "cooling off" period before proceeding to surgery

B. Recently, most experts advocate early cholecystectomy—within several days of the onset of symptoms—based on lower complication rates, reduced costs, and shortened recovery periods

ABNORMAL LIVER-ENZYME RESULTS

I. Definition: Elevated liver-enzyme levels in asymptomatic patients

II. Pathogenesis:

A. **Aminotransferases**: Both aminotransferases–aspartate aminotransferase and alanine aminotransferase–are normally present in serum in low concentrations; elevations in normal levels are sensitive indicators of liver cell injury and are important in identification of hepatocellular diseases such as hepatitis
   1. Aspartate aminotransferase (AST) is found primarily in the liver, cardiac muscle, skeletal muscle, and kidneys
   2. Alanine aminotransferase (ALT) is found in highest amounts in the liver making this enzyme a more specific indicator of liver injury than AST
   3. Both enzymes are released into the blood when the liver cell membrane is damaged; however, there is poor correlation between the degree of liver-cell damage and the level of aminotransferases as necrosis of liver cells is not required for the release of aminotransferases
   4. The most common causes of elevated aminotransferase levels are the following: alcohol-related liver injury, chronic hepatitis B and C, autoimmune hepatitis, hepatic steatosis (fatty infiltration of the liver), nonalcoholic steatohepatitis, hemochromatosis, Wilson's disease, alpha$_1$-antitrypsin deficiency, and celiac sprue

B. **Alkaline phosphatase**: Levels most often become elevated from two sources–liver and bone and can indicate a pathologic, and sometimes, a physiologic process

1. Pathologic conditions that cause elevations in alkaline phosphatase levels include liver disorders such as chronic cholestatic or infiltrative liver diseases and bone diseases

   a. Cholestatic diseases or conditions include partial obstruction of bile ducts, primary biliary cirrhosis, primary sclerosing cholangitis, adult bile ductopenia, and cholestasis induced by the use of substances such as anabolic steroids

   b. Infiltrative diseases include sarcoidosis, other types of granulomatous diseases, and, less often, unsuspected metastasis of cancer to the liver

2. An influx of placental alkaline phosphatase into the circulation of women in their third trimester of pregnancy commonly occurs

3. Persons with blood type O or B may experience increases in serum alkaline phosphatase levels after eating a fatty meal because of an influx of intestinal alkaline phosphatase

4. Alkaline phosphatase levels also vary with age; adolescents in a growth spurt can have serum alkaline phosphatase levels two times as high as healthy adults due to the leakage of bone alkaline phosphatase into the blood

5. In adults, age is a factor in defining normal levels of this enzyme; for example, levels normally begin to gradually increase between 40 and 65 years, especially in women so that the normal alkaline phosphatase level in an otherwise healthy woman at age 65 is more than 50 percent higher than the level in her 30-year-old counterpart

C. **γ-Glutamyltransferase**: Levels are a very sensitive indicator of the presence or absence of hepatobiliary disease; however, lack of specificity makes elevations difficult to interpret because increased levels can also occur in a wide variety of clinical conditions

1. Elevated levels can occur in pancreatic disease, myocardial infarction, renal failure, chronic obstructive pulmonary disease, diabetes, and alcoholism

2. In addition, elevated levels are also found in patients on medications such as phenytoin and barbiturates

3. Whereas the use of serum γ-glutamyltransferase measurements has been recommended by some to identify patients with unreported alcohol use, the lack of specificity of the test makes its use of questionable value

4. The best use of serum γ-glutamyltransferase may be to evaluate the meaning of elevations in other serum enzyme levels (see IV.E.4. below)

III. Clinical Presentation

A. Patients are asymptomatic and abnormal liver-enzyme results were unanticipated

1. As many as 6% of normal asymptomatic persons may have abnormal liver-enzyme levels

2. The overall prevalence of liver disease in the general population is about 1%

3. The normal range for any laboratory test is the average (mean) value in a group of healthy persons ±2 standard deviations; thus, 5% of results obtained from the norm group falls outside the defined "normal" range (2.5% below and 2.5% above)

B. Variable presentation depending on the underlying cause if one is eventually identified

IV. Diagnosis/Evaluation

A. The first step in the evaluation of patients with elevated liver-enzyme levels but no symptoms is to repeat the test to confirm the results

1. If the results of the repeat test are normal, no further evaluation is indicated; however, repeating the test again in 3-6 months is probably a good option

2. If the results of the repeat test remain abnormal, further evaluation is indicated beginning with a complete history and physical examination in an effort to identify the most common causes of liver-enzyme elevations

B. History

1. Inquire about any symptoms such as anorexia, weight loss, malaise

2. Ask about alcohol and drug use; ask patient, "Do you ever drink alcohol?" If yes, continue with frequency and amount questions. Do the same with drug use keeping in mind that many patients conceal information about alcohol and drug use

3. Obtain detailed medication history; a listing of medications, herbs, and drugs or substances of abuse reported to cause elevations in liver-enzyme levels are contained in the table below

4. Determine if the initiation of a medication (prescription or over-the-counter), or other substance use could be associated with the increase in liver-enzyme levels
5. Ask about previous medical history including any previous acute illnesses that could have been hepatitis, surgical history for any gastrointestinal problems, history of blood transfusions prior to 1990
6. Obtain detailed sexual history
7. Question patient about household/work/recreational exposures to chemicals such as carbon tetrachloride, vinyl chloride; ask about recent participation in strenuous exercise

---

MEDICATIONS, HERBS, AND DRUGS OR SUBSTANCES OF ABUSE REPORTED TO CAUSE ELEVATIONS IN LIVER-ENZYME LEVELS

Medications

Antibiotics
→ Synthetic penicillins
→ Ciprofloxacin
→ Nitrofurantoin
→ Ketoconazole and fluconazole
→ Isoniazid

Antiepileptic drugs
→ Phenytoin
→ Carbamazepine

Statins
→ Simvastatin
→ Pravastatin
→ Lovastatin
→ Atorvastatin

Nonsteroidal anti-inflammatory drugs

Sulfonylureas for hyperglycemia
→ Glipizide

Herbs and homeopathic treatments
→ Chaparral
→ Alchemilla (lady's mantle)
→ Senna
→ Shark cartilage
→ Scutellaria (Skullcap)

Chinese herbs
→ Ji bu huan
→ Ephedra (Ma-huang)

Drugs and substances of abuse
→ Anabolic steroids
→ Cocaine
→ MDMA ("Ecstasy")
→ Phencyclidine ("Angel dust")

Glues and solvents
→ Glues containing toluene
→ Trichloroethylene

Adapted from Pratt, D.S. (2000). Evaluation of abnormal liver-enzyme results in asymptomatic patients. *New England Journal of Medicine, 342*, 1268.

C. Physical Examination: Focus should be on searching for evidence of liver disease
   1. Skin exam for spider angioma, palmar erythema, jaundice
   2. Sclera for icterus
   3. Abdominal exam, checking for ascites, right upper quadrant tenderness, hepatomegaly, splenomegaly
   4. Complete other parts of the exam as necessary

D. Differential Diagnosis: Many conditions/diseases cause liver-enzyme elevations

E. Additional Diagnostic Testing (once repeat testing has confirmed the liver-enzyme elevation)
   1. A cause for the persistent elevation should be sought
   2. If elevations in aminotransferase levels are persistent, evaluate for the most common causes, based on patient history (**Note**: Only two of the most common causes are discussed here–patients in whom other causes are suspected [see II.A. above], should be referred to an expert for evaluation and management])
      a. **Alcohol-related liver injury**: A γ-glutamyltransferase level that is two times the normal level in patients with an aspartate aminotransferase:alanine aminotransferase ratio of at least 2:1 strongly suggests a diagnosis of alcohol abuse. Use of γ-glutamyltransferase level as a single test to diagnose alcohol abuse is not recommended because of its lack of specificity
      b. **Positive hepatitis A, B, or C serologies**: Positive hepatitis A IgM serology; management consists of observation of patient and symptomatic support; positive hepatitis B or C infection, follow clinically with serial liver chemistries and refer to hepatologist for management
   3. If elevations in alkaline phosphatase levels are persistent in a patient with no other symptoms, determination of the source of the evaluation–whether bone or liver–is the first step in the evaluation
      a. Levels of γ-glutamyltransferase and alkaline phosphatase are usually elevated in parallel in patients with liver disorders; thus such a pattern should prompt an evaluation for liver disorders such as cholestatic diseases or infiltrative liver diseases (see II.B. above)
      b. In bone disorders, an elevated serum alkaline phosphate level but a normal γ-glutamyltransferase level should prompt an evaluation for bone diseases
      c. Referral to an expert at this point is appropriate

4. Elevations in γ-glutamyltransferase levels are difficult to interpret because of the lack of specificity of such elevations
   a. The value of this test is its role in evaluating the meaning of elevations in other serum enzyme levels
   b. For example, it can be used to confirm the hepatic origin of elevated alkaline phosphatase levels and to support the diagnosis of alcohol abuse in patients with elevated aminotransferase levels

V. Plan/Management

   A. Diagnostic testing (including repeat testing of the initial test) as outlined above is the first step in management

   B. If alcohol abuse is found to be the underlying problem, manage patient according to recommendations in the section on ALCOHOL PROBLEMS and consult with a hepatologist; refer patients with drug abuse for management

   C. If chronic hepatitis (B or C) is diagnosed, refer patient to a hepatologist for further evaluation and management

   D. If medications are suspected to be the cause of elevated aminotransferase levels, the easiest way to determine whether a medication is responsible is to stop its use and see whether the test results return to normal (obviously, some medications, e.g., antiepileptic drugs cannot be abruptly discontinued but must be tapered; therefore, discontinuation of a medications must be done using caution and judgment)

   E. Patients whose underlying cause for the persistent elevations in liver-enzymes remains unclear should be referred to an expert for further evaluation and management

   F. Follow up: Variable depending on whether patient is being managed in a primary care setting (as may be the case when a medication has caused the elevations in aminotransferase levels) or by the specialist to whom patient was referred

VIRAL HEPATITIS

I. Definition: An inflammatory process of the liver caused by infection by one of six distinct viruses (A, B, C, D, E, and G); other causes of hepatitis are not considered here

II. Pathogenesis

   A. Hepatitis A (HAV): RNA virus which is classified as a member of the picornavirus group; replication appears to be limited to the liver; only one serotype of HAV has been recognized in humans

   B. Hepatitis B (HBV): DNA-containing hepadnavirus; important components include HBsAg, hepatitis B core antigen, and hepatitis B e antigen (HBeAg)

   C. Hepatitis C (HCV): Small, single-stranded RNA virus that belongs to the family of Flavivirus; the most closely related human viruses are hepatitis G virus, yellow fever virus, and dengue virus; natural targets of HCV are hepatocytes

   D. Hepatitis D (HDV): Small particle consisting of an RNA genome and a delta protein antigen, both of which are coated with hepatitis B surface antigen; requires HBV as a helper virus and cannot produce infection in absence of HBV

   E. Hepatitis E (HEV): Single-stranded RNA virus that is presently classified as an unassigned genus of "hepatitis E-like" viruses

   F. Hepatitis G (HGV): Single-stranded RNA virus that is included in the Flaviviridae family and shares a 27% homology with HCV

III. Clinical Presentation

    A.   Hepatitis A

1. In US, hepatitis A is one of the most frequently reported vaccine-preventable diseases; highest rates occur in children 5 to 14 years of age and lowest rates among adults >40 years of age; reported cases have had an unequal geographic distribution in the US with the highest rates occurring in a limited number of states and communities; prevalence rates in these areas consistently remain higher than average

2. Incidence displays a cyclic pattern, and most disease occurs in the context of community-wide outbreaks during which a large proportion of persons do not have a recognized risk factor but become infected nonetheless

3. **Mode of transmission** is primarily through fecal-oral route; spreads readily in households and child care centers, with risk of spread in such centers increasing with the number of children who wear diapers; young children, frequently asymptomatic when infected, play an important role in HAV transmission

4. Other identified sources of infection include international travel, food-borne or waterborne outbreak, male homosexual activity, and injection-drug use; in approximately 50% of reported cases, the source cannot be determined

5. Unlike other infectious diseases that spread in child care centers, children who are infected are either asymptomatic or have very mild, nonspecific symptoms; adult contacts of infected children who themselves become infected, on the other hand, usually are symptomatic

6. Illness is self-limited and includes jaundice, anorexia, nausea, vomiting, malaise, and fever

7. When acquired during infancy and early childhood, infections are likely to be mild without jaundice; adult infections are likely to be quite severe

8. Viral shedding and the contagious period last 1-3 weeks, with the infected person being **most** contagious 1-2 weeks before the onset of illness; risk of transmission diminishes and is minimal in the week after onset of jaundice (if present)

9. **Incubation period** is 15-50 days, with an average of 25-30 days

10. **Chronic infection does not occur**

11. **Diagnosis**: Anti-HAV IgM appears early in the disease, and usually disappears after four months, but may persist for 6 months or longer. Presence of serum IgM indicates current or recent infection. Anti-HAV IgG develop shortly after the appearance of IgM; the presence of total anti-HAV without IgM anti-HAV indicates past infection and immunity

    B.   Hepatitis B

1. The number of new infections per year has declined from an estimated 260,000 in the 1980s to about 78,000 in 2001
   a. Highest rate of disease occurs in 20-49 year olds
   b. Greatest decline has happened among children and adolescents due to routine hepatitis B immunization

2. **Transmission** occurs via contact with infected blood or body fluids such as semen, cervical secretions, wound exudates, and saliva (blood and serum contain the highest concentrations of virus and saliva contains the lowest)

3. **Modes of transmission** include
   a. Transfusion of blood or blood products (uncommon in US today; estimated to be 1 in 63,000)
   b. Needle-sharing
   c. Percutaneous or mucous membrane exposures to blood or body fluids
   d. Heterosexual and homosexual activity
   e. Person-to-person spread of HBV can occur in settings involving close (nonsexual) contact over extended period that occurs when a chronically ill person resides in a household
   f. Vertical transmission (during perinatal period)
   g. More than 30% of infected persons do not have a readily identifiable risk factor
   h. Not transmitted via fecal-oral route

4. The primary reservoir for infection is the HBV chronic carrier (defined as person with serum HBsAg-positive for 6 months or who is immunoglobulin [Ig] M anti-HBc [antibody to hepatitis B core antigen] negative and HBsAg-positive)

5. Hepatitis B causes a spectrum of illness ranging from an asymptomatic seroconversion, to acute illness with anorexia, nausea, malaise, and jaundice, to fatal hepatitis

6. Arthralgias, arthritis, and a macular skin eruption can also occur as part of the illness

7. Asymptomatic infection is most common in young children

8. Age of the person at initial HBV infection is the major determinant of chronicity; chronic HBV infection is much more likely to develop after prenatal or perinatal exposure than after exposure later in life
9. To illustrate the effect of age on chronic disease, chronic HBV infection develops in
   a. Up to 90% of infants infected by perinatal transmission
   b. Thirty percent of children 1-5 years of age
   c. Six percent of older children, adolescents, and adults
10. There are an estimated 1.25 million chronically infected persons in the US; 20-30% of that number acquired their infection in childhood
11. **Incubation period** is 45-160 days, with an average of 90 days
12. **Diagnosis**: Diagnostic tests are described in the table below

INTERPRETATION OF THE HEPATITIS B PANEL		
Tests	Results	Interpretation
HBsAg anti-HBc anti-HBs	negative negative negative	susceptible
HBsAg anti-HBc anti-HBs	negative positive positive	immune due to natural infection
HBsAg anti-HBc anti-HBs	negative negative positive	immune due to hepatitis B vaccination
HBsAg anti-HBc IgM anti-HBc anti-HBs	positive positive positive negative	acutely infected
HBsAg anti-HBc IgM anti-HBc anti-HBs	positive positive negative negative	chronically infected
HBsAg anti-HBc anti-HBs	negative positive negative	four interpretations possible*

* 1. May be recovering from acute HBV infection
2. May be distantly immune and test not sensitive enough to detect very low level of anti-HBs in serum
3. May be susceptible with a false positive anti-HBc
4. May be undetectable level of HBsAg present in the serum and the person is actually a carrier

Source: Centers for Disease Control and Prevention. National Center for Infectious Diseases.(2002). Viral hepatitis B. Retrieved October 21, 2002, from http://www.cdc.gov/ncidod/diseases/hepatitis/b/Bserology.htm.

C. Hepatitis C
1. Prevalence of HCV infection varies throughout the world, with the highest number of infections reported in Egypt; in the US 1.8% of the population is positive for HCV antibodies; given that 3 of every 4 seropositive persons also have viremia, an estimated 2.7 million persons in the US have active HCV infection
2. **Mode of transmission** is primarily through injection drug use and receipt of a blood transfusion prior to 1990; in some cases, no risk factors can be identified
3. Until the last decade, blood transfusion was a major risk of HCV infection in developed countries such as the US; with the introduction of improved blood-screening measures (in 1990 and 1992) based on detection of HCV antibodies, the risk of transfusion-associated HCV infection has dramatically declined (**Note**: Current risk from blood that is negative for HCV antibodies is less than 1 in 103,000 transfused units, with the residual risk a consequence of blood donations that occur in the interval between infection and the development of detectable antibodies [estimated to be less than 12 weeks])
4. Sexual transmission of the virus is an inefficient means, much less efficient than is the case for HIV-1 infection; reasons for this may be the low levels of the virus in genital fluids and tissues (of HCV infected persons) or to a lack of appropriate target cells in the genital tract; coinfection with HIV-1 appears to increase the risk of sexual transmission

5. Casual household contact and contact with the saliva of infected persons also appear to be very inefficient modes of transmission; nosocomial transmission has been documented (from patient to patient by a colonoscope, during dialysis, and during surgery)
6. Prevalence of HCV infection is not higher among healthcare workers than among the general population, but needle-stick injuries in the healthcare setting continue to result in nosocomial transmission
7. Estimate of the comparative risks of transmission through a needle stick based on the rule of threes
   a. HBV is transmitted in 30% of exposures
   b. HCV is transmitted in 3% of exposures
   c. HIV-1 is transmitted in 0.3% of exposures
8. Maternal-fetal transmission occurs infrequently and is most often associated with coinfection in HIV-1 in the mother
9. Signs and symptoms of acute infection are often indistinguishable from those of hepatitis A or B infection–jaundice, malaise, and nausea
10. HCV infection is infrequently diagnosed in the acute phase; the majority of persons have either no symptoms or only mild symptoms
11. Acute infection leads to chronic infection in the majority of persons; spontaneous clearance of the viremia once chronic infection has been established is rare
12. Most chronic infections result in hepatitis; cirrhosis of the liver occurs in 15-20% of those with chronic disease; in addition to hepatic disease, extrahepatic manifestations of HCV infection include autoimmune or lymphoproliferative states
13. The course of HCV infection is greatly accelerated by coinfection with HIV-1 or HBV; further, superinfection with hepatitis A virus in HCV persons can result in severe acute or fulminant hepatitis
14. All persons with HCV antibody and/or HCV-RNA in their blood are considered to be contagious
15. **Incubation period** ranges from 2 to 26 weeks with an average of 7 to 8 weeks
16. **Diagnosis**: Two types of tests are available for diagnosis of HCV

DIAGNOSTIC TESTS FOR HCV

Serologic assays for antibodies
⇨ Screening assays based on antibody detection have greatly reduced risk of transfusion-related infection; once persons seroconvert, they usually remain positive for HCV antibodies
⇨ Primary serologic screening assay for HCV is the enzyme immunoassay which has been greatly improved in sensitivity over the past few years; can detect antibodies within 4 to 10 weeks after infection
◆ Positive results are confirmed by a recombinant immunoblot assay (RIBA)
◆ With the availability of improved enzyme immunoassays and better RNA-detection assays, confirmation by recombinant immunoblot assay may become less important in the future

Molecular tests for viral particles
⇨ Qualitative HCV RNA tests are based on the PCR technique and have a lower limit of detection of fewer than 100 copies of HCV RNA per mL
⇨ Appropriate use for these tests include the following
◆ In patients with negative results on enzyme immunoassay in whom acute infection is suspected
◆ In patients who have hepatitis with no identifiable cause
◆ In patients with known reasons for false negative results on antibody testing
◆ For the confirmation of viremia and the assessment of treatment response

---

D. Hepatitis D
1. Occurs as either a **coinfection** with HBV (e.g., following inoculation with blood or secretions that contain both agents) or as a **superinfection** in established chronic HBV infection
2. **Mode of transmission** is via blood or blood products, injection drugs, or sexual contact providing HBV also is present
3. Transmission from mother to newborn is uncommon
4. Hepatitis D resembles hepatitis B in terms of when symptoms appear and period of infectivity
5. Hepatitis D can cause hepatitis only in persons with acute or chronic HBV infection
6. **Incubation period** for HDV superinfection is approximately 2-8 weeks; when both viruses (B and D) infect simultaneously, incubation period averages 90 days and ranges from 45-160 days
7. **Diagnosis**: Radioimmunoassay and enzyme immunoassay for anti-HDV antibody are available (methods for detection of HDV RNA area also available)

E. Hepatitis E
1. Occurs predominantly in India, South Central Asia, and the Middle East, but also occurs in the Western Hemisphere, including the US (rare)
2. There is a possibility of a zoonotic reservoir for HEV
3. **Mode of transmission** is the fecal-oral route
4. Causes an acute illness with jaundice, malaise, anorexia, abdominal pain, arthralgias, and fever
5. Occurs more commonly in adults than children and is most serious when it occurs in pregnant women
6. **Period of communicability** is unknown, but probably continues for at least 2 weeks after the acute phase
7. **Chronic infection does not seem to occur**
8. **Incubation period** ranges from 15-60 days, with an average of 40 days
9. **Diagnosis**: Serologic and PCR-based assay for the diagnosis of acute HEV infection are available in research and commercial laboratories

F. Hepatitis G
1. Reported in adults and children throughout the world; found in about 1.5% of blood donors in US
2. Infection with the virus causes mild, if any, disease; no treatment is indicated
3. Infection has been reported in up to 20% of adults with chronic HBV or HCV infection, indicating that coinfection is a common occurrence
4. **Mode of transmission** is through transfusions; also can be transmitted by organ transplantation
5. Other important risk factors include injection drug use, hemodialysis, and homosexual and bisexual contacts, indicating that sexual transmission can occur
6. Transplacental transmission seems to be rare
7. **Incubation period** is unknown
8. No evidence that HGV causes fulminant or chronic disease
9. **Diagnosis**: No serologic test is available; currently, can be diagnosed only by use of polymerase chain assay which is not readily available

G. The following table contains a comparison of viral hepatitis, A to E

COMPARISON OF VIRAL HEPATITIS, A TO E			
Form	**Primary Route of Transmission**	**Incubation Period**	**Chronicity**
Hepatitis A	Fecal-oral, contaminated food/water	15-50 days	None
Hepatitis B	Blood/body fluids	45-160 days	Yes
Hepatitis C	Blood/blood products	2 - 26 weeks	Yes
Hepatitis D	Blood/body fluids	2 - 8 weeks	Yes
Hepatitis E	Fecal-oral	(?) 2 - 9 weeks	None

H. Viral hepatitis, A to E, are similar in their clinical expression and therefore cannot be readily distinguished by clinical features

I. Clinical features include the following:
1. Fatigue, lassitude, anorexia, nausea, dark urine, low grade fever, right upper abdominal discomfort, myalgia, and arthralgias
2. Only a minority of persons who are infected develop jaundice
3. Many infected persons are asymptomatic

J. The characteristic laboratory abnormalities are elevated aminotransferase levels that are high early in the prodromal period, peak before jaundice is maximal, and fall slowly during the convalescent period
1. Aspartate aminotransferase (AST) and alanine aminotransferase (ALT) levels are typically 500-2000 IU/L
2. ALT is usually higher than AST (in alcoholic hepatitis, the reverse is usual)
3. Alkaline phosphatase is only modestly elevated
4. Degree of hyperbilirubinemia is variable
5. Urinary bile usually precedes jaundice
6. Increase in prothrombin time is uncommon; if present suggests severe illness
7. WBC count is usually low-normal, and blood smear may show a few atypical lymphocytes

K. Serologic testing determines the specific etiologic diagnosis

IV. Diagnosis/Evaluation

A. History
1. Question about onset and duration of symptoms (usual symptoms are general fatigue, malaise, joint and muscle pain, loss of appetite, nausea, vomiting, diarrhea, and low-grade fever; tenderness of right upper quadrant and jaundice may also occur)
2. Ask about darkened urine, light-colored stools
3. Inquire about similar illness in household contacts
4. Ask about sexual behaviors and similar illness in sexual partners
5. Ask about history of blood transfusions, IV drug use, alcohol abuse
6. Inquire about occupation
7. Obtain travel history, especially travel to Asia or Africa where hepatitis B is especially common
8. Obtain past medical history and medication history

B. Physical Examination
1. Examine skin, mucous membranes, and sclera for jaundice
2. Perform abdominal exam to determine size, surface characteristics, and tenderness of liver; determine if spleen is enlarged

C. Differential Diagnosis: Noninfectious causes of hepatitis including medications, acute alcohol induced injury

D. Diagnostic Tests
1. If acute viral hepatitis is suspected, order appropriate diagnostic tests recommended above based on type of hepatitis that is suspected (many insurance carriers will not pay for "hepatitis panels")
2. Serologic features of viral hepatitis (A to E) are summarized in the following table:

SEROLOGIC FEATURES OF VIRAL HEPATITIS		
Form of Infection	**Serologic Markers**	**Interpretation**
Hepatitis A	IgM anti-HAV	Acute disease
	IgG anti-HAV	Remote infection and immunity
Hepatitis B		See Interpretation of the Hepatitis B Panel above
Hepatitis C	Anti-HCV	Acute, chronic, or resolved disease
	HCV RNA	Qualitative tests to detect presence or absence of virus and quantitative tests to detect amount of virus
Hepatitis D	HBsAg and anti-HDV	Acute disease
	• IgM anti-HBc positive	Co-infection
	• IgG anti-HBc positive	Superinfection
Hepatitis E	IgM anti-HEV	Acute disease
	IgG anti-HEV	Remote infection and immunity
IgM, immunoglobulin M; anti-HAV, antibody to hepatitis A virus; IgG, immunoglobulin G; anti-HCV, antibody to hepatitis C virus; anti-HDV, antibody to hepatitis D virus; HBsAg, hepatitis B surface antigen; anti-HBc, antibody to hepatitis B core antigen; anti-HEV, antibody to hepatitis E virus		

3. If HBsAg is positive, obtain IgM anti-HBc to differentiate acute hepatitis B (IgM anti-HBc is positive) from chronic hepatitis B (IgM anti-HBc is negative). Chronic hepatitis B is also defined by 2 HBsAg-positive tests separated by at least 6 months
4. Testing for anti-HDV should be done in all persons with chronic hepatitis B to rule out coexisting hepatitis D
5. If all test results are negative, follow up testing for anti-HCV is appropriate because of delay in appearance of antibody
6. CBC, total and direct bilirubin, prothrombin time, liver enzymes, urinalysis should be obtained also
7. All persons with chronic hepatitis should have liver biopsy to determine extent of disease

V. Plan/Management

A. Hepatitis usually resolves spontaneously over 4-8 weeks

B. For acute infections for viral hepatitis (A, B, C, D, E), provide symptomatic treatment for symptoms such as myalgia, nausea, vomiting, and pruritus

C. Bed rest, special diets, vitamin supplements are not required; patient should abstain from alcohol and should not engage in strenuous activities or contact sports

D. If patient on hepatotoxic drugs, those should be discontinued until recovery has occurred

E. FDA-approved therapeutic options for treatment of chronic hepatitis B infection are interferon alfa-2b (Intron A), the nucleoside analog lamivudine (Epivir-HBV), and the nucleotide analog, adefovir (Hepsera)
    1. Adefovir and lamivudine are given PO in a once daily dose, and the cost for a one-month supply is $528 and $156, respectively
    2. Interferon alfa-2b is given either SC or IM and the cost for a one-month supply of a daily dose is $2,131, and for a 3x/week dose is $1,739 (based on AWP listings in *Drug Topics Red Book Update*, December 2002)
    3. Patients should be referred to an expert for management

F. All patients with chronic HCV infection are potential candidates for antiviral therapy but the risks and benefits of treatment must be assessed individually, especially given the typically slow course of natural infection
    1. Only a subgroup of persons with chronic infection will have a clear indication for therapy; patients with detectable levels of HCV RNA who have elevated alanine aminotransferase levels that are persistent and who have a liver biopsy positive for fibrosis or at least moderate necrosis and inflammation have a high risk of disease progression and should be treated provided there are no contraindications
    2. Combination therapy with interferon and ribavirin has proven to be very effective
    3. Patients with persistently normal alanine aminotransferase levels and no histologic evidence of pathologic changes in the liver have a very good prognosis without therapy
    4. Patients should be immediately referred to an expert for management

VI. Control measures: Hepatitis A

A. Improved sanitation and personal hygiene (especially good hand washing) are the keys to controlling spread of the virus

B. Postexposure prophylaxis for household and sexual contacts: Give 0.02 mL/kg of immune globulin (IG) as soon as possible after exposure (use of IG more than 2 weeks after last exposure in not indicated) **and** give HAV vaccine in dosage and schedule as described in table under VI.D. below

C. Hepatitis A vaccine: Havrix and Vaqta, both with pediatric and adult formulations are available in the US; these are inactivated vaccines prepared from cell culture-adapted HAV; Havrix contains a preservative and Vaqta is formulated without a preservative
    1. Currently, vaccination is recommended for adults with certain risk factors and for children who live in communities where the reported annual incidence exceeds two times the average annual rate in the US (high risk regions or states include the following–AK, AZ, CA, ID, NV, NM, OK, OR, SD, UT, WA)
    2. There is disagreement among the experts regarding whether to extend routine hepatitis A immunization to children outside these areas

RECOMMENDED DOSES AND SCHEDULES FOR INACTIVATED HEPATITIS A VACCINES*				
Age (years)	Vaccine	Volume per Dose	No. of Doses	Schedule
2-18	Havrix	0.5 mL	2	Initial and 6-12 mos later
2-17	Vaqta	0.5 mL	2	Initial and 6-18 mos later
19 and older	Havrix	1.0 mL	2	Initial and 6-12 mos later
18 and older	Vaqta	1.0 mL	2	Initial and 6 mos later

* Havrix is manufactured b SmithKline Beecham Biologicals, Rixensart, Belgium, and distributed by SmithKline Beecham Pharmaceuticals, Philadelphia, PA; Vaqta is manufactured and distributed by Merck & Co, Inc, West Point, PA

D. Hepatitis A vaccine should be given routinely to persons ≥2 years of age in the following groups
1. International travelers
2. Patients with chronic liver disease
3. Homosexual and bisexual men
4. Users of injection and noninjection illegal drugs
5. Persons with clotting-factor disorders
6. Persons with risk of occupational exposure
7. Any healthy person at least 2 years of age at discretion of health care provider (examples, child care center staff/attendees, custodial care workers, hospital workers, food handlers)

VII. Control measures: Hepatitis B

A. Prenatal screening for HBsAg can prevent perinatal transmission (for care of infant whose mother is HBsAg-positive, consult *Red Book* [2000] pp. 298-300, as these infants require special care including HBIG within 12 hours after birth)

B. Prevention of HBV transmission to medical personnel is possible through use of universal precautions for blood and body fluids; nonetheless, all health care workers and others with occupational exposure to blood are at high risk and should be immunized

C. Consult *Red Book* (2000) for complete listing of other high-risk groups who should receive pre-exposure hepatitis B immunization

D. Recommendations for Hepatitis B prophylaxis after percutaneous or permucosal exposure are contained in the following table

RECOMMENDED POSTEXPOSURE PROPHYLAXIS FOR EXPOSURE TO HEPATITIS B VIRUS

Vaccination and Anti-body Response Status of Exposed Workers	Treatment When Source Is		
	HBsAg Positive	HBsAg Negative	Source Not Tested or Status Unknown
Unvaccinated	HBIG x 1; initiate HB vaccine series	Initiate HB vaccine series	Initiate HB vaccine series
Previously vaccinated: Known responder*	No treatment	No treatment	No treatment
Known non-responder**	HBIG x 2 or HBIG x 1 and initiate re-vaccination[†]	No treatment	If known high-risk source, treat as if source were HBsAg positive
Antibody response unknown	Test exposed person for anti-HBs 1. If adequate,* no treatment 2. If inadequate,** HBIG x 1 and vaccine booster	No treatment	Test exposed person for anti-HBs 1. If adequate,* no treatment 2. If inadequate,** administer vaccine and booster and recheck titer in 1 to 2 months

HBsAg = hepatitis B surface antigen; HBIG = hepatitis B immune globulin; HB = hepatitis B; anti-HBs = antibody to HBsAg
* Responder is defined as a person with adequate levels of serum antibody to hepatitis B surface antigen (i.e., anti-HBs ≥10 ml U/mL)
**A non-responder is a person with inadequate response to vaccination (i.e., anti-HBs <10 mIU/mL)
[†] The option of giving one dose of HBIG and reinitiating the vaccine series is preferred for non-responders who have not completed a second 3-dose vaccine series; for persons who previously completed a second vaccine series but failed to respond, 2 doses of HBIG are preferred
Adapted from Centers for Disease Control and Prevention. (2001). Updated US Public Health Service guidelines for the management of occupational exposures to HBV, HCV, and HIV and recommendations for postexposure prophylaxis. *MMWR, 50*, No. RR-11, p. 22.

VIII. Control measures: Hepatitis C

A. Should be managed with the universal precautions for blood and body fluids as in hepatitis B

B. Immunoprophylaxis is not available

IX.   Control measures: Hepatitis D

    A.   Transmission is similar to that of HBV, so universal precautions for blood and body fluids should be observed

    B.   Cannot be transmitted in the absence of HBV, so prevention of HBV is key to prevention

    C.   Immunoprophylaxis not available; because HDV cannot be transmitted in the absence of HBV infection, hepatitis B immunization protects against HDV infection and thus should be obtained

X.   Control measures: Hepatitis E

    A.   Immunoprophylaxis not available

    B.   Prevention through good sanitation and hygiene

XI.   Control measures: Hepatitis G

    A.   Immunoprophylaxis not available

    B.   Should be managed with universal precautions for blood and body fluids as in hepatitis B

XII.   Follow Up

    A.   Variable depending on type of hepatitis

    B.   Hepatitis A does not have a chronic stage, so generally resolves without any long-term effects (Hepatitis E only found in developing countries and rarely in the US at this time)
        1.   Make sure post-exposure prophylaxis for household and sexual contacts as described under VI.B. above is given; contacts should then be appropriately immunized with HAV vaccine (see VI.D. above)
        2.   Emphasize control measures to prevent spread
        3.   Recheck patient after 2 weeks to evaluate condition

    C.   Hepatitis B, C, D should be referred for management because of development of high rate of chronic hepatitis

REFERENCES

Abramowicz, M. (2001). Proton pump inhibitors. *The Medical Letter, 43,* 36-37.

Abramowicz, M. (2002). Adefovir (Hepsera) for chronic hepatitis B infection. *The Medical Letter, 44,* 105-106.

Abramowicz, M. (2002). Alosetron (Lotronex) revisited. *The Medical Letter, 44,* 67-68.

Abramowicz, M. (2002). Tegaserod maleate (Zelnorm) for IBS with constipation. *The Medical Letter, 44,* 79-80.

Ahluwalia, J.P., Graber, M.A., & Silverman, W.B. (2002). Gastroenterology and hepatology. In M.A. Graber & M.L. Lanternier (Eds.), *University of Iowa: The family practice handbook* (pp. 151-204). St. Louis: Mosby.

Academy of Pediatrics. (2000). *Red book: Report of the Committee on Infectious Diseases* (25th ed.). Elk Grove Village, IL: Author.

American Gastroenterological Association. (1999) AGA medical position statement: Guidelines for the evaluation and management of chronic diarrhea. *Gastroenterology, 116,* 1461-1463.

American Gastroenterological Association. (1999). AGA technical review on the evaluation and management of chronic diarrhea. *Gastroenterology, 116,* 1464-1486.

American Gastroenterological Association. (2001). AGA technical review on nausea and vomiting. *Gastroenterology, 120,* 263-286.

American Gastroenterological Association. (2001). AGA medical position statement: Nausea and vomiting. *Gastroenterology, 120,* 261-262.

American Gastroenterological Association Clinical Practice Committee. (2002). AGA technical review on the evaluation of liver chemistry tests. *Gastroenterology, 123*, 1367-1384.

American Gastroenterological Association Clinical Practice Committee. (2003). Colorectal cancer screening and surveillance: Clinical guidelines and rationale—update based on new evidence. *Gastroenterology, 124,* 544-560.

Anand, C.A. (2002). Amebiasis. In R.E. Rakel & E.T. Bope (Eds.). *Conn's current therapy* (pp. 57-61). Philadelphia: WB Saunders.

Andres, J.M., & Francisco, M.P. (2001). Jaundice. In R.A. Hoekelman, H.M. Adams, N.M. Nelson, M.L. Weitzman, & M.H. Wilson (Eds.), *Pediatric primary care* (pp. 1170-1181). St. Louis: Mosby.

Ansdell, V. (2002). Intestinal parasites. In R.E. Rakel & E.T. Bope (Eds.). *Conn's current therapy* (pp. 537-544). Philadelphia: WB Saunders.

Arce, D.A., Ermocilla, C.A., & Costa, H. (2002). Evaluation of constipation. *American Family Physician, 65,* 2283-2290.

Bytzer, P., & Talley, N.J. (2001). Dyspepsia. *Annals of Internal Medicine, 134*, 815-822.

Centers for Disease Control and Prevention. (2001). Diagnosis and management of foodborne illnesses: A primer for physicians. *Morbidity and Mortality Weekly Report, 50*(No. RR-02), 1-69

Centers for Disease Control and Prevention. (2001). Updated US Public Health Service guidelines for the management of occupational exposures to HBV, HCV, and HIV and recommendations for postexposure prophylaxis. *Morbidity and Mortality Weekly Report, 50*(No. RR-11), 1-44.

Centers for Disease Control and Prevention. (2002). Outbreaks of gastroenteritis associated with noroviruses on cruise ships—United States, 2002. *Morbidity and Mortality Weekly Report, 51*, 1112-1115.

Chan, F.K.L., Hung, L.C.T., & Suen, B.Y. (2002). Celecoxib versus diclofenac and omeprazole in reducing the risk of recurrent ulcer bleeding in patients with arthritis. *New England Journal of Medicine, 247*, 2104-2110.

Colgan, R., Michocki, R., Greisman, L., & Moore, T.A. (2003). Antiviral drugs in the immunocompetent host. *American Family Physician, 67,* 757-762.

DeVault, K.R., & Castell, D.O., for the Practice Parameters Committee of the American College of Gastroenterology. (1999). Updated guidelines for the diagnosis and treatment of gastroesophageal reflux disease. *American Journal of Gastroenterology, 94*, 1434-1442.

Drossman, D.A. (1995). Diagnosing and treating patients with refractory functional gastrointestinal disorders. *Annals of Internal Medicine, 123,* 688-697.

Dunphy, R.C., & Verne, G.N. (2003). Progress report: Irritable bowel syndrome. *Emergency Medicine*, (Feb), 13-19.

Etzkorn, K.P., & Rodriquez, L. (2002). Constipation. In R.E. Rakel & E.T. Bope (Eds.). *Conn's current therapy* (pp. 18-21). Philadelphia: WB Saunders.

Flynn, C.A. (2001). The evaluation and treatment of adults with gastroesophageal reflux disease. *The Journal of Family Practice, 50*, 57-64.

Goroll, A.H., & Mulley, A.G. (2002). *Primary care medicine recommendations.* Philadephia: Lippincott Williams & Wilkins.

Goroll, A.H., & Mulley, Jr., A.G. (2000) Approach to the patient with an external hernia. In A.H. Goroll & A.G. Mulley, Jr. (Eds.), *Primary care medicine* (pp. 431-434). Philadelphia: Lippincott.

Graber, M.A. (1998). Dealing with acute abdominal pain: Part 1: Clues to the diagnosis. *Emergency Medicine, 30*, 74-100.

Hasler, W.L. (2002). The irritable bowel syndrome. *Medical Clinics of North America*, 1525-1551.

Horwitz, B., & Fisher, R.S. (2001). The irritable bowel syndrome. *New England Journal of Medicine, 344*, 1846-1850.

Infectious Diseases Society of America. (2001). Practice guidelines for the management of infectious diarrhea. *Clinical Infectious Diseases, 32*, 331-350.

Koch, K.L. (2002). Nausea and vomiting. In R.E. Rakel & E.T. Bope (Eds.). *Conn's current therapy* (pp. 6-9). Philadelphia: WB Saunders.

Lauer, G.M., & Walkers, B.D. (2001). Hepatitis C infection. *New England Journal of Medicine, 345*, 41-52.

McColl, I. (1998). More precision in diagnosing appendicitis. *New England Journal of Medicine, 338*, 190-191.

Meurer, L.A., & Bower, D.J. (2002). Management of *Helicobacter pylori* infection. *American Family Physician, 65*, 1327-1336, 1339.

Mittal, R.K., & Balaban, D.H. (1997). The esophagogastric junction. *New England Journal of Medicine, 336*, 924-932.

Morris, J.G. (2002). Food-borne illness. In R.E. Rakel & E.T. Bope (Eds.). *Conn's current therapy* (pp. 77-82). Philadelphia: WB Saunders.

National Institutes of Health Consensus Development Conference Statement. (2002). *Management of hepatitis C*: 2002. Bethesda, MD: Author.

Pandolfino, J.E. & Kahrilas, P.J. (2002). Gastroesophageal reflux disease. In R.E. Rakel & E.T. Bope (Eds.). *Conn's current therapy* (pp. 524-527). Philadelphia: WB Saunders.

Pratt, D.S. & Kaplan, M.M. (2000). Evaluation of abnormal liver-enzyme results in asymptomatic patients. *New England Journal of Medicine, 342*, 1266-1271.

Prystowsky, J.B. (2002). Cholelithiasis and cholecystitis. In R.E. Rakel & E.T. Bope (Eds.). *Conn's current therapy* (pp. 461-463). Philadelphia: WB Saunders.

Ravich, W.J. (2002). Dysphagia. In R.E. Rakel & E.T. Bope (Eds.). *Conn's current therapy* (pp. 471-476). Philadelphia: WB Saunders.

Rettenbacher, T., Hollerweger, A., Gritzmann, N., Gotwald, T., Schwamberger, K., & Ulmer, H. (2002). Appendicitis: Should diagnostic imaging be performed if the clinical presentation is highly suggestive of the disease? *Gastroenterology, 123*, 992-996.

Rivkina, A., & Rybalov, S. (2002). Chronic hepatitis B: Current and future treatment options. *Pharmacotherapy, 22*, 721-737.

Sack, D.A. (2002). Acute infectious diarrhea. In R.E. Rakel & E.T. Bope (Eds.). *Conn's current therapy* (pp. 12-18). Philadelphia: WB Saunders.

Shaheen, N., & Ransohoff, D.F. (2002). Gastroesophageal reflux, Barrett esophagus, and esophageal cancer: Scientific review. *JAMA, 287*, 1972-1981.

Shaheen, N., & Ransohoff, D.F. (2002). Gastroesophageal reflux, Barrett esophagus, and esophageal cancer: Clinical applications. *JAMA, 287*, 1982-1986.

Smith, J.C. (2001). Abdominal pain. In R.A. Hoekelman, H.M. Adams, N.M. Nelson, M.L. Weitzman, & M.H. Wilson (Eds.), *Pediatric primary care* (pp.965-970). St. Louis: Mosby.

Smoot, D.T. (2002). Gastritis and peptic ulcer disease. In R.E. Rakel & E.T. Bope (Eds.). *Conn's current therapy* (pp. 492-497). Philadelphia: WB Saunders.

Suerbaum, S., & Michetti, P. (2002). *Helicobacter pylori* infection. *New England Journal of Medicine, 347*, 1175-1185

Thompson, W.G., Longstreth, G.F., Drossman, D.A., Heaton, K.W., Irvine, E.J., & Muller-Lissner, S.A. (1999). Functional bowel disorders and functional abdominal pain. *Gut, 45*(Suppl II), II43-II47.

Trowbridge, R.L., Rutowski, N.K., & Shojania, K.G. (2003). Does this patient have acute cholecystitis? *JAMA, 289*, 80-86.

Willey, J., & Richter, J.E. (2002) Managing gastroesophageal reflux disease. *Women's Health in Primary Care, 4*, 665-671.

Genitourinary Problems

Constance R. Uphold

BENIGN PROSTATIC HYPERPLASIA

I.   Definition: Benign adenomatous hyperplasia of the periurethral prostate gland

II.   Pathogenesis

    A.   Enlarged prostate and/or an increase in smooth muscle tone of the prostate and bladder neck cause reduced or interrupted urinary flow, inability to empty bladder, and increased frequency of urination

    B.   The etiology of benign prostatic hyperplasia (BPH) is uncertain but several factors appear to play a role
        1.   Increased 5α-dihydrotestosterone (DHT), the active form of testosterone
        2.   Increased estrogen
        3.   Stimulation of α-adrenergic nerve endings interfering with the opening of the bladder neck internal sphincter
        4.   Smoking may have a protective effect

III.   Clinical Presentation

    A.   Commonly seen in men >50 years; 50% of all men have BPH identifiable histologically at 60 years of age with a 90% prevalence by age 85; approximately 1/4 of males in US will eventually require treatment for relief of symptoms of BPH

    B.   Most patients have a gradual worsening of the following symptoms:
        1.   Obstructive symptoms include a weak urinary stream, abdominal straining to void, hesitancy, intermittency, incomplete bladder emptying, and terminal dribbling
        2.   Irritative symptoms include frequency, nocturia, and urgency

    C.   Complications of BPH are variable:
        1.   Patients are often more susceptible to urinary tract infections
        2.   In long-standing BPH, urinary incontinence may be present
        3.   Severe prostate enlargement can block the urethra, causing acute urinary retention

IV.   Diagnosis/Evaluation

    A.   History
        1.   Determine onset and duration of symptoms
        2.   The American Urological Association (AUA) Symptom Index can be used to rate symptom severity
            a.   Self-administered 7-item questionnaire that rates the symptom severity on a scale from 0 (not at all) to 5 (almost always); items are then summed to obtain a total score
            b.   Men rate the following symptoms that they might have had over the past month: Sensation of not emptying their bladder after urination, occurrence of the need to urinate within 2 hours of last urination, episodes of having to start and stop during urination, difficulty postponing urination, weak urinary stream, occurrence of needing to push and strain to urinate, and the number of times got up from bed to urinate during the night
        3.   Ask about pain or discomfort as well as hematuria
        4.   Question about fevers and penile discharge
        5.   Possibly ask patient to record symptoms for a period of one week
        6.   Ask about recent onset of back or bone pain, anorexia, or weight loss which often accompanies malignancy
        7.   Obtain a complete medical history, specifically asking about genitourinary problems and surgeries, diabetes mellitus, and neurological diseases
        8.   Ask about history of indwelling urinary catheter
        9.   Gather a complete medication history:
            a.   Ask patients whether cold or sinus medications aggravate symptoms
            b.   Drugs such as anticholinergics can impair bladder contractility and sympathomimetics can increase outflow resistance

B. Physical Examination
    1. Perform an abdominal examination to detect a distended bladder, renal tenderness, or a mass
    2. Perform a digital rectal examination (DRE) to estimate the size, consistency, symmetry and tenderness of the prostate, to detect nodules or indurations that may be indicative of prostate cancer, and to evaluate anal sphincter tone (prostate size does not correlate well with complications of BPH)
        a. Normal prostate is about 2.5 x 3 cm in vertical and transverse diameters
        b. In BPH, the gland is often enlarged, firm, smooth, symmetrical, with an obliterated median sulcus
        c. In prostate cancer, the gland may be asymmetric and nodular with a hard and fixed mass
    3. Consider watching the patient void to determine size and force of urinary stream (normally, a man should be able to empty bladder of 300 mL of urine in 12-15 seconds)
    4. Perform a focused neurologic examination to detect diseases such as multiple sclerosis

C. Differential Diagnosis
    1. Other causes of bladder outlet obstruction
        a. Prostatic cancer (see IV.B.2.c. above)
        b. Urethral obstruction
        c. Vesical neck obstruction
    2. Impaired detrusor contractility related to neurogenic, myogenic or psychogenic factors
    3. Detrusor instability/hyper-reflexia from inflammatory or infectious conditions
        a. Cystitis
        b. Prostatitis
        c. Bladder cancer
    4. Any disease causing increased urinary frequency may mimic BPH such as diabetes mellitus, hypercalcemia, or nocturnal diuresis of congestive heart failure

D. Diagnostic Tests
    1. Urinalysis to rule out urinary tract infection, hematuria, and glycosuria
    2. Creatinine to assess renal function; elevated levels suggest urinary retention or underlying renal disease that necessitates early referral to urologist
    3. Consider ordering prostate-specific antigen (PSA) levels; digital rectal examination (DRE) together with the serum PSA is the best strategy for detecting prostate cancer
        a. Although not recommended by some major task forces, including the US Preventive Services Task Force (USPSTF), the American Urological Association recommends annual PSA testing beginning at age 50 in all men with a least a 10-year life expectancy and earlier in men with increased risk for prostate cancer
        b. Remember that BPH and prostate cancer as well as the following factors may elevate PSA levels: Prostatitis, physical activity, infection, prostate biopsy, cystoscopy
        c. Other factors decrease PSA levels: Medications such as finasteride (Proscar), surgical or medical castration, herbal medicines or compounds
    4. Consider performing a biopsy to rule-out a diagnosis of prostate cancer if the PSA level is 4.0 ng/mL or higher, if patient's PSA level increases significantly from one test to the next, or if DRE is abnormal
    5. Uroflowmetry to detect lower urinary tract obstruction is usually recommended
    6. Consider postvoid residual urine volume to detect obstruction and impaired detrusor function
    7. Order urine cytologic studies if irritative voiding symptoms are severe
    8. Optional tests:
        a. Imaging of the upper urinary tract (particularly in patients with history of urinary tract infection or urolithiasis with hematuria or renal insufficiency)
        b. Urethrocystoscopy (particularly in patients with hematuria, urethral stricture disease, bladder cancer, or previous lower urinary tract surgery)
        c. Pressure-flow studies to distinguish between obstruction and impaired detrusor contractility and in patients with a history of primary bladder dysfunction
        d. Filling cystometrography

V. Plan/Management

A. Refer men who have the following conditions to urologist:
    1. Refractory urinary retention who have failed at least one attempt at catheter removal
    2. Recurrent infections, recurrent retention, refractory hematuria, bladder stones, large bladder diverticula, or renal insufficiency clearly related to BPH
    3. Consider referral if complications exist or if patients have severe symptoms

B. The treatment of patients who have no absolute indications for surgery is usually based on the severity of symptoms; however, the risks and benefits of all options should be carefully discussed with the patient

C. Watchful waiting
1. Typically, men with mild symptoms (AUA score ≤7) prefer this strategy; however, probabilities of disease progression and development of complications are uncertain
2. Monitor patient's symptoms and clinical course semi-annually or annually
3. Discuss behavioral techniques to reduce symptoms
    a. Limit fluid intake after dinner
    b. Consider other behavioral techniques that may or may not prove helpful:
        (1) Frequent voiding and double voiding (urinate, wait 3 minutes, and void again)
        (2) Avoidance of sudden diuresis which often occurs after drinking caffeine or alcohol
        (3) Performance of prostatic massage after intercourse
    c. Avoid certain medications if possible (see following table)

MEDICATIONS THAT MAY WORSEN BPH SYMPTOMS

Class	Agents	Comments
ANTICHOLINERGICS		
→ **Antidepressants**	***Highest effects:*** amitriptyline (highest), amoxapine, clomipramine ***Moderate effects:*** bupropion, doxepin, imipramine, maprotiline, nortriptyline, trimipramine	Includes non-prescription and prescription medications which have anticholinergic properties; may worsen outflow obstruction
→ **Antiparkinson agents**	Benztropine, trihexyphenidyl	
→ **Antipsychotics**	***Highest effects:*** clozapine, mesoridazine, promazine, triflupromazine, thioridazine ***Moderate effects:*** chlorpromazine, pimozide	
→ **Antispasmodics**	Atropine, belladonna alkaloids, clidinium bromide, dicyclomine HCl, glycopyrrolate, hexocyclium, isopropamide, L-hyoscyamine, mepenzolate bromide, methantheline bromide, methscopolamine bromide, oxyphencyclimine HCl, propantheline bromide, tridihexethyl chloride	
→ **Cold preparations containing antihistamines**	***Highest effects:*** carbinoxamine, clemastine, diphenhydramine, methdilazine, promethazine, trimeprazine ***Moderate effects:*** azatadine, brompheniramine, chlorpheniramine, cyproheptadine, dexchlorpheniramine, phenindamine, triprolidine	
α-ADRENERGIC AGONISTS	Pseudoephedrine	Includes cold preparations that contain decongestants
DIURETICS	**Thiazides:** chlorthalidone, hydrochlorothiazide **Thiazide-like:** indapamide, metolazone **Loop Diuretics:** bumetanide, furosemide, torsemide	These medications do not worsen outflow obstruction, but may make symptoms of polyuria and frequency more bothersome. Thus, they are generally safe, but their influence on symptoms should be considered

Adapted from Hebel, S.K. (Ed.). (1996). *Drug facts and comparisons.* St. Louis: Facts and Comparisons, Inc.

D. α-adrenergic blockers are usually prescribed first, particularly for men with small prostates (<40 grams) and men with acute, mainly irritative symptoms
1. Three approved drugs (terazosin, doxazosin mesylate, tamsulosin HCl) have similar efficacies but tamsulosin is uroselective and has the fewest adverse effects and does not need dose titration
2. Significant benefits of α-blockers include the following:
    a   Reduce symptoms and increase uroflow by decreasing bladder outlet resistance
    b. Improve lipid levels
    c. Terazosin and doxazosin additionally decrease blood pressure in hypertensive men but do not alter blood pressure in normotensive men
3. Limited evidence that these drugs reduce complication rates or postpone future surgery

4. Prescribe one of the following long-acting agents; tamsulosin may be best in men who are normotensive, whereas terazosin and doxazosin may be best in hypertensive men (to avoid postural hypotension, both terazosin and doxazosin should be taken at bedtime and the dosages should be slowly increased; caution patients to carefully arise from bed at night and in the morning)
   a. Terazosin (Hytrin)
      (1) Begin with small initial doses such as 1 mg QD HS for 3 days, 2 mg for 11 days, 5 mg for 7 days and 10 mg once daily, thereafter
      (2) Maximum dose is 20 mg/day
   b. Doxazosin mesylate (Cardura)
      (1) Begin with 1 mg QD HS; double dose every 1-2 weeks if needed
      (2) Maximum dose is 8 mg/day
   c. Tamsulosin HCl (Flomax)
      (1) Fewest adverse effects, except for increased ejaculation problems
      (2) Offers no advantage to reducing B/P in hypertensive patients
      (3) Typically, prescribe 0.4 mg QD about 30 minutes before the same meal each day; does not require titration but may need to increase dosage to 0.8 if there is no response after 2-4 weeks
      (4) Do not crush, chew, or open caps; swallow whole
   d. A once-daily formulation of alfuzosin has been developed; has similar efficacies to other α-blockers and a good side effect profile like tamsulosin, but does not cause ejaculatory problems

E. Finasteride (Proscar), a 5α-reductase inhibitor, is the drug of choice for men with relatively large prostates (>40 grams), PSA values >2-4 ng/mL, and for men who have contraindications or failed treatment with α-adrenergic blockers; finasteride is also indicated for men with hematuria
   1. Prescribe 5 mg QD for at least 6 months; no titration is needed
   2. Effective in decreasing prostatic size, increasing peak urinary flowrate and reducing symptoms
   3. Reduces growth of prostate by inhibiting conversion of testosterone to the more active dihydrotestosterone
   4. Inform patient that full response to therapy may take 6-12 months; α-adrenergic blockers may be initially prescribed with finasteride to provide more rapid relief by relaxing prostatic smooth muscles; once finasteride becomes effective, the α-adrenergic blocker can be withdrawn
   5. Drug is usually well tolerated, but 5% of men complain of sexual dysfunction

F. Dutasteride (Avodart), a Type I and II 5α-reductase inhibitor, is a newer agent
   1. Reduces prostate size and improves symptoms
   2. Prescribe 0.5 mg PO QD
   3. Before prescribing, exclude other causes of BPH symptoms such as prostate cancer
   4. Symptoms typically improve in 3 months, but allow at least 6 months of therapy to assess drug's efficacy
   5. Monitor prostate specific antigen (PSA) after 3-6 months of treatment
   6. Inform patient to avoid donating blood for at least 6 months after last dose

G. Combination therapy with an α-adrenergic blocker and finasteride is becoming accepted as a therapy for men at higher risk of progression (large prostates, >50 years old, decreased urine flow)

H. Surgery has the best chance for relief of symptoms, but also has the greatest risks, even though most men have no problems with the following surgical procedures:
   1. Transurethral resection of prostate (TURP) is still the "gold standard" for treatment
      a. Special instrument is inserted into urethra and the inside of prostate is partially resected
      b. Long-term complications include retrograde ejaculation, erectile dysfunction, incontinence, and urethral stricture of bladder neck contracture
   2. Transurethral incision of the prostate (TUIP): Instrument makes one or two small incisions into prostate to reduce pressure on the urethra
   3. Open prostatectomy involves an incision into the lower abdomen to remove part of the medial portion of the prostate; this surgery is reserved for patients with very large prostates

I. Minimally invasive therapies treat patients without general or regional anesthesia
  1. It is hypothesized that these therapies will relieve symptoms without any surgical complications and have only minimal side effects
  2. Anejaculation has been associated with these therapies
  3. The following options offer promise, but there are no long-term data on their effectiveness:
    a. Transurethral needle ablation (TUNA)
    b. Transurethral microwave therapy (TUMT)
    c. Laser therapy
    d. High-intensity focused ultrasonography (HIFU)
    e. Transurethral vaporization of the prostate (TUVP)

J. Phytotherapy, the use of plants or plant extracts such as saw palmetto berry, is available in the US, but because of insufficient empirical data, this therapy is not currently recommended

K. Follow Up
  1. Teach patient to assess for signs and symptoms of retention and obstruction
  2. Patients who opt for the "watchful waiting" strategy should be followed every 6-12 months
  3. Patients on terazosin and doxazosin should be re-evaluated in 4-6 weeks; some clinicians titrate medications every 1-2 weeks; typically, clinical response is not seen for 4-6 weeks
  4. Patients on tamsulosin should be re-evaluated at 2-4 weeks for dosage adjustment if needed
  5. Patients on finasteride should be re-evaluated around 6 months to determine drug effectiveness
  6. Follow up is at the discretion of the urologist for patients who have surgery or minimally invasive therapies

CHRONIC KIDNEY DISEASE

I. Definition:

DEFINITION OF CHRONIC KIDNEY DISEASE

Kidney damage for ≥3 months, as defined by structural or functional abnormalities of the kidney, with or without decreased GFR*, manifest *by either*:

- Pathological abnormalities; or
- Markers of kidney damage, including abnormalities in the composition of the blood or urine, or abnormalities in imaging tests

OR

GFR* <60 mL/min/1.73 m^2 ≥3 months, with or without kidney damage

*GFR: glomerular filtration rate

Adapted from National Kidney Foundation Kidney Disease Outcome Quality Initiative Advisory Board. (2002). Executive summary. Clinical practice guidelines for chronic kidney disease. *American Journal of Kidney Diseases, 39*(Suppl 1), S17-S31.

II. Pathogenesis

A. Occurs with a decrease in glomerular filtration rate (GFR) and a reduction in the clearance of certain solutes principally excreted by the kidneys
  1. Initially the functioning nephrons blunt the drop in total glomerular filtration rate
  2. Eventually glomerular hyperfiltration and hypertension lead to progressive glomerular sclerosis and overt proteinuria
  3. Clinical manifestations result from disturbances in electrolyte and fluid balance, elimination of metabolic wastes and toxins, erythropoietin production, and blood pressure control
  4. When serum creatinine rises above 2 mg/dL or creatinine clearance falls to 60 mL, progression to end-stage renal disease (ESRD) is imminent

B. Diseases of the kidney are classified according to etiology and pathology
1. Diabetic kidney disease (type 1 and type 2 diabetes)
2. Nondiabetic kidney diseases
a. Glomerular diseases (autoimmune diseases, systemic infections, drugs, neoplasia)
b. Vascular diseases (large vessel disease, hypertension, microangiopathy)
c. Tubulointerstitial diseases (urinary tract infection, stones, obstruction, drug toxicity)
d. Cystic diseases (polycystic kidney disease)
3. Diseases in the transplant
a. Chronic reject
b. Drug toxicity (cyclosporine or tacrolimus)
c. Recurrent diseases (glomerular diseases)
d. Transplant glomerulopathy

III. Clinical Presentation

A. Risk factors for development of chronic kidney disease (CKD)

RISK FACTORS FOR DEVELOPMENT OF CHRONIC KIDNEY DISEASE

- Diabetes
- Hypertension
- Autoimmune disease
- Systemic infections
- Exposure to drugs or procedures associated with acute decline in kidney function
- Recovery from acute kidney failure
- Age >60 years
- Family history of kidney disease
- Reduced kidney mass (includes kidney donors and transplant recipients)

B. Patients with declining renal function are often asymptomatic until the very late stages of the disease, because of the compensatory ability of the remaining nephrons; often patients with CKD are discovered by accident with routine medical tests

C. The following table presents the stages of CKD with corresponding clinical presentations

STAGES OF CHRONIC KIDNEY DISEASE: CLINICAL PRESENTATIONS

Stage	Description	GFR Range (mL/min/1.73 m^2)	Clinical Presentation
	At increased risk	≥90 (without markers of damage)	CKD risk factors
1	Kidney damage with normal or ↑ GFR	≥90	Markers of damage (Nephrotic syndrome, nephritic syndrome, tubular syndromes, urinary tract symptoms, asymptomatic urinalysis abnormalities, asymptomatic radiologic abnormalities, hypertension due to kidney disease)
2	Kidney damage with mild ↓ GFR	60-89	Mild complications
3	Moderate ↓ GFR	30-59	Moderate complications
4	Severe ↓ GFR	15-29	Severe complications
5	Kidney Failure	<15 (or dialysis)	Uremia, cardiovascular disease

Adapted from National Kidney Foundation Kidney Disease Outcome Quality Initiative Advisory Board. (2002). Executive summary.

D. Initially symptoms are vague and may include fatigue, anorexia, and weakness

E. As the condition worsens, many patients develop pruritus, nausea, vomiting, diarrhea, constipation, nocturia, hypertension, and mild anemia

F. Late in the course of the disease, the following clinical manifestations occur:
1. Hyperphosphatemia, hypocalcemia, hyperkalemia, metabolic acidosis, and worsening anemia
2. Symptoms include pruritus, generalized malaise, lassitude, forgetfulness, loss of libido, weight loss, changes in sleep pattern, metallic taste in mouth, brown, dry tongue, hyper-reflexia, altered behavior, and cognitive changes
3. May have fluid overload and manifestations that accompany congestive heart failure
4. Peripheral neuropathy may be present and includes the following symptoms: Restless leg syndrome, asterixis (flapping of the hands when the arms are extended and hands are in dorsiflexion), myoclonus, and loss of vibratory sense
5. Ultimately, the patient may develop the following: Pale or yellow skin, uremic frost (rare today with use of dialysis), reversible hair loss, nail changes, coma, and seizures

G. Hypertension is a common problem in the majority of patients; uncontrolled hypertension as well as ingestion of nonsteroidal anti-inflammatory agents, infections, intercurrent diseases, and dehydration may hasten the course to end stage

H. Patients with CKD are at increased risk of cardiovascular disease, including coronary heart disease, cerebrovascular disease, peripheral vascular disease, and heart failure

IV. Diagnosis/Evaluation

A. History
1. Ask about symptoms related to abnormalities of the urinary tract such as dysuria, frequency, hesitancy, nocturia, urinary incontinence, and renal colic
2. Ask about other associated symptoms such as nausea, vomiting, fatigue, itching, restless legs, decreased attentiveness, weight change, dyspnea, and leg swelling
3. Obtain a complete medication history, particularly nonsteroidal anti-inflammatory agents and nephrotoxic antibiotics (aminoglycosides)
4. Ask about recent infections (potential diagnosis of post-infectious glomerulonephritis or HIV-associated nephropathy; infections can also cause marked decline in GFR)
5. Inquire about skin rash or arthritis (potential diagnosis of autoimmune disease)
6. Obtain a thorough medical history, with particular emphasis on discovering the presence of a systemic illness that can cause renal failure such as hypertension, diabetes mellitus, collagen vascular disease, and HIV infection
   a. Ascertain that patient has not had recent radiocontrast induced x-rays
   b. Inquire about GI problems and hemorrhage, dehydration, and bleeding
7. Carefully obtain medication use including over-the-counter products
8. Review family history for Alport's syndrome, renal disease, kidney disease, diabetes mellitus, or renal failure
9. Obtain dietary history and subjective global assessment (SGA) in patients with decreased GFR
10. Assess for cardiovascular disease (CVD) risk factors as patients with CKD are at increased risk
11. Health-related quality of life should be assessed regularly; use standardized, self-administered instruments such as SF-36 (Ware & Sherbourne, 1992)

B. Physical Examination
1. Measure vital signs including orthostatic blood pressure; regular, close monitoring of blood pressure is essential in patients with CKD or at risk for CKD
2. Do a complete eye exam, including funduscopy
3. Observe skin for rashes
4. Assess neck for carotid bruits and jugular venous distention (indicates volume overload)
5. Perform a complete cardiovascular examination
6. Auscultate lungs; particularly assess for rales
7. Perform a complete abdominal examination; carefully palpate for enlarged kidneys, masses and flank tenderness; auscultate for bruits
8. Pelvic or rectal examination should be done to evaluate for causes of lower urinary tract obstruction such as prostatic or cervical carcinoma
9. Examine lower extremities for edema
10. In men, perform a rectal exam (prostate)
11. Assess for signs of central and peripheral neurologic involvement
12. Complete a mental status examination
13. Because CKD is related to systemic diseases, a complete physical examination may be needed

C. Differential Diagnosis
  1. Ascertain that the CKD is not acute or involves conditions that can be treated; acute renal failure (ARF) is associated with the following:
     a. Blood urea nitrogen (BUN) is increased out of proportion to the increase in serum creatinine clearance
     b. Patients tend to be more symptomatic than patients with CKD
     c. Patients are less likely to have severe anemia, hypocalcemia, and hyperphosphatemia than patients with CKD
     d. See table FREQUENT CAUSES OF ACUTE DECLINE IN GFR in V.C.
  2. Also refer to pathogenesis II.B. for common causes of CKD
D. Diagnostic Tests: Ordered to establish the severity and etiology of the renal failure and to determine the presence of complicating abnormalities
  1. Individuals at increased risk for CKD (see table RISK FACTORS III.A.) should be screened with the following three tests to determine if they have chronic kidney disease
     a. Serum creatinine for estimation of glomerular filtration rate (GFR)
        (1) Estimates of GFR are the best overall indices of the level of kidney function
        (2) Estimate GFR level from prediction equations that take into account the serum creatinine concentration and age, gender, race, and muscle mass; see following table for formula

+--+
| **Cockcroft-Gault Formula** |
| |
| (140 - age) X (weight in kilograms) (in women X 0.85) |
| Creatinine Clearance = ─── |
| 72 X Serum Creatinine (in mg/dL) |
+--+

        (3) Measurement of creatinine clearance using timed (24 hour) urine collections is no better than prediction equations at predicting GFR but is useful in patients who are vegetarians, malnourished, who have muscle wasting, amputation, or may need to start dialysis
        (4) Normal level in young adults is about 125 mL/min per 1.73 m^2 and declines by about 1 mL/min per 1.73 m^2 per year thereafter
     b. Proteinuria and albuminuria are early and sensitive markers in many types of CKD
        (1) Gold standard tests are quantitative assessments such as measurement of excretion of total protein or albumin in a timed urine sample or measurement of protein-to-creatinine ratio or albumin-to-creatinine ratio
        (2) Alternative tests are measurements of the ratio of protein or albumin to creatinine in an untimed "spot" urine specimen or spot urine collection by dipsticks for protein or albumin (need albumin-specific dipstick)
        (3) Positive dipstick results need confirmation of proteinuria by a quantitative measurement within 3 months
     c. Urinary sediment or urine dipstick for red blood cells and white cells
  2. Additional tests are needed for selected patients, depending on risk factors:
     a. Ultrasound imaging for patients with symptoms of urinary tract obstruction, infection, renal calculi, or who have family history of polycystic kidney disease
     b. Serum electrolytes
     c. Urinary concentration or dilution (specific gravity or osmolality)
     d. Urinary acidification (pH)
     e. Diabetic patients should be followed for microalbuminuria by radioimmunoassay
     f. In patients over age 40 with unexplained renal failure, consider ordering a urine electrophoresis to exclude the possibility of multiple myeloma
  3. For patients with CKD the following tests are needed at least annually:
     a. Ratio of protein or albumin to creatinine in spot urine samples
     b. Measurement of serum creatinine for estimation of GFR should be done at least yearly in patients with CKD and more often in patients who have the following characteristics:
        (1) GFR <60 mL/min/1.73 m^2
        (2) Fast GFR decline in past year (greater than or equal to 4 mL/min/1.73 m^2)
        (3) Risk factors for faster progression
        (4) Ongoing treatment to slow progression
        (5) Exposure to risk factors for acute GFR
     c. Urine sediment of dipstick for red blood cells and white blood cells
     d. Imaging of kidneys, usually by ultrasound
     e. Serum electrolytes

4. In patients with GFR <60 mL/min/1.73 m^2 assess or measure the following:
   a. Hemoglobin
      (1) If anemic, order RBC indices, reticulocyte count, iron studies (serum iron, total binding capacity, percent transferrin saturation, ferritin) and test for occult blood in stool
      (2) Consider ordering tests to rule-out vitamin B$_{12}$ and folate deficiencies
   b. Nutritional status
      (1) Order serum albumin and serum total cholesterol
      (2) If malnourished, order 24-hour urine collection for urea nitrogen excretion and conduct food recall/records for protein and total energy intake
   c. Bone disease
      (1) Order serum parathyroid hormone, serum calcium, serum phosphorus
      (2) If abnormal serum levels, consider Vitamin D levels, bone x-rays, and DEXA scan
   d. Neuropathy
      (1) Serum electrolytes
      (2) Consider nerve conduction velocity
5. Blood urea nitrogen (BUN) (normal range, 11-23 mg/dL) and serum creatinine (normal range, 0.6-1.2 ml/dL) provide only crude estimates of renal function
   a. BUN is dependent on renal blood flow, volume expansion, and protein intake; conditions other than CKD may elevate BUN such as dehydration and gastrointestinal bleeding
   b. Creatinine is a better indicator of CKD than BUN but is high in persons with a great deal of muscle mass and reduced when intake of red meat is low
6. Renal biopsy may be needed for a definitive diagnosis of CKD

V. Plan/Management

A. A nephrologist is usually involved in the initial plans and consulted regularly as the patient's condition changes

B. Identify patients who have life-threatening conditions and require emergent or urgent intervention
   1. Fluid overload, especially pulmonary edema
   2. Hyperkalemia
   3. Metabolic acidosis
   4. Pericarditis
   5. Encephalopathy
   6. Uremic symptoms such as vomiting or anorexia

C. Institute mechanisms to prevent and correct acute decline of GFR (see following table for causes)

FREQUENT CAUSES OF ACUTE DECLINE IN GFR
➡ Volume depletion
➡ Intravenous radiographic contrast
➡ Selected antimicrobials such as aminoglycosides and amphotericin B
➡ Nonsteroidal anti-inflammatory agents including cyclo-oxygenase type 2 inhibitors
➡ Angiotensin-converting enzyme inhibitors and angiotensin-2 receptor blockers
➡ Cyclosporine and tacrolimus
➡ Obstruction of the urinary tract

D. Initiate treatments to slow the progression of CKD (see following table)

TREATMENTS TO SLOW THE PROGRESSION OF CHRONIC KIDNEY DISEASE IN ADULTS		
	Diabetic Kidney Disease	Nondiabetic Kidney Disease
Strict glycemic control	Yes	N/A
ACE-inhibitors or angiotensin-receptor blockers	Yes	Yes (greater effect in patients with proteinuria)
Strict blood pressure control	Yes <125/75 mm Hg	Yes <130/85 mm Hg (greater effect in patients with proteinuria) <125/75 mm Hg (in patients with proteinuria)
Dietary protein restriction	Inconclusive	Inconclusive

E. Consider treating other factors that may accelerate progression of CKD; effectiveness of these interventions is inconclusive
   1. Smoking cessation
   2. Lipid-lowering drugs and diet modification in patients with dyslipidemia
   3. A low-protein diet is probably not beneficial with moderate renal impairment; for patients with severe renal impairment, a low protein diet of 0.6 g/kg/day may slow progression; adequate calorie intake (35-50 kcal/kg/day) must be maintained to avoid endogenous protein catabolism
   4. Modify the dosage of many medications

F. Carefully select medications to treat concomitant conditions that do not impair the kidney function (see table)

CONSIDERATIONS IN SELECTING MEDICATIONS TO TREAT CONCOMITANT CONDITIONS

Drug	Comments
Antihypertensives	
Diuretics	Loop diuretics preferred because of superior efficacy in low glomerular filtration rate (GFR) states. Spironolactone and other K+ sparing diuretics should be used with caution to avoid hyperkalemia
Angiotensin converting enzyme inhibitors (ACE-Is)/ angiotensin receptor blockers (ARBs)	Beneficial effects in patients with diabetic nephropathy, heart failure, and some kidney diseases. May decrease GFR in some patients with kidney insufficiency or kidney artery stenosis. Serum K+ should be monitored
Beta-blockers	Metoprolol is the preferred beta-blocker due to hepatic excretion
Calcium antagonists	Generally safe to use in patients with kidney disease
Alpha-blockers	Beneficial in patients with prostatic hypertrophy
Clonidine	Generally safe to use in patients with kidney disease
Vasodilators	Generally safe to use in patients with kidney disease, though may cause sodium retention
Antibiotics	Dosage adjustments frequently required in kidney failure. Acyclovir, other antivirals, and sulfa drugs may cause crystalluria. Acyclovir/ganciclovir dose must be decreased to avoid encephalopathy. Trimethoprim can cause hyperkalemia. Aminoglycosides are nephrotoxic and dose adjustments required based on estimated GFR
Nonsteroidal anti-inflammatory drugs	Use with caution in patients with kidney disease. Frequent cause of acute kidney failure. Cyclooxygenase-2 agents are not kidney protective. Other adverse effects include worsening of hypertension, hyperkalemia, and sodium retention.
Lipid lowering agents	Avoid fibrates. May need to lower statin doses due to increased risk of myopathy
Hypoglycemic agents	
Insulin	Half-life prolonged in patients with kidney disease and dosage of insulin must be decreased accordingly
Oral agents	Biguanides (e.g., metformin): use with caution in patients with decreased GFR. Kidney insufficiency prolongs half-life of many agents, requiring dosage adjustment to avoid hypoglycemia
Cardiac glycosides	Half-life prolonged with kidney insufficiency, and dosage must be decreased.
Gout therapy	Allopurinol dosage should be decreased in patients with kidney insufficiency. Allopurinol may cause interstitial nephritis and should be stopped if kidney function deteriorates acutely. Colchicine should be used with caution in patients with kidney disease to avoid neutropenia and adverse gastrointestinal effects
Antiepileptics	Dosage adjustments often required with decreased GFR.
Over-the-counter medications	
Antacids	Avoid magnesium- or aluminum-containing antacids. In general, calcium carbonate or acetate is safe in kidney failure
Salt substitutes	Often contain potassium and may cause hyperkalemia
Decongestants/antihistamines	May be associated with worsening hypertension and urinary retention
Herbal remedies	Effects on kidney function and other organs unknown. Ephedrine-containing products worsen hypertension, and some weight loss therapies can cause volume depletion
Vitamins	Multivitamins and folate generally are beneficial in patients with kidney disease. Vitamin A and D usage should be monitored to avoid toxicity and hypercalcemia.

Adapted from VHA/DoD (2002). The VHA-DoD clinical practice guideline: Managing chronic and pre-end-stage kidney disease, Part 1. Federal Practitioner Supplement, August 1-29.

G. Treat complications
1. Sodium imbalance and fluid overload
    a. In early stages, do not restrict intake of sodium as this could accelerate renal damage
    b. In later stages, cautious sodium restriction (2-3 g/day) and fluid restriction if hyponatremia is present are necessary; intake of fluids should equal urine output and insensible losses
    c. Loop diuretics or combination diuretic therapy may be needed to control fluid overload
2. Renal osteodystrophy and secondary hyperparathyroidism with altered calcium and hyperphosphatemia
    a. In early CKD, cautious dietary phosphate restriction is usually sufficient (restrict ingestion of dairy products and cola-colored soft drinks)
    b. Oral phosphate binders may be needed to maintain serum phosphorus concentration below 4.5-5.5 mg/dL; prescribe one of the following:
        (1) Calcium supplement such as calcium carbonate: start with 500 mg BID/TID with meals and increase dose until phosphorus level falls to <5.5 mg/dL
        (2) Sevelamer (Renagel); dosage is based on serum phosphorus levels (serum phosphorus >6-<7.5 mg/dL: 800 mg TID; 7.5-9 mg/dL: 1.2-1.6 g TID; >9 mg/dL: 1.6 g TID)
3. Metabolic acidosis is usually mild and does not need treatment in early stages
    a. When the plasma bicarbonate concentration falls below 15 mEq/L, consider alkali supplements such as sodium bicarbonate tablets 600 mg BID initially, and titrate bicarbonate to the 16-20 mEq/L range
    b. Remove any external acid loads such as aspirin, vitamin C, or excess protein intake
    c. Regularly monitor serum potassium and calcium levels as both may fall during treatment for acidosis
4. Hyperkalemia rarely occurs until the late stages of CKD
    a. Cautiously use drugs which predispose to potassium retention such as potassium-sparing diuretics, potassium supplements, ACE inhibitors, ARBs, and NSAIDs
    b. Avoid salt substitutes
    c. Monitor potassium levels regularly as elevated levels can lead to electrocardiographic changes; K >6.5 mEq/L is a medical emergency
    d. Dietary potassium restriction to <1 mEq/kg/day and use of diuretics if patient has fluid overload are usually effective (see following table for potassium content of foods)
    e. Occasionally sodium polystyrene sulfonate (Kayexalate) may be needed (consult nephrologist)

POTASSIUM CONTENT OF FOODS	
Highest content	Dried figs, molasses, seaweed
Very high content	Dried fruit (dates, prunes), nuts, avocados, bran cereals, wheat germ, lima beans
High content	Vegetables: Spinach, tomatoes, broccoli, winter squash, beets, carrots, cauliflower, potatoes Fruits: Bananas, cantaloupes, kiwi, oranges, mango Meat: Ground beef, steak, pork, veal, lamb

5. Anemia is primarily due to a relative deficiency in erythropoietin (EPO)
    a. Iron, folate, and vitamin B_{12} deficiencies should be ruled-out or treated
    b. Early in course of disease, suggest a multivitamin regimen that includes folate
    c. Patients with severe debilitating anemia or patients with coronary artery disease of congestive heart failure are best candidates for treatment
    d. Recombinant human erythropoietin (Procrit, Epogen) treatment can be started at a dose of 50-100 Units per kg (usual maximum dose is 150 U/kg) administered subcutaneously three times a week; aim for target hemoglobin of 11-12 g/dL
        (1) Monitor B/P because erythropoietin can elevate blood pressure
        (2) Monitor iron stores and administer supplemental iron as needed; in many cases, intravenous iron will be required to achieve and/or maintain adequate iron stores
6. Symptoms of itching, hiccups, and nausea
    a. Reducing protein intake may lessen symptoms
    b. Order prochlorperazine (Compazine) 5-10 mg PO QID prn for nausea
    c. Itching may be minimized with menthol or phenol lotion or capsaicin cream
7. Volume overload
    a. Weigh patient at every visit and obtain measures of lean body mass
    b. Restrict dietary sodium to 2 g/day
    c. Consult with specialist about a diuretic regimen

8.   Most patients will progress to end-stage renal disease and will require dialysis or renal transplantation; early collaboration with a nephrologist is recommended

H.   Patient education
1.   Emphasize that adherence to medications and dietary and lifestyle changes may reduce the rate of kidney disease progression
a.   Healthy lifestyles such as smoking cessation, weight control, and limiting alcohol intake are beneficial
b.   Control of blood pressure is important
c.   In diabetics, the importance of blood glucose control should be emphasized
2.   Instruct patients about the possible adverse effects of NSAIDs, which are in many over-the-counter pain preparations

I.   Follow up is dependent on severity of condition
1.   Patients in early stages of CKD should be seen every 1-4 months
2.   Order hemoglobin levels every 1-2 weeks when patient starts erythropoietin therapy or after a major change in dose

ERECTILE DYSFUNCTION

I.   Definition: Persistent inability to achieve and maintain a penile erection sufficient for satisfactory sexual intercourse; the term, erectile dysfunction (ED), has replaced impotence

II.   Pathogenesis: Normal erectile function requires coordination of psychological, vascular, neurological, hormonal, and cavernosal factors; impairment of any of these factors may result in erectile dysfunction

A.   Common organic causes; as many as 90% of patients with ED have primary organic problems
1.   Vasculogenic disorders (most common cause): Hypertension, atherosclerosis, peripheral vascular disease, diabetes mellitus
2.   Neurogenic disorders: Parkinson's disease, stroke, multiple sclerosis, spinal cord injury
3.   Endocrine disorders: Hypogonadism, thyroid diseases, hyperprolactinemia
4.   Urologic disorders: Urological malignancy
5.   Penile disorders: Priapism, Peyronie's disease
6.   Other disorders: Renal failure, hepatic failure, chronic obstructive pulmonary disease
7.   Medications: antihypertensives, antidepressants such as SSRIs, antiandrogens, NSAIDs, benzodiazepines, gemfibrozil, digoxin, metoclopramide, H_2 receptor blockers, phenothiazines, ketoconazole
8.   Alcohol, tobacco, recreational drugs
9.   Injuries such as radiation, surgery, trauma, or bicycling

B.   Psychogenic factors may result in inhibitory sympathetic nervous system activity and ED
1.   Although only 10-20% of cases are due solely to psychogenic factors, many men have a psychogenic component secondary to an organic etiology
2.   Depression is related to ED; approximately 90% of severely depressed men report complete ED

C.   ED is not an inevitable consequence of aging, but rather results from repetitive neurovascular insults that increase likelihood of injury to the vascular supply to and within the corpora cavernosa

III.   Clinical Presentation

A.   About half of all men between 40 and 70 years of age have some degree of ED, but only a small percentage of affected males of all ages seek treatment

B.   ED is associated with loss of self-esteem, poor self image, increased anxiety, issues of masculinity, and affects interactions with families and associates

IV.   Diagnosis/Evaluation: ED may be the presenting symptom of a variety of diseases; a thorough history and physical examination, and battery of diagnostic tests to detect these diseases are needed

   A.   History
      1.   Because many men will not mention ED unless directly questioned, begin history with a question such as, "Are you having any concerns or problems about sexual intercourse?"
      2.   After erectile dysfunction is identified, ask the patient what he thinks is causing the problem
      3.   Inquire about the onset, duration, and evolution of the problem; a gradual onset suggests an organic problem, whereas a sudden onset indicates a psychogenic origin unless the patient has experienced trauma or surgery
      4.   Determine if problem is intermittent or constant; intermittent problems are usually associated with psychogenic causes
      5.   Ask the patient how the disorder affects his life
      6.   Ask the patient to rate his current degree of erection on a scale of 1-10 with "10" the fullest erection he can ever recall
      7.   Determine whether the problem is failure to attain or maintain an erection; problems with initiating an erection indicate a neurologic, endocrinologic or psychogenic cause whereas problems with sustaining an erection suggest a vascular problem
      8.   Determine whether patient can achieve any degree of penetration
      9.   Inquire whether patient has nocturnal or morning erections; inability to have nocturnal/morning erections suggests an organic cause
      10.   Explore whether other sexual problems exist such as changes in libido, difficulty having orgasms, premature ejaculation, or performance anxiety
      11.   Explore possible risk factors such as changes in medical status, injuries, surgery, and frequency of bicycling
      12.   Obtain a complete past medical history and review of symptoms
      13.   Obtain a complete medication history
      14.   Question about alcohol, tobacco, and recreational drug use
      15.   Explore associated situational factors such as overwork, stressors, marital tensions
      16.   Question about previous attempts to manage the problem
      17.   If patient has a partner, ask about the quality of the relationship and the health of the partner
      18.   If possible, involve the partner in the evaluation and encourage a joint discussion of how the problem is affecting the couple's relationship
      19.   A diary of the patient's erectile activity for 3-4 weeks may be helpful
      20.   The International Index of Erectile Function is a 15-item, self-administered questionnaire which can be used to assess erectile function prior to and during treatment (see Rosen, et al., 1997 in reference list)

   B.   Physical Examination
      1.   Observe general appearance, noting signs of depression and anxiety which may reveal a psychogenic cause
      2.   Measure vital signs with particular attention to blood pressure to uncover a vascular problem
      3.   Assess the distribution of facial, axillary, and pubic hair to check for hypogonadism
      4.   Palpate neck for thyromegaly to identify a thyroid problem
      5.   Examine breasts for gynecomastia and nipple tenderness to detect an endocrine problem
      6.   Perform a complete cardiovascular examination including peripheral pulses and auscultation for abdominal and inguinal bruits to detect a vascular cause
      7.   Inspect penis to detect deformities such as micropenis or hypospadias and signs of inflammation and infection
      8.   Palpate penis to uncover Peyronie's disease which involves plaques of dense fibrous tissues surrounding corpus cavernosum of penis, leading to deformity and painful erection
      9.   Examine testes for size, position, consistency, and abnormalities to detect a testicular problem
      10.   Perform a rectal exam to check for prostate hypertrophy, prostatitis, or malignancy
      11.   Perform a complete neurologic examination, including the following:
         a.   Deep tendon reflexes and a sensory motor examination of the lower extremities
         b.   Genital and perineal sensation
         c.   Anal sphincter tone and the bulbocavernosus reflex, which is performed by asking patient to squeeze the glans penis during a rectal examination (when the reflex is present, the anal sphincter contracts)

   C.   Differential Diagnosis: Premature ejaculation, sexual desire disorders, orgasmic disorders, and sexual arousal disorders are often confused with erectile dysfunction

D.   Diagnostic Tests
1.   To identify hypogonadism, obtain a morning serum testosterone level; if the test is abnormal, order the following:
a.   Serum prolactin level
b.   Serum gonadotropins (luteinizing hormone, follicle-stimulating hormone)
2.   Tests to exclude unrecognized diseases may be helpful: Lipid profile, thyroid function tests, fasting blood sugar, urinalysis, complete blood count, and creatinine
3.   A noninvasive device such as the RigiScan Plus System is often helpful
a.   At home, patient sleeps with a portable monitor attached to the penis and device records nocturnal erectile activity
b.   At the office, the RigiScan Plus System can be used to detect patient's response to visual erotic stimulation
4.   A less sophisticated and costly test to determine presence and quality of nocturnal erections is the Snap-gauge band which is placed on base of penis at bedtime and examined in the morning for breakage of three plastic filaments
5.   To detect a vascular problem, a diagnostic test injection of prostaglandin E_1, phentolamine, and papaverine is given intracorporeally and the response of the penis is observed
6.   Duplex ultrasonography, penile angiography, penile biothesiometry, and nerve conduction may be needed; referral to a specialist is recommended for these tests

V.   Plan/Management

A.   Refer to a specialist men who have the following:
1.   Certain diseases such as multiple sclerosis and uncontrollable diabetes mellitus
2.   Suspected urologic problem such as Peyronie's disease or prostate cancer
3.   Problems that fail to improve with standard primary care therapies
4.   Severe depression with psychogenic ED

B.   Treat the underlying cause of erectile dysfunction
1.   For example, if problems are due to bicycling, suggest changing body positioning, restricting riding intensity, and reducing the duration of the ride
2.   Treat associated medical problems; for example, treatment and prevention of hypertension may reduce ED
3.   Patients with substance abuse problems (smoking, alcohol, drugs) should be enrolled in specialized program to stop their habits and referred for counseling
4.   If possible, change medications if they have adverse effects on erectile functioning; for example substitution of SSRI with bupropion or nefazodone; or substitution of β-blocker with angiotensin-converting enzyme (ACE) inhibitor, alpha blocker, or calcium channel blocker
5.   Age is positively correlated with dysfunction; advise patients that behavioral modifications such as slowing down the pace of foreplay may counteract the effects of aging

C.   Several pharmacologic and physical interventions are available
1.   Discuss the advantages and disadvantages of each option with the patient and his partner
2.   The following table outlines the treatment options

TREATMENT OPTIONS		
First Line	Second Line	Third Line
Oral erectogenic medications	Intracavernosal self-injection	Penile prosthesis
Vacuum constriction devices	Intraurethral alprostadil	Penile revascularization
Counseling & couples/sexual therapy		

D.   The contribution of psychological factors should always be considered; referral to a sex therapist and/or a psychologist/psychiatrist/counselor may be useful for both organic and psychogenic problems and is often used in conjunction with pharmacologic and physical treatments

E.   Oral erectogenic medications
1.   Sildenafil (Viagra) is a phosphodiesterase inhibitor
a.   Although this drug is expensive it has advantages: Permits discreet administration, is well-tolerated, and is not invasive
b.   Enhances normal sexual response by preventing the inactivation of the potent second messenger molecules in the smooth muscle relaxation of erectile tissue; unlike other therapies, it augments rather than bypasses the normal erection process

c. Absolutely contraindicated in patients taking medications that contain nitrates; combination with inhaled nitrates such as amyl nitrates or "poppers" can be fatal (see table RECOMMENDATIONS OF AMERICAN HEART ASSOCIATION)

d. Use cautiously in patients with cardiovascular disease, patients on multidrug antihypertensives, and other drugs such as ritonavir, cimetidine, and erythromycin; half life may be prolonged in patients with liver or renal disease

e. Advise patient to take medication 1 hour before anticipated sexual activity; however, Viagra can be taken anywhere from 4 hours to 30 minutes before intercourse

f. Best taken without food to maximize rapid absorption

g. Dosage range is 25-100 mg/day; available in 25, 50, 100 mg tabs
   (1) For patients with low risk for adverse events, the recommended starting dose is 50 mg; in patients with high risk for adverse events start at 25 mg
   (2) Re-evaluate patients early and frequently and only change doses slowly

h. No more than one dose per day is recommended; initial prescription fills should give only limited supplies

i. Adverse effects include headache, indigestion, facial flushing, cardiovascular events, and visual abnormalities such as a bluish tinge to vision

j. Consider giving first dose in office with monitoring of vital signs

---

RECOMMENDATIONS OF THE AMERICAN HEART ASSOCIATION

✓ Sildenafil is absolutely contraindicated in men taking long-acting or short-acting nitrate drugs

✓ If the man has stable coronary disease and does not need nitrates regularly, the risks of sildenafil should be carefully discussed. If the man requires nitrates because of mild-to-moderate exercise limitation due to coronary disease, sildenafil should not be given

✓ All men taking an organic nitrate (including amyl nitrate) should be informed about the nitrate-sildenafil hypotensive interaction

✓ Men must be warned of the danger of taking sildenafil 24 hours before or after taking a nitrate preparation

✓ Before sildenafil is prescribed, treadmill testing may be indicated in some men with cardiac disease to assess the risk of cardiac ischemia during sexual intercourse

✓ Initial monitoring of blood pressure after the administration of sildenafil may be indicated in men with congestive heart failure who have borderline low blood pressure and low volume status and in men being treated with complicated, multidrug antihypertensive regimens

From Cheitlin, M.D., Hunter, A.M. Jr., Brindis, R.G., et al. (1999) Use of sildenafil (Viagra) in patients with cardiovascular disease. *Circulation*, *99*, 168-177.

---

2. Yohimbine (Yocon), an alpha-2 adrenoceptor (sympathetic) antagonist, is an extract of an African herbal root
   a. Studies found that yohimbine was more effective than placebo; positive effects were most noticeable in patients with psychogenic ED
   b. Although not recommended by most authorities, for patients with non-organic ED, some experts suggest using the drug on a trial basis for 1 month
   c. Usually well tolerated, but may cause mild blood pressure elevations, palpitations, nervousness, and irritability

3. Trazodone HCl (Desyrel), a serotonin antagonist and reuptake inhibitor, has been reported to improve ED, but its beneficial effects have not been substantiated in clinical trials

4. Oral agents under review by FDA include phentolamine (Vasomax), a vasodilator, and sublingual apomorphine (Uprima), a potent emetic

F. Vacuum/constriction devices are nonpharmacologic and noninvasive methods for treating ED
   1. A plastic cylinder is applied over the penis, creating a closed chamber; the cylinder is connected by tubing to a vacuum which withdraws air from around the penis and produces penile engorgement with blood; a constrictor ring is positioned as base of penis to trap the blood
   2. Device is inexpensive, reversible, and well tolerated
   3. Effective in approximately 95% of patients
   4. Adverse effects are minimal and include edema and ecchymosis
   5. Has no drug interactions which is a major advantage because many patients with ED have associated co-morbidities and use numerous medications
   6. Keeping the constrictor ring on for more than 30 minutes may cause permanent damage to the penis and is not recommended under any circumstances
   7. Some patients dislike the mechanical nature of the devices and others are bothered by the lack of spontaneity in sexual relations
   8. Most patient dissatisfaction is due to inadequate training in the use of the device; written materials and videotapes are available; use of certified representatives is a cost-effective method of providing education to the patient and his partner

G. Intracavernosal or penile injection therapy
   1. Injection produces erections in approximately 5-20 minutes by relaxing the penile muscle tissue and allowing blood to become trapped in the penile shaft; erections last about 1 hour
   2. Approximately 90% of patients have a functional erection with penile injection therapy
   3. Local complications of all medications include hematomas and edema
   4. Inform patient of the possibility of a prolonged erection which must be treated promptly
      a. Priapism is an infrequent complication and usually occurs when patient increases dose on his own
      b. Priapism may cause irreversible cellular damage and fibrosis
      c. Priapism is usually preventable with careful dose adjustment; to prevent fibrosis, instruct men to compress the injection site for 5 minutes
      d. An erection lasting for >4 hours is a medical emergency
      e. Treatment of injection-induced priapism involves corporal aspiration of blood or intracorporeal injection of phenylephrine HCl; long-term management involves decreasing medication so that erection lasts no longer than 1 hour
   5. Alprostadil (Caverject) is the drug of choice for initial penile injection therapy
      a. Determine optimal dose in office; on first trial, patient should stay in office until complete detumescence occurs
         (1) Initial dose is 2.5 mcg for vasculogenic, psychogenic, or mixed etiology; initial dose is 1.25 mcg for neurogenic etiology
         (2) If no response to first dose occurs, may give 2nd dose after 1 hour; if partial response occurs, wait 24 hours before 2nd dose
         (3) Maintenance dose range is 5 mcg to 60 mcg with most patients having doses ranging between 10-20 mcg
      b. Inject drug into dorsolateral aspect of the proximal third of the penis; visible veins should be avoided; the side injected and the site of injection should be alternated
      c. The erection lasts about 30-60 minutes
      d. Recommended frequency is no more than 3 times weekly, with 24 hours between each dose; reduce dose if erections last longer than one hour
      e. Contraindications include myeloma, leukemia, deformity of penis or penile implant, sickle cell anemia or carrier state, and patients for whom sexual activity is inadvisable
      f. Needle for injection is very fine and causes little pain; an autoinjector is available for patients with needle phobia, poor vision, or suboptimal manual dexterity
   6. If alprostadil fails other drugs such as papaverine and phentolamine have been tried as single agents or in combination
      a. Papaverine causes less pain and is less expensive than alprostadil
         (1) Increased risks of priapism and fibrosis
         (2) Highly effective in men with psychogenic and neurogenic dysfunction; less effective in men with vasculogenic ED
      b. Phentolamine is another, less frequently used drug; adverse effects include hypotension and reflex tachycardia
   7. A three-drug mixture of papaverine, phentolamine, and alprostadil may be the most effective

H. Intraurethral treatments are effective in about 40% of patients
   1. Patient inserts an applicator into the distal urethra (about 1 inch) which allows for placement of the drug suppository, prostaglandin E_1 (alprostadil [MUSE]); insert after urination
   2. Drug is absorbed into surrounding tissue called corpus spongiosum and relaxes the smooth muscle within the penis which allows blood to enter and become trapped in the penis
   3. Erection occurs within 5-10 minutes of insertion
   4. Dosage is based on extent of patient's erectile dysfunction and his response to titration in the office; initial dose is 125 or 250 mcg; maximum dose is 1000 mcg
   5. Available in four standard dosages of 125, 250, 500, and 1,000 mcg
   6. Maximum is 2 suppositories per day
   7. Adverse effects include local discomfort, urethral bleeding, dizziness, and hypotension; priapism is an uncommon adverse effect; partners may have vaginal burning or itching
   8. Advantages are local application, minimal systemic effects, and rarity of drug interactions
   9. Disadvantages are penile pain and inconsistent efficacy

I. Surgery is recommended usually only after other treatments have failed
  1. Penile prosthesis surgery
     a. A semirigid malleable or hydraulic inflatable device is implanted into two sides of the penis, allowing erections as often as desired
     b. Inform patient of the possibility of infection, erosion, mechanical failure and the need for possible reoperation; also discuss that an implant will preclude use of other therapies in the future
     c. Not used in patients with psychogenic ED unless a psychiatrist or psychologist participates in preoperative evaluation and agrees with the need for implantation
  2. Penile vascular surgery is considered investigational; optimal candidate is a young man without vascular disease

J. Hormonal replacement therapy is considered for patients with clearly documented hypogonadism
  1. Prior to beginning therapy it is important that a PSA level and a digital rectal examination be done to evaluate for possible prostate disease; testosterone may enhance prostatic hyperplasia and stimulate the growth of occult prostate cancer
  2. Intramuscular injections or transdermal formulations of testosterone are available
     a. Intramuscular injections of 200 mg testosterone cypionate or testosterone enanthate are given every 14-21 days
     b. Testoderm: Apply 5 mg patch every 24 hours to clean, dry area of arm, back, or upper buttocks
     c. Monitor testosterone, liver function, hemoglobin, hematocrit, PSA, cholesterol, and lipids every six months
     d. During therapy measure serum testosterone levels to determine attainment of therapeutic blood levels

K. Patient Education
  1. Emphasize that there is strong relationship between ED and vasculogenic problems such as hypertension, diabetes mellitus, and peripheral vascular disease; lifestyle modifications (diet, exercise, reduction in stress and alcohol intake, and smoking cessation) are recommended
  2. With any pharmacological method, teach patients to use drugs as prescribed; to enhance performance, patients sometimes take drugs in higher doses and more frequently than advised which can lead to serious consequences
  3. With all therapies, it is important to provide an integrated educational plan which stresses the importance of the emotional and sexual relationship between the patient and his partner
  4. Caution patients with cardiovascular disease, particularly elderly patients, that there is a degree of risk with sexual intercourse like other forms of physical activity; intercourse increases heart rate and cardiac workload; patients should report any chest pain and cardiac symptoms
  5. Remind patients that therapies enhance sexual satisfaction but do not protect them against STDs, including HIV infection
  6. See following table for internet resources

INTERNET RESOURCES FOR PATIENTS	
The Canadian Erectile Difficulties Resource Center	http://www.edhelp.ca
The National Kidney & Urologic Diseases Information Clearinghouse	http://www.niddk.nih.gov/health/urolog/pubs/ impotnce/impotnce.htm
Men's Health.com Impotence Risk Quiz	http://www.menshealth.com/sex2/impotence_quiz.shtml

L. Follow Up:
  1. When starting new therapies, evaluate patient in one to two weeks to assess adverse effects of therapy and to ascertain if patient understands and is using the method correctly
  2. Re-evaluate patients approximately every 3 months or more frequently if there are problems or patient lacks confidence or has additional concerns about therapy

HEMATURIA

I.   Definition: Presence of red blood cells (RBCs) in urine

A.   More than 3 RBCs per high-power field on microscopic evaluation of the urinary sediment from two of three properly collected urinalysis specimens is the diagnostic criteria for hematuria

B.   However, in patients at risk for significant disease (see following table), 1 or 2 RBCs are suspicious and deserve further evaluation

RISK FACTORS FOR SIGNIFICANT DISEASE IN PATIENTS WITH MICROSCOPIC HEMATURIA
✓ Analgesic abuse such as acetaminophen, aspirin compounds
✓ Cigarette smoking
✓ Male gender
✓ Age >40 years
✓ Occupational exposures: Individuals working in printing, leather, rubber, and dye industries
✓ Cyclophosphamide use
✓ History of gross hematuria
✓ History of urologic disorder or disease
✓ History of irritative voiding symptoms
✓ History of urinary tract infection
✓ Pelvic irradiation
✓ Family history of urologic cancer

II. Pathogenesis: RBCs can enter the genitourinary tract at any site from the glomerulus to the urethral meatus and the causes can be categorized as prerenal, renal, postrenal, or false

A.   Prerenal
1.   Coagulopathy such as hemophilia or thrombocytopenic purpura
2.   Drugs such as warfarin sodium, heparin sodium, or aspirin
3.   Sickle cell disease or trait
4.   Collagen vascular disease such as systemic lupus erythematosus
5.   Wilm's tumor

B.   Renal
1.   Nonglomerular
a.   Pyelonephritis
b.   Polycystic kidney disease
c.   Granulomatous disease such as tuberculosis
d.   Malignant neoplasm
e.   Congenital and vascular anomalies
2.   Glomerular
a.   Glomerulonephritis
b.   Berger's disease
c.   Lupus nephritis
d.   Benign familial hematuria
e.   Vascular abnormalities such as vasculitis
f.   Alport's syndrome (familial nephritis)

C.   Postrenal
1.   Renal calculi
2.   Ureteritis
3.   Cystitis
4.   Prostatitis
5.   Benign prostatic hyperplasia

6. Epididymitis
7. Urethritis
8. Malignant neoplasm

D. False
1. Menstrual bleeding
2. Hemoglobinuria
3. Intake of certain foods such as beets, rhubarb, blackberries, fava beans
4. Intake of certain medications such as quinine sulfate, phenazopyridine, phenytoin, phenindione, phenothiazine, rifampin, sulfasalazine
5. Excretion of porphyrins

E. Miscellaneous causes
1. Strenuous exercise
2. Fever
3. Trauma
4. Viral infections
5. Schistosomiasis (travel)

F. Hematuria may be a complaint in patients with factitious hematuria such as narcotic seekers complaining of kidney stones or individuals in families with Munchausen syndrome

G. Essential hematuria occurs when no definable cause can be found

III. Clinical Presentation

A. Hematuria may be gross (visible to naked eye) or microscopic (detected on dipstick or microscopic exam)
1. Gross hematuria is commonly associated with infections and neoplasms
2. Microscopic hematuria is most commonly associated with infection and benign prostatic hypertrophy

B. Clinical manifestations are variable; painless hematuria is often associated with a malignancy

IV. Diagnosis/Evaluation

A. History
1. Question about timing and appearance of hematuria
   a. Hematuria seen at onset of urination often indicates bleeding in the urethra
   b. Terminal hematuria seen in the last few drops of urine often indicates the bladder neck or prostate as the source
   c. Hematuria seen throughout urination suggests that a lesion could be located anywhere from the upper urinary tract to the bladder
2. Ask about associated symptoms:
   a. Colicky flank pain radiating to groin suggests a kidney stone
   b. Dysuria and frequency suggest cystitis, especially in females
   c. Hesitancy and dribbling suggest benign prostatic hypertrophy
   d. Hemoptysis, hematuria, and acute renal failure in an anemic patient suggest Goodpasture's syndrome
   e. Loin-pain and hematuria in a young woman taking oral contraceptives may indicate small-vessel occlusive vascular disease
   f. In a systemic disease, fever, joint pains, and rash are typical manifestations
3. Ask patient to describe any blood clots that have occurred
   a. Large, thick clots suggest the bladder as the bleeding source
   b. Specks or thin, stringy clots suggest the upper urinary tract as the source
4. Determine whether hematuria is transient or persistent
   a. In persons <40 years, transient hematuria is common and seldom secondary to significant disease
   b. In persons >40 years, persistent and transient hematuria may be due to malignancy
5. Ask whether the patient bruises easily or has extended bleeding after a minor cut or dental work (coagulopathy or bleeding dyscrasia may be present)
6. In females, inquire about the last menstrual period
7. Obtain a complete medication history

8. Inquire about a history of pharyngitis with an impetiginous skin rash followed by hematuria, edema and hypertension (presentation of glomerulonephritis)
9. Ask about recent trauma and strenuous exercise
10. Question about risk factors for developing uroepithelial cancer (see preceding table I.B.)
11. Explore previous medical history, making certain to inquire about sickle cell disease and trait, previous urinary tract infections, metabolic and endocrine diseases, and surgeries
12. Inquire about exposure to tuberculosis
13. Explore patient's family history; kidney stone disease, Alport's syndrome, benign familial hematuria, and familial nephritis are common across generations of families

B. Physical Examination
1. Measure vital signs; elevated temperature suggests infection, neoplasm, or systemic disease; elevated blood pressure suggests glomerulonephritis or renal parenchymal disease
2. Observe skin for signs of exanthems, pallor, ecchymosis, or purpura
3. Examine for systemic infection such as tonsillar enlargement, lymphadenopathy, and exanthems
4. If Alport's syndrome is suspected, perform a hearing test, as this syndrome is associated with hearing defects
5. Auscultate heart
6. Perform complete abdominal exam, noting tenderness, organomegaly, bladder distention, masses, or bruits
7. Assess for costovertebral angle tenderness which suggests pyelonephritis or urinary tract obstruction
8. Examine extremities for edema which may be associated with glomerulonephritis
9. In adult males, perform a prostate and rectal exam; a swollen, tender prostate suggests prostatitis; prostate nodule suggests prostatic carcinoma
10. In males, examine testes, spermatic cord, and vas deferens for tenderness and masses
11. In males, examine penis for condyloma acuminatum, meatal stenosis, foreign body
12. In females, perform a pelvic examination
    a. Inspect vulva and urethral meatus, noting signs of atrophic vaginitis, urethral carbuncle, or urethral irritation
    b. Bimanual exam may uncover a uterine or ovarian mass which may secondarily involve the genitourinary tract

C. Differential Diagnosis
1. Essential hematuria is a diagnosis of exclusion
2. The majority of cases of hematuria will present with symptoms, signs, or laboratory test results that pinpoint a specific diagnosis
3. For those patients with asymptomatic, isolated hematuria for whom a cause cannot be identified always consider neoplasm (see table RISK FACTORS I.B.)

D. Diagnostic Tests
1. Always obtain a urinalysis (UA) and a subsequent culture to confirm findings on the UA (best to obtain a freshly voided, morning specimen and examine it within 30 minutes); dipstick can give false-positive results and should always be used in conjunction with a microscopic examination
    a. Alkaline pH and positive nitrite and leukocyte esterase reactions suggest urinary tract infections
    b. Hematuria with pyuria but no bacteria suggest a sexually transmitted disease (chlamydia, gonorrhea), viral infection, or, less commonly, tuberculosis
    c. Protein suggests glomerulonephritis
    d. If the dipstick test is negative for RBCs but the urine appears red, pigmenturia caused by endogenous substances that change color of urine is the likely cause
    e. Microscopic examination of urinary sediment can help determine the site of bleeding
        (1) RBC casts suggest glomerulonephritis
        (2) Crystals suggest renal calculi
    f. If exercise hematuria is suspected, patient should refrain from active participation in sports for at least 48 hours prior to urinalysis
2. If bacterial infection is detected, treat patient and repeat urinalysis in 6 weeks
3. Serum creatinine should be ordered if there is isolated microscopic hematuria in absence of bacterial infection

4. Complete evaluation for primary renal disease (see table that follows) or referral to nephrologist is needed in the following patients:
   a. Patients whose microscopic hematuria is accompanied by significant proteinuria (+1 or greater on dipstick urinalysis should prompt 24-hour collection to quantify degree of proteinuria), dysmorphic red blood cells, red cell casts, or elevated serum creatinine levels
   b. Patients who have risk factors for significant disease (see table RISK FACTORS, I.B.)

TESTS TO EVALUATE FOR PRIMARY RENAL DISEASE

I. Imaging Tests (order one of the following):

	Advantages
A. Intravenous urography	First choice; inexpensive; widely available
B. Ultrasonography	Good for detection of renal cysts
C. Computed tomography	Highest efficacy for the range of possible underlying pathologies and shortens diagnostic work-up

II. Cystoscopy to visualize bladder mucosa, urethra, and urethral orifices to exclude bladder cancer

III. Cytology to detect urothelial cancers; three first-morning voiding urine specimens should be obtained on three separate days

---

5. Order additional tests depending on clinical presentation of the patient
   a. Flat plate and upright films of abdomen to assess renal size and detect renal calculi
   b. Complete blood count to document blood loss and presence of systemic involvement
   c. 24-hour urine specimen for determination of the concentration of calcium, uric acid, and creatinine
   d. African American patients should be screened for sickle cell disease or trait
   e. Clotting studies (i.e., prothrombin time, partial thromboplastin time, platelet count, bleeding time) if a coagulopathy or a bleeding disorder is suspected
   f. Administer a purified protein derivative (PPD) and order urine culture for acid-fast bacillus when tuberculosis is a possibility
   g. In patients who have proteinuria in addition to hematuria order a 24-hour collection of creatinine and protein
   h. Order erythrocyte sedimentation rate (ESR) for patients with suspected secondary glomerular disease such as endocarditis and systemic lupus erythematosus
   i. An immunologic survey consisting of titers of IgG, IgA, IgM, and IgE are helpful if Schönlein-Henoch purpura or glomerular disease is suspected
   j. Voiding cystourethrography can reveal congenital anomalies, stone formation, or foreign bodies
   k. Angiography is not usually performed, but is the only test to detect arteriovenous malformations and may be considered in patients with gross, painless hematuria after other studies have excluded carcinoma and other renal disease
6. A renal biopsy is performed when no cause is apparent

V. Plan/Management

   A. Consider referring the following patients to a specialist:
      1. Patients with gross, painless hematuria throughout the voiding process
      2. Patients with risk factors for malignancy such as older age and smoking
      3. Patients with urologic trauma
      4. Patients with microscopic hematuria accompanied with significant proteinuria, red blood cells, red cell casts, or elevated serum creatinine levels

   B. Treat infections with appropriate antibiotics (see section on URINARY TRACT INFECTIONS)

   C. Exercise-induced hematuria and benign familial hematuria require no treatment, as they are self-limited conditions

   D. Treatment of renal calculi
      1. Once ureteral obstruction is excluded and the acute episode has passed, small stones which can be passed may be managed with hydration (maintain urine flow rate of 3-4 L/day) and analgesia; refer patients with large stones to specialist
      2. Patients can be considered for lithotripsy
      3. A low-purine diet and uricosuric agents may prevent recurrence of uric acid stones

E. Follow Up
1. Because patients who are treated for uncomplicated infections may also have underlying disorders such as a malignancies, close follow up is needed; repeat urinalysis 2-3 times in a 4-6 week period to determine that hematuria has abated
2. Patients with a negative initial workup for asymptomatic microscopic hematuria should have repeat urinalysis, voided urine cytology, and blood pressure measurements at 6, 12, 24, and 36 months
3. Additional evaluation with repeat imaging and cystoscopy is needed in patients with persistent hematuria who are at risk for underlying disease; particularly for patients with gross hematuria, abnormal urinary cytology, and irritative voiding symptoms in the absence of infection
4. Further evaluation or referral to a nephrologist is recommended if hematuria persists and hypertension, proteinuria, or evidence of glomerular bleeding develops

INTERSTITIAL CYSTITIS

I. Definition: Chronic bladder syndrome characterized by pelvic pain and irritative voiding symptoms

II. Pathogenesis: Unknown but probably related to many factors, including autoimmune, allergic, and infectious etiologies

III. Clinical presentation

A. Epidemiology
1. Most common in women; approximately 10% of diagnosed patients are men
2. Onset usually occurs between 30 and 70 years of age

B. The most common type of IC is nonulcerative; the more severe form involves ulcers in the layers of the bladder wall

C. Symptoms include frequency, urgency, nocturia, dyspareunia, and chronic pelvic pain in the absence of known infectious and/or neoplastic disease
1. The most typical symptom is pain; pain is usually relieved by voiding small amounts of urine, but quickly recurs as the bladder fills
2. An uncomfortable, constant urge to void is a common complaint
3. In women, the symptoms may worsen in the week before menstruation

D. IC is a debilitating disease that is marked by flare-ups and remissions; the chronic pain and resultant sleep deprivation can lead to stress and depression; suicidal ideation is 3-4 times more common in patients with IC than in general population

IV. Diagnosis/Evaluation

A. History
1. Ask about voiding patterns and associated symptoms such as frequency, urgency, nocturia
2. Question if patient has pain during voiding and, if so, whether pain is increased or relieved by filling and emptying bladder
3. Ask if patient has increased pain during sexual intercourse
4. Question about vaginal/urethral discharge and hematuria
5. Determine if symptoms are worse during menstruation
6. Carefully explore how condition is affecting patient's work, school, social activities, and family life; complete a health-related quality of life assessment
7. Obtain history of previous failed and successful treatments
8. Ask patient to keep log of voiding activity and patterns

B. Physical Examination
1. Perform complete abdominal examination
2. In women, perform pelvic examination to rule out vaginitis and vulvar lesions; patients with IC have tenderness at bladder base and on anterior vaginal wall
3. In men, prostate examination is needed

C. Differential Diagnosis
1. Urinary tract infections such as cystitis and prostatitis
2. Gynecological conditions such as vaginitis and endometriosis
3. Neuropathic bladder dysfunction
4. Neoplasm
5. Overactive bladder

D. Diagnostic Tests
1. Order urinalysis and urine culture to exclude infectious disease (patients with IC may have normal UA or microscopic hematuria or pyuria; culture should be negative unless patient has concomitant infection)
2. Cystoscopy and hydrodistention under anesthesia confirms the diagnosis; always order if patient has significant microscopic hematuria
3. Consider biopsies and urine cytology to rule out carcinoma of bladder
4. If tuberculosis is suspected, order urine testing for acid-fast bacillus
5. Urodynamic testing is not required for diagnosis, but may be useful in excluding detrusor instability as the cause of symptoms
6. Potassium chloride sensitivity test is available, but further research is needed before this test can be recommended

V. Plan/Management

A. Patient education
1. Discuss that IC is not a malignancy nor a risk factor for a more serious disease
2. Explain to patient that IC has an organic basis
3. Counsel patient that there is no specific cure and that disease is chronic; treatment is to relieve symptoms and to help patient gain control of his/her condition
4. Discuss possible precipitating factors such as acidic food, caffeine, alcohol, soy sauce, citrus fruits, artificial sweeteners, and chocolate that can be avoided to see if they aggravate symptoms
5. Remind that cigarette smoking can irritate bladder
6. Teach patient the importance of adequate nonirritating fluid intake
7. Bladder retraining and methods to increase bladder capacity may be helpful

B. Oral pharmacological treatments may be effective; may use drugs in combination for greater efficacy
1. First-line medication is one of the following:
    a. Tricyclic antidepressants such as amitriptyline (Elavil), doxepin (Sinequan) and imipramine (Tofranil), prescribe 25-75 mg at bedtime; start with low dose and gradually titrate upwards until relief is obtained or side effects become bothersome
    b. Antihistamines such as hydroxyzine (Atarax) 25-75 mg at bedtime
    c. Pentosan polysulfate (Elmiron) 100 mg TID; take with water 1 hour before or 2 hours after meals
    d. Aspirin or nonsteroidal anti-inflammatory drugs may relieve pain
2. Other possible medications are phenazopyridine (Pyridium), oxybutynin chloride (Ditropan), nifedipine (Procardia), or gabapentin (Neurontin)
3. Patients with severe pain require long-acting opioids

C. Intravesicular treatments provide high local concentrations in the bladder; most commonly used agent is dimethyl sulfoxide (Rimso-5)
1. Instillations of Rimso-5 are given every 1-2 weeks for total of 4-8 treatments
2. Patients can be taught how to instill agent by self-catheterization

D. Adjuvant treatments
1. Transcutaneous electrical nerve stimulation may improve symptoms
2. Physical therapy with biofeedback for pelvic floor relaxation is beneficial in some patients

E. Follow up is variable; in early course of disease, appointments should be scheduled every 1-3 months
1. Instillations of Rimso-5 are given every 1-2 weeks for total of 4-8 treatments
2. Patients can be taught how to instill agent by self-catheterization

URINARY INCONTINENCE

I. Definition: Involuntary loss of urine

II. Pathogenesis: Results from pathologic, anatomic, or physiologic factors

   A. Overactive bladder is a clinical syndrome that includes urge incontinence (the inability to delay urination with an abrupt and strong desire to void) as well as urgency, frequency, dysuria, and nocturia
       1. Due to detrusor instability, detrusor hyperactivity, or to a hypersensitive bladder which may be associated with any of the following:
           a. Lower urinary tract problems: Carcinoma, infection, atrophic vaginitis-urethritis, obstruction
           b. Central nervous system disorders: Stroke, multiple sclerosis, or Parkinson's disease
           c. Drugs: Hypnotics or narcotics
       2. Most cases result from idiopathic inability to suppress detrusor contractions

   B. Stress incontinence is leakage of urine during activities that increase abdominal pressure such as coughing, sneezing, laughing, or other physical activities
       1. In females, condition is due to hypermobility of the base of the bladder and urethra associated with poor pelvic support often due to vaginal childbirth; infrequently it is due to intrinsic urethral weakness from previous surgery or radiation
       2. In males, condition is due to an overflow from an underactive or acontractile detrusor associated with one of the following: Prostate gland problems, urethral stricture, neurological problems, or idiopathic detrusor failure

   C. Overflow incontinence occurs with overdistention of the bladder due to the following:
       1. Underactive or acontractile detrusor secondary to drugs, fecal impaction, or neurologic conditions such as diabetic neuropathy or low spinal cord injury
       2. Bladder outlet or urethral obstruction secondary to prostatic hyperplasia, prostatic carcinoma, or urethral stricture in men; cystoceles or uterine prolapse in women
       3. Detrusor external sphincter dyssynergia associated with multiple sclerosis or spinal cord injury

   D. Functional incontinence is mainly caused by factors outside the lower urinary tract such as dementia or immobility that hinder the patient from appropriate toileting

   E. Mixed incontinence occurs in women with stress incontinence and overactive bladder

   F. Lack of continuity or deformity (fistulas, ectopic ureter, and diverticulae) can also cause urinary incontinence (UI)

III. Clinical Presentation

   A. Epidemiology
       1. Approximately 15-35% of all noninstitutionalized individuals older than 60 years have UI
       2. Women have twice the prevalence of men
       3. Often goes undetected, because <50% of affected patients report episodes to clinician

   B. Social, psychological, and financial ramifications are enormous
       1. Often a major factor in the decision to place persons in nursing homes
       2. Patients have extreme embarrassment and stress due to odor and appearance
       3. UI increases the risk of falls in elderly persons

   C. Associated urinary symptoms are irritative (frequency, urgency, nocturia) or obstructive (hesitancy, weak stream, straining to void)

   D. Incontinence is associated with decubitus ulcers, urinary tract infections, sepsis, renal failure, and increased mortality

   E. Patients with overactive bladder often have a sensation of bladder fullness with little warning before passage of urine

F.   Stress incontinence is the most prevalent type of incontinence; common in women who have borne children and postmenopausal women

G.   Overflow incontinence is characterized by frequent passage of small amounts of urine

IV.   Diagnosis/Evaluation

A.   History
1.   The following single question may be helpful: "Do you consider this accidental loss of urine a problem that interferes with your day-to-day activities or bothers you in other ways?"
2.   Ask about onset and duration of incontinence
3.   Ask about dysuria, hesitancy, nocturia, frequency, hematuria, pain
4.   To determine severity, ask about the amount and frequency of urine loss and daily voids; assess the number and types of protection devices used per day
5.   To determine the type of UI, ask the following questions
   a.   Do you leak urine when you cough, laugh, sneeze, or exercise? (stress UI)
   b.   Does the urge to urinate awaken you from sleep? (overactive bladder)
   c.   Do you leak urine during sex? (overactive bladder)
   d.   Do you feel that you are unable to completely empty your bladder? (outlet obstruction, interstitial cystitis, or urinary tract infection)
6.   Obtain a complete past medical history to identify contributing factors such as diabetes, stroke, fecal impaction, cognitive impairment, depression, and neuromuscular disorders
7.   A complete obstetric and gynecologic history should include gravity, parity, types of deliveries; previous surgeries, radiotherapy treatments, trauma, and estrogen status
8.   Obtain a complete list of all medications, including nonprescription drugs
9.   Determine fluid intake such as drinking of caffeine-containing and/or other diuretic fluids
10. Explore precipitants such as cough, surgery, childbirth, menopause, trauma, new onset of illness, or new medications
11. With frail or functionally impaired persons, also ask about environmental factors such as access to toilets and social factors such as living arrangements and caregiver involvement
12. Explore types and results of previous treatments
13. Ask patient to complete a "voiding" record or diary to monitor the frequency, timing, amount of voiding, and factors associated with UI

B.   Physical Examination
1.   Perform a complete abdominal exam to detect masses, suprapubic tenderness, or fullness
2.   In men, perform genital exam to detect abnormalities of the foreskin, glans penis, and perineal skin
3.   In women, perform a pelvic exam to assess perineal skin, pelvic prolapse (cystocele, uterine prolapse), pelvic mass, perivaginal muscle tone, atrophic vaginitis, and to estimate post-voiding residual (PVR) urine by abdominal palpation and percussion and/or bimanual examination; also assess the vaginal wall and urethra
4.   Perform a rectal exam to assess for perineal sensation, resting and active sphincter tone, rectal mass, and fecal impaction; in men, also assess the consistency and contour of the prostate and check for bulbocavernosus reflex
5.   Complete a neurological exam including deep tendon reflexes, soft and sharp sensation
6.   Assess mental status
7.   Perform a musculoskeletal exam to uncover secondary causes of incontinence such as occurs with functional incontinence due to weakness and problems ambulating
8.   Measure PVR:
   a.   After patient has voided, catheterize patient (use Coudé tip catheters in men to ease insertion) or assess by pelvic ultrasound; ultrasound is best approach in men with suspected prostate obstruction
   b.   PVR <50 mL is adequate bladder emptying; PVR >200 mL is inadequate emptying; PVRs between 50-200 mL are considered equivocal, and test should be repeated
9.   Consider additional tests
   a.   Provocative stress testing can be performed
      (1)   Ask patient to relax and then cough vigorously
      (2)   Watch for urine loss from the urethra

b. Marshall test
(1) During pelvic exam, patient bears down or coughs with a full bladder
(2) If the examiner can stop the observed stress incontinence by manually elevating and supporting the anterior vaginal wall, then the test is considered positive for anatomic stress incontinence
c. Observe voiding to detect problems with hesitancy, dribbling or interrupted stream

C. Differential Diagnosis
1. Important to differentiate transient incontinence from other types of incontinence; transient incontinence usually has an acute onset with the following identifiable precipitating factors:
a. Delirium, hypoxia, urinary tract infections, atrophic urethritis or vaginitis, recent prostatectomy, glycosuria, excessive urine production such as in congestive heart failure, restricted mobility, psychological factors such as depression or stool impaction
b. Ingestion of certain medications such as sedatives, hypnotics, diuretics, anticholinergic agents, alpha-adrenergic agents, calcium channel blockers, alcohol, caffeine, or narcotics
2. Vaginal reflux is a common problem that is often misdiagnosed as UI; usually occurs in overweight individuals
a. Voided urine becomes trapped in vagina; later, as female stands and moves, the urine dribbles out of urethra
b. Treatment is patient education on ways to avoid trapped urine in vagina
(1) Spread legs wide apart when urinating
(2) Reverse sitting position on toilet to spread labia may be helpful

D. Diagnostic Tests
1. Obtain a urinalysis (UA) to detect contributing conditions such as hematuria, pyuria, bacteriuria, glycosuria, and proteinuria (dipstick is acceptable for screening, but microscopic exam is usually needed)
2. Order a urine culture if bacteria is detected from the UA
3. Simple cystometry can be performed in the office as a substitute for the expensive gold standard, cystometrography
a. Catheter is inserted into bladder
b. After bladder empties, the plunger is removed from a bayonet-tipped 50 mL syringe and tip is inserted into end of catheter
c. 50 mL of sterile water is poured into the open end of the syringe which is held 15 cm above the urethra
d. Continue instilling water in 50 mL increments until patient experiences urge to urinate
e. At this point, instill water in 25 mL increments until patient complains of severe urgency or until bladder contractions occur (contractions can be detected with rise and fall of fluid level in syringe)
f. Severe urgency or bladder contractions <300 mL of bladder volume leads to diagnosis of urge incontinence
4. In a patient suspected of having obstruction, noncompliant bladder, or urinary retention, order blood urea nitrogen (BUN) and creatinine levels
5. In patients with polyuria in absence of diuretic drugs, order fasting serum glucose levels and serum calcium levels
6. In patients with hematuria and possible malignancy or recent onset of irritative voiding, perform urine cytology
7. Consult specialist about further testing of patients who meet one of the following criteria:
a. Uncertain diagnosis and trouble developing a treatment plan based on basic diagnostic tests
b. Failure to respond to adequate therapeutic trial and thus a candidate for further treatment
c. Presence of other comorbid conditions such as severe pelvic prolapse and prostate nodule
8. Specialized tests are not routinely required to make diagnosis of UI but may be ordered and include urodynamic tests, endoscopic tests, cystoscopy, multichannel or subtracted cystometrography, urethral pressure profiles, urethral sphincter electromyography, and imaging tests of the upper and lower tract with and without voiding

V. Plan/Management

A. Refer patients with the following problems to a specialist: Previous pelvic or anti-incontinence surgery, incontinence associated with recurrent urinary tract infections, prostate nodule or prostate asymmetry, gross pelvic prolapse, neurologic abnormality, hematuria without infection, significant persistent proteinuria, failure to respond to treatment of presumptive diagnosis

B. Important to quickly identify and treat transient incontinence or reversible causes of UI such as urinary tract infection

C. Behavioral techniques are first-line options for patients with overactive bladder, stress, and mixed UI, because they reduce symptoms and have no reported side effects; behavioral techniques do not benefit patients with overflow UI

1. **Bladder training** (or bladder drills) is best for patients with overactive bladder; involves three components: Education, scheduled voiding, and positive reinforcement
   a. Patients are required to resist or inhibit the sensation of urgency, to postpone voiding, and to void according to a schedule
   b. Initially the voiding schedule is set between 2-3 hours and then progressively increased to improve bladder capacity and control
   c. Treatment may continue for several months with frequent health care contacts

2. For patients not motivated or unable to do bladder training, try habit training
   a. A scheduled toileting is planned at regular intervals
   b. Unlike bladder training, there is no systematic plan to motivate the patient to delay voiding and resist the urge to void

3. For the dependent or cognitively impaired incontinent patient, prompted voiding which teaches patients to discriminate their incontinence status and to request toileting assistance from caregivers may be beneficial
   a. Prompted voiding is often used as a supplement to habit training
   b. Steps in prompted voiding are the following:
      (1) Patient is regularly checked by caregiver and asked to verbally report if wet or dry
      (2) Patient is asked to attempt to use toilet
      (3) Patient is praised for dryness and trying to use toilet

4. **Pelvic floor muscle exercises** or Kegel exercises improve urethral resistance through active exercise of the periurethral and pelvic muscles; best approach for patients with stress or mixed UI and men who recently had transurethral prostatectomy
   a. First, teach the correct technique of contracting and differentiating the periurethral and pelvic muscles with palpation and verbal feedback to assure correct performance
   b. Teach to "draw in" muscles as if to control urination, but do not contract abdominal, buttocks or inner thigh muscles
   c. Teach how to sustain contractions for up to 10 seconds followed by an equal period of relaxation
   d. Exercises should be done about 30-80 times a day for at least 6 weeks; may need to be done indefinitely

5. Electrical stimulation alone or with pelvic floor exercises is effective
   a. A vaginal or anal probe is used to produce a contraction of the levator ani muscle
   b. Stimulation is typically performed at home once or twice daily for 1-2 hours to keep the pelvic floor muscles contracted

6. Vaginal cones may be used along with pelvic muscle training in women
   a. Patient uses cones that are of identical shape and volume but of increasing weight
   b. Woman inserts cone into vagina and rests cone on the superior surface of the perineal muscle
   c. Twice daily woman tries to retain cone by doing pelvic muscle exercise for up to 15 minutes
   d. As muscles get stronger, the weight of the cone is increased

7. Biofeedback can be used in conjunction with other behavioral therapies

D. Pharmacologic treatment should be based on type of incontinence (see following table)

PHARMACOLOGIC TREATMENT FOR INCONTINENCE			
Drug	**Dosage**	**Side Effects**	**Comments**
Drugs for Overactive Bladder			
Anticholinergic and smooth muscle relaxant			
Extended release oxybutynin (Ditropan XL)	Initially 5 mg QD, may increase weekly in 5 mg increments (swallow whole with fluids); usual dose is 5-30 mg daily	Anticholinergic effects	Both Ditropan XL and Detrol LA can be used as first-line treatment; these drugs have replaced generic oxybutynin as the first drug choice because of favorable side effect profiles
Oxybutynin (Oxytrol) Patch	Apply twice a week, rotating sites on abdomen, hip, buttocks	Causes less dry mouth but is more expensive than oral oxybutynin	
Tolterodine long acting (Detrol LA)	4 mg QD; may decrease to 2 mg QD; swallow whole	Anticholinergic effects	
Drugs for Stress Incontinence			
α-Adrenergic agonist			
Pseudoephedrine* (Sudafed 12 Hour)	120 mg in sustained release form BID	Anxiety, insomnia, headache	Use cautiously in patients with hypertension, hyperthyroidism, cardiac problems
Local estrogen therapy*			
Estrogen cream (Premarin vaginal cream) OR	Apply daily for first 3 weeks, then once or twice weekly thereafter	Continuous use may increase risk of uterine cancer in women with intact uteri	May also benefit patients with urge incontinence
Estradiol vaginal ring (Estring)	7.5 micrograms/24 hours; Insert 1 ring into vagina; replace after 90 days	Use very cautiously in women, especially those with intact uteri; risks include neoplasm and thromboembolism	
Alternative Drug for Overactive Bladder and Stress Incontinence			
Tricyclic agent			
Imipramine (Tofranil)	10-25 mg QD/BID/TID; max total daily dose: 25-100 mg	Nausea, insomnia, postural hypotension	Research is limited on this drug

*Combined α-adrenergic agonist such as pseudoephedrine and estrogen supplementation may be effective when initial single drug fails

E. Promising new therapies to treat overactive bladder
   1. Neuromodulation of the sacral nerve roots through electrodes implanted in the sacral foramina
   2. Extracorporeal magnetic innervation is a noninvasive procedure in which the patient sits in pulsating magnetic chair that stimulates the pelvic floor

F. Other techniques and devices may be beneficial, particularly for stress UI; emphasize that any device which decreases urine outflow should be used cautiously; warn patient to never delay voiding >4 hours
   1. Pessaries are soft pieces of plastic or rubber that women put into their vaginas to hold up prolapsed bladders or uteri
      a. Patients must be individually fitted
      b. Teach patient how to insert and remove pessary
      c. Reinforce that patient should remove pessary each night and should reinsert it in the morning
      d. Pessary should be washed with soap and water prior to insertion
   2. Periurethral injections
      a. Agent is injected into tissues surrounding the urethra to add bulk to tissues and to close the passage to prevent leakage
      b. Repeated injections are sometimes required
      c. Glutaraldehyde cross-linked bovine collagen (Contigen Bard Collagen Implant) and carbon-coated beads (Durasphere, Advanced Uroscience) are injectable agents
   3. Other types of occlusive devices such as urethral plugging or stenting have not been widely accepted by women and many of these devices are no longer available on the market
   4. Surgery to correct genuine stress incontinence is another option; retropubic urethropexies, and suburethral slings are often performed; a new minimally invasive suburethral sling is gaining favor

G. Consult specialist for patients with stress UI and overactive bladder who fail to respond to behavioral training and initial drug treatment

H. Treatment of overflow incontinence may require intermittent (first choice), indwelling or suprapubic catheterization; before catheterization, an exhaustive evaluation to identify the cause of retained urine and to exclude conditions that require surgical or alternative interventions is needed

I. Surgery is an option for patients with UI due to bladder neck or urethral obstruction, detrusor overactivity, intrinsic and sphincter deficiency, and urethral hypermobility in females

J. Absorbent pads and garments should be used **only** as an adjunct to other therapies during the period of evaluation and for long-term care in patients with chronic intractable UI

K. Physical and environmental devices can be installed to facilitate patient's toileting

L. Patient education
   1. Dietary modifications may be helpful and include decrease or elimination of alcohol, sweetener substitutes, caffeine, and possibly citrus juices and fruits, highly spicy foods, carbonated beverages, sugar, honey, milk, and milk products
   2. Discuss ways to eliminate constipation
   3. Teach the importance of adequate fluid intake (1500 mL of water per day)
   4. Weight reduction may decrease pressure on bladder, thereby improving UI
   5. Smoking cessation may decrease urine leakage; nicotine is irritating to the detrusor muscle
   6. Recommend double voiding to anyone with post voiding residual (PVR); urinate, wait 3 minutes, and void again (double voiding also reduces risk of urinary tract infections)
   7. Encourage patients to urinate on a regular schedule (every 2-4 hours); avoid urinating too frequently, or postponing urinating when bladder is full
   8. Provide patient resources (see following table)

RESOURCES ON URINARY INCONTINENCE	
Organization	**Website**
Access to Continence Care & Treatment	http://www.wellness.com/INCONT/acct/contents.htm
International Continence Society	http://www.icoffice.org
National Association for Continence	http://www.nafc.org
National Bladder Foundation	http://www.bladder.org

M. Follow Up: Frequent contact via the phone or with office visits is needed to provide support and positive reinforcement

CYSTITIS AND PYELONEPHRITIS

I. Definition: Bacteria in urine that have the potential to injure tissues of the urinary tract and adjacent structures. Urinary tract infections (UTIs) are often classified as upper and lower tract infections

   A. Cystitis, infection of the bladder, is an example of a common lower tract infection

   B. Pyelonephritis is the main upper tract infection and involves infection of the renal parenchyma

II. Pathogenesis of cystitis and pyelonephritis

   A. In women, the major cause is invasion of the urinary tract by bacteria that ascend the urethra from the introitus. Females have a short urethra that is in close proximity to the perirectal area making colonization possible

   B. Currently, researchers are exploring whether there is a genetic link for women who are prone to frequent UTIs; studies are underway to develop a blood test to identify high-risk females

C. In males, cystitis and pyelonephritis are uncommon
   1. In the past, these problems were considered the result of an underlying abnormality; currently it is believed that isolated cystitis in young, healthy males may be due to endogenous bacteria without an underlying abnormality or related to a subclinical case of prostatitis
   2. In older men over age 50 years, a broad range of pathogens may be involved, and these infections are often related to structural abnormalities such as benign prostatic hypertrophy

D. Pathogens in community-acquired infections: Bacteria adhere to uroepithelial cells
   1. Gram negative bacilli are most common; 75-90% of infections are due to *Escherichia coli*
      a. Other gram negative bacilli organisms include *Klebsiella pneumoniae* or *Proteus mirabilis*
      b. A wide range of gram-negative bacilli and other microorganisms may be causative agents in men; particularly in older men
   2. Gram-positive cocci account for 5-15% of infections; *Staphylococcus saprophyticus* is the second most common pathogen and often occurs in young, sexually active females
   3. In postmenopausal women *E. coli* infection is common, but other bacteria are also prevalent due to the increased pH of the vagina that occurs with estrogen deficiency
   4. Rates of ampicillin resistance among pathogens is approximately 40%, whereas rates of trimethoprim-sulfamethoxazole resistance range from 10-20%

E. In hospital settings, *E. coli* is less prevalent with Proteus, Klebsiella, Enterobacter, Pseudomonas, Staphylococci, and Enterococci species being more common

F. Risk factors in both genders
   1. Diabetes mellitus: Not necessarily an increased risk for developing infection but often there is a disorder of bladder emptying which makes UTI more difficult to eradicate
   2. Urinary instrumentation and catheterization
   3. Obstruction of normal flow of urine resulting from calculi, tumors, urethral strictures
   4. Neurogenic bladder disease from strokes, multiple sclerosis, spinal cord injuries
   5. Vesicoureteral reflux as a result of a congenital abnormality or more often from bladder overdistention from obstruction

G. Risk factors in females
   1. Increased sexual activity, diaphragm and spermicide use, and failure to void after intercourse
   2. Pregnancy
   3. History of recent urinary infection
   4. Postponing urination or incomplete voiding in women
   5. Shorter distance between urethra and anus
   6. Tampons and wiping from back to front after a bowel movement are **not** risk factors

H. Risk factors in males
   1. Homosexuality
   2. Lack of circumcision
   3. Having a sexual partner with vaginal colonization by uropathogens
   4. HIV infection with CD4+ T-lymphocyte counts of less than 200/mm^3
   5. Obstruction of normal flow resulting from prostatic hypertrophy and urethral strictures

III. Clinical Presentation

A. Epidemiology
   1. After puberty, the prevalence of UTIs increases significantly in females, but remains low in males
   2. After age 65, UTIs are more common with an equal incidence in males and females

B. In the elderly, UTIs are the most common cause of sepsis; elderly patients may present with changes in mental status, decreased appetite, somnolence, and mild fever

C. Cystitis
   1. Adults, particularly the elderly, may be asymptomatic
   2. Typical symptoms include abrupt onset of dysuria, urgency, frequency, nocturia, suprapubic heaviness or discomfort; fever is uncommon

D. Pyelonephritis
   1. Acute onset of chills, fever, flank pain, headache, malaise, costovertebral angle tenderness, and possibly hematuria
   2. Often occurs concurrently or after a lower urinary tract infection
   3. May be associated with renal calculi, ureteral obstruction, or neurogenic bladder.

IV. Diagnosis/Evaluation

A. History
   1. Determine onset and duration of urinary symptoms
   2. Ask about strength and character of urine stream when voiding, particularly in older men
   3. Determine whether dysuria occurs during urination or after urine begins to pass over inflamed labia as with herpes simplex infections
   4. Inquire about associated symptoms such as fever, chills, nausea, vomiting, diarrhea, constipation, abdominal and back pain, hematuria
   5. Ask about onset, duration, and characteristics of vaginal or urethral discharge
   6. Always query females about recent sexual activity, method of birth control, and date of last menstrual period
   7. Past medical history should include drug allergies, chronic diseases such as diabetes mellitus or multiple sclerosis, previous genitourinary problems
   8. Ask patient to count number of previous UTIs and discuss results of previous treatments

B. Physical Examination
   1. Assess vital signs, particularly noting elevated temperature and signs of orthostatic hypotension
   2. Perform a complete abdominal exam to detect tenderness, a distended bladder, or a mass
   3. Palpate back for costovertebral tenderness
   4. In females may need to inspect perineum and do complete pelvic, speculum, and rectal exams
   5. In males inspect and palpate external genitalia and scrotum; perform prostate and rectal exams
   6. Consider performing a neurologic examination to detect diseases such as multiple sclerosis

C. Differential Diagnosis
   1. Males
      a. Gonococcal and nongonococcal urethritis in males (often asymptomatic, but may have mucoid or purulent urethral discharge)
      b. Prostatitis (a tender prostate on rectal exam is usually present)
      c. Epididymitis (testicular tenderness and erythema are present)
      d. Benign prostatic hypertrophy (symptoms include changes in urinary stream and nocturia)
      e. Prostatodynia (presents with perineal or back pain accompanied by unilateral testicular pain or dysuria; urinalysis and urine culture are negative)
   2. Females
      a. Dysuria without accompanying symptoms is a poor indicator of UTI; four symptoms (dysuria, frequency, hematuria, and back pain) and one sign (costovertebral angle tenderness) increase the probability of UTI
      b. Interstitial cystitis is characterized by suprapubic pain that is relieved by bladder emptying
      c. Urethral syndrome
         (1) Patient has irritative voiding symptoms with an absence of objective findings
         (2) There is no cure; treatment is symptomatic
      d. Vulvovaginitis (external dysuria, vulvar erythema, and vulvar lesions are often present)
      e. Vaginitis
         (1) Patients deny urinary urgency and frequency
         (2) Usually there are no bacteria in the urine unless vaginal discharge contaminates urine specimen
         (3) Vaginal discharge, odor, and pruritus may be present
      f. Cervicitis (cervix will be abnormal on pelvic exam)
      g. Atrophic vaginitis in menopausal and postmenopausal women
      h. Urethral trauma due to sexual intercourse, physical activity (horseback riding, bicycling), and sensitivity to scented creams, bath products, and toilet paper
   3. Both genders
      a. Urinary calculi (usually patient has severe pain and hematuria)
      b. Bladder outlet obstruction (changes in urinary stream occur)
      c. Renal tuberculosis (hematuria is common)
      d. Tumors and carcinoma (hematuria is common)

D. Diagnostic Tests
   1. Urine collection
      a. Clean catch voided specimens are usually acceptable for adults
         (1) First morning specimen is the best voided specimen
         (2) If urine specimen is obtained later in the day, bladder should not be emptied for at least 2 hours and patients should avoid high fluid intake which would dilute sample
      b. Single in-and-out catheterization of the bladder should be done on patients who are unable to give a clean midstream urine specimen (i.e., elderly patients who are incontinent or demented)
   2. Urinalysis
      a. Dipstick urinalysis; findings of UTIs are the following:
         (1) Leukocyte esterase test is positive and denotes pyuria or WBCs in the urine; false positive esterase tests occur with kidney stones, tumors, urethritis, and poor collection techniques; false negative test may occur early in course of UTI
         (2) Nitrites are positive with gram negative infections; false negatives occur with use of diuretics early in course of UTI, and inadequate levels of dietary nitrate or presence of bacteria that do not produce nitrate reductase (*Staphylococcus saprophyticus*, *Enterococcus, Pseudomonas*)
      b. Microscopic analysis: Examine urine sediment under high power (40X) to count WBCs and perform Gram's stain to identify type of bacteria
         (1) Significant pyuria is >2-5 leukocytes per high power field or if using a counting hemocytometer, 10 or more white blood cels/mm^3 are used as the criterion
         (2) Gram's stain is done to identify whether bacteria are gram negative or positive and the shape and pattern of bacteria; it is not helpful to count bacteria on a Gram's stain
   3. Urine culture and sensitivity (urine C&S)
      a. The traditional standard for significant bacteriuria was 10^5 colony-forming units (cfu) of a uropathogen per mL of urine; today the criterion that is used is 10^2 in symptomatic females or 10^3 in symptomatic males
      b. Bacterial identification and determination of antibiotic susceptibilities or urine C&S are not necessary in most uncomplicated UTIs
      c. Bacterial identification or urine C&S is important in infections in males, females who have complicated UTIs, and females who are symptomatic but pyuria is absent
   4. With systemic symptoms order CBC with differential and in severely ill and, possibly, elderly patients order blood cultures; consider ordering erythrocyte sedimentation rate
   5. In females with symptoms associated with sexually transmitted disease (STD), perform wet mount of vaginal secretions and order *N. gonorrhoeae* (GC) cultures and chlamydia test; also gram stain cervical secretions
   6. In a male with a possible STD, gram stain urethral secretion and order GC culture and chlamydia tests
   7. Other studies are usually not needed; consider additional tests such as renal ultrasound, voiding cystourethrogram, intravenous pyelogram (IVP), renal scan, renal biopsy, or cystoscopy in patients with repeat infections, slow resolution of symptoms, and atypical features such as persistent hematuria

V. Plan/Management

A. Acute uncomplicated bacterial cystitis in women (see table ANTIBIOTICS FOR TREATING CYSTITIS)
   1. In females with uncomplicated UTIs (young, immunocompetent, nonpregnant, non-diabetic women without structural problems, previous UTIs, or history of indwelling urinary catheter or urinary tract instrumentation), urine cultures are not indicated before treatment or post-treatment
   2. Trimethoprim-sulfamethoxazole for 3 days is considered the current standard therapy; shorter courses of therapy are not recommended
   3. Trimethoprim alone is equivalent to trimethoprim-sulfamethoxazole
   4. Fluoroquinolones are more expensive, and, to postpone emergence of resistance to these drugs, they should be used as initial empirical therapy only in communities with high resistance to trimethoprim-sulfamethoxazole; some experts also recommend a fluoroquinolone as first choice when the woman has used trimethoprim-sulfamethoxazole within the past 6 months or for women who have been recently hospitalized
   5. Nitrofurantoin and fosfomycin tromethamine (Monurol) may become more useful if resistance to trimethoprim-sulfamethoxazole increases
   6. β-lactams are less effective in treatment of cystitis
   7. Phenazopyridine HCl (Pyridium) may be prescribed 100 mg TID for three days if the patient is experiencing bladder spasms; warn patient that urine will turn orange

ANTIBIOTICS FOR TREATING CYSTITIS			
Trimethoprim/sulfamethoxazole (Bactrim)	160 mg/800 mg	1 DS tab	BID
Trimethoprim (Trimpex)	100 mg	1 tab	BID
Ofloxacin (Floxin)*†	200 mg	1 tab	BID
Norfloxacin (Noroxin)*†	400 mg	1 tab	BID
Ciprofloxacin (Cipro) or Ciprofloxacin extended release (Cipro XR)	100-250 mg; 500 mg	1 tab 1 tab	BID QD
Nitrofurantoin (Macrodantin)§	100 mg	1 tab	QID
Fosfomycin tromethamine (Monurol)	3 g	1 sachet with 3-4 oz. of H_2O	Single dose

*Take on an empty stomach
†Take with full glass of water
§Take with food

B. Complicated bacterial cystitis in women
1. Treat with an oral fluoroquinolone for 14 days (see table above) or if the organism is known to be susceptible, trimethoprim-sulfamethoxazole
2. If a gram-positive bacterium is the likely pathogen, prescribe amoxicillin (Amoxil) or amoxicillin/clavulanic acid (Augmentin); for both drugs, prescribe 875 mg every 12 hours or 500 mg every 8 hours
3. Order pretreatment and post-treatment urinalyses and urine cultures and sensitivities

C. Recurrent infections in females (must repeat urine culture and sensitivity each time patient has symptoms)
1. Relapse (uncommon and caused by original infecting pathogen)
   a. Occurs within two weeks of completion of therapy
   b. Treat for 2-6 weeks longer
   c. Seek occult source of infection or urologic abnormality; consider renal function tests (BUN & creatinine), an intravenous pyelogram (IVP), and referral to a specialist
2. Reinfection (cystitis) in premenopausal females: Most recurrent UTIs are due to reinfection with a new organism rather than a relapse of the same initial infection; risk factors are history of UTI in childhood, sexual intercourse, and spermicide exposure
   a. If patient has ≤2 UTIs in one year:
      (1) Recommend patient-initiated therapy for symptomatic episodes (give patient a written prescription which she may fill when symptoms occur)
      (2) Prescribe 3-day regimen (see preceding table on ANTIBIOTICS) based on patient's past culture results and clinical success
   b. If patient has ≥3 UTIs in one year
      (1) If UTIs occur only after intercourse recommend a single-dose antibiotic after coitus such as trimethoprim/sulfamethoxazole 160 mg/800 mg (2 double strength tablets) or nitrofurantoin (Macrodantin) 200 mg
      (2) If UTIs are not related to intercourse, prophylactic antimicrobials should be used for 6 months after the infection has been eradicated
         (a) Urine cultures should be done every 1-2 months
         (b) Extend prophylactic therapy to 1-2 years if reinfection occurs at end of 6-month period.
         (c) One of the following prophylactic antimicrobials should be prescribed for 6 months (may take daily or thrice weekly): Nitrofurantoin (Furadantin) 50 mg tablet HS; trimethoprim/sulfamethoxazole (Bactrim) 40/200 mg tablets, half tablet of regular strength at HS; cephalexin (Keflex) 250 mg tablet at HS
   c. Explore whether patient is using diaphragms, spermicides, and not voiding after intercourse which may be causing reinfections
3. Reinfections in perimenopausal women may occur due to residual urine after voiding which is associated with bladder or uterine prolapse and also due to lack of estrogen which changes vaginal microflow allowing increased colonization by E. coli; risk factors for reinfection in elderly women are catheterization, incontinence, antimicrobial exposure, and impaired functional status
   a. Aforementioned antimicrobial prophylaxis may be beneficial
   b. Alternatively, prescribe topical estradiol cream (see section on ATROPHIC VAGINITIS for dosage)

  c. Oral intake of at least 300 mL/day of cranberry juice may prevent infections although recent clinical trials have not found this therapy effective

  d. Teach patient to double void (urinate completely, wait 3 minutes, and then urinate again)

 4. Vaccines to protect against recurrent *E. coli* infections are being studied

D. Pyelonephritis in females (consider consultation with a specialist)

 1. Urine cultures are always indicated to definitively identify the invading organism and its antimicrobial sensitivity before treatment

 2. Hospitalization and intravenous antibiotics are recommended for certain cases:

  a. Women with signs and symptoms suggestive of bacteremia (high fever, high WBC count), vomiting, dehydration

  b. Women who are pregnant, have a chronic disease, have abnormal urinary tracts, who have a history of nonadherence to therapies, and who fail to improve during the initial outpatient period

  c. Recommended treatment is parenteral fluoroquinolone, an aminoglycoside with or without ampicillin, or an extended-spectrum cephalosporin with or without an aminoglycoside

 3. For patients with moderate or severe infections, stabilize patient in emergency room or clinic with parenteral antibiotics (third-generation cephalosporin or fluoroquinolone); discharge to home with a prescription for an oral fluoroquinolone

 4. Milder cases can be treated on an outpatient basis but close monitoring is needed

  a. Recommended treatment is an oral fluoroquinolone for 14 days (see table ANTIBIOTICS FOR TREATING CYSTITIS, V.A.) or if the organism is known to be susceptible, trimethoprim-sulfamethoxazole

  b. If a gram-positive bacterium is the likely pathogen, prescribe amoxicillin (Amoxil) or amoxicillin/clavulanic acid (Augmentin); for both drugs, prescribe 875 mg every 12 hours or 500 mg every 8 hours or

 5. If the 2-week regimen fails, a longer course of 4-6 weeks should be considered because renal parenchymal disease is more difficult to eradicate than bladder mucosal infections

 6. Patient's symptoms should improve within 12-48 hours; if not, consider consultation with a specialist and look for deeper infections (imaging studies are often done to exclude obstruction, calculi, and formation of intrarenal abscesses)

 7. Schedule return visits or contact patient by phone in 12-24 hours

 8. Follow up cultures should be ordered at 2 weeks and 3 months post-treatment

 9. Consult specialist for patients with recurrences of pyelonephritis (recommended that these patients need further urologic investigation such as an excretory urography)

E. Treatment of uncomplicated bacterial cystitis in healthy males <50 years

 1. In the past all cases of bacterial cystitis in males were believed to be due to underlying structural problems such as prostatic hypertrophy; today, some, but not all experts, recommend that the first UTI can be treated with 7-14 day regimen of fluoroquinolone (first choice for men), trimethoprim-sulfamethoxazole, or trimethoprim (see table ANTIBIOTICS FOR TREATING CYSTITIS, V.A.) for doses

 2. Shorter treatments are not recommended

 3. Pretreatment and post-treatment urine cultures are recommended

 4. Some authorities recommend reculturing urine at 4-6 weeks as prostatitis may be a related cause

F. In males over age 50 years, a broad range of bacteria may be causing the infection

 1. Consider ordering renal function tests (blood urea nitrogen [BUN], creatinine) and consider urological consult and intravenous pyelogram (IVP)

 2. Prescribe extended 10-14 day course of one of antibiotics (see table ANTIBIOTICS FOR TREATING CYSTITIS, V.A.); a fluoroquinolone is often recommended as first-line antibiotic

 3. Always do urine culture prior to starting drug therapy and after therapy has been completed

 4. Because many men have relapse infection, a follow up visit in 4-6 weeks is recommended; consider ordering a segmented urine collection to detect bacterial prostatitis which often causes subsequent infections (see section on PROSTATITIS for procedure)

G. Persistent or recurrent bladder infections in males: Consult urologist

H.   Pyelonephritis in males (consultation with a specialist is recommended)
1.   In men, pyelonephritis usually suggests a structural problem and is an indication for hospitalization, parenteral antibiotic therapy, and an IVP
2.   Close follow up is essential
3.   Occasionally, outpatient therapy is an acceptable alternative in healthy, young men; outpatient treatment is similar to that in the adult woman

I.   Patient education may help prevent future recurrent infections
1.   Avoid a full bladder
2.   Do not postpone urinating or rush during urination
3.   Increase fluid intake at first signs of infection
4.   Void after intercourse
5.   For women, consider other types of birth control if using a diaphragm or spermicides
6.   Call clinician if symptoms are not resolved at end of therapy or if new symptoms develop

J.   Catheter-associated UTI
1.   Diagnosis can be made when the urine culture shows 100 or more cfu per ml
2.   Infections are usually polymicrobic
3.   For mild to moderate infections, treat with an oral fluoroquinolone for 10-14 days
4.   For severe infections, treat with an oral or parenteral fluoroquinolone for 14-21 days
5.   Patients with asymptomatic bacteriuria do not need treatment except for following cases: Patients who are immunosuppressed after organ transplant, patients at risk for bacterial endocarditis, and patients who are scheduled for urinary tract instrumentation

K.   Asymptomatic bacteriuria
1.   Defined as reproducible growth of at least 10^5 cfu of the same species of bacteria per milliliter of urine in a patient who has no signs or symptoms of UTI (need 2 positive urine specimens)
2.   Routine screening and treatment are not recommended; treatment is recommended for pregnant women and adults prior to invasive procedures and for renal transplant recipients
a.   Order pretreatment and 2-week post-treatment urinalyses and urine cultures and sensitivities
b.   Treat with seven-day course of antibiotics based on culture and sensitivity results; fluoroquinolones are not recommended during pregnancy; nitrofurantoin or trimethoprim-sulfamethoxazole should be used cautiously in third trimester of pregnancy
3.   If bacteriuria is found by chance, further investigation to exclude predisposing structural and functional abnormalities of the urinary tract may be beneficial

L.   Referral
1.   In women consider referral for upper tract illness, recurrent multiple infections, and infections with unusual organisms
2.   Consider referring all males with UTIs with exception of young, healthy men who do not have recurrent infections

M.   Follow up is variable depending on age, gender, and condition of patient
1.   For uncomplicated cystitis in treated females, no follow-up or urine testing is needed; for complicated cystitis in treated women, follow-up urine culture is needed
2.   For cystitis in males, follow up urine culture is needed after treatment; some recommend following these patients with repeat urine testing and a segmented urine collection to detect prostatitis in 4-6 weeks
3.   Reinfections need close follow up with urine cultures every 1-2 months
4.   Patients with pyelonephritis should be contacted within 12-24 hours after treatment is begun; then, reschedule visits 2 weeks and 3 months post-treatment for urine cultures

PROSTATITIS

I. Definition: Inflammation or infection of the prostate gland (see following table for classification)

CLASSIFICATION AND DEFINITION OF PROSTATITIS	
Classification	**Definition**
• Type I (acute bacterial prostatitis)	Acute infection of the prostate gland
• Type II (chronic bacterial prostatitis)	Chronic or recurrent infection of the prostate
• Type III (chronic nonbacterial prostatitis/chronic pelvic pain syndrome [CPPS])	Chronic genitourinary pain in absence of infection and uropathogenic bacteria localized in the prostate gland
• Type IIIA (inflammatory CPPS)	WBCs in semen, expressed prostatic secretions, or post-prostatic massage urine
• Type IIIB (noninflammatory CPPS)	No WBCs in semen, expressed prostatic secretions, or post-prostatic massage urine
• Type IV (asymptomatic inflammatory prostatitis)	No subjective symptoms; detected by prostate biopsy or by presence of WBCs in expressed prostatic secretions, or semen during evaluation for other disorders

Adapted from National Institutes of Health. (1995). National Institutes of Health summary statement. National Institutes of Health/National Institute of Diabetes and Digestive and Kidney Diseases workshop on chronic prostatitis. Executive summary. Bethesda, MD: NIH.

II. Pathogenesis

    A. Etiology
        1. Bacterial prostatitis may result from an ascending urethral infection, reflux of infected urine, extension of a rectal infection, or from hematogenous spread
        2. Chronic nonbacterial prostatitis has an unknown etiology; may be associated with an autoimmune process, an allergic reaction, neuromuscular dysfunction, psychological factors, or disorders of the bladder outlet, detrusor hyperreflexia, or pelvic floor tension myalgia
        3. Asymptomatic inflammatory prostatitis is related to other disorders

    B. Pathogens
        1. Acute and chronic bacterial prostatitis: Gram-negative bacilli (predominantly *Escherichia coli*), followed by species of *Proteus* and *Proventia,* and less commonly, *Enterobacter, Klebsiella, Pseudomonas, and Serratia*
        2. Chronic nonbacterial prostatitis: *Gardnerella vaginalis*, Chlamydia species, *Ureaplasma urealyticum*, or mycoplasma may cause this type, but most studies do not support this view

III. Clinical Presentation

    A. In all types of prostatitis except Type IV, pain is the predominant complaint, with varying degrees of voiding symptoms and sexual dysfunction

    B. In all types of chronic prostatitis, there is a significant, negative impact on quality of life similar to the impact of unstable angina, a recent myocardial infarction, and active Crohn's disease

    C. Acute bacterial prostatitis is a serious and severe illness
        1. Least common type of prostatitis
        2. Usually occurs in men aged 40-60 years
        3. Characterized by systemic illness with fever, chills, and malaise
        4. Intense symptoms with acute onset of dysuria, frequency, inhibited urinary voiding, low back pain, suprapubic discomfort, and perineal pain
        5. May have painful sexual intercourse and pain when defecating
        6. Initial, terminal, or less often, total hematuria may be present
        7. May have significant edema that results in acute urinary retention
        8. Prostatic abscess is another complication; consider this in men who do not respond to prolonged courses of antibiotics

D. Chronic bacterial prostatitis
   1. Uncommon type
   2. Occurs in men 50-80 years
   3. Systemic illness is not usually present
   4. Symptoms are slow in onset and include varying degrees of bladder outflow obstruction such as dribbling, hesitancy, loss of stream volume and force
   5. Hematuria, hematospermia, or painful ejaculations may be present
   6. Hallmark feature is recurrent urinary tract infections; patient is typically asymptomatic and urine is sterile between episodes

E. Chronic nonbacterial prostatitis/chronic pelvic pain syndrome (CPPS)
   1. Most common type of prostatitis
   2. Occurs in men 30-50 years
   3. Symptoms are indistinguishable from chronic bacterial prostatitis (type II); patients have pain with ejaculation and voiding as well as variable irritative and obstructive voiding symptoms
   4. In men with noninflammatory type (IIIB), pelvic pain is typically the predominant complaint

F. Asymptomatic inflammatory prostatitis (diagnosed incidentally during an evaluation for other disorders); limited research on the natural history and clinical presentation of this type of prostatitis

G. All types of prostatitis can have dangerous sequelae and lead to urinary retention, renal parenchymal infection, or bacteremia; chronic infection may produce prostatic stones

IV. Diagnosis/Evaluation

A. History
   1. Ask about onset and course of illness
   2. Inquire about associated symptoms such as urethral discharge, urethral meatal itching, fever, perineal pain, hematuria, hesitancy, decreased stream, painful ejaculation, incontinence, back pain, and weight loss
   3. Ask patient about the number of previous urinary tract infections and the successes and failures of previous treatments
   4. Ask if sexual partner is having symptoms such as dysuria
   5. Explore whether the patient has had new sexual partners
   6. The nine-question NIH Chronic Prostatitis Symptom Index (NIH-CPSI) addresses four important domains: pain, voiding symptoms, impact, and quality of life; it is a useful tool for initial assessment as well as an outcome measure following treatment (see Litwin, et al., 1999)

B. Physical Examination
   1. Observe general appearance for signs of systemic illness
   2. Measure vital signs
   3. Perform a complete abdominal exam; bladder distention may be present
   4. Assess external genitalia and scrotum
   5. Carefully and gently palpate prostate because vigorous massage can disseminate bacteria in the bloodstream, resulting in bacteremia
      a. Acute bacterial: Prostate is tender, warm, swollen, and boggy
      b. Chronic bacterial: Prostate is enlarged and boggy
      c. Chronic nonbacterial (inflammatory): Prostate examination is highly variable
      d. Chronic nonbacterial (noninflammatory): Prostate is usually normal
      e. Asymptomatic inflammatory prostatitis: Variable findings

C. Diagnostic Tests
   1. For patients with acute symptoms, order a urinalysis and urine culture; diagnosis of acute prostatitis is based on clinical findings and a positive urinalysis and culture; do **not** collect segmented urine culture if acute prostatitis is suspected due to danger of septicemia
   2. The Stamey-Meares four-glass localization method is the gold standard for diagnosis of chronic prostatitis, but it is infrequently used by primary care clinicians (see table INTERPRETATION OF DIAGNOSTIC TESTS)
      a. **Do not perform** if there is evidence of acute prostatitis, urethritis, urinary tract infection, if patient has been taking antibiotics within one month, if patient has ejaculated within 2 days, or if patient has a distended bladder
      b. First step: Collect 10 mL of voided urine and label VB_1 (first specimen of bladder voiding)
      c. Ask patient to void but stop in midstream and collect 50-100 mL of urine; VB_2 (classic midstream voiding)

d. Massage prostate from each lateral lobe to the midline, about 6-7 times on each side; milk urethra to produce secretion; collect secretions on a swab, slide, or in a cup and label EPS (expressed prostatic secretion)
e. Then ask patient to void another 5-10 mL of urine; label VB$_3$ (voided urine post prostatic massage)
f. Perform microscopic analysis and order cultures on all specimens

3. An alternative test to the four-glass localization test is the pre- and postmassage test (PPMT) (see table INTERPRETATION OF DIAGNOSTIC TESTS)
a. Test is simple, easy to perform, and cost-effective
b. Patient obtains midstream urine sample, then examiner massages prostrate, and a second urine sample is obtained; both specimens are sent for microscopy and culture

INTERPRETATION OF DIAGNOSTIC TESTS

Test	Test Components			
Pre- and post-massage test (PPMT)		Midstream urine specimen	Expressed prostatic massage (EPS)	
Stamey-Meares four-glass test	Premassage urine specimen (VB$_1$)	Midstream urine specimen (VB$_2$)	Expressed prostatic massage (EPS)	Postmassage urine specimen (VB$_3$)
Condition	**Test Findings***†			
Cystitis	+ bacteria + WBC	+ bacteria + WBC	- bacteria - WBC	- bacteria - WBC
Acute Bacterial (I)	+ bacteria + WBC	+ bacteria + WBC	Avoid massage	Avoid massage
Chronic bacterial prostatitis (II)	- bacteria ± WBC	- bacteria ± WBC	+ bacteria + WBC	+ bacteria + WBC
Chronic nonbacterial prostatitis/CPPS inflammatory (IIIA)	- bacteria ± WBC	-bacteria ± WBC	- bacteria + WBC	- bacteria + WBC
Chronic nonbacterial prostatitis/CPPS noninflammatory (IIIB)	- bacteria - WBC	- bacteria - WBC	- bacteria - WBC	- bacteria - WBC
Asymptomatic prostatitis (IV)	± bacteria ± WBC	± bacteria ± WBC	+ bacteria + WBC	+ bacteria + WBC

*Negative bacteria is no bacterial growth; positive bacteria is growth of a single bacterial species (>100,000 colony forming units per mL)
† Negative WBCs is <10 white blood cells per high-power field; positive WBCs is >10 to 20 white blood cells per high-power field

4. If chronic bacterial prostatitis is suspected, order blood urea nitrogen, creatinine, and consider ordering a intravenous pyelogram and a transrectal ultrasound to discover prostate calculi
a. In men over 45 years, consider ordering a serum prostate specific antigen, although it will probably be above normal in men with prostatic inflammation
b. Consider urodynamic testing for men with chronic nonbacterial prostatitis
c. If abscess is suspected, transrectal ultrasound can usually provide adequate image of the prostate
d. In older men, consider ordering urine cytologies to rule out bladder malignancy

D. Differential Diagnosis
1. Acute prostatitis is usually apparent from the characteristic presentation
2. Chronic bacterial and nonbacterial prostatitis often have a less clear presentation and may resemble other disorders such as the following:
a. Benign prostatic hyperplasia (see section on BPH)
b. Urethral stricture
c. Bladder carcinoma
d. Cystitis (see section on CYSTITIS)
e. Nongonococcal urethritis (see section on URETHRITIS)

V. Plan/Management

A. Treatment of acute bacterial prostatitis
1. Patients with severe symptoms require hospitalization and parenteral antibiotics; aggressive therapy is needed if an abscess is present
2. Initial empiric outpatient treatment is trimethoprim/sulfamethoxazole (Bactrim) 160/800 mg, one double strength tablet BID until the culture sensitivity report is available, treatment should last 4-6 weeks (some clinicians treat for 14-21 days)
3. Alternative therapy is norfloxacin (Noroxin) 400 mg tablets BID for 4-6 weeks or ciprofloxacin (Cipro) 500 by BID
4. Symptomatic treatment such as bed rest and sitz baths for 20-30 minutes BID/TID may be beneficial
5. For pain, prescribe analgesic or anti-inflammatory agent and a stool softener
6. Patients who fail to improve within 48 hours of antibiotic treatment, who are >50 years, or who have recurrent infections, need referral to a urologist because of the likelihood of associated benign prostatic hypertrophy

B. Chronic bacterial prostatitis is often difficult to cure
1. Prescribe 3-4 month course of double-strength trimethoprim-sulfamethoxazole (Bactrim) BID or norfloxacin (Noroxin) 400 mg tab BID or ciprofloxacin (Cipro) 500 mg tablets BID (duration of treatment is controversial, some clinicians treat for only 6 weeks)
2. Consider prophylactic drugs if infection persists: 1 regular tablet (80 mg trimethoprim/400 mg sulfamethoxazole [Bactrim]) HS for an indefinite period or nitrofurantoin (Macrodantin) 100 mg HS, indefinitely
3. Patients with refractory prostatitis should be evaluated for prostatic stones with an x-ray of kidneys, ureters, and bladder
4. Segmented cultures should be obtained 4-6 weeks after therapy is initiated
5. Prostatic massage once or twice a week for 4 weeks may be helpful

C. Chronic nonbacterial prostatitis; no universally effective treatments are available
1. Although not supported by existing evidence, many experts recommend a trial of antibiotics such as doxycycline (Vibramycin) 100 mg BID, erythromycin (E-mycin) 500 mg QID, or trimethoprim-sulfamethoxazole (Bactrim) 1 DS tablet BID for 6 weeks (some clinicians treat for 14-21 days)
2. In small studies, thermal therapy was shown to be beneficial
3. Reassurance that the condition is noninfectious, not contagious, and not related to cancer may relieve anxiety
4. Counseling and approaches used for patients who have chronic pain syndromes may help
5. Other therapies have been suggested, but are not evidence-based
   a. Nonsteroidal anti-inflammatory drugs
   b. Antispasmodic agent, oxybutynin (Ditropan)
   c. Alpha-adrenergic blocking drugs such as prazosin or tamsulosin
   d. Finasteride
   e. Diazepam alone or in combination with prazosin
   f. Anticholinergic agents to reduce irritative urinary symptoms
   g. Nutritional supplements (saw palmetto or zinc sulfate)
   h. Allopurinol
   i. Pentosan polysulfate, an anti-inflammatory glycosaminoglycan
   j. Prostate massage, particularly after sexual activity
   k. Frequent ejaculations

D. Asymptomatic inflammatory prostatitis
1. Limited research is available to guide treatment choices
2. If patient has chronic asymptomatic prostatitis that is known to elevate the prostate specific antigen (PSA) levels, some experts recommend 14-day course of antibiotics; it may be wise to treat before drawing subsequent PSA levels

E. The following patient education is not evidence-based, but may be helpful
1. Teach patients to avoid alcohol, coffee, or tea
2. Instruct patient to discontinue all over-the-counter drugs with anticholinergic properties such as antihistamine/decongestants

F. Follow Up
    1. For acute and chronic bacterial prostatitis return in 4-6 weeks for urinalysis and culture of urine and expressed prostate secretions; consider further diagnostic tests to exclude a structural cause for the infection
    2. For chronic nonbacterial prostatitis, follow up will depend on patient's symptoms and response to therapy

EPIDIDYMITIS

I. Definition: Inflammation of the epididymis

II. Pathogenesis:

    A. Pathogens apparently reach the epididymis through the lumen of the vas deferens from infected urine, the posterior urethra, or seminal vesicles
        1. In postpubertal boys and males under 35 years, infection is often sexually transmitted
        2. Most often caused by *Chlamydia trachomatis* or *Neisseria gonorrhoeae*
        3. *Escherichia coli* may be a pathogen in men who are the insertive partner during anal intercourse

    B. Epididymitis may be nonsexually transmitted
        1. Typically due to coliform bacteria that usually cause urinary tract infections
        2. Usually associated with urinary tract infections in men >35 years with urinary tract instrumentation, surgery, or anatomical abnormalities

    C. Uncommon causes are due to trauma, tuberculosis epididymitis, systemic fungal infections; antiarrhythmic drug, amiodarone, may cause infection confined to the head of the epididymitis

III. Clinical Presentation

    A. Most common cause of acute scrotal pain in postpubertal males
        1. Usually patients have a history of sexual activity
        2. Sexually transmitted epididymitis usually is associated with urethritis

    B. Commonly, there is a gradual onset of unilateral testicular pain and tenderness, dysuria, and urethral discharge

    C. Fever occurs in approximately 50% of patients; nausea and vomiting are unusual

    D. Scrotum is tender on palpation and usually accompanied with a hydrocele and palpable swelling of the epididymis

    E. Uncommon complications include testicular necrosis, testicular atrophy, and infertility

IV. Diagnosis/Evaluation

    A. History
        1. Determine onset, duration, and course of symptoms
        2. Ask about scrotal pain, dysuria, urinary frequency and urgency, and color, amount, and consistency of urethral discharge
        3. Inquire about possible associated symptoms such as fever, nausea, and vomiting
        4. Explore sexual history and condom use; ask about new sexual partners and if sexual partners have complained of dysuria or urinary frequency
        5. Question about previous urinary tract infections and treatments
        6. Inquire about previous genitourinary surgery, urinary tract instrumentation, and anatomic abnormalities
        7. Inquire about recent trauma to testes

B.   Physical Examination
1.   Inspect scrotum, noting edema and erythema which are typical
2.   Palpate scrotum
a.   In epididymitis, testes are tender but the position, size, and consistency of testes is entirely normal
b.   Palpable swelling of epididymis is usually present
3.   Passive elevation of testis may relieve pain in epididymitis (Prehn's sign)
4.   Perform rectal exam (this exam may elicit prostatic tenderness and result in expression of urethral discharge)

C.   Differential Diagnosis
1.   Must differentiate testicular torsion, which is an emergent condition, from epididymitis (see following table)

DIFFERENTIATION OF EPIDIDYMITIS AND TESTICULAR TORSION		
	Epididymitis	**Testicular Torsion**
History		
Onset of pain	Gradual	Acute
Nausea and vomiting	Rare	50%
Voiding symptoms	50%	No
Urethral discharge	50%	No
Physical Examination		
Epididymal swelling only	Early	10%
Scrotal edema	Most	Most
Scrotal erythema	Most	Most
Fever	50%	Rare

2.   Orchitis (patient usually has recently had parotitis or mumps)
3.   Testicular tumor (usually presents with painless swelling)
4.   Trauma (usually elicited on history)
5.   Skin pathology such as insect bites or folliculitis

D.   Diagnostic Tests
1.   Emergency testing for testicular torsion may be necessary when the onset of pain is sudden and severe or if there is uncertainty about the diagnosis; consult a specialist and consider ordering one of the following: Doppler ultrasound, scrotal ultrasound (operator-dependent), or radionuclide scrotal imaging (not operator-dependent)
2.   Obtain urinalysis (in about 20-95% of epididymitis cases there is pyuria compared to 0-30% in cases with testicular torsion)
3.   Collect urine culture and sensitivity and gram-stained smear of uncentrifuged urine for gram-negative bacteria
4.   In men who may have a sexually transmitted disease obtain the following:
a.   Gram-stained smear of urethral exudate or intraurethral swab specimen to detect urethritis (≥5 polymorphonuclear leukocytes per oil immersion field) and for presumptive diagnosis of gonococcal infection
b.   Culture of urethral exudate or intraurethral swab specimen or nucleic acid amplification test (either by first-void urine or intraurethral swab) for *N. gonorrhoeae* and *C. trachomatis*
c.   Collect first-void urine and examine for leukocytes if the urethral Gram stain is negative; culture and Gram-stained smear of uncentrifuged mid-stream urine specimen should be collected
d.   Syphilis serology and HIV counseling and testing
5.   In older men, a culture of expressed prostatic secretions should be obtained and a search should be made for an obstruction at the bladder outlet with tests such as an intravenous pyelography

V. Plan/Management

    A.   Most patients can be treated on outpatient basis; consider hospitalization for men with severe pain suggesting other diseases (i.e., torsion, abscess), or when men are febrile or noncompliant

    B.   For active heterosexual men <35 years of age, most likely cause is a sexually transmitted disease
        1.   For epididymitis most likely due to gonococcal or chlamydial infection, treat empirically before culture results are available with the following: doxycycline (Vibramycin) 100 mg PO BID for 10 days <u>and</u> ceftriaxone (Rocephin) 250 mg IM in a single dose
        2.   For epididymitis most likely caused by enteric organisms or in patients allergic to tetracyclines and/or cephalosporins, treat empirically with ofloxacin (Floxin) 300 mg PO BID for 10 days or levofloxacin (Levaquin) 500 mg QD for 10 days
        3.   Treat sexual partners if their contact with the index patient was within 60 days preceding onset of symptoms in the patient
        4.   Instruct patients to avoid sexual intercourse until they and their sex partners are cured or until treatment is completed and patients and partners are asymptomatic

    C.   For men >35 years, for men allergic to cephalosporins and/or tetracyclines, and for cases most likely caused by enteric organisms, prescribe one of the following:
        1.   Ofloxacin (Floxin) 300 mg BID for 10 days
        2.   Levofloxacin (Levaquin) 500 mg BID for 10 days

    D.   Symptomatic treatment of bed rest, scrotal support, scrotal elevation, sitz baths, pain medication, and ice packs may be beneficial

    E.   Follow Up
        1.   For patients whose symptoms fail to improve within 3 days, re-evaluate both the diagnosis and treatment
            a.   Swelling and tenderness that persist after antimicrobial therapy require comprehensive evaluation
            b.   Differential diagnosis includes tumor, abscess, infarction, testicular cancer, and tuberculosis or fungal epididymitis
        2.   For men <35 years, no follow up or test of cure is needed if symptoms resolve
        3.   In older men, repeat urine cultures are needed after completion of the therapy and further diagnostic tests can also be scheduled at this time

TESTICULAR TORSION

I.   Definition: Twisting of spermatic cord which results in compromised testicular blood flow

II.   Pathogenesis

    A.   Occurs when the free-floating testis rotates on the spermatic cord and occludes its blood supply

    B.   May occur spontaneously (may occur in sleep) or after activity or trauma

III.   Clinical Presentation

    A.   Commonly occurs between 6-12 years, but a significant number of patients are over the age of 21 years

    B.   If not surgically treated, there will be ischemic injury and necrosis of the testis
        1.   Many patients have an anatomic defect known as "bell-clapper" deformity
        2.   Typical history is sudden onset of testicular pain which radiates to groin; but in some cases there is minimal swelling and little or no pain
        3.   May also have lower abdominal pain which leads to erroneous diagnosis of appendicitis or gastroenteritis

4. Nausea and vomiting occur in about half of the patients; usually there is no fever, urethral discharge, or dysuria
5. Degree of injury is determined by the severity of the arterial compression and the interval between the onset and surgical intervention (for severe torsion, must intervene within 4-8 hours to salvage the testis)

IV. Diagnosis/Evaluation

A. History: Testicular torsion is a urological emergency so rapidly gather a focused history
1. Ask about onset and circumstances surrounding onset
2. Ask about accompanying symptoms such as nausea, vomiting, fever, dysuria, urethral discharge
3. Determine any occurrence of trauma or unusual physical activity
4. To rule out epididymitis, question about recent change in sexual partners and symptoms of dysuria and urethral discharge

B. Physical Examination: Perform a rapid but systematic exam
1. Observe general appearance (patients with testicular torsion are in acute distress, have pain on ambulation, and prefer to lie quietly on the examination table)
2. Inspect scrotal skin (often skin is erythematous, taut, and without normal rugae with torsion)
3. Palpate testes (testis may be located high in the scrotum as a result of shortening of the cord by twisting)
4. Palpate the epididymis which normally is located on the posterolateral surface of the testis and is smooth, discrete, and nontender (with testicular torsion the epididymis will not be in this typical position as a result of cord twisting and will be extremely tender)
5. Palpate vas deferens from the testicle to the inguinal ring (normally vas deferens is smooth, discrete and nontender)
6. Try to elicit the cremasteric reflex; positive reflex is testicular retraction when the upper, medial thigh is stroked (usually absent in torsion, but present in epididymitis)
7. Perform a complete abdominal exam

C. Differential Diagnosis
1. Epididymitis is the most difficult condition to differentiate (see table in section on EPIDIDYMITIS, differentiating epididymitis from torsion)
2. Torsion of the testicular appendage
a. Pain is usually less severe than with torsion of the entire testis; pain and swelling develop gradually
b. "Blue dot" sign at superior aspect of testis is diagnostic of this problem
c. Management is bedrest and scrotal elevation
d. With appropriate management, symptoms resolve within a week
3. Orchitis
4. Incarcerated inguinal hernia
5. Vasculitis
6. Tumor
7. Trauma
8. Henoch-Schönlein purpura is a systemic vasculitic syndrome characterized by nonthrombocytopenic purpura, arthralgia, renal disease, gastrointestinal pain, and bleeding
9. Idiopathic scrotal edema

D. Diagnostic Tests: When clinical presentation is typical, surgical exploration is usually carried out without further testing. When torsion is unlikely, but confirmation of clinical diagnosis is sought, consider ordering the following:
1. Doppler ultrasound (absent testicular artery pulsations with torsion); the development of color Doppler imaging with pulsed Doppler has improved accuracy of this test
2. Nuclear testicular scanning allows evaluation of blood flow to the scrotal contents (decreased perfusion with torsion)
3. Scrotal ultrasonography can be ordered; does not distinguish torsion from epididymitis but is helpful in evaluating scrotal masses and trauma
4. Urinalysis (will be normal in 90% of patients with testicular torsion, but will often be abnormal in epididymitis)

V.   Plan/Management:

A.   Immediate consultation and surgical intervention; this is a urological emergency; salvage of endocrine function requires detorsion within 4-8 hours

B.   Manual detorsion may be successful when performed by an experienced clinician, but surgical exploration is still needed to confirm complete detorsion

C.   Follow Up: Surgeon should arrange follow up to determine response to operation

VARICOCELE

I.   Definition: Dilated plexus of scrotal veins situated above the testis in the scrotum

II.   Pathogenesis: Due to valvular incompetence of the spermatic vein

A.   Varicoceles on left side in adolescents are usually of unknown etiology; new left-sided and right-sided varicoceles in older men may be renal tumors

B.   Varicoceles on the right side may represent acute venous obstruction from a tumor or intra-abdominal pathology

III.   Clinical Presentation

A.   Usually found in older adolescents but can occur at any age (onset in prepubertal males and in adult males is often associated with pathology)

B.   Approximately 15% of all adult males have a varicocele

C.   Varicoceles occur almost exclusively on the left side; a unilateral right varicocele is rare; bilateral varicoceles are more common than previously thought

D.   Testis resembles a bag of worms with a bluish discoloration that is visible through the scrotum (see Figure 13.1)

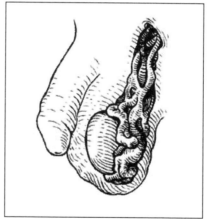

Figure 13.1. Varicocele

E.   Varicocele is most prominent when the patient is standing; tends to collapse when the patient is sitting or supine

F.   Patient is usually asymptomatic and testis is nontender, but may have mild pain or a feeling of heaviness in the scrotum

G.   Varicoceles are associated with a time-dependent decline in testicular function; decreased sperm counts, infertility, and testicular atrophy are associated in about 65%-75% of patients with varicoceles

IV.   Diagnosis/Evaluation

A.   History
1.   Ask when patient first noticed varicocele
2.   Determine the rate the scrotum is enlarging
3.   Ask if the varicocele collapses upon sitting or standing
4.   Inquire about testicular pain or discomfort
5.   Question about problems with infertility

B.   Physical Examination
1.   If varicocele is not visible, ask patient to stand and perform a Valsalva maneuver
2.   Palpate testes, epididymis, and vas deferens first in standing then supine positions
3.   Perform a rectal examination to assess prostate size since the prostate may shrink with testosterone deficiency that may occur with varicoceles

C.   Differential Diagnosis
1.   Hydrocele
2.   Spermatocele
3.   Testicular tumor
4.   Epididymal cyst

D.   Diagnostic Tests
1.   For right-sided varicoceles, suddenly appearing left-sided varicoceles, new onset varicoceles in adults, consult specialist about ordering the following:
a.   Venography is the gold standard for diagnosing varicoceles in adults; also used to detect venous obstruction or renal carcinoma associated with varicoceles
b.   Doppler ultrasound, thermography, and scrotal scintigraphy are nonspecific for diagnosing varicoceles, but may be beneficial in some cases
2.   Consider ordering a minimum of two semen analyses
a.   Infertile young men with varicoceles and abnormal semen analyses should be offered the option of varicocele repair
b.   Young men with normal semen analyses should be followed with semen analyses every one to two years
3.   Consult specialist about other tests for assessing reproductive function in adults such as testis biopsy and fine needle aspiration with flow cytometry

V.   Plan/Management

A.   Refer the following patients to a surgeon:
1.   All patients with right-sided varicoceles
2.   All adult males with new onset of varicoceles
3.   The following adolescent males:
a.   When varicocele is voluminous, rapidly increasing in size, or does not disappear in sitting and supine positions
b.   When pain is present
c.   When there is evidence of testicular atrophy, defined as two standard deviations in testicular size when compared with normal testicular growth curves
d.   When there is greater than a 2 mL difference in testicular volume as noted on serial ultrasonography examination

B.   If surgery is not recommended, explain that patient needs to monitor the growth and symptoms related to the varicocele

C.   Follow Up: If surgery is not performed, explain to patient the need to return to clinic if he experiences increasing discomfort or if scrotum changes in size and shape

REFERENCES

Akduman, B., & Crawford, E.D. (2001). Terazosin, doxazosin, and prazosin: Current clinical experience. *Urology, 58*(Suppl. 6A), 49-54.

American Association of Clinical Endocrinologists. (1998). AACE clinical practice guidelines for the evaluation and treatment of male sexual dysfunction. *Endocrine Practice, 4,* 219-235.

American Urological Association. (1999). Prostate specific antigen (PSA): Best practice policy. *Oncology, 14,* 267-286.

American Urological Association. (2001). Evaluation of asymptomatic microscopic hematuria in adults: The American Urological Association best practice policy. Parts I and II. *Urology, 57,* 599-610.

Anderson, J.E. (1997). Hematuria. In L. Dornbrand, A.J. Hoole, & R.H. Fletcher (Eds.). *Manual of clinical problems in adult ambulatory care* (3rd ed.). Philadelphia: Lippincott-Raven.

Andriole, V.T. (2002). Asymptomatic bacteruria in patients with diabetes – enemy or innocent visitor. *New England Journal of Medicine, 347,* 1617-1618

Appell, R.A. (2002). Urinary incontinence. In R.E. Rakel & E.T. Bope (Eds.). *2002 Conn's current therapy.* Philadelphia: Saunders.

Bent, S., Nallamothu, B.K., Simel, D.L., Fihn, S.D., & Saint, S. (2002). Does this woman have an acute uncomplicated urinary tract infection? *JAMA, 287,* 2701-2710.

Berns, J.S. (2002). Chronic renal failure. In R.E. Rakel & E.T. Bope (Eds.). *2002 Conn's current therapy.* Philadelphia: Saunders.

Blute, M.L., & Larson, T. (2001). Minimally invasive therapies for benign prostatic hyperplasia. *Urology, 58*(Suppl. 61), 33-41.

Bremnor, J.D., & Sadovsky, R. (2002). Evaluation of dysuria in adults. *American Family Physician, 65,* 1589-1596.

Cheitlin, M.D., Hutter, A.M. Jr., Brindis, R.G., Ganz, P., Kaul, S., Russell, R.O. Jr., et al. (1999) Use of sildenafil (Viagra) in patients with cardiovascular disease. *Circulation, 99,* 168-177.

Collins, M.M., MacDonald, R., & Wilt, T.J. (2000). Diagnosis and treatment of chronic abacterial prostatitis: A systematic review. *Annals of Internal Medicine, 133,* 367-381.

Collins, M.M., MacDonald, R., & Wilt, T.J. (2002). Interventions for chronic abacterial prostatitis (Cochrane Review). In *The Cochrane Library, Issue 2.* Oxford: Update Software Ltd.

Collins, M.M., MacDonald, R., & Wilt, T.J. (2002). Allopurinol for chronic prostatitis (Cochrane Review). In *The Cochrane Library, Issue 2.* Oxford: Update Software Ltd.

Culligan, P.J., & Heit, J. (2000). Urinary incontinence in women: Evaluation and management. *American Family Physician, 62,* 2433-2444, 2447, 2452.

Department of Veteran Affairs. (1999). *The primary care management of erectile dysfunction.* Washington DC: Department of Veterans Affairs.

Fang, L.S-T. (2000). Evaluation of the patient with hematuria. In A.H. Goroll, & A.G. Mulley, Jr. (Eds.). *Primary care medicine: Office evaluation and management of the adult patient* (4th ed.). Philadelphia: Lippincott.

Fang, L.S-T. (2000). Management of patient with chronic renal failure. In A.H. Goroll, & A.G. Mulley, Jr. (Eds.). *Primary care medicine: Office evaluation and management of the adult patient* (4th ed.). Philadelphia: Lippincott.

Fromer, D.L., & Kaplan, S.A. (2002). Benign prostatic hyperplasia. In R.E. Rakel & E.T. Bope (Eds.). *2002 Conn's current therapy.* Philadelphia: Saunders.

Goodson, J.D. (2000). Approach to incontinence and other forms of lower urinary tract dysfunction. In A.H. Goroll, & A.G. Mulley, Jr. (Eds.). *Primary care medicine: Office evaluation and management of the adult patient* (4th ed.). Philadelphia: Lippincott.

Gupta, K., Hooton, T.M., & Stamm, W.E. (2001). Increasing antimicrobial resistance and the management of uncomplicated community-acquired urinary tract infections. *Annals of Internal Medicine, 135,* 41-50.

Hanno, P.M., & Sant, G.R. (2001). Clinical highlights of the National Institute of Diabetes and Digestive and Kidney Diseases/Interstitial Cystitis Association scientific conference on interstitial cystitis. *Urology, 57*(Suppl 6AO), 2-6.

Hebel, S.K. (Ed.). (1996). *Drug facts and comparisons.* St. Louis: Facts and Comparisons, Inc.

Hoffman, R.M., MacDonald, R., Slaton, J.W., & Wilt, T.J. (2003). Laser prostatectomy versus transurethral resection for treating benign prostatic obstruction: A systematic review. *Journal of Urology, 169,* 210-215.

Jepson, R.G., Mihaljevic, L., & Craig, J. (2002). Cranberries for preventing urinary tract infection (Cochrane Review). *The Cochrane Library, Issue 2.*

Jones, S.R. (2002). Bacterial infections of the urinary tract in men. In R.E. Rakel & E.T. Bope (Eds.). *2002 Conn's current therapy*. Philadelphia: Saunders.

Junnila, J., & Lassen, P. (1998). Testicular masses. *American Family Physician, 57,* 685-692.

Kaplan, S.A. (2001). 5α-reductase inhibitors: What role should they play? *Urology, 58*(Suppl 6A), 65-70.

Krieger, J.N. (2002). Urinary tract infections: What's new? *Journal of Urology, 168,* 2351-2358.

Levine, L.A. (2002). Erectile dysfunction. In R.E. Rakel & E.T. Bope (Eds.), *2002 Conn's current therapy.* Philadelphia: Saunders.

Levy, A.S. (2002). Nondiabetic kidney disease. *New England Journal of Medicine, 347,* 1505-1511.

Litwin, M.S., McNaughton-Collins, M., Fowler, F.J. Jr., Nickel, J.C., Calhoun, E.A., Pontari, M.A., et al. (1999). The National Institutes of Health chronic prostatitis symptom index: Development and validation of a new outcome measure. Chronic Prostatitis Collaborative Research Network. *Journal of Urology, 162,* 369-375.

Lipsky, B.A. (1999). Prostatitis and urinary tract infection in men: What's new; what's true? *American Journal of Medicine, 106,* 327-334.

Lowe, F.C., & Ku, J.C. (2001). Phytotherapy in management of benign prostatic hyperplasia. *Urology, 58* (Suppl. 6A), 71-77.

Lue, T.F. (2000). Erectile dysfunction. *New England Journal of Medicine, 342,* 1802-1813.

Metts, J.F. (2001). Interstitial cystitis: Urgency and frequency syndrome. *American Family Physician, 64,* 1199-1206, 1212-1214.

Miller, T.A. (2000). Diagnostic evaluation of erectile dysfunction. *American Family Physician, 61,* 95-104, 109-110.

Medical Society for the Study of Venereal Diseases (1999). National guidelines for the management of prostatitis. *Sexually Transmitted Infections, 75*(Suppl. 1), S46-S50.

National Kidney Foundation Kidney Disease Outcome Quality Initiative Advisory Board. (2002). Clinical practice guidelines for chronic kidney disease. Executive summaries of 2000 updates, anemia, chronic kidney disease. *American Journal of Kidney Diseases, 39*(Suppl 1), S17-S31.

Nickel, J.C. (1999). Research guidelines for chronic prostatitis: Consensus report from the First National Institutes of Health International Prostatitis Collaborative Network. *Urology, 54,* 229-233.

Nickel, J.C. (2002). Prostatitis. In R.E. Rakel & E.T. Bope (Eds.), *2002 Conn's current therapy.* Philadelphia: Saunders.

National Institutes of Health. (1995). National Institutes of Health summary statement. National Institutes of Health/National Institute of Diabetes and Digestive and Kidney Diseases workshop on chronic prostatitis. Executive summary. Bethesda, MD: NIH.

Nickel, J.C., Nyberg, L.M., & Hennenfent, M. for the International Prostatitis Collaborative Network. (1999). Research guidelines for chronic prostatitis: Consensus report from the First National Institutes of Health International Prostatitis Collaborative Network. *Urology, 54,* 229-233.

Obrador, G.T., & Pereira, B.J.G. (2002). Systemic complications of chronic kidney disease: Pinpointing clinical manifestations and best management. *Postgraduate Medicine, 111,* 115-122.

O'Leary, M.P. (2001). Tamsulosin: Current clinical experience. *Urology, 58*(Suppl. 6A), 42-48.

Orenstein, R., & Wong, E.S. (1999). Urinary tract infections in adults. *American Family Physician, 59,* 1225-1234.

Rahman, J., & Smith, M.C. (1998). Chronic renal insufficiency: A diagnostic and therapeutic approach. *Archives of Internal Medicine, 158,* 1743-1751.

Remuzzi, G., Ruggenenti, P., & Perico, N. (2002). Chronic renal diseases: Renoprotective benefits of renin-angiotensin system inhibition. *Annals of Internal Medicine, 136,* 604-615.

Roehrborn, C.G. (2002). Alfuzosin: Overview of pharmacokinetics, safety, and efficacy of a clinically uroselective α-blocker. *Urology, 58* (Suppl. 6A), 55-64.

Roehrborn, C.G. (2002). Are all α-blockers created equal? An update. *Urology, 59*(Suppl. 2A), 3-6.

Roehrborn, C.G., Bartsch, G., Kirby, R., Andriole, G., Boyle, P., de la Rosette, J., et al. (2001). Guidelines for the diagnosis and treatment of benign prostatic hyperplasia: A comparative international review. *Urology, 58,* 642-650.

Rosen, R.C., Riley, A., Wagner, G., Osterloh, I.H., Kirkpatrick, J., & Mishra, A. (1997). The International Index of Erectile Function (IIEF): A multidimensional scale for assessment of erectile dysfunction. *Urology, 49,* 822-830.

Sant, G.R., & Hanno, P.M. (2001). Interstitial cystitis: Current issues and controversies in diagnosis. *Urology, 57*(Suppl 6A), 82-88.

Schnelle, J.F., & Smith, R.L. (2001). Quality indicators for the management of urinary incontinence in vulnerable community-dwelling elders. *Annals of Internal Medicine, 135,* 752-758.

Scientific Committee of the First International Consultation on Incontinence. (2000). Assessment and treatment of urinary incontinence. *Lancet, 355,* 2153-2158.

Stevermer, J.J., & Easley, S.K. (2000). Treatment of prostatitis. *American Family Physician, 61,* 3015-3022, 3025-3026.

US Preventive Services Task Force (2002). Screening for prostate cancer: Recommendations and rationale. *Annals of Internal Medicine, 137,* 915-916.

Van Haarst, E.P., van Andel, G., Heldeweg, E.A., Schlatmann, T.J.M., & van der Horst, H.J.R. (2001). Evaluation of the diagnostic workup in young women referred for recurrent lower urinary tract infections. *Urology, 57,* 1068-1072.

VHA/DoD. (2002). The VHA/DoD clinical practice guideline: Managing chronic and pre-end-stage kidney disease, Part I. *Federal Practitioner Supplement, August,* 1-29.

Ware, J.E., & Sherbourne, C.D. (1992). The MOS 36-item short-form health survey (SF-36): A conceptual framework and item selection. *Medical Care, 30,* 473-483.

Warren, J.W., Abrutyn, E., Hebel, J.R., Johnson, J.R., Schaeffer, A.J., & Stamm, W.E. (1999). Guidelines for antimicrobial treatment of uncomplicated acute bacterial cystitis and acute pyelonephritis in women. *Clinical Infectious Diseases, 29,* 745-758.

Workowski, K.A., & Levine, W.C. (2002). Sexually transmitted diseases treatment guidelines — 2002. *MMWR,* 51(RR06), 1-80.

Gynecology

MARY VIRGINIA GRAHAM & SYLVIA WORDEN

ABNORMAL PAPANICOLAOU (PAP) SMEAR

I.   Definition: Cervical cytological abnormalities interpreted and reported by cytologists using the 2001 Bethesda System

II.   Pathogenesis

    A.   Evidence linking human papillomavirus (HPV) with cervical cancer and its precursors is very strong
        1.   Oncogenic strains include HPV types 16, 18, 31, 33, 35, 39, 45, 51, 52, 56, and 58; types 16 and 18 are present in more than 80% of cervical cancers
        2.   Incidence of infection with HPV is directly related to sexual activity; the greater the number of partners, the greater the risk of HPV infection
        3.   Infection with an oncogenic strain does not mean that a woman will inevitably develop intraepithelial lesions

    B.   Other cofactors that have a role in development of cervical neoplasia include smoking, sexual behavior (early onset and multiple partners), and immunological status of the woman

III. Clinical Presentation

    A.   Approximately 13,000 women in the US develop cervical cancer each year, and about 4,500 women die of the disease

    B.   Most women who develop cervical cancer have never had a Pap smear or have not had one in the past 5 years

    C.   Of the more than 50 million women who undergo Pap testing in the US each year, approximately 3.5 million (7%) are diagnosed with a cytological abnormality requiring additional follow-up or evaluation

IV.   Diagnosis/Evaluation/Plan/Management

    A.   Cervical cytology is primarily a screening test that in some instances may serve as a medical consultation by providing an interpretation that contributes to a diagnosis

    B.   The 2001 Bethesda System for reporting the results of cervical cytology is in the table below

BETHESDA SYSTEM 2001

SPECIMEN TYPE: *Indicate conventional smear (Pap smear) versus liquid-based versus other*

SPECIMEN ADEQUACY
- Satisfactory for evaluation (*describe presence or absence of endocervical/transformation zone component*)
- Unsatisfactory for evaluation *(specify reason)*
  - ❖ Specimen rejected/not processed *(specify reason)*
  - ❖ Specimen processed and examined, but unsatisfactory for evaluation of epithelial abnormality because of *(specify reason)*

GENERAL CATEGORIZATION *(optional)*
- Negative for Intraepithelial Lesion or Malignancy
- Epithelial Cell Abnormality: See Interpretation/Result (*specify 'squamous' or 'glandular' as appropriate*)
- Other: See Interpretation/Result (*e.g., endometrial cells in a woman ≥40 years of age*)

AUTOMATED REVIEW
- *If case examined by automated device, specify device and result*

ANCILLARY TESTING
- *Provide a brief description of the test methods and report the result so that it is easily understood by the clinician*

INTERPRETATION/RESULT
- **_NEGATIVE FOR INTRAEPITHELIAL LESION OR MALIGNANCY_** (*when there is no cellular evidence of neoplasia, state this in the General Categorization above and/or in the Interpretation/Result section of the report, whether or not there are organisms or other non-neoplastic findings*)
  - ❖ ORGANISMS:
    - ➢ *Trichomonas vaginalis*
    - ➢ Fungal organisms morphologically consistent with *Candida* spp
    - ➢ Shift in flora suggestive of bacterial vaginosis
    - ➢ Bacteria morphologically consistent with *Actinomyces* spp
    - ➢ Cellular changes consistent with Herpes simplex virus
  - ❖ OTHER NON-NEOPLASTIC FINDINGS *(Optional to report; list not inclusive):*
    - ➢ Reactive cellular changes associated with
      - inflammation (includes typical repair)
      - radiation
      - intrauterine contraceptive device (IUD)
    - ➢ Glandular cells status post hysterectomy
    - ➢ Atrophy
- **_OTHER_**
  - ❖ Endometrial cells (*in a woman ≥40 years of age*) (*Specify if 'negative for squamous intraepithelial lesion'*)
- **_EPITHELIAL CELL ABNORMALITIES_**
  - ❖ SQUAMOUS CELL
    - ➢ Atypical squamous cells
      - of undetermined significance (ASC-US)
      - cannot exclude HSIL (ASC-H)
    - ➢ Low grade squamous intraepithelial lesion (LSIL) encompassing: HPV/mild dysplasia/CIN 1
    - ➢ High grade squamous intraepithelial lesion (HSIL) encompassing: moderate and severe dysplasia, CIS/CIN 2 and CIN 3
    - ➢ Squamous cell carcinoma
  - ❖ GLANDULAR CELL
    - ➢ Atypical
      - endocervical cells (NOS *or specify in comments*)
      - endometrial cells (NOS *or specify in comments*)
      - glandular cells (NOS *or specify in comments*)
    - ➢ Atypical
      - endocervical cells, favor neoplastic
      - glandular cells, favor neoplastic
    - ➢ Endocervical adenocarcinoma *in situ*
    - ➢ Adenocarcinoma
      - endocervical
      - endometrial
      - extrauterine
      - not otherwise specified (NOS)
- **_OTHER MALIGNANT NEOPLASMS_:** *(specify)*

EDUCATIONAL NOTES AND SUGGESTIONS *(optional)*
  Suggestions should be concise and consistent with clinical follow-up guidelines published by professional organizations (references to relevant publications may be included)

C. Components of the 2001 Bethesda System are further described in the following tables to assist in clinical decision-making

D. An explanation of **Specimen Type/Specimen Adequacy** is contained in box below

> **Specimen Type:** In this first section of the report, the type specimen that was submitted is identified—conventional smear (Pap smear) versus liquid-based versus other
>
> **Specimen Adequacy:** In the second section of the report, specimen adequacy is addressed; considered by many to be the single most important quality assurance component of the report, there are **two** mutually exclusive categories that are possible (**one** will be checked)
> - First category is *Satisfactory for evaluation*
>   - A notation is made regarding the presence or absence of an endocervical/transformation zone component for specimens with adequate squamous cellularity
>   - Further comments on quality indicators may be added to the *Satisfaction for evaluation* designation such as when the specimen is "partially obscured" (50-75% of epithelial cells cannot be visualized)
> - Second category is *Unsatisfactory for evaluation* (reason is specified; there are **two** possibilities)
>   - Specimen rejected/not processed (reason will be specified, and includes such things as an unlabelled specimen; specimens in this category will not have been evaluated microscopically)
>   - Specimen processed and examined, but unsatisfactory for evaluation of epithelial abnormality because of (reason will be specified here, and includes such things as ">75% of epithelial cells obscured")

E.   A description of **General Categorization** is contained in the box below

> **General Categorization:** The third section of the report is an **optional** component of the Bethesda System and its aim is to allow clinicians/office staff to triage reports easily
>
> Three mutually exclusive categories in this section
> - *Negative for Intraepithelial Lesion or Malignancy*
>   - Specimens for which no epithelial abnormality is identified are reported here
> - *Epithelial Cell Abnormality*
>   - Abnormality was detected and clinician is directed to "See Interpretation/Result"
> - *Other*
>   - This category is for cases in which there are no morphological abnormalities in the cells per se, but the findings may indicate some increased risk (e.g., benign-appearing "endometrial cells in a woman ≥40 years of age")
>
> Note that because the categories are mutually exclusive, selection of the general category is based on the **most** clinically significant result when several findings are present

F.   The Automated Review/Ancillary Testing components are summarized in the box below

> **Automated Review:** The fourth section of the report. For slides scanned by automated computer systems, the instrumentation used and review results are included in the cytology report
>
> **Ancillary Testing:** If ancillary molecular test was performed, the type of assay as well as the results are reported here in the fifth section of the report

G.   **Interpretation/Result:** In this category, the sixth section of the report, there are three possibilities (1) *Negative for Intraepithelial Lesion or Malignancy*; (2) *Other*, and; (3) *Epithelial Cell Abnormalities* (**Note:** In the 2001 Bethesda System the term "diagnosis" has been replaced by "interpretation" or "result" to convey that cervical cytology provides an interpretation of findings that must be interpreted within the context of clinical findings)

H.   **Interpretation/Result:** *Negative for Intraepithelial Lesion or Malignancy* is the first reporting category and is described in the box below

> **Negative for Intraepithelial Lesion or Malignancy**
>
> In this first category, specimens for which no epithelial abnormality is identified are reported here
>
> In addition, if certain non-neoplastic conditions are present, a notation is made regarding the presence of such conditions here. Non-neoplastic conditions that are identified are under two headings: (1) Organisms, and (2) Other non-neoplastic findings (optional to report)
>
> Organisms that are listed here include the following:
>> Trichomonas vaginalis
>> Fungal organisms morphologically consistent with *Candida* spp
>> Shift in flora suggestive of bacterial vaginosis
>> Bacteria morphologically consistent with *Actinomyces* spp
>> Cellular changes consistent with Herpes simplex virus
>
> Other non-neoplastic findings (optional to report; list not inclusive)
>> Reactive cellular changes associated with
>>> Inflammation (includes typical repair)
>>> Radiation
>>> Intrauterine contraceptive device (IUD)
>> Glandular cells status post-hysterectomy
>> Atrophy
>
> **Note:** Findings of non-neoplastic condition causing reactive changes does not alter the status of a specimen that has been reported as *Negative for Intraepithelial Lesion or Malignancy*

I. **Interpretation/Result:** *Other* is the second reporting category and is described in the box below

> **Other**
>
> In this second category, endometrial cells are noted if the woman is ≥40 years of age, regardless of the date of the LMP, because menstrual/menopausal status, exogenous hormone therapy, and other clinical risk factors are often unknown
>
> Identification of endometrial cells if not associated with menses or after menopause may indicate risk for an endometrial abnormality, although most often this is a benign finding
>
> **Note:** Cervical cytology, primarily a screening test for squamous epithelial lesions and squamous cancer, is unreliable for detection of endometrial lesions and should not be used to evaluate suspected endometrial abnormalities

J. **Interpretation/Result:** *Epithelial Cell Abnormalities* is the third reporting category and is described in the box below

> **Epithelial Cell Abnormalities**
>
> Epithelial cell abnormalities are of two types: Squamous Cell and Glandular Cell
>
> - **Squamous Cell**
>   - ❖ Atypical squamous cells (ASC) are subdivided into two categories: atypical squamous cells of undetermined significance (ASC-US) and atypical squamous cells, cannot exclude high-grade squamous intraepithelial lesion (ASC-H)
>   - ❖ Squamous intraepithelial lesions (SIL) are defined by a two-tiered system using the terms low-grade squamous intraepithelial lesion (LSIL), and high-grade intraepithelial lesion (HSIL) to refer to cervical cancer precursors. Further, a two-tiered terminology for the histopathological classification of cervical intraepithelial neoplasia (CIN) has also been adopted with CIN 1 referring to low-grade precursors and CIN 2,3 denoting high-grade precursors. Current emphasis in the US has shifted to detection and treatment of histologically confirmed high-grade disease; thus it is logical for the ASC category qualifiers to emphasize the importance of detecting high-grade SIL (HSIL)
>   - ➢ Dichotomous division of SIL is based on evidence that LSIL is generally a transient infection with HPV while HSIL is more often associated with viral persistence and higher risk for progression
>   - ➢ Detection of HSIL has emerged as the central purpose of screening
> - **Glandular Cell**
>   - ❖ The classification of glandular abnormalities has been substantially revised in the 2001 Bethesda System. Glandular cell abnormalities are classified into three categories: (1) *Atypical glandular cells, either endocervical, endometrial, or "glandular cells" not otherwise specified [AGC NOS]*; (2) *Atypical glandular cells, either endocervical cells or "glandular cells" favor neoplasia [AGC "favor neoplasia"]*; and (3) *endocervical adenocarcinoma in situ (AIS)*
>   - ❖ In a majority of cases, morphological features permit differentiation between atypical endometrial and endocervical cells. The finding of atypical glandular cells (AGC) is important clinically because the percentage of cases associated with underlying high-grade disease is higher than for ASC-US

K. Recommended management of women with squamous cell and glandular cell abnormalities are contained in the tables below

---

RECOMMENDED MANAGEMENT OF WOMEN WITH ATYPICAL SQUAMOUS CELLS OF UNDETERMINED SIGNIFICANCE (ASC-US)

There are three acceptable approaches to management of women with ASC-US: (1) A program of repeat cervical cytological testing; (2) Colposcopy; or (3) DNA testing for high-risk types of HPV. **(Note:** HPV-DNA testing is the preferred approach when liquid-based cytology is used at the initial screening visit; called "reflex testing," HPV DNA testing of the original sample is initiated only if the cytology test yields an interpretation of ASC-US)

- When a program of repeat cervical cytological testing is used to manage women with ASC-US
  - ❖ Patients should have repeat testing (using either conventional or liquid-based cytology) at 4- to 6-month intervals until 2 consecutive "negative for intraepithelial lesion or malignancy " results are obtained; at that point, patient can return to routine screening program
  - ❖ Women diagnosed with ASC-US or greater cytological abnormality on the repeat tests should be referred for colposcopy
- When immediate colposcopy is used to manage women with ASC-US
  - ❖ Women who are found not to have cervical intraepithelial neoplasia (CIN) should be followed up with repeat cytological testing at 12 months
  - ❖ Women who are found to have biopsy confirmed CIN should be referred without delay for treated by a specialist
- When DNA testing for high-risk types of HPV using a sensitive molecular test is used to manage women with ASC-US
  - ❖ Women who test positive for high-risk HPV DNA should be referred for colposcopic evaluation
  - ❖ Women who test negative for high-risk HPV DNA can be followed up with repeat cytological testing at 12 months

---

RECOMMENDED MANAGEMENT OF WOMEN WITH ASC-US IN SPECIAL CIRCUMSTANCES— POSTMENOPAUSAL, IMMUNOSUPPRESSED, PREGNANT

- Postmenopausal women
  - ➢ Provide a course of intravaginal estrogen (if evidence of genital atrophy and no contraindications to estrogen use)
  - ➢ Repeat cervical cytology test approximately one week after completing regimen; if the first repeat test is "negative for intraepithelial lesion or malignancy" a second repeat test should be done in 4 to 6 months; if this second repeat test is also "negative," patient can return to routine screening
  - ➢ If either repeat test is reported as ASC-US or greater, the patient should be referred for colposcopy
- Immunosuppressed women
  - ➢ Refer for colposcopy
- Pregnant women
  - ➢ Manage in the same manner as nonpregnant women

RECOMMENDED MANAGEMENT OF WOMEN WITH ATYPICAL SQUAMOUS CELLS, CANNOT EXCLUDE HIGH-GRADE SQUAMOUS INTRAEPITHELIAL LESION (ASC-H)

All women with ASC-H obtained using either conventional or liquid-based cervical cytology must be referred for colposcopic evaluation

---

RECOMMENDED MANAGEMENT OF WOMEN WITH LOW-GRADE SQUAMOUS INTRAEPITHELIAL LESION (LSIL)

Women with LSIL should be referred for colposcopy; subsequent management options depend on whether a lesion is identified, whether the colposcopic exam is satisfactory, and whether the patient is pregnant

Rationale: Whereas the majority of women with LSIL have either no cervical lesion or CIN 1 (which regress in most cases without treatment or are completely excised with biopsy); management of these women with repeat cytological studies is problematic for the following reasons

- ➢ Rates of loss to follow-up for repeat testing are usually very high
- ➢ There is a 53% to 76% likelihood of abnormal follow-up cytology results requiring eventual colposcopy
- ➢ There is a small risk of delaying identification of invasive cancers

RECOMMENDED MANAGEMENT OF WOMEN WITH LISL IN SPECIAL CIRCUMSTANCES— POSTMENOPAUSAL, ADOLESCENT, PREGNANT

- Postmenopausal women
  - ➤ Follow-up without an initial colposcopy is an acceptable option when one of the two protocols below are used
    - ❖ May follow-up with repeat cytological testing at 6 and 12 months with a threshold of ASC-US or greater for referral for colposcopy (see MANAGEMENT OF WOMEN WITH ASC-US IN SPECIAL CIRCUMSTANCES— POSTMENOPAUSAL, IMMUNOSUPPRESSED, PREGNANT above)
    - ❖ A second option is to follow up with HPV DNA testing at 12 months with referral for colposcopy if testing is positive for high-risk HPV DNA
- Adolescents
  - ➤ Follow-up without initial colposcopy is an acceptable option; if this option is chosen, select one of the following approaches:
    - ❖ Repeat cytological testing at 6 and 12 months with a threshold of ASC for referral for colposcopy, OR
    - ❖ Follow up with HPV DNA testing at 12 months with referral for colposcopy if testing is positive for high-risk HPV DNA
- Pregnant women
  - ➤ See MANAGEMENT OF WOMEN WITH HISL IN SPECIAL CIRCUMSTANCES section below

RECOMMENDED MANAGEMENT OF WOMEN WITH HSIL

Colposcopy with endocervical assessment is the recommended management of women with HSIL; subsequent management options depend upon whether a lesion is identified, whether the colposcopic examination is satisfactory, whether the patient is pregnant, and whether immediate excision is appropriate

Rationale: A cytological diagnosis of HISL is **not common**; women with a cytological diagnosis of HSIL have about a 70-75% chance of having biopsy confirmed cervical intraepithelial neoplasia (CIN) 2 or 3 and a 2% chance of having invasive cervical cancer

RECOMMENDED MANAGEMENT OF WOMEN WITH HISL IN SPECIAL CIRCUMSTANCES— PREGNANT, YOUNG WOMEN OF REPRODUCTIVE AGE

- Pregnant women
  - ➤ Refer for colposcopic evaluation by clinicians who are experienced in the evaluation of colposcopic changes characteristic of pregnancy
- Young women of reproductive age
  - ➤ Refer for colposcopic evaluation and biopsy of lesions suspicious for high-grade disease or cancer; when biopsy-confirmed CIN 2, 3 is not identified in a young woman with cytology-confirmed HSIL, observation with colposcopy and cytology at 4- to 6-month intervals for 1 year is acceptable, provided colposcopic findings are satisfactory, endocervical sampling is negative, and the patient accepts the risk of occult disease

RECOMMENDED MANAGEMENT OF WOMEN WITH ATYPICAL GLANDULAR CELLS (AGC) OR ADENOCARCINOMA IN SITU (AIS)

- ➤ Women with all subcategories of AGC should be referred for colposcopy with endocervical sampling, with the exception of women with atypical endometrial cells, who should initially be evaluated with endometrial sampling; endometrial sampling should be performed in conjunction with colposcopy in women >35 years with AGC and in younger women with AGC who have unexplained vaginal bleeding
- ➤ Women with a cytological test result of AIS should also be referred for colposcopy with endocervical sampling
- ➤ Management of women with initial AGC or AIS using a program of repeat cervical cytological testing is **unacceptable**

L. **Educational Notes and Suggestions:** This is the final section of the 2001 Bethesda System and is optional. In this section, written comments regarding the validity and significance of a cytology result are directed to the clinician who requested the test. If used, the format and style may vary depending on preferences of the laboratory and its clinicians and must be based on follow-up guidelines published by professional organizations (e.g., American College of Obstetricians and Gynecologists, American Society for Colposcopy and Cervical Pathology)

M. For more detailed information, consult the 2001 Bethesda System dedicated web site (http://bethesda2001.cancer.gov) or download the guidelines at www.ama-assn.org

ABNORMAL UTERINE BLEEDING

I. Definition: Bleeding not associated with normal menses, i.e., deviations in the amount, duration, or frequency of bleeding

   A. Normal menstrual cycle lasts about 28 days
      1. Polymenorrhea refers to an abnormally shortened cycle with bleeding occurring every 21 days or sooner
      2. Oligomenorrhea refers to an abnormally lengthened cycle with bleeding occurring every 35 days or later

   B. Blood loss during normal menses totals about 60 mL over a maximum of 7 days (mean duration of flow is 4 days)
      1. Menorrhagia refers to total blood loss of >80 mL and bleeding for >7 days, occurring at regular intervals
      2. Hypomenorrhea refers to blood loss of <60 mL

   C. Other abnormal bleeding patterns are the following:
      1. Intermenstrual bleeding is bleeding that occurs between regular menstrual periods
      2. Metrorrhagia is bleeding that is frequent and irregular
      3. Menometrorrhagia is a pattern of frequent and irregular bleeding that becomes prolonged

II. Pathogenesis

   A. Dysfunctional uterine bleeding (DUB) results from persistent stimulation of endometrium by estrogen which is unopposed by periodic influence of progesterone; 80-90% of DUB is associated with anovulation
      1. When ovulation does not occur, progesterone is not produced, and the effects of estrogen predominate
      2. Unopposed estrogen causes endometrium to become thicker and more vascular (hyperplasia); without progesterone the structural support needed to sustain vascularity is absent which results in randomly occurring spontaneous superficial hemorrhages
      3. Alterations in prostaglandin synthesis and release are believed to play a central role in anovulatory DUB (also in ovulatory DUB which is much less common)

   B. Anovulatory DUB most often occurs in women at the extremes of reproductive life--postmenarcheal (adolescent) and perimenopausal women; pathophysiology of DUB varies with age
      1. In adolescent years there is an immaturity of the hypothalamic-pituitary-gonadal axis
      2. In perimenopausal women, DUB is due to decreased sensitivity of the ovary to follicle stimulating hormone (FSH) and luteinizing hormone (LH) stimulation
      3. May be associated with significant obesity; female adipose tissue produces estrogen and the level may rarely dip low enough to allow normal menses to occur
      4. DUB is a diagnosis of exclusion

   C. Reproductive tract disorders frequently cause abnormal vaginal bleeding
      1. Abnormal pregnancy (e.g., threatened, incomplete, missed abortions; ectopic pregnancies; trophoblastic disease; abnormalities of placental location)
      2. Anatomic abnormalities of the uterus (e.g., polyps, uterine myomas, adenomyosis, endometriosis)
      3. Trauma or presence of foreign body
      4. Infection of the lower or upper genital tract
      5. Malignancies involving the cervix, endometrium, vagina, vulva, or ovaries (more common in postmenopausal women)

   D. Systemic diseases, including coagulation defects, liver failure, prolactinemia, and thyroid dysfunction, can manifest as abnormal vaginal bleeding

   E. Iatrogenic causes include medications that contain estrogen and progesterone, phenytoin, anticoagulants, corticosteroids

III. Clinical Presentation: Age of the patient, pattern of bleeding, and associated signs and symptoms provide clues to the possible etiology

A. In adolescents, the following are likely causes
1. DUB is the most frequent cause of bleeding in this age group, accounting for about 75% of cases
   a. Some 50% of cycles are anovulatory for the first 1-2 years after menarche
   b. External forces can disrupt the often slow maturation of the hypothalamic-ovarian axis
      (1) Physical and mental stress can interfere with normal ovulation
      (2) Excessive exercise in ballet dancers, gymnasts, and other athletes results in low body fat and can interrupt ovulation
      (3) Eating disorders such as anorexia and bulimia can disrupt ovulation even in women of normal or excess weight
2. Thyroid dysfunction is relatively more frequent in this age group; chlamydial infection is common
3. Disorders of early pregnancy, particularly abortion and ectopic pregnancy, are important factors causing bleeding
4. Chlamydial infection as well as breakthrough bleeding associated with oral contraceptive use are common
5. Coagulation disorders are a less common cause
6. Among adolescent females the most frequent foreign body that is retained is a tampon; bleeding is usually accompanied by foul-smelling discharge

B. In young adult women, the most common causes are disorders of early pregnancy, infection, and abnormalities of the uterus; less common are DUB, malignancies of the reproductive tract, thyroid disorders (nonthyroid endocrine disorders or blood dyscrasias seldom manifest for the first time in this age group)
1. Anovulatory DUB is **less** frequent cause of sustained menstrual irregularity in this age group as compared with adolescents and older women
2. Most women will experience occasional anovulatory cycles that may be identified by delayed or increased flow

C. In perimenopausal women (>35 years to menopause), the most common cause is anovulatory DUB; other causes include the following
1. Anatomic abnormalities of the uterus
2. Disorders of early pregnancy
3. Endometrial hyperplasia
4. Infection of the lower or upper genital tract
5. Thyroid dysfunction (not uncommon in this age group)
6. Malignancies of the reproductive tract (more common in postmenopausal women)

D. In all postmenopausal women who have an intact uterus, bleeding is most often caused by atrophic changes of the endometrium (45%), but malignancy must **always** be ruled out

E. Pattern of bleeding and associated signs and symptoms provide additional clues to possible causes
1. DUB results in irregularity of menstrual interval, episodes of amenorrhea, and periods of heavy, prolonged bleeding
2. Women with coagulation disorders may have signs of petechiae, ecchymoses, or epistaxis
3. Disorders of early pregnancy have variable spotting due to hemorrhage, usually with pelvic pain, cramping and possibly signs and symptoms of pregnancy
4. Infection is usually associated with vaginal discharge, lower abdominal pain, and dyspareunia
5. Leiomyomas are a common cause of bleeding and result in uterine enlargement; abdominal exam may be positive for a large mass if the leiomyoma is larger than a 12 week pregnant uterus
6. In cervical carcinoma, bleeding is often postcoital, intermenstrual, and described as spotting
7. Both hypothyroidism and, less commonly, hyperthyroidism can cause menstrual abnormalities
8. Endometrial carcinoma begins with intermenstrual discharge, which is watery with small amounts of blood and then progresses to heavier bleeding

IV.   Diagnosis/Evaluation

    A.   History

       1.   **Data relating to LMP**: Inquire about timing and duration of last **normal** menses and ask woman if she has kept a menstrual calendar

       2.   **Timing amount and pattern of abnormal bleeding**: Ask when bleeding begins, whether it is spotting or heavy, how long bleeding lasts, whether it is daily spotting, and how heavy the heavy days (**Note**: Daily spotting is suggestive of a polyp or infectious cause; heavy flow tapering to spotting, with no bleeding for several days, then returning to heavy flow again is characteristic of anovulatory bleeding)

       3.   **Determine if menstrual cycles are associated with premenstrual molimina that accompanies ovulatory cycles**: Ask about symptoms of breast fullness/tenderness, abdominal bloating, mood changes, edema, weight gain, and menstrual cramps

       4.   **Associated signs and symptoms**: Ask about presence of abdominal/pelvic pain, vaginal discharge, pain on intercourse, pain with urination or defecation, or pelvic heaviness (**Note**: Pelvic pain/heaviness may indicate an ovarian cyst [functional, dermoid, corpus luteum], endometriosis, or myoma)

       5.   **Contraceptive use and sexual practices/history**: Obtain this essential information

       6.   **Drugs and medications**: Ask about medications, including oral contraceptives and long-acting contraceptives such as Depo-Provera and Norplant

       7.   **Past medical history**: Inquire about past/present problems including endocrine, hematological, and gynecological problems (**Note**: Ask: "Are you seeing or have you recently seen a healthcare provider for any other problem?") Ask about family history of bleeding disorders

       8.   **Gynecologic/obstetric history**: Obtain complete history in these areas

> Obstetric history includes number of pregnancies (gravidity) and outcome of each (parity); by convention, this information is recorded as follows:
>
> **Gravida (G) a, Para (P) b, c, d, e**
>
> a = number of pregnancies
> b = number of term pregnancies (≥37 weeks)
> c = number of preterm pregnancies (viability through 36 weeks)
> d = number of abortions (spontaneous and induced) and ectopic pregnancies
> e = number of living children

       9.   **Behavior/lifestyle**: Ask about recent changes in weight, life, activity, exercise patterns

    B.   Physical Examination

       1.   First, perform rapid assessment of hemodynamic stability (determine if patient is hypotensive or has orthostatic hypotension)

       2.   Inspect skin for bruising, petechia, or purpura

       3.   Always do pelvic and speculum examinations

          a.   Insure that bleeding is uterine and not from urethra, rectum, or superficial surface of cervix

          b.   Assess for foreign body in vault, examine cervical os for erosion, polyps, and mucopurulent discharge

          c.   Evaluate the uterus for tenderness, size, and shape

          d.   Carefully assess the adnexa

       4.   Assess thyroid and check for abdominal masses and tenderness

    C.   Differential Diagnosis: Rule out all conditions noted under Pathogenesis

    D.   Diagnostic Tests

       1.   If ectopic pregnancy is suspected, obtain an immediate pelvic ultrasound; refer to emergency OB/GYN care if confirmed

       2.   Always obtain pregnancy test (βhCG) to determine if bleeding is due to a complication of pregnancy [may be the most important test!]

       3.   In adolescents, obtain a coagulation profile (women in this age group are at significant risk for coagulopathy and are at very low risk for an endometrial lesion or atypia)

       4.   Obtain complete blood count and platelet count

       5.   Papanicolaou (Pap) smear if not done within past year

       6.   Test for sexually transmitted diseases (gonorrhea and chlamydia)

7. In women over the age of 35, an endometrial biopsy must be performed (some experts recommend that a transvaginal ultrasound be performed first)
8. A transvaginal ultrasound is indicated in all women in whom intracavitary lesions are suspected (allows for the detection of intracavitary polyps or submucous fibroids, measurement of the endometrial stripe, and the identification of ovarian masses); this test could be performed prior to endometrial biopsy and then only women at high risk for endometrial hyperplasia or cancer would require an endometrial biopsy (**Note:** Women at high risk are the following: Premenopausal women who are 35 years of age or older, those who are 30 or more years of age with a history of chronic anovulation and the associated long-term exposure to unopposed estrogen, obese women who produce increased estrogen from androgen precursors in adipose tissues, post-menopausal women not taking HRT as well as those taking HRT who experience break-through bleeding)
9. If symptoms suggest, TSH to evaluate for thyroid dysfunction

V. Plan/Management

A. Patients who are hemodynamically unstable should be referred to the ED for emergent management

B. Patients with complications of pregnancy should be referred to the ED for emergent management

C. Adolescents with excessive uterine bleeding who are found to have an abnormal coagulation profile require further testing and should be referred to a hematologist for further evaluation and management

D. Treat obvious benign causes of vaginal bleeding such as the following
1. Removal of foreign body from the vagina (most often impacted tampon)
    a. Under good visualization, and with the patient in the lithotomy position, grasp the tampon with a pair of sponge holding forceps (May also perform bimanual exam and sweep tampon out)
    b. Place a basin of water as close to the introitus as possible (to minimize malodor)
    c. Quickly immerse the tampon under water without releasing the forceps
    d. Flush the tampon and water down toilet
    e. **Note:** The unpleasant odor that envelopes the room is the most problematic; immersing the removed tampon into water the instant it is removed from the vagina reduces the malodor and the embarrassment to the patient
    f. May provide antibiotics 7-10 days if tampon in place for several days or has caused cervical erosion (Doxycycline 100 mg BID x 7-10 days)
2. For breakthrough bleeding from oral contraceptives
    a. Counsel that breakthrough bleeding decreases dramatically after first 3 months of pills
    b. Instruct to take pills at same time each day
    c. Last, change oral contraceptive to one with a higher progestational activity (usually effective regardless of when bleeding occurs in the cycle) such as Desogen, Loestrin 1.5/30, or Yasmin

E. Women who are not pregnant, who are hemodynamically stable, and who have a benign endometrium (biopsy reveals endometrial proliferation or hyperplasia without atypia or with a normal TVUS and low-risk for having endometrial hyperplasia) should be managed according to recommendations outlined in the table that follows

TREATMENT OF DUB	
Progestins are the cornerstone of treatment of chronic, recurrent bleeding episodes when an organic cause has been excluded	
Progestins can be used to halt a moderate to heavy episode of bleeding and continued monthly use can regulate cycles and prevent recurrences	
Progestins stop growth of endometrium and promote the support and organization of estrogen-primed endometrium	
When progestin is later withdrawn, sloughing of tissue occurs; bleeding may be initially heavy, but rapidly diminishes	
Medication	**Dosing**
Medroxyprogesterone acetate (Provera) [MPA]	10 mg daily for 10-12 days each month
Can be administered on menstrual cycle days 12-21 or the first 10 days of the month for women with anovulatory DUB	
Alternatives: Low dose combination OCs may also be used and are considered by many clinicians to be first-line agents. This option can be used in otherwise healthy nonsmoking women with no contraindications to OC use; re-evaluate in 3 months, and then annually (**Note:** No combination estrogen-progestin formulation is FDA-approved for the treatment of abnormal uterine bleeding in perimenopausal or other women)	

F. Nonsteroidal anti-inflammatory drugs (NSAIDs) are prostaglandin synthetase inhibitors that have been shown to decrease bleeding in women with menorrhagia
   1. Prescribe mefenamic acid (Ponstel) 250 orally TID for 5 days starting with menses to correct relative prostaglandin overproduction
   2. Other NSAIDS that may be helpful include:
      a. Naproxen 250-500 mg BID for 5 days beginning with onset of menses
      b. Ibuprofen 600-1200 mg per day (in divided doses) for 5 days beginning with onset of menses

G. Follow up: In 3 months to assess clinical response to therapy and to repeat endometrial biopsy

AMENORRHEA

I. Definition: Absence of menses for at least 3 months duration at any age when menstrual function should be present

II. Pathogenesis

   A. An intact hypothalamic-pituitary-ovarian-axis, a hormonally responsive uterus, and an intact outflow tract need to function in a coordinated manner for menstruation to occur

   B. If any part of the system functions incorrectly, withdrawal menses do not occur and amenorrhea is the symptom

III. Clinical Presentation

   A. Diagnostic Criteria: Primary Amenorrhea
      1. No bleeding by age 14 in the absence of growth and development of secondary sexual characteristics
      2. Failure to have menses by age 16, regardless of presence of normal growth and development with the appearance of secondary sexual characteristics

   B. Diagnostic Criteria: Secondary Amenorrhea
      1. Woman must have had at least one spontaneous menstrual period
      2. Six months of amenorrhea (some say 3)

   C. Common causes of primary amenorrhea along with usual presenting signs are the following
      1. Gonadal dysgenesis--there is a lack of mature (stages 4 or 5) breast/pubic hair development, but small amounts of development (stages 2 or 3) may be present secondary to only adrenal hormone secretion
      2. Müllerion (uterovaginal) anomalies--normal breast/pubic hair development occurs
      3. Hypothalamic/pituitary disorders--normal breast/pubic hair development does not occur
      4. Constitutional delay secondary to an immature hypothalamic-pituitary axis--short stature (under 5 feet at age 14) is found

   D. Common causes of secondary amenorrhea
      1. Pregnancy (most common cause)
      2. Prolactin-secreting pituitary tumors
      3. Hypothalamic hypofunction secondary to excessive stress, weight loss, and/or strenuous exercise (as many as half of all competitive female athletes may experience some menstrual abnormality, with luteal phase deficiency, anovulation, and amenorrhea the three most common)
      4. Hyperandrogenism and polycystic ovary syndrome
      5. Premature ovarian failure; endocrine disorders such as thyroid disease and diabetes mellitus
      6. Medications such as oral and injectable contraceptive steroids

IV. Diagnosis/Evaluation

    A.   History: Primary Amenorrhea
        1.   Question about growth and development; occurrence of growth spurt (ask: "Was there a period of 6 months - 1 year when you grew out of all your clothes, shoes?")
        2.   Ask questions about puberty (breasts and pubic hair--when development began and how far it has advanced)
        3.   Ask about diet, exercise patterns, stress

    B.   Physical Examination: Primary Amenorrhea
        1.   Height, weight
        2.   Observe for common anomalies associated with gonadal dysgenesis
            a.   Neck folds, low setting of ears
            b.   Chest configuration, whether 4th metacarpal is short, cubitus, valgus
        3.   Assess breast and pubic hair development using Tanner stages
        4.   Speculum exam for imperforate hymen, presence of vagina and uterus, and bimanual exam for adnexal masses
            a.   Estrogen exposed vaginal mucosa is thick, with rugae
            b.   Presence of cervix at end of canal is sufficient evidence that uterus is present
            c.   Clear cervical mucus in os is good indication that estrogen is present
            d.   Bimanual exam to confirm presence, size of uterus, and any masses

    C.   Differential Diagnosis: Primary amenorrhea is a symptom. There are numerous etiologies for this symptom

    D.   Diagnostic Tests: Primary Amenorrhea (should be ordered by the specialist to whom patient was referred)

    E.   History: Secondary Amenorrhea
        1.   Question patient regarding the following
            a.   Age at menarche, cycle regularity, duration of menstrual flow (was it fairly constant month to month?) (**Note**: The presence of cycle regularity leads to a strong presumption of ovulation)
            b.   Presence of symptoms suggesting ovulation--mittelschmerz, bloating, breast tenderness
            c.   When and how deviation from prior menstrual cyclicity occurred
            d.   Number and outcomes of pregnancies, postpartal course
            e.   Type of contraception and possibility of pregnancy
        2.   Obtain past medical history, medications currently taking (and recently discontinued such as oral contraceptives—" post-pill amenorrhea")
        3.   Question regarding growth of excess hair on face, chest, abdomen, upper back; ask about presence of acne
        4.   Ask about galactorrhea (breast milk). Persistent galactorrhea, even slight and unilateral, is significant
        5.   Question regarding weight changes, skin texture, energy level, bowel habits, and temperature tolerance
        6.   Take social history including exercise, eating habits and patterns, and stress at home, school, and work
        7.   If woman is competitive athlete, obtain information about intensity and duration of training (**Note**: A triad of disordered eating, amenorrhea, and osteoporosis occurs in the elite athlete)

    F.   Physical Examination: Secondary Amenorrhea
        1.   Vital signs, height and weight, and calculate BMI (see OBESITY section for how to calculate and interpret BMI)
        2.   Examine skin for signs of androgen excess--acne and hirsutism
        3.   Examine thyroid for size, presence of nodularity
        4.   Assess breast development for Tanner staging and presence of galactorrhea
        5.   Speculum exam for degree of vaginal rugation, type of cervical mucus (amount, stretchability, ferning pattern when dried on glass slide)
        6.   Bimanual exam for masses; for example, a unilateral ovarian enlargement can mean a steroid-producing tumor. Assess deep tendon reflexes as index of thyroid status

    G.   Differential Diagnosis: Secondary amenorrhea is a symptom. There are numerous etiologies for this symptom

H. Diagnostic Tests: Secondary Amenorrhea
1. Focused diagnostic tests based on history and physical examination findings are useful to isolate the underlying cause to the hypothalamic/pituitary, ovarian, or uterine/vaginal compartments, or to other organ systems
2. First, measure βhCG to rule out the most common cause (pregnancy); also order serum prolactin, TSH, FSH, and estradiol level (refer to V. Plan/Management for test interpretation)
3. CBC, serum chemistries, and urinalysis should also be ordered to rule out systemic disease

V. Plan/Management

A. Primary Amenorrhea: Refer all patients with primary amenorrhea to specialist for further work-up

B. Secondary Amenorrhea: Consult the table below

INTERPRETATION OF DIAGNOSTIC TESTING

➢ If sensitive thyroid-stimulating hormone (TSH) is abnormal, an asymptomatic thyroid disorder is present; refer for evaluation

➢ If prolactin is elevated, refer for a diagnostic evaluation of the etiology of the hyperprolactinemia

➢ If prolactin and FSH levels are normal, and history and physical exam suggest androgen excess, order a free testosterone level and refer patient for sonography to evaluate for evidence of polycystic ovary syndrome (PCOS); [women with this disorder do not always display clinical evidence of androgen excess]; refer for evaluation

➢ If estradiol is <40 pg/mL, and FSH is >30 mIU/mL, in a women <40 years of age, suspect premature ovarian failure

   • If woman is <25 years, refer to obtain karyotype and for further evaluation

   • If woman is <35 years, an autoimmune disease should be considered (additional tests are TSH [should have already been obtained], antinuclear antibodies, rheumatoid factors, 24 hour urine cortisol; refer for evaluation)

➢ If estradiol is <40 pg/mL, FSH is normal or decreased, and patient has history of severe dietary weight loss or anorexia nervosa, a BMI < 17, engages in highly strenuous exercise, or has severe stress, hypothalamic dysfunction is the likely cause; decreased gonadotropin levels are failing to stimulate sufficient estradiol production to produce endometrial proliferation

   • Screen for eating disorders and refer appropriately

   • Refer for dietary counseling for prudent diet, high in calcium rich food,

   • Counsel regarding risks of estrogen deficiency

   • Prescribe calcium and vitamin D supplements (see section on MENOPAUSE)

   • Prescribe low-dose oral contraceptives (if no contraindications)

C. Follow-up: Variable depending on the diagnosis

BARTHOLIN'S GLAND CYSTS AND ABSCESSES

I. Definition: An occlusion and/or infection of a Bartholin's gland or its ducts

II. Pathogenesis:

A. Bartholin's glands are bilateral vulvovaginal structures located at about the 4 and 8 o'clock positions on the posteriolateral aspect of the vestibule (area enclosed by the labia at the mouth of the vagina) (see Figure 14.1)

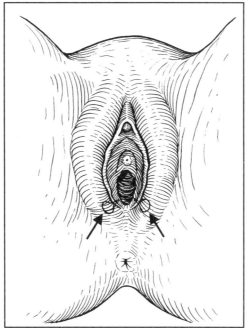

Figure 14.1. Bartholin's Glands

B. These vestibular glands are normally about the size of a pea and are made up of mucin-producing and excreting acini that drain into transitional and squamous epithelium-lined ducts about 2.5 cm long; the ducts exit into a fold between the hymen and labium

C. Obstruction of a Bartholin's duct occurs most commonly near the orifice
1. The exact etiology is usually unknown although infection with inflammation probably plays a major role
2. The duct becomes closed, while the mucus-secreting gland continues to produce fluid

D. An enlargement in the absence of inflammation is a cyst

E. With acute inflammation, an abscess develops
1. Bartholin's duct abscesses may be caused by gonococcal or chlamydial infections
2. However, other organisms such as *Staphylococcus aureus*, *Streptococcus fecalis*, and *Escherichia coli* also commonly cause the infection

III. Clinical Presentation

A. Dilatation of a Bartholin's duct due to obstruction is probably the most common finding in women complaining of vulvar masses and tends to be recurrent in some women

B. A normal Bartholin's gland and duct are nonpalpable, and any cystic swelling in the labia minora on the posteriolateral aspect of the vestibule usually represents a cyst or abscess

575

C. Cysts are generally 1 to 3 cm in size and are usually asymptomatic
    1. The patient may notice a bulge in the labia or mass may be found during routine clinical exam
    2. Cysts tend to grow slowly and noninfected cysts are normally sterile (see Figure 14.2)

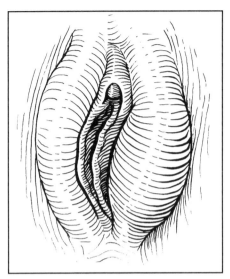

Figure 14.2. Bartholin's Gland Cyst

D. With acute inflammation, an abscess develops with symptoms of swelling, tenderness, and erythema; patient may be unable to engage in sex or sports due to pain

IV. Diagnosis/Evaluation

A. History
    1. Ask about onset, duration of cyst/abscess
    2. Ask about presence of associated symptoms such as pain, swelling, erythema and ask if presence of cyst/abscess has limited normal activities
    3. Determine if there are any symptoms present that might indicate presence of a sexually transmitted disease--discharge, irregular bleeding, dyspareunia
    4. Ask about trauma to the site
    5. Ask about history of recurrent cysts/abscesses

B. Physical Examination
    1. Inspect external genitalia for presence of lesions and masses, other abnormalities
    2. Carefully palpate the vaginal introitus with the thumb and forefinger for presence of swelling/masses, presence of fluctuance, areas of tenderness
    3. Palpate inguinal nodes for enlargement

C. Differential Diagnosis
    1. Sebaceous cyst
    2. Vaginal inclusion cyst
    3. Fibromas
    4. Lipomas
    5. Hematoma

D. Diagnostic Tests: None indicated unless abscess is recurrent; then perform culture and sensitivity testing of discharge from abscess

V. Plan/Management

A. Asymptomatic Bartholin's gland cysts in patients under age 40 may not require treatment
    1. Many small ductal cysts do not interfere with intercourse, or cause discomfort with walking, sitting, or other activities, and usually wax and wane in size. Treatment consists of daily sitz baths or warm compresses applied to area and spontaneous resolution of the cyst usually occurs
    2. Over time, some cysts eventually become symptomatic and require treatment

3. Referral to specialist for drainage of cyst and placement of Word catheter in the cavity is recommended
4. Word catheter is left in place for up to 4 weeks to allow drainage and formation of an epithelized outflow tract

B. Asymptomatic Bartholin's gland cysts in patients over 40 are usually excised because of concern about Bartholin's gland carcinoma (rare)

C. Patients experiencing severe pain due to a Bartholin's abcess should be referred immediately for incision and drainage with placement of catheter

D. Most ductal abscesses will eventually "point" and spontaneously rupture resulting in immediate relief; the process will be hastened with frequent sitz baths
1. Because of the polymicrobial nature of most abscesses, broad-spectrum antibiotic coverage is recommended (Doxycycline 100 mg po BID x 7-10 days; or Augmentin 875 mg PO BID x 7-10 days; or Keflex 500 mg. PO BID x 10 days)
2. Advise patient to continue with frequent sitz baths to provide relief and facilitate healing
3. Abscess may recur and definitive treatment with placement of a Word catheter may be necessary

E. Early abscesses (that have not ruptured) should be treated with sitz baths until the abscess points, which makes incision and definitive treatment easier; broad-spectrum antibiotics (see above) should also be prescribed
1. Refer the patient for incision, drainage, and placement of a Word catheter for up to 4 weeks to facilitate drainage and formation of an epithelized outflow tract
2. This procedure usually results in complete resolution of the condition

F. Follow Up: None indicated unless cyst/abscess fails to resolve

BREAST MASS

I. Definition: Benign and malignant lesions of the breast

II. Pathogenesis

A. Common benign lesions
1. Fibrocystic changes of the breast (FCB)
   a. Abnormal restructuring in the layering of the parenchyma most likely related to estrogen/progestin imbalance resulting in excessive ductal stimulation and proliferation
   b. Result of restructuring is atrophic epithelial segments and fibrous replacement
2. Fibroadenoma
   a. Originates from the terminal duct--lobular unit, and believed to be hormonally induced
   b. Composed of fibrous and epithelial elements
3. Cysts
   a. Believed to arise from dilatation or obstruction of collecting ducts
   b. Microcysts are nonpalpable, and macrocysts are usually palpable

B. Breast cancer
1. Arises from transformed epithelium that originates within ducts or lobules
2. For a period of time, these transformed cells are non-invasive; if undisturbed, eventually there is local, lymphatic, and hematogenous spread

III. Clinical Presentation

A. The existence of a "dominant" area (lump, nodule, mass, or thickening) that is different from surrounding tissue or asymmetric compared to the opposite breast constitutes an abnormal finding
1. The basic question is whether a dominant area exists; issues of smoothness, hardness, distinctness from surrounding tissue are secondary
2. Causes of a specific dominant area must be determined by means other than physical examination

B. Benign lesions
1. Fibrocystic changes of the breast (FBC)
   a. Most common of all benign breast conditions
   b. Occurs in about 50% of women with highest incidence among women in their 20s and 30s who are in reproductive, premenopausal years; symptoms cease with menopause (unless hormone replacement is begun)
   c. Risk factors include nulliparity, late age of natural menopause, middle class, and Caucasian race
   d. Condition is characterized by cyclic bilateral breast pain (mastalgia), which usually worsens premenstrually and resolves after onset of menses
   e. Thickened symmetrical plaques of glandular breast tissue that feel rubbery, lack discreteness, and blend into the surrounding breast tissue
2. Fibroadenoma
   a. The second-most common form of benign breast disease occurring in about 10% of women, most often in 20-30 year age group (median age at diagnosis is 30 years)
   b. May be stimulated by pregnancy and regress with menopause
   c. Usually presents as single, smooth, round, mobile lumps which are usually painless (**Note**: Can feel firm or "rubbery"); commonly located in upper-outer quadrants
   d. Difficult to distinguish from cysts
3. Cysts
   a. Tend to occur around the fourth decade of life and in the perimenopausal period
   b. Round or oval, usually well demarcated from surrounding tissue
   c. Smooth, firm, and mobile

C. Breast cancer
1. An estimated 182,800 new invasive cases of breast cancer occurred among women in the US during 2000
2. Rare in women under 25; 48% of new breast cancer cases and 56% of breast cancer deaths occur in women age 65 and over
3. Approximately 32% of all newly diagnosed cancers in women are cancers of the breast
4. Risk factors include the following:
   a. Female gender, residence in North America or northern Europe and older age
   b. Family history of breast cancer in first-degree relative, especially if bilateral and/or premenopausal in onset
   c. Menarche occurrence before age 11 or after age 14
   d. Onset of menopause after age 55 or more than 35 years duration of menses
5. Usually presents as a painless, firm, fixed mass that does not change with menstruation; most common in upper, outer-quadrant (50%), but they can appear anywhere

D. Spontaneous unilateral nipple discharge that is clear/bloody may be associated with malignancy

E. Age is an important factor with most women <25 years of age with masses having benign conditions and 75% of women >70 years of age with palpable masses having cancer

IV. Diagnosis/Evaluation

A. History
1. Question regarding presence/location of mass, characteristics of mass--tenderness, mobility, size, single or multiple. Ask if any lymph nodes have seemed enlarged
2. If presenting complaint is mastalgia, ask regarding frequency, severity, duration, location (localized, diffuse, or bilateral). Ask if the pain is cyclic occurring during the premenstrual phase or noncyclic. Determine if the pain is due to **trauma**
3. Inquire about changes in breast mass with menstruation (if not postmenopausal), presence of nipple discharge (spontaneous rather than elicited), type of discharge (bloody, serous, clear, milky), and laterality (one or both nipples)
4. Obtain detailed menstrual history including age at menarche, dates of last period, and age at menopause (if appropriate). Determine the phase of menstrual cycle the patient is in at presentation (**Note**: Clinical breast exam is best performed a week or so after onset of menses when tissue is least congested)
5. Question about medication history, including current and past use of oral contraceptives and hormone replacement therapy

6.   Obtain history of risk factors for breast cancer (see above), as well as information relating to previous breast masses, biopsies, and breast surgery
7.   Determine and document in chart date of last clinical breast exam, when last mammogram was done and results, and breast self-examination practices

B.   Physical Examination
1.   With patient sitting on table
a.   Inspect for symmetry, contour, and vascular pattern variation
b.   Inspect skin, noting discoloration, retraction, dimpling, edema
2.   Have patient raise arms above head and place hands on hips
3.   Palpate the axillary, supraclavicular, and infraclavicular nodes for adenopathy
4.   With patient supine and arm extended and slightly bent on side being examined
a.   Inspect breast and skin as in the upright position
b.   Palpate the breast tissue, supraclavicular region, and chest wall following a vertical strip pattern
c.   Gently palpate the entire nipple-areolar complex; do not squeeze the nipple unless the patient has complained of nipple discharge
5.   Consider teaching patient how to perform BSE during exam; advise patient that the USPSTF has concluded there is insufficient evidence to recommend for or against performing routine breast self-examination
6.   If a dominant area (i.e., lump, mass, nodule, or thickening different from surrounding tissue or asymmetric compared to the opposite breast) is found, the area should be assessed and then described
a.   Use tip of forefinger as a ruler
b.   Do simultaneous mirror image palpation bilaterally
c.   Chart description of dominant area with drawing that is appropriately labeled

C.   Differential Diagnosis: Benign versus malignant tumor

D.   Diagnostic Tests: Patients under age 30 may be rescheduled after their next menstrual period for re-evaluation of the mass, to assess whether it has gotten smaller or gone away before proceeding with diagnostic tests listed here
1.   Bilateral diagnostic mammography is the initial test to evaluate a breast mass; however, in women younger than 40 years, sensitivity of test is greatly reduced because of dense glandular breast tissue and ultrasound is the preferred study
2.   Breast ultrasonography complements diagnostic mammography in evaluation of palpable mass; a primary role is to differentiate between solid and cystic lesions
3.   Fine needle aspiration with biopsy (FNAB) may be performed in office procedure when mass is easily palpable and cyst-like, without an initial mammogram or ultrasound
a.   If cyst, aspiration of fluid (benign cystic fluid appears clear yellow, straw colored, green, or brown) results in resolution of mass; repeat clinical breast exam in 4-6 weeks
b.   Recurrence of mass requires prompt evaluation with mammography and ultrasonography
c.   Blood-tinged aspirate requires cytological evaluation
d.   Failure to aspirate fluid by FNA suggests mass is solid; aspirated cells should be sent for cytological evaluation
4.   Excisional biopsy is the definitive step in determining if a breast mass is malignant

V.   Plan/Management

A.   If abnormalities are found on mammography or ultrasonography, refer patient for management

B.   If fibrocystic breast changes are diagnosed via FNA, the aspiration itself may be therapeutic for benign cysts and may relieve localized pain

C.   Patients may be managed as follows to control symptoms

- Counsel patient that no cure exists for FBC but symptomatic therapy will control symptoms in most cases
- Instruct to wear support bra to stabilize the breasts
- Advise that dietary modifications are controversial but reduction in caffeine intake and salt intake may help some patients
- Prescribe oral contraceptives (if no contraindications) that are low dose estrogen (20 mcg); patient usually has reduction in pain after a few months of therapy
- Low-dose danazol (Danocrine), a synthetic androgen, is the only FDA-approved drug for treatment of severe mastalgia (works by blocking midcycle surges of LH and FSH; also reduces estrogen effects) [rarely prescribed in US for this indication because of high cost and side effects]
  - ➢ Dosing: 50-200 mg BID x 4-6 months (**Note**: Begin therapy during menses or perform appropriate tests to ensure patient is not pregnant); dose can be reduced to 100 mg every other day
  - ➢ Several months of use may be needed before drug becomes effective
  - ➢ **Note**: Drug can cause alterations in the lipid profile and hepatic dysfunction
- Premenstrual use of NSAIDs and vitamin E may be helpful in some patients
  - ➢ Ibuprofen, 400 mg tabs, Q 4-6 hours for 2-3 days at time of maximal engorgement
  - ➢ Vitamin E (150-600 IU/day) taken daily
- Patients whose breast pain does not resolve with above measures should be referred to a specialist for management

D. If fibroadenoma is diagnosed via fine needle aspiration biopsy (FNAB) or ultrasonography, conservative management is usually indicated in women <40 years of age
1. In past, routine practice was excision
2. Monitor size of mass with serial ultrasounds, unless patient desires excision

E. If cyst is diagnosed via FNA, aspiration itself provides both diagnosis and treatment

F. Follow Up: Variable depending on diagnosis

CONTRACEPTION

I. Definition: Prevention of pregnancy by reversible or irreversible methods used by either or both sexual partners

II. Pathogenesis: Not applicable

III. Clinical Presentation

A. Requests for contraceptives and contraceptive counseling are among the most frequent reasons women visit a healthcare clinician

B. The proportion of never-married women currently in a sexual relationship has increased for all age categories over the past decade

C. Pregnancy rates among teens are greater in the US than in any other developed country in spite of a very small declining trend in teen pregnancy

D. Almost one half of pregnancies in the US are unintended in spite of the fact that there are many safe contraceptive methods available

E. Female sterilization, oral contraceptives, male condoms, and male sterilization are the dominant contraceptive methods in the US today

IV.   Diagnosis/Evaluation

   A.   History
      1.   **Obtain a menstrual history** including age at menarche, duration of, frequency of, and interval between menstrual periods, the last menstrual period (LMP, which is dated from the first day of last normal menses), any intermenstrual bleeding, pain with menses, and perimenstrual symptoms
      2.   **Obtain an obstetric history**, including number of pregnancies and outcome of each (see section on ABNORMAL UTERINE BLEEDING [IV.A.] for information on taking an obstetric history)
      3.   **Obtain a gynecologic history** including breast history, previous gynecologic surgery, infectious diseases involving the reproductive tract, any history of infertility, use of douching/feminine hygiene products, and diethylstilbestrol (DES) exposure in utero
      4.   **Obtain a sexual history** eliciting age at first intercourse; present sexual partner(s) and their gender; number of lifetime partners; types of sexual practices; level of satisfaction with sex life
      5.   **Obtain a contraceptive history** including contraceptive method currently used and reason for its choice; when begun, any problems, and satisfaction with method; inquire about previous methods used and why discontinued
      6.   **Inquire about** past or present **sexual abuse** or assault; screen for intimate-partner violence
      7.   **Obtain a complete medical and surgical history**, including information about cardiovascular disease, thromboembolic disease, liver problems, diabetes mellitus, blood transfusions, and migraine headaches
      8.   **Inquire about substance use** including tobacco, alcohol, and drug use; ask what medications are currently being taken
      9.   **Question about allergies** and any history of adverse drug reactions
      10.   **Determine childhood diseases** and immunization status
      11.   **Obtain family history**, asking about stroke, CVD, cancer, DM in first-degree relative

   B.   Physical Examination
      1.   **General Principles**: Hormonal contraception can safely be provided based on careful review of medical history and blood pressure measurement; for most women, no further evaluation is necessary
      2.   Measure blood pressure
      3.   If pelvic examination is performed (e.g., woman requests to be fitted for a diaphragm, or Pap smear screening or chlamydia screening are required [based on US Preventive Services Task Force (USPSTF) recommendations]), the following components should be considered
         a.   Inspection and examination of external genitalia
         b.   Speculum examination of the internal structures
         c.   Pap smear and specimens as appropriate
         d.   Bimanual examination of the pelvic organs
         e.   Rectovaginal exam of posterior aspect of pelvic organs (if indicated)
      4.   Consider clinical breast examination (the USPSTF recommends screening mammography, with or without clinical breast examination every 1-2 years for women aged 40 and older). Consider instruction in breast self-exam (BSE); patient should be advised that benefits of breast self-examination have not been established and that the USPSTF has no recommendations for or against teaching or performing routine BSE

   C.   Differential Diagnosis: Not applicable

   D.   Diagnostic Tests
      1.   Variable depending on findings from history and physical examination/blood pressure evaluation
      2.   Type of contraceptive method selected by patient also influences which diagnostic testing is required (e.g., pregnancy test may be required, depending on the method selected by the patient)

V.   Plan/Treatment

   A.   All patients should be counseled regarding the following and counseling must be documented in the chart
      1.   Anatomy and physiology of reproduction
      2.   Contraceptive methods, including how they work, effectiveness, advantages, and disadvantages
      3.   The need to use condoms to prevent STDs, regardless of contraceptive method selected
      4.   Risks and benefits of all methods, as well as informed consent that is signed by patient and placed in chart when IUD, implants, injections, or other hormonal contraceptives are chosen by patient

   B.   Assist patient to select one of the methods contained in the following overview of commonly used contraceptive methods, and provide counseling appropriate to the method selected

VI.   Brief Overview of Commonly Used Contraceptive Methods

A.   **Spermicides** contain nonoxynol-9 (N-9), which disrupt integrity of sperm membrane; available as creams, gels, foams, film, tablets, and suppositories and should be placed deep in vagina near cervix prior to intercourse
1.   **Effectiveness:** About 5-50% of women experience an unintended pregnancy during a year of typical use; there is no significant difference among various forms
2.   **Advantages:** Inexpensive, easily available, convenient with infrequent intercourse, few side effects or user risk; provides some protection against some STDs
3.   **Disadvantages:** May cause local irritation (**Note:** Use of N-9 has become controversial recently after studies of prostitutes in Africa using large amounts of spermicide vaginally with the aim of reducing transmission of HIV were actually found to have a greater risk of seroconversion than the control group who was not using spermicide. The relevance of these studies to patient groups in the US remains unclear, but it may be wise for women at extremely high risk [prostitutes; partners of HIV+ individuals] to avoid any substance, including large amounts of N-9, that can irritate and disrupt vaginal mucosal integrity)

B.   **Male condoms** are more commonly used today to prevent transmission of STDs than for pregnancy prevention. They are thin sheaths made from latex or polyurethane which serve as a physical barrier (patients should be advised to avoid "skin" condoms). The Centers for Disease Control and Prevention (CDC) no longer recommends condoms lubricated with the spermicide N-9
1.   **Effectiveness:** There is a 3% probability of pregnancy during a year of perfect use; causes of failure include slippage and breakage during intercourse and improper application
2.   **Advantages:** Inexpensive, easy to use, easily available, reduce risk of STDs
3.   **Disadvantages:** May decrease tactile sensation; condoms made of polyurethane are compatible with oil-based lubricants, but those made from latex are not

C.   **Female condoms (Reality)** have been in use since 1992 and are the first barrier contraceptive for women offering some protection against STDs. Composed of a thin polyurethane sheath that is 7.8 cm in diameter and 17 cm in length, the sheath has two polyurethane rings. The inner ring is at the closed end of the sheath that is placed inside the vagina and a larger ring remains outside the vagina providing some protection to the labia and the base of the penis. The inner ring provides stability for the condom, which is prelubricated with a dry silicone-based lubricant. The condom can be inserted up to 8 hours prior to intercourse and is intended for one-time use
1.   **Effectiveness:** About 5% of women have an unintended pregnancy during a year of perfect use
2.   **Advantages:** Controlled by woman and provides some STD protection
3.   **Disadvantages:** Anatomy of woman may make stable placement difficult

---

Patient Education Relating to Use of Spermicides and Condoms

The correct way to use spermicides and condoms (appropriate lubricants to use with condoms, and how to put on and remove both male and female condoms) should be discussed
➢   Follow Up: In 1 year for annual exam
➢   Discuss emergency contraception and offer prescription

D.   **Diaphragms** are dome-shaped rubber caps with flexible rims that fit over the cervix and block the passage of sperm; spermicides are applied to the inner aspect of the dome, which is placed against the cervix
1.   **Effectiveness:** About 6% of women have an unintended pregnancy during a year of perfect use
2.   **Types:** Three types are commonly used
a.   Flat spring rim: A thin rim with gentle spring strength, appropriate for use in women with normal vaginal size, contour, a shallow arch behind the symphysis pubis and normal vulvar tone
b.   Arching spring rim: A sturdy rim with considerable strength, used in women with less than optimal vaginal support (indicated for women who have had a vaginal delivery which usually causes some amount of first degree cystocele) [**Note:** This type is the most commonly used]
c.   Coil spring rim: A thin but sturdy rim useful in women with normal vaginal size, contour, and with an average or deep arch behind the symphysis pubis

3. **Goal** for fitting is to find the largest size that remains comfortable for the patient; most common problem in diaphragm fitting is selecting a size that is **too small**
    a. Generally, a nulliparous woman will be fitted with sizes 65, 70, or 75
    b. A multiparous woman, with sizes 75, 80, or 85
    c. A grand multiparous woman, with size 85 or larger
4. **Procedure** for fitting with diaphragm
    a. May use fitting rings or sets of various sizes of diaphragms (for the purpose of this explanation, a diaphragm will be used)
    b. Begin with a size in the middle of the probable range or estimate diaphragm size by using technique described below

DIAPHRAGM FITTING
• Insert your index and middle fingers into vagina until middle finger reaches vaginal posterior wall
• With tip of your thumb, mark the place where your index finger touches the pubic bone
• Remove your fingers
• Diaphragm is sized appropriately if it fits between mark on index finger and tip of middle finger

    c. After selecting the size believed to be appropriate, introduce the diaphragm into the vagina (first, lubricate the rim of the diaphragm; then compress the sides with fingers and thumbs of one hand, and place in vagina as one would place a speculum--inserting downward and inward)
    d. Check placement to make certain that the lower rim is in the posterior fornix, the circumference is against the lateral vaginal walls, and the upper rim is secured behind the symphysis pubis
    e. Determine if the size is right by referring to the table below

IS THE DIAPHRAGM TOO SMALL, TOO LARGE, OR JUST RIGHT?
It's Too Small if
• it moves around in the vagina
• it can't be stabilized behind the symphysis pubis
• it is loose
• it comes out when woman coughs/bears down
• there is more than enough space to place your fingertips between rim and symphysis pubis
It's Too Large if
• rim buckles forward against the vaginal walls
• woman feels discomfort when the diaphragm is in place
• there is not enough space to place your fingertips between rim and symphysis pubis
It's Just Right if
• it fits snugly in the vagina without buckling forward
• it covers the cervix
• it fits both into posterior fornix and up behind symphysis pubis
• woman cannot feel the diaphragm and it does not cause discomfort
• there is just enough space to place your fingertips between rim and symphysis pubis

    f. Teach the woman how to insert, place, check, and remove the diaphragm; give woman detailed instructions on how to use and care for diaphragm
    g. Should be refitted after childbirth or a significant weight loss/gain.
5. **Advantages:** May be inserted up to 6 hours prior to intercourse; reduced risk of STDs and a reduced risk of cervical cancer; works well with infrequent intercourse
6. **Disadvantages:** UTIs are more common; some women are sensitive to contraceptive jelly; use has been associated with toxic shock syndrome (TSS), so should be avoided during menses and left in place no longer than 24 hours; requires fitting by a healthcare clinician and yearly replacement

E. **Cervical caps** are soft rubber cups with a firm, round rim (Prentif Cavity Rim Cervical Cap) that fit snugly around the base of the cervix. Spermicide is placed inside the cap prior to insertion
    1. **Effectiveness:** About 9-26% of women experience an unintended pregnancy during a year of perfect use (nulliparous women are less likely than parous women to become pregnant)
    2. **Advantages:** Provides continuous contraception protection for 48 hours with no need to remove for additional spermicide

3. **Disadvantages:** Must be removed after 48 hours because of possible risk of TSS; some women experience odor problems with use for more than a few hours. Device must be fitted by a health care clinician and thus requires a visit and replacement every year at annual exam

---

Patient Education Relating to Use of Diaphragm and Cervical Cap
- Provide patient with insertion and removal instructions and how to care for devices
- Include information on application of spermicidal jelly or cream when using the devices and when to remove
- Follow up: In 1 year for annual exam
- Discuss emergency contraception and offer prescription

F. **Intrauterine devices (IUDs)** are inserted into the uterus and their mechanisms of action are believed to prevent sperm from fertilizing ova
    1.   **Effectiveness:** About 0.6 to 1.5% of women experience unintended pregnancy in first year of use with perfect use
    2.   **Types:** Presently there are two intrauterine contraceptive devices marketed in the US: the Copper T-380A (ParaGard) and the intrauterine levonorgestrel-releasing system (Mirena) [Production of Progestasert has been suspended]
        a.   The ParaGard is a T-shaped polyethylene device whose stem is wrapped with copper wire, and whose cross-arms are partly covered by copper tubing; fertilization is prevented primarily through creation of an intrauterine environment that is spermicidal; it is approved for 10 years of use
        b.   Mirena is a plastic T-shaped device that releases 20 mcg of levonorgestrel daily; it is approved for 5 years of use. The levonorgestrel produces a contraceptive effect in a number of ways—by thickening cervical mucus and by inhibiting sperm mobility and endometrial growth; there is minimal systemic absorption of the progestin
        c.   IUDs are not abortifacients
    3.   **Precautions** to IUD use are outlined in following table

---

PRECAUTIONS TO IUD USE

Refrain from providing an IUD for women with the following diagnoses (World Health Organization [WHO] category #4)
- Known or suspected pregnancy
- Active, recent (within past 3 months), or recurrent pelvic infection
- Severely distorted uterine cavity caused by anatomical abnormalities of the uterus including:
  - Leiomyomata
  - Endometrial polyps
  - Cervical stenosis
  - Bicornuate uterus
  - Small uterus

Exercise caution if an IUD is used or considered in the following situations and carefully monitor for adverse effects (WHO category #3)
- Risk factors for pelvic inflammatory disease
  - Purulent cervicitis, until treated
  - Any history of gonorrhea or chlamydia (especially recent infections)
- Risk factors for sexually transmitted diseases, including multiple sexual partners or a partner who has multiple partners
- Impaired response to infection
- Risk factors for infection with HIV and AIDS
- Undiagnosed, irregular, heavy or abnormal uterine bleeding, cervical or uterine malignancy, unresolved Pap smear
- Previous problems with IUD (any and all)
- Past history of severe vasovagal reactivity or fainting
- Difficulty in obtaining emergency follow-up care and treatment for PID

Adapted from Hatcher, R.A., Trussel, J., Stewart, F., Cates, W., Stewart, G., Guest, F., & Kowal, D. (1998). *Contraceptive Technology*, 17th edition, New York: Ardent Media, Inc., pp 517-518.

    4.   **Timing of insertion:** Usually recommended during menses to avoid pregnancy
    5.   Provide a copy of the FDA-approved and manufacturer-supplied leaflet or pamphlet to each IUD user; consent forms can be written to include a statement such as "I have been given a copy of (title) and have been encouraged to read it carefully"
    6.   **Follow up** after patient's next menses (3-6 weeks after insertion) to make certain IUD is in place and that there are no signs of infection; further routine visits are not required. Continue annual exam schedule
    7.   **Advantages:** High efficacy, which is sustained over 10 years for the ParaGard and 5 years for the Mirena; absence of systemic metabolic effects; method is not related to coitus; immediately reversible

8. **Disadvantages:** Risk of uterine perforation, increase in spontaneous abortion, ectopic pregnancy, uterine bleeding and pain, pelvic infection; need for clinician to insert and remove

---

Patient Education Relating to Use of IUDs: "PAINS"

- P   Period: late (pregnancy), abnormal spotting or bleeding
- A   Abdominal pain, pain with intercourse, severe cramping
- I   Infection exposure (STD); abnormal vaginal discharge
- N   Not feeling well; fever, chills
- S   String missing, shorter or longer

Adapted from Nelson, A,, Hatcher, R.A., Zieman, M., Watt, A., Darney, P.D., & Creinin, M.D., et al. (2000) *Managing Contraception*, Tiger, GA: Bridging the Gap Foundation

G. **Combination oral contraceptives** prevent pregnancy by a number of effects of estrogen and progestin: they inhibit ovulation, presumably as a result of gonadotropin suppression induced by the estrogen and progestin effects on the hypothalamic/pituitary axis; they act directly on the cervical mucus, making it thicker which inhibits sperm penetration; they act directly on the endometrium, inhibiting its development into a state favorable for implantation

1. **Effectiveness:** About 0.1% of women experience an unintended pregnancy within the first year of use with perfect use (combined pills); the figure is 0.5% with progestin-only pills

2. **Advantages:** Easy to use, convenient, rapidly reversible, use controlled by woman, many noncontraceptive benefits such as prevention of gynecologic malignancies (endometrial and ovarian), prevention of benign conditions such as fibrocystic breast changes

3. **Disadvantages:** Dependent on user adherence to daily use, provides no protection against STDs, expensive, prescription needed, many possible side effects

4. World Health Organization (WHO) precautions to the use of oral contraceptives are contained in the following table

---

REFRAIN FROM PROVIDING COMBINED OCs

Refrain from providing combined oral contraceptives for women with the following diagnoses (World Health Organization [WHO] category #4)

- Deep vein thrombosis or pulmonary embolism, or history thereof
- CVA, coronary artery or ischemic heart disease, or history thereof
- Structural heart disease, complicated by pulmonary hypertension, atrial fibrillation, or history of subacute bacterial endocarditis
- Diabetes with vascular disease of >20 years duration
- Breast cancer
- Pregnancy
- Lactation (<6 weeks postpartum)
- Liver problems (all types)
- Headaches, including migraine with focal neurologic symptoms
- Major surgery with prolonged immobilization or any leg surgery
- Over 35 years of age and currently a heavy smoker (15 or more cigarettes a day)
- Hypertension, 160+/100+ or with vascular disease

Exercise caution if combined oral contraceptives are used or considered in the following situations and carefully monitor for adverse effects (WHO category #3)

- Postpartum <21 days
- Lactation (6 weeks to 6 months)
- Undiagnosed abnormal vaginal/uterine bleeding
- Over 35 years of age and light smoker (fewer than 15 cigarettes/day)
- Past history of breast cancer but no evidence of recurrence for 5 years
- Use of drugs that affect liver enzymes (Consult PDR)
- Gallbladder disease

Adapted from Hatcher, R.A., Trussel, J., Stewart, F., Cates, W., Stewart, G., Guest, F., & Kowal, D. (1998). *Contraceptive Technology*, 17th edition, New York: Ardent Media, Inc., pp 517-518.

5. Whereas some experts (see Hatcher et al., 1998) believe that no single OC in the sub-50 mcg (estrogen content) is clearly superior to another, other experts (see Vandenbroucke et al., 2001) recommend that third-generation progestins in combination preparations **not** be the first choice for new users because of the increase in the extent of adverse hemostatic changes and the associated risk of thrombosis associated with this class of progestins

a. One approach is to start with low-dose (estrogen content) combination OCs without regard to the progestin used in the preparation (see table that follows for product examples)

b. Another approach is to **avoid** third-generation progestins in combination preparations as the **first choice for new users** (third generation progestins used in combination OCs are desogestrel and, outside the US, gestodene) [see table that follows for product examples]

6. The newest progestin, drospirenone, is an analogue of spironolactone, an aldosterone antagonist with antimineralocorticoid and antiandrogenic activities (see table that follows for product example)

7. Women who are not candidates for estrogen-containing OCs should be considered for progestin-only pills such as Micronor or others listed in table of oral contraceptives categorized according to composition, or may consider other highly effective non-estrogen contraceptives

8. **Body weight and oral contraceptive failure**: A number of studies have demonstrated that women weighing 70.5 kg or more have an increased risk of OC failure, a risk that is particularly elevated in women using very low dose OCs

   a. This effect could be due to differences in metabolism in higher body weight women or because of decreased circulating levels of lipophilic contraceptive steroids

   b. Body weight should thus be a consideration in recommending oral contraceptive use for women with a body weight of 70.5 kg or more

9. **Contraception in perimenopause** is a concern for many women; over half of pregnancies among women aged 40 years of age or older are unintended

   a. Combined oral contraceptives can help maintain regular bleeding cycles and a consistent hormonal pattern up to menopause

   ---

   <u>**Women over 40 who are candidates for OCs**</u>

   - Nonsmokers, who have no cardiovascular disease
   - Negative family history of premature cardiovascular disease
   - History of normal mammograms (must be done yearly)
   - Normal cholesterol, HDL/LDL, triglycerides, and fasting blood sugar
   - Weight within healthy range
   - No risk factors other than age
   - No contraindications to OC use

   ---

   b. Prescribe the lowest dose that is effective (those containing 20 mcg EE can help minimize estrogen-related side effects) [See table for product examples]

To determine when a woman who is near 50 years of age is menopausal and no longer in need of contraception, do the following

- Woman should be advised to stop taking active pills; after a period of at least 2 weeks of not taking active pills, obtain FSH. If level is 30 or greater, she can be considered menopausal and no longer in need of contraception
- By age 50, 75% of women are either a few months away from their final menstrual period, or they have already experienced their final menstrual period

---

10.   The following table lists oral contraceptives categorized according to composition:

ORAL CONTRACEPTIVES CATEGORIZED BY COMPOSITION				
Type	Drug	Estrogen (mcg)	Progestin (mg)	Color of active tablets
COMBINATION ESTROPHASIC				
Ethinyl estradiol/norethindrone acetate	Estrostep Fe	(5 tabs) 20 (7 tabs) 30 (9 tabs) 35	1 1 1	white (triangle) white (square) white (round)
COMBINATION TRIPHASIC				
Ethinyl estradiol/norethindrone	Ortho-Novum 7/7/7	(7 tabs) 35 (7 tabs) 35 (7 tabs) 35	0.5 0.75 1	white light peach peach
	Tri-Norinyl	(7 tabs) 35 (9 tabs) 35 (5 tabs) 35	0.5 1 0.5	blue yellow-green blue
Ethinyl estradiol/norgestimate	Ortho Tri-Cyclen	(7 tabs) 35 (7 tabs) 35 (7 tabs) 35	0.18 0.215 0.25	white light blue blue
	Ortho Tri-Cyclen Lo	(7 tabs) 25 (7 tabs) 25 (7 tabs) 25	0.18 0.215 0.25	white light blue dark blue
Ethinyl estradiol/levonorgestrel	Tri-Levlen	(6 tabs) 30 (5 tabs) 40 (10 tabs) 30	0.05 0.075 0.125	brown white light yellow
	Triphasil	(6 tabs) 30 (5 tabs) 40 (10 tabs) 30	0.05 0.075 0.125	brown white light yellow
	Enpresse	(6 tabs) 30 (5 tabs) 40 (10 tabs) 30	0.05 0.075 0.125	pink white orange
Ethinyl estradiol/desogestrel	Cyclessa	(7 tabs) 25 (7 tabs) 25 (7 tabs) 25	0.1 0.125 0.15	yellow orange red
COMBINATION BIPHASIC				
Ethinyl estradiol/norethindrone	Ortho-Novum 10/11	(10 tabs) 35 (11 tabs) 35	0.5 1	white peach
	Jenest-28	(7 tabs) 35 (14 tabs) 35	0.5 1	white peach
Ethinyl estradiol/desogestrel	Mircette	(21 tabs) 20 (5 tabs) 10	0.15 0	white yellow
				(Continued)

ORAL CONTRACEPTIVES CATEGORIZED BY COMPOSITION *(CONTINUED)*

Type	Drug	Estrogen (mcg)	Progestin (mg)	Color of active tablets
COMBINATION MONOPHASIC				
Ethinyl estradiol/norethindrone	Loestrin 1/20	20	1	white
	Loestrin (Fe) 1/20	20	1	white
	Loestrin 1.5/30	30	1.5	green
	Loestrin (Fe) 1.5/30	30	1.5	green
	Brevicon	35	0.5	blue
	Norinyl 1+35	35	1	light yellow
	Nortrel 0.5/35	35	0.5	yellow
	Nortrel 1/35	35	1	yellow-green
	Ortho-Novum 1/35	35	1	peach
	Ovcon-35	35	0.4	peach
	Ovcon-50	50	1	yellow
Ethinyl estradiol/levonorgestrel	Alesse	20	0.1	Pink
	Aviane	20	0.1	orange
	Lessina	20	0.1	pink
	Levlite	20	0.1	pink
	Levlen	30	0.15	light orange
	Nordette	30	0.15	light orange
	Portia	30	0.15	pink
Ethinyl estradiol/norgestrel	Cryselle	30	0.3	white
	Lo/Ovral	30	0.3	white
	Ovral	50	0.5	white
Ethinyl estradiol/ Ethynodiol diacetate	Demulen 1/35	35	1	white
	Demulen 1/50	50	1	white
Mestranol/norethindrone	Norinyl 1/50	50	1	white
	Ortho-Novum 1/50	50	1	yellow
Ethinyl estradiol/desogestrel	Apri	30	0.15	rose
	Desogen	30	0.15	white
	Ortho-Cept	30	0.15	orange
Ethinyl estradiol/norgestimate	Ortho-Cyclen	35	0.25	blue
Ethinyl estradiol/drospirenone	Yasmin	30	3	yellow
PROGESTIN-ONLY				
Norethindrone	Micronor	---	0.35	lime
	Nor-QD		0.35	yellow
Norgestrel	Ovrette	---	0.075	yellow

Adapted from Murphy, J.L. (2003, January). Tables: Oral contraceptives. *Monthly prescribing reference.* New York: Prescribing References, Inc.

Patient Education Relating to Use of Oral Contraceptives

➤ Instruct to use a backup method of birth control during first pack of pills

➤ Provide instructions on when to start the pills based on information in the table that follows

➤ Instruct patient to contact you if she does not have a menstrual period when expected while taking OCs

➤ Teach the patient the OC danger signs and symptoms that signal that the OC should be discontinued immediately. Use the acronym ACHES (*A*bdominal pain, *C*hest pain, *H*eadaches, *E*ye problems, *S*evere leg pain) and also include teaching on unilateral numbness, weakness, or tingling, slurring of speech (possible stroke), hemoptysis (possible pulmonary embolism)

➤ Provide a copy of the FDA-approved and manufacturer-supplied leaflet or pamphlet to each oral contraceptive user; consent forms can be written to include a statement such as "I have been given a copy of (title) and have been encouraged to read it carefully"

➤ When starting a woman on OCs for the first time, give her a 3 month supply and have her return for a BP check and for evaluation on how she is doing on the OCs; then give her enough OCs to last for the remainder of the year

➤ Follow Up: In 1 year for annual exam

RETIMING MENSES FOR CONVENIENCE

➤ Many patients are interested in skipping placebo pills to retime or skip menses
➤ Users of monophasic 30 mcg EE OCs may take as many as 3 packs of pills without using the placebo pills, which establishes a menstrual cycle with bleeding every 10th week rather than every 4th week (works less effectively with triphasic OCs)
➤ Patients should be cautioned to never take active OCs for less than 21 days when they retime menses for convenience

DRUG INTERACTIONS

➤ Drug interactions involving oral contraceptives are of two types
  ▪ Effects of other drugs on OC efficacy
  ▪ Effects of OCs on efficacy of other drugs
➤ **Selected interactions only are listed here!**
➤ **Consult PDR** for possible interactions when prescribing medications for patients taking oral contraceptives; advise patients to remind other health care providers to whom they present for care to do the same
➤ As a general rule, patients should use condoms throughout any cycle during which they receive antibiotic therapy (especially rifampin) and some antiseizure medications as these medications interfere with OC efficacy (may need pill with higher estrogen component to prevent BTB and pregnancy)
➤ Fluconazole, a medication frequently taken by women of childbearing age, does not interfere with OC effectiveness

INSTRUCTIONS FOR STARTING ORAL CONTRACEPTIVES

➤ Advise woman to start OCs on the first day of her menstrual cycle or on the first Sunday after her period begins (if period begins Sunday, she should take the first pill on that day)
➤ Instruct patient to take 1 pill a day until pack is finished, then
➤ If on 28-day pack, begin a new pack immediately; skip no days
➤ If using 21-day pack, stop for 7 days, and then restart (**Note**: Caution patient not to wait until period starts, but to wait 7 days after completing pack, and then start next pack)
➤ Instruct to take at the same time each day and to associate with something that is done regularly at same time of day (going to bed, brushing teeth, etc.)
➤ Explain that a backup method such as condoms or foam should be used for first seven days during the first few cycles

Adapted from Dickey, R.P. (2002). *Managing contraceptive pill patients.* 11th Edition, Durant, OK: EMIS, Inc.

INSTRUCTIONS ABOUT EARLY SIDE EFFECTS

➤ Advise that some side effects are common during the first few cycles of use, but that they should disappear after that time
➤ Side effects to expect include the following
  • Breakthrough bleeding (BTB) and spotting
  • Symptoms associated with early pregnancy, especially nausea
➤ Encourage patient to delay making a decision about discontinuing the pill until after 3rd cycle to give side effects a chance to resolve

Adapted from Dickey, R.P. (2002). *Managing contraceptive pill patients.* 11th Edition, Durant, OK: EMIS, Inc.

INSTRUCTIONS FOR DEALING WITH MISSED PILLS

First, explain to patients the difference between the 21-pill pack and the 28-pill pack (first 21 pills in 28-pill pack contain hormones and the last 7 contain no hormones)

Patients who are taking the 28-pill pack and miss any of the last 7 (reminder pills) pills can discard the missed pill(s), and take the remaining "reminder" pills as scheduled to finish the pack
They should then start the next pack on usual schedule

Patients who miss any of the 21 hormonal pills must do the following

Use back-up contraception even if one pill was missed, or even if a pill was taken as much as 12 hours late (if only 1 pill was missed or taken late, back-up contraception such as condoms should be used for 7 days or patient should abstain from sex for 7 days)

Advise Patient to Get Back on Schedule by Following These Guidelines

If patient is <24 hours late in taking a pill	Take the missed pill immediately and return to the daily pill-taking routine making sure to take the next pill at the regular time
If patient is 24 hours late in taking a pill	Take both the missed pill and today's pill at the same time
If patient is >24 hours late in taking one pill, and is late for or completely missed a second pill as well	Take the last pill that was missed immediately; take the next pill on time; throw out the other missed pills, and take the rest of the pills in pack right on schedule. Use condoms for 7 days or abstain from sex for 7 days

If a pill was completely missed during the third week of pills (pills 15-21), advise the patient to do the following
- Finish the remainder of the hormonal pills in pack (take through pill 21 if using a 28-pill pack)
- Do not take a week off pills if using a 21-day pill pack OR do not take the last 7 pills (the nonhormonal pills) in the 28-pill pack
- Begin taking a new pack of pills as soon as the hormonal pills in the current pack have been taken
- Advise patient that she might not have a period until the end of the second pack of pills, but missing a period is not harmful
- In all cases, back-up contraception for at least 7 days must be used

Adapted from Hatcher, R.A., Trussel, J., Stewart, F., Cates, W., Stewart, G., Guest, F., & Kowal, D. (1998). *Contraceptive Technology*, 17th edition, New York: Ardent Media, Inc., pp 517-518.

H.   **Norplant** is a long-acting subdermal contraceptive implant that is currently not available in the US

I.   **Depo-Provera** is an injectable form of long-acting progesterone with a mechanism of action similar to that of other progestin-only contraceptives; a good choice for women in whom estrogen-containing OCs are contraindicated, barrier methods are inadvisable because of compliance problems, and in women older than age 35 who smoke

1.   **Effectiveness**: About 0.3% of women experience an unintended pregnancy within the first year with perfect use

2.   **Advantages**: Easy to use, decreased menstrual flow and avoidance of the rare but serious complications attributable to estrogen use

3.   **Disadvantages**: Unpredictable vaginal bleeding, adverse changes in lipids, patients are more likely to experience weight gain than patients using combined hormonal methods

4.   How Administered: Usual dose is 150 mg, given IM every 12 weeks

a.   Initial dose should be administered by the 5th day of menses in nonpostpartum women

b.   In non-nursing postpartum women, initial dose should be given within first 5 days postpartum and at 6 weeks postpartum for breastfeeding mothers

c.   Approximately half of women using this method experience amenorrhea after a year of injections (a harmless side effect that may be desired by the patient)

Patient Education Relating to Use of Depo-Provera

➤   Advise to use a backup form of contraception for the first seven days after the initial injection (may not be necessary if first injection given during first 5 days after the beginning of a normal menstrual period)

➤   Remind to return every 12 weeks for a repeat injection

➤   Explain that unpredictable menstrual bleeding, most often decreased blood flow, is common

➤   Review "red flags" with patient--repeated, very painful headaches, heavy bleeding, depression, severe pain in the lower abdomen, prolonged pain or bleeding at injection site

➤   Remind patients that this method provides no protection against sexually transmitted diseases

➤   Back-up methods of contraception must always be used when >one week late for injection

➤   For patients who are late for their injection and have unprotected intercourse, advise them to contact healthcare clinician regarding options; one option is emergency contraception; by calling (1-888-NOT-2-LATE) patients can be provided with phone numbers of 5 providers of emergency contraception in the area

---

J.   **Lunelle** is an injectable contraceptive administered every 28 days (may be given up to 33 days after the previous injection). Each 0.5 cc dose contains 25 mg medproxyprogesterone acetate and 5 mg estradiol cypionate. The injection is given intramuscularly into the deltoid or gluteus maximus; the initial dose is given within the first 5 days of the menstrual cycle. Suitable candidates for the use of Lunelle include women who prefer regular cycles to amenorrhea and who find monthly injection acceptable and accessible (**Note:** Lunelle [in the pre-filled syringe deliver system] has been voluntarily recalled by the manufacturer, Pharmacia, because of a production error that may have resulted in insufficient dosing. Lunelle packaged in vials is not affected by this recall. For more information, healthcare clinicians may call 800-323-4204 and patients may call 800-691-6813)

1.   **Effectiveness:** Failure rate within the first year is 0.1-0.4/100 women
2.   **Advantages:** Menstrual regularity, decreased ovulatory and menstrual pain, convenient, a good method for women who are forgetful with daily pills; does not disrupt spontaneity of intercourse; rapidly reversible; may have less adverse effects on lipid profile than combined OCs.
3.   **Disadvantages:** Possible increased spotting in the first month of use, side effects such as depression, anxiety, irritability, fatigue and other mood changes. Not suitable for women who fear injections
4.   **Precautions**: See precautions for combined OCs
5.   **Patient teaching**: Advise patients to be alert for "ACHES," as with Combined OCs

K.   **Ortho Evra** is a new transdermal contraceptive patch that is changed weekly for three weeks, then reapplied after a 7-day patch-free interval during which a withdrawal bleed will occur (i.e., a new patch is applied weekly for 3 weeks; week 4 is patch-free). The thin matrix-type transdermal patch contains three layers; the middle layer holds and releases the active hormones norelgestromin (150 mcg/day) and ethinyl estradiol (20 mcg/day). Evra is similar to combined OCs in contraceptive effectiveness and cycle control, and may be considered as a contraceptive option for women who are eligible to take combined OCs and other estrogen-containing contraceptives

1.   **Advantages:** Ortho Evra may be a good method for women who are forgetful with daily pill-taking or fearful of injections; highly effective; rapidly reversible
2.   **Disadvantages:** Visibility of the patch decreases user privacy; site reactions; may come off with exercise or swimming (detachment is uncommon); shares similar side effects with combined OCs; may be less effective in women weighing greater than 198 pounds
3.   **Precautions:** See precautions for Combined OCs.
4.   **Patient teaching** should include:
        a.   Apply the patch to the abdomen, upper chest (not the breasts), upper outer arm, or buttocks at the beginning of the menstrual cycle
        b.   A new patch is applied weekly for three weeks; week four is patch-free
        c.   No decals, stickers, or other decorations should be applied to the patch
        d.   Patients should be instructed to rotate the application site (may use the same anatomical area but rotate the site)
        e.   Dispensed in packages of 3 patches for use in 1 cycle; single replacement patches are also available
        f.   Patients should be alert for "ACHES" as with combined OCs

L.   **NuvaRing** is a combined contraceptive vaginal ring containing the progestin etonogestrel and ethinyl estradiol (EE). It is inserted by the patient and worn within the vagina for a three-week period, then discarded. After 7 days, during which a withdrawal bleed occurs, a new ring is inserted. Contraceptive efficacy is similar to combination OCs. This is another good method for women who are candidates to use combined OCs but worry about forgetting daily pills

1.   **Advantages:** No fitting by healthcare clinician is needed; good for patients who dislike taking pills; may be removed for short intervals (i.e. during sexual intercourse); highly effective
2.   **Disadvantages:** May not be a suitable method for women with uterine prolapse; may forget to re-insert ring if taken out for intercourse; may forget to take ring out and insert a new one after menses

3. **Precautions:** See precautions for Combined OCs
4. **Patient teaching** should include:
   a. The ring may be removed for short periods of time but should be inserted again without undue delay (no longer than 3 hours)
   b. Patients should mark their calendars when a ring should be removed and when the next one should be inserted
   c. Patients should be alert for "ACHES", as with combined OCs

---

Patient Education Relating to Use of All Contraceptive Methods

➢ **Always** remind patients that condoms must be used with each sexual encounter to provide protection against STDs regardless of the method used for contraception

---

M. **Postcoital emergency contraception** (EC) for patients who have unintended unprotected intercourse can be provided via two hormonal regimens—combined estrogen-progestin (Preven and Yuzpe) and progestin only (Plan B). Both Preven and Plan B are **dedicated** products specifically marketed for emergency contraception; however, the products listed in the following table have been declared safe and effective by the FDA for use as emergency contraception (Yuzpe method)
   1. The Preven kit utilizes a combined estrogen-progestin regimen
      a. Contains 4 tabs with a combination of ethinyl estradiol 50 mcg and levonorgestrel 250 mcg as well as a home pregnancy test and a patient education booklet
      b. Dosing: 2 tabs PO within 72 hours of unprotected intercourse or a contraceptive failure and 2 tabs 12 hours later **(see M.8.b. below for comments on the 72-hour time limit)**
   2. The Plan B kit utilizes a progestin-only regimen
      a. Contains 2 doses of 0.75 mg levonorgestrel and patient education booklet; no pregnancy test is included
      b. Dosing: 1 tab PO as soon as possible or within 72 hours of unprotected intercourse followed by the second tab 12 hours later **(see M.8.b. below for comments on the 72-hour time limit)**
   3. The Yuzpe regimen, standard therapy for EC for many decades utilizes large doses of ethinyl estradiol plus levonorgestrel or norgestrel per dose
      a. These hormones are found in many brands of combined oral contraceptives available in the US
      b. The following table presents selected regimens for administering these drugs for emergency contraception

---

REGIMENS FOR ORAL EMERGENCY CONTRACEPTIVE USE IN THE UNITED STATES

Brand	Pills per dose	Ethynyl estradiol per dose (mg)	Progestin per dose (mg)
Ovral	2 white pills	100	0.50
Alesse	5 pink pills	100	0.50
Nordette	4 light-orange pills	120	0.60
Levlen	4 light-orange pills	120	0.60
Lo/Ovral	4 white pills	120	0.60
Triphasil	4 yellow pills	120	0.50
Tri-Levlen	4 yellow pills	120	0.50

The treatment schedule is one dose within 72 hours after unprotected intercourse, and another dose 12 hours later

Adapted from *Brands of Oral Contraceptives That Can Be Used For Emergency Contraception in the United States.* Available at http://www.not-2-late.com Accessed March 11, 2002.

✓ No laboratory testing including a pregnancy test is necessary before prescribing EC

✓ Assessment can be done entirely by history; examination and laboratory tests are not necessary

✓ A strong medical and legal case exists for prescribing EC over-the-counter as is done in many other countries

✓ Patient will report whether she had unprotected/inadequately protected intercourse; the determination of whether the act was not adequately protected should be left to her judgment

4. Clinicians should use encounters for emergency contraception as an opportunity to counsel patients about contraceptive options and avoidance of unintended pregnancies
5. **Effectiveness**: Reduces the risk of pregnancy by about 75% (**Note**: Risk of becoming pregnant during unprotected intercourse during 2nd or 3rd week of cycle is about 8 of every 100 women; with ECs, this is reduced to about 2 out of every 100 women, which represents a 75% reduction)
6. **Side effects**: About 42% of women who take ECs have nausea and about 16% have vomiting; patients can minimize nausea and vomiting by using the levonorgestrel regimen (Plan B); in addition, pretreatment with the antiemetic drug meclizine can significantly reduce the chance of these side effects. Once nausea occurs, antiemetics are unlikely to be effective (Note: Advising patient to take with food to reduce nausea and vomiting lacks merit with these particular drugs)
    a. Preferred patient management when vomiting occurs shortly after taking EC is unknown
    b. Some experts believe that vomiting indicates that sufficient quantities of steroid have been absorbed and the dose need not be repeated
    c. Others recommend repeating the dose, particularly if vomiting occurs shortly after the dose is taken (within 1 hour)
7. **Safety**: Almost all women can safely use ECs
    a. Not indicated for women with a suspected or confirmed pregnancy because the treatment will not work if the woman is already pregnant (however, evidence suggests that no harm would occur to her, the course of her pregnancy, or the fetus if emergency contraception were used in error)
    b. Treatment may not be appropriate in women with active migraine or marked neurologic symptoms
    c. In women with a history of stroke or blood clots in the lungs or legs, treatment with progestin-only pills may be preferable (Plan B)
8. Some data indicate that emergency contraceptive hormones are more effective the sooner after intercourse they are taken
    a. In a large WHO clinical trial, pregnancy was prevented in 77% of cases if the Yuzpe regimen was used on the first day after intercourse, but only 31% of cases if it was used on the third day—other studies have found no decrease in effectiveness with delay of treatment
    b. The 72-hour time limit should be considered a guideline only; women should be advised to use the treatment as soon as possible after unprotected intercourse, but treatment should **not be withheld** from those women who present past the 72-hour time limit
    c. To avoid delays in treatment, consideration should be given to prescribing over the telephone, having after-hours systems in place, and providing prescriptions for EC to patients at their annual examination
9. The Copper-T IUD has also been approved for emergency contraception and can be inserted up to five days after unprotected intercourse; reduces the risk of pregnancy following unprotected intercourse by more than 99%

Patient Education Relating to Use of Emergency Contraception -- Counsel patient as follows:

➡ Hormonal contraception is very safe
  - Prevents pregnancy from starting which is fundamentally different from interruption of an already established pregnancy
  - Probably works via multiple mechanisms (e.g., inhibition of ovulation, alterations in endometrium, changes to the cervical mucus, alterations in transport of sperm or egg through the reproductive tract, interference with corpus luteum function, and direct inhibition of fertilization) that may depend on timing of administration
  - Should not be confused with medical abortion—six to seven days elapse between a coital act and establishment of pregnancy, defined as implantation—EC acts in the interval to prevent pregnancy
➡ EC cannot interrupt an established pregnancy—by the time a pregnancy is established, EC will no longer be effective
➡ EC is not intended for regular use—unlike regular contraceptive methods—because it is less effective and has more side effects than other methods
➡ Repeated need for EC is a sign that the currently used approach to contraception is not working well and other approaches should be considered–options that are appropriate should be identified with the help of the healthcare clinician
➡ For more information relating to emergency contraception, consult the following emergency contraception web sites:
  - www.not-2-late.com (also found at e.Princeton.edu)
  - www.backupyourbirthcontrol.org

DYSMENORRHEA

I.   Definition: Pain that occurs in lower abdomen/pelvis around the time of menses that has no anatomic cause

II.   Pathogenesis

    A.   Primary dysmenorrhea results from a cascade of events precipitated by increased levels of prostaglandin $F_2\alpha$ ($PGF_2\alpha$), leukotrienes, and vasopressin
        1.   These hormones lead to alterations in uterine basal tone, and increases in uterine contraction strength and frequency, resulting in vasospasm and reductions in uterine blood flow
        2.   Pain occurs as a result of tissue hypoxia and ischemia

    B.   Secondary dysmenorrhea is painful uterine contractions due to a clinically identifiable cause, and may be classified as follows:
        1.   External to the uterus (examples are endometriosis, tumors, adhesions, and nongynecologic causes)
        2.   Within the wall of the uterus (examples are adenomyosis, leiomyomas)
        3.   Within the cavity of the uterus (examples are polyps and infection)

III. Clinical Presentation

    A.   Approximately 25% of women of childbearing age in the US have dysmenorrhea, with about 10% having levels of discomfort that cause absence from school or work

    B.   Incidence of primary dysmenorrhea is as follows
        1.   Greatest in women in teens and early 20s
        2.   Declines in women in their 30s and 40s
        3.   Uncommon during initial 3-6 menstrual periods when ovulation is not yet well established

    C.   Secondary dysmenorrhea increases in incidence as women grow older due to the increased prevalence of processes that cause the condition among older women

    D.   Pain of primary dysmenorrhea is characterized by the following
        1.   Onset is within 6-12 months after menarche and occurs only during ovulatory cycles
        2.   Occurs within a few hours before or at the onset of menstruation (lasts 24-72 hours each month)
        3.   Located in suprapubic area and radiates to back, upper thighs
        4.   Associated with diarrhea, nausea, and vomiting in some women

    E.   Women with secondary dysmenorrhea usually experience pain consistent with the underlying pathology such as the following
        1.   GI symptoms, UTI symptoms, and so on suggest nongynecologic causes
        2.   Dyspareunia and pelvic pain unrelated to menses (but also occurring with menses) suggest causes such as endometriosis, infection (PID), adenomyosis, and leiomyomas

IV.   Diagnosis/Evaluation

    A.   History
        1.   Obtain a complete menstrual history and contraceptive history
        2.   Question patient about location of pain, when it begins, if it radiates, if there are associated symptoms of nausea, vomiting, or diarrhea
        3.   Inquire if pain occurs independently of menses in addition to occurring with menses. Ask if there is dyspareunia
        4.   Ask if there are urinary tract symptoms, if there is any vaginal discharge
        5.   Question patient about treatments tried and results

    B.   Physical Examination
        1.   Measure blood pressure, pulse rate, temperature
        2.   Evaluate heart and lungs
        3.   Perform abdominal exam, evaluating for bowel sounds, tenderness, masses, rigidity, guarding, rebound tenderness

4. Perform pelvic exam; inspect cervix for mucopurulent discharge from the endocervix; gently scrape cervix to test for friability

5. Perform bimanual exam to check for adnexal tenderness, uterine tenderness, and cervical motion tenderness

C. Differential Diagnosis
1. For primary dysmenorrhea, the most important differential diagnosis to consider is that of secondary dysmenorrhea
2. For secondary dysmenorrhea, must consider the following
   a. Intrauterine causes such as adenomyosis, myomas, polyps, IUDs, infection
   b. Extrauterine causes such as endometriosis, tumors, inflammation, adhesions, and nongynecologic causes

D. Diagnostic Tests
1. For primary dysmenorrhea, none indicated
2. For secondary dysmenorrhea, H & P should guide test selection

V. Plan/Management

A. For secondary dysmenorrhea, treatment of the underlying cause is indicated; if no obvious cause is uncovered, refer to expert for management

B. For primary dysmenorrhea, drugs that suppress the production of prostaglandins (PGs) are indicated; best accomplished by using nonsteroidal anti-inflammatory drugs (NSAIDs) at scheduled intervals to prevent re-formation of prostaglandin metabolites and pain recurrence

C. NSAIDs inhibit prostaglandin synthesis and exhibit antiinflammatory and analgesic activity
1. The most commonly used NSAIDs for dysmenorrhea come from two classes: fenamates and propionic acids. Important to remind patient to take at scheduled intervals and not PRN
2. Fenamates are considered the best choice of NSAIDs because they act as antiprostaglandins preventing both the production of PGs and binding of PG to its receptor
   a. Mefenamic acid (Ponstel) 500 mg initial dose, then 250 mg Q 6 H
   b. Has the advantage of more rapid onset and longer duration of activity (naproxen has the same advantage)
3. Propionic Acids are also a good choice
   a. Naproxen (Naprosyn) 500 mg initial dose, then 250 mg Q 6-8 H, OR
   b. Ibuprofen (Motrin) 400-800 mg Q 4-8 H, OR
   c. Naproxen sodium (Anaprox) 550 mg initial dose, then 275 mg Q 8-12 H
4. Drug that is selected for treatment should be tried over the course of 2-4 cycles before success or failure is judged
5. If treatment failure occurs with one class, the second trial should utilize the other class
6. Patients almost always respond to this therapy; because this treatment is very successful, a failure to achieve pain relief in the patient should prompt a reevaluation of the diagnosis of primary dysmenorrhea

D. The newest class of NSAIDs, the cyclooxygenase-2 (COX-2) specific inhibitor, includes several drugs that have been approved for treatment of primary dysmenorrhea: one example is rofecoxib (Vioxx)
1. Dosing is 25-50 mg once daily x 2-3 days each month for women 18 years of age and older; adolescents <18 years, not recommended
2. May or may not be beneficial in treatment of women with history of GI bleeding or ulceration (but with short course of NSAID treatment needed each month, this is usually not an issue); use in healthy women may not be warranted because of the very high cost (about $3/tablet) and the reluctance of some insurance companies to pay for the medication unless need can be clearly demonstrated (patient must have failed treatment with other, much cheaper, NSAIDs)

E. Oral contraceptives are also highly effective and may be used in addition to or instead of NSAIDs if NSAIDs prove inadequate or if the patient also has contraceptive needs
1. Oral contraceptives prevent fluctuations of endogenous progesterone levels and are first-line therapy for patients who also desire contraception
2. Almost all patients with primary dysmenorrhea achieve good pain relief with use of OCs
3. Low dose combination oral contraceptives should be prescribed if there are no contraindications

F. Nonpharmacologic management
1. A regular aerobic exercise program may be helpful and should be recommended
2. Use of acupuncture and acupressure on a weekly basis may also be helpful
3. Use of a transcutaneous electrical nerve stimulation (TENS) unit is effective in some patients

G. Follow Up
1. In 3-6 months to evaluate treatment efficacy
2. If neither NSAIDs nor hormonal therapy provide relieve after 3-6 months of therapy, refer patient for workup for causes of secondary amenorrhea

PREMENSTRUAL SYNDROME

I. Definition: A recurrent cyclical symptom complex that occurs with greatest frequency and severity in the late luteal phase (5-11 days prior to onset of menses) and abates within 1-2 days of the onset of menses

II. Pathogenesis

A. No single etiology has been identified and several mechanisms for pathogenesis have been described

B. Most evidence suggests that normal fluctuations in ovarian gonadal steroids result in aberrant responses to target tissues, particularly those located in the brain
1. Among the many mechanisms that have been postulated to explain these aberrant responses are
a. Altered metabolism of progesterone by the CNS, resulting in altered CNS reactivity and transmission, or
b. Preexisting or induced alterations in CNS transmission that result in altered responsivity to normal gonadal steroid fluctuations
2. The underlying brain dysfunction is triggered in a high-estrogen or high-estrogen and high-progesterone milieu—the milieu at ovulation or during the luteal phase

III. Clinical Presentation

A. Incidence of PMS is reported to be as high as 40% of women of reproductive age; however, only about 5% experience symptoms severe enough to limit daily functioning

B. Disorder is more prevalent in women from 30-40 years of age, and is more frequent in women with history of postpartum depression or affective illness

C. PMS presents as irritability, depression, crying spells, mood swings, sleep disturbance, appetite changes, and changes in libido; this presentation is similar to that seen in mood disorders and anxiety

D. Patients with true PMS will have symptoms in the luteal phase only

E. PMS is associated only with **ovulatory** menstrual cycles

F. Diagnosis is made on the basis of history of a symptom-free follicular phase in contrast to emotional and physical disturbances that characterize the luteal phase

G. Diagnostic criteria for premenstrual dysphoric disorder (PMDD) are contained in the table below, adapted from the fourth edition of the *Diagnostic and Statistical Manual of Mental Disorders*. Focus is on psychological symptoms rather than on physical symptoms

H. Clinically, the two conditions--PMS and PMDD--overlap
1. Many women with PMS meet the diagnostic criteria for PMDD
2. PMDD is a much more narrowly defined disorder than PMS
3. Presently, PMS and PMDD appear to be two points on a continuum, but further research is needed

IV. Diagnosis/Evaluation

   A. History: (**Note**: Be cautious in accepting patient's self-diagnosis of PMS)
      1. Ask about age at onset of symptomatology; when in cycle symptoms are experienced; most significant symptoms; degree of severity
      2. Inquire about variations from cycle to cycle
      3. Using the diagnostic criteria for PMDD, ask patient if the 11 symptoms listed are present during last week of luteal phase (define luteal phase for patient) during menstrual cycles (**Note**: This is the best approach to the patient who reports significant impairment)
      4. Inquire about previous history of depression; previous treatment for PMS and results
      5. Determine if patient is experiencing dysmenorrhea (many women confuse PMS with dysmenorrhea), situational depression, or an eating disorder
      6. Obtain data regarding drug and alcohol use; obtain medication history
      7. Use the SAFE Questions to screen for spousal abuse (see DOMESTIC VIOLENCE: INTIMATE PARTNER ABUSE section)

   B. Physical Examination: No specific physical findings aid in diagnosis; physical and pelvic exams as part of a general health survey may be completed, however

   C. Differential Diagnosis
      1. Depression
      2. Anxiety disorder
      3. Relationship discord/domestic violence
      4. Drug/alcohol abuse
      5. Eating disorder
      6. Dysmenorrhea
      7. Hypothyroidism

   D. Diagnostic Tests: None indicated unless hypothyroidism is suspected (**Note**: Make certain patient understands that laboratory testing is not helpful in most cases)

V. Plan/Management

   A. Prospective data collection by the patient for at least 2 menstrual cycles must be done to establish pattern of symptoms and establish diagnosis

   B. Several commercially available checklists can be used by the patient to record occurrence and severity of symptoms on a daily basis throughout entire cycle. Available forms are the *Menstrual Distress Questionnaire* (Moos, 1969) and the *Premenstrual Syndrome Symptomatology Questionnaire* (Vargyas, 1986) [see reference list]

C. After 2 months of data collection related to occurrence and severity of symptoms, interpretation of data can be made
    1. The suspected diagnosis of PMS is confirmed if other disorders (see differential diagnosis) are ruled out, and patient's symptomatology is limited to luteal phase
    2. Patients who report a high degree of symptomatology throughout menstrual cycle should be referred for further evaluation, as PMS is unlikely

D. Treatment must be individualized based on symptoms

CONSERVATIVE MEASURES FOR SYMPTOM MANAGEMENT

- **Support and reassurance**: Patient should know that her problems are not uncommon
- **Stress reduction**: Many women benefit from formal instruction in stress management techniques such as relaxation exercises, biofeedback, and reflexology
- **Education**: Monitoring daily symptoms will help patient obtain a degree of control in life and will allow her to avoid making major decisions when symptoms are worse
- **Diet**: Advise to eat a well-balanced diet (see NUTRITION)
- **Caffeine**: Suggest that patient attempt a trial of caffeine elimination to determine if this alleviates her symptoms (**Note**: Suggest that use be tapered to avoid caffeine-withdrawal headaches)
- **Exercise**: Personal preferences should be taken into account, but some type of regular daily activity should be undertaken (**Note**: Exercise is a great stress-reducer)
- **Vitamin Supplementation**: Studies to date suggest that calcium and magnesium supplementation may be helpful (1,200 mg/day of calcium carbonate and 200-400 mg/day of magnesium)
- **Herbal and other therapies**: Women should not be discouraged from trying therapies such as teas and herbs so long as ingredients are clearly identified, the products are safe, and the patient's symptoms are not severe; ask patient to bring in product for you to evaluate the ingredients

---

E. Pharmacologic therapies may also be used in conjunction with the conservative measures listed above

---

PHARMACOLOGIC THERAPIES FOR SYMPTOM RELIEF

- NSAIDs can be prescribed for those patients with premenstrual and menstrual pain including headache, cramping, low back pain, breast tenderness. See section on DYSMENORRHEA for appropriate NSAIDs and dosages
- Selective serotonin reuptake inhibitors are often used for treating PMS particularly in patients whose symptoms are severe or who fail to respond to conservative measures listed above
  - Fluoxetine (Prozac, Sarafem) 10-20 mg PO QD in AM; may be appropriate for women with complaints of depression
  - Sertraline hydrochloride (Zoloft) 50-100 mg PO QD; may be appropriate for women who complain of fatigue or insomnia
  - Paroxetine (Paxil) 10 mg PO QD
  - Advise patient about common side effects, be aware of drug interactions and monitor response at 3 months
- Oral contraceptives work well for some women; most effective when symptoms of PMS are primarily physical – less helpful when mood symptoms are the central complaint
  - This method is most appropriate in women needing contraception

---

F. Follow Up
    1. In 2 months to review diary
    2. Every 3-6 months until symptoms controlled

MENOPAUSE

I.   Definition: Physiologic cessation of menses for 12 consecutive months as a result of follicular depletion; other important definitions include the following:

    A.   Perimenopause: Changes in ovarian function that occur in the years preceding the permanent cessation of menstruation (average duration is about 5 years); ovulation occurs irregularly as a result of fluctuations in the hormones of the hypothalamic-pituitary-ovarian axis as menopause approaches

    B.   Postmenopause: Period of time dating from the last menstrual period regardless of whether the menopause was induced or spontaneous

    C.   Premature menopause: "Natural" ovarian failure before age 40

    D.   Artificial menopause: Cessation of menses following surgical removal of ovaries

    E.   Delayed menopause: Cessation of menses after age 54

    F.   Climacteric: Refers to the entire transition from the reproductive to the postreproductive interval in a woman's life

II.   Natural History

    A.   A major factor in the onset of menopause is failure of ovarian follicular development and subsequent ovarian hormone depletion

    B.   There is decreased negative feedback on the hypothalamic-pituitary unit with increased levels of follicle stimulating hormone (FSH) and luteinizing hormone (LH)

    C.   When ovaries no longer produce estrogen and cannot respond to FSH, ovulation ceases and menstruation ends

III. Clinical Presentation

    A.   Average age of onset is 51 years; in the US today, approximately 50 million women are 50 years of age and older

    B.   Women who smoke cigarettes experience menopause 1-2 years earlier than nonsmokers

    C.   Approximately 5 years prior to menopause, the length of the menstrual cycle becomes more variable
        1.   Patients may experience a combination of long, short, normal, and anovulatory cycles during this time period
        2.   All women, however, do not go through the same transition of regular menses to irregular menses to amenorrhea as they approach menopause

    D.   The main clinical consequence of menopause is the cessation of secretion of ovarian hormones that accompany folliculogenesis—the two main hormones made by the follicle and corpus luteum during a menstrual cycle are estradiol and progesterone (ovaries also secrete androgens, but the decline in secretion is usually not clinically apparent at the time of menopause)

E. Certain physiologic changes are the consequence of decreased secretion of ovarian steroid hormones, primarily estrogen; withdrawal of estrogen as well as the hypoestrogenism (which becomes chronic over time) are responsible for the presenting signs and symptoms which begin during perimenopause and produce long-term consequences during postmenopause

    1. The most common symptoms relate to vasomotor instability; >75% of women at menopause report hot flashes ("flushes") and/or night sweats (thought to be caused by a combination of fluctuating estradiol levels and a narrowing of the thermoneutral zone)

        a. The first physical manifestation of ovarian failure

        b. Skin of face and anterior chest becomes flushed for about 90 seconds; may feel cool with resolution of flush and experience sweats (commonly occurs at night)

        c. Caused by declining estradiol-17β secretion by the ovarian follicles

    2. Other common symptoms that may or may not be directly related to estrogen deficiency (but which often occur at this time) include insomnia (probably related to vasomotor symptoms), mood swings, and depression (Note: As a group, postmenopausal women **do not** experience more depression than women in younger age groups)

    3. Atrophy of the genitourinary tract eventually occurs over a period of 5-10 years due to chronic hypoestrogenism

        a. Vulvar epithelium thins and pubic hair becomes sparse

        b. Labia majora and minora become flattened

        c. Vaginal mucosa atrophies (atrophic vaginitis) and becomes thin and pale with loss of rugae; vaginal pH increases to >5; consequences of these changes include vaginal dryness leading to dyspareunia which impacts sexual desire and response

        d. Uterus and cervix become smaller; uterine prolapse is more common at this time

        e. Paravaginal tissues supporting the bladder and rectum become atrophic resulting in loss of support for the bladder (cystocele) and rectum (rectocele)

        f. Lining of the urinary tract atrophies and may cause symptoms of dysuria and frequency

    4. Breasts eventually change in size and contour due to atrophy of epithelial glands and ducts; breasts droop, flatten, and nipples become smaller and flatter over a period of 5-10 years (from chronic hypoestrogenism)

    5. Bone loss, which begins slowly at about age 35, greatly accelerates at menopause

        a. Bone demineralization is a natural consequence of aging (occurs in both genders)

        b. Onset occurs 15 to 20 years earlier in women than in men due to acceleration after ovarian failure

F. Cardiovascular disease is the major cause of death after menopause, with almost 50% of women developing coronary artery disease and about 30% dying from it; the possible cardioprotective effects of hormone-replacement therapy has led to enthusiasm for its use in recent years but that enthusiasm was greatly dampened in 2002

IV. Diagnosis/Evaluation

A. History

    1. Determine severity, onset, and duration of symptoms

    2. Obtain complete gynecologic histories (include menstrual, pregnancy, vaginal or pelvic infections, gynecologic surgical procedures, pelvic pain/discomfort, vaginal bleeding not related to menses, sexual and contraceptive histories)

    3. Inquire about birth control methods currently using (in perimenopausal women)

    4. Obtain a complete medical and medication history

    5. Assess risk status for coronary heart disease, osteoporosis, breast cancer, and endometrial cancer

B. Physical Examination

    1. Measure vital signs and make a general evaluation of appearance

    2. Measure height and weight

    3. Perform clinical breast examination and consider review of breast self-exam with the patient; keep in mind that evidence is insufficient to recommend for or against teaching or performing routine breast self-examination, according to the US Preventive Services Task Force (2002)

    4. Auscultate heart and palpate peripheral pulses

    5. Auscultate lungs

    6. Perform abdominal examination to rule out masses and organomegaly

    7. Perform pelvic and speculum examinations

        a. Examine vulvar skin and mucous membranes for abnormalities. The characteristic changes of postmenopause occur only after 5-10 years of estrogen deprivation; thus such changes are not apparent in perimenopausal and recently menopausal women)

b. Examine vagina (signs of chronic hypoestrogenism should not be present for 5-10 years postmenopause)

c. Examine cervix, noting size and shape

d. Perform a bimanual examination

    (1) Eventually the postmenopausal uterus becomes about half the size of a woman's fist (this is a long-term consequence of estrogen depletion, and is **not** found in women who are in early menopause)

    (2) Consider a malignancy, endometrial hyperplasia, or a fibroid when the uterus size or shape is abnormal

    (3) Ovaries are often not palpable in menopausal women, so any adnexal mass should prompt further evaluation

e. Perform a rectovaginal examination; colon cancer is the fourth most common cancer in women; obtain stool for occult blood in women 50 and older (see section on PERIODIC HEALTH EVALUATION for screening recommendations relating to colorectal cancer)

C. Differential Diagnosis

1. Thyroid disorders

2. Clinical depression

3. Any cause of secondary amenorrhea (see section on AMENORRHEA)

4. Always consider pregnancy

D. Diagnostic Tests

1. Consider TSH to rule out thyroid disorder (if suspected based on history and physical examination findings)

    a. Hyperthyroidism often presents with flushing, sweating, heat intolerance, heart palpitations, and insomnia

    b. Hypothyroidism often presents with menstrual disorders, fatigue, dry skin, mood swings, and weight gain

2. Diagnosis of menopause can be made with relative certainty by confirmation of estrogen deficiency via measurement of the primary premenopausal estrogen 17-β estradiol (E_2) and serum follicle stimulating hormone (FSH)

    a. Elevation of serum FSH level above 30-40 mIU/mL is diagnostic

    b. 17-β estradiol (E_2) level less than 30 pg/mL (Note: premenopausal women frequently have low levels of estradiol during menses; thus this test is not diagnostic in women who are menstruating at time of test)

    c. Maturation index of vaginal smear (vaginal hormonal cytology) was used in past as index of estrogen deficiency but is not often used today

3. Obtain Pap smear (if one has not been done in past 12 months)

4. Order mammogram if one has not been done in past 1-2 years

5. Based on woman's age and risk factors, other diagnostic testing related to prevention may be indicated (consult section on PERIODIC HEALTH EVALUATION for recommendations)

V. Plan/Management

A. Provide general counseling related to the transition to menopause; offer educational materials as appropriate

B. Review commonly experienced menopausal symptoms as well as health risks of women in this age group—specifically, cardiovascular disease and osteoporosis; review the health risks of this particular patient

C. Encourage lifestyle and nonpharmacologic therapies for health promotion such as exercise, smoking cessation, prudent diet, use of alcohol in moderation (no more than one drink per day) [for patients who ever drink alcohol], calcium and vitamin D intake (see section on NUTRITION for recommended intake of vitamin supplements)

D. Explain current recommendations relating to benefits and risks of postmenopausal hormone-replacement therapy (see table that follows); assess patient's interest in HRT

HRT: DEFINITE BENEFITS AND RISKS, PROBABLE RISKS, AND AREAS OF UNCERTAINTY RELATED TO USE

All women should be counseled regarding the definite benefits, definite risks, probable increase in risk, and areas of uncertainty related to the use of hormone-replacement therapy. Information in table is based on expert opinion at the time of this book's publication; clinicians are urged to stay abreast of current developments

Definite Benefits

Symptoms of Menopause
> Menopause-related symptoms reported most often (50-80% of women) include hot flashes, night sweats, vaginal dryness, insomnia, mood swings, and depression
> Strong evidence that hormone-replacement therapy is highly effective in controlling vasomotor and genitourinary symptoms

Osteoporosis
> Bone loss greatly accelerates at menopause
> Use of estrogen reduces risk of vertebral fractures by about 50% and risk of hip fracture by about 25%

Definite Risks

Endometrial cancer
> Long-term use of unopposed estrogen (without a progestin) increases the risk of endometrial cancer by a factor of 8 to 10
> Women with an intact uterus must be given a sufficient dose of a progestin to oppose effects of estrogen on endometrium

Venous Thromboembolism
> Postmenopausal use of estrogen increases risk of DVT by a factor of 2 to 3.5

Breast Cancer
> HRT (estrogen and progestin) increases the risk of breast cancer. In July 2002, the estrogen plus progestin arm of the Women's Health Initiative (WHI), a clinical trial with more than 27,000 predominantly healthy women (primary prevention) randomized to ERT alone, HRT, or placebo was halted after a mean of 5.2 years of follow-up when interim results showed the rates of invasive breast cancer were unacceptably high (risk decisively outweighed benefit)

Probable Increase in Risk

Gallbladder Disease
> In the Heart and Estrogen/Progestin Replacement Study (HERS), risk of gallbladder disease was 38% higher in women who received hormone therapy versus placebo

Areas of Uncertainty

Coronary Heart Disease
> HERS was specifically designed to compare effects of estrogen and progestin with placebo in 2,763 women with established CVD. HRT was expected to reduce the combined incidence of nonfatal myocardial infarction (MI) and coronary heart disease (CHD) death in women in the intervention group; instead, there was no difference in the outcomes in the two groups after an average of 4.1 years of follow-up. Moreover, there was a 52% increase in cardiovascular events in the first year in the HRT group compared with placebo; in the later years of the study, there was a nonsignificant trend toward fewer events in the treatment versus placebo group (**Note:** There have been other studies focusing on **secondary prevention** with similar results and more studies are underway)
> The WHI found an unexpected increase in the number of cardiovascular events and stroke in women taking either ERT or HRT in the first 2 years of the trial; the increase was not deemed large enough to stop the trial which was scheduled to end in 2005. The HRT arm of the trial has now been halted because of an unacceptable increase in breast cancer risk. However, a sufficient number of CHD events had occurred by 5.2 years of average follow-up to suggest to the researchers that continuation to the planned end would have been unlikely to yield a favorable result

Colorectal Cancer
> Inconclusive whether HRT impacts risk of colorectal cancer; results from the WHI showed a reduction in colorectal cancer in the hormone group which is consistent with findings from observational studies which have consistently suggested that users of HRT/ERT may be at lower risk of colorectal cancer. Mechanisms by which this reduction in risk occurs are unclear; results of other trials of postmenopausal hormone use will help resolve this area of uncertainty

Cognitive Dysfunction
> Inconclusive whether HRT has a positive impact on cognitive dysfunction

Adapted from:
Manson, J.E., & Martin, K.A. (2001). Postmenopausal hormone-replacement therapy. *New England Journal of Medicine, 345*, 34-40.
Mosca, L., Collins, P., Herrington, D.M., Mendelsohn, M.E., Pasternak, R.C., Robertson, R.M., et al. (2001). Hormone replacement therapy and cardiovascular disease: A statement for Healthcare Professions from the American Heart Association. *Circulation, 104*, 499-503.
Writing Group for the Women's Health Initiative (2002). Risks and benefits of estrogen plus progestin in healthy postmenopausal women. *Journal of American Medicine Association, 288*, 321-333.
HERS Research Group. (2002). Cardiovascular disease outcomes during 6.8 years of hormone therapy: Heart and estrogen/progestin replacement study follow-up (HERS II). *Journal of American Medicine Association, 288*, 49-57.

E. **Patients with an interest in relief of menopausal symptoms** including vasomotor symptoms (hot flashes, night sweats), genitourinary symptoms (vaginal dryness, dyspareunia, urgency, frequency, and dysuria), or symptoms of insomnia, mood swings, and dysphoria (that may or may not be related to fluctuations in estrogen levels) may be managed according to information in table that follows and also may be candidates for treatment with short-term use of HRT

Vasomotor Symptoms (hot flashes and night sweats)

Counsel Patients About Hot Flashes and Night Sweats
- Occur spontaneously but may be triggered by the following:
  o Warm environment
  o Caffeine or alcohol-containing beverages
  o Spicy foods
  o Emotional upset
- Rapid onset and resolution; usually <3 minutes in duration
- Described as waves of heat flushing skin of face and upper chest
- With resolution, woman feels cold and breaks into "cold sweat"
- Often occur in the evening or during the night
- Hot flashes/night sweats contribute to insomnia in some women
- Usually resolve spontaneously after 2-3 years

Advice for Patients for Keeping Cool
- Avoid triggers when possible
- Dress in layers to make removal of clothing easy
- Keep house/office cool; keep a small fan handy
- Keep well hydrated (at least 64 oz of water/day)

Recommend soy foods. Soybeans, in the phytoestrogen plant class, contain high-quality protein, essential fatty acids, and isoflavones (substances whose chemical structure is very similar to that of estradiol, and which are linked to many beneficial health effects). Soybeans are low in fat and contain no cholesterol. Eating whole soy foods is healthier and safer than taking soy supplements—the table below lists several types of soy foods. (**Note:** Keep in mind [and counsel patients accordingly] that evidence for use of soy and other phytoestrogens to relieve menopausal symptoms is either inconclusive or minimal; however, the FDA has authorized a health claim allowing food manufacturers to label certain soy protein food products as heart healthy)

Types of Soy Foods	Recommended Intake
Soy milk	Most experts recommend consuming about 25 grams of
Tofu, a soybean curd	soy protein/day within the context of a healthy diet
Tempeh, cooked and fermented soybeans	4 oz of firm tofu = 13 g of protein
Miso, a fermented soy paste	8 oz of soy milk = 10 g of protein
Soy or isoflavone supplements (capsules/pills) are **not** recommended	
For a free guide of soy-based recipes, refer patients to www.soyfoods.com or call 1-800-TALKSOY	

Recommend other sources of phytoestrogens, contained in whole grains, some fruits (pears, plums, strawberries) and vegetables (garlic, broccoli, carrots, sweet potatoes), and oily seeds such as flaxseed (meal and flour), sunflower seeds, and peanuts
Recommend black cohosh (Cimicifuga racemosa), traditionally used by Native Americans for gynecologic and other conditions, for hot flashes on a short-term basis (no more than 6 months). Available as Remifemin (Glaxo SmithKline); long-term use cannot be presumed to be safe because appropriate clinical studies have not been conducted. The National Institutes of Health is now supporting a clinical trial to test black cohosh and red clover, which contains isoflavones, but results are not yet available

Remind patients that not all herbs and dietary supplements are risk-free and should therefore be used cautiously
Consider use of one of the following medications to treat patients with moderate to severe vasomotor symptoms: **Note** that all are off-label uses and should therefore be prescribed cautiously
- Clonidine, a central alpha-adrenergic agonist commonly used as an antihypertensive agent. Usual dose: Patch, extended release, 0.1 mg/24 hours
- Serotonin Reuptake Inhibitor Drugs (SSRIs): Consider use of one of the following: paroxetine (Paxil) 10 mg/day, OR fluoxetine (Prozac), 20 mg/day, OR sertraline (Zoloft), 25 mg/day
- Venlafaxine (Effexor), 12.5 mg BID
- Megace (megestrol), 20 mg BID
- Consult PDR for contraindications/precautions, dosing, interactions, and adverse reactions for all medications listed here

Genitourinary Symptoms

Recommend products to increase vaginal moisture and alleviate dyspareunia: Astroglide, Replens, Lubrin, Vagisil Intimate Moisturizer, and Moist Again (all over-the-counter products)

Advise patients to stay sexually active. Caution patients regarding the use of dietary supplements of the hormone dehydroepiandrosterone (DHEA) to boost desire/responsivity. DHEA supplements, made mostly from yams and available in health food stores, can have serious side effects including liver damage (**NOTE:** There are no FDA approved products on the market for treatment of female sexual dysfunction)

Recommend intravaginal estrogen in the form of creams or rings for patients with vaginal dryness/atrophic vaginitis (over a period of years with estrogen deficiency, vaginal dryness may progress to atrophic vaginitis—see III.D.3 above for description of vaginal changes due to hypoestrogenism that result in atrophic vaginitis)

(Continued)

Genitouriary Symptoms *(continued)*

Transvaginal Estrogen Preparations

Creams
- Premarin vaginal cream, 0.625 mg/g
  Dosing: ½-1 g intravaginally QD cyclically (3 weeks on, 1 week off). Discontinue or taper after 3 months
- Estrace vaginal cream, 0.1 mg/g
  Dosing: 2 g/day x 1-2 weeks, then reduce to 1 g/day x 1-2 weeks; maintenance dose is 1 g, 1 to 3 x/week. Discontinue or taper after 3 months

Vaginal Ring
- Estring vaginal ring, releases 7.5 mcg/24 hours
  Instruct patient to insert ring deeply into upper 1/3 of vaginal vault; remove and replace after 90 days. Reassess at 3-6 month intervals

Vaginal estrogen should be used with caution as these products may cause small but measurable increases in circulating estrogen and may cause proliferative endometrial changes

---

Mood Swing, Insomnia, Dysphoria

Consider trial of SSRIs (See specifics above under *Vasomotor Symptoms*) [**Note**: Not FDA approved for this indication] Consult PDR for warnings/precautions, dosing, interactions, and adverse reactions]. Black cohosh has also been reported to be useful in stabilizing emotions

---

F. **Women who wish to manage their menopausal symptoms with HRT** and who are without contraindications may be considered for use of HRT (**NOTE:** Some experts consider menopausal symptoms a valid indication for short-term [<5 years] use of HRT in selected women without contraindications.) The US Preventive Services Task Force did not evaluate the use of HRT to treat symptoms of menopause, but did recommend that the balance of benefits and harms for an individual woman will be influenced by her personal preferences, individual risks for specific chronic diseases, and the presence of menopausal symptoms. See table below which lists selected HRT preparations and prescribing information including contraindications and precautions

G. **Women at increased risk for osteoporosis** should be managed according to section on OSTEOPOROSIS (see for screening, prevention, and treatment recommendations); the US Preventive Services Task Force recommends against the routine use of estrogen and progestin for the prevention of chronic conditions such as osteoporosis in postmenopausal women

H. **Healthy women** who are concerned about preventing cardiovascular disease should be advised that HRT should not be initiated or continued for the express purpose of primary prevention of CVD. These women should be counseled that lifestyle approaches including smoking avoidance, proper nutrition, and regular exercise are important for all women

I. **Women with multiple coronary risk factors** should be advised that HRT should not be initiated for the secondary prevention of CVD; these women should be counseled regarding lifestyle approaches as above. Lipid lowering and blood pressure control with pharmacotherapy are indicated in women who do not meet target lipid or blood pressure levels with lifestyle interventions

J. **Women with documented heart disease** should be advised that HRT does not appear to reduce the risk of cardiovascular events in women with established heart disease, and may pose an increased risk of CVD events in the first year of treatment with HRT

K. **Women with documented heart disease who have been taking HRT** for more than one or two years and who are doing well, do not necessarily need to discontinue the short-term use of HRT (less than 5 years)

OVERVIEW OF HORMONE REPLACEMENT THERAPY

In women with an intact uterus, include progestin in addition to estrogen to avoid development of endometrial hyperplasia and cancer

Oral route is most commonly used for HRT administration

Combined HRT regimens given the oral route are of **two types**: Sequential (also called cyclic) and continuous combined
- **Sequential regimen:** Estrogen is administered daily and progestin is administered on 10-14 days of each month
  Monthly withdrawal bleeding usually occurs on a regular basis
  Over time, pattern of bleeding usually remains fairly stable (withdrawal bleeding continues to occur in about 75% of women even after 1 year of therapy)
- **Continuous combined regimen**: Both estrogen and progestin are administered continuously
  Usually associated with unpredictable but infrequent bleeding in early cycles
  Amenorrhea may occur after the first year of therapy due to endometrial atrophy
  Is the **preferred regimen** in most cases because of the eventual amenorrhea that usually develops

COMMONLY USED ORAL ESTROGEN AND PROGESTIN PREPARATIONS: SEQUENTIAL REGIMEN AND CONTINUOUS COMBINED REGIMEN

For use with either the Sequential or Continuous Combined Regimens	
Estrogen Preparations	*Usual Daily Dose*
Conjugated equine estrogens (CEE)	
Premarin	0.625 mg
Esterified estrogen (EE)	
Estratab	0.625 mg
Menest	0.625 mg
Micronized estradiol	
Estrace	1.0 mg
Estropipate	
Ortho-Est	0.625 mg
For Use with Sequential Regimen	
Progestin Only Preparations	*Usual Daily Dose*
Medroxyprogesterone (MPA)	
Provera	5-10 mg (Added first 10-14 days of calendar month)
Amen	5-10 mg (As above)
Cycrin	5-10 mg (As above)
Micronized progesterone	
Prometrium	100-200 mg (Added first 10-14 days of calendar month)
For Use with Continuous Combined Regimen	
Progestin Only Preparations	*Usual Daily Dose*
Medroxyprogesterone (MPA)	
Provera	2.5 mg (daily dose)
Cycrin	2.5 mg (daily dose)

USING THE SEQUENTIAL OR CONTINUOUS COMBINED REGIMENS

Women with an intact uterus using the Sequential Regimen
Prescribe one of the estrogen preparations from the above list (daily dosing) and one of the progestin preparations listed under Sequential Regimen from above list for the **first 10-14 days** of the calendar month. Continue this regimen without interruption

Women with an intact uterus using the Continuous Combined Regimen
Prescribe one of the estrogen preparations from the above list (daily dosing) and one of the progestin preparations listed under Continuous Combined Method from above list (daily dosing) **OR**
Select a product from the table below which lists preparations combining estrogen and progesterone in a single tablet

ORAL ESTROGEN AND PROGESTIN COMBINATIONS FOR USE IN THE CONTINUOUS COMBINED REGIMEN

Product Name	Supplied As	Dosing
Prempro	Tabs containing 0.625 mg CEE and 2.5 mg MPA	1 tab PO QD
Premphase	Two packets of 14 tabs each First packet: 14 tabs each containing 0.625 mg CEE Second packet: 14 tabs each containing 0.625 mg CEE plus 5 mg MPA	1 tab PO QD
Ortho-Prefest	Tabs delivering pulsed therapy; Daily low-dose 17β-estradiol and intermittent bursts of norgestimate combined with estradiol (3 day cycle that is repeated continuously)	1 tab PO QD
Activella	Tabs containing 1 mg 17β-estrdiol and 0.5 mg norethindrone	1 tab PO QD
FemHRT	Tabs containing 5 mcg ethinyl estradiol and 1 mg norethindrone	1 tab PO QD

L. Women who are candidates for the transdermal route for estrogen replacement (women without a uterus) or estrogen-progestin replacement are those with significant liver function abnormalities (transdermal estrogen avoids first-pass liver metabolism); in addition, transdermal estrogen has a more favorable effect on serum triglycerides

Commonly Used Patches for ERT/HRT
ERT: Climara, Esclim, Vivelle   HRT: CombiPatch

M. Contraindications to HRT use are contained in the box that follows

> **Contraindications**
> Unexplained vaginal bleeding
> Active liver disease
> History of venous thromboembolism
> History of endometrial cancer
> History of breast cancer
>
> **Relative Contraindications**
> Familial hyperlipidemia
> Active gallbladder disease

N. Make certain patient understands the risks and benefits of HRT and the fact that the harms of estrogen-progestin therapy outweigh the chronic disease prevention benefits for postmenopausal women

O. Review danger signs of HRT: vaginal bleeding that does not follow the usual pattern associated with HRT, calf pain, chest pain, shortness of breath, hemoptysis, severe headache, vision problems, breast changes, abdominal pain, and jaundice

P. Follow Up
  1. Reassess at 3-6 months to determine response to therapy, whether pharmacologic or nonpharmacologic
  2. Yearly annual visit may be needed for history, physical examination, Pap smear and other diagnostic testing as well as counseling based on recommendations of the US Preventive Services Task Force (see HEALTH MAINTENANCE chapter)

VULVOVAGINAL CANDIDIASIS

I. Definition: Infection of the vulvar area and vagina by *Candida albicans* and other *Candida* sp. or yeasts

II. Pathogenesis

    A. Little is known about factors that contribute to the overgrowth of normal flora in the vagina

    B. When the complex balance of microorganisms changes, however, potentially pathogenic endogenous microorganisms that are part of the normal flora such as *Candida albicans* proliferate to numbers that cause symptoms

    C. Usually caused by *C. albicans* but occasionally caused by other *Candida* sp. or yeasts

III. Clinical Presentation

    A. Approximately 25% of all vaginal infections are due to vulvovaginal candidiasis (VVC); this condition is not transmitted sexually but is often diagnosed in women being evaluated for STDs

    B. An estimated 75% of women will have at least one episode of VVC, and 45% will have two or more episodes; approximately 10-20% of women will have complicated VVC (see box below for definition)

    C. Vulvar pruritus is the cardinal symptom and a white discharge may also be present; vulvar erythema is the most often observed sign, with edema and excoriation of the vulva also often observed; vaginal secretions have a normal pH (3.5-4.5)

    D. Primarily a disease of the childbearing years; pregnancy is the most common predisposing factor

    E. Depressed cell-mediated immunity (such as with HIV+ status, chemotherapy) also is risk factor

    F. Most healthy women with uncomplicated VVC have no precipitating factors; in a minority of women with asymptomatic *Candida* colonization, antibiotic use precipitates VVC

    G. On the basis of clinical presentation, microbiology, host factors, and response to therapy, VVC can be classified as either uncomplicated or complicated

Uncomplicated VVC	Complicated VVC

• Sporadic or infrequent vulvovaginal candidiasis
   OR
	• Recurrent vulvovaginal candidiasis
	   OR

• Mild-to-moderate vulvovaginal candidiasis
   OR
	• Severe vulvovaginal candidiasis
	   OR

• Likely to be *C. albicans*
   OR
	• Non-albicans candidiasis
	   OR

• Non-immunocompromised women	• Women with uncontrolled diabetes, debilitation, or immunosuppression or those who are pregnant

Source: Centers for Disease Control and Prevention (CDC). (2002) Sexually transmitted diseases treatment guidelines 2002. *MMWR 51* (No. RR-6) p. 45

IV. Diagnosis/Evaluation

    A. History
        1. Question about vulvar itching, discharge, odor, dysuria, dyspareunia
        2. Ask about previous occurrences of yeast infections
        3. Ask about predisposing factors such as pregnancy, recent antibiotic or estrogen therapy, history of diabetes, HIV+ status
        4. Ask about douching and use of feminine hygiene products (regular douching should always be discouraged; patients often try douching to relieve symptoms of vaginal infection that instead should be diagnosed and properly treated)

B. Physical Examination
    1. Examine vulva for erythema, edema, and excoriation
    2. Perform pelvic exam and examine vagina for erythema, white patches/plaques; note odor of secretions (should not be malodorous)

C. Diagnostic Tests
    1. Obtain sample of vaginal secretions from anterior or lateral vaginal walls on a dry swab and apply to pH paper. In candidiasis, pH of vaginal secretions is ≤4.5 (normal pH of vagina is 3.5-4.5)
    2. Microscopic examination of slide containing vaginal secretions mixed with 10% potassium hydroxide (KOH) shows typical hyphae and budding yeast

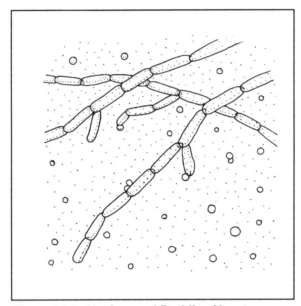

Figure 14.3. Hyphae and Budding Yeast

D. Differential Diagnosis
    1. Other common causes of vaginitis--bacterial vaginosis and trichomoniasis
    2. Common causes of cervicitis--chlamydia and gonorrhea which can sometimes cause a vaginal discharge

V. Plan/Management

A. Short-course topical formulations (i.e., single dose and 1-3 day regimens) effectively treat uncomplicated VVC

608

RECOMMENDED REGIMENS FOR TREATMENT OF UNCOMPLICATED VULVOVAGINAL CANDIDIASIS

Intravaginal Agents:

Butoconazole 2% cream 5 g intravaginally for 3 days, ***

OR

Butoconazole 2% cream 5 g (Butoconazole 1-sustained release), single intravaginal application,

OR

Clotrimazole 1% cream 5 g intravaginally for 7-14 days, ***

OR

Clotrimazole 100 mg vaginal tablet for 7 days,

OR

Clotrimazole 100 mg vaginal tablet, two tablets for 3 days,

OR

Clotrimazole 500 mg vaginal tablet, one tablet in a single application,

OR

Miconazole 2% cream 5 g intravaginally for 7 days,***

OR

Miconazole 100 mg vaginal suppository, one suppository for 7 days,***

OR

Miconazole 200 mg vaginal suppository, one suppository for 3 days,***

OR

Nystatin 100,000-unit vaginal tablet, one tablet for 14 days,

OR

Tioconazole 6.5% ointment 5 g intravaginally in a single application.

OR

Terconazole 0.4% cream 5 g intravaginally for 7 days,

OR

Terconazole 0.8% cream 5 g intravaginally for 3 days,

OR

Terconazole 80 mg vaginal suppository, one suppository for 3 days.

Oral Agent:

Fluconazole 150 mg oral tablet, one tablet in single dose

*** Over-the-counter (OTC) preparations

NOTE: The creams and suppositories in this regimen are oil-based and may weaken latex condoms and diaphragms. Refer to condom product labeling for further information

Source: Centers for Disease Control and Prevention (CDC). (2002) Sexually transmitted diseases treatment guidelines 2002. *MMWR 51* (No. RR-6) p. 45

B. Self-medication with OTC products should be used only in women who have previously been diagnosed with VVC and who experience a recurrence of the same symptoms
1. Persistence of symptoms after self-treatment signals need to seek health care
2. Recurrence within 2 months of self-treatment also indicates need to seek health care

C. Treatment of sexual partners is not necessary unless candidal balanitis is present

D. Follow-up of patients with uncomplicated VVC: Return visits only for those patients in whom symptoms persist or who experience a recurrence within 2 months of onset of initial symptoms

E. **Complicated VVC includes the following categories**: Recurrent VVC (RVVC), severe VVC, non-*albicans* VVC, compromised host, pregnancy, and HIV infection; treatment considerations for each of these categories are considered below

F. **Recurrent VVC (RVVC)** [defined as *four* or more episodes of symptomatic VVC in a 12-month period] affects a small percentage of women (<5%)
1. Pathogenesis of RVVC is poorly understood and most women with RVVC have no apparent predisposing conditions
2. Vaginal cultures should be obtained to confirm the clinical diagnosis and to identify unusual species; *Candida glabrata* does not form pseudohyphae or hyphae and is not easily recognized on microscopy
3. Conventional antimycotic therapies are not as effective against these species as against *C. albicans*
4. Routine treatment of sex partners is controversial
5. Recommended regimens for both initial and maintenance therapy are contained in the table that follows

RECOMMENDED REGIMENS FOR RECURRENT VULVOVAGINAL CANDIDIASIS
Initial Therapy: A longer duration of initial therapy is recommended
7-14 days of topical therapy (see table RECOMMENDED REGIMENS FOR TREATMENT OF UNCOMPLICATED VULVOVAGINAL CANDIDIASIS for medications)
OR
150 mg oral dose of fluconazole repeated 3 days later
This regimen is designed to achieve mycologic remission before initiating a maintenance antifungal regimen
Maintenance Therapy: Long-term treatment with antifungals is recommended for RVVC Ketoconazole, 100 mg dose once daily OR Fluconazole, 100-150 mg dose once weekly OR Itraconazole, 400 mg dose once monthly OR Itraconazole, 100 mg dose once daily
All maintenance regimens should be continued for 6 months (30%-40% of women will have recurrent disease after maintenance therapy is stopped)
Note: Patients receiving long-term ketoconazole therapy should be monitored for liver toxicity

Source: Centers for Disease Control and Prevention. (2002). Sexually transmitted diseases treatment guidelines 2002. *MMWR, 51* (No. RR-6), p. 46

G.   **Severe VVC** is defined as extensive vulvar erythema, edema, excoriation, and fissure formation
1. Clinical response rates are lower in these patients when treatment is with short courses of topical or oral therapy
2. Either 7-14 days of topical azole or 150 mg of fluconazole in two sequential doses (second dose 72 hours after initial dose) is recommended

H.   Optimal treatment of patients with **non-*albicans* VVC** remains unknown
1. Longer duration therapy (7-14 days) with a non-fluconazole azole drug is recommended as first-line therapy
2. If recurrence occurs, 600 mg of boric acid in a gelatin capsule is recommended, administered vaginally once daily for 2 weeks; this regimen has clinical and mycologic eradication rates of about 70%
3. Referral to a specialist is advised if recurrences continue

I.   Treatment of patients with VVC and an underlying debilitating medical condition (**compromised host**)
1. Efforts to correct modifiable conditions should be made
2. More prolonged (i.e., 7-14 days) conventional antimycotic treatment is necessary as these patients usually have poor response to short-term therapies

J.   Treatment of **pregnant women** with VVC: Only topical azole therapies, applied for 7 days, are recommended for use among pregnant women

K.   Treatment of **HIV-infected women** with VVC should not differ from that for seronegative women
1. Symptomatic VVC is more frequent in seropositive women and correlates with severity of immunodeficiency
2. Although long-term prophylactic therapy with fluconazole at a dose of 200 mg weekly has been effective in reducing *C. albicans* colonization and symptomatic VVC, it is not recommended for routine primary prophylaxis in HIV-infected women in the absence of recurrent VVC

L.   Follow-up of women with complicated VVC is variable, depending on patient diagnosis and recurrence rate

REFERENCES

Abramowicz, M. (2002). Ortho Evra: A contraceptive patch. *The Medical Letter, 44*, 5-8.

Abramowicz, M. (2002). Yasmin—an oral contraceptive with a new progestin. *The Medical Letter, 44*, 55-57.

Ballagh, S.A. (2001). Vaginal ring hormone delivery systems in contraception and menopause. *Clinical Obstetrics & Gynecology, 44*, 106-113.

Barbieri, R.L. (1999). Amenorrhea. In R.L. Barbieri, S.L. Berga, A.H. DeCherney, J. Hade, & E.F. Sheets (Eds.), *Gynecology in primary care: A step-by-step approach* (pp. 1-6). New York: Scientific American, Inc.

Bastian, L.A., Smith, C.M., & Nanda, K. (2003). Is this woman perimenopausal? *Journal of the American Medical Association, 289*, 895-902.

Beckman, C.R., Ling, F.W., Laube, D.W., Smith, R.P, Barzansky, B.M., & Herbert, W.N. (2002). *Obstetrics and gynecology* (4th ed.). Philadelphia: Lippincott Williams & Wilkins.

Berga, S.L. (1999). Premenstrual syndrome. In R.L. Barbieri, S.L. Berga, A.H. DeCherney, J. Hade, & E.F. Sheets (Eds.), *Gynecology in primary care: A step-by-step approach* (pp. 11-15). New York: Scientific American, Inc.

Burkman, R.T. (2001). Oral contraceptives: Current status. *Clinical Obstetrics & Gynecology, 44*, 62-72.

Centers for Disease Control and Prevention. (2002). Sexually transmitted diseases treatment guidelines 2002. *MMWR, 51*(No.RR-6), 1-78.

Chan, P.D., & Winkle, C.R. (2002). *Current clinical strategies: Gynecology and obstetrics.* Laguna Hills, CA: CCPS Publishing.

Chen, C., Weiss, N.S., Newcomb, P., Barlow, W., & White, E. (2002). Hormone replacement therapy in relation to breast cancer. *Journal of the American Medical Association, 287*, 734-741.

DeCheney, A.H., & Hade, J. (1999). Abnormal vaginal bleeding. In R.L. Barbieri, S.L. Berga, A.H. DeCherney, J. Hade, & E.F. Sheets (Eds.), *Gynecology in primary care: A step-by-step approach* (pp. 7-11). New York: Scientific American, Inc

Dickey, R.P. (2002). *Managing contraceptive pill patients* (11th ed.). Durant, OK: Emis Medical Publishers

Greydanus, D.E., Patel, D.R., & Rimsza, M.E. (2001). Contraception in the adolescent: An update. *Pediatrics, 107*, 562-573.

Grimes, D.A. (2001). Contraception for women in the perimenopause. *The Contraception Report, 12*, 4-12.

Grimes, D.A. (2002). Switching emergency contraception to over-the-counter status. *New England Journal of Medicine, 347*, 846-848.

Grimes, D.A., & Raymond, E.G. (2002). Emergency contraception. *Annals of Internal Medicine, 137*, 180-189.

Gruber, C.J., Tschugguel, W., Schneeberger, C., & Huber, J.C. (2002). Production and actions of estrogens. *New England Journal of Medicine, 346*, 340-352.

Hatcher, R.A., Trussell, J., Stewart, F., Cates, W., Stewart, G., Guest, F., & Kowal, D. (1998). *Contraceptive technology.* New York: Adrent Media.

Henshaw, S.K. (1998). Unintended pregnancy in the United States. *Family Planning Perspectives, 30,* 329-336.

HERS Research Group. (2002). Cardiovascular disease outcomes during 6.8 years of hormone therapy. *Journal of the American Medical Association, 288*, 49-57.

Hill, D.A., & Lense, J.S. (1998). Office management of Bartholin gland cysts and abscesses. *American Family Physician 57*, 1611-1616.

Humphrey, L.L., Chan, B.K., & Sox, H.C. (2002). Postmenopausal hormone replacement therapy and the primary prevention of cardiovascular disease. *Annals of Internal Medicine, 137, 273-284*.

Kaunitz, A.M. (2001). Injectable long-acting contraception. *Clinical Obstetrics & Gynecology, 44*, 73-91.

Kovalevsky, G., & Barnhart, K.T. (2001). Norplant and other implantable contraceptives. *Clinical Obstetrics & Gynecology, 44*, 92-100.

Krattenmacher, R. (2000). Drospirenone: Pharmacology and pharmacokinetics of a unique progestogen. *Contraception, 62*, 29-38.

Krauss, R.M. (2002). Individualized hormone replacement therapy? *New England Journal of Medicine, 346*, 1017-1018.

Kronenberg, F., & Fugh-Berman, A. (2002). Complementary and alternative medicine for menopausal symptoms: A review of randomized, controlled trials. *Annals of Internal Medicine, 137*, 805-815.

LeBlanc, E.E., Janowsky, J., Chan, B.K., Nelson, H.D. (2001). Hormone replacement therapy and cognition. *Journal of the American Medical Association. 285,* 1489-1495.

Manson, J.E., & Martin, K.A. (2001). Postmenopausal hormone-replacement therapy. *New England Journal of Medicine, 345,* 34-40.

Miller, J., Chan, B.K., & Nelson, H.D. (2002). Postmenopausal estrogen replacement and risk for venous thromboembolism: A systematic review and meta-analysis for the US Preventive Services Task Force. *Annals of Internal Medicine, 136,* 680-690.

Mishell, D.R., Goodwin, T.M., & Brenner, P.F. (2002). *Management of common problems in obstetrics and gynecology.* United Kingdom: Blackwell Publications.

Mitka, M. (2001). New advice for women patients about hormone therapy and the heart. *Journal of the American Medical Association. 286:* 907.

Moos, R.H. (1969). The development of a premenstrual distress questionnaire. *Psychosomatic medicine, 30,* 850-855.

Mosca, L., Collins, P., Herrington, D.M., Mendelsohn, M.E., Pasternak, R.C., Robertson, R.M., Schenck-Gustafsson, K., Smih, S.C., Taubert, K.A., & Wenger, N.K. (2001). Hormone replacement and cardiovascular disease: A statement for healthcare professionals from the American Heart Association. *Circulation, 104,* 499-503.

Mulders, T.M. & Dieben, T.O. (2001). Use of the novel combined contraceptive vaginal ring NuvaRing for ovulation inhibition. *Fertility & Sterility, 75,* 865-70

Munro, M.G. (2000). Medical management of abnormal bleeding. *Obstetrics and Gynecology Clinics of North America, 27,* 287-301.

Nelson, A., Hatcher, R.A., Zieman, M., Watt, A., Darney, P.D., & Creinin, M.D. (2000). *Managing contraception.* Tiger, GA: Bridging the Gap Foundation.

Nelson, H.D. (2002). Assessing benefits and harms of hormone replacement therapy: Clinical applications. *Journal of the American Medical Association, 288,* 882-888.

Nelson, H.D., Humphrey, L.L., Nygren, P., Teutsch, S.M. & Allen, J.D. (2002). Postmenopausal hormone replacement therapy: Scientific review. *Journal of the American Medical Association, 288,* 872-881.

Nuovo, J. (2002). Evaluation and management of abnormal pap smear. *Primary Care Reports, 8,* 29-36.

Nyirjesy, P. (2001). Chronic vulvovaginal candidiasis. *American Family Physician, 63,* 697-702.

Pena, K.S., & Rosenfeld, J.A. (2001). Evaluation and treatment of galactorrhea. *American Family Physician, 63,* 1763-1775.

Pennachio, D.L. (2001). New approaches to emergency contraception. *Patient Care,* (March 15), 19-27.

Petrozza, J.C., & Poley, K. (1999). Dysfunctional uterine bleeding. In M.G. Curtis & M.P. Hopkins (Eds.), *Glass's office gynecology,* (pp. 241-264). Baltimore: Williams & Wilkins.

Raab, S.S. (2001). Subcategorization of Papanicolaou tests diagnosed as atypical squamous cells of undetermined significance. *American Journal of Clinical Pathology, 116,* 631-634.

Rodriguez, C., Patel, A.V., Calle, E.E., Jacob, E.J., Thun, M.J. (2001). Estrogen replacement therapy and ovarian cancer mortality in a large prospective study of US women. *Journal of the American Medical Association. 285,* 1460-5.

Sawaya, G.R., Brown, A.D., Washington, A.E., & Garber, A.M. (2001). Current approaches to cervical-cancer screening. *New England of Medicine, 344,* 1603-1610.

Schwetz, B.A. (2002). New contraceptive patch. *Journal of the American Medical Association, 287,* 1006-1007.

Smallwood, G.H., Meador, M.D., Lenihan, J.P., et al. (2001). Efficacy and safety of a transdermal contraceptive system. *Obstetrics & Gynecology, 96,* 799-805.

Solomon, D., Davey, D., Kuman, R., Moriarty, A., O'Connor, D., Prey, et al. (2002). The 2001 Bethesda system: Terminology for reporting results of cervical cytology. *Journal of the American Medical Association, 287,* 2114-2119.

Stennchever, M.A., Droegmueller, W., Herbst, A., & Mishell, D.R. (2001). *Comprehensive gynecology* (4th ed.). St. Louis: Mosby.

Stephenson, J. (2000). Widely used spermicide may increase, not decrease, risk of HIV transmission. *Journal of the American Medical Association. 284,* 949.

Stewart, F.H., Harper, C.C., Ellertson, C.E., Grimes, D.A., Sawaya, G.F., Trussell, J. (2001). Clinical breast and pelvic examination requirements for hormonal contraception: Current practice vs. evidence. *Journal of the American Medical Association. 285,* 2232-2239.

Torgerson, D.J. & Bell-Syer, S.E. (2001). Hormone replacement therapy and prevention of nonvertebral fractures: A meta-analysis of randomized trials. *Journal of the American Medical Association. 285,* 2891-2897.

Tsourounis, C. (2001). Clinical effects of phytoestrogens. *Clinical Obstetrics and Gynecology, 44,* 836-842.

US Preventive Services Task Force. (1996). *Guide to clinical preventive services.* Baltimore: Williams & Wilkins.

US Preventive Services Task Force. (2002). Hormone replacement therapy for primary prevention of chronic conditions: Recommendations and rationale. *Annals of Internal Medicine, 137,* 834-839.

US Preventive Services Task Force. (2002). Screening for breast cancer: Recommendations and rationale. *Annals of Internal Medicine, 137,* 344-346.

Vandenbroucke, J.P., Rosing, J., Bloemenkamp, K.W., Middeldorp, S., Helmerhorst, F.M., Bouma, B.N., et al. (2001). Oral contraceptives and the risk of venous thrombosis. *New England of Medicine, 344,* 1527-1535.

Vargyas, J.M. (1986). Premenstrual syndrome. In D.R. Mishell, & V. Davajan (Eds.), *Infertility, contraception, and reproductive endocrinology.* Cambridge, MA: Blackwell Scientific Publications.

Varila, E., Wahlstrom, T., Rauramo, I. (2001). A 5-year follow-up study on the use of a levonorgestrel intrauterine system in women receiving hormone replacement therapy. *Fertility & Sterility, 76,* 969-973.

Villareal, D.T., Binder, E.G., Williams, D.B., Schechtman, K.B., Yarasheski, K.E., Kohrt, W.M. (2001). Bone mineral density response to estrogen replacement in frail elderly women. *Journal of the American Medical Association. 286, 815-820.*

Viscoli, C.M., Brass, L.M., Kernan, W.N., Sarrel, P.M., Suissa S, Horwitz, R.I. (2001). A clinical trial of estrogen-replacement therapy after ischemic stroke. *New England Journal of Medicine, 345,* 1243-1249.

Wagner, J.D., Anthony, M.S., & Cline, J.M. (2001). Soy phytoestrogens: Research and benefits and risks. *Clinical Obstetrics and Gynecology, 44,* 843-852.

Wright, T.C., Cox, J.T., Massad, S., Twiggs, L.B., & Wilkinson, E.J. (2002). 2001 consensus guidelines for the management of women with cervical cytological abnormalities. *Journal of the American Medical Association, 287,* 2120-2129.

Writing Group for the Women's Health Initiative. (2002). Risks and benefits of estrogen plus progestin in healthy postmenopausal women. *Journal of the American Medical Association, 288,* 321-333.

Sexually Transmitted Diseases

MARY VIRGINIA GRAHAM

Bacterial Vaginosis
Figure: Clue Cell, White Blood Cell (WBC), and Trichomonas Vaginalis
Table: Recommended & Alternative Regimens for Nonpregnant Women
Table: Recommended Regimens for Pregnant Women

Trichomoniasis

Chlamydial Infection
Table: Special Considerations: Management During Pregnancy

Gonorrhea
Table: Recommended Regimens: Uncomplicated Gonococcal Infections
Table: Recommended Regimens: Uncomplicated Gonococcal Infections of the Pharynx

Mucopurulent Cervicitis

Nongonococcal Urethritis
Table: Recommended & Alternative Regimens for Management of Patients with NGU
Table: Recommended Regimens for Management of Recurrent/Persistent Urethritis

Pelvic Inflammatory Disease
Table: Diagnostic Criteria for PID
Table: Situations When Hospitalization of Patients with Acute PID is Indicated
Table: Recommended Regimens for Ambulatory Treatment of Acute PID

Syphilis
Table: Recommended Treatment of Syphilis in Adults
Table: Management of Sex Partners
Table: Guidelines for Follow-Up of Patients with Syphilis

Genital Herpes Simplex Virus (HSV) Infection
Table: Recommended Regimens: First Clinical Episode
Table: Counseling for Management of Patients with Genital Herpes
Table: Episodic Therapy for Recurrent Genital Herpes
Table: Suppressive Therapy for Recurrent Genital Herpes
Table: Recommended Regimens for Episodic Infection in Persons Infected with HIV
Table: Recommended Regimens for Daily Suppressive Therapy in Persons Infected with HIV

Human Papillomavirus Infection (Genital Warts)
Table: Overview of Treatment
Table: External Genital Warts: Recommended Regimens
Table: Education and Counseling of Patients with Genital Warts

BACTERIAL VAGINOSIS

I. Definition: Clinical syndrome resulting from replacement of the normal H_2O_2-producing *Lactobacillus sp.* in the vagina with high concentrations of anaerobic bacteria (e.g., *Prevotella* sp. and *Mobiluncus* sp.), *Gardnerella vaginalis*, and *Mycoplasma hominis*

II. Pathogenesis

    A. Cause of the microbial alteration is not fully understood

    B. Bacterial vaginosis (BV) is associated with having multiple sex partners, douching, and lack of vaginal lactobacilli

    C. Remains unclear whether BV results from acquisition of a sexually transmitted pathogen

    D. Women who have never been sexually active are rarely affected

III. Clinical Presentation

    A. BV is the most prevalent cause of vaginal discharge and malodor in women

    B. Approximately half of the women with BV may not report symptoms of BV

    C. Clinical criteria require three of the following symptoms or signs
        1. Homogenous, white, noninflammatory discharge that smoothly coats the vaginal walls
        2. Presence of clue cells on microscopic examination
        3. Vaginal fluid pH >4.5
        4. Fishy odor of vaginal discharge before or after addition of 10% KOH (whiff test)

    D. Although it is unclear whether BV is transmitted sexually, this vaginal infection is included in this section because it is often diagnosed in women being evaluated for STDs

IV. Diagnosis/Evaluation

    A. History
        1. Question about onset of symptoms, description of discharge—whether malodorous, its appearance, and amount
        2. Ask if other signs and symptoms are present
        3. Ask if woman uses frequent douching, feminine hygiene products to control odor
        4. Obtain complete menstrual history and history of contraceptive use including condom use

    B. Physical Examination
        1. Examine introitus for homogenous, white discharge
        2. Perform speculum exam and look for homogenous discharge coating vaginal walls; vaginal walls should not appear inflamed; note odor for characteristic foul, fishy odor and obtain specimens for diagnostic testing (see IV.D. below)
        3. Inspect cervix (should be normal) and perform bimanual exam

    C. Differential Diagnosis
        1. Other common cause of vaginitis—trichomoniasis and vulvovaginal candidiasis
        2. Common causes of cervicitis—chlamydia and gonorrhea

    D. Diagnostic Tests
        1. Obtain sample of vaginal secretions from anterior or lateral wall on a dry swab and apply to pH paper. In bacterial vaginosis, pH of vaginal secretions is >4.5 (normal pH of vagina is 3.5-4.5)
        2. Microscopic examination of slide containing vaginal secretions mixed with saline shows clue cells. Secretions have an amine odor before or after being mixed with a drop of 10% KOH (positive whiff test)
        3. Figure 15.1 depicts a clue cell, which is an epithelial cell to which many bacteria are attached

4. When a Gram stain is used to diagnose BV, a determination of the relative concentration of the bacterial morphotypes characteristic of the altered flora of BV is an acceptable laboratory method
5. Culture of *G. vaginalis* is not recommended as a diagnostic tool because it is not specific
6. A DNA probe based test for high concentrations of *G. vaginalis* (Affirm VP III, manufactured by Becton Dickinson, Sparks, MD) may have clinical utility
7. Other commercially available tests that may be useful for diagnosing BV include a card test for the detection of elevated pH and trimethylamine (FemExam test card, manufactured by Cooper Surgical, Shelton, CT) and prolineaminopeptidase (Pip Activity TestCard, manufactured by Litmus Concepts, Inc., Santa Clara, CA)

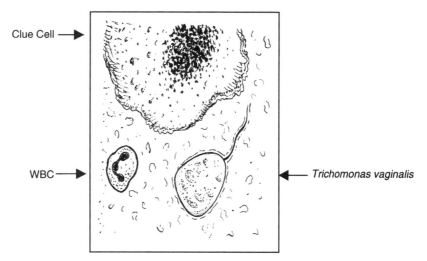

Figure 15.1. Clue Cell, WBC, & *Trichomonas vaginalis*

V. Plan/Management

A. The principal goals of therapy in non-pregnant women are to a) relieve vaginal symptoms and signs of infection and b) reduce the risk for infectious complications after abortion or hysterectomy

B. All women with symptomatic disease require treatment

C. All **symptomatic** pregnant women should be tested and treated: BV during pregnancy is associated with adverse outcomes, including premature rupture of the membranes, preterm labor, preterm birth, and postpartum endometritis

D. Because treatment of BV in **asymptomatic** pregnant women at high-risk for preterm delivery with a recommended regimen has reduced preterm delivery in several clinical trials, some specialists recommend the screening and treatment of these women
    1. Optimal treatment regimens have not been established
    2. Screening (if conducted) and treatment should be performed at the first prenatal visit

E. Data are conflicting regarding whether treatment of asymptomatic pregnant women at low risk for preterm delivery reduces adverse outcomes of pregnancy; therefore consultation/referral to a specialist is recommended

RECOMMENDED REGIMENS FOR NONPREGNANT WOMEN
Metronidazole 500 mg orally twice a day for 7 days, OR Metronidazole gel 0.75%, one full applicator (5 g) intravaginally once a day for 5 days, OR Clindamycin cream 2%, one full applicator (5 g) intravaginally at bedtime for 7 days
ALTERNATIVE REGIMENS FOR NONPREGNANT WOMEN
Metronidazole 2 g orally in a single dose, OR Clindamycin 300 mg orally twice a day for 7 days, OR Clindamycin ovules 100 mg intravaginally once at bedtime for 3 days

Source: Centers for Disease Control and Prevention. (2002). Sexually transmitted diseases treatment guidelines 2002. *MMWR, 51*(No.RR-6), pp. 43-44

F.   Patients should be advised to avoid consuming alcohol during treatment with metronidazole and for 24 hours thereafter. Clindamycin cream and ovules are oil-based and might weaken latex condoms and diaphragms. Advise patients to refer to condom product labeling for additional information

G.   Routine treatment of sex partners is **not** recommended

H.   Patients who have BV and also are infected with HIV should receive the same treatment regimen as those who are HIV-negative

I.   Follow Up
   1.   Follow-up visits are not necessary if symptoms resolve
   2.   Use alternative treatment regimens for treatment of recurrent disease
   3.   Recurrence of BV is common but no long-term maintenance regimen is recommended
   4.   Asymptomatic pregnant women who are at high risk for preterm delivery should receive follow-up one month after completion of therapy to evaluate efficacy of treatment

TRICHOMONIASIS

I.   Definition: Infection of the vagina by *Trichomonas vaginalis*. May also involve Skene's ducts and lower urinary tract in women, and the lower genitourinary tract in men

II.   Pathogenesis

   A.   *Trichomonas vaginalis*, a unicellular flagellated protozoan, causes this primarily STD

   B.   Incubation period is 4-28 days with the average being 1 week

III.   Clinical Presentation

   A.   Trichomoniasis comprises about 10% of all vaginal infections and is observed primarily in women with normal estrogen levels

   B.   Infection is frequently asymptomatic. If symptomatic, symptoms are usually worse immediately after menstruation and during pregnancy

   C.   Cardinal symptoms are a diffuse, malodorous, yellow-green discharge and vulvar irritation

   D.   Diffuse edema and redness is usually apparent in vulvar and vaginal tissue; the cervix may be inflamed and friable. Rarely, punctate lesions on the cervix give a "strawberry" appearance

   E.   Flagellated protozoa are seen in wet prep of vaginal secretions. Vaginal secretions have a pH of >4.5 (normal pH of the vagina is 3.5-4.5)

   F.   Most men who are infected with *T. vaginalis* do not have symptoms; others have nongonococcal urethritis (NGU)

IV. Diagnosis/Evaluation

    A. History
        1. Question about presence of discharge, characteristics of discharge (odor, color, amount), and associated symptoms (vulvar irritation, dysuria, dyspareunia)
        2. Obtain menstrual history and ask if menstruation makes symptoms worse
        3. In males, question about dysuria
        4. Obtain history of previous STDs; ask about condom use

    B. Physical Examination
        1. Examine external genitalia for signs of vulvar irritation, discharge pooling at introitus or posterior fourchette
        2. Perform pelvic exam to determine if vagina has erythema, edema; note type, color, and amount of discharge; examine cervix for erythema, friability, discharge
        3. Obtain specimens for diagnostic testing (see IV.D. below)

    C. Differential Diagnosis
        1. Other common causes of vaginitis—bacterial vaginosis and vulvovaginal candidiasis
        2. Common causes of cervicitis—chlamydia and gonorrhea

    D. Diagnostic Tests
        1. Obtain sample of vaginal secretions from anterior or lateral wall on a dry swab and apply to pH paper. In trichomoniasis, pH of vaginal secretions is >4.5 (normal pH of the vagina is 3.5-4.5)
        2. Microscopic examination of slide containing vaginal secretions mixed with saline solution shows organisms with whip-like flagellae that are motile and slightly larger than WBCs (see Figure 15.1 of trichomonad)
        3. In men, collect the first 5-30 mL of an early morning specimen of urine. Examine under microscope for trichomonads (this test should be reserved for situations in which this infection is suspected [e.g., contact with trichomoniasis])
        4. Culture is the most sensitive commercially available method of diagnosis
        5. No FDA-approved PCR test for *T.vaginalis* is available in US

V. Plan/Management

    A. Recommended regimen is metronidazole 2 g orally in a single dose

    B. Alternative regimen is metronidazole 500 mg twice daily for 7 days

    C. Management of treatment failure
        1. If treatment failure occurs with either regimen, retreat with metronidazole 500 mg twice daily for 7 days
        2. If treatment failure occurs again, patient should be treated with a 2 g dose of metronidazole once daily for 3-5 days
        3. Patients with laboratory-documented infection who do not respond to the 3-5 days treatment regimen and who have not been reinfected should be managed in consultation with a specialist; consultation is available from CDC (tel.770-488-4115; website: http://www.cdc.gov/std/)

    D. Sex partners should be treated and patients should be instructed to avoid sex until they have been cured (after therapy has been completed and patient and partner are asymptomatic)

    E. Patients should be advised to avoid consuming alcohol during treatment with metronidazole and for 24 hours thereafter

    F. Pregnant women who are symptomatic with trichomoniasis should be treated to ameliorate symptoms with 2 g of metronidazole in a single dose

    G. Data have not indicated that treating asymptomatic trichomoniasis during pregnancy lessens the association between vaginal trichomoniasis and adverse pregnancy outcomes

    H. Patients who have trichomoniasis and also are infected with HIV should receive the same treatment regimen as those who are HIV-negative

I.	Follow Up: None indicated for men and women who become asymptomatic after treatment (or who are initially asymptomatic) [See V.C. above for management of treatment failures]

CHLAMYDIAL INFECTION

I.	Definition: A sexually transmitted disease caused by *Chlamydia trachomatis*

II.	Pathogenesis

A.	*C. trachomatis,* a bacterial agent with at least 18 serologic variants (serovars) divided between the following two biologic variants: oculogenital (serovars A-K) and LGV (serovars L1-L3); genital infections are usually caused by serovars B and D through K

B.	Infects the genital tract of women most commonly at the transition zone of the endocervix and infects the urethra in men

C.	Incubation period is variable but is usually at least 1 week

III.	Clinical Presentation

A.	A frequent cause of cervicitis in women and urethritis in men, particularly among sexually active adolescents and young adults

B.	Asymptomatic sexually active women aged 25 and under should be routinely screened for chlamydial infection; other asymptomatic women at risk for infection should also be screened

C.	In women, chlamydial infection can cause mucopurulent cervicitis, urethritis, salpingitis, and proctitis; several important sequelae can result from infection including pelvic inflammatory disease (PID), ectopic pregnancy, and infertility

D.	In men, chlamydial infection can cause nongonococcal urethritis (NGU) and acute epididymitis (see NGU and EPIDIDYMITIS)

E.	Women may complain of abnormal vaginal discharge, dysuria, abnormal vaginal bleeding, and pelvic pain; commonly they are asymptomatic

F.	Men may complain of discharge of mucopurulent or purulent material from the urethra and burning during urination; commonly they are asymptomatic

IV.	Diagnosis/Evaluation

A.	History
1.	In women, ask about presence of abnormal vaginal discharge, dysuria, abnormal bleeding, pelvic pain, and dyspareunia
2.	In women, obtain menstrual history and contraceptive history
3.	In men, ask about presence of mucopurulent/purulent discharge from urethra, presence of burning on urination
4.	Inquire about sexual history including age at first intercourse, number of partners in past year, types of sexual practices, use of condoms
5.	Ask about past history of STDs including types, frequency, and treatment

B.	Physical Examination
1.	In women, perform speculum exam to inspect cervix for mucopurulent discharge from the endocervix. Obtain specimens for diagnostic testing and gently scrape cervix to test for friability
2.	Bimanual exam to check for adnexal tenderness, uterine tenderness, and cervical motion tenderness
3.	In men, examine the urethra for mucopurulent/purulent discharge and obtain specimens for diagnostic testing

C.   Differential Diagnosis
1.   PID in women
2.   Gonorrhea

D.   Diagnostic Tests
1.   Nucleic acid amplification tests (NAATs) enable detection of *N. gonorrhoeae* and *C. trachomatis* on all specimens; these tests are more sensitive than traditional culture techniques and are the preferred method of detection of *C. trachomatis*
2.   Perform microscopic analysis of vaginal secretions in women (wet-prep and/or Gram stain) to detect coexisting vaginal infections

V.   Plan/Management

A.   Chlamydia is a reportable disease in every state; such reports are kept strictly confidential, and in most jurisdictions, such reports are protected by statute from subpoena
1.   Reporting can be provider-and/or laboratory-based
2.   Clinicians who are unsure of local reporting requirements should seek advice from local health departments or state STD programs

B.   Recommended regimens for treatment of chlamydial infection are azithromycin 1 g orally in a single dose OR doxycycline 100 mg orally twice a day for 7 days

C.   Alternative regimens: Erythromycin base 500 mg orally four times a day for 7 day, OR erythromycin ethylsuccinate 800 mg orally four times a day for 7 days, OR ofloxacin 300 mg orally twice a day for 7 days, OR levofloxacin 500 mg orally for 7 days

D.   Selecting a treatment
1.   Doxycycline has the advantage of low cost and a long history of safety and efficacy
2.   Azithromycin has the advantage of single-dose administration and may be more cost effective in patients in whom compliance is an issue (single-dose, directly observed therapy [DOT] in the clinical setting is possible)
3.   Ofloxacin is similar in efficacy to doxycycline and azithromycin, but it is more expensive to use and offers no advantage with regard to the dosage regimen
4.   Erythromycin is less efficacious than either azithromycin or doxycycline; in addition, gastrointestinal side effects frequently discourage patients from complying with this regimen
5.   Levofloxacin has not been evaluated for treatment of *C. trachomatis* infection in clinical trials, but its pharmacology and in vitro microbiologic activity are similar to that of ofloxacin

E.   To maximize compliance with recommended therapies, medications for chlamydial infections should be dispensed on site, and the first dose should be directly observed

F.   To minimize further transmission of infection, patients treated for chlamydia should be instructed to abstain from sexual intercourse for 7 days after single-dose therapy or until completion of a 7-day regimen

G.   To minimize the risk for reinfection, patients also should be instructed to abstain from sexual intercourse until all of their sex partners are treated

H.   Treatment of sex partners: Patients should be instructed to refer their sex partners for evaluation, testing, and treatment, based on the following guidelines
1.   Sex partners should be evaluated, tested, and treated if they had sexual contact with the patient during the 60 days preceding onset of symptoms in the patient or diagnosis of chlamydia
2.   The most recent sex partner should be evaluated and treated even if the time of the last sexual contact was >60 days before symptom onset or diagnosis

SPECIAL CONSIDERATIONS: MANAGEMENT DURING PREGNANCY
Recommended Regimens
• Erythromycin base 500 mg orally four times a day for 7 days, OR amoxicillin 500 mg orally three times a day for 7 days
Alternative Regimens
• Erythromycin base 250 mg orally four times a day for 14 days, OR
• Azithromycin 1 g orally in a single dose
Doxycycline and ofloxacin are contraindicated in pregnant women
Repeat testing, preferably by culture, 3 weeks after completion of therapy is recommended for all pregnant women, because these regimens may not be highly efficacious and the frequent side effects of erythromycin might discourage patient compliance

Adapted from: Centers for Disease Control and Prevention. (2002). Sexually transmitted diseases treatment guidelines 2002. *MMWR, 51*(No.RR-6), p. 34.

I. Patients who have chlamydia and also are infected with HIV should receive the same treatment regimen as those who are HIV-negative

J. Follow Up
1. Patients do not need to be retested for chlamydia after completing treatment with doxycycline or azithromycin unless symptoms persist or reinfection is suspected
2. A test-of-cure (TOC) may be considered 3 weeks after completion of treatment with erythromycin; the CDC makes no recommendations relating to retesting for chlamydia after completing treatment with either ofloxacin or levofloxacin
3. Most post-treatment infections result from reinfection, often occurring because sex partners were not treated or because the patient resumed sex among a network of persons with a high prevalence of infection
4. Consider advising all women with chlamydial infection to be rescreened 3-4 months after treatment; rescreening is especially a high priority for adolescents (Note: Rescreening is different from early retesting to detect therapeutic failure [TOC])
5. Rescreen all women treated for chlamydia whenever they next present for care within the following 12 months; regardless of whether patient believes her sex partners were treated
6. See above table, SPECIAL CONSIDERATIONS: MANAGEMENT DURING PREGNANCY for follow-up recommendations for pregnant women

GONORRHEA

I. Definition: A sexually transmitted disease caused by *Neisseria gonorrhoeae,* a Gram-negative diplococcus that prefers columnar and pseudo-stratified epithelium

II. Pathogenesis

A. *N. gonorrhoeae* organisms are Gram-negative diplococci present in exudate and secretions of infected mucous surfaces

B. Transmission results from intimate contact, such as sexual acts and parturition; incubation period is usually 2-7 days

III. Clinical Presentation

A. In the US, an estimated 600,000 new *N. gonorrhoeae* infections occur each year, with the highest rate of infection in sexually active young adults

B. Transmission risk from an infected male to a woman is 70% after one exposure; from infected woman to male is as low as 20% with one exposure but rises to 60-90% with four exposures

C. At least 20% of neonates of infected women delivered vaginally acquire the disease

D. Most infections among men produce symptoms that cause them to seek treatment before serious sequelae develop; however, this may not be soon enough to prevent transmission to others

E. Many infections among women, on the other hand, do not produce symptoms until complications (e.g., PID) have occurred

F. In women, common sites of infection are the urethra, endocervix, upper genital tract, pharynx, and rectum
   1. Presenting symptoms include increased vaginal discharge, abnormal uterine bleeding, and dysuria
   2. Up to 40% of pelvic inflammatory disease (PID) is caused by gonorrhea
   3. Disseminated disease occurs most often when gonorrhea is acquired during menses or pregnancy; common features of disseminated disease include tenosynovitis, petechial or pustular acral skin lesions, fever, and asymmetrical arthralgias
   4. A primary measure for controlling gonorrhea is the screening of high-risk women

G. In men, common sites of infection are the urethra, epididymis, prostate, rectum, and pharynx; disseminated disease may also occur

IV. Diagnosis/Evaluation

A. History
   1. Inquire about onset and duration of symptoms
   2. In women, ask about presence of vaginal discharge, dysuria, abnormal bleeding, abdominal/pelvic pain, and dyspareunia; obtain menstrual history and contraceptive history
   3. In men, ask about dysuria, urethral discharge, rectal pain or discharge
   4. Inquire about sexual history including age at first intercourse, number of partners in past year, types of sexual practices, and use of condoms
   5. Ask about past history of STDs, including types, frequency, treatments

B. Physical Examination
   1. Take temperature to determine if febrile
   2. In women, perform pelvic exam; inspect Bartholin's and Skene's glands for tenderness and enlargement and the urethra for discharge; inspect cervix for mucopurulent discharge and obtain specimens for diagnostic testing (see IV. D. below); gently scrape cervix to test for friability
   3. In women, perform a bimanual exam to check for adnexal tenderness and masses, for uterine tenderness, and cervical motion tenderness
   4. In men, examine for urethral discharge and obtain specimens for diagnostic testing (see IV. D. below); if anal sex practiced, perform rectal exam for tenderness and discharge

C. Differential Diagnosis: Chlamydia and pelvic inflammatory disease in women

D. Diagnostic Tests
   1. Microscopic examination of Gram-stained smears (for Gram-negative intracellular diplococci) of exudate from the endocervix in females and the urethra in males is helpful in the initial evaluation
   2. A number of nonculture gonococcal tests are available which enable detection of both *N. gonorrhoeae* and *C. trachomatis* on specimens—direct fluorescent antibody (DFA) tests, enzyme immunoassays (EIA), and nucleic acid amplification tests (NAATs)

V. Plan/Treatment

A. Gonorrhea is a reportable disease in every state; such reports are kept strictly confidential, and in most jurisdictions, such reports are protected by statute from subpoena
   1. Reporting can be provider-and/or laboratory-based
   2. Clinicians who are unsure of local reporting requirements should seek advice from local health departments or state STD programs

B. Recommended regimens for treatment of adults and adolescents with uncomplicated gonococcal infections of the cervix, urethra, and rectum are contained in the following table

---

RECOMMENDED REGIMENS: UNCOMPLICATED GONOCOCCAL INFECTIONS
OF THE CERVIX, URETHRA, AND RECTUM

Cefixime 400 mg orally in a single dose*
OR
Ceftriaxone 125 mg IM in a single dose
OR
Ciprofloxacin 500 mg orally in a single dose[1]
OR
Ofloxacin 400 mg orally in a single dose[1]
OR
Levofloxacin 250 mg orally in a single dose[1]
PLUS
IF CHLAMYDIAL INFECTION IS NOT RULED OUT
Azithromycin 1 g orally in a single dose
OR
Doxycycline 100 mg orally twice a day for 7 days

---

* In July 2002, WYETH PHARMACEUTICALS discontinued manufacturing cefixime (Suprax) in the US—no other pharmaceutical company manufactures or sells cefixime tablets or suspension in the US. Cefixime is the only CDC-recommended oral antimicrobial agent to which *N. gonorrhoeae* has not developed significant resistance. In the absence of cefixime, the primary recommended treatment option for gonorrhea if the infection was acquired in Asia, the Pacific Islands (including Hawaii), or California is ceftriaxone

[1] Quinolones should not be used for infections acquired in Asia, the Pacific Islands, (including Hawaii) or California.

Source: Centers for Disease Control and Prevention. (2002). Sexually transmitted diseases treatment guidelines 2002. *MMWR, 51* (No.RR-6), p. 37

C.   Alternative Regimens: Spectinomycin 2 g in a single IM dose, OR ceftizoxime 500 mg in a single IM dose, OR cefotaxime 500 mg in a single IM dose

D.   Many other antimicrobials are active against *N. gonorrhoeae*, but none have substantial advantages over the recommended regimens

E.   **Dual therapy** for gonococcal and chlamydial infections
   1.   Routine dual therapy without testing for chlamydia can be cost-effective for populations in which chlamydial infection accompanies 10%-30% of gonococcal infections (cost of therapy is less than cost of testing)
   2.   However, in geographic areas in which the rates of coinfection are low, some clinicians might prefer a highly sensitive test for chlamydia rather than treating presumptively
   3.   Presumptive treatment is indicated for patients who may not return for test results

F.   Gonococcal infections of the pharynx are more difficult to eradicate than infections at urogenital and anorectal sites. Recommended regimens for treatment of adults with uncomplicated gonococcal infections of the pharynx are contained in the table below

---

RECOMMENDED REGIMENS: UNCOMPLICATED GONOCOCCAL INFECTIONS OF THE PHARYNX

Ceftriaxone 125 mg IM in a single dose
OR
Ciprofloxacin 500 mg orally in a single dose
PLUS
IF CHLAMYDIAL INFECTION IS NOT RULED OUT
Azithromycin 1 g orally in a single dose
OR
Doxycycline 100 mg orally twice daily for 7 days

Source: Centers for Disease Control and Prevention. (2002). Sexually transmitted diseases treatment guidelines 2002. *MMWR, 51* (No.RR-6), pp. 37-38

G.   Pregnant women should be treated with a recommended or alternate cephalosporin as listed above. Pregnant women who cannot tolerate a cephalosporin should be administered a single, 2-g dose of spectinomycin IM . Either erythromycin or amoxicillin is recommended for treatment of presumptive or diagnosed *C. trachomatis* infection (see CHLAMYDIAL INFECTIONS section above for treatment of pregnant women) [**Note: Pregnant women should not be treated with quinolones or tetracyclines**]

H. Treatment of sex partners: Patients should be instructed to refer their sex partners for evaluation, testing, and treatment, based on the following guidelines
   1. All sex partners of patients who have *N. gonorrhoeae* infection should be evaluated and treated for *N. gonorrhoeae* and *C. trachomatis* infections if their last sexual contact with the patient was within 60 days before onset of symptoms or diagnosis of infection in the patient
   2. If the patient's most recent sexual encounter was >60 days before onset of symptoms or diagnosis, the patient's most recent sex partner should be treated

I. Patients should be instructed to avoid sexual intercourse until therapy is completed and until they and their sex partners no longer have symptoms

J. Persons with disseminated gonococcal infection (bacteremia) should be hospitalized for initial parenteral antibiotic therapy

K. Patients who have gonorrhea and also are infected with HIV should receive the same treatment regimen as those who are HIV-negative

L. Follow Up
   1. Patients with uncomplicated gonorrhea and who are treated with any of the recommended regimens need not return for a test of cure
   2. Patients with persistent symptoms after treatment need to be re-evaluated for antimicrobial susceptibility
   3. Persistence of symptoms usually results from reinfection rather than treatment failure (indicates need to improve patient education and partner referral)

MUCOPURULENT CERVICITIS

I. Definition: A sexually transmitted syndrome in which there is purulent or mucopurulent endocervical exudate visible in the endocervical canal or in an endocervical swab specimen

II. Pathogenesis

   A. Mucopurulent cervicitis (MPC) can be caused by *Chlamydia trachomatis* and *Neisseria gonorrhoeae*, but in **most cases** neither organism can be isolated

   B. Other non-microbiologic determinants (e.g., inflammation in the zone of ectopy) may be involved

III. Clinical Presentation

   A. MPC is often asymptomatic, but some women have an abnormal vaginal discharge and vaginal bleeding (e.g., after sexual intercourse)

   B. Speculum examination of cervix reveals a purulent or mucopurulent endocervical exudate visible in the endocervical canal or in an endocervical specimen examined under the microscope

   C. MPC can persist despite repeated courses of antimicrobial therapy

   D. Some experts consider an increased number of polymorphonuclear leukocytes (PMNs) on Gram stain of endocervical secretions as being helpful in the diagnosis of MPC; however, this criterion has not been standardized and is not available in some settings

IV. Diagnosis/Evaluation

   A. History
      1. Inquire about the onset and duration of symptoms, if present
      2. Ask about presence of vaginal discharge, dysuria, abnormal bleeding particularly after sexual intercourse
      3. Obtain menstrual history and contraceptive history

4. Inquire about sexual history including age at first intercourse, present partner(s), types of sexual practices, and use of condoms
5. Inquire about past history of STDs, including types, frequency, treatments

B. Physical Examination
1. Determine if febrile
2. Perform speculum exam to inspect cervix, to sample secretions for purulent or mucopurulent discharge, and to obtain specimens for diagnostic testing (see IV.D. below); assess for cervical motion tenderness and gently scrape cervix to determine friability
3. Perform bimanual exam, checking for adnexal tenderness, masses

C. Differential Diagnosis
1. Urinary tract infection
2. Chlamydia
3. Gonorrhea
4. Trichomonal vaginitis

D. Diagnostic Tests
1. Gram stain of endocervical secretions looking for PMNs and intracellular Gram-negative diplococci
2. Perform nucleic acid amplification tests (NAATs) or other nonculture tests which enable detection of both *C. trachomatis* and *N. gonhrrhoeae*
3. Wet mount exam for trichomonas
4. Urine for culture and sensitivity (if symptomatic)

V. Plan/Management

A. Results of sensitive tests for *C. trachomatis* and *N. gonorrhoeae* should determine the need for treatment

B. Empiric treatment should be considered for patients suspected of having ghonorrhea and/or chlamydia if a) the prevalences of these infections are high in the patient population, and b) the patient might be difficult to locate for treatment

C. Sex partners of women with MPC should be notified, examined, and treated for the STD identified or suspected in the index patient
1. A microbiologic test of cure is usually not recommended
2. Patients and their sex partners should be counseled to abstain from sexual intercourse until therapy is completed (i.e., 7 days after a single-dose regimen or after completion of a 7-day regimen)

D. Patients who have MPC and who also are infected with HIV should receive the same treatment regimen as those who are HIV-negative

E. Follow Up
1. Should be as recommended for the infections for which the woman is being treated
2. If symptoms persist, woman should be instructed to return for reevaluation and to abstain from sexual intercourse even if the course of prescribed therapy has been completed

NONGONOCOCCAL URETHRITIS (NGU)

I. Definition: Inflammation of the urethra not caused by gonococcal infection and characterized by a mucoid or purulent urethral discharge

II. Pathogenesis

A. *Chlamydia trachomatis* is a frequent cause of NGU (15%-55% of cases); however, the prevalence differs by age group with lower prevalence of this organism among older men

B. Etiology of most cases of nonchlaymdial NGU is unknown; *Ureaplasma urealyticum* and *Mycoplasma genitalium* have been implicated as causes in some studies

C. *Trichomonas vaginalis* and herpes simples virus (HSV) sometimes cause NGU

III. Clinical Presentation

A. Most common STD syndrome in males living in industrialized countries

B. NGU is substantially more common than gonococcal urethritis in most areas of US

C. Many men are entirely asymptomatic; primary complaints are urethral discharge (yellow, white, or cloudy), dysuria, or urethral itching

D. Urethritis can be documented by the presence of **any** of the following signs:
1. Mucopurulent or purulent discharge
2. Gram stain of urethral secretions demonstrating ≥5 WBCs per oil immersion field; Gram stain is the preferred rapid diagnostic test for evaluating urethritis
3. Positive leukocyte esterase test on first-void urine, or microscopic examination of first-void urine demonstrating ≥10 WBCs per high power field

IV. Diagnosis/Evaluation

A. History
1. Ask about onset, duration of symptoms
2. Inquire about presence and color of discharge, presence of dysuria, and urethral itching
3. Inquire about sexual history including age at first intercourse, number of partners in the past year, types of sexual practices, use of condoms
4. Inquire about past history of STDs, including types, frequency, and treatments

B. Physical Examination: Examine urethra for mucopurulent discharge and obtain specimens for diagnostic testing (see IV.D. below)

C. Differential Diagnosis: Gonorrhea

D. Diagnostic Tests
1. Gram-stain urethral smear (≥5 WBCs per oil immersion field PLUS no intracellular Gram-negative diplococci are expected findings)
2. Positive leukocyte esterase test on first void urine, or microscopic examination of first-void urine demonstrating ≥10 WBCs per high power field
3. Test for *N. gonorrhoeae* and *C. trachomatis* using nonculture tests such as nucleic acid amplification tests (NAATs), which enable detection of both organisms

V. Plan/Management

A. Treatment should be initiated as soon as possible after diagnosis; to improve compliance, medication should be provided in the clinic/office

B. Recommended regimens and alternative regimens are contained in the tables that follow

RECOMMENDED REGIMENS FOR MANAGEMENT OF PATIENTS WITH NGU
Azithromycin 1 g orally in a single dose   OR   Doxycycline 100 mg orally twice a day for 7 days

Source: Centers for Disease Control and Prevention. (2002). Sexually transmitted diseases treatment guidelines 2002. *MMWR, 51*(No.RR-6), p. 31.

ALTERNATIVE REGIMENS FOR MANAGEMENT OF PATIENTS WITH NGU
Erythromycin base 500 mg orally four times a day for 7 days
OR
Erythromycin ethylsuccinate 800 mg orally four times a day for 7 days
OR
Ofloxacin 300 mg twice a day for 7 days
OR
Levofloxacin 500 mg once daily for 7 days

Source: Centers for Disease Control and Prevention. (2002). Sexually transmitted diseases treatment guidelines 2002. *MMWR, 51*(No.RR-6), p. 31.

C. If none of the criteria for confirming urethritis are met (see III.D. above), treatment should be deferred until the diagnostic test results for *N. gonorrhoeae* and *C. trachomatis* are obtained
   1. If the results are positive for either infection, the appropriate treatment should be given and sex partners referred for evaluation and treatment
   2. Empiric treatment of symptoms without documentation of urethritis is recommended only for patients at high risk for infection who are unlikely to return for follow-up (such patients should be treated for both gonorrhea and chlamydia) [see GONORRHEA and CHLAMYDIA for treatment recommendations]
   3. Partners of patients empirically treated should be evaluated and treated

D. Management of sex partners: Patients should refer for evaluation and treatment all sex partners within the preceding 60 days. Because a specific diagnosis may facilitate partner referral, testing for gonorrhea and chlamydia is encouraged

E. Recurrent and persistent NGU may be due to a lack of compliance, or more often, reinfection by untreated sex partner
   1. Men with persistent or recurrent urethritis should be re-treated with the initial regimen if they failed to comply with the treatment regimen or if they were re-exposed to an untreated sex partner
   2. Otherwise, a culture of an intraurethral swab specimen and a first-void urine specimen for *T. vaginalis* should be performed
   3. If the patient was compliant with the initial regimen and re-exposure can be excluded, the following regimen is recommended

RECOMMENDED REGIMENS FOR MANAGEMENT OF PATIENTS WITH RECURRENT/PERSISTENT URETHRITIS (FOR USE IN PATIENTS WHO WERE COMPLIANT WITH INITIAL THERAPY AND RE-EXPOSURE CAN BE EXCLUDED)		
		Erythromycin base 500 mg PO four times a day for 7 days
Metronidazole 2 g orally in a single dose	**PLUS**	**OR**
		Erythromycin ethylsuccinate 800 mg PO four times a day for 7 days

Source: Centers for Disease Control and Prevention. (2002). Sexually transmitted diseases treatment guidelines 2002. *MMWR, 51* (No.RR-6), p. 31

   4. Refer for evaluation by an expert if objective signs of urethritis continue after adequate treatment

F. Patients who have NGU and also are infected with HIV should receive the same treatment regimen as those who are HIV-negative

G. Follow Up
   1. Patients should be instructed to return for evaluation if symptoms persist or recur after completion of therapy
   2. Patients should be instructed to abstain from sexual intercourse until 7 days after therapy is initiated

PELVIC INFLAMMATORY DISEASE (PID)

I. Definition: A spectrum of inflammatory disorders of the upper female genital tract, including any combination of endometritis, salpingitis, tubo-ovarian abscess, and pelvic peritonitis

II. Pathogenesis

   A. Sexually transmitted organisms, especially *Neisseria gonorrhoeae* and *Chlamydia trachomatis*, are implicated in many cases

   B. Microorganisms that can be part of the vaginal flora (e.g., anaerobes, *G. vaginalis*, *H. influenzae*, enteric Gram-negative rods, and *S. agalactiae*) also have been associated with PID

   C. In addition, cytomegalovirus (CMV), *M. hominis* and *U. urealyticum* may be etiologic agents in some cases of PID

III. Clinical Presentation

   A. Incidence of PID is highest among sexually active adolescents

   B. Variables that **increase** risk of PID include adolescence, multiple sex partners, previous episode of STD, use of an intrauterine device, and douching

   C. Variables that **decrease** risk include use of oral contraceptives and barrier contraceptives

   D. Most typical presentation is continuous bilateral lower abdominal or pelvic pain that may be accompanied by fever, nausea, and vomiting

   E. In many patients the infection is asymptomatic (silent PID) or symptoms are vague and mild with abnormal vaginal bleeding, dyspareunia, or change in vaginal discharge as the only signs and symptoms (atypical PID); many episodes of PID go unrecognized

   F. PID symptoms most often begin within one week of onset of menses

   G. The diagnosis of PID usually is based on clinical findings; no single historical, physical, or laboratory finding is both sensitive and specific for the diagnosis

   H. The following recommendations for diagnosing PID are made by the CDC to help healthcare providers recognize when PID should be suspected and when there is a need to obtain additional information to increase diagnostic certainty

DIAGNOSTIC CRITERIA FOR PID

Minimum Criteria

Empiric treatment of PID should be instituted in sexually active young women and others at risk for STDs if all the following **minimum criteria** are present and no other cause(s) for the illness can be identified
- Uterine/adnexal tenderness or
- Cervical motion tenderness

Additional Criteria

More elaborate diagnostic evaluation often is needed because incorrect diagnosis and management may cause unnecessary morbidity. These additional criteria may be used to increase the specificity of the minimum criteria listed above
- Oral temperature >101F (>38.3C)
- Abnormal cervical or vaginal mucopurulent discharge
- Presence of white blood cells (WBCs) on saline microscopy of vaginal secretions
- Elevated erythrocyte sedimentation rate
- Elevated C-reactive protein
- Laboratory documentation of cervical infection with *N. gonorrhoeae* or *C. trachomatis*

Definitive Criteria

The **most specific criteria** for diagnosing PID include the following
- Endometrial biopsy with histopathologic evidence of endometritis
- Transvaginal sonography or magnetic resonance imaging techniques showing thickened fluid-filled tubes with or without free pelvic fluid or tubo-ovarian complex, and
- Laparoscopic abnormalities consistent with PID

Adapted from: Centers for Disease Control and Prevention. (2002). Sexually transmitted diseases treatment guidelines 2002. *MMWR, 51*(No.RR-6), pp. 48-49

IV. Diagnosis/Evaluation

    A. History
        1. Ask about presence of lower abdominal/pelvic pain, including onset, duration, location, and character or pain
        2. Ask the patient if she has had fever
        3. Inquire about presence of vaginal discharge, postcoital bleeding, spotting between menstrual periods, and gastrointestinal symptoms
        4. Obtain sexual history including age at first intercourse, number of partners in past year, types of sexual practices, and contraceptive history (ask if IUD is used)
        5. Inquire about past history of STDs, including type, frequency, treatments; ask about HIV+ status
        6. Obtain complete menstrual history including pattern of recent menstrual cycles and a description of the last menses (Ask: "Did onset of pain coincide with LMP?")

    B. Physical Examination
        1. Determine if febrile
        2. Examine abdomen for tenderness, masses, signs of peritonitis
        3. On speculum exam, inspect cervix for inflammation; insert swab(s) into cervix to sample mucus in order to obtain specimens for diagnostic testing, and to examine gross appearance of cervical secretions (a transparent discharge similar to clear hair styling gel is normal; secretions that appear yellow or green on swab are not normal)
        4. Perform bimanual exam to check for adnexal masses, uterine tenderness, and for cervical motion tenderness (pain that occurs when cervix is moved from side to side)

    C. Differential Diagnosis
        1. Appendicitis
        2. Ectopic pregnancy
        3. Tubo-ovarian abscess
        4. Ovarian cyst
        5. Pyelonephritis

D. Diagnostic Tests
1. Pregnancy Test
2. Nonculture tests such as nucleic acid amplification tests (NAATs) which enable detection of both *N. gonorrhoeae* and *C. trachomatis* should be obtained before treatment
3. CBC with differential and sedimentation rate
4. Wet prep or Gram stain of endocervical secretions
   a. If number of epithelial cells > than number of WBCs per high-powered field, then patient almost certainly does not have PID
   b. If WBCs outnumber epithelial cells per high powered field, patient may have PID
5. VDRL or RPR

V. Plan/Management

A. PID treatment regimens must provide empiric, broad-spectrum coverage of likely pathogens. Antimicrobial coverage should include *N. gonorrhoeae, C. trachomatis*, anaerobes, Gram-negative facultative bacteria, and streptococci

B. Inpatient therapy for every case of PID is unrealistic. The CDC has made recommendations for when to select inpatient therapy and these recommendations are contained in the following table

SITUATIONS WHEN HOSPITALIZATION OF PATIENTS WITH ACUTE PID IS INDICATED
• Surgical emergencies such as appendicitis and ectopic pregnancy cannot be excluded • Patient has a tubo-ovarian abscess • Patient is pregnant • Patient has severe illness, nausea and vomiting, or high fever • Patients is unable to follow or tolerate an outpatient oral regimen • Patient fails to respond clinically to oral antimicrobial therapy

Adapted from: Centers for Disease Control and Prevention. (2002). Sexually transmitted diseases treatment guidelines 2002. *MMWR, 51* (No.RR-6), p. 49

C. Outpatient therapy for PID is described in the table below

RECOMMENDED REGIMENS FOR AMBULATORY TREATMENT OF ACUTE PID
Regimen A Ofloxacin 400 mg orally twice a day for 14 days **OR** Levofloxacin 500 mg orally once daily for 14 days ***WITH OR WITHOUT*** Metronidazole 500 mg orally BID for 14 days
Regimen B Cefoxitin 2 g IM <u>plus</u> Probenecid 1 g orally in a single dose concurrently, **OR** ceftriaxone 250 mg IM in a single dose, **OR** other parenteral third-generation cephalosporin (e.g., ceftizoxime or cefotaxime) ***PLUS*** Doxycycline 100 mg orally twice a day for 14 days ***WITH or WITHOUT*** Metronidazole 500 mg orally twice a day for 14 days

Source: Centers for Disease Control and Prevention. (2002). Sexually transmitted diseases treatment guidelines 2002. *MMWR, 51*(No.RR-6), p. 51-52

D. Management of sex partners:
1. Male sex partners of women with PID should be examined and treated if they had sexual contact with patient during the 60 day period preceding onset of symptoms in patient
2. Evaluation and treatment are imperative because of the risk of reinfection of the patient and the strong likelihood of urethral gonococcal or chlamydial infection in the sex partner
3. Sex partners should be treated empirically with regimens effective against both *C. trachomatis* and *N. gonorrhoeae* regardless of the apparent etiology of PID

E. Pregnant women who have suspected PID should be hospitalized and treated with parenteral antibiotics

F. Whether the management of immunodeficient HIV-infected women with PID requires more aggressive interventions (e.g., hospitalization or parenteral antimicrobial regimens) has not been determined

G. Follow Up
1. Patients treated on an ambulatory basis need to be monitored closely and reevaluated within 72 hours for clinical improvement (**Note**: Clinical improvement is defined as defervescence; reduction in direct or rebound abdominal tenderness; reduction in uterine, adnexal, and cervical motion tenderness within 72 hours of initiation of therapy)
2. Patients who do not demonstrate improvement within 72 hours usually require hospitalization, additional diagnostic tests, and surgical intervention
3. Some experts recommend rescreening for *C. trachomatis* and *N. gonorrhoeae* 4-6 weeks after therapy is completed in women with documented infection with these pathogens

SYPHILIS

I. Definition: A systemic sexually transmitted disease involving multiple organ systems and caused by *Treponema pallidum*, a spirochete

II. Pathogenesis

A. *T. pallidum* is a thin, delicate organism with humans as the sole host

B. Organism penetrates intact skin or mucous membrane during sexual contact, multiplies, and rapidly spreads to regional lymph nodes

C. Spirochetes enter the blood stream within hours and are transported to other tissues

D. Congenital syphilis results from transplacental passage of the organism

E. Incubation period for acquired primary syphilis is about 3 weeks, but ranges from 10-90 days after exposure

III. Clinical Presentation

A. The pattern of syphilis infection in the US has changed during recent years; although the South continues to have the highest rate (56.2% in 2001) of primary and secondary (P&S) syphilis, rates actually decreased in the South over the two-year period (2000-2001) by 8.1%
1. In the West, rates increased 40% and in the Northeast rates increased 57.1% over that same time period
2. Racial/ethnic disparities in syphilis rates are decreasing because of declining rates among non-Hispanic blacks and increasing rates among non-Hispanic whites
3. The number of P&S cases increased among men during 2000-2001, ending the decade-long trend characterized by annual declines in syphilis cases among both men and women
4. This increase in syphilis cases among men is associated with reports in several cities of syphilis outbreaks among men having sex with men (MSM); these outbreaks were characterized by high rates of HIV co-infection and high-risk sexual behavior among subpopulations of MSM

B. To guide therapeutic decisions and disease intervention strategies, acquired syphilis has been divided into the following stages: primary, secondary, latent, and tertiary

C. Primary syphilis: Characterized by appearance of ulcer or chancre at site of inoculation, usually on genitals 3-4 weeks after exposure
1. Genital lesions are usually indurated and painless
2. Extragenital lesions (e.g., lips, breast) are often painful
3. Regional lymphadenopathy usually present
4. Chancre persists for 1-5 weeks and heals spontaneously

D. Secondary syphilis: Occurs about 6-8 weeks later and is characterized by flu-like symptoms—headache, generalized arthralgia, malaise, fever, and lymphadenopathy, followed by a generalized rash
1. Rash is macular, papular, annular, or follicular; often involves the palms and soles
2. Rash persists for 2-6 weeks then spontaneously heals
3. Mucous patches often occur in mouth, throat, on cervix; flat, papular lesions (condylomata lata) occur in intertriginous areas

4. About 25% of infected persons have at least one cutaneous relapse
5. Secondary syphilis is the most contagious state of the disease
6. Even without treatment, signs of first 2 stages resolve spontaneously, and infected persons enter the next state: the latent state

E. Latent syphilis: Defined as those infections characterized by seroactivity without other evidence of disease
   1. Patients can be diagnosed as having early latent syphilis if, within the year preceding the evaluation, they had
      a. A documented seroconversion,
      b. Unequivocal symptoms of primary or secondary syphilis, or
      c. A sex partner documented to have primary, secondary, or early latent syphilis
   2. All other cases of latent syphiilis are either late latent syphilis or latent syphilis of unknown duration
   3. Difficult to make this distinction in practice, because exact date of infection is usually difficult to establish
   4. Nontreponemal serologic titers usually are higher during early latent syphilis than late latent syphilis; this characteristic cannot be relied upon as the sole distinguishing factor
   5. About 1/3 of persons with latent syphilis are little inconvenienced by the disease
   6. After a variable period of latency, about 1/3 of untreated cases go on to develop tertiary syphilis, and about 28% of these will die because of the disease

F. Tertiary syphilis: Refers to gumma and cardiovascular syphilis, but not to all neurosyphilis (when there is evidence of central nervous system infection); since the advent of penicillin therapy, all forms of tertiary syphilis have become uncommon

G. Congenital syphilis involves multiple organ systems with the stage of syphilis in the mother determining the effects on the fetus
   1. Early congenital syphilis occurs from birth to age 2 and is characterized by mucocutaneous lesions, rhinitis, and other symptoms
   2. Congenital syphilis can be asymptomatic, especially in the first weeks of life
   3. Late congenital syphilis is characterized by bone and joint disorders, cranial neuropathies, and interstitial keratitis which causes blindness if untreated

IV. Diagnosis/Evaluation

A. History
   1. Question about onset, duration of symptoms
   2. Ask about presence or history of chancre (when it appeared, where located, if symptomatic, when healed)
   3. Inquire about presence (or history of) rash, mucous patches, condylomata lata
   4. Ask about sexual behavior, use of condoms
   5. Determine if sex partner has had similar symptoms
   6. Obtain past history of STDs, including types, frequency, duration, treatment; establish HIV status
   7. Obtain past medical history, medication history, drug and alcohol use, allergies

B. Physical Examination
   1. Examine genital area and other skin surfaces (breast, buttocks) for characteristic chancre (primary syphilis)
   2. Look for mucocutaneous lesions of secondary syphilis

C. Differential Diagnosis
   1. Primary syphilis: Syphilis can mimic all lesions that appear to be genital ulcers: genital herpes, chancroid, lymphogranuloma venereum, scabies, balanitis should all be suspect
   2. Secondary syphilis: Syphilis can mimic many skin disorders: all undiagnosed mucous or cutaneous eruptions should be suspect

D. Diagnostic Tests
   1. Darkfield microscopy and direct fluorescent antibody tests of lesion exudate or tissue are the definitive methods for diagnosing early syphilis
   2. A presumptive diagnosis is possible with the use of two types of serologic tests for syphilis
      a. Nontreponemal-specific tests: Rapid Plasma Reagin (RPR) test and Venereal Disease Research Laboratory (VDRL) test

b. Treponemal-specific tests: Fluorescent treponemal antibody absorbed (FTA-ABS) and *T. pallidum* particle agglutination (TP-PA)

c. Use of only one type of serologic test is insufficient for diagnosis, because false-positive nontreponemal test results may occur secondary to some medical conditions

3. VDRL and RPR are used for initial screening, to monitor disease activity, and to determine efficacy of treatment

a. A fourfold change in titer, equivalent to a change of two dilutions (e.g., from 1:16 to 1:4 or from I:8 to 1:32) is considered necessary to demonstrate a clinically significant difference between two nontreponemal test results that were obtained using the same serologic test

b. A decline in titers equivalent to a change of two dilutions indicates effective treatment, and a failure of test titers to decline fourfold by 6 to 12 months after therapy indicates treatment failure

c. RPR is test most often used today, but the tests are comparable

4. For sequential serologic tests, the same test (VDRL or RPR) should be used

5. Treponemal tests are used to confirm diagnosis of syphilis in persons with reactive VDRL or RPR

a. Usually remain reactive for life regardless of treatment or disease activity

b. About 15%-25% of patients treated during primary stage revert to being serologically nonreactive after 2-3 years

6. Nontreponemal tests usually become nonreactive with time after treatment; in some patients, nontreponemal antibodies can persist at a low titer for a long period of time; response is referred to as the "serofast reaction"

V. Plan/Treatment

A. Report all cases of syphilis to appropriate public health authorities so that case finding can be performed

B. Treatment is based on clinical and serologic staging of the disease and is summarized in the following table

RECOMMENDED TREATMENT OF SYPHILIS IN ADULTS	
Stage	**Treatment***
Primary and Secondary Syphilis	Benzathine penicillin G 2.4 million units IM in a single dose *Other Management Considerations:* Always test for HIV infection. If symptoms or signs of neurologic or ophthalmic disease are present, refer for evaluation (invasion of CSF by *T. pallidum* is common among adults with primary or secondary syphilis; however, CSF analysis is not recommended for routine evaluation of patients unless clinical signs or symptoms are present)
Latent syphilis: Early latent syphilis and late latent syphilis (syphilis of unknown duration)	**Early Latent:** Benzathine penicillin G 2.4 million units IM in a single dose **Late Latent (or when duration is unknown):** Benzathine penicillin G 7.2 million units total, given as three doses of 2.4 million units IM each at 1-week intervals *Other Management Considerations:* Always test for HIV infection. All patients who have latent syphilis should be evaluated clinically for evidence of tertiary disease (e.g., aortitis, gumma, and iritis) and for evidence of neurologic involvement (e.g., cognitive dysfunction, motor or sensory deficits). Some experts recommend performing a CSF examination on all patients with latent syphilis and a nontreponemal serologic test of ≥1:32
Tertiary disease (no evidence of neurosyphilis)	As for **late latent** disease, with appropriate management of complications (refer to infectious diseases [ID] specialist)
Neurosyphilis	Aqueous crystalline penicillin G, 18-24 million units/day given as 3-4 million units IV every 4 hours for 10-14 days, or procaine penicillin 2-4 million units IM a day PLUS Probenecid 500 mg orally QID both for 10-14 days (refer to ID specialist)

*For patients allergic to penicillin, see alternatives under V.D. below

Adapted from Centers for Disease Control and Prevention. (2002). Sexually transmitted diseases treatment guidelines 2002. *MMWR,51* (No.RR-6), pp. 20-23

C. The Jarisch-Herxheimer reaction is an acute febrile reaction frequently accompanied by headache, myalgia, and other symptoms that usually occur within the first 24 hours after any therapy for syphilis

1. Patients should be informed about this possible adverse reaction
2. Occurs most often among patients who have early syphilis
3. Antipyretics may be used, but they have not been shown to prevent the reaction

D. Management of nonpregnant, penicillin-allergic patients who have primary and secondary syphilis

1. Data to support the use of alternatives to penicillin in the treatment of primary and secondary syphilis are limited

2. Doxycycline (100 mg twice daily for 14 days) and tetracycline (500 mg four times daily for 14 days) are regimens that have been used for many years; compliance is usually better with doxycycline as it causes fewer gastrointestinal side effects than tetracycline
3. Some experts recommend ceftriaxone 1 g daily either IM or IV for 8-10 days
4. Also, preliminary data suggest that azithromycin 2 g may be effective as a single oral dose
5. Patients with penicillin allergy whose compliance with alternative therapies or follow-up cannot be ensured should be desensitized and treated with benzathine penicillin (consult expert)

E. Management of nonpregnant, penicillin-allergic patients who have latent syphilis—early latent and late latent syphilis or syphilis of unknown duration
1. Effectiveness of alternatives to penicillin in the treatment of latent syphilis has not been well documented
2. **Early latent:** Should respond to therapies recommended as alternatives to penicillin for the treatment of primary and secondary syphilis (under V.D. above)
3. **Late latent syphilis or latent syphilis of unknown duration:** The only acceptable alternatives for treatment of this stage of the disease are doxycycline 100 mg orally twice daily for 28 days, **or** tetracycline 500 mg orally four times daily for 28 days
4. These therapies should be used only in conjunction with close serologic and clinical follow-up

F. Management of nonpregnant, penicillin-allergic patients who have tertiary syphilis: Treat according to alternative regimens for **late latent** syphilis (refer to ID specialist for management)

G. Patients with neurosyphilis require expert management (refer to ID specialist)

H. Management of sex partners should be guided by the following recommendations

---

MANAGEMENT OF SEX PARTNERS

Sexual transmission of *T. pallidum* occurs only when mucocutaneous syphilitic lesions are present; such manifestations are uncommon after the first year of infection. **However, patients exposed sexually to a patient who has syphilis in any stage should be evaluated both clinically and serologically as follows:**

Persons exposed within the 90 days preceding the diagnosis of primary, secondary, or early latent syphilis in a sex partner might be infected even if seronegative--**Treat presumptively**

Persons exposed >90 days before the diagnosis of primary, secondary, or early latent syphilis in a sex partner and in whom serologic test results are not available immediately and the opportunity for follow-up is uncertain--**Treat presumptively**

For purposes of **partner notification and presumptive treatment of exposed sex partners**, patients with syphilis of unknown duration with high nontreponemal serologic test titers (defined as ≥1:32) can be assumed to have early syphilis. However, serologic titers should not be used to differentiate early from late latent syphilis for the purpose of determining treatment for the index case

Long-term sex partners of patients who have latent syphilis should be evaluated clinically and serologicaly for syphilis and treated on basis of findings

---

Adapted from Centers for Disease Control and Prevention. (2002). Sexually transmitted diseases treatment guidelines. 2002. *MMWR,51* (No.RR-6), p. 20

I. Congenital syphilis
1. Infants born to mothers who have reactive nontrepnemal and treponemal test results should be evaluated with a quantitative nontreponemal serologic test (RPR or VDRL)
   a. Test should be performed on infant serum
   b. Umbilical cord blood may be contaminated with maternal blood and might yield a false-positive result
   c. A treponemal test of a newborn's serum is not necessary
2. Evaluation of infant includes the following
   a. Complete physical exam of neonate for evidence of congenital syphilis
   b. Pathologic examination of the placenta or umbilical cord using specific fluorescent antitreponemal antibody staining
   c. Darkfield microscopic examination or direct fluorescent antibody staining of any suspicious lesions or body fluids (example, nasal discharge)
3. Consult expert regarding therapy decisions and treatment guidelines for all infants born to seroreactive mothers

J.   Special Considerations: Management of Syphilis in Pregnancy
1.   All women should be screened serologically for syphilis at the first prenatal visit (with additional screening at 28 weeks and at delivery for high-risk patients)
2.   Seropositive pregnant women should be referred for expert care

K.   Syphilis in HIV infected persons
1.   Diagnostic considerations
a.   Both treponemal and non-treponemal serologic tests for syphilis can be interpreted in usual manner for most patients who are coinfected with *T. pallidum* and HIV (aberrant serologic responses do occur, but are uncommon)
b.   When clinical findings suggest syphilis, but serologic tests are nonreactive or unclear, alternate tests such as biopsy of lesion, darkfield examination or direct fluorescent antibody staining of lesion material may be helpful
2.   Treatment
a.   The recommended treatment is the same as that for HIV-negative patients
b.   HIV-infected patients who have either late latent syphilis or syphilis of unknown duration should have a CSF examination before treatment
c.   Refer these patients for expert care if available

3.   Follow Up
a.   HIV infected persons should have clinical follow-up and serologic testing at 3, 6, 9, 12, and 24 months after therapy
b.   If at any time clinical symptoms develop or nontreponemal titers rise fourfold, a repeat CSF examination should be performed (refer to expert for management)

L.   Treatment failure can occur with any regimen. Assessing response to treatment is often difficult, and definitive criteria for cure or treatment failure have not been established; follow-up guidelines for patients with primary, secondary, latent, and tertiary syphilis are contained in the following table

---

GUIDELINES FOR FOLLOW-UP OF PATIENTS WITH PRIMARY, SECONDARY, LATENT, AND TERTIARY SYPHILIS

Patients with Primary and Secondary Syphilis
- Patients in this category should be examined clinically and serologically at 6 months and 12 months; more frequent evaluation may be prudent if follow-up is uncertain
  - ✓ Patients who have a fourfold or greater decline in titers (e.g., A 1:32 titer that declines to 1:8 or lower) at 6 and 12 months has received effective treatment
  - ✓ Patients who have signs or symptoms that persist or recur or who have a sustained fourfold increase in nontreponemal test titer (i.e., compared with the maximum or baseline titer at the time of treatment) most probably either failed treatment or were reinfected
  - ✓ Such patients should be re-treated and also reevaluated for HIV infection; because treatment failure usually cannot be reliably distinguished from reinfection with *T. pallidum*, a CSF analysis also should be performed
  - ✓ Re-treatment (as recommended by most experts): 3 weekly injections of benzathine penicillin G 2.4 million units IM [unless CSF examination indicates neurosyphilis is present]

Patients with Latent Syphilis: Early Latent and Late Latent Syphilis or Latent Syphilis of Unknown Duration
- Quantitative nontreponemal serologic tests should be repeated at 6, 12, and 24, months
- Patients with a normal CSF examination should be retreated for latent syphilis if
  - ✓ Titers increase fourfold
  - ✓ An initially high titer (≥1:32) fails to decline at least fourfold; a fourfold change in titer is equivalent to a change of two dilutions (e.g. from 1:32 to 1:8) within 12-24 months of therapy, or
  - ✓ Signs or symptoms attributable to syphilis develop

Patients with Tertiary Syphilis
- Patients require CSF examinations to assess treatment response (refer to expert for management)

Adapted from Centers for Disease Control and Prevention. (2002). Sexually transmitted diseases treatment guidelines. 2002. *MMWR, 51* (No.RR-6), p. 20-25

GENITAL HERPES SIMPLEX VIRUS INFECTION

I. Definition: Infection with herpes simplex viruses (HSV). Two serotypes of HSV have been identified: HSV-1 and HSV-2. Most cases of recurrent genital herpes are caused by HSV-2. (see SKIN PROBLEMS IN CHILDREN AND ADULTS for herpes simplex infections of the skin and mucous membranes)

II. Pathogenesis

    A. HSV-1 and HSV-2 are epidermotropic viruses with infection occurring within keratinocytes

    B. Transmission is only by direct contact with active lesions, or by virus-containing fluid such as saliva or cervical secretions in persons with no evidence of active disease

    C. Inoculation of the virus into skin or mucosal surfaces produces infection, with an incubation period of 2-14 days

    D. About 48 hours after entering the host, the virus transverses afferent nerves to find host ganglion
        1. The trigeminal ganglia are the target of the oral virus--primarily HSV-1
        2. The sacral ganglia are the target of the genital virus--most often HSV-2

    E. Upon reactivation, the virus retraces its route, causing recurrence in the cutaneous area affected by the same nerve root, but not necessarily in the original site

    F. Generally HSV-1 is associated with infection of the lips, face, buccal mucosa, and throat; HSV-2, with the genitalia

    G. In spite of the distinctive sites of herpetic lesions with each serotype, there is overlap in site of infection in approximately 25% of individuals who are infected
        1. Type 1 strains can be recovered from the genital tract
        2. Type 2 strains probably can be recovered from the pharynx as a result of oral-genital activity
        3. Whereas type 1 HSV genital infections in children also can result from autoinoculation of virus from the mouth, sexual abuse must always be considered in prepubertal children with genital herpes

III. Clinical Presentation

    A. Genital herpes is a recurrent, life-long viral infection; at least 50 million persons in the U.S. have genital HSV infection

    B. Most HSV-2 infected persons have not been diagnosed
        1. Infections are either mild or unrecognized with the virus shed intermittently in the genital tract
        2. Most infections are transmitted by persons unaware that they are infected or asymptomatic when transmission occurs

    C. The usual sequence of disease in which signs/symptoms occur is painful papules followed by vesicles, ulceration, crusting, and healing

    D. First clinical episode of genital herpes
        1. Symptoms of primary infection that is symptomatic often consists of hyperesthesia, burning, itching, dysuria, pain, and tenderness in the genital area
        2. Fever and lymphadenopathy are frequently present
        3. More systemic manifestations are present than with recurrent episodes
        4. Viral shedding is prolonged (average 12 days) and healing of lesions takes 21 days on average
        5. Persons with genital infection with HSV-1 (about 30% of patients with first episode herpes) have a much lower risk of symptomatic recurrent outbreaks

    E. Recurrent episodes of HSV infection
        1. Most patients (about 50%) with symptomatic first episode HSV-2 infection will have recurrent episodes within 6 months after the first clinical episode
        2. Frequently have prodrome with recurrences

3. Lesions often localized in recurrent episodes
4. Length of viral shedding reduced compared to primary episode (average 7 days)
5. Healing of lesions is also faster (5 days on average)

IV. Diagnosis/Evaluation

A. History
1. Question regarding location, onset, duration, and appearance of lesions; ask if pain, burning, or paresthesia present prior to eruption
2. Ask about associated symptoms of fever, myalgia, malaise
3. Ask regarding previous occurrence of similar lesions, symptoms
4. Inquire about exposures to infected persons and use of condoms

B. Physical Examination
1. Examine genital area for characteristic location, distribution, appearance of lesions
2. Check for enlarged lymph nodes in inguinal area

C. Differential Diagnosis
1. Syphilis
2. Chancroid
3. Folliculitis
4. Molluscum contagiosum

D. Diagnostic Tests
1. Isolation of HSV in cell culture is the preferred virologic test in patients who present with genital ulcers or other mucocutaneous lesions (**Note:** Sensitivity of culture declines rapidly as lesions begin to heal, usually within a few days of onset)
   a. Unroof vesicle and scrape the material with Dacron-tipped swab
   b. Place swab in viral transport media
   c. Virus grows rapidly and cultures may be positive within 2-3 days (can take longer)
2. Because false-negative HSV cultures are common, particularly in patients with healing lesion or recurrent infections, type-specific serologic tests are useful in confirming a clinical diagnosis of genital herpes; additionally, such tests can be used to diagnose persons with unrecognized infection and to manage sex partners of persons with genital herpes
   a. Currently, the FDA-approved gG-based type-specific assays include POCkit HSV-2 (manufactured by Diagnology); HerpeSelect-1 ELISA IgG or HerpeSelect-2 ELISA IgG (manufactured by Focus Technology, Inc.); and HerpeSelect 1 and 2 Immunoblot IgG (manufactured by Focus Technology, Inc.)
   b. The POCkit HSV-2 assay is a point-of-care test that provides results for HSV-2 antibodies from capillary blood or serum during a clinic visit
   c. The Focus Technology assays are laboratory-based
   d. Sensitivities of these tests for detection of HSV-2 antibody vary from 80% to 90%
   e. Specificities of these assays are ≥96%
3. The CDC does not recommend the Tzanck test for diagnosing HSV infection

V. Plan/Management

A. Healthcare providers often must treat patients before test results are available because early treatment decreases the possibility of transmission and because successful treatment of genital herpes depends upon prompt initiation of therapy
1. Treat for the diagnosis considered most likely on basis of clinical presentation and epidemiologic circumstances
2. Even after complete diagnostic evaluation, at least 25% of patients who have genital ulcers have no laboratory-confirmed diagnosis

B. Many patients with first-episode genital herpes present with mild clinical manifestations but later develop severe or prolonged symptoms. Most patients with initial genital herpes should receive antiviral therapy as outlined in the following table

RECOMMENDED REGIMENS: FIRST CLINICAL EPISODE

Select one of the following regimens

Acyclovir 400 mg orally 3 times a day for 7-10 days, OR

Acyclovir 200 mg orally 5 times a day for 7-10 days, OR

Famciclovir 250 mg orally 3 times a day for 7-10 days, OR

Valacyclovir 1 g orally twice a day for 7-10 days

Note: Treatment may be extended if healing is incomplete after 10 days of therapy

Adapted from Centers for Disease Control and Prevention. (2002). Sexually transmitted diseases treatment guidelines 2002. *MMWR, 51*(No.RR-6), p. 14

COUNSELING FOR MANAGEMENT OF PATIENTS WITH GENITAL HERPES

Two main goals of counseling are to help patient cope with infection and to prevent sexual and perinatal transmission

Information and Lifestyle Counseling

✓ Counsel patient regarding natural history of disease emphasizing recurrent episodes, asymptomatic viral shedding, and sexual transmission; partner notification should be encouraged

✓ Sexual and perinatal transmission can occur during asymptomatic periods; sex partners of infected persons should be advised that they might be infected even if they have no symptoms

✓ Type-specific serologic testing of asymptomatic partners of persons with genital herpes can determine whether risk for HSV acquisition exists

✓ Asymptomatic viral shedding occurs more frequently in persons with genital HSV-2 than HSV-1 and also occurs more frequently in those with infection <12 months

✓ Latex condoms when used consistently and correctly, can reduce risk for genital herpes when infected areas are covered by condom

✓ Need to abstain from all sexual activity when lesions or prodromal symptoms are present

Counseling Relating to Role of Antiviral Drugs

✓ Systemic antiviral drugs partially control the signs and symptoms when used to treat initial and recurrent episodes or when used as daily suppressive therapy

✓ Episodic and suppressive therapy is effective in preventing or shortening the duration of recurrent episodes

Resources Available for Patients

✓ Refer to educational resources: CDC National STD/HIV Hotline (800-227-8922); web site http://www.ashastd.org

Adapted from Centers for Disease Control and Prevention. (2002). Sexually transmitted diseases treatment guidelines 2002. MMWR, 51(No.RR-6), p. 15

C. Patients with recurrent episodes of HSV infection can be managed in one of two ways--either episodically, to shorten the duration of lesions, or continuously with the use of suppressive therapy to reduce the frequency of recurrences

    1. Options for treatment of recurrent episodes should be discussed with all patients

    2. The following tables outline episodic therapy and suppressive therapy for recurrent HSV disease

EPISODIC THERAPY FOR RECURRENT GENITAL HERPES

Select <u>one</u> of the following regimens

- Acyclovir 400 mg orally three times a day for 5 days
- Acyclovir 200 mg orally 5 times a day for 5 days
- Acyclovir 800 mg orally twice a day for 5 days
- Famciclovir 125 mg orally twice a day for 5 days
- Valacyclovir 500 mg orally twice a day for 3- 5 days
- Valacyclovir 1.0 g orally once a day for 5 days

<u>About Episodic Therapy</u>

✓ Treatment is most efficacious when begun during the prodrome or within 1 day after onset of lesions

✓ If episodic therapy for recurrence is chosen, patient should be provided with antiviral therapy, or a prescription for the medication, so that treatment can be initiated at the first sign of prodrome or genital lesions

Adapted from Centers for Disease Control and Prevention. (2002). Sexually transmitted diseases treatment guidelines 2002. *MMWR, 51*(No.RR-6), p. 14

SUPPRESSIVE THERAPY FOR RECURRENT GENITAL HERPES

Select one of the following regimens

- Acyclovir 400 mg orally twice a day
- Famciclovir 250 mg orally twice a day
- Valacyclovir 500 mg orally once a day*
- Valacyclovir 1.0 gram orally once a day

About Suppressive Therapy
- ✓ Daily suppressive therapy reduces the frequency of genital herpes recurrences by ≥75% among patients who have frequent recurrences (defined as 6 or more recurrences per year)
- ✓ Suppressive therapy with acyclovir reduces but does not eliminate asymptomatic viral shedding
- ✓ Suppressive therapy has not been associated with emergence of acyclovir resistance among immunocompetent patients
- ✓ After 12 months of continuous suppressive therapy, discontinuation should be discussed with patient
- ✓ Famciclovir and valacyclovir should not be used for over 12 months
- ✓ Safety and efficacy have been documented among patients using daily acyclovir for as long as 6 years

*May be less effective than other valacyclovir or acyclovir dosing regimens in patients who have very frequent recurrences (≥10 outbreaks per year)

Adapted from Centers for Disease Control and Prevention. (2002). Sexually transmitted diseases treatment guidelines 2002. *MMWR, 51*(No.RR-6), p. 14

D. Management of sex partners
  1. Partners can usually benefit from evaluation and counseling
  2. Symptomatic partners should be evaluated and treated
  3. Asymptomatic partners should be questioned concerning history of genital lesions, educated to recognize symptoms of herpes, and offered type-specific serologic testing for HSV infection

E. Lesions caused by HSV are common among HIV-infected patients and may be severe, painful and atypical. Episodic or suppressive therapy with oral antiviral agents is often beneficial; see recommendations in the tables that follow

RECOMMENDED REGIMENS FOR EPISODIC INFECTION IN PERSONS INFECTED WITH HIV
Acyclovir 400 mg orally three times a day for 5-10 days
OR
Acyclovir 200 mg five times a day for 5-10 days
OR
Famciclovir 500 mg orally twice a day for 5-10 days
OR
Valacyclovir 1.0 g orally twice a day for 5-10 days

Source: Centers for Disease Control and Prevention. (2002). Sexually transmitted diseases treatment guidelines. *MMWR, 51*(No.RR-6), p. 16

RECOMMENDED REGIMENS FOR DAILY SUPPRESSIVE THERAPY IN PERSONS INFECTED WITH HIV
Acyclovir 400-800 mg orally two to three times a day
OR
Famciclovir 500 mg orally twice a day
OR
Valacyclovir 500 mg orally twice a day

Source: Centers for Disease Control and Prevention. (2002). Sexually transmitted diseases treatment guidelines 2002. *MMWR, 51*(No.RR-6), p. 16

F. If lesions persist or recur in patients receiving antiviral treatment, resistance should be suspected and patients should be referred to a specialist for management; patients should also be referred to a specialist if lesions are severe as hospitalization and IV therapy may be necessary

G. Pregnant women with genital herpes should be referred to a specialist for management (**Note:** The safety of acyclovir, valacyclovir, and famciclovir therapy in pregnant women has not been established)

H. Infants exposed to HSV during birth, as proven by virus isolation or presumed by observation of lesions should be followed by a specialist

I. Follow Up: Variable depending on clinical needs of patient

HUMAN PAPILLOMAVIRUS INFECTION (GENITAL WARTS)

I. Definition: A sexually transmitted disease caused by certain types of the human papillomavirus (HPV) that produces epithelial tumors of the skin and mucous membranes

II. Pathogenesis

   A. More than 30 types of HPV can infect the genital tract

   B. The virus enters the body via an epithelial defect and infects the stratified squamous epithelium of the lower genital tract

   C. Visible genital warts usually are caused by HPV types 6 or 11

   D. Other HPV types in the anogenital region--types 16, 18, 31, 33, and 35--have been strongly associated with cervical neoplasia

III. Clinical Presentation

   A. Most HPV infections are asymptomatic, unrecognized, or subclinical

   B. Clinical HPV infections develop following an incubation period of unknown length but it is estimated to range from 3 months to several years; depending on the size and anatomic location, genital warts can be painful, friable, and pruritic

   C. In addition to the external genitalia, (i.e., the penis, vulva, scrotum, perineum, and perianal skin), genital warts can occur on the uterine cervix and in the vagina, urethra, anus, and mouth

   D. Intra-anal warts are seen predominantly in patients who have had receptive anal intercourse; these warts are distinct from perianal warts, which can occur in men and women without a history of anal sex

   E. In addition to the genital area, HPV types 6 and 11 have been associated with conjunctival, nasal, oral, and laryngeal warts

   F. Individual warts may become confluent and appear as a single, large fleshy lesion

   G. Growth of warts may be stimulated by pregnancy, oral contraceptive use, immunosuppression, and local trauma

IV. Diagnosis/Evaluation

   A. History
      1. Question about location, onset, duration, and presence of any associated symptoms
      2. Inquire about exposures to sexually transmitted diseases (unprotected intercourse)
      3. Ask if partner has similar lesions
      4. Inquire about past history of HPV
      5. Question regarding pregnancy, use of oral contraceptives, and immune status

   B. Physical Examination
      1. Examine external genitalia and rectal areas for characteristic lesions
      2. To assist in visualization of warts, apply 3-5% acetic acid to the vulva (women), penis (men) and perianal areas to reveal acetowhitening
      3. Perform Pap smear to detect cervical dysplasia in women who have not had a Pap test within the past year

C. Differential Diagnosis
1. Herpes simplex
2. Syphilis
3. Molluscum contagiosum

D. Diagnostic Tests: Visible anogenital warts are diagnosed by clinical inspection; no data support the use of type-specific HPV nucleic acid tests in the routine diagnosis or management of visible genital warts

V. Plan/Management

A. Primary goal of treating visible warts is the removal of symptomatic warts
1. Treatment can induce wart-free periods in most patients; most patients have fewer than 10 warts with a total wart areas of 0.5-1.0 cm^2
2. Currently available treatments do not affect the natural history of HPV infection
3. Most genital warts are asymptomatic and, left untreated, often resolve on their own
4. Existing data indicate that currently available therapies for genital warts may reduce, but probably do not eradicate, infectivity
5. Patients should be advised that no available treatment is superior to the others; no single treatment is ideal for all patients or all warts
6. A treatment protocol is important because many if not most patients require a course of therapy rather than a single treatment

---

OVERVIEW OF TREATMENT

Treatment of Genital Warts Should be Guided by
- Preference of the patients after they have been informed of the options
- Available resources
- Experience of healthcare provider

Factors that Influence Selection of Treatment
- Wart size, morphology, number, and anatomic site (in general, warts located on moist surfaces and/or intertriginous areas respond better to topical treatment than do warts on drier surfaces)
- Patient preference and provider experience
- Convenience, cost of treatment, and adverse treatment effects

Treatment Modality Should be Changed if
- Patient has not improved substantially after 3 provider-administered treatments, OR
- Warts have not cleared after 6 treatments

Avoid overtreatment: Risk/benefit ratio of treatment should be evaluated throughout course of therapy

To Increase Efficiency and Efficacy, Clinicians Should be Knowledgeable about
- At least one patient-applied treatment
- At least one provider-administered treatment that is available

Note: Opinion is divided regarding the practice of employing combination therapy (i.e., the simultaneous use of two or more modalities on the same wart at the same time). Because of the limitations of currently available treatments, some providers employ combination therapy; others believe that combining modalities may increase complications without improving efficacy

---

Adapted from Centers for Disease Control and Prevention. (2002). Sexually transmitted diseases treatment guidelines 2002. *MMWR, 51*(No.RR-6), p. 53-55

EXTERNAL GENITAL WARTS: RECOMMENDED REGIMENS

Patient-Applied
(Note: For patient-applied treatments, patient must be able to identify and reach warts)

Podofilox 0.5% solution or gel (relatively inexpensive, easy to use, safe, antimitotic drug) **Not for use in pregnancy**
- Dosing:
  - ✓ Apply BID x 3 days, followed by 4 days of no therapy
  - ✓ May repeat cycle as necessary for a total of 4 cycles
- Instruction to patient: Apply solution with cotton swab, gel with finger to visible genital warts
- Comments:
  - ✓ Most patients experience mild/moderate pain or local irritation after treatment
  - ✓ If possible, provider should apply initial treatment to demonstrate proper application technique and identify which warts should be treated
  - ✓ Total wart area treated should be ≤10 cm^2, and total volume of podofilox should be ≤0.5 mL per day

Imiquimod 5% cream (immune enhancer that stimulates production of interferon and other cytokines) **Not for use in pregnancy**
- Dosing: Apply QD at bedtime, 3 times/week for up to 16 weeks
- Instructions to patient: Apply cream with a finger at bedtime and wash off with mild soap/water after 6-10 hours
- Comment: Many patients may be clear of visible warts by 8-10 weeks

Follow up: Traditionally, follow-up visits are not required for patients using self-administered therapy; however, follow-up may be useful several weeks into therapy to determine appropriateness of medication use and response to treatment

Provider-Administered

Select **one** of the following
Cryotherapy with liquid nitrogen or cryoprobe (destroys warts by thermal-induced cytolysis)
- Repeat applications Q 1-2 weeks
- Pain after application, followed by necrosis and sometimes blistering, is common

  Note: Major limitation of this modality is that proper use requires substantial training; most warts are overtreated or undertreated by providers who have not been trained resulting in poor efficacy or increased complications

Podophyllin resin 10-25% in compound tincture of benzoin (contains several compounds including antimitotic podophyllin lignans)
- Apply small amount (thin layer) to each wart and allow to air dry
- Limit application to ~0.5 mL of podophyllin or an area of ≤10 cm^2 of warts per session
- Instruct patient to thoroughly wash preparation off 1-4 hours after application (to reduce local irrittion)
- Repeat weekly if necessary
  Note: Not for use in pregnancy

Trichloroacetic acid (TCA) or bichloroacetic acid (BCA) 80%-90% (caustic agents that destroy warts by chemical coagulation of the proteins)
- Apply sparingly to warts only (TCA has low viscosity comparable with that of water and can spread rapidly)
- Allow to dry--a white "frosting" develops
- Powder with talc or sodium bicarbonate to neutralize acid (if acid is applied excessively, can damage adjacent tissues)
- Repeat weekly if necessary

Surgical removal either by tangential scissor excision, tangential shave excision, curettage, or electrosurgery

Adapted from Centers for Disease Control and Prevention. (2002). Sexually transmitted diseases treatment guidelines 2002. *MMWR, 51*(No.RR-6), p. 54-55

B. Alternative regimens for treatment of external genital warts are intralesional interferon or laser surgery

C. For treatment of cervical and vaginal warts, referral to an expert is recommended

D. For treatment of urethral meatus warts, referral to an expert is recommended

E. For treatment of external anal warts, use of cryotherapy with liquid nitrogen or TCA or BCA 80%-90%; apply as directed above under EXTERNAL GENITAL WARTS: RECOMMENDED REGIMENS

F. Management of warts on rectal mucosa and on oral mucosa should be by an expert

G. Management of pregnant women: Refer to expert for management

H. Management of immunodeficient patients: Refer to expert for management (increased incidence of squamous cell carcinoma arising in or resembling genital warts may occur more frequently among immunosuppressed persons, thus requiring biopsy for confirmation of diagnosis)

Adapted from Centers for Disease Control and Prevention. (2002). Sexually transmitted diseases treatment guidelines 2002. *MMWR, 51*(No.RR-6), p. 56-57

I. Management of sexual partners of patients with visible warts
  1. Examination of partners not necessary for the management of genital warts because no data indicate that reinfection plays a role in recurrences
  2. The value to treatment in reducing infectivity is not known
  3. Use of condoms reduces, but does not eliminate risk of transmission

J. Subclinical genital HPV infection (without exophytic warts)
  1. Subclinical genital HPV infection is a term used to refer to manifestations of infection in the absence of visible genital warts, including situations where infection is detected on the cervix by Pap test, colposcopy, or biopsy; on the penis, vulva, or other genital skin by the appearance of white areas after application of acetic acid; or on any genital skin by a positive test for HPV
  2. Subclinical genital HPV infection occurs more frequently than visible warts in both men and women
  3. Screening for subclinical genital HPV infection using DNA or RNA tests is not recommended
  4. In the absence of coexistent squamous intraepithelial lesion (SIL), treatment is not recommended for subclinical genital HPV infection diagnosed by colposcopy, biopsy, acetic acid soaking of genital skin/mucous membranes, or the detection of HPV by laboratory tests
  5. The diagnosis of subclinical genital HPV infection is often not definitive, and no therapy has been identified that eradicates infection

K. Management of sexual partners of patients with subclinical genital HPV infection
  1. Examination of sex partners is unnecessary
  2. Most sex partners of infected patients probably are already infected subclinically with HPV
  3. No screening tests for subclinical infection are available
  4. Whether patients who have subclinical HPV infection are as infectious as patients who have exophytic warts is unknown

L. Recommendations relating to cervical cancer screening for women who attend STD clinics or have a history of STDs
  1. Precursor lesions for cervical cancer occur about five times more frequently among women attending STD clinics than among women attending family planning clinics
  2. If woman has not had a Pap smear during previous 12 months, a Pap smear should be obtained as part of the routine pelvic examination in the STD clinic
    a. The sequence of Pap testing in relation to collection of other cervicovaginal specimens does not appear to influence Pap test results/interpretation
    b. Thus, when other cultures or specimens are collected for STD diagnosis, the Pap test can be obtained last
  3. Provide woman with printed information about Pap smears and a report containing a statement that a Pap smear was obtained during her clinic visit
  4. A copy of the Pap smear result should be provided to the patient for her records
  5. Counsel woman about need for an annual Pap smear, and provide her with names of local clinics/providers where Pap smears can be obtained on an annual basis and adequate follow-up is available

6. Women who have external genital warts do not need to have Pap tests more frequently than women who do not have warts, unless otherwise indicated
7. See ABNORMAL CERVICAL CYTOLOGY section for information on management of patients with cervical cytological abnormalities

M. Follow Up
1. After visible warts have cleared (which may require several visits for provider-administered treatments), a follow-up evaluation is not mandatory but may be helpful
2. Patient should be advised to watch for recurrences, which occur most frequently during first 3 months after treatment; patients concerned about recurrences should be offered a follow-up evaluation 3 months after treatment
3. Women should be counseled to undergo regular Pap screening as recommended for women without genital warts (see screening for cervical cancer in HEALTH MAINTENANCE chapter)

REFERENCES

Centers for Disease Control and Prevention. (2002). Discontinuation of cefixime tablets—United States. *Morbidity and Mortality and Weekly Report, 51*, 1052.

Centers for Disease Control and Prevention. (2002). Increases in fluoroquinolone-resistant *Neisseria gonorrhoeae*—Hawaii and California, 2001. *Morbidity and Mortality and Weekly Report, 51*, 1041-1044.

Centers for Disease Control and Prevention. (2002). Primary and secondary syphilis—United States. *Morbidity and Mortality and Weekly Report, 51*, 971-973.

Centers for Disease Control and Prevention. (2002). Sexually transmitted diseases treatment guidelines 2002. *Morbidity and Mortality Weekly Report, 51*(No. RR-6).

Centers for Disease Control and Prevention. (2003). HIV/STD risks in young men who have sex with men who do not disclose their sexual orientation—six US cities, 1994-2000. *Morbidity and Mortality Weekly Report, 52*, 81-86.

Hatcher, R.A., Trussell, J., Stewart, F., Cates, W., Stewart, G., Guest, F., & Kowal, D. (1998). *Contraceptive technology.* New York: Ardent Media.

Hill, Y.L., & Brio, F.M. (2001, March). Adolescents and sexually transmitted infections. *Medical Aspects of Human Sexuality*, 7-13.

Hook, E.W., & Marra, C.M. (1992). Acquired syphilis in adults. *New England Journal of Medicine, 326*, 1060-1067.

Obata-Yasuoka, M. (2002). Bacterial vaginosis: Making the diagnosis and reducing the incidence. *Obstetrics and Gynecology, 100*, 759-764.

Roddy, R.E. Zekeng, L., Ryan, K.A., Tamoufe, U., & Tweedy, K.G. (2002). Effect of nonoxynol-9 gel on urogenital gonorrhea and chlamydial infection: A randomized controlled trial. *JAMA, 287*, 1117-1122.

Turner, C.F., Rogers, S.M., & Miller, H.G. (2002). Untreated gonococcal and chlamydial infection in a probability sample of adults. *Journal of the American Medical Association, 287*, 726-733.

16 Human Immunodeficiency Virus Infection and Acquired Immunodeficiency Syndrome

CONSTANCE R. UPHOLD

HUMAN IMMUNODEFICIENCY VIRUS (HIV) INFECTION AND ACQUIRED IMMUNODEFICIENCY SYNDROME (AIDS) IN ADULTS AND ADOLESCENTS

I. Definitions:

A. HIV infection: Infection with human retrovirus, Human Immunodeficiency Virus (HIV)

B. AIDS: Disease characterized by opportunistic infections (see following table for case definition)

CONDITIONS INCLUDED IN THE 1993 AIDS SURVEILLANCE CASE DEFINITION

- HIV+ persons with CD4 cell counts <200/μL or a CD4 percent <14%*
- Candidiasis of bronchi, trachea, or lungs
- Candidiasis, esophageal
- Cervical cancer, invasive*
- Coccidioidomycosis, disseminated or extrapulmonary
- Cryptococcosis, extrapulmonary
- Cryptosporidiosis, chronic intestinal (>1 mo duration)
- Cytomegalovirus disease (other than liver, spleen, or nodes)
- Encephalopathy, HIV-related
- Herpes simplex: Chronic ulcer(s) (>1 mo duration); or bronchitis, pneumonitis, or esophagitis
- Histoplasmosis, disseminated or extrapulmonary
- Isosporiasis, chronic intestinal (>1 mo duration)
- Kaposi's sarcoma
- Lymphoma, Burkitt's (or equivalent term)
- Lymphoma, immunoblastic (or equivalent term)
- Lymphoma, primary, of brain
- *Mycobacterium avium* complex or *M. kansasii*, disseminated or extrapulmonary
- *Mycobacterium tuberculosis*, any site (pulmonary* or extrapulmonary)
- *Mycobacterium*, other species or unidentified species, disseminated or extrapulmonary
- *Pneumocystis carinii* pneumonia
- Pneumonia, recurrent*
- Progressive multifocal leukoencephalopathy
- *Salmonella* septicemia, recurrent
- Toxoplasmosis of brain
- Wasting syndrome due to HIV

*Added January 1993

Source: Center for Communicable Diseases. 1992. 1993 revised classification system for HIV infection and expanded surveillance case definition of AIDS among adolescents and adults. *MMWR, 41* (RR-17)

II. Pathogenesis

A. HIV invades the body and may enter any cell, but it has a propensity to infect and kill cells of the immune system, particularly the CD4+ T-cells (T-lymphocytes)

B. HIV actively replicates which leads to immune system damage and results in susceptibility to opportunistic infections (OIs), cancer, neurologic diseases, wasting, and death

C. Transmission occurs by direct contact of a person's blood or body secretions with the blood or body secretions of a person infected with HIV virus
   1. Body fluids considered to be infectious include blood, tissues, cerebrospinal fluid, synovial fluid, peritoneal fluid, pleural fluid, pericardial fluid, amniotic fluid, semen, and vaginal secretions
   2. Body fluids that are **not** considered infectious include feces, nasal secretions, sputum, sweat, tears, urine, vomitus, and saliva (unless contaminated with blood)
   3. Certain activities are associated with high risk of infection such as unprotected anal, oral, or vaginal sex with multiple partners; unprotected sex with an HIV positive person; IV drug abuse; blood transfusions outside the US or during 1977-1985; unprotected sex with a person who has recent or past history of sexually transmitted diseases
   4. Highest percentage of HIV transmissions occurs during sex acts where body fluids are exchanged
   5. IV drug use is the second most frequent route of transmission

III. Clinical Presentation

A. Epidemiology
   1. The first AIDS cases were reported in 1981
   2. Seroprevalence of HIV in US is 0.3%
   3. Highly active antiretroviral therapy (HAART), defined as a combination of three or more antiretroviral drug therapy (ART) agents, has revolutionized HIV/AIDS care with substantial decreases in AIDS-defining complications, hospitalizations, and deaths
   4. The largest decline in cases of HIV/AIDS occurred among persons aged 25-44 years
   5. Increasing proportions of individuals living with AIDS are black or Hispanic, female, residents of the South, and individuals exposed to HIV through heterosexual contact
   6. Approximately one fourth of individuals living with HIV infection are unaware of their infection
   7. Rising drug resistance to all three classes of ART has been found in new HIV infections

B. Viral load and CD4+ T-cell counts help to assess the prognosis of HIV-infected patients
   1. Viral load measures the level of circulating plasma HIV-RNA; the greater the number of virus, the more active the infection, and the worse the prognosis
   2. CD4+ T-cell counts assess the general level of immunity or the extent of HIV-induced immune damage already suffered; the lower the CD4+ T-cell count the greater the risk for OIs
   3. A decrease in viral load of one log is associated with an average increase in CD4+ T-cells of about 85/mm^3

C. The natural history of HIV infection encompasses a wide spectrum of disease but infection is always harmful and true long-term survival free of major immune damage is uncommon

D. The acute retroviral syndrome develops after HIV exposure and a 1-3 week incubation period
   1. Symptoms resemble those of infectious mononucleosis and are self-limited, lasting 1-3 weeks
      a. Fever, fatigue, lymphadenopathy, pharyngitis, and arthralgias are typical
      b. Rash, diarrhea, nausea, vomiting, hepatosplenomegaly, thrush, weight loss, and neurological disorders (aseptic meningitis, Guillain-Barré) are less common problems
   2. Best diagnostic tests to detect disease are p24 antigen or plasma HIV RNA (viral load)
   3. Syndrome is associated with rapid HIV replication or high viral load
   4. Seroconversion occurs 3-5 weeks after transmission and is accompanied by sharp drop in viral load

E. Early HIV disease: Period between seroconversion to 4 months following HIV transmission
   1. At approximately 4 months, the plasma levels of HIV RNA reach a set point that shows a very gradual increase, averaging 7% a year over several years in the absence of antigenic stimuli such as intercurrent illness or immunizations or antiretroviral therapy; this set point predicts the subsequent rate of progression
      a. High concentrations (>100,000 copies/mL) are associated with median survival of 4.4 years
      b. Low concentrations (<5,000 copies/mL) are associated with median survival >10 years

2. Patients in early course of disease are usually asymptomatic, but may have the following:
   a. Lymphadenopathy and dermatologic abnormalities (seborrheic dermatitis, psoriasis, eosinophilic folliculitis)
   b. Oral lesions such as aphthous ulcers, herpes simplex labialis, and oral hairy leukoplakia usually occur later but may present
3. As the disease progresses, patients have more frequent skin disorders, oral lesions, and infections as well as diarrhea, intermittent fevers, night sweats, chills, unexplained weight loss, myalgias, arthralgia, headache, and fatigue

F. Symptomatic HIV disease: Complications are due to direct effects of the virus or to immunosuppression which occurs after a significant quantity of CD4+ T-cells has been destroyed
   1. Direct effect of HIV: Persistent generalized lymphadenopathy, HIV-associated dementia, lymphocytic interstitial pneumonia, HIV-associated nephropathy, and progressive immunosuppression; other possible consequences are anemia, neutropenia, thrombocytopenia, cardiomyopathy, myopathy, peripheral neuropathy, chronic meningitis, polymyositis, and Guillain-Barré syndrome
   2. Immunosuppression results in opportunistic infections and tumors, primarily from compromised cell-mediated immunity; see tables in V.F., V.G., V.H., V.I. for further clinical presentation of OIs
   3. Only about 2% or less of HIV-infected patients can maintain CD4+ T-cell counts in the normal range for lengthy periods of time (>12 years) without antiretroviral therapy
   4. In untreated patients, CD4+ T-cells average a 40-60/mm^3 decrease per year
   5. OIs, particularly pneumocystic pneumonia, occur when CD4+ T-cell counts fall below 200/mm^3
   6. Risk for opportunistic infections increases dramatically as CD4+ T-cell counts drop below 50/mm^3

G. HAART has extended patients' life expectancies but has potential adverse effects
   1. Lactic acidosis and hepatic steatosis occur from treatment with NRTIs (nucleoside reverse transcriptase inhibitor); syndrome is associated with high mortality rate
      a. Patients are considered to have lactic acidemia if they are asymptomatic with lactate >10 mmol/L or if they are symptomatic with lactate 5-10 mmol/L
      b. Clinical manifestations include unexplained onset and persistence of nausea, abdominal pain and distention, vomiting, diarrhea, anorexia, dyspnea, weakness, ascending neuromuscular weakness, myalgias, paresthesias, weight loss, and hepatomegaly
      c. Laboratory evaluation reveals increased serum lactate and may include increased anion gap, decreased serum bicarbonate, elevated aminotransferases, creatine phosphokinase, lactic dehydrogenase, lipase, and amylase
      d. Echotomography and computed tomography scans may detect enlarged fatty liver, and histologic examination may detect microvesicular steatosis
      e. If NRTI treatment continues, patients may have mitochondrial toxicity with severe lactic acidosis resulting in tachypnea, dyspnea, and ultimately respiratory failure
   2. Hepatotoxicity
      a. Defined as 3-5 times increase in serum transaminases with or without clinical hepatitis
      b. Typically, patients are asymptomatic
      c. Nevirapine has the greatest potential for causing clinical hepatitis and fatal hepatotoxicity
      d. Fatal hepatotoxicity was reported in 3 pregnant women using didanosine/stavudine
      e. Other risk factors include protease inhibitor (PI) use (major), hepatitis C infection (major), hepatitis B infection, alcohol abuse, baseline elevated liver enzymes, stavudine use, and use of other hepatotoxic agents
   3. Hyperglycemia, glucose intolerance, insulin resistance, new-onset diabetes mellitus, diabetic ketoacidosis, and exacerbation of pre-existing diabetes mellitus are strongly associated with PI use; conditions may also occur with PI-sparing regimens
   4. Fat maldistribution syndrome; often referred to as lipodystrophy or as lipodystrophy syndrome when combined with metabolic abnormalities including insulin resistance and hyperlipidemia
      a. Occurs primarily in association with PIs, but may occur in non-PI regimens
      b. The abdomen, dorsocervical fat pad, and breasts are sites for fat accumulation
      c. The face and extremities are most often affected by fat atrophy
   5. Hyperlipidemia with elevation of total serum cholesterol, low-density lipoprotein, and fasting triglycerides
      a. Occurs primarily with use of PIs; strongest association with ritonavir
      b. Association with NNRTIs (nonnucleoside reverse transcriptase inhibitor) is unclear and contradictory
      c. Very high triglycerides may be associated with pancreatitis
   6. Increased spontaneous bleeding episodes may occur with patients with hemophilia A and B

7. Osteonecrosis, osteopenia, and osteoporosis are other metabolic complications that have a definitive association with HIV itself; association with ART and PIs is unclear
    a. Factors associated with decreases in bone mineral density include alcohol abuse, hemoglobinopathies, corticosteroid treatment, hyperlipidemia, and hypercoagulability states
    b. Patients typically complain of pain in affected site of bone loss, but about 5% of those affected are asymptomatic
8. Skin rash
    a. Occurs most commonly with NNRTI class of drugs (predominantly with nevirapine); abacavir is the NRTI and amprenavir is the PI most often associated with rashes
    b. Most cases are mild to moderate and occur within first weeks of initiating therapy
    c. Serious manifestations include Stevens-Johnson syndrome, toxic epidermal necrosis (TEN), and a life-threatening syndrome with drug rash, eosinophilia, and systemic symptoms (DRESS)
    d. Abacavir may cause fatal hypersensitivity reaction that occurs with or without rash plus fever, fatigue, myalgia, nausea/vomiting, diarrhea, abdominal pain, pharyngitis, cough, dyspnea

IV. Diagnosis/Evaluation

A. History
    1. Determine risk factors for HIV (see following table); many primary care clinicians miss opportunities to identify and test persons at high risk for HIV infection

---

SCREENING STRATEGIES TO IDENTIFY PATIENTS AT RISK FOR HIV INFECTION

- Did you ever receive a transfusion of blood products outside the US or between 1977 and 1985?

- Open-ended question by provider, "What are you doing now or what have you done in the past that you think may put you at risk for HIV infection?"

- Screening questions* -- "Since your last HIV test (if ever), have you
    ✓ injected drugs and shared equipment (e.g., needles, syringes, cotton, water) with others?"
    ✓ had unprotected intercourse with someone that you think might be infected (e.g., a partner who injected drugs, has been diagnosed or treated for a sexually transmitted disease [STD] or hepatitis, has had multiple or anonymous sex partners, or has exchanged sex for drugs or money)?"
    ✓ had unprotected vaginal or anal intercourse with more than one sex partner?"
    ✓ been diagnosed or treated for an STD, hepatitis, or tuberculosis?"
    ✓ had a fever or illness of unknown cause?"
    ✓ been told you have an infection related to a 'weak immune system'?"

---

* Clients who respond affirmatively to ≥1 of these questions should be considered at increased risk for HIV

Adapted from Centers for Disease Control and Prevention. (2001). Revised guidelines for HIV counseling, testing, and referral. Technical Expert Panel Review of CDC Counseling, Testing and Referral Guidelines. *MMWR 50* (RR-9), 1-58.

    2. History at initial visit after the diagnosis is confirmed; patient's health status may range from asymptomatic to advanced immunodeficiency; this first encounter sets the stage for a partnership with the patient that may last for years
        a. Explore the duration of HIV positivity as well as when and how the patient was infected
        b. Document when the patient was first diagnosed with HIV infection
        c. Inquire about testing (when and where was it done?; what led to testing?)
        d. Ask about results of prior diagnostic tests
        e. Inquire about medications, treatments (including complementary therapies), responses to treatments, and history of adherence to medications
        f. Obtain past risk history (see preceding table)
        g. Inquire about sexual history such as number of partners within last year, use of condoms, history of other sexually transmitted diseases
        h. Ask about previous medical care including immunization status (pneumococcal, influenza, tetanus, hepatitis A and B, varicella) and prior TB skin tests
        i. Document significant past medical history (opportunistic infections, hospitalizations, surgeries, chickenpox, and chronic diseases, particularly tuberculosis, hepatitis, shingles, anemia, heart disease, neuromuscular conditions, alcoholism, and psychiatric disorders)
        j. Explore risk for cardiovascular disease such as obesity, smoking, hypertension, diabetes, family history, blood lipids
        k. In women, obtain a gynecological history including use and type of contraception, pregnancy history, current menstrual pattern, date of last pelvic exam and pap smear, history of abnormal pap smear, and history of vaginal bleeding; ask about desire for pregnancy

l.   Inquire about travel to Ohio and Mississippi River valleys (risk of histoplasmosis) and to Southwestern desert (risk of coccidioidomycosis)

m.   Assess patient's and family's knowledge about HIV

n.   Obtain a detailed social and mental health history to determine psychosocial assets/needs

o.   Screen for domestic violence (see section on DOMESTIC VIOLENCE for questions)

p.   Perform an HIV-related review of systems (ROS) directed toward uncovering symptoms of infection (fevers, night sweats, weight change, lymphadenopathy, visual changes, skin changes, new headaches, memory problems, mouth lesions, difficulty swallowing, cough/chest pain, diarrhea, nausea, vomiting, vaginitis, peripheral neuropathy, weakness, insomnia, depression)

3.   History on subsequent visits

a.   Document most recent CD4+ T-cell count and HIV viral load

b.   Document medications used for treating HIV infection

    (1)   Inquire about adverse effects from medications

    (2)   Always ask about adherence; a simple, direct question such as "How many doses have you missed in the past 24 hours?" may be nonthreatening

c.   Inquire about new or worsening symptoms

d.   Perform an HIV-related ROS (see IV.A.2.p.)

B.   Physical Examination

1.   Vital signs (fever is a sign of opportunistic infections and neoplasms)

2.   Measure weight (important in detecting "wasting syndrome" and determining the type of dietary intervention that is needed)

3.   Observe general appearance, noting signs of distress and depression

4.   Inspect for signs of weight maldistribution syndrome and measure waist/hip (or waist alone); measure breasts in women

5.   Examine skin for color, lesions, ecchymosis, and signs of dehydration

6.   Inspect nails for discoloration (e.g. due to zidovudine use or fungal infection)

7.   Carefully assess the eyes, including ophthalmoscopy for retinopathy

8.   Examine oropharynx, noting thrush, hairy oral leukoplakia, herpes simplex, periodontal problems, ulcerations

9.   Palpate for lymphadenopathy as generalized lymphadenopathy is frequently present; localized lymphadenopathy may indicate carcinoma

10.   Perform pulmonary and cardiac exams for pneumonia and cardiomyopathy

11.   Perform a complete breast examination; protease inhibitors and ketoconazole can cause gynecomastia in men

12.   Perform examination of abdomen, noting organomegaly

13.   Examine anal area for detection of sexually transmitted diseases, ulcerations, and fissures

14.   Perform pelvic and speculum exams on women for cervical dysplasia, vaginal candidiasis, and sexually transmitted diseases; perform a complete genitourinary examination on men

15.   Perform a musculoskeletal exam, noting muscle mass, strength, and tenderness (to detect myositis that may be associated with antiretroviral therapy [ART])

16.   Perform complete neurologic exam, including testing of cranial nerves, cerebellar function, reflexes, sensory function, and mental status for dementia and neuropathy

17.   Perform a psychiatric examination

C.   Differential diagnosis

1.   Mononucleosis

2.   Chronic fatigue syndrome

3.   Cancer

4.   Anemia

5.   Infections

6.   Autoimmune diseases

7.   Adrenal insufficiency

D.   Diagnostic tests

1.   **Testing to determine the diagnosis of HIV**

a.   **Antibody testing** uses enzyme-linked immunoabsorbent assay (ELISA) and a Western blot to make the diagnosis (both tests must be positive to confirm the diagnosis)

    (1)   ELISA, the initial test, is sensitive but not highly specific (may have false positives)

    (2)   Either a Western blot (WB) or an immunofluorescence assay (IFA) is used for confirmation of positive ELISA tests; WB and IFA are specific but labor intensive

b. Other tests for detection of antibodies
    (1) Calypte HIV-1 Urine EIA uses urine for screening; positive results require confirmation by standard serology
    (2) OraSure can detect antibodies from a sample of oral saliva
    (3) Home Access Express Test is an anonymous, finger-stick blood test for antibodies which can be done by an individual at home and purchased over-the-counter
c. SUDS and OraQuick are FDA-approved rapid tests
    (1) Tests are definitive if negative; positive results need confirmation with standard serology
    (2) Advantageous in settings in which there are occupational exposures and where reliable follow-up is unlikely such as in emergency rooms and STD clinics
d. Persons with positive antibody tests are considered HIV seropositive; however, a negative antibody test does not guarantee that an individual is seronegative
    (1) A window period exists; it may take 1-3 months after HIV exposure for seroconversion or for antibodies to form in sufficient amounts to be detectable by antibody tests
    (2) Because of this window period, persons with initial negative antibody tests and low risks should be retested at 6 months and high risk persons should be retested at 6 months and 1 year
e. **Antigen tests** can determine diagnosis by direct detection of virus, but they are expensive; useful in diagnosing persons with acute retroviral syndrome which occurs before antibody tests become positive
    (1) Viral load testing (RNA polymerase chain reaction [RT-PCR] and branched DNA [bDNA] assays) can measure the amount of HIV RNA in the plasma
    (2) p24 antigen can identify the presence of the HIV protein, but cannot quantify the amount of HIV; useful for diagnosing acute retroviral syndrome if RNA testing is unavailable
    (3) Diagnosis of HIV infection based on HIV RNA testing should be confirmed by standard methods (Western blot serology performed 2-4 months after the initial indeterminate or negative test)

2. **Tests to monitor disease progress**: CD4+ T-cells and HIV RNA (viral load)
    a. Recommended schedule for ordering CD4+ T-cell and viral load tests:
        (1) At time of diagnosis and after initiation of therapy at 4, 8-12, and 16-24 weeks to assess response to therapy
        (2) Once viral suppression (2 sequential viral load measurements below the limit of detection of the most sensitive assay available) has been attained, monitor every 8-12 weeks
        (3) Consider more frequent monitoring in cases of intercurrent illness, change of antiretroviral therapy (ART), if adherence is questionable, or for patients with discordant responses (CD4+ T-cells that do not increase with successful viral suppression)
    b. Measurement of CD4+ T-cell counts
        (1) Determine effectiveness of antiretroviral therapy, prognosis of disease, and need for prophylaxis of opportunistic infections
        (2) Typically, counts increase by more than 50 cells/mm^3 at 4-8 weeks after ART has been started or changed; additional increase of 50-100 cells/mm^3 per year thereafter
        (3) A substantial decrease in CD4+ T-cells is a decrease of >30% from baseline for absolute cell numbers
    c. Measurement of HIV RNA levels or viral loads
        (1) RNA polymerase chain reaction (RT-PCR) and branched DNA (bDNA) assays can measure the amount of HIV RNA in the plasma; results with RT-PCR are twice the levels with bDNA
        (2) Effective therapy reduces viral load by more than 90% (a 1-log$_{10}$, or 10-fold, reduction) within 8 weeks of treatment; consider poor adherence, viral resistance, or inadequate drug exposure (e.g., malabsorption) if viral load fails to decrease to these levels
        (3) After 16-24 weeks of ART, plasma viral levels should be undetectable
        (4) Rates of viral load decline are affected by baseline CD4+ T-cells, the initial viral load, potency of drug regimen, medication adherence, previous exposure to ART, and presence of any opportunistic infections

      (5)   A threefold or 0.5-$\log_{10}$ increase or decrease in viral levels is considered a minimal change

      (6)   Viral load results may be inaccurate during or within 4 weeks after successful treatment of any intercurrent infection, resolution of symptomatic illness, or immunization because of the immune activation of virus associated with these events

3.   **Tests to screen for concomitant diseases, immunity status, and as a base-line before drugs are administered;** ordered at first visit after diagnosis is confirmed and thereafter as recommended

    a.   Mantoux method using the purified protein derivative (PPD) to screen for tuberculosis and annually for high-risk patients (anergy testing is no longer recommended)

      (1)   Do not order if patient has history of positive PPD or history of TB treatment

      (2)   Positive PPD for person with HIV is >5 mm of induration

    b.   Rapid plasma reagin (RPR) or the Venereal Disease Laboratories (VDRL) to screen for syphilis which occurs in approximately 20% of patients with HIV infection; for patients with high-risk of developing STDs, order annually

    c.   Pap smear for women to screen for cervical dysplasia at baseline and at 6 months; then, annually if negative

    d.   Chemistry panel including liver function tests and renal profile; useful as baseline measures since patient may be receiving drugs with potential hepatic or renal toxicities

    e.   Hepatitis screen

      (1)   Anti-HBc to determine hepatitis immunity and need for HBV vaccine

      (2)   HBsAg and anti-HCV to detect active hepatitis if patient has unexplained elevated transaminase levels; obtain anti–HCV in all injection drug users

      (3)   Positive anti-HCV should be verified with recombinant immunoblot assay (RIBA) or reverse transcriptase-polymerase chain reaction (RT-PCR)

    f.   Toxoplasmosis serology (anti-toxoplasma antibody or IgG titer)

      (1)   Patient is at risk for reactivation toxoplasmosis when CD4+ T-cells drop below 100/mm^3

      (2)   Consider repeating in seronegative patients when their CD4+ T-cell counts are <100/mm^3

    g.   CBC with differential and platelet count; anemia, leukopenia, or thrombocytopenia are common in HIV infection and can also result from drug therapy; order every 3-6 months

    h.   Order lipid profile and glucose at baseline before antiretroviral therapy and at switch of therapy, 3-6 months after starting or switching therapy, and at least annually thereafter

    i.   The following are optional tests:

      (1)   Chest x-ray to screen for latent TB and as a baseline test

      (2)   Cytomegalovirus (CMV) IgG; CMV retinitis is a common complication and develops in seropositive patients when CD4+ T-cell drops below 50-75/mm^3

      (3)   Glucose-6-phosphate dehydrogenase deficiency (G-6-PD), particularly for high risk patients (African Americans and men of Mediterranean heritage): If test is positive, patient has a deficiency and should not use dapsone and possibly should not use a sulfonamide

      (4)   Varicella IgG to determine need for post-exposure prophylaxis with varicella zoster immune globulin

      (5)   Gonorrhea and chlamydia screens for women

      (6)   CD4+ cell subset determinations to enumerate memory and naive cells are used primarily in clinical trials to help define the degree of immune reconstitution

4.   **Therapeutic drug monitoring**

    a.   In patients on zidovudine, order CBC at least every 3 months

    b.   Closely monitor liver enzymes after ART initiation; after nevirapine initiation monitor every 2 weeks for first month, then monthly for first 12 weeks, then every 1-3 months

    c.   Order routine fasting blood glucose tests at baseline and then every 3-6 months when PIs are used, particularly in patients with preexisting diabetes

    d.   Closely monitor lipid levels in patients with risk for atherosclerotic disease; in all patients assess at baseline, 3-6 months after ART is started or changed, and annually thereafter

    e.   Routine measurements of lactate levels and bone density (dual energy X-ray absorptiometry or quantitative ultrasound) among asymptomatic patients are not currently recommended; patients with symptoms of avascular necrosis should have CT ordered

    f.   There are no clear recommendations for monitoring body fat composition abnormalities; serial waist/hip (or waist alone) and breast measurement in women may be helpful

5. **Drug-resistance testing**
   a. Considered standard of care in management of treatment failure
      (1) Provides guidance on which drugs to exclude or include in new regimens
      (2) Perform testing when patient is on ART
   b. Strongly consider testing in patients who may have been infected with a resistant viral strain, particularly patients with a recent infection or when the initial response to ART is suboptimal despite excellent drug adherence
   c. Resistance testing is **not** recommended in following circumstances
      (1) Chronic infection in treatment naïve patients
      (2) After patient has discontinued ART for >2 weeks
      (3) When viral load is <1000 copies/mL
   d. Order either genotypic or phenotypic assays; for patients with complex treatment history, both assays may provide important and complementary information
      (1) Both assays measure only the dominant HIV species and thus some resistant strains may not be detected; assays are best at identifying drugs that will be ineffective rather than drugs that will work
      (2) Genotypic assays measure mutations on the reverse transcriptase or protease gene; results are available in 1-2 weeks
      (3) Phenotypic assays are more analogous to conventional antibacterial sensitivity tests; these assays are more costly and take 2-3 weeks to run
6. **Drug concentration monitoring**
   a. Not universally recommended
   b. May be beneficial in cases of treatment failure or when salvage therapy with a ritonavir-enhanced PI-based regimen has been started (particularly if other drugs have known pharmacological interactions such as efavirenz)

V. Plan/Management (care should be supervised by infectious disease specialist); because treatment of HIV infection changes rapidly consult following websites for updated information: CDC Clearinghouse (http://www.cdc.org) and the HIV Information Network (http://www.hivatis.org)

   A. Provide **patient education and counseling** at each visit; adjust amount and complexity of teaching and counseling based on patient's degree of stress, prior knowledge, readiness to learn, and cognitive abilities
      1. Provide information about transmission and how to prevent spread of infection such as not sharing razors or toothbrushes, carefully cleaning up blood spills, disposing of used feminine sanitary products
      2. Discuss lifestyle choices and safe sex practices such as latex barriers including condoms, female vaginal pouches, and dental dams
         a. Even patients with undetectable viral loads should be considered infectious and should practice safe sex
         b. HIV-infected males should wear condoms even when engaging in sexual activity with other HIV-infected individuals to prevent transmission of drug-resistant strains of HIV and other sexually transmitted diseases
         c. Spermicides containing *nonoxynol-9* are not effective means of HIV prevention
      3. Provide education and support to stop injecting drugs; for patients that continue to inject discuss safety issues such as never sharing needles, disposing of syringes after use, and using sterile injection equipment
      4. Discuss ways to avoid exposure to infection from opportunistic infections
         a. Recommend that patient wash hands after changing diapers, handling pets, and gardening or having other contact with soil
         b. Avoid changing cat liter box due to risk of toxoplasmosis; avoid rough play with kittens due to risk of cat scratch disease
         c. Avoid animals aged <6 months when obtaining a pet
         d. Discuss susceptibility to contagious disease and how to protect self
         e. Travel, specifically to developing countries, may be hazardous due to high risk for food-borne and waterborne infections
            (1) Antimicrobial prophylaxis is not routinely recommended, but may be warranted in patients with high risk (consider ciprofloxacin 500 mg daily for high risk persons)
            (2) All travelers to developing countries should have a supply of antibiotics (e.g. ciprofloxacin 500 mg BID for 3-7 days) to take empirically if diarrhea occurs
            (3) Consult specialist in travel medicine for advice concerning immunizations, chemoprophylaxis against malaria, and protection against arthropod vectors

  f. Teach about food safety
   (1) Foods should be well done and thoroughly cooked; avoid raw/rare meat, fish and poultry, raw eggs, or unpasteurized dairy products
   (2) Wash hands after contact with raw meat
   (3) Wash fruits and vegetables before eating
   (4) Avoid foods from delicatessen counters or heat/reheat these foods until steaming
   (5) Consider using filtered or bottled water

5. Discuss ways to handle notification of partners and others; the local health department can assist with anonymous partner notification/elicitation

6. Discuss healthy diet; referral to nutritionist is beneficial
  a. Recommend eating a variety of foods from different food groups
  b. Encourage nutrient density or making every bite of food count; avoid foods with little protein, vitamins, and minerals
  c. Choose foods that are as close to their natural states as possible; use whole wheat instead of white bread or brown rice instead of white
  d. Use olive and canola oils instead of margarine and vegetable oils which are rich in polyunsaturated fatty acids and may suppress the immune system
  e. Recommend low-fat diets to reduce risk of developing hyperlipidemia
  f. To prevent decreased bone density, suggest an adequate intake of calcium and vitamin D
  g. One or two daily multivitamin/mineral supplement(s) is(are) recommended

7. Encourage smoking cessation and decreasing or eliminating other types of substance abuse (alcohol, recreational drugs)

8. Reinforce the importance of healthy lifestyles such as good oral hygiene, good sleep habits, and ways to reduce stress such as exercise, relaxation techniques, and guided imagery; massage therapy and referral to a psychologist may be beneficial

9. Exercise, including weight-bearing exercise, helps prevent adverse effects of HAART such as hyperlipidemia and bone density problems

10. Provide information on prognosis and future therapy plans; emphasize that advances in HIV therapy have dramatically improved outcomes and that patients who adhere to therapy can usually lead fairly normal lives and have a long life (however, remind that cure of HIV is unlikely)

11. Discuss what to do if an emergency arises and which symptoms require immediate attention

12. Help empower patients to become actively involved in their care through support groups, learning about the disease and treatments, and developing a partnership with the clinician

13. For patients in the late stage of disease offer information on advance directives; discuss living wills, health care surrogates; consider referral for home care or hospice care

14. Provide information on community resources and website resources (see following table)

WEB SITE RESOURCES	
HIV Prevention	http://hivinsite.ucsf.edu
Medical information	www.hopkins-aids.edu
Medical information	www.medscape.com

B. For patients on ART, medication adherence is crucial; nonadherence is the strongest predictor of virologic failure
 1. Determine patient's readiness before initiating ART
 2. Effective communication and trust between patient and clinician is essential
 3. Negotiate a treatment plan that the patient understands and to which he/she can commit
 4. Reinforce the need to adhere at every visit; emphasize that 90-95% of doses must be taken for optimal viral suppression
 5. Inform patient of potential side effects, ways to manage side effects, and possible adverse drug interactions
 6. Enlist support of friends/family, provide written drug schedules, pill boxes, or alarm clocks
 7. Factors to consider in improving adherence are pill volume, pill size, dietary restrictions, and toxic adverse effects

C. **Immunization** recommendations
1.   Influenza vaccine should be administered annually; pneumococcal, Hepatitis A and B vaccines should be administered to susceptible patients according to recommended guidelines (see table PROPHYLAXIS TO PREVENT FIRST EPISODE OF OPPORTUNISTIC DISEASE)
2.   *Haemophilus influenzae* type B vaccine is no longer recommended as most infections in HIV-infected persons involve nontypeable strains
3.   Administer tetanus-diphtheria, mumps, rubella, measles vaccines identical to patients without HIV
4.   If polio vaccine is needed, use enhanced inactivated polio vaccine (eIPV)
5.   Do **not** use any of the following vaccines: Live polio, varicella zoster, BCG, or any live or attenuated vaccine except measles, mumps, and rubella

D. **Health maintenance referrals** are optional
1.   Twice-yearly dental examinations
2.   Periodic ophthalmology examinations: screening for CMV retinitis by a trained ophthalmologist or optometrist should be considered every 4-6 months once the patient's CD4+ T-cell count falls below 75-100/mm^3

E. Medications should be given to **prevent opportunistic infections** when a person's CD4+ T-cell counts fall to certain levels or after exposure to certain pathogens (see following table)

PROPHYLAXIS TO PREVENT FIRST EPISODE OF OPPORTUNISTIC DISEASE

Pathogen	Indication Discontinuing/Restarting Primary Prophylaxis	Preventive regimens	
		First Choice	Alternative
I. Strongly recommended as standard of care			
Pneumocystis carinii pneumonia (PCP)*	CD4+ count <200 cells/μL or oropharyngeal candidiasis; also consider prophylaxis for persons with a CD4+ percentage of <14% or for persons with a history of AIDS-defining illness and possibly for those with CD4+ counts of >200 cells/μL but <250 cells/μL Discontinue in patients who have responded to HAART with an increase in CD4+ count >200 cells/μL for ≥3 mos; restart if CD4+ count decreases to <200 cells/μL or if PCP recurs	Trimethoprim-sulfamethoxazole (TMP-SMZ), 1 DS PO QD or TMP-SMZ, 1 SS PO QD*	TMP-SMZ, 1 DS PO three times a week; dapsone, 50 mg PO BID or 100 mg PO QD; dapsone, 50 mg PO QD plus pyrimethamine, 50 mg PO weekly plus leucovorin, 25 mg PO weekly; dapsone, 200 mg PO plus pyrimethamine, 75 mg PO plus leucovorin, 25 mg PO weekly; or aerosolized pentamidine, 300 mg every month via Respirgard II nebulizer
Mycobacterium tuberculosis Isoniazid-sensitive†	Tuberculin skin test (TST) reaction ≥5 mm or prior positive TST result without treatment or contact with case of active tuberculosis, regardless of TST result	Isoniazid, 300 mg PO plus pyridoxine, 50 mg PO QD x 9 mos or isoniazid, 900 mg PO plus pyridoxine, 100 mg PO twice a week x 9 mos	Rifampin, 600 mg PO QD x 4 mos or rifabutin, 300 mg PO QD X 4 mos; pyrazinamide, 15-20 mg/kg PO QD X 2 mos plus either rifampin, 600 mg PO QD X 2 mos or rifabutin, 300 mg PO QD X 2 mos
Isoniazid-resistant	Same as above	Rifampin, 600 mg PO QD or rifabutin, 300 mg PO QD X 4 mos	Pyrazinamide, 15-20 mg/kg PO QD X 2 mos plus either rifampin, 600 mg PO QD X 2 mos or rifabutin, 300 mg PO QD X 2 mos
Multidrug-resistant	Same as above	Consult Public Health authorities	----
Toxoplasma gondii	IgG antibody to *Toxoplasma* and CD4+ count <100/μL Discontinue when CD4+ count increases to >200 cells/μL for ≥3 mos; restart prophylaxis when CD4+ count decreases to <100-200 cells/μL	TMP-SMZ, 1 DS PO QD	TMP-SMZ, 1 SS PO QD; dapsone, 50 mg PO QD plus pyrimethamine, 50 mg PO weekly plus leucovorin, 25 mg PO weekly; atovaquone, 1,500 mg PO QD with or without pyrimethamine, 25 mg PO QD plus leucovorin, 10 mg PO QD *(Continued)*

PROPHYLAXIS TO PREVENT FIRST EPISODE OF OPPORTUNISTIC DISEASE *(CONTINUED)*

Pathogen	Indication Discontinuing/Restarting Primary Prophylaxis	Preventive regimens	
		First Choice	**Alternative**
Mycobacterium avium complex	CD4+ count <50 cells/μL Discontinue when CD4+ count increases to >100 cells/μL for ≥3 mos; restart when CD4+ count <50-100 cells/μL	Clarithromycin, 500 mg PO BID or azithromycin, 1,200 mg PO weekly	Rifabutin, 300 mg PO QD; azithromycin, 1,200 mg PO QD plus rifabutin, 300 mg PO QD
Varicella-zoster virus (VZV)	Significant exposure to chickenpox or shingles for patients who have no history of either condition or, if available, negative antibody to VZV	Varicella-zoster immune globulin (VZIG), 5 vials (1.25 mL each) IM administered ≤96 h after exposure, ideally within 48 hours	None

II. Usually recommended

Pathogen	Indication	First Choice	Alternative
Streptococcus pneumoniae	CD4+ count of ≥200 cells/μL; also consider prophylaxis for persons with CD4+ counts of <200 cells/μL	23-valent polysaccharide vaccine, 0.5 mL IM (Revaccination ≥5 years after the first dose is optional; consider revaccinating sooner if the initial vaccination was administered when the CD4+ count was <200 cells/μL and the CD4+ count has increased to >200 cells/μL while on HAART)	None
Hepatitis B virus[§]	All susceptible patients (i.e., antihepatitis B core antigen-negative)	Hepatitis B vaccine: 3 doses	None
Influenza virus	All patients (annually, before influenza season)	Inactivated trivalent influenza virus vaccine: one annual dose (0.5 mL) IM	Oseltamivir, 75 mg PO QD (influenza A and B); rimantadine, 100 mg PO BID, or amantadine, 100 mg PO BID (influenza A); reduce doses in patients with decreased renal or hepatic function or who have seizure disorders
Hepatitis A virus[§]	All susceptible patients at increased risk for hepatitis A infection (i.e., antihepatitis A virus-negative) (e.g., illegal drug users, men who have sex with men, hemophiliacs) or patients with chronic liver disease, including chronic hepatitis B or C	Hepatitis A vaccine: two doses	None

III. Evidence for efficacy but not routinely indicated

Pathogen	Indication	First Choice	Alternative
Bacteria	Neutropenia	Granulocyte-colony-stimulating factor (G-CSF), 5-10 μg/kg SQ QD X 2-4 weeks or granulocyte-macrophage colony-stimulating factor (GM-CSF), 250 μg/m^2 SQ QD X 2-4 weeks	None
Cryptococcus neoformans	CD4+ count <50 cells/μL	Fluconazole, 100-200 mg PO QD	Itraconazole, 200 mg PO QD
Cytomegalovirus (CMV)	CD4+ count <50 cells/μL and CMV antibody positivity	Oral ganciclovir, 1 g PO TID	None
Histoplasma capsulatum	CD4+ count <100 cells/μL, endemic geographic area	Itraconazole, 200 mg PO QD	None

* TMP-SMZ reduces the frequency of toxoplasmosis and some bacterial infections. Patients receiving dapsone should be tested for glucose-6 phosphate dehydrogenase deficiency.

[†]Directly observed therapy (DOT) is recommended for isoniazid (e.g. 900 mg twice weekly); isoniazid regimens should include pyridoxine to prevent peripheral neuropathy. If rifampin or rifabutin is administered concurrently with protease inhibitors or nonnucleoside reverse transcriptase inhibitors, potential pharmacokinetic interactions may occur. Fatal and severe liver injury associated with treatment of latent tuberculosis infection among HIV patients treated with 2 month regimen of daily rifampin and pyrazinamide has occurred.

[§]For persons requiring vaccination against both hepatitis A and B, a combination vaccine is available.

Adapted from Centers for Disease Control and Prevention. (2002). Guidelines for preventing opportunistic infections among HIV-infected persons – 2002: Recommendations of the U.S. Public Health Service and the Infectious Diseases Society of America. *MMWR, 51*(RR-8), 1-52.

F.	It is important to recognize the signs and symptoms of **opportunistic diseases**, diagnose and treat appropriately, and then provide prophylaxis to prevent recurrences (**see V.K . for prevention of recurrences**) (see following table for diagnosis and treatment of bacterial infections)

ASSESSMENT, DIAGNOSIS, AND TREATMENT OF COMMON BACTERIAL OPPORTUNISTIC INFECTIONS

Transmission	Clinical Characteristics	Diagnosis	Treatment
Mycobacterium Avium Intracellulare (MAI) or M. Avium Complex Infections			
Widely dispersed in environment and found in most water supplies	Diarrhea, abdominal pain, organomegaly, high fevers, weight loss, fatigue, enlarged nodes, elevated alkaline phosphatase	Cultures of blood, stool, or bone marrow; lymph node and liver biopsy	Clarithromycin 500 mg BID **plus** ethambutol (EMB)15-25 mg/kg/day ± rifabutin (RFB) 300 mg QD; alternatively, azithromycin 600 mg QD plus EMB ± RFB; duration is indefinite in absence of immune reconstitution; with HAART may discontinue when MAC treatment is >1 year and CD4+ T-cell count is >100/mm^3 for 3-6 months, and patient is asymptomatic
Mycobacterium Tuberculosis			
Spread through droplet nuclei coughed up by persons with untreated TB	Productive, prolonged cough; fever, chills, night sweats, fatigue, weight loss, hemoptysis, lymphadenopathy	PPD skin test, chest x-ray, sputum smear and culture	**+ PPD but no active disease:** If patient is not receiving HAART: rifampin (RIF) 600 mg QD plus pyrazinamide (PZA) 20 mg/kg/day x 2 months; if patient is on HAART: Isoniazid (INH) 300 mg QD plus pyridoxine 50 mg QD x 9 months **Active disease: 12 months treatment;** If patient is not taking PI or NNRTI: INH/RIF/PZA/EMB (or streptomycin [SM]) daily x 2 months then INH/RIF daily or 2-3 times/week x 18 weeks (other regimens are available) If patient is receiving PI or NNRTI: INH/RFB/PZA/EMB daily x 8 weeks, then INH/RFB daily or 2 times per week x 18 weeks (other regimens are available)
Syphilis			
Caused by *Treponema pallidum*; Sexually transmitted disease	Primary: chancre Secondary: Rash on palms and soles Tertiary: No outward signs Neurosyphilis: CNS problems	RPR or VDRL and then FTA-ABS; lumbar puncture recommended with neurologic symptoms, treatment failure, and late latent syphilis	**Primary, secondary and early latent (<1 year):** benzathine penicillin G 2.4 mil units IM x 1 with follow-up 2, 3, 6, 9 & 12 months, if titer fails to decrease 4-fold at 6-12 months or patient is symptomatic, retreat with benzathine penicillin G 2.4 mil units IM once a week x 3 weeks **Latent and tertiary, not neurosyphilis:** benzathine penicillin G 2.4 mil units IM weekly x 3 weeks **Neurosyphilis:** aqueous penicillin G 18-24 mil units/day IV x 10-14 days (3-4 mil units q 4 hours); retreat if CSF WBC fails to decrease at 6 mos or CSF still abnormal at 2 years

G.   See following table for diagnosis and treatment of fungal infections

ASSESSMENT, DIAGNOSIS, AND TREATMENT OF COMMON FUNGAL OPPORTUNISTIC INFECTIONS

Transmission	Clinical Characteristics	Diagnosis	Treatment
Candidiasis			
Caused by *candida albicans* when CD4+ T-cells drop below 500/mm^3	Oral: White plaques anywhere in oral cavity, burning sensation, absence of taste, pain when swallowing	Swab lesion: KOH prep	Clotrimazole 10 mg troches; dissolve in saliva, 1 troche 5 times daily for 14 days; or - fluconazole 100 mg PO QD for 7-14 days
	Vaginal: Thick white vaginal discharge; itching, burning, redness in vaginal area	Swab vagina: KOH prep	Miconazole vaginal suppository 200 mg: 1 suppository HS X 3 nights; or - fluconazole 150 mg tab PO single dose
	Esophageal: Dysphagia, odynophagia	Diagnosed empirically or with endoscopy	Fluconazole 200 mg tab PO QD; up to 400 mg/day x 2-3 weeks
Cryptococcal Meningitis			
Yeast-like fungus found widely in environment, especially in soil contaminated with bird excrement	Fever, headache, fatigue, nausea, memory loss, confusion, problems with coordination	Cryptococcal serum antigen; lumbar puncture: India ink, cryptococcal antigen, culture	Amphotericin B 0.7 mg/kg/day IV plus flucytosine 100 mg/kg/day PO x 14 days, then fluconazole 400 mg/day for 8-10 weeks; lifelong suppressive therapy with fluconazole 200 mg/day

H.   See following table for diagnosis and treatment of protozoal infections:

ASSESSMENT, DIAGNOSIS, AND TREATMENT OF COMMON PROTOZOAL OPPORTUNISTIC INFECTIONS

Transmission	Clinical Characteristics	Diagnosis	Treatment
Pneumocystis Carinii Pneumonia (PCP) (Has characteristics of both protozoa & fungi)			
Believed to infect most humans during childhood, and then remains dormant	Dry, non-productive cough; shortness of breath, fever, fatigue, weight loss	Chest X-ray; Induced sputum; Broncho-alveolar lavage	Mild-Moderate Disease: TMP/SMX* PO 15 mg/kg/day, TMP equivalent in 3-4 divided doses x 21 days (usually 2 DS tabs TID or IV x 21 days); or - TMP 15 mg/kg/day PO plus dapsone 100 mg/day times 21 days for sulfa allergy Severe Disease:TMP/SMX PO 15 mg/kg TMP equivalent/day in 4 divided doses for 21 days with prednisone 40 mg PO BID x 5 days, then 40 mg QD x 5 days, then 20 mg QD to completion
Toxoplasmic Encephalitis			
30% U.S. adults infected with parasite which remains dormant until immune system is damaged	Fever, headache, neurological problems such as seizures, changes in mental status, coma	CT scan or MRI of brain for ring enhancing lesions; Positive toxoplasma IgG in serum	Pyrimethamine 100-200 mg PO loading dose, then 50-100 mg QD with sulfadiazine or trisulfapyrimidine 4-8 g PO QD plus folinic acid 10 mg PO QD for at least 6 weeks
Cryptosporidiosis			
Transmitted to humans via contact with feces, contaminated water or food	Chronic watery diarrhea, abdominal cramps, nausea, fever, weight loss, headache	Modified acid fast stain of stool; endoscopy with biopsy or bowel biopsy	Treatment is difficult – consider referral to specialist; sometimes paromomycin 500 mg PO TID or 1000 mg PO BID with food x 14-28 days then 500 mg BID may be effective

*Trimethoprim/sulfamethoxazole

I. See following table for diagnosis and treatment of viral infections:

ASSESSMENT, DIAGNOSIS, AND TREATMENT OF COMMON VIRAL OPPORTUNISTIC INFECTIONS

Transmission	Clinical Characteristics	Diagnosis	Treatment
Cytomegalovirus Retinitis			
High percentage of US adults are infected with virus which remains dormant until immune system is damaged	Cytomegalovirus may infect GI tract, brain, and other organs but common site is the eye with blurred vision, floaters, flashing lights, loss of peripheral vision	Diagnosis of CMV retinitis made with indirect funduscopy by a trained ophthalmologist	Consult ophthalmologist; ganciclovir (IV, oral, implant), valganciclovir (oral), foscarnet (IV, intraocular injection), cidofovir (IV), fomivirsen (injection into vitreous) are effective therapies
Oral Hairy Leukoplakia			
Caused by Epstein-Barr virus	White, non-removable lesion with a corrugated surface on lateral margins of tongue	Clinical presentation	None usually needed; may treat with acyclovir 800 mg PO 5 times a day x 2-3 weeks
Progressive Multifocal Leukoencephalopathy (PML)			
Caused by J.C. virus; most people are infected by 2 years of age, but virus remains latent in brain until immune system is sufficiently damaged	Insidious onset with rapid progression; confusion, lack of energy, loss of balance, memory and speech problems, blurred or double vision, hallucinations, seizures, paralysis and eventual death	CT scan or MRI which may reveal focal brain lesions which do not enhance or cause surrounding edema	HAART may be effective; treatment with cidofovir is questionable; consult with specialist
Herpes Simplex, Herpes Zoster, and Molluscum Contagiosum (see chapter on SKIN PROBLEMS)			

J. See following table for diagnosis and treatment of cancers:

ASSESSMENT, DIAGNOSIS, AND TREATMENT OF CANCERS ASSOCIATED WITH HIV INFECTION

Transmission	Clinical Characteristics	Diagnosis	Treatment
Kaposi's Sarcoma			
May be sexually transmitted and is caused by herpes virus, HHV-8	Red, brown or pink blotches on skin which change to hard, raised purplish-red lesions; can be on internal organs as well as common places of arms, legs, and chest	Visual examination or skin biopsy	Referral to specialist; generally responds to HAART; often left untreated or can treat with topical liquid nitrogen, alpha interferon, radiation, laser therapy, chemotherapy
Lymphomas			
Cancers of lymphoid cells; B-cell non-Hodgkin's lymphoma is most common	Spreads quickly, occurs in brain and outside of the lymph nodes	Depending on site; biopsy, CT/MRI, bone marrow biopsy, lumbar puncture	Refer to specialist

K. Patients who have a history of opportunistic diseases should be administered chemoprophylaxis to prevent recurrence (see following table)

PROPHYLAXIS TO PREVENT RECURRENCE OF OPPORTUNISTIC DISEASE AFTER CHEMOTHERAPY FOR ACUTE DISEASE

Pathogen	Indication Discontinue/Restart Prophylaxis	Preventive Regimens	
		First choice	Alternatives
I. Recommended as standard of care			
Pneumocystis carinii	Prior *P. carinii* pneumonia Discontinue when CD4+ count has increased to >200 cells/μL for ≥3 mos; Restart if CD4+ count decreases to <200 cells/μL or if PCP recurred at a CD4+ count of >200 cells/μL	Trimethoprim-sulfamethoxazole (TMP-SMZ), 1 DS PO QD or TMP-SMZ, 1 SS PO QD	Dapsone, 50 mg PO BID or 100 mg PO QD; dapsone 50 mg PO QD plus pyrimethamine, 50 mg PO weekly plus leucovorin, 25 mg PO weekly; aerosolized pentamidine, 300 mg every mo via Respirgard II nebulizer; atovaquone, 1,500 mg PO QD; TMP-SMZ, 1 DS PO three times a week
*Toxoplasma gondii**	Prior toxoplasmic encephalitis Discontinue with patients who complete initial therapy, remain asymptomatic, and have sustained (e.g., ≥6 mos) increase in CD4+ count >200 cells/μL; restart if CD4+ count decreases to <200 cells/μL	Sulfadiazine 500-1000 mg PO QID plus pyrimethamine 25-50 mg PO QD plus leucovorin 10-25 mg PO QD	Clindamycin, 300-450 mg PO Q 6-8 h plus pyrimethamine, 25-50 mg PO QD plus leucovorin, 10-25 mg PO QD; atovaquone, 750 mg PO Q 6-12 hours with or without pyrimethamine, 25 mg PO QD plus leucovorin, 10 mg PO QD
Mycobacterium avium complex**	Documented disseminated disease Discontinue when patient has completed a course of ≥12 months of treatment, remains asymptomatic, and has a sustained (≥6 mos) increase in CD4+ counts to >100 cells/μL; restart if CD4+ count decreases to <100 cells/μL	Clarithromycin,** 500 mg PO BID plus ethambutol, 15 mg/kg PO QD with or without rifabutin, 300 mg PO QD	Azithromycin, 500 mg PO QD plus ethambutol, 15 mg/kg PO QD with or without rifabutin, 300 mg PO QD
Cytomegalovirus	Prior end-organ disease Consult ophthalmologist; discontinue when CD4+ count has sustained (≥6 mos) increases to >100-150 cells/μL, and no evidence of active disease; restart if CD4+ count decreases to 100-150 cells/μl	Valganciclovir, 900 mg PO QD; ganciclovir, 5-6 mg/kg IV 5-7 days/wk or 1,000 mg PO TID; or foscarnet, 90-120 mg/kg IV QD; or (for retinitis) ganciclovir sustained-release implant every 6-9 mos plus ganciclovir, 1.0-1.5 g PO TID	Cidofovir, 5 mg/kg IV every other week with probenecid 2 g PO 3 hours before the dose followed by 1 g PO 2 hours after the dose, and 1 g PO 8 hours after the dose (total of 4 g); fomivirsen 1 vial (330 μg) injected into vitreous, then repeated every 2-4 weeks; valganciclovir 900 mg PO QD
Cryptococcus neoformans	Documented disease Discontinue when patient has completed a course of initial therapy, remains asymptomatic, and has a sustained increase (≥6 mos) in CD4+ count to >100-200 cells/μL; restart if CD4+ count decreases to 100-200 cells/μL	Fluconazole, 200 mg PO QD	Amphotericin B, 0.6-1.0 mg/kg IV weekly-- three times weekly; itraconazole, 200 mg PO QD
Histoplasma capsulatum	Documented disease; no recommendation to discontinue prophylaxis	Itraconazole, 200 mg PO BID	Amphotericin B, 1.0 mg/kg IV weekly
Coccidioides immitis	Documented disease; no recommendation to discontinue prophylaxis	Fluconazole 400 mg PO QD	Amphotericin B, 1.0 mg/kg IV weekly; itraconazole, 200 mg PO BID
Salmonella species	Bacteremia	Ciprofloxacin, 500 mg PO BID for ≥2 mos	Antibiotic chemoprophylaxis with another active agent

(Continued)

| | Indication | Preventive Regimens | |
Pathogen	Discontinue/Restart Prophylaxis	First choice	Alternatives
II. Recommended only if subsequent episodes are frequent or severe			
Herpes simplex virus	Frequent/severe recurrences	Acyclovir, 200 mg PO TID or 400 mg PO BID; famciclovir, 250 mg PO BID	Valacyclovir, 500 mg PO BID
Candida (oral, vaginal, or esophageal)	Frequent/severe recurrences	Fluconazole, 100-200 mg PO QD	Itraconazole solution, 200 mg PO QD

*Pyrimethamine-sulfadiazine confers protection against PCP as well as toxoplasmosis; clindamycin-pyrimethamine does not offer protection against PCP

**Drug interactions can be problematic (e.g. those observed with clarithromycin and rifabutin); rifabutin has been associated with uveitis, chiefly when administered at daily doses of >300 mg or concurrently with fluconazole or clarithromycin

Adapted from Centers for Disease Control and Prevention. (2002). Guidelines for preventing opportunistic infections among HIV-infected persons – 2002: Recommendations of the U.S. Public Health Service and the Infectious Diseases Society of America. *MMWR, 51(*RR-8), 1-52.

L. **Antiretroviral drug therapy (ART)** or **highly active antiretroviral therapy (HAART)** should be individualized; see the following table for principals of therapy; also see V.P. through V. R. for discussion of specific drug classes, drug interactions, etc

PRINCIPLES OF THERAPY
1. Treatment decisions must be individualized using a number of criteria: Efficacy and durability of antiretroviral activity, tolerability and adverse effects, convenience of regimen, drug-drug interactions, and potential salvageability of the initial regimen
2. Because currently available antiretroviral regimens do not eradicate HIV, the goal of therapy is to durably inhibit viral replication, to enable patient to attain and maintain an effective immune response to most potential microbial pathogens, and to improve quality of life
3. Simultaneous initiation of combinations of effective anti-HIV drugs that the patient has not previously received and that are not cross-resistant with antiretroviral agents that the patient has previously received is the most effective method to achieve durable suppression of HIV replication
4. Drug monotherapy is **NOT** a recommended option as it presents risk for development of drug resistance and potential development of cross-resistance to related drugs
5. Each antiretroviral drug should be used according to optimum schedules and dosages
6. Any change in antiretroviral therapy increases future therapeutic constraints
7. Women need optimal antiretroviral therapy regardless of pregnancy status
8. Structured, supervised, or strategic treatment interruptions are not currently recommended
9. If ART needs to be discontinued, stop all antiretroviral agents simultaneously
10. Patient adherence is extremely important as intermittent use leads to resistance; emphasize that patient should not stop any medications without consulting clinician

M. Recommendations for **initiating antiretroviral therapy in treatment-naïve individuals** (see following table)
1. CD4+ T-cell count is the major determinant of when to initiate therapy
2. Viral loads offer additional information to help make timing decisions; CD4+ T-cell counts decrease more rapidly in untreated patients with high viral loads
3. Be aware of risk of immune reconstitution that may occur concomitantly with increase in CD4+ T-cell counts in patients starting ART when there is confirmed or suspected opportunistic infection
4. In collaboration with the patient, consider both the benefits and risks of early initiation of ART when the CD4+ count is in the >200 cells/mm^3 – 350 cell/mm^3 range (see table BENEFITS AND RISKS)
5. When initiating ART, start all drugs simultaneously and at full dose with the following exceptions: Dose escalation regimens are recommended for ritonavir, nevirapine, and for certain patients, ritonavir plus saquinavir

6. Dosages of ART must be altered when used with certain medications (see tables under V.Q. and V.R.)
7. Always consider overlapping toxicities when prescribing ART with other medications (consult drug manual) (see table HIV-RELATED DRUGS WITH OVERLAPPING TOXICITIES)

RECOMMENDATIONS FOR INITIATING THERAPY IN TREATMENT-NAÏVE INDIVIDUALS

Disease Type	Recommendation
Symptomatic HIV disease	Treatment recommended
Asymptomatic HIV disease ≤200 CD4+ cells/μL	Treatment recommended
Asymptomatic HIV disease, >200 CD4+ cells/μL	Treatment decision should be individualized; recommendations are based on: • CD4+ cell count and rate of decline* • HIV RNA level in the plasma** • Patient interest in and potential to adhere to therapy • Individual risks of toxicity and drug-drug pharmacokinetic interaction

* Some clinicians and guidelines use a CD4+ count threshold of 350 cells/μL to initiate therapy, a high rate of CD4+ cell count decline is >100 cells/μL per annum
** A high viral load is >50,000-100,000 copies/mL. The frequency of CD4+ cell measurements before therapy is initiated may be guided by the plasma HIV RNA level

Adapted from Yeni, P.G., Hammer, S.M., Carpenter, C.C.J., Cooper, D.A., Fischl, M.A., Gatell, J.M., et al. (2002). Antiretroviral treatment for adult HIV infection in 2002: Updated recommendations of the International AIDS Society—USA Panel. *JAMA, 288,* 222-235.

BENEFITS AND RISKS OF EARLY INITIATION OF ANTIRETROVIRAL THERAPY

Potential Benefits:
✓ Easier control of viral replication and mutation
✓ Preservation of immune function
✓ Delayed progression to AIDS
✓ Decreased risk of increased HIV genetic complexity
✓ Decreased risk for selection of resistant virus
✓ Decreased risk for drug toxicity
✓ Decreased risk for immune reconstitution syndrome
✓ Decrease in risk of viral transmission

Potential Risks:
✓ Reduction in quality of life from adverse drug effects
✓ Limitation of future choices of ART agents
✓ Unknown long-term toxicity of drugs
✓ Inconvenience of drug administration
✓ Earlier development of drug resistance if viral suppression is suboptimal
✓ Unknown duration of effectiveness of current antiretroviral agents

HIV-RELATED DRUGS WITH OVERLAPPING TOXICITIES

Bone Marrow Suppression	Peripheral Neuropathy	Pancreatitis	Nephrotoxicity	Hepatotoxicity	Rash	Diarrhea	Ocular Effects
Cidofovir	Didanosine	Cotrimoxazole	Adefovir	Azithromycin	Abacavir	Atovaquone	Didanosine
Cotrimoxazole	Isoniazid	Didanosine	Aminoglycosides	Clarithromycin	Amprenavir	Didanosine	Ethambutol
Cytotoxic chemo-therapy	Stavudine	Lamivudine (children)	Amphotericin B	Fluconazole	Atovaquone	Clindamycin	Rifabutin
Dapsone	Zalcitabine	Pentamidine	Cidofovir	Isoniazid	Cotrimoxazole	Nelfinavir	Cidofovir
Flucytosine		Ritonavir	Foscarnet	Itraconazole	Dapsone	Ritonavir	
Ganciclovir		Stavudine	Indinavir	Ketoconazole	Delavirdine	Lopinavir/ritonavir	
Hydroxyurea		Zalcitabine	Pentamidine	Nucleoside reverse transcriptase inhibitors	Efavirenz	Tenofovir	
Interferon-α				Nonnucleoside reverse transcriptase inhibitors	Nevirapine		
Pegylated interferon-α				Protease inhibitors	Sulfadiazine		
Primaquine				Rifabutin			
Pyrimethamine				Rifampin			
Ribavirin							
Rifabutin							
Sulfadiazine							
Trimetrexate							
Valganciclovir							
Zidovudine							

Adapted from Centers for Disease Control and Prevention. (2002) Guidelines for the use of antiretroviral agents among HIV-infected adults and adolescents: Recommendations of the Panel on Clinical Practices for Treatment of HIV. *MMWR, 51*(RR-7), 1-55.

8.   Choose one of the following preferred combination regimens when initiating therapy; discuss advantages and disadvantages of each regimen with the patient (see table that follows)

PREFERRED INITIAL COMBINATION REGIMENS FOR TREATMENT-NAÏVE PATIENTS*

Regimen	Possible Advantages	Possible Disadvantages	Drug-interaction Complications	Impact on Future Options
NNRTI-sparing regimen PI (with or without low-dose ritonavir** with 2 NRTIs)	• Clinical, virologic, and immunologic efficacy well-documented • Continued benefits despite viral breakthrough • Resistance requires multiple mutations • Targets HIV at 2 steps of viral replication (reverse transcriptase and PI)	• Might be difficult to use and adhere to • Long-term side effects might include lipodystrophy,§ hyperlipidemia, and insulin resistance	• Mild to severe inhibition of cytochrome P450 pathway; ritonavir is most potent inhibitor, but this effect can be exploited to boost levels of other PIs	• Preserves NNRTIs for use in treatment failure • Resistance primes for cross-resistance with other PIs
PI-Sparing regimen NNRTI with 2 NRTIs	• Spares PI-related side effects • Easier to use and adhere to, compared with PIs	• Comparability to PI-containing regimens regarding clinical results unknown • Resistance conferred by a single or limited number of mutations	• Fewer drug interactions compared with PIs	• Preserves PIs for later use • Resistance can lead to cross-resistance throughout entire NNRTI class

* PI = Protease inhibitor; NNRTI = nonnucleoside reverse transcriptase inhibitor; NRTI = nucleoside reverse transcriptase inhibitor
** Low-dose ritonavir can boost saquinavir, indinavir, amprenavir, or lopinavir; nelfinavir is not sufficiently enhanced by low-dose ritonavir to justify this combination
§ Certain side effects being attributed to PI therapy (e.g., lipodystrophy) have not been reported to be associated strictly with using PI-containing regimens. Lipodystrophy has also been described among patients on NRTIs alone and among patients not on antiretroviral therapy

Adapted from Centers for Disease Control and Prevention. (2002) Guidelines for the use of antiretroviral agents among HIV-infected adults and adolescents: Recommendations of the Panel on Clinical Practices for Treatment of HIV. *MMWR, 51*(RR-7), 1-55.

9.   Other combination regimens when initiating therapy may be selected (see following table)

OTHER COMBINATION REGIMENS WHEN INITIATING THERAPY

Regimen	Comment
PI-sparing/NNRTI-sparing regimens 3 NRTIs	• National Institutes of Allergy and Infectious Diseases (NIAID) (2003) study found that in treatment-naïve patients, a combination of three NRTIs, Trizivir, was inferior to two other efavirenz-containing treatment regimens • Not routinely recommended as initial therapy for patients with high viral loads (>100,000 copies/mL) or with low CD4+ T-cells • Preserves both PI and NNRTI classes for later use • Limited cross-resistance within the NRTI class
PI (with or without low-dose ritonavir) with an NNRTI plus 1 or 2 NRTIs	• Not routinely recommended due to risks of multiclass drug resistance and high toxicity, but may be beneficial for patients with advanced disease for which no effective therapy exists, and for cases in which *in vitro* resistance testing suggests regimen may be effective
NRTI-sparing regimen PI (with low-dose ritonavir) plus NNRTI	• Limited information available on this regimen

10. Carefully select specific ART agents for combination regimens (see following table for acceptable antiretroviral combinations); monotherapy and dual therapy regimens should **not** be selected

ACCEPTABLE ANTIRETROVIRAL COMBINATIONS FOR INITIAL TREATMENT*

Recommendation	Column A	Column B
Strongly Recommended	Efavirenz Indinavir Nelfinavir Ritonavir plus indinavir Ritonavir plus lopinavir (coformulated as Kaletra) Ritonavir plus saquinavir (soft-gel capsule[†] or hard-gel capsule[†])	Didanosine plus lamivudine Stavudine plus didanosine** Stavudine plus lamivudine Zidovudine plus didanosine Zidovudine plus lamivudine
Recommended as alternatives	Amprenavir Delavirdine Nelfinavir plus saquinavir (soft-gel capsule) Nevirapine Ritonavir Saquinavir (soft-gel capsule)	Zidovudine plus zalcitabine
No recommendation because of insufficient data	Hydroxyurea in combination with antiretroviral drugs Ritonavir plus amprenavir Ritonavir plus nelfinavir Tenofovir[§]	---
Not recommended and should not be offered (all monotherapies whether from column A or B)	Saquinavir (hard-gel capsule)***	Stavudine plus zidovudine Zalcitabine plus didanosine Zalcitabine plus lamivudine Zalcitabine plus stavudine

* ART drug regimens include one choice each from columns A and B of this table; drugs are listed in alphabetical, not priority order
[†] Saquinavir (soft-gel capsule) refers to Fortovase; Saquinavir (hard-gel capsule) refers to Invirase
** Pregnant women might be at increased risk for lactic acidosis and liver damage when treated with stavudine plus didanosine. This combination should be used for pregnant women only when the potential benefit outweighs the potential risk
*** Use of saquinavir (hard-gel capsule) (i.e., Invirase) is only recommended in combination with ritonavir
[§] Data from clinical trials are limited to use in salvage. Data from trials of tenofovir as initial therapy should be available in the future

Adapted from Centers for Disease Control and Prevention. (2002) Guidelines for the use of antiretroviral agents among HIV-infected adults and adolescents: Recommendations of the Panel on Clinical Practices for Treatment of HIV. *MMWR, 51*(RR-7), 1-55.

11.   New antiretroviral agents with clinical data (see table)

NEW DRUGS WITH CLINICAL DATA	
Drug	**Comment**
Enfuvirtide (Fuzeon)	• Interferes with entry of HIV-1 into cells by inhibiting fusion of viral and cellular membranes; blocks HIV's ability to infect healthy CD4+ T-cells • Indicated for therapy in treatment-experienced patients with evidence of HIV-1 replication despite ongoing antiretroviral therapy • Adverse events include local injection site reactions (occur commonly), increased rate of bacterial pneumonia, and potential hypersensitivity reactions • Dose is 90 mg (1 mL) twice daily injected subcutaneously into upper arm, anterior thigh, or abdomen • Does not interact with other antiretroviral agents or rifampin
Atazanavir	• Protease inhibitor • Once-a-day dosing • Less lipid problems than other PIs
Emtricitabine (ETC)	• Drug similar to, but more potent than lamivudine
Amdoxovir (DAPD)	• Nucleoside active against NRTI resistant strains

N.   Consider discontinuing ART for patient who began ART at CD4+ T-cell >350/mm^3; closely monitor patients who discontinue ART as they may have rebound in viral replication and renewed immunologic decline

O.   Considerations for **changing an antiretroviral regimen** (see following table)
1.   If change is due to drug toxicity or inability to comply with regimen, substitute one or more alternative drugs of same potency from the same class of agents as causing suspected toxicity
2.   If change is due to failure to achieve acceptable viral suppression or immune response, use ≥2 or ≥3 new drugs

GUIDELINES FOR CHANGING AN ANTIRETROVIRAL REGIMEN BECAUSE OF SUSPECTED DRUG FAILURE

➡ Criteria for changing therapy include 1) a suboptimal reduction in plasma viremia after initiation of therapy, 2) reappearance of viremia after suppression to undetectable levels, 3) substantial increases in plasma viremia from the nadir of suppression, and 4) declining CD4+ T-cell numbers

➡ Before deciding to change therapy on the basis of viral load, a second test should be used to confirm viral load determination

➡ Clinicians should distinguish between the need to change a regimen because of drug intolerance or inability to comply with the regimen versus failure to achieve sustained viral suppression; single agents can be changed for patients with drug intolerance

➡ Usually a single drug should not be changed or added to a failing regimen; using ≥2 new drugs or using a new regimen with ≥3 new drugs is preferable. If susceptibility testing indicates resistance to one agent only in a combination regimen, replacing only that drug is possible; however, this approach requires clinical validation

➡ In some cases treatment failure is not associated with viral resistance, particularly if virus remains detectable at lower levels after several months of ART; if there is no evidence of resistance or nonadherence, regimen intensification is acceptable; addition of ritonavir, abacavir, or tenofovir disoproxil fumarate may be used; do not use NNRTIs and lamivudine alone as intensification agents

➡ Certain patients have limited options for new regimens of desired potency; in selected cases, continuing the previous regimen if partial viral suppression was achieved is a rational option

➡ In certain situations, regimens identified as suboptimal for initial therapy because of limitations imposed by toxicity, intolerance, or nonadherence are rational options, including in late-stage disease. For patients with no rational options who have virologic failure with return of viral load to baseline (i.e., pretreatment levels) and declining CD4+ T-cell counts, discontinuing antiretroviral therapy should be considered, but continuing regimens that maintain selective pressure on virus is preferred

➡ Experience is limited regarding regimens that use combinations of two protease inhibitors or combinations of protease inhibitors with NNRTIs; for patients with limited options because of drug intolerance or suspected resistance, these regimens provide alternative options

➡ Tenofovir may have a role in management of treatment-experienced patients

(Continued)

GUIDELINES FOR CHANGING AN ANTIRETROVIRAL REGIMEN BECAUSE OF SUSPECTED DRUG FAILURE (CONTINUED)

➡ Information is limited regarding the value of restarting a drug that the patient has previously received. Susceptibility testing might be useful if clinical evidence indicating emergence of resistance is observed; however, testing for phenotypic or genotypic resistance in peripheral blood virus might fail to detect minor resistant variants. Thus, the presence of resistance is more useful information in altering treatment strategies than the absence of detectable resistance

➡ Clinicians should avoid changing from ritonavir to indinavir or vice versa for drug failure because high-level cross-resistance is probable

➡ Clinicians should avoid changing among NNRTIs for drug failure because high-level cross-resistance is probable

➡ Decisions to change therapy and choices of new regimens require the clinician to have substantial experience and knowledge regarding the care of persons living with HIV infection. Clinicians who are less experienced are strongly encouraged to obtain assistance through consultation with or referral to a knowledgeable clinician

Adapted from Centers for Disease Control and Prevention. (2002). Guidelines for using antiretroviral agents among HIV-infected adults and adolescents: Recommendations of the Panel on Clinical Practices for Treatment of HIV. *MMWR, 51*(RR-7). 1-55.

3. Possible regimens following initial antiretroviral regimen failure (see following table)

TREATMENT OPTIONS WHEN CHANGING ANTIRETROVIRAL REGIMENS

Initial Regimen	Predicted Early Resistance Pattern*	Possible Interventions
	Generally Recommended	
NNRTI-sparing regimen PI (with/without low-dose ritonavir) plus 2 NRTIs	M184V** if regimen includes lamivudine	Revise/strengthen NRTI/NtRTI component Ritonavir boost PI component, if not part of initial regimen Change to NNRTI-based regimen
PI-sparing regimen NNRTI plus 2 NRTIs	M184V** with/without NNRTI-associated mutation, if regimen includes lamivudine	Revise/strengthen NRTI/NtRTI component Change to PI-based regimen if NNRTI resistance present
PI-sparing/NNRTI-sparing regimen 3 NRTIs (including abacavir)	M184V** if regimen includes lamivudine	Change to PI- or NNRTI-based regimen with revision or strengthening of NRTI component or consider adding NtRTI
	Special Circumstances	
PI (with/without low-dose ritonavir) plus NNRTI plus 1 or 2 NRTIs	M184V** with/without NNRTI-associated mutation, if regimen includes lamivudine	Revise/strengthen NRTI component Ritonavir boosts PI component if not part of initial regimen Eliminate NNRTI if associated mutation present
	Under Investigation	
NRTI-sparing regimen PI (with low-dose ritonavir) plus NNRTI	NNRTI-associated mutation	Eliminate NNRTI and add 2 NRTIs or consider adding NtRTI

* The likely drug resistance patterns are listed for illustrative purposes assuming virological failure is detected early. Drug-resistance testing is recommended to determine the actual genotype or phenotype profile of the patient's viral strain
** The M184V mutation confers high-level resistance (500- to 1000-fold decrease in susceptibility) to lamivudine and low-level resistance (2- to 4-fold decrease in susceptibility) to abacavir

Adapted from Yeni, P.G., Hammer, S.M., Carpenter, C.C.J., Cooper, D.A., Fischl, M.A., Gatell, J.M., et al. (2002). Antiretroviral treatment for adult HIV infection in 2002: Updated recommendations of the International AIDS Society—USA Panel. *JAMA, 288,* 222-235.

P.   Nucleoside or nucleotide reverse transcriptase inhibitors (NRTIs): Block the conversion of virus RNA into viral DNA through inhibition of reverse transcriptase; inhibit viral spread to uninfected cells rather than eradicating the virus (see following table of factors to consider when selecting a NRTI)

NUCLEOSIDE OR NUCLEOTIDE REVERSE TRANSCRIPTASE INHIBITORS

Generic Name/ Trade Name	Form	Dosing Recommendations	Adverse Effects	Contraindications/ Precautions	Comments
Zidovudine/ Retrovir	100 mg capsules, 300 mg tablets, 10 mg/mL intravenous solution, or 10 mg/mL oral solution Each Combivir tab contains 300 mg zidovudine and 150 mg lamivudine Each Trizivir tab contains 300 mg zidovudine, 150 mg lamivudine, and 300 mg abacavir	200 mg TID or 300 mg BID or with lamivudine as Combivir, 1 dose BID or with abacavir and lamivudine as Trizivir, 1 dose BID	✓ Major: bone marrow suppression with anemia and/or neutropenia ✓ Common subjective: nausea, headaches, insomnia, fatigue, malaise, vomiting, GI pain ✓ Less common: myopathy and muscle pain ✓ Long-term: nail pigmentation ✓ Rare but life-threatening: lactic acidosis with hepatic stenosis	Consider dose adjustment in patients with liver dysfunction	✓ Take without regard to food ✓ Cautiously use with ganciclovir or other marrow-suppressing drugs ✓ Do **not** use with stavudine, doxorubicin, ribavirin ✓ Consider discontinuing if hemoglobin falls below 7.5 g/dL ✓ Monitor CBC 2-4 weeks after initiating and then periodically ✓ Superior CNS effects compared to other NRTIs
Didanosine/ Videx or Videx EC	25, 50, 100, 150, 200 mg chewable/ dispersible buffered tablets; 100, 167, 250 mg buffered powder for oral solution; 125, 200, 250, or 400 mg enteric coated capsules	Body weight >60 kg: 200 mg BID (buffered tablets), 250 mg BID (buffered powder) or 400 mg QD (buffered tablets or enteric coated capsules) Preferred dosing is BID; once-daily dosing reserved for patients who need simplified regimen	✓ Pancreatitis (potentially fatal) ✓ Peripheral neuropathy ✓ Diarrhea and GI problems ✓ Rare but life-threatening: lactic acidosis with hepatic stenosis	Consider dose adjustment in patients with renal and liver dysfunction; do not prescribe to alcoholics, patients with history of pancreatitis, and possibly those with poor seizure control	✓ Take ½ hour before or 2 hours after meals ✓ Do not give within two hours following drugs requiring an acid environment (ketoconazole, dapsone, tetracyclines, quinolones, cimetidine) ✓ Monitor amylase levels and assess for abdominal pain, nausea, and vomiting ✓ Separate dosing of delavirdine, indinavir, tenofovir by 1-2 hours ✓ Use cautiously with alcohol, stavudine, pentamidine, hydroxyurea, allopurinol, ganciclovir
Zalcitabine/ HIVID	0.375, 0.75 mg tablets	0.75 mg TID	✓ Peripheral neuropathy ✓ Aphthous ulcers ✓ Pancreatitis (less frequently than with didanosine) ✓ Rare but life-threatening: lactic acidosis with hepatic stenosis	Extreme caution when given to patients with hepatitis B; consider dose adjustment in patients with renal and liver disease Avoid in patients with peripheral neuropathy or history of pancreatitis	✓ Take without regard to food ✓ Less efficacious than other NRTIs ✓ Numerous drug interactions *(continued)*

NUCLEOSIDE OR NUCLEOTIDE REVERSE TRANSCRIPTASE INHIBITORS *(CONTINUED)*

Generic Name/ Trade Name	Form	Dosing Recommendations	Adverse Effects	Contraindications/ Precautions	Comments
Lamivudine/ Epivir	150 mg tablets or 10 mg/mL oral solution	150 mg BID; or with zidovudine as Combivir, 1 dose BID or with zidovudine and abacavir as Trizivir, 1 dose BID	✓ Minimal toxicity but may have headache, nausea, diarrhea, abdominal pain, insomnia ✓ Rare but life-threatening: lactic acidosis with hepatic stenosis	Consider dose adjustment in patients with renal dysfunction	✓ Take without regard to food ✓ Increased drug absorption when given with trimethoprim/ sulfamethoxazole ✓ Delays or reverses resistance of zidovudine ✓ Resistance develops rapidly if not given with another antiretroviral ✓ Not recommended with ddC and ddI ✓ Do not add as single agent to a failing regimen ✓ Has activity against Hepatitis B
Stavudine/Zerit	15, 20, 30, 40 mg capsules or 1 mg/mL oral solution	Body weight >60 kg: 40 mg BID; body weight <60 kg: 30 mg BID	✓ Pancreatitis (possibly fatal) ✓ Peripheral neuropathy ✓ Neuromuscular weakness (possibly fatal) ✓ Rare but life-threatening: lactic acidosis with hepatic stenosis	Consider dose adjustment in patients with renal and liver dysfunction	✓ Take without regard to food ✓ Do not take with zidovudine ✓ Use cautiously with other drugs that cause peripheral neuropathy
Abacavir/ Ziagen	300 mg tablets or 10 mg/mL oral solution	300 mg BID or with zidovudine and lamivudine as Trizivir, 1 dose BID	✓ Hypersensitivity reaction that can be fatal: fever, rash, nausea, vomiting, malaise, fatigue, anorexia, or possibly respiratory symptoms (sore throat, cough, SOB) ✓ Rare but life-threatening: lactic acidosis with hepatic stenosis	Use cautiously in patients with liver disease	✓ Take without regard to meals ✓ <u>Discontinue</u> if hypersensitivity reaction occurs and do <u>not</u> restart ✓ Do not add as a single agent to a failing regimen ✓ Alcohol increases abacavir levels ✓ May antagonize methadone
Tenofovir disoproxil fumarate/Viread	300 mg tablets	300 mg daily for patients with creatinine clearance ≥60 mL/min; not recommended for patients with creatinine clearance <60 mL/min	✓ Asthenia, headache, diarrhea, nausea, vomiting, and flatulence ✓ Rare but life-threatening: lactic acidosis with hepatic stenosis	Contraindicated in patients with renal insufficiency	✓ Take with food to increase bioavailability ✓ Separate 1-2 hours from didanosine ✓ Limited information about efficacy

Adapted from Centers for Disease Control and Prevention. (2002) Guidelines for the use of antiretroviral agents among HIV-infected adults and adolescents: Recommendations of the Panel on Clinical Practices for Treatment of HIV. *MMWR, 51*(RR-7), 1-55.

Q. Protease inhibitors (PI) (see following table)
   1. Mechanisms of action: Inhibit HIV replication in cells that are chronically infected with HIV; competitively inhibit the HIV protease enzyme, a necessary enzyme for formation of the protein capsule surrounding the viral RNA in mature virions
   2. Toxicities of PIs sometimes limit their use; elevated glucose, serum triglycerides, and cholesterol are often reported along with changes in body habitus
   3. Always check drug manual and drug insert before prescribing PI
   4. Certain drugs should not be used with PIs (see table DRUGS THAT SHOULD NOT BE USED WITH PIs)
   5. When PIs are used with other PIs or NNRTIs, dosage modifications must be made (See tables DOSAGE CHANGES WITH OTHER PIS AND DOSAGE CHANGES WITH NNRTIs)

6. PIs interact with numerous medications and require dose modifications or cautious use (See table DOSAGE ADJUSTMENTS WHEN PRESCRIBING PIs)

PROTEASE INHIBITORS (PIS)

Name/Form	Dosing Recommendations	Food Effect	Adverse Events	Comments
Indinavir/Crixivan 200, 333, 400 mg capsules	800 mg every 8 hours; separate dosing with didanosine buffered preparation by 1 hour, Videx EC and indinavir can be administered together	Take 1 hour before or 2 hours after meals; may take with skim milk or low-fat meal	Nephrolithiasis; gastrointestinal intolerance and nausea; increased indirect bilirubinemia (inconsequential); transaminase elevation; headache, asthenia, blurred vision, dizziness, rash, metallic taste, thrombocytopenia, alopecia, hyperglycemia, hemolytic anemia; fat redistribution and lipid abnormalities, possible increased bleeding episodes among patients with hemophilia	✓ Drink >48 ounces of fluid to reduce risk of nephrolithiasis ✓ Can use oral contraceptives ✓ Separate dosing of didanosine by 1-2 hours
Ritonavir/Norvir 100 mg capsules 600 mg/7.5 mL solution by mouth	600 mg every 12 hours; separate dosing with didanosine by 2 hours Dose escalation: Days 1&2: 300 mg BID Days 3-5: 400 mg BID Days 6-13: 500 mg BID Day 14: 600 mg BID	Take with food, if possible; this might improve tolerability	Gastrointestinal intolerance, nausea, vomiting, diarrhea; paresthesias (circumoral and extremities); hepatitis; pancreatitis, asthenia; taste perversion; triglycerides increase >200%; elevated creatinine phosphokinase and uric acid; hyperglycemia, fat redistribution and lipid abnormalities, possible increased bleeding episodes among patients with hemophilia	✓ Refrigerate capsules; capsules can be left at room temperature for ≤30 days ✓ Capsule and liquid contain alcohol ✓ Coadministration with certain other drugs can be fatal ✓ Combination regimen with saquinavir is 400 mg BID plus ritonavir 400 mg BID ✓ Antagonizes oral contraceptives
Nelfinavir/Viracept 250 mg tablets 50 mg/g oral powder	750 mg TID or 1,250 mg BID	Take with meal or snack	Diarrhea; hyperglycemia, fat redistribution and lipid abnormalities, possible increased bleeding episodes among patients with hemophilia; transaminase elevation	✓ May crush or dissolve tabs and mix in small amount water ✓ Powder may be mixed with non-acidic food or beverage ✓ Antagonizes oral contraceptives
Saquinavir/ Invirase 200 mg hard-gel capsules	400 mg BID with ritonavir; **otherwise Invirase is not recommended**	No food effect when taken with ritonavir	Gastrointestinal intolerance, nausea, and diarrhea; headache; elevated transaminase; hyperglycemia, fat redistribution and lipid abnormalities; possible increased bleeding episodes among patients with hemophilia	✓ Use only in combination with ritonavir
Saquinavir/ Fortovase 200 mg soft-get capsules	1200 mg TID (1600 mg BID is **not** recommended)	Take with large meal	Gastrointestinal intolerance, nausea, diarrhea, abdominal pain, and dyspepsia; headache; elevated transaminase; hyperglycemia; fat redistribution and lipid abnormalities; possible increased bleeding episodes among patients with hemophilia	✓ Refrigerate or store at room temperature (≤3 months)
Amprenavir/ Agenerase 50 mg, 150 mg capsules or 15 mg/mL oral solution (Capsules and solution are not interchangeable on mg/mg basis)	Body weight >50 kg: 1200 mg BID (capsules) or 1400 mg BID (oral solution) Body weight <50 kg: 20 mg/kg BID (capsules) maximum 2400 mg daily total; 1.5 mL/kg BID (oral solution) maximum 2800 mg daily total; With ritonavir: amprenavir 600 mg BID plus ritonavir 100 mg BID or amprenavir 1200 mg QD plus ritonavir 200 mg QD	Can be taken with or without food, but high-fat meal should be avoided	Gastrointestinal intolerance, nausea, vomiting, diarrhea; rash; oral paresthesias; transaminase elevation; hyperglycemia; fat redistribution and lipid abnormalities; possible increased bleeding episodes among patients with hemophilia; oral solution contains propylene glycol; therefore, contraindicated among pregnant women, children aged <4 years, patients with hepatic or renal failure, and patients treated with disulfiram or metronidazole	✓ Do not take with vitamin E supplements ✓ Separate dosing of didanosine, antacids by 1-2 hours ✓ Reduces effectiveness of oral contraceptives ✓ Contraindicated in patients with renal or hepatic failure, pregnant patients treated with disulfiram or metronidazole

(Continued)

PROTEASE INHIBITORS (PIs) *(CONTINUED)*

Name/Form	Dosing Recommendations	Food Effect	Adverse Events	Comments
Lopinavir plus ritonavir/Kaletra 133.3 mg lopinavir plus 33.3 mg ritonavir capsules, 80 mg lopinavir plus 20 mg ritonavir per mL oral solution	400 mg lopinavir plus 100 mg ritonavir BID	Take with food	Gastrointestinal intolerance, nausea, vomiting, diarrhea; asthenia; elevated transaminase enzymes; hyperglycemia; fat redistribution and lipid abnormalities; possible increased bleeding episodes among patients with hemophilia	✓ Separate dosing of didanosine by 1-2 hours ✓ May antagonize oral contraceptive ✓ Refrigerated capsules are stable until expiration date on label; if stored at room temperature, stable for 2 months ✓ Oral solution contains alcohol

DRUGS THAT SHOULD NOT BE USED WITH PIs

Drug Category	Calcium Channel Blocker	Cardiac	Lipid-lowering Agents	Antimyco-bacterial	Anti-histamine	GI Drugs	Neuroleptic	Psychotropic	Ergot Alkaloids (Vasoconstrictor)	Herbs
Protease Inhibitors										
Indinavir	None	None	Simvastatin Lovastatin	Rifampin	Astemizole Terfenadine	Cisapride	None	Midazolam Triazolam	Dihydroergotamine (D.H.E.45) Ergotamine (various forms)	St. John's wort
Ritonavir	Bepridil	Amiodarone Flecainide Propafenone Quinidine	Simvastatin Lovastatin	None	Astemizole Terfenadine	Cisapride	Pimozide	Midazolam Triazolam	Dihydroergotamine (D.H.E.45) Ergotamine (various forms)	St. John's wort
Saquinavir	None	None	Simvastatin Lovastatin	Rifampin	Astemizole Terfenadine	Cisapride	None	Midazolam Triazolam	Dihydroergotamine (D.H.E.45) Ergotamine (various forms)	St. John's wort
Nelfinavir	None	None	Simvastatin Lovastatin	Rifampin	Astemizole Terfenadine	Cisapride	None	Midazolam Triazolam	Dihydroergotamine (D.H.E.45) Ergotamine (various forms)	St. John's wort
Amprenavir	Bepridil	None	Simvastatin Lovastatin	Rifampin	Astemizole Terfenadine	Cisapride	None	Midazolam Triazolam	Dihydroergotamine (D.H.E.45) Ergotamine (various forms)	St. John's wort
Lopinavir plus Ritonavir	None	Flecainide Propafenone	Simvastatin Lovastatin	Rifampin	Astemizole Terfenadine	Cisapride	Pimozide	Midazolam Triazolam	Dihydroergotamine (D.H.E.45) Ergotamine (various forms)	St. John's wort

Suggested Alternatives
Simvastatin, lovastatin: Atorvastatin, pravastatin, fluvastatin, cerivastatin (alternatives should be used with caution)
Rifabutin: Clarithromycin, azithromycin (*Mycobacterium avium-intracellulare* prophylaxis); clarithromycin, ethambutol (*Mycobacterium avium-intracellulare* treatment)
Rifampin: Rifabutin (*Mycobacterium tuberculosis*)
Astemizole, terfenadine: Loratadine, fexofenadine, cetirizine
Midazolam, triazolam: Temazepam, lorazepam

Adapted from Centers for Disease Control and Prevention. (2002) Guidelines for the use of antiretroviral agents among HIV-infected adults and adolescents: Recommendations of the Panel on Clinical Practices for Treatment of HIV. *MMWR, 51*(RR-7), 1-55.

DOSAGE CHANGES WHEN PIs ARE PRESCRIBED WITH OTHER PIs

Drug affected	Ritonavir	Saquinavir	Nelfinavir	Amprenavir	Lopinavir/ritonavir
Protease inhibitors					
Indinavir	Indinavir 400 mg BID plus ritonavir 400 mg BID; or indinavir 800 mg BID plus ritonavir 100 or 200 mg BID	No changes	Indinavir 1200 mg BID plus nelfinavir 1250 mg BID	No change	Indinavir 600 mg BID; lopinavir, standard dose
Ritonavir	---	Invirase or Fortovase 400 mg BID plus ritonavir 400 mg BID; or Invirase or Fortovase 800 mg BID plus ritonavir 200 mg BID	Ritonavir 400 mg BID plus nelfinavir 500-750 mg BID	Amprenavir 600 mg BID plus ritonavir 100 mg BID or amprenavir 1200 mg QD plus ritonavir 200 mg QD	Lopinavir is coformulated with ritonavir as Kaletra
Saquinavir	---	---	Standard nelfinavir; Fortovase 800 mg TID or 1200 mg BID	No change	Saquinavir 800 mg BID; lopinavir, standard dose
Nelfinavir	---	---	---	No change	---
Amprenavir	---	---	---	---	Amprenavir 600-750 mg BID; lopinavir, increase to 500 mg BID

Adapted from Centers for Disease Control and Prevention. (2002) Guidelines for the use of antiretroviral agents among HIV-infected adults and adolescents: Recommendations of the Panel on Clinical Practices for Treatment of HIV. *MMWR, 51*(RR-7), 1-55.

DOSAGE CHANGES WHEN PIs AND NNRTIs ARE PRESCRIBED TOGETHER

Drug affected	Nevirapine	Delavirdine	Efavirenz
Protease inhibitors and nonnucleoside reverse transcriptase inhibitors			
Indinavir	Indinavir 1000 mg every 8 hours; nevirapine, standard dose	Indinavir 600 mg every 8 hours; delavirdine, standard dose	Indinavir 1000 mg every 8 hours; efavirenz, standard dose
Ritonavir	Standard dose	Delavirdine, standard dose; ritonavir, data unavailable	Ritonavir 600 mg BID (500 mg BID for intolerance); efavirenz, standard dose
Saquinavir	Data unavailable	Fortovase 800 mg TID; delavirdine, standard but monitor transaminase levels	Coadministration not recommended when saquinavir is used as a single PI
Nelfinavir	Standard dose	Data unavailable but monitor for neutropenic complications	Standard dose
Amprenavir	Data unavailable	---	Amprenavir 1200 mg TID as single protease inhibitor or 1200 mg BID plus ritonavir 200 mg BID; efavirenz, standard dose
Lopinavir/ritonavir	Consider lopinavir 533/133 mg BID for protease inhibitor-experienced patients; nevirapine, standard dose	Insufficient data	Consider lopinavir 533/133 mg BID for protease inhibitor-experienced patients; efavirenz, standard dose
Nevirapine	---	---	Standard dose
Delavirdine	---	---	---

Adapted from Centers for Disease Control and Prevention. (2002) Guidelines for the use of antiretroviral agents among HIV-infected adults and adolescents: Recommendations of the Panel on Clinical Practices for Treatment of HIV. *MMWR, 51*(RR-7), 1-55.

DOSAGE ADJUSTMENTS WHEN PRESCRIBING PIS AND OTHER DRUGS*

| Drugs affected | Antifungals Ketoconazole | Antimycobacterials | | Clarithromycin | Miscellaneous |
		Rifampin	Rifabutin		
Protease Inhibitors					
Indinavir	Indinavir 600 mg TID	Contraindicated	Decrease rifabutin to 150 mg daily or 300 mg 2-3 times/week; indinavir, 1,000 mg TID	No dose adjustment	Grapefruit juice decreases levels Do not exceed 25 mg of sildenafil in 48-hour period
Ritonavir	Use with caution: do not exceed 200 mg/day of ketoconazole	No data; increased liver toxicity possible	Decrease rifabutin to 150 mg every other day or dose three times/week; ritonavir: standard dose	Adjustment for renal insufficiency	Multiple interactions (always check drug manual)
Saquinavir	Standard dose of saquinavir	Contraindicated, unless using ritonavir plus saquinavir, then use rifampin 600 mg daily or 2-3 times/week	No dose adjustment unless using ritonavir plus saquinavir; then use rifabutin 150 mg 3 times/week	No dose adjustment	Grapefruit juice increases levels; Dexamethasone decreases levels; Use sildenafil 25 mg starting dose
Nelfinavir	No dose adjustment	Contraindicated	Decrease rifabutin to 150 mg QD or 300 mg 2-3 times/week; increase nelfinavir dose to 1000 mg TID	---	Do not exceed 25 mg of sildenafil in 48-hour period
Amprenavir	No data available	Avoid concomitant use	Decrease rifabutin to 150 mg QD or 300 mg 3 times/week	No dose adjustment	Do not exceed 25 mg of sildenafil in 48-hour period
Lopinavir	Do not exceed 200 mg/day of ketoconazole	Avoid concomitant use	Decrease rifabutin dose to 150 mg every other day; lopinavir: standard dose	---	Do not exceed 25 mg of sildenafil in 48-hour period

* Lipid lowering agents and anticonvulsants frequently interact with PIs; check package insert and drug manual before prescribing drugs from these classes

Adapted from Centers for Disease Control and Prevention. (2002) Guidelines for the use of antiretroviral agents among HIV-infected adults and adolescents: Recommendations of the Panel on Clinical Practices for Treatment of HIV. *MMWR, 51*(RR-7), 1-55.

R. Nonnucleoside reverse transcriptase inhibitors (NNRTI) (see following table)
   1. Act on a nonsubstrate binding site of the enzyme which alters the shape of the active site (see following table)
   2. Always check drug manual or drug insert before prescribing NNRTI
      a. Certain drugs should not be used with NNRTIs (see table DRUGS THAT SHOULD NOT BE USED WITH NNRTIs)
      b. NNRTIs often interact with other medications and require dose modifications or cautious use (see table DOSAGE ADJUSTMENTS WHEN PRESCRIBING NNRTIs)
      c. Some NNRTI dosages should be modified when used with PIs (see table DOSAGE CHANGES WHEN PIS AND NNRTIs ARE PRESCRIBED TOGETHER in V.Q.)

NONNUCLEOSIDE REVERSE TRANSCRIPTASE INHIBITORS (NNRTIs)

Generic/Trade Name	Form	Dosing Recommendations	Food effect	Adverse Events
Nevirapine/Viramune	200 mg tablets or 50 mg/5mL oral suspension	200 mg by mouth daily for 14 days; thereafter, 200 mg by mouth BID	Take without regard to meals	✓ Rash* ✓ Severe, life-threatening hepatotoxicity including hepatic necrosis (monitor patients intensively during first 12 weeks of therapy)
Delavirdine/Rescriptor	100 mg tablets or 200 mg tablets	400 mg by mouth TID; 4, 100 mg tablets can be dispersed in ≥3 oz water to produce slurry; 100 mg tablets should be taken as intact tablets; separate buffered preparations dosing with didanosine or antacids by 1 hour	Take without regard to meals	✓ Rash* ✓ Increased transaminase levels ✓ Headaches
Efavirenz/Sustiva	50, 100, 200 mg capsules or 600 mg tablets	600 mg by mouth daily on an empty stomach, preferably at bedtime	Take on empty stomach	✓ Rash* ✓ Central nervous system symptoms** ✓ Increased transaminase levels ✓ False-positive cannabinoid test

* During clinical trials, NNRTI was discontinued because of rash among 7% of patients taking nevirapine, 4.3% of patients taking delavirdine, and 1.7% of patients taking efavirenz. Rare cases of Stevens-Johnson syndrome have been reported with the use of all three NNRTIs
** Adverse events can include dizziness, somnolence, insomnia, abnormal dreams, confusion, abnormal thinking, impaired concentration, amnesia, agitation, depersonalization, hallucinations, and euphoria

DRUGS THAT SHOULD NOT BE USED WITH NNRTIs

Drug Category	Calcium Channel Blocker	Cardiac	Lipid-lowering Agent	Anti-mycobacterial	Antihistamine	GI Drugs	Neuroleptic	Psychotropic	Ergot Alkaloids (Vasoconstrictor)
Nevirapine	None	None	None	Insufficient data	None	None	None	None	None
Delavirdine	None	None	Simvastatin Lovastatin	Rifampin Rifabutin	Astemizole Terfenadine	Cisapride Hydrogen-2 blockers Proton pump inhibitors	None	Midazolam Triazolam	Dihydroergotamine (D.H.E.45) Ergotamine (various forms)
Efavirenz	None	None	None	None	Astemizole Terfenadine	Cisapride	None	Midazolam Triazolam	Dihydroergotamine (D.H.E.45) Ergotamine (various forms)

Suggested Alternatives

Simvastatin, lovastatin: Atorvastatin, pravastatin, fluvastatin, cerivastatin (alternatives should be used with caution)
Rifabutin: Clarithromycin, azithromycin (*Mycobacterium avium-intracellulare* prophylaxis); clarithromycin, ethambutol (*Mycobacterium avium-intracellulare* treatment)
Rifampin: Rifabutin (*Mycobacterium tuberculosis*)
Astemizole, terfenadine: Loratadine, fexofenadine, cetirizine
Midazolam, triazolam: Temazepam, lorazepam

DOSAGE ADJUSTMENTS WHEN PRESCRIBING NNRTIs*

Drugs affected	Antifungals	Antimycobacterials			Miscellaneous
	Ketoconazole	Rifampin	Rifabutin	Clarithromycin	
Nonnucleoside reverse transcriptase inhibitors					
Nevirapine	Not recommended	Use only if clearly indicated	No dose adjustment	No dose adjustment	Methadone levels decreased
Delavirdine	No data available	Contraindicated	Not recommended	Adjust dose for renal failure	May increase levels of dapsone, warfarin, quinidine; do not exceed 25 mg of sildenafil in 48-hour period
Efavirenz	No data available	Unknown	Increase rifabutin dose to 450-600 mg QD or 600 mg 3 times/week; efavirenz: standard dose	Alternative recommended	Methadone levels decreased. Monitor warfarin when used concomitantly

* Lipid-lowering agents and anticonvulsants may interact with NNRTIs; check package insert and drug manual before prescribing drugs from these classes

Above tables adapted from Centers for Disease Control and Prevention. (2002) Guidelines for the use of antiretroviral agents among HIV-infected adults and adolescents: Recommendations of the Panel on Clinical Practices for Treatment of HIV. *MMWR, 51*(RR-7), 1-55.

S. Adjuvant therapy to antiretroviral drugs
1. Approaches that augment (interleukin 2) or dampen (cyclosporin A, corticosteroids, hydroxyurea, and mycophenolic acid) immune response may prove beneficial, but at present there is insufficient clinical data to recommend their use
2. Hydroxyurea has significant toxicities which also limit its use

T. Treatment regimen for **primary HIV infection** (acute retroviral syndrome)
1. When suspicion of acute infection is high, a test for HIV RNA should be performed; positive results should have confirmatory testing performed (Western blot serology)
2. Aggressive treatment of primary HIV infection may be best time to alter disease course, however some experts believe the risks of ART are too great to recommend drug therapy to all patients
3. If patient and clinician agree, prescribe a combination antiretroviral regimen (see table, INITIAL COMBINATION REGIMENS FOR TREATMENT-NAÏVE PATIENTS [V.M.8.])
4. Testing for plasma HIV RNA levels and CD4+ T-cell counts should be performed on initiation of therapy, and then after 4, 8-12, 16-24 weeks on ART
5. The optimal duration and composition of therapy is unknown but because of latently infected CD4+ T-cells, several years of treatment may be needed (some experts recommend that treatment should be indefinite whereas others treat for 1 year and then provide close monitoring)

U. Treatment of **patients with HIV- and HCV-coinfection**
1. Advise to avoid (best) or limit alcohol intake
2. Vaccinate against hepatitis A and possibly hepatitis B if susceptible
3. Regularly evaluate for liver disease and treat as these patients experience liver disease in a shorter time course than patients infected with only HCV

V. Considerations for ART among **HIV-infected adolescents**; medication dosages used to treat HIV and OIs should be based on Tanner staging of puberty and not specific age
1. For patients in early puberty (Tanner stages I and II) prescribe dosages based on pediatric guidelines
2. For patients in late puberty (Tanner stage V) prescribe dosages based on adult guidelines
3. For patients in the midst of growth spurt (Tanner stage III females and Tanner stage IV males) choose either adult or pediatric dosing guidelines and closely monitor for medication efficacy and toxicity

W. **Treatment of HAART-associated adverse clinical events**
1. Lactic acidosis
   a. Immediately discontinue ART: Lactate >5 mmol/L with symptoms or lactate >10 mmol/L
   b. Consider discontinuing ART: Lactate >5 mmol/L with or without symptoms
   c. Carefully monitor lactate levels if asymptomatic and lactate is 2-5 mmol/L
   d. Although there is limited empirical data, thiamine and riboflavin may be helpful

2. Hepatotoxicity
   a. Closely monitor liver enzymes after ART is initiated; for example, after nevirapine initiation monitor every 2 weeks for first month, then monthly for first 12 weeks; then every 1-3 months
   b. Discontinue the drug causing the adverse event
3. Hyperglycemia (see section on DIABETES MELLITUS)
   a. Closely monitor patients when PIs are used; some clinicians recommend routine fasting blood glucose tests every 3-6 months
   b. Avoid use of PI as initial therapy in patients with pre-existing glucose intolerance or diabetes
   c. Teach patients the warning signs of hyperglycemia (polydipsia, polyphagia, polyuria)
   d. Most clinicians recommend continuation of ART in absence of severe diabetes
   e. Emphasize diet, exercise, weight loss; antidiabetic drug therapy should follow guidelines for non-HIV infected population (preference should be given to insulin sensitizing agents such as metformin [except those with history of renal disease or lactic acidemia] or thiazolidinediones [except those with liver disease])
4. Fat accumulation
   a. No effective therapy is available but some clinicians switch antiretrovirals or switch to another class of drugs
   b. Carefully evaluate for cardiovascular events and pancreatitis
5. Hyperlipidemia (also see section on HYPERLIPIDEMIA)
   a. Recommend low-fat diets, regular exercise, control of blood pressure, and smoking cessation
   b. Avoid use of PI, if possible, in patients with preexisting cardiovascular risk factors, family history of hyperlipidemia
   c. Hypercholesterolemia may respond to statins; with continuing high cholesterol levels, fibrates may be added to statin therapy after 3-4 months of treatment
      (1) Remember that certain statins interact with PIs
      (2) Atorvastatin is probably the best statin to use with PIs, but should be used cautiously and in reduced doses
   d. Isolated triglyceride elevations respond best to low-fat diets and fibrates
   e. If lipid elevations are severe and unresponsive to above therapies, consider modifying antiretroviral therapy; switching PI component to nevirapine or abacavir may be effective
6. Osteonecrosis, osteopenia, and osteoporosis
   a. No recommendations are made for routine measurement of bone density or for prophylaxis or treatment to prevent decreases in bone density
   b. Teach patients to have an adequate intake of calcium and vitamin D and to engage in appropriate weight-bearing exercises
   c. If osteoporotic fractures occur, more aggressive therapies with bisphosphonates, raloxifene, or calcitonin may be prescribed
   d. Surgical resection of involved bone is only effective therapy for symptomatic osteonecrosis
7. Skin rashes
   a. Discontinue nevirapine and do not use another NNRTI if patient has severe skin reaction
   b. Discontinue abacavir if skin rash occurs as this may be a symptom of abacavir-associated systemic hypersensitivity
   c. For mild skin rashes from NNRTI, some clinicians manage with antihistamines and do not discontinue drug, but this practice has been questioned

X. **Symptom management**
   1. Wasting syndrome was previously defined as otherwise unexplained loss of 10% of body weight; proposed new definition is presented in following table

---

PROPOSED NEW DEFINITION OF HIV-ASSOCIATED WASTING

Patient must meet one of following criteria:

- 10% unintentional weight loss over 12 months
- 7.5% unintentional weight loss over 6 months
- 5% body cell mass (BCM) loss within 6 months
- In men: BCM <35% of total body weight and body mass index (BMI) <27 kg/m^3
- In women: BCM <23% of total body weight and BMI <27 kg/m^3
- Body mass index (BMI) <20 kg/m^3

Adapted from Polsky, B., Kotler, D., & Steinhart, C. (2001). HIV-associated wasting in the HAART era: Guidelines for assessment, diagnosis, and treatment. *AIDS Patient Care, 15,* 411-423.

a. Causative factors include
  (1) Decreased food intake due to mouth or esophageal ulcers, anorexia (often related to depression), early satiety, nausea, or financial problems
  (2) Decreased absorption from loss of enzymes causing lactose intolerance; to avoid this problem teach patient to avoid all milk products by reading labels
  (3) Increased metabolic demand from infection, fever, and malignancies
  (4) Malabsorption due to infections and bacterial overgrowth
  (5) In rare cases may be due to lactic acidosis; with this condition, wasting is accompanied by abdominal pain, fatigue, and exercise-induced dyspnea
b. Order following diagnostic tests to rule-out infection and treat as needed: Stool culture, blood culture, cryptococcal serum antigen, and other tests based on patient's clinical presentation; consider lactic acid levels and liver enzymes if lactic acidosis is suspected
c. Treat cause (i.e., infection), but if etiology is unclear, consider the following:
  (1) Daily multivitamin
  (2) If patient has anorexia, consider prescribing one of the following appetite stimulants:
    (a) Megestrol acetate (Megace) 40 mg/mL susp.; 800 mg/day; adverse effects include impotence, decreased libido, hypertension
    (b) Dronabinol (Marinol): 2.5 mg BID before lunch and supper, may gradually increase to maximum of 20 mg/day; adverse effects include abuse potential, euphoria, psychomimetic reactions, altered mental status
  (3) Recommend nutritional supplements (10 cans per day are needed for total daily caloric needs)
    (a) If patient needs to gain weight and can tolerate milk use Carnation Instant Breakfast
    (b) If the patient needs to gain weight but cannot tolerate milk give Ensure or Sustacal
    (c) If patient has severe malabsorption state use an elemental diet (with easily absorbed nutrients) such as Vivonex TEN
d. Consider other beneficial therapies such as growth hormone (Serostim) 6 mg subcutaneous injection QD X 12 weeks, thalidomide 50-300 mg/day PO x 2-12 weeks with starting dose of 100 mg/day, or anabolic steroids such as oxandrolone (men: 20-40 mg/day PO and women: 5-20 mg/day PO)
2. Testosterone failure may cause wasting as well as a decrease in energy levels and muscle mass
  a. To diagnose, order serum testosterone level
  b. Treatment is testosterone enanthate or testosterone cypionate IM injections 200-400 mg every 2 weeks or 100-200 mg every week or testosterone patch (Testoderm TTS), apply 5 mg patch every 22-24 hours to arm, back or upper buttocks (application site rotation is not necessary)
3. Diarrhea
  a. Acute diarrhea is often due to medications, anxiety, irritable bowel syndrome, or untreatable viral agents such a Norwalk agent; presence of severe diarrhea, fever, and fecal leukocytes and/or blood increase the likelihood of a treatable pathogen
  b. Chronic diarrhea is often due to infections; about 20-30% of chronic diarrhea cases are idiopathic
  c. Initially, order following diagnostic tests to rule-out parasites or infection: Stool for ova and parasites, bacterial stool culture, *C-difficile* toxin, acid-fast bacterial smear of stool can sometimes detect *Mycobacterium avium* and cryptosporidiosis; consult specialist for further tests such as CT, colonoscopy, endoscopy
  d. If infection is ruled-out, prescribe one of following
    (1) Loperamide (Imodium) 2 mg caps, two in AM and one after each BM up to maximum of 8 caps
    (2) Alternative: Diphenoxylate (Lomotil) 2.5 mg; 2 tabs or 10 mL QID
  e. Patient education
    (1) Increase fluids
    (2) Follow a low lactose, low fat, high fiber diet
    (3) Use LactAid instead of milk
    (4) Avoid caffeine, fried foods, carbonated beverages, cabbage, broccoli
4. Nausea and vomiting
  a. Rule out infections
  b. Symptomatically treat with prochlorperazine (Compazine) 5-10 mg QID, or ondansetron (Zofran) 4-10 mg QID
5. Pain is a common symptom (see section on PAIN)

6. Fever without focal symptoms
   a. Common causes are *Mycobacterium avium complex*, tuberculosis, lymphoma, cytomegalovirus infection, secondary syphilis
   b. Following diagnostic tests should be obtained: Blood culture for conventional bacteria and for acid-fast bacteria, cryptococcal serum antigen, CBC; consider PPD, RPR, chest x-ray, liver enzymes, LDH, urinalysis, blood gases for PCP, urine culture
   c. Symptomatic treatment (see section on FEVERS)
7. Anemia may be caused by numerous factors
   a. Order the following diagnostic tests to identify cause of anemia:
      (1) CBC: if patient has normal WBCs but decreased RBCs consider infection with parvovirus
      (2) Bleeding (stool guaiac), hemolysis (smear), iron deficiency (serum iron, transferrin, % saturation, ferritin, reticulocyte count), B_{12} and folate deficiencies (serum B_{12}, serum folate)
   b. If patient is on zidovudine, consider switching to another NRTI
   c. If cause of anemia cannot be corrected and if hemoglobin is <9 g/dL, prescribe erythropoietin (Epogen, Procrit); some experts recommend erythropoietin should be given when patients have mild symptomatic anemia (13 g/dL in men & 11 g/dL in women) or moderate anemia (12 g/dL in men and 10 g/dL in women)
      (1) Measure ferritin levels; patient must have adequate iron stores to respond to drug
      (2) Initially administer 100 units/kg SQ 3 times per week to maximum of 300 units/kg 3 times per week or 40,000 units subcutaneous injection every week (investigational dosing schedule, but increasingly used in practice)
         (a) If hemoglobin increases by >1 g/dL at 4 weeks, continue same dose and continue to monitor response; when hemoglobin is >11-13 g/dL, hold erythropoietin or decrease by 10,000 units per week
         (b) If hemoglobin increase is <1 g/dL at 4 weeks, increase to 60,000 units a week; if hemoglobin increase is <1 g/dL at week 12, discontinue
8. Neutropenia
   a. May be due to drugs such as zidovudine or ganciclovir or to HIV infection
   b. Prescribe G-CSF (Neupogen) or GM-CSF (Leukine) 1-10 μg/kg/day; usual initial dose of G-CSF is 1μg/kg/day SQ with increases of 1μg/kg/day at 5-7 day intervals to maintain absolute neutrophil count (ANC) at 1000-2000 cells/mm^3; usual maintenance dose is 300 μg given 3-7 times per week
9. Mouth ulcers are common, particularly if patient is on zalcitabine (See sections on APHTHOUS ULCERS, HERPES SIMPLEX, CANDIDIASIS)
10. Dermatological problems: Common causes are infection, neoplastic diseases, and reaction to medications
    a. Eosinophilic folliculitis or red, itchy bumps is a common manifestation
       (1) Generally disappears when CD4+ T-cells rise above 200/mm^3 and viral load is undetectable
       (2) For symptomatic treatment, prescribe cetirizine (Zyrtec) 5-10 mg QD or loratadine (Claritin) 10 mg QD and one of following:
          (a) Camphor 0.5/Menthol 0.5 lotion (Sarna)
          (b) Topical steroids
          (c) Ultraviolet light
    b. See treatment of other dermatological conditions in SKIN chapter
11. Peripheral neuropathy: discontinue implicated NRTIs and treat with one of following:
    a. Nortriptyline (Pamelor) 10 mg HS; increase dose by 10 mg q 5 days to maximum of 75 mg HS or 10-20 mg TID
    b. Ibuprofen 600-800 mg TID
    c. Capsaicin-containing ointments (Zostrix) for topical application
12. Mental health problems are common (see sections on DEPRESSION, INSOMNIA, and ANXIETY)

Y. Follow Up: Adjust follow-up to clinical condition of patient
1. Patients who are asymptomatic and not on antiretroviral therapy should be seen every 3-6 months
2. Patients who begin antiretroviral therapy or begin a new antiretroviral regimen should be re-evaluated in one month
3. Patients who are stable and on antiretroviral therapy should be seen every 1-3 months depending on their clinical situations

OCCUPATIONAL EXPOSURE TO BLOOD AND OTHER BODY FLUIDS THAT MAY CONTAIN HUMAN IMMUNODEFICIENCY VIRUS (HIV)

I. Definitions:

    A. Health care personnel (HCP) are persons (employees, students, contractors, attending clinicians, public-safety workers, or volunteers) whose activities involve contact with patients or with blood or other body fluids from patients in a health care, laboratory setting, or public-safety setting

    B. An exposure that may place the HCP at risk for HIV infection includes incidents involving blood, tissue or other body fluids contaminated with visible blood; semen, vaginal, cerebrospinal, synovial, pleural, peritoneal, pericardial, and amniotic fluids have an undetermined risk; examples include the following:
        1. Percutaneous injury such as a needlestick or cut with a sharp object
        2. Contact of mucous membrane or nonintact skin (e.g., exposed skin that is chapped, abraded or has dermatitis) with blood, tissues, or other potentially infectious body fluids
        3. Any direct contact with concentrated HIV in a research laboratory or production facility
        4. Human bites; possibility of infection for both the person bitten and the person who inflicted bite

II. Pathogenesis: (see section on HIV/AIDS in Adults and Adolescents)

III. Clinical Presentation

    A. As of December 2001, 57 US HCP have reported documented occupationally acquired HIV infection (negative HIV-antibody tests at the time of exposure and subsequent seroconversion); another 138 HCP have possible occupationally acquired HIV infection (lack of documented seroconversion as result of exposure)

    B. Nurses are the most commonly exposed professional group

    C. Risk after a needlestick when the source patient is HIV positive is approximately 0.3%; risk of mucocutaneous transmission is approximately 0.09%

IV. Diagnosis/Evaluation

    A. History
        1. Evaluate exposure (determine type of incident, amount of fluid involved, and duration of exposure)
        2. Evaluate exposure source person
            a. Explore prior HIV testing results and CD4+ T-cell levels
            b. History of possible HIV exposures such as IV drug use, sexual contact with a known HIV infected partner, unprotected sexual contact with multiple partners, etc.
            c. Ask exposure source about clinical symptoms that may suggest acute syndrome or undiagnosed HIV infection
            d. If exposure source is HIV positive, determine current HIV RNA levels, CD4+ T-cells, and current and previous antiretroviral therapies; resistance to antiretroviral agents should be suspected in source persons with clinical progression of disease or persistently increasing viral loads or decreasing CD4+ T-cell counts
        3. For purposes of considering postexposure prophylaxis (PEP), ask HCP about current use of medications and underlying medical conditions

    B. Physical Examination
        1. Thoroughly assess site of wound
        2. Explore mental status and anxiety level of HCP

C. Differential Diagnosis: None

D. Diagnostic Test
    1. Evaluation of occupational exposure source
        a. Test for HIV antibody; consider rapid HIV-antibody test such as Single Use Diagnostic System HIV-1 Test (Abbott-Murex Diagnostics)
        b. For exposure sources whose infection remains unknown (exposure source refuses testing), consider medical diagnoses, clinical symptoms, and history of risk behaviors when making management decisions
    2. Evaluation of HCP
        a. Perform HIV antibody testing to establish serostatus at time of exposure if the source person is HIV infected or has recently engaged in high risk behaviors; routine use of direct virus assays (HIV p24 antigen EIA or tests for HIV RNA) are not recommended
        b. Consider using a rapid HIV-antibody test (see above IV.D.1.a.)
        c. Perform follow-up HIV antibody testing at 6 weeks, 12 weeks, and 6 months if the exposure source person is HIV infected or has high risk for HIV infection; extended follow-up (12 months) is needed for HCP who become infected with HCV following exposure to an exposure source coinfected with HIV and HCV; extended follow-up should be individually considered for all HCP depending on type of exposure, etc.
        d. Pregnancy testing should be offered to all nonpregnant women of childbearing age if pregnancy status is unknown
        e. See section "Follow-Up" (V.D.2.) for monitoring of drug toxicity if PEP is used

V. Plan/Management

A. Wound and skin sites should be washed with soap and water; flush mucous membranes with water

B. Postexposure prophylaxis (PEP)
    1. Discuss risks and benefits of PEP
    2. Selection of type of PEP regimen should involve consideration of the comparative risk of the exposure (see table POSTEXPOSURE PROPHYLAXIS)
    3. Selection of drug regimens (see table POSTEXPOSURE PROPHYLAXIS DRUG REGIMENS)
        a. Two-drug regimens are used for most exposures but three-drug regimens should be used for exposures that have increased risk
        b. Drug selection should also be based on whether the exposure source person's virus is known or suspected to be resistant to one of more the potential drugs for PEP
    4. If indicated, PEP should be started as soon as possible
    5. Re-evaluation of HCP should be considered within 72 hours postexposure, especially as additional information about exposure source person or exposure becomes available
    6. PEP should be administered for 4 weeks, if tolerated
    7. If PEP is taken and the source is later determined to be HIV negative, discontinue PEP

POSTEXPOSURE PROPHYLAXIS FOR PERCUTANEOUS INJURIES, MUCOUS MEMBRANE EXPOSURES, AND NONINTACT SKIN EXPOSURES

Exposure Type	Infection Status of Source			
	HIV-Positive Class 1*	HIV-Positive Class 2*	Source of Unknown HIV Status**	Unknown Source†
Percutaneous (less severe: solid needle and superficial injury) -or- Mucous membrane or skin (small volume: few drops)	Recommend basic 2-drug PEP	Recommend expanded 3-drug PEP	Generally, no PEP warranted; however, consider basic 2-drug PEP for source with HIV risk factors	Generally, no PEP warranted; however, consider basic 2-drug PEP in settings where exposure to HIV-infected persons is likely
Percutaneous (more severe: large-bore needle, deep puncture, visible blood on device, needle used in artery or vein) -or- Mucous membrane or skin (large volume: major blood splash)	Recommend expanded 3-drug PEP	Recommend expanded 3-drug PEP	Generally, no PEP warranted; however, consider basic 2-drug PEP for source with HIV risk factors	Generally, no PEP warranted; however, consider basic 2-drug PEP in settings where exposure to HIV-infected persons is likely

* HIV-Positive, Class 1 – asymptomatic HIV infection or known low viral load (e.g., <1,500 RNA copies/mL). HIV-Positive, Class 2 – symptomatic HIV infection, AIDS, acute seroconversion, or known high viral load. If drug resistance is a concern, obtain expert consultation. Initiation of postexposure prophylaxis (PEP) should not be delayed pending expert consultation, and, because expert consultation alone cannot substitute for face-to-face counseling, resources should be available to provide immediate evaluation and follow-up care for all exposures
** Source of unknown HIV status (e.g., deceased source person with no samples available for HIV testing)
† Unknown source (e.g., a needle from a sharps disposal container)

Adapted from Center for Disease Control. (2001). Updated U.S. Public Health Service guidelines for the management of occupational exposures to HBV, HCV, and HIV and recommendations for postexposure prophylaxis. *MMWR, 50*(RR11), 1-42

POSTEXPOSURE PROPHYLAXIS DRUG REGIMENS*

Regimen Category	Drug Regimen
Basic Regimen	Zidovudine, 600 mg per day in two or three divided doses plus lamivudine 150 mg BID; available as Combivir (one tab BID)
Alternate Basic Regimen	Lamivudine 150 mg BID plus stavudine 40 mg BID (if body weight is <60 kg, 30 mg BID)
Alternate Basic Regimen	Didanosine 400 mg QD on empty stomach if a buffered tablet is used (if body weight is <60 kg, 125 mg BID) or 250 mg QD if a delayed-release capsule is used plus stavudine 40 mg BID (if body weight is <60 kg, 30 mg BID)
Expanded Regimen	Basic regimen plus one of the following: indinavir 800 mg every 8 hours, nelfinavir 750 mg TID, nelfinavir 1250 mg BID, efavirenz 600 mg QD HS, abacavir 300 mg BID (available as Trizivir, a combination of zidovudine, lamivudine, and abacavir [1 tab BID])

*Ritonavir, saquinavir, amprenavir, delavirdine, lopinavir/ritonavir are agents that can used as PEP with expert consultation; nevirapine is generally not recommended for use as PEP

Adapted from Center for Disease Control. (2001). Updated U.S. Public Health Service guidelines for the management of occupational exposures to HBV, HCV, and HIV and recommendations for postexposure prophylaxis. *MMWR, 50*(RR11), 1-42

C.   Counseling and education
1.   The emotional effect of exposure is great; HCP need social support and accurate information
2.   Advise HCP to use the following measures to prevent secondary transmission: Practice sexual abstinence or use condoms, refrain from donating blood, plasma, organs, tissue, or semen; refrain from breastfeeding, if applicable
3.   Counsel on importance of completing the prescribed drug regimen
4.   Inform of possible drug toxicities and the need for monitoring and possible drug interactions
5.   Advise to seek medical evaluation for any acute illness that occurs during follow-up period as this may indicate acute HIV infection, a drug reaction, or another medical problem needing attention
6.   Resources for guidance on management of occupation exposures (see table)

RESOURCES FOR OCCUPATION EXPOSURES	
National Clinician's Postexposure Prophylaxis Hotline	http://www.ucsf.edu/hivcntr
Needlestick (management of blood exposures)	http://www.needlestick.mednet.ucla.edu
US Public Health Service (guidelines)	http://www.cdc.gov/mmwr/preview/mmwrhtml/rr5011a1.htm

D.   Follow Up
1.   HCP need counseling, postexposure testing and medical evaluation regardless of whether they receive PEP; HIV antibody testing should be performed at 6 weeks, 12 weeks, and 6 months
2.   If PEP is used, monitor for drug toxicity at baseline and again 2 weeks after starting PEP
    a.   Select tests based on medical conditions of exposed person and toxicity of drugs
    b.   Minimally order CBC and renal and hepatic function tests
    c.   Order serum glucose if regimens include a protease inhibitor
    d.   If indinavir is used, monitor for crystalluria, hematuria, hemolytic anemia, and hepatitis

REFERENCES

Bartlett, J.G. (2001). *The Johns Hopkins Hospital 2002 guide to medical care of patients with HIV infection* (10th ed.). Philadelphia: Lippincott, Williams & Wilkins.

Center for Communicable Diseases. (1992). 1993 revised classification system for HIV infection and expanded surveillance case definition of AIDS among adolescents and adults. *MMWR, 41* (RR-17).

Centers for Disease Control and Prevention. (2001). Revised guidelines for HIV counseling, testing, and referral. Technical Expert Panel Review of CDC Counseling, Testing and Referral Guidelines. *MMWR 50* (RR-9), 1-58.

Centers for Disease Control and Prevention. (2001). Updated U.S. Public Health Service guidelines for the management of occupational exposures to HBV, HCV, and HIV and recommendations for postexposure prophylaxis. *MMWR, 50*(RR11), 1-42

Centers for Disease Control and Prevention. (2002). Approval of a new rapid test for HIV antibody. *MMWR, 51,* 1051-1052.

Centers for Disease Control and Prevention. (2002). Guidelines for using antiretroviral agents among HIV-infected adults and adolescents: Recommendations of the Panel on Clinical Practices for Treatment of HIV. *MMWR, 51*(RR-7). 1-55.

Centers for Disease Control and Prevention. (2002). Guidelines for preventing opportunistic infections among HIV-infected persons – 2002: Recommendations of the U.S. Public Health Service and the Infectious Diseases Society of America. *MMWR, 51*(RR-8), 1-52.

Centers for Disease Control and Prevention. (2002). Update: AIDS—United States, 2000. *MMWR, 51,* 592-595.

Ferri, R.S., Adinolfi, A., Orsi, A.J, Sterken, D.J., Keruly, J.C., Davis, S., et al. (2001). Treatment of anemia in patients with HIV infection, Part 1: The need for adequate guidelines. *Journal of the Association of Nurses in AIDS Care, 12,* 39-51.

Ferri, R.S., Adinolfi, A., Orsi, A.J, Sterken, D.J., Keruly, J.C., Davis, S., et al. (2002). Treatment of anemia in patients with HIV infection, Part 2: Guidelines for management of anemia. *Journal of the Association of Nurses in AIDS Care, 13,* 50-59.

Gerberding, J.L. (2003). Occupational exposure to HIV in health care settings. *New England Journal of Medicine, 348,* 826-833.

Green, M.L. (2002). Evaluation and management of dyslipidemia in patients with HIV infection. *Journal of General Internal Medicine, 17,* 797-810.

Joffe, B.I., Panz, V.R., & Raal, F.J. (2001). From lipodystrophy syndromes to diabetes mellitus. *Lancet, 351,* 1379-1381.

Keithley, J.K. (2001). Management of antiretroviral-related nutritional problems: State of the science. *Journal of the Association of Nurses in AIDS Care, 12*(Suppl), 67-74.

Little, S.J., Holte, S., Routy, J.P., Daar, E.S., Markowitz, M., Collier, A.C., et al., (2002). Antiretroviral-drug resistance among patients recently infected with HIV. *New England Journal of Medicine, 347,* 385-394.

Moyle, G.J., Datta, D., Mandalia, S., Asbol, D., & Gazzard, B.G. (2001). Hyperlactataemia and lactic acidosis during antiretroviral therapy. *Antiretroviral Therapy, 6*(Suppl), 66.

National Institute of Allergy and Infectious Diseases. (2003). Important interaction results from a phase III, randomized, double-blind comparison of three protease inhibitor-sparing regimens for initial treatment of HIV infection (AACTG Protocol A5095). Available at http:www.nlm.nih.gov/databases/alerts/hiv.html

Piscitelli, S.C., & Gallicano, K.D. (2001). Interactions among drugs for HIV and opportunistic infections. *New England Journal of Medicine, 344,* 984-996.

Polsky, B., Kotler, D., & Steinhart, C. (2001). HIV-associated wasting in the HAART era: Guidelines for assessment, diagnosis, and treatment. *AIDS Patient Care, 15,* 411-423.

Schambelan, M., Benson, C.A., Carr, A., Currier, J.S., Dubé, M.P., Gerber, J.G., et al. (2002). Management of metabolic complications associated with antiretroviral therapy for HIV-1 infection: Recommendations of an International AIDS Society – USA Panel. *Journal of Acquired Immune Deficiency Syndrome, 31,* 257-275.

Smith, K. Y. (2002). Selected metabolic and morphologic complications associated with highly active antiretroviral therapy. *Journal of Infectious Disease, 185*(Suppl 2), S123-S127.

Steinhart, C., Orrick, J.J., & Simpson, K. (2002). *HIV/AIDS primary care guide.* Gainesville, FL: University of Florida.

US Food and Drug Administration. (2003). FDA approves first drug in new class of HIV treatments for HIV infected adults and children with advanced disease. Available at: http://www.fda.gov/bbs/topics/NEWS/2003/NEW00879.html

Yeni, P.G., Hammer, S.M., Carpenter, C.C.J., Cooper, D.A., Fischl, M.A., Gatell, J.M., et al. (2002). Antiretroviral treatment for adult HIV infection in 2002: Updated recommendations of the International AIDS Society—USA Panel. *JAMA, 288,* 222-235.

17 Musculoskeletal Problems

CONSTANCE R. UPHOLD

Ankle Sprain
Table: Classification of Ankle Sprains
Figure: Anatomical Structures of the Ankle
Figure: Anterior Drawer Sign
Figure: Talar Tilt Test
Figure: Resistance Exercises

Elbow Pain
Figure: Anatomical Structures of the Elbow
Figure: Palpation of the Lateral Epicondyle with the Thumb
Figure: Palpation of the Medial Epicondyle with the Thumb

Fibromyalgia
Table: The American College of Rheumatology 1990 Criteria for Classification of Fibromyalgia
Figure: Tender Points Identified by American College of Rheumatology
Table: Websites for Fibromyalgia Syndrome Organizations

Gout

Joint Pain
Table: Classification of Systemic Lupus Erythematosus

Knee Injury, Acute
Figure: Anatomical Structures of the Knee
Figure: Testing for Fluid in the Knee Joint
Figure: Collateral Ligament Testing
Figure: Lachman's Test
Figure: McMurray Maneuver
Table: Ottawa Knee Rule
Table: Pittsburgh Decision Rules

Low Back Problems, Acute
Table: Causes of Acute Low Back Pain in Adults
Figure: Common Disc Syndromes: Neurologic Findings
Figure: Straight Leg Raise
Figure: Patrick's Test
Figure: Gaenslen's Sign
Table: Red Flags for Potentially Serious Conditions
Table: Strategies to Minimize Stress to the Back

Lower Extremity Pain, Overuse Injuries
Figure: Measurement of Q-Angle or the Patellofemoral Angle

Osteoarthritis
Table: Criteria for Osteoarthritis of the Hip and Knee
Table: Technique for Quadriceps Strengthening Exercises

Osteoporosis

Plantar Fasciitis

Rheumatoid Arthritis

Shoulder Pain

Wrist Pain

ANKLE SPRAIN

I. Definition: Injury to the ligaments of the ankle

II. Pathogenesis

    A. Due to sudden stress on one or more of the supporting ligaments of the ankle

    B. Often occurs from stepping off a curb or into a hole

    C. If injury is sports-related, it is often due to jumping or falling on outstretched ankle; basketball, football, and cross-country running are the sports in which sprains occur most frequently

    D. Inversion injuries which involve the anterior talofibular or the calcaneofibular ligaments occur most often
        1. Occurs when the foot is plantarflexed and inverted
        2. Physical findings include anterolateral swelling, tenderness over anterior talofibular ligament, and, with severe sprains, a positive anterior drawer sign

    E. Eversion injuries which usually involve the deltoid ligament are the second most common type
        1. Occurs when foot is dorsiflexed and everted
        2. Location of maximal pain, swelling, and tenderness is medial rather than lateral

III. Clinical Presentation

    A. Most common musculoskeletal injury; approximately 85% of all ankle injuries in adults are due to sprains

    B. Classification of sprains (see table the follows)

CLASSIFICATION OF ANKLE SPRAINS	
Grade	**Clinical Manifestations**
I. First degree: Partial tear of ligament	Joint is stable with minimal pain, swelling, and ecchymosis Slight or no functional loss (able to bear weight with minimal pain)
II. Second degree: Incomplete tear of ligament, with moderate functional loss	Ligament appreciably torn but the joint remains stable Severe swelling (>4 cm about the fibula) and severe ecchymosis
III. Third degree: Complete tear and loss of integrity of ligament	Loss of function and motion (unable to bear weight); unstable joint

    C. Immediate pain is noticed and swelling over the injured ligament often occurs within 1 hour of the injury

    D. Persons with previous ankle injuries have increased risk of reinjuring the same ankle

    E. Characteristics of severe ankle injuries
        1. Eversion injury
        2. Syndesmosis sprain: Mechanism of injury is excessive dorsiflexion and eversion of the ankle joint with internal rotation of the tibia (suspect this injury if swelling or ecchymosis occurs above the malleolus)
        3. Immediate diffuse swelling which may indicate bleeding
        4. Inability to bear weight immediately
        5. Sensation of a "pop", "snap", locking of joint, or kick into the heel
        6. On physical exam, patient often has a positive drawer sign and a positive squeeze test

IV. Diagnosis/Evaluation

    A. History
        1. Ask patient to precisely describe how the injury occurred
        2. Ask patient to describe the foot position at the time of injury
        3. Ask patient to point to the location of the maximum pain
        4. Determine whether the patient was able to bear weight after injury

5.   Determine whether the patient had a sensation of a "pop," a "snap," or had any locking of the joint which may indicate a partial- or full-tendon rupture
6.   Question when and where the swelling and ecchymosis were first noticed
7.   Ascertain whether there is any associated pain in the leg, knee, or foot
8.   Inquire about previous musculoskeletal injuries
9.   Inquire about self-treatment

B.   Physical Examination
1.   Always compare injured side with unaffected side; examine most painful area last
2.   Observe ankle, concentrating on the lateral and medial aspects of the foot and ankle, for swelling, ecchymosis, and deformity
3.   Assess neurovascular status of foot; evaluate distal pulses (tibialis posterior and/or dorsalis pedis) and dermatomes for sensation
4.   Palpation should be systematic (see Figure 17.1 of anatomical structures)
    a.   Start with bony structures: Shaft of fibula, distal fibula over lateral malleolus, medial malleolus, base of the fifth metatarsal, all the tarsals, metatarsals, and phalanges
    b.   Next palpate the ligamentous structures:
       (1)   Anterior tibiofibular ligament
       (2)   Anterior talofibular ligament
       (3)   Calcaneofibular ligament
    c.   Palpate tendons including the Achilles, the peroneal tendons, and the anterior tibial tendon

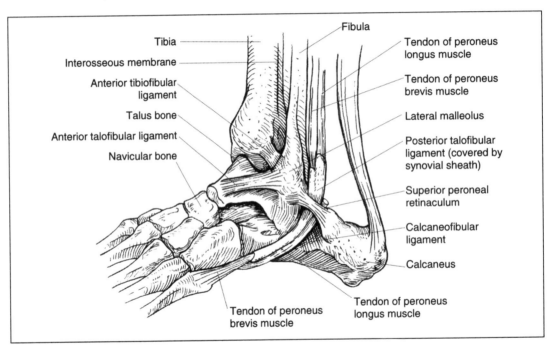

Figure 17.1. Anatomical Structures of the Ankle.

5.   Perform active range of motion and assess the limits of unassisted movement
6.   Perform passive range of motion and assess the limits of manipulation by the examiner without effort of the patient
7.   Perform resisted range of motion to determine muscular strength by measuring the patient's active movement against resistance
8.   Perform three special tests:
    a.   Anterior drawer test is used to assess the anterior talofibular and other ligaments of the lateral side of the ankle (see Figure 17.2)

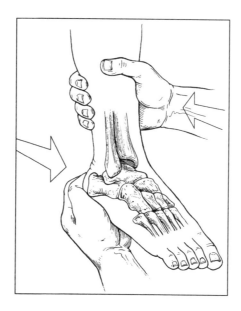

Figure 17.2. Anterior Drawer Sign.

Examiner grasps distal tibia with one hand and heel with other hand; patient's foot is held firmly while backward force is applied to tibia; Positive test is graded 1+ for slight movement, 2+ for moderate movement, and 3+ for marked movement

      b.   Talar tilt test is used to assess stability of the calcaneofibular ligament (see Figure 17.3)

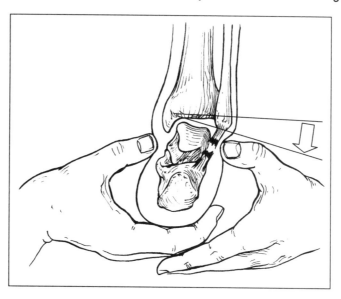

Figure 17.3. Talar Tilt Test.

Grasping the distal tibia and heel with other hand, apply gentle inversion force to affected ankle; ligaments are probably damaged if the talar tilt around the ankle is 5-10° greater around injured than around uninjured ankle

            c.   Squeeze test should be done if medial or severe lateral injury has taken place
                 (1)   Examiner's hands are placed 6 inches inferior to the knee with thumbs on the fibula and fingers on the medial tibia
                 (2)   Leg is squeezed as if to bring fibula and tibia together
                 (3)   Pain with this test denotes syndesmotic injury which is a severe injury
      9.   Assess joints above and below injury

   C.   Differential Diagnosis
      1.   Strains: Injuries to the tendons and muscles; usually have gradual onset of pain due to overuse rather than trauma
      2.   Tendonitis presents with pain with active stretching and plantar flexion against resistance; pain is worse with hill running (see section LOWER EXTREMITY PAIN)

3. Tendon ruptures such as Achilles have a sudden onset of shooting pain in calf, followed by weakness in leg and inability to walk on toes (see section LOWER EXTREMITY PAIN)
4. Fractures often occur in persons who engage in high velocity, high impact sports
   a. Four basic injury mechanisms for fractures: Lateral displacement of talus (most common), medial displacement of talus, axial compression of talus, and repetitive microtrauma
   b. Refer to orthopedist
5. Gout, arthritis, or infection may present with a painful ankle, but examination findings and history are inconsistent with trauma

D. Diagnostic Tests
   1. When to order x-rays is controversial; some authorities suggest x-rays should be routinely ordered to rule out bony involvement whereas the recently-developed Ottawa rules recommend the following:
      a. Order ankle series if there is pain near the malleoli and either inability to bear weight both immediately and in the emergency department, or bone tenderness at the posterior edge or tip of either malleolus
      b. Order foot x-ray series if there is pain in the midfoot and either inability to bear weight both immediately and in emergency department, or bone tenderness at the navicular or the base of the fifth metatarsal
   2. Consider ordering stress films when the ankle cannot be easily manipulated to test for stability or when the patient has chronically unstable ankles
   3. Consider computed tomography (CT) scan or magnetic resonance imaging (MRI) for the following: Ankle sprains that remain symptomatic for >6 weeks, injuries that involve crepitus or catching and locking, and suspected syndesmosis sprains (see III.E.2.)

V. Plan/Management

A. Refer to orthopedist patient with Grade III sprains, injuries with neurovascular compromise, tendon rupture or subluxation, a wound that penetrates the joint, injuries with mechanical "locking" of the joint, and injuries to the syndesmosis; consider orthopedist referral for all eversion injuries

B. Early treatment (approximately first 48 hours) of less severe sprains focuses on regaining range of motion, early mobilization of joints, limiting soft-tissue effusion while protecting ankle against reinjury; follow the **PRICE** therapy (**P**rotection, **R**est, **I**ce, **C**ompression, **E**levation)
   1. Protected weight-bearing with an orthosis is permitted with weight bearing to tolerance as soon as possible following the injury; crutches can be used until painless-weight bearing is achieved
      a. Taping the ankle, a lace-up splint, a thermoplastic ankle stirrup splint, a functional walking orthosis, or a short-leg cast will protect ankle and allow mobility
      b. For severe injuries initial immobilization is required and a simple plaster posterior splint or plastic ankle-foot orthosis may facilitate early rehabilitation and prevent the ankle from stiffening in a plantar flexed, slightly inverted position; air-filled or gel-filled ankle braces that restrict flexion-dorsiflexion may also help
      c. Generally, protected range of motion is superior to rigid immobilization with a cast
   2. Apply ice to injury as many times as possible a day for 20 minutes for the first 48 hours or until edema and inflammation have stabilized
   3. Compression can be accomplished by using an Ace wrap to hold ice in place and after ice application to prevent swelling (when wrapping ankle, make sure to include heel)
   4. Elevate ankle above the level of heart
   5. For pain, prescribe a nonsteroidal anti-inflammatory agent (NSAID) such as ibuprofen (Motrin) 400 mg every 4-6 hours prn or a COX-2 selective nonsteroidal anti-inflammatory drug (NSAID) such as celecoxib (Celebrex) 100 mg BID or rofecoxib (Vioxx) 25 mg QD if the patient is elderly or has a history of gastrointestinal, liver, or kidney problems

C. Functional rehabilitation is critical regardless of grade of injury (consider referral to physical therapist)
   1. The exact time to begin exercising varies with the severity of the sprain; generally the following exercises can be started after first 48 hours if the patient's pain and swelling are resolving normally
      a. Toe alphabet in which entire foot and ankle trace letters of alphabet in air
      b. Isometrics in which side of injured foot/ankle is placed against an immovable object and pressed
      c. Toe raising in which patient raises up and down on toes while holding onto object to maintain balance
   2. Approximately 2 weeks post-injury begin the following:
      a. Resistive exercises with surgical or bicycle tubing (see Figure 17.4)

    b.   Remind patient that once an injury has occurred, the joint will never be as strong which will increase likelihood of reinjury unless strengthening exercises are continued

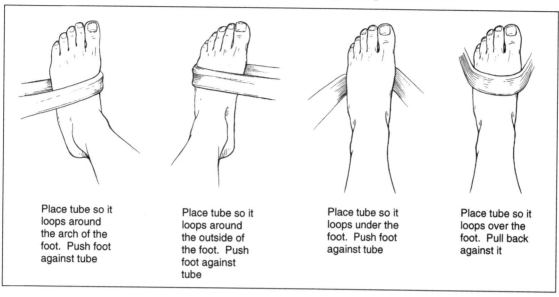

Place tube so it loops around the arch of the foot. Push foot against tube

Place tube so it loops around the outside of the foot. Push foot against tube

Place tube so it loops under the foot. Push foot against tube

Place tube so it loops over the foot. Pull back against it

Figure 17.4. Resistance Exercises

    3.   Last phase of functional rehabilitation
        a.   When the patient achieves full weight-bearing without pain, proprioceptive training should be started for the recovery of balance and postural control (i.e., walk on normal or in heel-to-toe fashion over various surfaces and progress from hard, flat floor to uneven surfaces)
        b.   There should be full resolution of swelling, normal joint motion, strength, and proprioception before the patient begins running; start with 50% walking and 50% jogging and gradually increase percentage of jogging until pain is no longer present

D.   In all phases of recovery and rehabilitation, protect the ankle from further injuries by taping ankle or using high-top lace-up shoes or a combination of proper shoes with a lace-up brace underneath

E.   Follow Up
    1.   Examine ankle in 7-10 days or sooner if pain and swelling do not decrease
    2.   If there is little improvement or the condition has worsened in 2-3 weeks, consider referral to orthopedist or the ordering of additional films or bone scans

ELBOW PAIN

I.   Definition: Chronic or recurrent pain or discomfort of the elbow caused by selected common problems

II.   Pathogenesis (see Figure 17.5. of anatomical structures of the elbow)

    A.   Lateral epicondylitis or "tennis elbow"
        1.   Inflammation of the common tendinous origin of the extensor muscles of the forearm on the humeral lateral epicondyle
        2.   Exact mechanism of injury is uncertain but activities that combine excessive pronation and supination of the forearm with an extended wrist are probably responsible

    B.   Medial epicondylitis or "golfer's elbow"
        1.   Inflammation of the common forearm flexor origin at the humeral medial epicondyle
        2.   Occurs in persons performing repetitive pronation activities

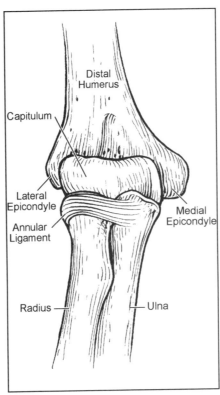

Figure 17.5. Anatomical Structures of the Elbow

III. Clinical Presentation

    A.   Lateral epicondylitis is one of the most common syndromes affecting the upper extremities
        1.   Commonly occurs in patients who frequently play tennis, badminton, or bowl
        2.   Also occurs in persons who engage in occupations that require using a wrench or screwdriver repetitively
        3.   The commonality among these activities is use of a strong grasp during wrist extension
        4.   Onset of symptoms is usually gradual with the patient complaining of tenderness on the lateral aspect of the elbow; swelling may occasionally be present

    B.   Medial epicondylitis is similar in presentation to "tennis elbow" described above but occurs less commonly
        1.   Occurs in golfers, but more commonly associated with certain manual activities such as the frequent carrying of objects with elbows flexed
        2.   Clinical presentation is similar to that of lateral epicondylitis except that the pain is located in the area of the medial, rather than the lateral epicondyle
        3.   Inflammation can involve the ulnar nerve and compression of the nerve may cause numbness in the little and ring fingers on the affected side

IV. Diagnosis/Evaluation

    A.   History
        1.   Inquire about onset, duration, and location of pain
        2.   Determine mechanism of injury
        3.   Determine what activities exacerbate the pain
        4.   Determine if associated symptoms of swelling, numbness and tingling of hand/fingers, or loss of strength in arm or hand are present
        5.   Inquire about participation in activities, either occupational or recreational, that require the following:
            a.   Strong grasp during wrist extension (if lateral epicondylitis is suspected)
            b.   Repetitive pronation of the arm or the carrying of heavy objects with elbows flexed (if medial epicondylitis is suspected)

6. Inquire about what makes the pain better or worse
7. Determine what treatments (either by the patient or another clinician) have been tried and their results
8. Ask about past medical history and medication history

B. Physical Examination
   1. If lateral epicondylitis is suspected, examine the elbow to determine the following
      a. Assess for tenderness over the lateral epicondyle or over the radiohumeral joint
      b. Assess range of motion (flexion and extension should be normal although extension may cause minimal pain)
      c. Evaluate motor function of the hand by asking patient to abduct the thumb, index, and little fingers against resistance
      d. Evaluate sensation at the dorsal web space between thumb and index finger (radial nerve), the tip of the long finger (median nerve), and the tip of the little finger (ulnar nerve)
      e. Have the patient perform supination (palms up) and pronation (palms down) against resistance
      f. To reproduce the patient's symptoms, perform the maneuver in Figure 17.6.; sharp, localized tenderness in area of palpation or just distal is diagnostic of tennis elbow

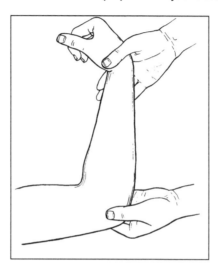

Figure 17.6. Palpation of the Lateral Epicondyle with the Thumb

   2. If medial epicondylitis is suspected, examine the elbow to determine the following:
      a. Assess for point tenderness over the medial epicondyle
      b. Assess range of motion (flexion and extension should be normal although extension may cause minimal pain)
      c. Evaluate motor function of the hand by asking patient to abduct the thumb, index, and little fingers against resistance
      d. Evaluate sensation at the dorsal web space between thumb and index finger (radial nerve), the tip of the long finger (median nerve), and the tip of the little finger (ulnar nerve)
      e. Palpate the medial epicondyle (see Figure 17.7) to determine degree of tenderness
      f. Valgus stress applied to the elbow may reproduce pain

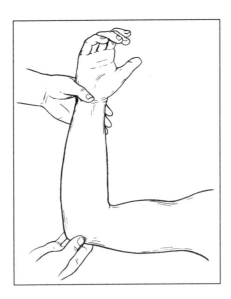

Figure 17.7. Palpation of the Medial Epicondyle with the Thumb

C. Differential Diagnosis for lateral and medial epicondylitis in adults includes nerve entrapment syndrome, olecranon bursitis, arthritis, fracture, gout/pseudogout, and infection

D. Diagnostic Tests
1. No tests are indicated when the history and physical examination are consistent with the suspected diagnosis
2. Order x-rays if atypical findings are noted on history or physical examination

V. Plan/Management

A. Lateral epicondylitis
1. Focus is on reduction of the inflammation, strengthening the involved muscle, and avoidance of further injury
2. Rest (immobilization in a sling for several days), ice, and use of rapidly acting NSAIDs (such as naproxen 375 mg BID or ibuprofen 600 mg TID) are helpful in reducing the inflammation
3. Referral to physical therapy can reduce symptoms and strengthen the involved muscle groups in the forearm and wrist through an appropriate exercise program, possibly preventing recurrences
4. Avoidance of the activity that caused the problem for several weeks or months is necessary
5. Use of an elbow strap (available at sporting goods stores) in the area of the muscle mass of the proximal portion of the forearm can be helpful, but is usually of limited value
6. Physiotherapy that includes massage, ultrasound therapy, and exercises may be helpful
7. Patients who fail to respond to conservative therapy should be referred to a specialist for management; local steroid injections may eventually be needed

B. Medial epicondylitis
1. Treatment is the same as described under V.A.
2. If ulnar nerve involvement is suspected based on history and physical examination, prompt orthopedic referral is indicated

C. Follow Up: Schedule return visit within one month to determine treatment effectiveness and to assess whether referral to a specialist is warranted

FIBROMYALGIA

I.   Definition: Complex syndrome involving fatigue and widespread, nonarticular musculoskeletal pain

II.   Pathogenesis

    A.   Etiology is unknown

    B.   The following mechanisms have been hypothesized to trigger fibromyalgia (FMS): Dysregulation of the autonomic and neuroendocrine systems, metabolic processes, immunological abnormalities, sleep disturbances, stress and trauma from accidents or surgery, and infection due to Epstein Barr virus, cytomegalovirus, human herpesvirus 6, enteroviruses, or *B. burgdorferi*

III. Clinical presentation

    A.   Age of onset is typically between 20-40 years; prevalence increases with age but can occur in childhood

    B.   Females are affected 8-10 times more than men

    C.   Most common symptoms are diffuse musculoskeletal pain, sleep disturbance, and persistent fatigue

    D.   Other symptoms include swelling of hands and feet, morning stiffness, headaches, paresthesias, sensitivity to cold and/or hot, dyspnea, chest pain, night sweats, visual problems, dizziness, painful menses, gastrointestinal complaints, memory impairment, anxiety, and depression

    E.   Patients may have associated conditions or comorbidities such as mitral valve prolapse, episodic hypoglycemia, Raynaud's disease, irritable bowel syndrome, myofascial pain syndrome, migraine headaches, depression, and chronic fatigue

    F.   Symptoms can be severe and patients may become functionally disabled

    G.   Because patients have chronic, multiple, vague complaints and no outward signs, they are often misdiagnosed as hypochondriacs and relationships with family and friends may deteriorate

    H.   Patients often have disturbance of stage 4 of sleep; disturbance of this stage for 2-3 consecutive nights can produce physical symptoms of FMS even in normal controls

    I.   Tender points (localized areas of muscle tenderness that result in pain when pressure is applied) are essential to the diagnosis; trigger points (pain is elicited at initial site of palpation as well as in a linear or circumferential pattern surrounding the site or at a distant site) are also common

    J.   The American College of Rheumatology (ACR) established clinical criteria for diagnosing FMS (see table AMERICAN COLLEGE OF RHREUMATOLOGY 1990 CRITERIA FOR CLASSIFICATION OF FIBROMYALGIA and Figure 17.8. TENDER POINTS IDENTIFIED BY AMERICAN COLLEGE OF RHEUMATOLOGY)

*1. History of widespread pain

Definition. Pain is considered widespread when all of the following are present: pain in the left side of the body, pain in the right side of the body, pain above the waist, and pain below the waist. In addition, axial skeletal pain (cervical spine or anterior chest or thoracic spine or low back) must be present. In this definition, shoulder and buttocks pain are considered as pain for each involved side. "Low back" pain is considered lower segment pain.

2. *Definition.* Pain, on digital palpation, must be present in at least 11 of the following 18 tender point sites:
  - Occiput: Bilateral, at the suboccipital muscle insertions
  - Low cervical: Bilateral, at the anterior aspects of the intertransverse spaces at C5-C7
  - Trapezius: Bilateral, at the midpoint of the upper border
  - Supraspinatus: Bilateral, at origins, above the scapula spine near the medial border
  - Second rib: Bilateral, at the second costochondral junctions, just lateral to the junctions on upper surfaces
  - Lateral epicondyle: Bilateral, 2 cm distal to the epicondyles
  - Gluteal: Bilateral, in upper outer quadrants of buttocks in anterior fold of muscle
  - Greater trochanter: Bilateral, posterior to the trochanteric prominence
  - Knee: Bilateral, at the medial fat pad proximal to the joint line

Note: For a tender point to be considered "positive" the subject must state that the palpation was painful

*For classification purposes, patients must satisfy both criteria. Widespread pain must have been present for at least 3 months

Source: Wolfe, F., Smythe, H.A., Yunus, M.B., Bennett, R.M., Bombadier, C., Goldenberg, D.L., et al. (1990). The American College of Rheumatology 1990 criteria for the classification of fibromyalgia. *Arthritis and Rheumatism, 33*, 160-173.

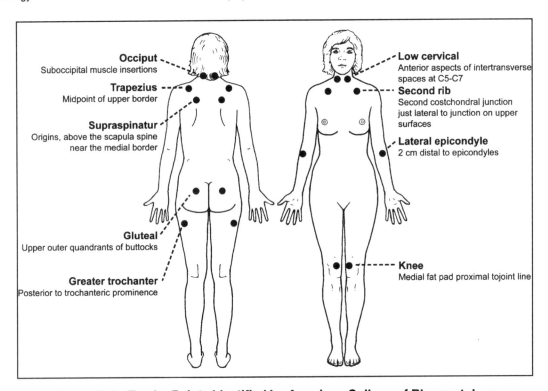

Figure 17.8. Tender Points Identified by American College of Rheumatology

IV. Diagnosis/Evaluation

    A. History: Obtain a thorough history and carefully listen to the patients describe their symptoms
        1. Question about associated symptoms such as headaches, diarrhea, lack of concentration
        2. Ask about factors that precipitate symptoms
        3. Explore how the disease has impacted on the patient's family, interpersonal relationships, work, school, and activities of daily living

    B. Physical Examination
        1. Measure vital signs
        2. Observe general appearance
        3. Assess neck for thyromegaly

4. Perform bilateral digital palpation using a force of about 4 kg/cm$_2$ which is approximately equal to pressing finger on bathroom scale until it registers 10 pounds, or until the nail bed just begins to blanch; to meet criteria of a positive tender point, patient must label the palpation as "painful," not just tender
5. Perform a complete musculoskeletal examination, particularly assess each joint
6. Assess mental status and perform a mental health assessment

C. Differential Diagnosis
1. Chronic fatigue syndrome: These patients have vague, systemic symptoms but do not usually complain of pain as is characteristic of FMS (see section on FATIGUE)
2. Rheumatoid arthritis, in contrast to FMS, presents with warm, erythematous joints in addition to pain
3. Systemic lupus erythematosus (SLE): Patients with FMS may present with mildly elevated ANA but other criteria of SLE are absent (see section on RHEUMATOID ARTHRITIS for SLE criteria)
4. Somatization and depression often accompany FMS but are not the primary diagnoses; patients with psychological problems do not have characteristic tender points
5. Myofascial pain syndrome presents with referred trigger points and occurs more frequently in men than women, which is not characteristic of FMS
   a. Trigger points, in contrast to tender points found in FMS, are usually nodular-type areas and cause radiating pain and muscle twitching
   b. To complicate the situation, myofascial pain syndrome may occur in patients with FMS
6. Drug-induced myopathies: Particularly consider this problem in patients taking statins to lower lipids
7. Polymyalgia rheumatica can be diagnosed by an elevated erythrocyte sedimentation rate (ESR)
8. Severe hypothyroidism mimics FMS but usually these patients have signs such as lid lag, dry skin, and an elevated thyroid stimulating hormone
9. Sleep apnea often goes undiagnosed; this disorder presents with loud snoring and thrashing in bed

D. Diagnostic Tests: No tests are available to detect FMS, consider the following tests to exclude other possible diagnoses
1. Complete blood count
2. Erythrocyte sedimentation rate (order in all persons >50 years who present with symptoms)
3. Measurement of muscle enzymes
4. Thyroid stimulating hormone
5. Rheumatoid factor

V. Plan/Management: A multifaceted approach with an interdisciplinary team is ideal; clinical trials of FMS therapies are limited

A. Patient Education
1. Provide reassurance that patient has a distinct, recognizable disease and that symptoms are real and can be managed
2. Explain to patient that complete resolution of pain and associated symptoms is unlikely, but that therapies can reduce pain and improve quality of life
3. Discuss ways to improve sleep (see section on INSOMNIA)
4. Help patient shift from a sense of helplessness and frustration to a sense of self-efficacy and hope
   a. Self-management courses to control symptoms and promote health are effective
   b. Cognitive behavioral therapy such as helping patients to prioritize their time and activities to include meaningful work and enjoyable leisure is beneficial
   c. Social support interventions may be beneficial; support groups may be located through a local chapter of the Arthritis Foundation (AF); find support groups on the AF website (see table for helpful FMS websites)

WEBSITES FOR FIBROMYALGIA SYNDROME ORGANIZATIONS	
Arthritis Foundation	http://www.arthritis.org
Fibromyalgia Network	http://www.fmnetnews.com
National Fibromyalgia Awareness Campaign	http://www.fmaware.com
National Fibromyalgia Partnership, Inc.	http://www.fmpartnership.org
American Chronic Pain Association	http://www.theacpa.org

B. Exercise: A program which includes pain reduction techniques of stretching, proper posture, and body mechanics with careful and gentle exercise such as walking, bicycling, and swimming is helpful
   1. Strenuous or excessive exercise should be avoided
   2. Referral to a physical therapist can be beneficial

C. Pharmacological treatment
   1. Medications to help the patient receive a restful sleep may be helpful; dosages should be individualized and are typically lower than those needed to treat depression
      a. Amitriptyline (Elavil) is commonly used; this drug increases non-REM stage 4 sleep by increasing serotonin levels in the FMS patient; prescribe amitriptyline 10 mg at HS and increase to 50-75 mg over a few weeks if needed
      b. Zolpidem (Ambien) 10 mg HS is an alternative drug to treat sleep problems; limit to 2-3 nights per week
      c. To help combat the concomitant fatigue and depression, a serotonin reuptake inhibitor like fluoxetine (Prozac) 20 mg can be given in the morning; a combination of amitriptyline and Prozac has been found to be more effective than either drug alone
   2. To treat muscle spasms muscle relaxants may be helpful; prescribe one of the following:
      a. Cyclobenzaprine (Flexeril) 10 mg TID; do not use more than three weeks
      b. Tizanidine (Zanaflex): 1-2 mg about 1 hour before bedtime; gradually increase 1-2 mg every 3-7 days; maintenance dose is 4-12 mg; do not use more than three weeks
   3. Tramadol (Ultram) 50-100 mg every 4-6 hours and topical anesthetics such as capsaicin (Zostrix) may be effective in relieving pain
   4. Gabapentin (Neurontin) may provide pain relief; initially prescribe 100 mg/day and increase to 200-800 mg/day
   5. Because of chronic nature of FMS, use narcotic agents only for patients with severe pain who have functional impairments and do not respond to other therapies
   6. Nonsteroidal anti-inflammatory drugs are not effective

D. Massage therapy, acupuncture, hypnosis, local infiltration of trigger points with 1% solution of lidocaine, stress management, relaxation techniques, transcutaneous electrical nerve stimulation, visualization, and meditation are additional effective therapies

E. Follow-up is variable and depends on the severity of symptoms as well as coping abilities and resources of the patients and their support systems

GOUT

I. Diagnosis: Inflammatory disease of peripheral joints caused by monosodium urate crystal deposition

II. Pathogenesis: Alteration in purine metabolism, the end product of which is uric acid

   A. Primary gout is due to inborn error in production or excretion of uric acid (90% have an underexcretion problem)

   B. Risk for developing primary gout is directly proportional to degree and duration of hyperuricemia

   C. Secondary gout is due to the following:
      1. A variety of acquired diseases such as myeloproliferative disease, lymphoproliferative disease, hemolytic anemia, glycogen storage disease, psoriasis, renal insufficiency, sarcoidosis
      2. Obesity, starvation, lead intoxication, and ingestion of drugs (salicylates, diuretics, pyrazinamide, ethambutol, nicotinic acid, alcohol)

III. Clinical Presentation

   A. Men over age of 30 years are most affected; disease is rare in women until after menopause

   B. Symptoms occur after 15-20 years of sustained, asymptomatic hyperuricemia

C. Acute phase
1. Sudden onset of joint inflammation and excruciating pain; one joint, often the metatarsophalangeal joint of great toe (referred to as podagra) is involved, but other common sites are instep of foot, ankle, knee, wrist, or elbow; older persons are more likely to have involvement of upper extremities or polyarticular presentations
2. First attack often begins at night or early morning and pain peaks in 24-36 hours; even without treatment symptoms subside in few days to weeks
3. Signs include a warm, tender, erythematous joint and possible fever
4. Attacks may be precipitated by minor trauma, illnesses causing hospitalization, surgery, or excessive ethanol intake

D. Intercritical period: Between attacks patient is asymptomatic without abnormal physical findings

E. Chronic gout
1. Asymptomatic intervals become shorter and more joints become involved as disease progresses
2. Over time persistent symptoms such as morning stiffness, synovial tissue thickening, and joint deformity occur
3. Tophi, chalky deposits of sodium urate, can develop at sites of irritation such as Achilles tendon, joints of hand, pinnae of ears; tophi seldom become visible until 10 years after the onset of gout
4. Extra-articular manifestations include low grade fever, chronic gouty nephropathy, nephrolithiasis, and acute uric acid nephropathy

IV. Diagnosis/Evaluation

A. History
1. Ask about aspirin intake, diuretic and alcohol use, recent changes in dietary intake
2. Ask about family history of gout
3. Carefully determine number, duration, and characteristics of previous attacks
4. For patients with chronic gout, explore associated symptoms such as fever, back pain, nausea

B. Physical Examination
1. Measure vital signs, noting elevated temperature and blood pressure
2. Observe and palpate painful joints
3. Observe for tophi and chronic joint deformity

C. Differential Diagnosis
1. Pseudogout due to presence of calcium pyrophosphate dihydrate (CPPD) in the joints
   a. Affects the elderly
   b. Has three phases (acute, asymptomatic, and chronic) similar to gout but rarely has tophuslike collections
   c. Affected joints are often the knees, wrists, MCP joints, elbows, and shoulders
   d. Symptomatic treatment with NSAIDs and colchicine is recommended during the acute phase
   e. In chronic cases, NSAIDs are recommended; no medication is known to prevent CPPD crystal formation
2. Cellulitis
3. Septic arthritis
4. Rheumatoid arthritis
5. Bursitis related to a bunion
6. Gout associated with hypertension, hyperlipidemia, renal disease, obesity, and alcohol overuse

D. Diagnostic tests
1. Aspirate joint fluid for smear and culture (to rule out infection) and to identify urate crystals (remember that gout and infection can coexist in the same joint)
2. Order serum uric acid levels
   a. A level >7.0 mg/dL supports the diagnosis of gout but is not specific; patients with chronic use of low-dose aspirin, renal insufficiency, and diuretic use may have elevated uric acid
   b. Serum uric acid levels also can be used to assess the risk for urate stones and the need for aggressive therapy
3. Consider 24-hour urine to measure uric acid excretion which is normally between 600-900 mg on a regular diet; levels >900 mg suggest overproduction of urate
4. During attacks, sedimentation rate and white blood cell count may be elevated

5. To rule out rheumatoid arthritis order rheumatoid factor titer
6. X-rays can rule out other conditions, but cannot differentiate gout from other diseases except in advanced cases when affected joints show punched out lesions in subchondral bone

V. Plan/Management: Goal is to abort acute attacks and prevent future attacks

A. General principles of pharmacological management
1. Initiate medications early in disease course to enhance likelihood of response
2. Drugs that affect serum urate levels should never be changed during an acute attack
3. Acute attacks usually resolve within 48 hours if properly managed; seek other diagnoses if symptoms are not improved in this time frame

B. Acute phase
1. Joint immobilization and decreased weight-bearing
2. Analgesics
   a. Non-steroidal anti-inflammatory drugs (NSAIDs) are considered the first line drugs; start drugs at high dose and then gradually reduce; consider one of the following:
      (1) Indomethacin (Indocin) 50 mg every 8 hours for 6-8 doses, then reduce to 25 mg every 8 hours until attack resolved (usually give high dose for 2-3 days and then taper dose over next 3-5 days); not a good choice in the elderly
      (2) Naproxen (Naprosyn), initially 750 mg followed by 250 mg every 8 hours
      (3) COX-2 selective NSAIDs (celecoxib, rofecoxib, meloxicam) are safer than nonselective NSAIDs, but their efficacy has not been established in treating gout
   b. Colchicine is used less frequently today due to potential adverse effects
      (1) Dosage depends on the severity of symptoms and individual characteristics of patient: Traditionally 0.5 mg tablet was given every hour until total dose of 7.0 mg or 14 doses was reached, symptoms abated, or patient had diarrhea, abdominal cramping, nausea and vomiting; today, colchicine is usually titrated based on pain, but the maximum dosage should not be exceeded
      (2) A better tolerated regimen in patients with normal renal function is 0.6 mg every 3-4 hours on day 1, followed by 0.6 mg daily or BID
      (3) For patients with severe gout who are unable to use NSAIDs or oral colchicine, intravenous colchicine is available but has caused fatal bone marrow suppression, mainly in older patients with renal/hepatic insufficiency
   c. Low-dose oral corticosteroids (30 mg of prednisone given daily for 2-3 days then tapered over 5-7 days) and intra-articular injections of steroids may also be beneficial once infection has been ruled out

C. Intercritical phase: **Daily prophylaxis** with NSAID or colchicine is often all that is needed to prevent development of frequent attacks and chronic gout
1. Prescribe indomethacin 25 mg BID or naproxen 250 mg TID
2. Alternatively, prescribe colchicine 0.5-0.6 mg BID; if the serum creatinine is greater than 1.6 mg/dL, the dose should not exceed 0.6 mg/day
3. Patients may also take 1 or 2 tablets of colchicine when they sense an impeding attack

D. Chronic gout
1. Treatment with a urate lowering agent or hypouricemic treatment (allopurinol or probenecid) is indicated in patients who have the following:
   a. Frequent (more than 3 attacks/year) and disabling attacks
   b. Tophaceous deposits in soft tissues
   c. Destructive gouty joint disease as seen by erosions on x-rays
   d. Recurrent urolithiasis; most recent stone within last 2 years
   e. Severe hyperuricemia (>13 mg/dL in males; >10 mg/dL in females; >15 mg/dL in patients with renal failure)
   f. Severe uric acid overproduction (urinary uric acid excretion >1100 mg/day)
   g. Gout with renal damage, urate nephropathy
   h. High tumor burden of leukemia-lymphoma about to receive cytotoxic treatment
2. If patient meets above criteria, begin urate lowering agent regimen that follows:
   a. Continue low doses of colchicine or NSAIDs for 2-12 months as prophylaxis to avoid fluctuation of uric acid levels which may precipitate an acute attack
   b. Do not start urate-lowering agent until at least one month after acute attack
   c. Order blood urea nitrogen (BUN), serum lipid levels, and CBC before drug therapy

d. To decrease synthesis of uric acid, if patient is secreting too much uric acid (>900 mg/day in 24-hour urine) or in patients with nephrolithiasis, creatinine clearance <50 mL/minute or tophaceous deposits prescribe allopurinol (Zyloprim). Give allopurinol 100 mg QD for 1 week, then raise by 100 mg at weekly intervals until maintenance dose of 300 mg/day is attained; however, a few patients may need doses as high as 800 mg/day; patients with renal insufficiency should have reduced dose

    (1) Goal is to keep uric acid <6.0 mg/dL

    (2) Allopurinol hypersensitivity reaction may be fatal and consists of fever, rash, decreased renal function, liver damage, and leukocytosis

    (3) Allopurinol potentiates the effects of warfarin and theophylline; decreases the metabolism of azathioprine

e. Alternatively, use probenecid (Benemid) (start low at 250 mg BID for 1 week then increase to 500 mg BID) to increase renal excretion of uric acid

    (1) Always encourage high fluid intake (>3 L/day)

    (2) Patients at risk for stones should be given trisodium citrate 5 gm TID for urine alkalinization

f. A uricosuric combination tablet of probenecid 500 mg and colchicine 0.5 mg given BID, as a maintenance dose is available

E. Patient education
1. Gradual weight reduction
2. Reduce alcohol consumption and reduce purine intake (anchovies, gravies, liver)
3. Avoid salicylates
4. Increase fluid intake to 3 L/day
5. Advise patients with chronic gout on hypouricemic treatment that control of disease is a lifelong commitment

F. Asymptomatic hyperuricemia
1. Search for causes
2. Generally asymptomatic hyperuricemia is not treated but followed closely

G. Follow Up
1. Patient with acute gout should be contacted or seen in 24 hours and return in 4 weeks to discuss maintenance therapy
2. Follow-up for patients with chronic gout should be individualized, however, yearly uric acid levels are recommended

JOINT PAIN

I. Definition: Discomfort or tenderness in one or more joints

II. Pathogenesis: See clinical presentation for common causes

III. Clinical presentation of common forms of joint pain

A. Pain involving multiple joints
1. Rheumatoid arthritis (RA): Chronic inflammatory polyarthritis with symmetric joint involvement and rheumatoid factor positivity (see section on RHEUMATOID ARTHRITIS)
2. Osteoarthritis: Joint pain and stiffness, usually lasting less than 30 minutes with lack of systemic symptoms (see section on OSTEOARTHRITIS)
3. Systemic lupus erythematosus (SLE): American Rheumatism Association Classification (1982) (see following table)

CLASSIFICATION OF SYSTEMIC LUPUS ERYTHEMATOSUS

- Malar rash: Fixed, erythematous, flat, or raised rash over malar eminences
- Discoid rash: Erythematous raised patches with scaling
- Photosensitivity
- Oral ulcers
- Arthritis involving 2 or more peripheral joints
- Serositis involving either pleuritis or pericarditis
- Renal disorder involving persistent proteinuria or cellular casts
- Neurologic disorder involving seizures or psychosis
- Hematologic disorders of hemolytic anemia, leukopenia, lymphopenia, or thrombocytopenia
- Immunologic disorder such as positive lupus erythematosus cell preparation or anti-DNA antibody to native DNA in abnormal titer or anti-Sm or false positive serologic test for syphilis for at least 6 months
- Abnormal titer of antinuclear antibody

* A person is said to have SLE if 4 or more of 11 criteria are present

Adapted from Tan, E.M., Cohen, A.S., Fries, J.F., Masi, A.T., McShane, D.J., Rothfield, W.F., et al. (1982). The 1982 revised criteria for the classification of systemic lupus erythematosus. *Arthritis and Rheumatology, 25*, 1275-1277.

4. Polymyalgia rheumatica usually presents in patients over age 50 with shoulder pain, hip-girdle stiffness and increased erythrocyte sedimentation rate

5. Systemic sclerosis or scleroderma initially involves arthralgia and inflammation of the hands; skin thickening, a hallmark of the disease, develops several months later

6. Fibromyalgia is a poorly understood syndrome involving widespread musculoskeletal pain and accompanied by fatigue, nonrestorative sleep, reduced functional ability, and sometimes accompanied by headaches, irritable bowel syndrome, paresthesias, restless leg syndrome, and cold sensitivity (see section on FIBROMYALGIA)

7. Reiter's syndrome, primarily a disease of young men, involves classic triad of arthritis, urethritis, and conjunctivitis

8. Psoriatic arthritis often presents with asymmetric joint involvement and characteristic nail and skin lesions

9. Gonococcal arthritis presents as migratory polyarthritis, tendinitis, and often has vesicular-pustular skin lesions

10. Lyme arthritis usually has classic history of tick bite and rash with arthritis in the knees (see section on LYME DISEASE)

11. Rheumatic heart disease presents in a migratory pattern of joint involvement with evidence of antecedent streptococcal infection

12. Inflammatory bowel disease such as ulcerative colitis and Crohn's disease is associated with gastrointestinal complaints

13. Ankylosing spondylitis affects young men most severely and presents with back pain and stiffness

14. Sickle cell disease causes pain, swelling, tenderness, and effusion in large joints

15. Vasculitic syndromes such as Henoch-Schönlein and polyarteritis nodosa usually have associated physical findings such as a purpuric rash

16. Malignancies such as leukemia and lymphoma sometimes affect the joints; bone pain, fever, and weight loss are typically present

17. Infections such as subacute bacterial endocarditis, influenza, rubella, mumps, chickenpox, infectious mononucleosis, hepatitis, Rocky Mountain-spotted fever, tularemia, and rat-bite fever can also involve joints

B. Pain involving single joint
   1. Infection
      a. Septic arthritis due to disseminated gonorrhea or gram positive bacteria, especially *Staphylococcus aureus,* is a serious condition, presenting with fever, chills, necrotic skin lesions, joint pain, and swelling
      b. Gram-negative bacterial infections and infections due to anaerobes are becoming frequent causes of monoarthritis due to the rising number of persons who are parenteral drug users and immunosuppressed persons
      c. Tuberculous arthritis with subsequent periarticular bone lesions and synovial involvement may occur even if pulmonary tuberculosis is not present
      d. Monoarthritis can herald the onset of HIV infection

2. Gout: First attack usually involves only 1 joint, often metatarsophalangeal joint of great toe, which is painful, warm and red; subsequent attacks may involve one or several joints (see section on GOUT)
3. Pseudogout resembles gout but primarily affects a knee or wrist joint; results from crystals of calcium pyrophosphate inducing joint inflammation and is often associated with hyperparathyroidism and hemochromatosis in the older patient
4. Trauma and foreign-body reactions may present with sudden pain and swelling in one joint
5. Osteomyelitis involves localized swelling, limitation of joint mobility, erythema, and tenderness over the involved area, fever, and and/or an associated ulcer or skin lesion with possibly a sinus tract draining infected fluid; risk factors include history of bacteremia, peripheral vascular disease, diabetes mellitus, trauma, or surgery in the affected area
6. Localized tumors (e.g., osteogenic sarcoma) and metastatic processes (e.g., neuroblastoma) may cause solitary joint pain; typically accompanied by fever and weight loss

C. Rheumatoid arthritis, osteoarthritis, systemic lupus erythematosus, arthritis of inflammatory bowel disease, Lyme disease, psoriatic arthritis, Behçet's disease, Reiter's syndrome, and hemarthrosis (bleeding into a joint commonly due to a clotting abnormality) can result in pain in single or multiple joints

IV. Diagnosis/Evaluation

A. History
1. Ascertain pain characteristics, onset, location at onset, what aggravates pain, and what functional loss has occurred
2. Ask about distribution of involved joints (symmetric involvement of metacarpophalangeal joints [MCP] and wrists suggests rheumatoid arthritis [RA], whereas involvement of distal interphalangeal joints [DIP] suggests osteoarthritis [OA])
3. Determine severity of pain by asking if it awakens patient at night or hinders activities of daily living
4. Explore history of previous attacks; past episodes lend support for a crystalline or other noninfectious cause
5. Inquire about previous trauma to joint or surrounding tissues
6. Question about tick bites, fever, sexual risk factors, intravenous drug use, alcohol abuse, immunosuppression, and travel in foreign countries -- all of which suggest an infectious cause
7. Inquire about rash, diarrhea, urethritis, or uveitis which supports a diagnosis of arthritides
8. Explore systemic symptoms such as fatigue, fever, sleep problems which suggest rheumatoid arthritis, SLE, fibromyalgia
9. Ask about history of gastrointestinal problems and determine whether there is a history of an ulcer, because this will affect choice of analgesic medication
10. A complete family history is important
11. Often a complete review of systems is needed to determine other involved organs

B. Physical Examination
1. Measure temperature and other vital signs (fever suggests infection such as septic arthritis)
2. Observe gait and general appearance
3. Examine joints for presence of tenderness, erythema, warmth, effusion, bony enlargement, and mechanical abnormalities
    a. Assessment must distinguish an arthritis, which involves the articular space, from conditions involving the periarticular area, such as bursitis, cellulitis, or tendinitis; painful limitation of motion probably indicates joint involvement
    b. Helpful to compare paired joints
    c. Remember to inspect, palpate, perform range of motion activities, and perform special tests as needed
4. Assess for muscle atrophy
5. Detailed physical examination is often needed to detect extra-articular manifestations
    a. Observe skin for malar and discoid lesions of SLE, exanthem of gonococcal arthritis, tophi of gout, and nodules of rheumatoid arthritis
    b. Observe nails for pitting (psoriatic arthritis)
    c. Examine eyes for conjunctivitis of Reiter's syndrome and also observe eyes, nose, and mouth for dryness as occurs with sicca syndrome which suggests Sjögren's syndrome that often accompanies rheumatoid arthritis
    d. Inspect mouth for ulcers in Behçet's syndrome, Reiter's syndrome, and SLE
    e. Auscultate heart and lungs noting pleural rubs and heart murmurs from RA , SLE, and rheumatic diseases

   f. Palpate elbows, Achilles tendons, and pinnae for nodules and tophi (rheumatoid arthritis and gout, respectively)

   g. Examine spine for restriction of motion and tenderness that indicates spondylitis

   h. Urethral or cervical discharge suggests gonococcal arthritis

  C. Differential Diagnosis: Rule out all conditions listed in section III.

  D. Diagnostic tests: No standard battery of tests exists; base selection of tests on history and physical examination

   1. Order x-rays if trauma or focal bone pain is present

   2. Joint aspiration with fluid cell count is done if signs of inflammation are present to differentiate inflammatory from non-inflammatory joint disease and to determine whether a joint is infected

   3. Complete cell count (CBC) and erythrocyte sedimentation rate (ESR) are useful as screens for inflammatory disease

   4. Rheumatoid factor may be helpful in confirming the diagnosis of RA, but is also often positive when the patient has other conditions

   5. Antinuclear antibody (ANA) is sensitive but not specific in diagnosing SLE

   6. Uric acids levels are often elevated in gout

   7. Magnetic resonance imaging can sometimes localize an infectious or inflammatory process in a joint, tissue, or bone; best utilized in soft tissue evaluation

   8. Tests for HIV antibodies should be ordered when risk factors for this disease are present

   9. Blood cultures are needed when sepsis is suspected

   10. Bone biopsy or culture is needed when osteomyelitis is suspected

V. Plan/Management

  A. Determine severity of disease and the need for hospitalization; rapid onset of pain, heat, swelling, and erythema of joint should be evaluated immediately for septic arthritis or osteomyelitis which can lead to rapid joint destruction and sepsis

  B. Treat known causes. For example, ceftriaxone (Rocephin) should be used to treat gonococcal arthritis

  C. Immobilization and rest of the involved joint, and hot and/or cold therapy are often helpful

  D. Pharmacological therapy for pain

   1. Anti-inflammatory pain agents should be postponed for at least 12-24 hours so that cultures can grow and joint aspiration can be repeated if needed; If pain is unbearable use acetaminophen or codeine which do not have anti-inflammatory effects

   2. Later aspirin (not with gout) or NSAIDs can be used (see section on PAIN)

  E. Follow up is variable

KNEE INJURY, ACUTE

I. Definition: Injury to the knee from acute trauma (also see sections LOWER EXTREMITY PAIN, OVERUSE INJURIES, and JOINT PAIN)

II. Pathogenesis: Injuries are due to trauma but excessive pronation of the foot or misalignment of an extremity can cause inappropriate stress on structures of the knee and predispose the knee to injury

  A. Strains and sprains of the collateral and cruciate ligaments are caused by forces that create abduction of the leg at the knee, hyperextension of the knee, or a direct blow to the knee

   1. Grade I sprains involve stretching fibers without significant structural damage

   2. Grade II sprains involve partial disruption of fibers with increased laxity

   3. Grade III sprains involve complete tearing of ligamentous tissues

    a. Anterior cruciate ligament (ACL) tear typically occurs when the foot is planted, the knee is flexed, and the individual suddenly changes direction, applying a rotational force to the knee

    b. Posterior cruciate ligament tear (PCL) usually occurs from a blow to the anterior proximal tibia with the knee flexed

      c.   Medial collateral ligament (MCL) injuries result from valgus stress or external rotational force with the legs firmly planted; occurs frequently in sports such as football or basketball; often associated with an ACL injury

      d.   Lateral collateral ligament (LCL) injuries are caused by varus stress or rotational force sustained when the feet are planted or hyperextended

B.   Tears of the medial and lateral meniscus are common and typically involve a simple twisting motion or a rotary force applied to a flexed knee joint; often caused by a noncontact injury

C.   Patellar subluxation or dislocation usually occurs with knee near extension and the tibia externally rotated or may result from a direct blow to knee; may accompany an anterior cruciate ligament (ACL) injury

D.   Fractures are found in about 6% of patients with acute knee trauma
1.   Patella: Result from falls, direct blows to the knee, or a powerful contraction of the quadriceps muscle
2.   Femoral condyles: Common causes are falls and motor vehicle accidents
3.   Tibial plateau: Due to compression forces, twisting forces, or a combination of both

III.   Clinical Presentation

A.   Ligament injuries
1.   Most frequently injured ligament is the medial collateral ligament, followed by the anterior cruciate ligament
2.   Patients have variable amounts of pain, stiffness, tenderness, and swelling depending on severity of ligament damage
3.   Anterior cruciate ligament injury is serious and the diagnosis is often missed
      a.   Patient typically falls to the ground and is unable to arise without assistance
      b.   An audible pop and "giving way" sensation may occur
      c.   A large, hemorrhagic effusion develops within first few hours
      d.   A positive Lachman test or anterior drawer test indicates instability of the ACL
4.   Posterior cruciate ligament injuries are relatively uncommon
      a.   Patient usually has a positive posterior drawer test and observation of knee may reveal hyperflexion
      b.   Patients typically present with less instability and swelling than patients with ACL injuries
5.   Collateral ligament injury (medial and lateral ligaments) involves local swelling, ecchymosis, laxity, localized medial or lateral tenderness; effusion is usually minimal

B.   Meniscus injury
1.   Often occurs in combination with injuries of the ACL or MCL
2.   Medial meniscus injuries are more common than lateral meniscus injuries
3.   Patient often recalls a twisting flexion injury of the knee following by pain with rotational movements and difficulty flexing the knee and bearing weight
4.   May have clicking, locking, catching, or giving way of knee
5.   Knee joint effusion and tenderness over the joint line are often noted
6.   Inability to squat or hop because of pain is characteristic

C.   Patellar subluxation or dislocation occurs more frequently in females than males
1.   Involves severe pain, medial tenderness, effusion, and inability to move knee
2.   On pivoting and running, patients often complain of "locking" or "popping" of knees

D.   Fractures are difficult to differentiate from other injuries; may result in severe pain, inability to bear weight, swelling, limited range of motion, and unequal leg length
1.   Crepitus is palpable with patellar fractures; pain increases with active knee extension
2.   Neurovascular compromise may occur with femoral condylar fractures
3.   Pain with compression of the side of joint may occur with tibial plateau fractures

IV. Diagnosis/Evaluation

    A. History
        1. Ask patient to precisely describe circumstances surrounding injury and mechanism of the injury; particularly ask if injury involved hyperextension of the knee, a direct blow to knee, or a twisting injury
        2. Inquire about location of pain, tenderness, and swelling in knee as well as hip, thigh, shin, ankle and foot
        3. Inquire about sensations of locking, clicking, catching, giving way or buckling of the knee
        4. Ask if there was an audible "pop"
        5. Ask patient to point to site of greatest pain
        6. Ask how quickly after the injury the swelling developed; swelling in the joint within 24 hours suggests hemarthrosis
        7. Ask about previous musculoskeletal injuries; important to determine if this is an acute problem or a pre-existing condition which has been aggravated
        8. Inquire about systemic symptoms such as fever, chills, night sweats
        9. Determine patient's occupation and job requirements
       10. Determine whether patient is involved in leisure or competitive athletics which will affect decisions about management
       11. Inquire about self treatments

    B. Physical Examination
        1. Always compare injured side with unaffected side during observation, palpation, range of motion, and special tests
        2. Observe gait and stance, noting lower extremity alignment
        3. Examination of the entire lower extremity is required
        4. Observe knee while standing for deformity, discoloration, swelling, and abrasions
        5. With patient seated and knee flexed at 90°, look for bulge of fluid on either side of patellar ligament
        6. Palpate in a proximal to distal direction with patient sitting and supine (see Figure 17.9. for anatomical structures)
           a. Begin with thigh, palpating quadriceps, hamstrings, and articular surfaces of the femoral condyles; consider measuring thigh girth to detect disuse atrophy
           b. Palpate patella and all around the joint line (tenderness at joint line suggests meniscal tear, whereas tenderness slightly above or below joint line suggests ligament damage)
           c. Palpate muscles around patella and collateral ligaments
           d. Palpate tibial plateau and tibial tuberosity

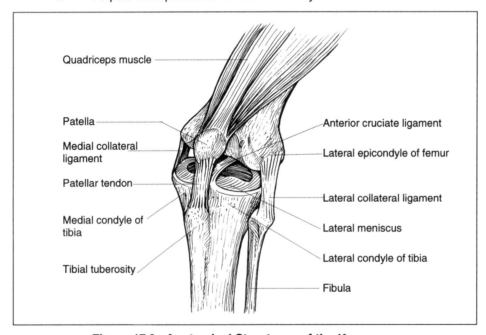

Figure 17.9. Anatomical Structures of the Knee.

7. Assess for effusion or fluid in knee joint (see Figure 17.10.)

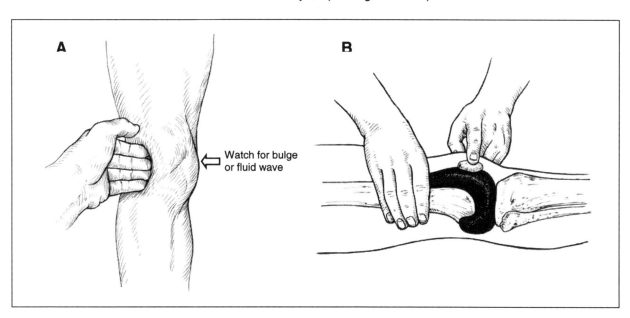

Figure 17.10. Testing for Fluid in the Knee Joint
A. The bulge sign. B. The patellar tap will suggest fluid in the knee as the patella clicks against the femur. With greater amounts of knee fluid, the patella will be ballottable.

8. Perform range of motion of knee
9. Assess mobility of patella by flexing knee 30° and applying medial and lateral pressure to determine amount of subluxation that is possible
10. Determine the quadriceps or Q angle (see Figure 17.18. in section on LOWER EXTREMITY PAIN)
   a. This angle is formed by lines drawn from center of patella to the tibial tubercle and from the center of patella to anterior superior spine
   b. When angle exceeds 15° it is abnormal and may be associated with patellar subluxation and dislocation
11. Determine ligament stability (see Figure 17.11.)
   a. Apply valgus (medial) or varus (lateral) stress when knee is at full extension and then at 30° flexion to assess stability of medial and lateral collateral ligaments
      (1) In first-degree sprains, end point is solid
      (2) In second-degree sprains, laxity is evident at 30° flexion but not at full extension
      (3) In third-degree sprains, there are no solid end points at either 30° flexion or full extension

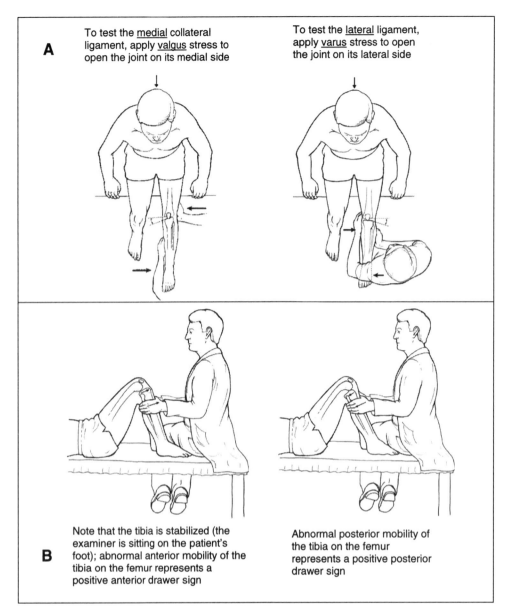

A:

To test the <u>medial</u> collateral ligament, apply <u>valgus</u> stress to open the joint on its medial side

To test the <u>lateral</u> ligament, apply <u>varus</u> stress to open the joint on its lateral side

B:

Note that the tibia is stabilized (the examiner is sitting on the patient's foot); abnormal anterior mobility of the tibia on the femur represents a positive anterior drawer sign

Abnormal posterior mobility of the tibia on the femur represents a positive posterior drawer sign

Figure 17.11. Collateral Ligament Testing

A: Collateral ligament testing. B: The "drawer" sign for cruciate ligament testing

b.   Assess stability of cruciate ligaments with the drawer test by applying anterior (see aforementioned illustration) and posterior forces to the proximal tibia when the knee is flexed and the foot is stabilized

c.   Lachman's test can also test cruciate ligaments and is performed with knee flexed to 30°; anterior drawer force is applied to the proximal tibia with one hand while the other hand stabilizes the femur (see Figure 17.12.)

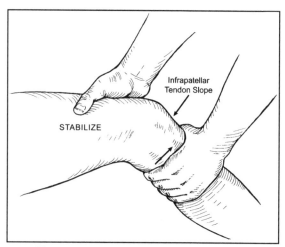

Figure 17.12. Lachman's Test

12. Assess meniscus
    a. Flex knee to 90° and palpate joint line
    b. Perform McMurray's test (see Figure 17.13.)

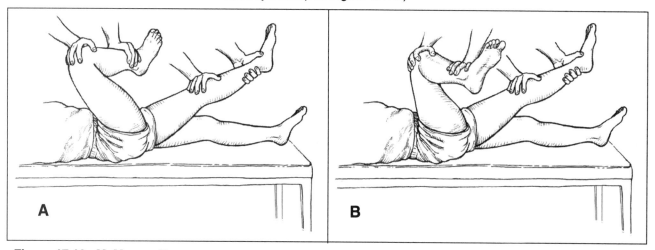

Figure 17.13. McMurray Maneuver.

A. Extension in internal rotation: Maximally flex knee, externally rotate tibia and apply varus stress as the knee is extended to test for lateral meniscus injury. A palpable or audible snap suggests a lesion in the lateral meniscus

B. Extension in external rotation: Perform flexion, external rotation as above but then apply valgus stress to test medial meniscus injury. A palpable or audible snap suggests a lesion in the medial meniscus

13. The apprehensive test is performed to detect patella dislocation
    a. Extend the knee but in a slightly flexed position
    b. Attempt to displace the patella laterally
    c. The test is positive and indicates patella dislocation if the patient becomes apprehensive about the procedure
14. Assess neurovascular status of extremity
15. Assess hip and back whenever a history of knee pain is combined with normal findings on the knee exam

C. Differential Diagnosis: Important to differentiate acute injuries from overuse injuries, inflammatory processes, infection, and neoplasms (see sections, LOWER EXTREMITY PAIN and JOINT PAIN)
    1. Overuse injuries have insidious onset and usually result from repetitive stress
        a. Chondromalacia patellae
        b. Osgood-Schlatter disease
        c. Patellar tendinitis
        d. Stress fractures
    2. Consider osteochondritis dissecans (see section LOWER EXTREMITY PAIN) for patients who have clinical findings of torn meniscus without a history of meniscal injury

3. Hemarthrosis or blood collecting in joint is a serious injury and results from extensive trauma and is often associated with ACL injuries
4. Inflammatory processes, infections, autoimmune diseases, and neoplasms are typically associated with systemic symptoms
5. Hip problems should be considered; referred pain from the hip occurs, especially in children and older patients who are at risk for metastatic disease, osteoarthritis, and fractures

D. Diagnostic Tests
1. To rule out knee fractures, consider ordering x-rays of the knee including anteroposterior, lateral and sunrise patella views; the Ottawa Knee and Pittsburgh Decision Rules are helpful in deciding when to use radiography (see following tables)

OTTAWA KNEE RULE

Order knee x-ray series for patients with the following findings:

1) Age 55 years or older
   Or
2) Isolated tenderness of patella*
   Or
3) Tenderness at head of fibula
   Or
4) Inability to flex to 90°
   Or
5) Inability to bear weight immediately or walk more than four steps immediately after injury

---

*No bone tenderness of knee other than patella

Adapted from Stiell, I.G., Wells, G.A., Hoag, R.H., Sivilotti, M.L., Cacciotti, T.F., Verbeek, P.R., et al. (1997). Implementation of the Ottawa Knee Rule for the use of radiography in acute knee injuries. *JAMA, 278,* 2075-2079.

PITTSBURGH DECISION RULES

Blunt trauma or a fall as mechanism of injury plus either of the following:

- Age younger than 12 years or older than 50 years
- Inability to walk four weight-bearing steps in the emergency department

---

Adapted from Bauer, S.J., Hollander, J.E., Fuchs, S.H., & Thode, H.C., Jr. (1995). A clinical decision rule in the evaluation of acute knee injuries. *Journal of Emergency Medicine, 13,* 611-615.

2. Although ligament injuries can usually be detected based on history and physical examination, joint laxity and rupture may be missed; magnetic resonance imaging (MRI) is accurate in diagnosing ligamentous injuries; ultrasound examination is inexpensive and may be useful; arthroscopy of the knee is the gold standard test for detection of ruptured anterior cruciate ligaments
3. MRI is accurate in diagnosing meniscal injuries
4. Patellar subluxation: Order knee x-rays (AP, lateral, obliques, and sunrise views); consider an arteriogram
5. Perform arthrocentesis for patients with knee effusion who do not have history of trauma or in whom infection is a possible diagnosis; order cell count, Gram's stain, and culture
6. Injuries that do not heal after 2 weeks of conservative treatment may require magnetic resonance imaging or in the case of a meniscus injury, an arthrogram which is less accurate

V. Plan/Management

A. With all types of injuries, the initial treatment is immobilization of the knee in a splint or rigid knee immobilizer, ice, compression, and elevation

B. Refer patients with the following conditions to an orthopedist; surgery or special therapeutic procedures and/or braces are often needed
1. Neurovascular compromise
2. Suspected fractures
3. Dislocation and subluxation of the patella
4. Suspected growth plate injury
5. Torn ligaments (Grade II and III sprains)

710

6. Suspected ACL injuries
7. Locked knee which is unable to be manipulated into place
8. Torn meniscus
9. Hemarthrosis
10. Suspected infection or tumor

C. Treatment for grade I sprains and minor injuries of the meniscus; management depends on the patient's age, athletic participation, occupation, and lifestyles
1. Rest depending on extent of injury; minor injuries may need only 1-2 days of rest
2. Apply ice (never directly to skin) 20 to 30 minutes with at least 10 minute breaks in application as often as possible during first 48 hours after injury
3. Elevate extremity
4. Consider prescribing NSAIDs such as ibuprofen (Motrin) 200-800 mg TID every 6 to 8 hours; some clinicians believe that NSAIDs hamper early healing and should be used conservatively
5. Teach crutch walking and the need to avoid weight-bearing until acute inflammation subsides
6. For injuries with pronounced symptoms, immobilize knee in brace for a minimal period of time
7. Exercise is important
   a. For minor injuries, exercise can be permitted within 1-2 days, but patient should be cautioned to gradually increase activity
   b. For more extensive injuries, activity should initially consist of isometric quadriceps tensing exercises
   c. Begin isotonic quadriceps exercises and range of motion exercises after acute inflammation subsides
8. Incision and drainage of large and fluctuant hematomas may be needed

D. Follow Up
1. For extensive injuries, schedule return visit in 24 hours
2. For less extensive injuries, return visits should be scheduled in two weeks or sooner if problems occur
3. Consult specialist for patients with ligament and meniscus injuries that improved only minimally after 2 weeks of conservative treatment
4. At the return visit, all patients should be taught ways to prevent further injuries to their knees particularly by proper exercising and conditioning and possibly the use of prophylactic braces

LOW BACK PROBLEMS, ACUTE

I. Definition: Activity intolerance due to lower back or back-related leg symptoms of less than 3 months duration

II. Pathogenesis

A. Acute low back pain in adults may be caused by mechanical factors, systemic diseases, or visceral diseases (see following table)

CAUSES OF ACUTE LOW BACK PAIN IN ADULTS		
Mechanical Low Back Pain or Leg Pain (~97%)	**Nonmechanical Spinal Disorders (~1%)**	**Visceral Disease (~2%)**
Lumbosacral strain	Neoplasia such as multiple myeloma, metastatic cancer, tumors	Diseases of pelvic organs such as pelvic inflammatory disease, prostatitis
Degenerative processes		
Herniated disk	Infections	
Spinal stenosis	Inflammatory arthritis such as ankylosing spondylitis, Reiter's syndrome	Renal diseases such as pyelonephritis, nephrolithiasis
Osteoporotic compression fractures		
Traumatic fractures	Paget's disease of bone	Aortic aneurysm
Spondylolisthesis		Gastrointestinal diseases such as penetrating ulcer, pancreatitis, cholecystitis
Spondylolysis		
Congenital diseases such as kyphosis & scoliosis		

Adapted from Deyo, R.A., & Weinstein, J.N. (2001). Low back pain. *New England Journal of Medicine, 344,* 363-370.

B. Pathogenesis of common causes of mechanical low back pain ("mechanical" refers to an anatomic or functional abnormality without an underlying malignant, neoplastic, or inflammatory disease)

    1. Lumbosacral strain

        a. Etiology is often unclear but results from stretching or tearing of muscles, tendons, ligaments, or fascia of back secondary to trauma or chronic mechanical stress

        b. Predisposing factors include chronic occupational strain, obesity, exaggerated lumbar lordosis, abnormal forward tipped-pelvis, weak paraspinal and/or abdominal muscles, leg length discrepancy, chronic poor posture, inadequate/inappropriate conditioning, and sub-optimal lifting habits

    2. Herniated intervertebral disk

        a. Intervertebral disks are composed of collagenous annulus fibrosis and gelatinous nucleus pulposus

        b. Herniation occurs with tears in annulus fibrosis which allows contents of nucleus pulposus to protrude

        c. When nerve roots are compressed by these contents, pain and other neurological signs and symptoms develop

    3. Spondylolysis is a break of the pars interarticularis; found in 5% of people over age 7

    4. Spondylolisthesis is a slip of the vertebrae (after spondylolysis) which allows one vertebral body to slide forward on its neighbor (usual site is L5 or S1); most common cause of back pain in persons <26 years, especially athletes

    5. Degenerative processes such as osteoarthritis are usually age-related

    6. Spinal stenosis results from soft tissue and bony encroachment of the spinal canal and nerve roots

    7. Osteoporotic compression fractures are related to normal aging, decrease in gonadal functioning, or secondary causes such as corticosteroid use or systemic diseases

III. Clinical presentation of common syndromes of acute low back problems

A. Lumbosacral strain is the most common cause of acute low back pain (~70% of cases)

    1. Most patients recover spontaneously within 4 weeks

    2. Occurs frequently between 20-40 years of age

    3. Typically, patient experiences minimal discomfort during or immediately after injury or activity with stiffness and pain occurring 12-36 hours later as soft tissue swells

    4. Pain is located in back, buttocks, or in one or both thighs

    5. Pain is aggravated by standing and flexion; is relieved with rest and reclining

B. Herniated intervertebral disk

    1. Occurs most frequently in young and middle-aged adults; in older persons the nucleus pulposus becomes more fibrotic and dehydrated resulting in a lower incidence of disk herniation compared with the incidence of degenerative disk disease

    2. Most patients begin to improve within 6 weeks; with time, the herniated portion of disk regresses and about 2/3s of the patients have either partial or complete recovery after 6 months

    3. Characterized by radicular pain, which is described as shooting, sharp, electric-type pain, associated with foot and leg pain and worsened with Valsalva maneuvers

    4. Paresthesia or numbness may occur in sensory distribution of nerve root

    5. Deep tendon reflexes are absent or depressed in distribution of nerve root

    6. Muscular weakness and atrophy may result

    7. Most common disk ruptures affect L-5 or S-1 nerve roots

8. Cauda equina involvement (compression of the lower portion of the nerve roots inferior to spinal cord proper) may occur secondary to central disk herniation and presents as insidiously worsening rectal and/or perineal pain with decreased perineal sensation, loss of sphincter control, and disturbances in bowel and bladder functions

9. Signs and symptoms depend on level of herniation (see Figure 17.14. on Common Disc Syndromes)

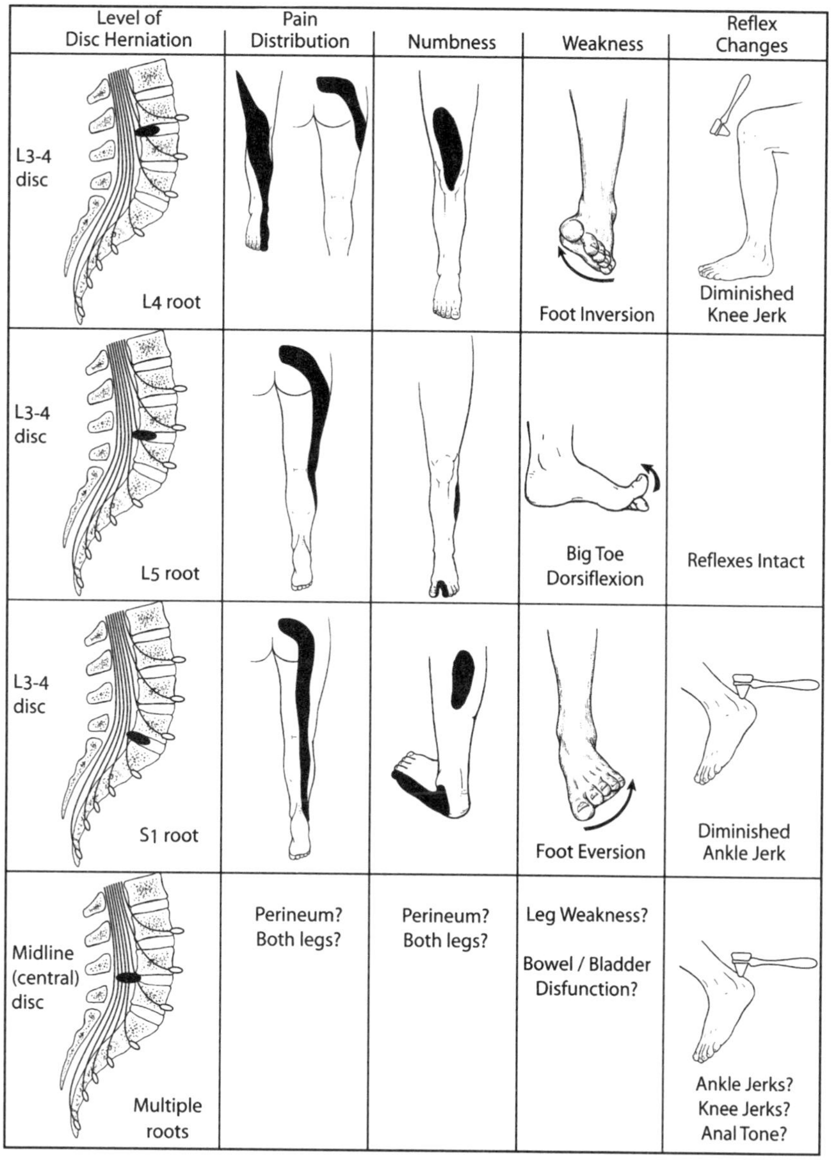

Level of Disc Herniation	Pain Distribution	Numbness	Weakness	Reflex Changes
L3-4 disc / L4 root			Foot Inversion	Diminished Knee Jerk
L3-4 disc / L5 root			Big Toe Dorsiflexion	Reflexes Intact
L3-4 disc / S1 root			Foot Eversion	Diminished Ankle Jerk
Midline (central) disc / Multiple roots	Perineum? Both legs?	Perineum? Both legs?	Leg Weakness? Bowel / Bladder Disfunction?	Ankle Jerks? Knee Jerks? Anal Tone?

Figure 17.14. Common Disc Syndromes: Neurologic Findings

C. Spondylolysis and spondylolisthesis
1. Often occurs from a stress fracture of the posterior vertebral elements or from hyperextension sports such as gymnastics, diving, or weight lifting
2. Family history for spondylolysis is often positive
3. Neurologic examination is usually normal, but patients may have tight hamstrings, and hyperextension (back bending) often reproduces pain at L5 or just below the iliac crests
4. If spondylolysis is suspected x-rays are ordered; if x-rays are negative and suspicion is still high, a bone scan is ordered

D. Degenerative process: Patients typically have gradual, insidious onset of pain accompanied by morning stiffness or stiffness after prolonged immobility

E.   Spinal stenosis
     1.   Occurs in middle-aged and older adults
     2.   Gradual onset of bilateral neurogenic claudication (leg pain and/or leg paresthesias and weakness) when walking; neurogenic claudication may also present as cramping in the buttocks with ambulation
          a.   Differentiate neurogenic claudication from vascular claudication in which symptoms of vascular insufficiency can be relieved by stopping activity or standing
          b.   Neurogenic claudication is usually relieved when patient flexes lumbar spine or sits
     3   Unlike lumbosacral strain, the pain does not remit, but remains stable or gradually worsens
     4.   In severe cases, patient may have bowel and bladder disturbances

F.   Osteoporotic compression fractures cause chronic pain and fatigue, particularly in the middle back; signs include spinal deformity (kyphosis, scoliosis) and loss of height

IV.   Diagnosis/Evaluation

   A.   History should uncover whether there is systemic disease, neurologic involvement that may require surgery, and social or psychological disease that can intensify and prolong the pain
        1.   Ask patient to point with one finger where he/she feels pain and then to describe pain and/or radiation of pain
        2.   Determine mechanism of onset; acute onset without trauma may signal serious conditions such as dissecting aortic aneurysm
        3.   Specifically ask about duration of pain; pain is considered chronic if it persists >6-9 weeks
        4.   Differentiate whether pain is mechanical and worsens after bending or lifting or is nonmechanical, occurring at rest, and related to extraspinal disorders such as pelvic or intra-abdominal conditions
        5.   Determine whether pain and paresthesia occur after walking which typically indicate neurologic involvement
        6.   Ask if sneezing, coughing, or performance of Valsalva maneuver intensifies pain (suggests disk herniation)
        7.   Inquire about pattern of symptoms; ask whether symptoms are constant or intermittent
        8.   Ask if patient has night-time pain which could suggest cancer or infection
        9.   Explore occurrence of systemic symptoms, such as weight loss and fever which could signal malignant disease or a serious infection
        10.   Ask about possible associated symptoms such as dysuria, bowel or bladder incontinence, muscle weakness, paresthesia, and loss of sensations
        11.   Obtain careful past medical history, noting previous trauma, TB, cancer, immunosuppression, urinary infection, osteoporosis, previous back problems, back surgery, and mental health problems
        12.   Inquire about steroid and other drug use
        13.   Determine patient's limitations and the effects of pain on occupational, social, recreational, and family activities
        14.   Use of pain drawings or visual analog scales may augment history

   B.   Physical Examination
        1.   Observe gait and general appearance
             a.   Patients with herniated disks usually are uncomfortable sitting and gait is cautious and awkward
             b.   Limping or coordination problems suggest a possible neurological problem
             c.   Severe guarding of lumbar motion may indicate spinal infection, tumor, or fracture
        2.   Determine temperature; fever is an ominous sign
        3.   Observe spine for alignment and abnormalities; observe skin overlying spine for signs of trauma or infection
        4.   Perform range of motion
             a.   Increased pain with extension often indicates osteoarthritis
             b.   Increased pain with flexion most often indicates strain or injured or herniated disk
        5.   Palpate spine and paraspinal structures noting point tenderness and paravertebral muscle spasm
        6.   If patient fell on tailbone, perform a rectal exam checking for stability of coccyx
        7.   Palpate ischial tuberosity and greater trochanter to rule out bursitis

8.   Perform traction maneuvers
    a.   Straight leg raise (SLR): Elevate each leg passively with flexion at hip and extension of knee (see Figure 17.15)
        (1)   Positive SLR is radicular symptoms (involving the leg and/or foot) when leg is raised to 45° (A)
        (2)   Dorsiflexion of foot sometimes exaggerates SLR responses (B)
        (3)   Crossed leg raise is very diagnostic for disk injury; positive when patient complains of pain in leg that is not raised (C)

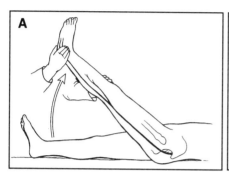 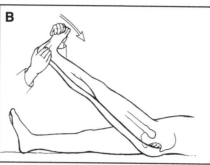 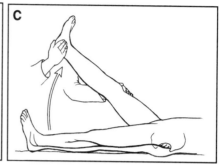

Figure 17.15. Straight Leg Raise

    b.   Patrick's test: Heel is placed on opposite knee and lateral force is exerted on knee and pressure is exerted on anterior superior iliac spine of the opposite side; increased pain indicates hip or sacroiliac disease (see Figure 17.16)

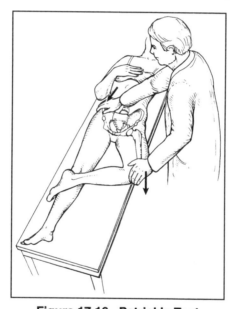

Figure 17.16. Patrick's Test

c.   Gaenslen's sign: Ask patient to lie supine on the table and draw both legs onto chest; then shift patient to side of table and allow unsupported leg to drop over edge while opposite leg is flexed; pain upon execution of this maneuver indicates pathology of the sacroiliac joint (see Figure 17.17)

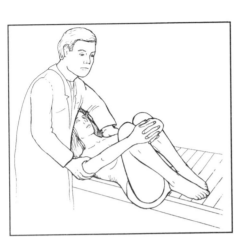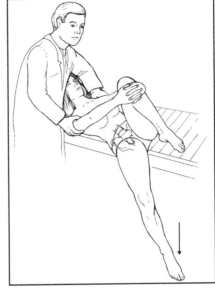

Figure 17.17. Gaenslen's Sign

9.   Check for malingering
   a.   Observe for overreaction
   b.   Perform axial loading (apply slight pressure to top of head); this test should not produce pain unless malingering is present
   c.   Perform pelvic rotation which should not elicit pain except with malingering
   d.   Perform distracted straight leg raise; inconsistent responses suggest malingering
   e.   Observe for nonanatomical motor or sensory regional disturbances
10.   Perform complete neurological examination
   a.   Determine pain and sensation distribution; pain and diminished or absent sensation should follow nerve root distribution (see Figure "Dermatomes" in HERPES ZOSTER in SKIN chapter)
   b.   Do complete motor strength assessment, including dorsiflexion of great toe (only abnormality of the common L4-5 disk protrusion may be great toe weakness)
      (1)   Ask patient to toe walk which tests calf muscles and mostly S1 nerve root
      (2)   Ask patient to heel walk which tests ankle and toe dorsiflexor muscles, L5, and some L4 nerve roots
      (3)   Ask patient to perform a single squat and rise which tests quadriceps muscles, mostly L4 nerve root
   c.   Circumferential measurements of calf and thigh bilaterally can detect muscle atrophy; differences of greater than 2 cm in measurements of the two limbs often indicate an abnormality
   d.   Deep tendon reflex testing
      (1)   Ankle jerk tests mostly the S1 nerve root
      (2)   Knee jerk tests mostly the L4 nerve root
      (3)   Up-going toes in response to stroking the plantar footpad (Babinski or plantar response) may indicate motor-neuron abnormalities such a myelopathy or demyelinating disease
11.   Check sensation of perineum to rule out cauda equina syndrome (compression of the lower portion of the nerve roots inferior to the spinal cord proper)
12.   Examine abdomen, noting masses or bruits
13.   Assessment of the legs and feet is necessary to differentiate spinal stenosis from vascular insufficiency
   a.   Inspect legs and feet for loss of hair and color changes that may accompany vascular insufficiency
   b.   Palpate legs and feet for temperature and tenderness
   c.   Palpate femoral, popliteal, and pedal pulses
14.   Consider pelvic and rectal examinations

15. Consider measuring chest expansion (measurement of <2.5 cm may indicate ankylosing spondylitis)

C. Differential diagnosis (also see table under PATHOGENESIS II.A.)
   1. Important to rule out red flags for potentially serious conditions (see following table)

RED FLAGS FOR POTENTIALLY SERIOUS CONDITIONS			
Possible Fracture	*Possible Tumor or Infection*	*Possible Cauda Equina Syndrome*	*Acute Abdominal Aneurysm*
Major trauma such as vehicle accident or fall from a high place	Age >50 and <20 years	Saddle anesthesia	Age >60 years
Minor trauma with even strenuous lifting (in older or potentially osteoporotic patient)	History of cancer	Recent onset of bladder dysfunction such as urinary retention, increased frequency, or overflow incontinence	Abdominal pulsating mass
	Constitutional symptoms such as fever, chills, or unexplained weight loss		Other atherosclerotic vascular disease
Use of corticosteroids	Risk factors for infection: Recent bacterial infection, IV drug abuse, or immunosuppression	Severe or progressive neurologic deficit in legs	Resting or night pain; tearing pain
Age greater >70 years or history of osteoporosis		Unexpected laxity of anal sphincter	
	Pain that worsens when supine; severe nighttime pain; rest pain; pain that fails to improve with therapy	Perianal/perineal sensory loss	
		Major motor weakness such as knee extension weakness or foot drop	

Adapted from Bigos, S., Bowyer, O., Braen, G., Brown, K., Deyo, R.A., Haldeman, S., et al. (1994). *Acute low back problems in adults. Clinical practice guideline No. 14.* AHCPR Publication No. 95-0642. Rockville, MD: Agency for Health Care Policy and Research, Public Health Service, U.S. Department of Health and Human Services.

   2. Differential diagnosis is extensive; always consider nonspinal pathology that occurs with systemic diseases and referred back pain that occurs with visceral diseases
   3. Psychosocial pathology may complicate the diagnosis and management of low back pain; consider malingering (see IV.B.9.)
   4. Pseudosciatica with a normal neurologic exam includes simple mechanical back pain, disorders of hip, thigh, pelvis, rectum, and vascular claudication
   5. True radicular pain (sciatica or shooting, sharp pain down to the lower leg and foot) includes herniated intervertebral disk, spondylolisthesis, compression fracture, degenerative spondylosis, herpes zoster, and neoplasm

D. Diagnostic Tests
   1. X-rays are useful in only a minority of cases
      a. For patients with low back pain less than 4-6 weeks and in the absence of signs and symptoms of dangerous conditions (see preceding table on RED FLAGS FOR POTENTIALLY SERIOUS CONDITIONS), no tests are needed
      b. If spinal fracture is a possibility, order plain x-ray of lumbosacral spine; if x-ray is negative and fracture is still suspected after 10 days or there are multiple sites of pain, consider bone scan or consultation
   2. If cancer and/or infection are/is suspected, particularly in patient >50 years, order CBC, erythrocyte sedimentation rate, urinalysis; if after these tests, there is still suspicion consider consultation or order bone scan, magnetic resonance imaging (MRI), or computed tomography (CT)
      a. MRI is best at imaging soft tissue (herniated disks, tumors; infections); poor choice of test to visualize fractures
      b. CT is better at imaging cortical bone (osteoarthritis)
      c. Bone scans with radioactive compounds are useful when radiographs of spine are normal, but patient has suspicious clinical findings for osteomyelitis, spondylolysis, neoplasm, metastatic disease, or occult fracture
   3. For patients whose back pain does not improve over 4 weeks:
      a. If symptoms are primarily in the low back consider ordering CBC, ESR, x-rays, CT, MRI, or bone scan depending on symptomatology and risk factors
      b. If spinal stenosis is suspected, spinal x-ray (not diagnostic, but may demonstrate degenerative changes), MRI, or CT should be considered

     c.   If sciatica symptoms are present >4 weeks, consult surgeon about choice of imaging study (MRI, CT) to define nerve root compression **or** order electromyography (EMG) if the level of nerve root dysfunction is not obvious from the physical examination; sensory evoked potentials may be added if spinal stenosis or spinal cord myelopathy is suspected

V.   Plan/Management of common mechanical low back pain disorders

    A.   Immediately consult specialist and arrange for emergency care and studies for patients with cauda equina or rapidly progressing neurologic deficits

    B.   Management of lumbosacral strain and probable herniated intervertebral disk
        1.   **Pharmacological therapy**
            a.   Generally, drugs should be prescribed on a regular rather than on as-needed basis
            b.   Safest effective medication is acetaminophen which may be used safely in combination with non-steroidal anti-inflammatory drugs (NSAIDs) or physical therapeutics
            c.   NSAIDs including aspirin are also effective but can cause gastrointestinal, renal, or allergic problems; COX-2 selective nonsteroidal anti-inflammatory drugs (NSAIDs) such as celecoxib (Celebrex) and rofecoxib (Vioxx) have better safety profiles than nonselective NSAIDs and are becoming the drugs of choice (see section on PAIN)
            d.   Muscle relaxants are a treatment option but are no more effective than NSAIDs in relieving low back symptoms and have adverse effects including drowsiness; cautiously consider prescribing cyclobenzaprine HCl (Flexeril) 10 mg QD to TID, or methocarbamol (Robaxin) initially 1.5 gm (2 tabs, 750 mg each) QID, then 750-1000 mg QID
            e.   Opioids should be avoided if possible, and if selected, used only for a short time
            f.   For some patients with herniated intervertebral disks, epidural corticosteroids injections provide relief
            g.   Patients with chronic back pain may benefit from antidepressant drug therapy
            h.   The following therapies are not recommended: Long-term oral steroids and colchicine
        2.   **Physical methods**
            a.   Referral for manipulation (manual loading of the spine using short or long leverage methods) may be beneficial
                (1)   Often reserved for patients who have pain for >3 weeks, because half of all patients improve spontaneously without any treatment within this time period
                (2)   Safe and effective for patients if they do NOT have radiculopathy
                (3)   Stop manipulation if there is no symptomatic or functional improvement after 4 weeks
            b.   Self application of heat and cold therapy may provide temporary symptom relief
                (1)   Cold therapy for 20-30 minutes several times a day for first 24 hours
                (2)   Topical heat 20-30 minutes several times a day after first day
             c.   Massage therapy has not been well studied; preliminary results have been promising
            d.   The following are ineffective: Traction, diathermy, ultrasound, biofeedback, shoe lifts, transcutaneous electrical nerve stimulation, acupuncture, back corsets, back belts
        3.   **Activity**
            a.   For most patients, bed rest is not needed; prolonged bed rest may have debilitating consequences
            b.   For patients with severe limitations, 2-4 days of bed rest may be beneficial
            c.   Low-stress, aerobic exercise (walking, riding bike, swimming, and eventually jogging) can be gradually and incrementally started within the first 2 weeks of symptoms; conditioning exercises for trunk muscles are not recommended during the first few weeks of symptoms
            d.   For patients with chronic back pain, intensive exercise reduces pain and improves functioning
        4.   **Surgery** should not be performed for patients with lumbosacral strain and most patients with probable herniated disks within the first 4 months; consider surgery if the patient has any of the following:
            a.   Cauda equina syndrome
            b.   Progressive or severe neurologic deficit
            c.   Persistent neuromotor deficit after 4-6 weeks of nonoperative treatment
            d.   Radicular pain for 4-6 weeks (surgery is elective); even patients with clinical findings of nerve root dysfunction due to disk herniation may recover activity tolerance within one month; no research has found that delaying surgery for one month worsens outcomes
        5.   **Patient education**
            a.   Discuss the natural history of the disorder; typically patients make a slow but complete recovery with conservative therapy, but problems often recur

b. Explain that diagnostic tests and special therapies are not needed unless red flags are present or symptoms markedly worsen or persist
c. Teach patient to minimize stress to the back (see table that follows)

STRATEGIES TO MINIMIZE STRESS TO THE BACK

- Avoid jerky, hurried movements when lifting
- Lift with legs by straddling the load; bend knees to pick up load; keep back straight (do not bend back)
- Keep objects close to the body at navel level when lifting
- Avoid twisting, bending, reaching while lifting
- Avoid prolonged sitting
- Change positions often while sitting
- A soft support at small of back, armrests to support some body weight, a slight recline in chair back may make sitting more comfortable
- Firm mattress/bed board, lying supine with hips and knees flexed on pillows is beneficial when sleeping

---

C. Management of spondylolysis
1. Begin with rest, analgesics, and hamstring stretching exercises
2. Back muscle strengthening exercises are recommended when the pain has subsided
3. Immobilization with back braces may be needed to achieve healing of fractures or to relieve irritation if patient is not responding to analgesics and exercises
4. Surgical fusion is rarely required

D. Management of spondylolisthesis
1. Begin with an adequate trial of conservative, symptomatic therapy
2. Progressive or severe neurologic deficit with severe functional impairments that persist for a year or longer are indications for surgery

E. Management of spinal stenosis
1. Symptomatic treatment should be used for first three months
2. Use of an exercise bicycle or walking and rest when pain occurs is recommended
3. Consider surgery which is usually a complete laminectomy for posterior decompensation for patients who cannot manage activities of daily living or who have new signs of bowel or bladder dysfunction

F. Management of degenerative disease (see section OSTEOARTHRITIS) and osteoporotic compression fractures (see section OSTEOPOROSIS)

G. Prevention of further back problems
1. Discuss that low back pain, like other chronic conditions, will get worse unless preventive measures are taken
2. Exercises to condition specific trunk muscles can be added a few weeks after acute symptoms; encourage patient to do exercises such as partial sit-ups or extension exercises such as lying prone and lifting legs off floor or upper torso off floor for at least 5 minutes a day
3. Instruct patient in proper lifting, sleeping position, and body mechanics (see table in V.B.5.)
4. Weight loss and smoking cessation may be beneficial

H. Follow Up
1. Re-evaluate patients with severe pain which does not improve in 24 hours
2. If patient is in moderate pain, re-evaluate in 7-10 days
3. For patients with mild pain, re-evaluate in 4-6 weeks; instruct patient to return sooner if neurological symptoms worsen or bowel/bladder dysfunction occurs

LOWER EXTREMITY PAIN, OVERUSE INJURIES

I. Definition: Acute or chronic discomfort or pain in the foot, leg, or hip due to overuse and repetitive stress (also see sections ANKLE SPRAIN and KNEE INJURY, ACUTE)

II. Pathogenesis: Overuse injuries are a result of extrinsic factors such as improper footwear and poor athletic training and intrinsic factors such a structural abnormalities, malalignment, or poor flexibility

   A. Shin splints: Microtears and inflammation of the sites of origin of the muscles originating from the shaft of the tibia; often due to overactivity

   B. Stress fractures are due to repetitive forces being applied to the lower leg during strenuous activity that causes the bony architecture to exceed a given threshold; a malaligned lower leg may be a predisposing factor

   C. Patellofemoral pain syndrome (PFPS) is due to one or both of the following:
      1. Mild malalignment of the extensor mechanism of the knee
      2. Repetitive microtrauma from overuse

   D. Chondromalacia patellae is due to degeneration of the cartilage on the articular surface of the patella; overuse and malalignment of the lower leg predispose individuals to this condition

   E. Iliotibial band syndrome is caused by overuse and excessive friction between the iliotibial band and the lateral femoral condyle, resulting in inflammation; related to change in footwear, increase in running schedule, or prolonged downhill running

   F. Slipped capital femoral epiphysis is a disorder of the growth and development of the upper femur due to a sudden or gradual dislocation of the head of the femur from its neck and shaft at the upper epiphyseal plate level; may be associated with endocrinopathies and heredity

   G. Tendonitis occurs from a direct blow or overuse with repetitive overloads or faulty technique; tendon ruptures may occur while exercising or with trauma

   H. Bursitis may be caused by acute trauma, contusion over bursae, overuse, or acute or chronic intra-articular inflammation (Baker's cyst)

   I. Plantar fasciitis results from small tears near the origin of the plantar fascia and causes foot pain, particularly on dorsiflexion of toes or when taking first steps in the morning (see section on PLANTAR FASCIITIS)

   J. Injuries from acute trauma such as sprains, fractures, tenosynovitis, subluxations, dislocations, ligament injuries, etc. occur (see sections on ANKLE SPRAINS and KNEE INJURY, ACUTE)

   K. Other important causes of lower extremity pain include rheumatoid arthritis, osteomyelitis, neoplasms, fractures, sprains, fibromyalgia, sickle cell anemia, septic arthritis, thyroid disorders, and conditions with psychosocial origins

III. Clinical Presentation

   A. Shin splints
      1. Most often develop in persons who undergo exercise and are not properly conditioned, do not warm up properly, run on hard or uneven surfaces, wear improper shoes, and/or have anatomical abnormalities
      2. Achy pain over the medial tibia that increases with exercise and improves with rest
      3. Tenderness over the medial tibia; may also have warmth

   B. Stress fractures of the lower extremities (metatarsal, tibial, fibular, femoral, and pelvic); most fractures heal in approximately 4-12 weeks
      1. Metatarsal stress fractures typically involve the second and third metatarsals and are common in athletes and military personnel who are frequently on their feet

2. Tibial stress fractures occur primarily in athletes
   a. Fractures most often occur in distal third of bone; fractures in the middle third of the tibia are of more concern because they are prone to nonunion
   b. Initially the pain occurs at the start of running activity and resolves with rest; eventually the pain lasts longer after running and finally persists even at rest
   c. Diffuse tenderness over medial aspect of tibia is typical
3. Fibular stress fractures are found primarily in runners; symptoms are similar to those found in tibial stress fractures
4. Femoral neck stress fractures occur primarily in long-distance runners and dancers
   a. Pain occurs in the groin, initially with activity and ultimately also at rest
   b. May result in long-term disability; complications include avascular necrosis, non-union, varus deformity, and bone displacement
5. Pelvic stress fractures are most common in long-distance runners
   a. Pain occurs in the inguinal, perineal, or adductor region after an increase in training activity
   b. Patient may be unable to stand unsupported on the affected side
   c. Healing may take longer than other stress fractures (i.e., 3-5 months)

C. Patellofemoral pain syndrome (PFPS)
   1. Most common complaint in sports medicine clinics, particularly for the running athlete
   2. Females are affected more than males, probably due to females having increased width of the gynecoid pelvis which results in an exaggerated Q angle (see IV.B.7.); also associated with femoral anteversion, external tibial torsion, ankle valgus, and excessive foot pronation
   3. Insidious onset of dull, achy knee pain sometimes associated with clicking or popping of knee on movement; pain is often poorly localized and bilateral
   4. Pain is exacerbated with extended sitting and activity involving knee flexion such as running and climbing and descending stairs
   5. A positive patellar apprehension test (patient experiences pain when trying to contract the patella by tightening the quadriceps) is often present
   6. Knee is stable without swelling and erythema
   7. May lead to chondromalacia patellae and patellofemoral degenerative arthritis

D. Chondromalacia patellae
   1. Occurs mainly in adults, infrequent incidence in adolescents
   2. Diffuse pain especially with climbing stairs or getting up from a squatting position
   3. Usually has a greater degree of malalignment than occurs with PFPS

E. Iliotibial band syndrome: Typically involves mild pain over lateral side of knee

F. Slipped capital femoral epiphysis
   1. Condition is a surgical emergency and requires immediate nonweight-bearing status to prevent further slippage
   2. Commonly affects sedentary, obese male adolescents
   3. Limp and varying degrees of achy pain in the groin or referred pain in the knee are typical
   4. May have sudden dislocation of the head of the femur resulting in severe pain with associated inability to bear weight or gradual dislocation resulting in increasing dull pain
   5. Abduction, internal rotation, and flexion of the hip are the movements most limited
   6. Most cases are stable with a good prognosis if diagnosed early
   7. Unstable cases have a poorer prognosis because of high risk of avascular necrosis

G. Tendonitis and tendon ruptures
   1. Common sites: Achilles tendon (above its insertion into the calcaneus), tibialis posterior (behind medial malleolus), tibialis anterior (dorsum of foot, under the extensor retinaculum), peroneal tendon (behind lateral malleolus, at the insertion into the base of the fifth metatarsal), patella
   2. Signs and symptoms include pain with active movement (aggravated in weight bearing) and passive stretching; localized swelling; morning stiffness; and possibly swelling or thickening in the tendon
   3. Achilles tendonitis is a common example and presents with pain on palpation of tendon and pain which is worse with active stretching and plantar flexion against resistance; tenderness is worse with hill running

4.	Patients with tendon ruptures such as Achilles have a sudden onset of shooting pain in calf
	a.	Pain is followed by weakness in leg and inability to stand or walk on toes
	b.	Signs include swelling, ecchymosis over the posterior aspect of the leg and heel, gap in tendon (approximately 5 cm proximal to its insertion), absence of normal plantar reflex, absence of active plantar flexion with good strength, and a positive Thompson test (with patient prone, flex the affected leg 90° at knee and squeeze calf; if foot doesn't move, the tendon is ruptured)

H.	Bursitis
	1.	Typically has swelling and pain over respective bursae (prepatellar, infrapatellar, and anserine bursae)
	2.	May be associated with a Baker's cyst
	3.	Because there usually is no joint involvement, range of motion is not limited

IV.	Diagnosis/Evaluation

A.	History
	1.	Inquire about mode of onset, duration, frequency, location, and characteristics of pain; night pain or pain that wakes the patient from sleep is a possible indicator of a malignant process
	2.	Question about discomfort in areas above and below the stated location of pain
	3.	Ask about joint pain, especially without a history of trauma, as joint pain is often related to rheumatologic diseases and needs to be ruled out
	4.	Query patient about recent trauma involving the lower leg
		a.	Determine how injury occurred
		b.	Ask patient to specifically describe the position and movement of his/her leg during the trauma
	5.	Inquire about a history of a fever, limp, joint stiffness, joint redness, grinding, or any audible popping or snapping sound
	6.	Inquire about exercise without pretraining, change in intensity or duration of exercise, recent viral infections, previous musculoskeletal problems, or repetitive activity
	7.	Ask about medication use, particularly steroid use, and recent immunizations such as rubella
	8.	Inquire about recent infections and family history of musculoskeletal problems, autoimmune diseases, and sickle cell disease
	9.	Inquire about self-treatments and what aggravates and relieves pain
	10.	Perform a review of systems to rule-out systemic disease

B.	Physical Examination
	1.	Assess vital signs, as increased temperature may point to a systemic disease
	2.	Observe gait
	3.	Observe for misalignment of bones such as femoral anteversion and external tibial torsion
	4.	Observe for signs of trauma, development of muscles, deformities, swelling, and erythema
	5.	May need to measure limb length
	6.	Compare opposite limb for swelling, muscle wasting, color, mobility, strength, pulses, and sensation
	7.	Determine quadriceps angle (Q angle) if PFPS and chondromalacia patellae are suspected (see Figure 17.18. MEASUREMENT OF Q ANGLE OR THE PATELLOFEMORAL ANGLE)

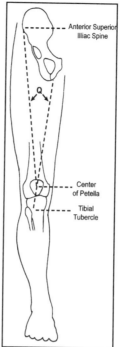

Figure 17.18: Measurement of Q-Angle or the Patellofemoral Angle

Q angle is measured as the angle between a line drawn from the center of the patella to the anterior superior iliac spine and a line drawn from the center of the patella to the tibial tubercle. Average Q angle is 10-13° in males and 15-18° in females. Any angle less than or greater than average angles may be associated with PFPS.

8. Palpate limb and joints for tenderness, swelling, and warmth
9. Perform range of motion of affected joints, noting any limitation in movement, crepitus, and tenderness
10. Assess muscle strength (distal weakness is often due to a neurological problem and proximal weakness is often due to a muscular problem)
11. Evaluate joint stability
12. Assess hamstring flexibility by having patient lie on back with hips flexed to 90° and then extend leg; failure to extend knee completely indicates hamstring tightness and may be a contributing factor in the extremity pain
13. If tendon rupture is suspected, perform the Thompson test (see III.G.4.b.)
14. Assess peripheral vascular status by palpating pulses and determining capillary refill time distal to site of pain
15. Perform a focused neurological examination of the affected extremity, assessing for sensation and deep tendon reflexes; observe patient walking on toes, heels, and hopping on one foot
16. A complete physical examination is often needed to rule out rheumatologic diseases

C. Differential Diagnosis (see conditions listed under Pathogenesis, II.A.-K.); other conditions include the following:
1. Septic arthritis often involves abrupt onset of fever, malaise, pain, and a tense, hot joint effusion
2. Inflammatory arthritis presents with warm, swollen, tender joints
3. Osteomyelitis commonly has extremity pain along with systemic signs of infectious disease such as fever and a septic appearance
4. Neoplasms are rare causes of limb pain; usually the pain is deep and "boring" and patient has systemic complaints such as weight loss and fever
5. Acute injuries due to trauma (see sections on ANKLE SPRAIN and KNEE INJURY)

D. Diagnostic Tests
1. If there is suspicion of systemic or infectious disease, or if pain has a longer duration than expected, is not relieved by common therapies, or is more intense than usually expected, the following tests may be helpful
    a. CBC
    b. Erythrocyte sedimentation rate
    c. Sickle cell preparation or hemoglobin electrophoresis

2. Consider rheumatologic studies for chronic pain
3. X-rays are usually ordered for the following:
    a. Pain due to trauma
    b. Suspected pathologic fractures, tumors, or metabolic defects
    c. Pain lasting longer than 4-6 weeks
    d. Any history of swelling
4. Bone scan is often ordered if stress fractures or osteomyelitis is suspected
5. Diagnostic tests are usually ordered for suspected common causes of extremity pain:
    a. Shin splints: Order x-ray or bone scan if uncertain about diagnosis
    b. For suspected tibial and fibular stress fractures, x-rays (AP, lateral, and both oblique views of leg) are usually ordered; x-rays may be negative in early stages; technetium-99m bone scans and MRI are most helpful
    c. PFPS: Order x-rays if pain lasts longer than 4-6 weeks
    d. Chondromalacia patellae: Order knee x-rays which include a tangential or sunrise view to look for lateral subluxation of the patella
    e. Iliotibial band syndrome: None usually needed
    f. Slipped capital femoral epiphysis: Order x-rays
    g. Tendonitis: none usually needed
    h. Bursitis
        (1) Arthrography is ordered to definitively diagnose a Baker's cyst; otherwise no tests are needed
        (2) If there is swelling, warmth, erythema, and tenderness in the bursa, aspirate fluid from bursa and examine with a Gram's stain and send sample for leukocyte count and culture

V. Plan/Management

A. Shin splints
    1. Rest: Unless the pain is severe, the athlete does not need to completely stop exercising but needs to reduce intensity and duration of exercise
    2. Ice should be applied to reduce swelling and inflammation
    3. Anti-inflammatory medication such as naproxen (Naprosyn) 250-500 mg every 6-8 hours
    4. May need to treat concomitant hyperpronation of foot with flexible orthotics or sturdy, well-fitting footwear
    5. Instruct patient to run on soft, flat surfaces; begin a program of pre-activity conditioning exercises

B. Stress fractures
    1. Consider referral to orthopedic surgeon for patients who have fractures that have a potential to result in delayed union or nonunion and bone displacement (i.e., tibial stress fractures in middle third anterior cortex, femoral neck stress fractures, pelvic stress fractures)
    2. Initial treatment is rest until there is no longer point tenderness on palpation or pain with activity (usually takes 6-8 weeks for tibial and fibular fractures to resolve; whereas femoral neck fractures and pelvic stress fractures take much longer)
    3. Ice is helpful in tibial and fibular fractures
    4. Anti-inflammatory medication may relieve pain
    5. Usually fractures heal without casting or surgery
    6. Activities such as biking and swimming typically produce less pain and help to maintain conditioning
    7. In female athletes, obtain a menstrual history, looking for amenorrhea which is associated with osteopenia and a higher incidence of stress fractures

C. PFPS
    1. Modify activities to avoid full flexion of the knee and stress on the patellofemoral joint
    2. After a brief period of rest, ice, and NSAIDs, begin stretching and strengthening program for quadriceps muscles (perform three sets of 10 repetitions each day during the acute phase)
        a. Quadriceps setting: Patient lies supine with affected knee fully extended, dorsiflexes foot, then tightens the thigh muscles or pushes the thigh into the floor
        b. Straight leg raise: Patient sits on floor, leans back on elbows with one leg fully extended and the other leg flexed to 90°; the extended leg is raised until it is parallel with the thigh of the flexed leg and held in this position for 5 seconds
        c. Terminal-arc extension: Patient lies on floor with knees in about 20° of flexion over a rolled towel of about 6 inches in diameter; patient then extends knee fully and holds for 5 seconds

      d.   After the acute phase, progressive resistance with ankle weights should be initiated

      e.   Encourage flexibility exercises as well

3.   Consider flexible orthotics for malalignment of lower extremities

4.   For exacerbations, use ice and anti-inflammatory medication

5.   Teach that pain tends to be chronic with exacerbations and remissions, but pain can be controlled; swimming or walking are better sports to participate in than running, basketball, and volleyball

D.   Chondromalacia patellae: Plan is similar to treatment for PFPS (see above)

E.   Iliotibial band syndrome: Rest for approximately 1-2 weeks (may take as long as 6 weeks), ice, limited use of NSAIDs, and gradual resumption of full activities with rehabilitation (quadriceps strengthening exercises); consider one-eighth-inch lateral heel wedge

F.   Slipped capital femoral epiphysis: Refer to orthopedic surgeon

G.   Tendonitis and tendon ruptures

1.   Initial treatment includes rest, ice, NSAIDs, and gentle stretching exercises

2.   Early referral to a physical therapy program to improve flexibility, resolve strength deficits, and correct foot biomechanical problems is recommended

3.   Heel lifts or orthotics may be helpful for tendonitis about the ankle

4.   Refer patients with tendon ruptures to an orthopedist

H.   Bursitis

1.   Rest (couple days to weeks), ice for 24 hours, and limited use of NSAIDs

2.   Aspirate tense, inflamed bursa or Baker's cyst to relieve pressure and pain

3.   Consider injecting corticosteroid solution if infection has been ruled-out or injecting a local anesthetic such as lidocaine

4.   Apply a bulky, compressive dressing for protection and comfort

5.   If a bacterial infection is present, prescribe antibiotics; infections tend to be gram-positive cocci and respond well to cephalexin (Keflex) or dicloxacillin (Dynapen)

I.   Follow up for extremity pain is variable depending on patient's problem

OSTEOARTHRITIS

I.   Definition: Degenerative disease of the cartilage of joints with loss of the joint surface

II.   Pathogenesis

A.   Natural history

1.   Progressive structural breakdown of articular cartilage that lines joint surfaces occurs

2.   Dense, smooth-surfaced bone forms at the base of cartilage lesion and marginal osteophytes develop

3.   Variable synovial inflammation results

B.   Factors associated with development of osteoarthritis (OA): Joint trauma, aging, obesity, occupational overuse, weak muscles around joints, congenital musculoskeletal disorders, metabolic disorders (i.e., Wilson's disease), endocrine disorders (i.e., diabetes mellitus), and crystalline deposit disease

C.   Contrary to common belief, active exercise without trauma is not associated with the development of secondary OA and may actually prevent development of the condition by strengthening muscles surrounding joints

D.   Theories of pathogenesis include biomechanical stress affecting articular cartilage and subchondral bone, biochemical changes in the articular cartilage and synovial membrane, and genetic factors

III. Clinical Presentation

    A. OA is the most common form of chronic arthritis and affects one-fourth of the adult population; by age 40, 90% of all persons have some joint problems; however, few people have major symptoms until 60 years or older

    B. Clinical manifestations
        1. Often presents with insidious, gradual onset of joint pain that worsens with weight bearing and activity and improves with rest
        2. Morning stiffness or stiffness after prolonged immobility usually lasts less than 30 minutes
        3. Crepitus on motion, joint tenderness on palpation, and limitation of joint motion are typical
        4. Joint deformity such as subluxation and formation of bony cysts may occur; Heberden's nodes in distal interphalangeal (DIP) joints appear in later stage
        5. Erythema and swelling, if present, are usually mild and localized to affected joint

    C. Joints most affected are the following: DIP, proximal interphalangeal (PIP), first metacarpophalangeal, knees, hip, cervical spine, and lumbar spine
        1. OA of hip is the most disabling and painful
        2. Knees are the most common symptomatic joints

    D. Although there is no criteria for the general diagnosis of OA, criteria have been established for OA of the hip and knee (see table that follows)

CRITERIA FOR OSTEOARTHRITIS OF THE HIP AND KNEE

<u>Hip</u>

Hip pain **and** radiographic femoral or acetabular osteophytes
    OR
Hip pain **and** radiographic joint space narrowing **and** erythrocyte sedimentation rate <20 mm/hour

<u>Knee</u>

Knee pain **and** radiographic osteophytes
    OR
Knee pain **and** age ≥40 years **and** morning stiffness ≤30 minutes in duration **and** crepitus on motion

---

Adapted from Hochberg, M.C., Altman, R.D., Brandt, K.D., Clark, B.M., Dieppe, P.A., Griffin, M.R., Moskowitz, R.W. & Schnitzer, T.J. (1995). Guidelines for the medical management of osteoporosis, Part I: Osteoarthritis of the hip, Part II: Osteoarthritis of the knee. *Arthritis and Rheumatism, 38,* 1535-1541.

IV. Diagnosis/Evaluation

    A. History
        1. Question about location of joint pain which is usually asymmetric and poorly localized
        2. Inquire about joint stiffness which usually lasts less than 30 minutes
        3. Ask about systemic symptoms which are usually absent
        4. Inquire about occupational activities related to overuse
        5. Explore factors such as trauma and extremity malalignment which predispose persons to more serious degenerative changes
        6. Obtain a complete past medical history, focusing on endocrine, musculoskeletal, and metabolic diseases
        7. Determine the degree to which joint problems are affecting activities of daily living and health-related quality of life

    B. Physical Examination
        1. Observe gait; patients with OA of hip may have a "lurching" gait or favor the affected joint
        2. Inspect affected joints for deformities, swelling, and color
        3. Assess joint range of motion
        4. Palpate for crepitus, warmth, edema, and tenderness
        5. Observe muscles for atrophy, particularly inspect the quadriceps muscles
        6. Evaluate muscle strength
        7. Assess joint stability

C. Differential Diagnosis: Atypical joint involvement, acute onset of symptoms, history of significant inflammation, and severe focal rest pain that occurs with malignancies are flags indicating alternative diagnoses
   1. Bone disease such as osteopenia, osteoporosis, malignancy
   2. Periarticular soft tissue abnormalities such as tendinitis, bursitis
   3. Neuromuscular disease such as neuropathy, Parkinson's Disease
   4. Vascular disease such as vasculitis
   5. Rheumatoid disease such as rheumatoid arthritis and gout
   6. Consider hemochromatosis in patients <60 years with OA and those with MCP involvement or chondrocalcinosis (calcification of cartilage)

D. Diagnostic Tests
   1. Consider ordering CBC, erythrocyte sedimentation rate (ESR), chemistry profile, urinalysis, serum calcium, serum phosphorus, uric acid, alkaline phosphatase (all normal with OA)
   2. Rheumatoid factor may or may not be present
   3. In younger patients (<60 years), order iron saturation or ferritin to rule out hemochromatosis
   4. X-rays are often ordered as baseline to determine progression of disease; typically there is narrowed joint space, sclerosis of subchondral bone, bony cysts, and osteophytes

V. Plan/Management: Goals are to control pain, improve function and health-related quality of life, maximize independence, and minimize complications

A. Patient education is an essential part of the plan
   1. The Arthritis Foundation website provides valuable information: http://www.arthritis.org
   2. Assistive and adaptive devices may be beneficial
      a. Lessen weight-bearing by purchasing elevated toilet seats and high chairs
      b. The use of a properly selected cane may reduce hip loading; top of cane's handle should reach the proximal wrist crease when the patient is standing with arms at side; cane should be placed in hand contralateral to the affected knee
      c. Wedge insoles may be helpful in correcting abnormal biomechanics due to varus deformity of the knee
      d. Splints and braces help control instability and pain; referral to occupational and physical therapists is beneficial
      e. Velcro fasteners on clothing can help maintain independence
      f. Built-up longer handles on toothbrush, hairbrush, and cooking utensils are helpful
   3. Self-help classes and community support groups have been reported to decrease pain, decrease health care visits, and improve quality of life

B. An exercise program is important; exercise improves strength and function, reduces pain, promotes a sense of well being, prevents contractures and deformities
   1. Recommend at least 30 minutes of moderate physical activity on most days of the week
   2. Refer patients to a physical therapist or an occupational therapist if they have difficulty maintaining minimum levels of physical activity
   3. Recommend eliminating or reducing the following aggravating factors: Strenuous activity, stair climbing, prolonged sitting, jogging
   4. Low impact and low torsional loading (twisting motion) exercises are best; swimming or water exercise decreases stress on joints and allows flexibility
   5. As strength builds, progressive resistance exercises can be added
   6. Alternate exercise activities to decrease the amount of repetition and burden on joints
   7. For OA of the knee, quadriceps strengthening exercises may reduce pain and improve function (see table below for exercise technique)

TECHNIQUE FOR QUADRICEPS STRENGTHENING EXERCISES

❖ Lie on back with one knee bent and the other leg straight with ankle dorsiflexed to 90°

❖ Tighten quadriceps muscle of straight leg and lift straight leg 25-50 cm off the ground

❖ Hold position for 10 seconds

❖ Lower leg and relax muscle

❖ Repeat exercise at least 10 times, alternating legs

C. Dietary supplements and nutrition
1. Although not recommended by some experts, the American Pain Society (2002) advises that patients should take 1,500 mg of oral glucosamine daily; this supplement may stimulate the production of cartilage matrix and provide nonspecific protection as an antioxidant against chemical damage; found to delay progression of knee osteoarthritis
2. Chondroitin 4-sulfate is sometimes combined with glucosamine preparations or may be taken as a separate supplement; because data on efficacy are preliminary, most authorities do not recommend using this supplement except on a trial basis
3. Advise patients to maintain an ideal body weight and to consume a balanced diet containing adequate amounts of protein, fats, vitamins, and minerals; patients whose body mass index (BMI) is greater than 30 kg/m^2 should follow a weight management program

D. Pharmacologic management of pain is important; a step-wise approach is recommended
1. Pain can often be controlled with analgesics that do not have anti-inflammatory properties; drug of choice for mild pain is acetaminophen 325 mg tabs (Tylenol), 2 tabs every 4-8 hours; do **not** exceed 4,000 mg per day
    a. Carefully monitor prothrombin time in patients taking warfarin sodium as acetaminophen can prolong the half-life of this drug
    b. Use acetaminophen cautiously in patients with existing liver disease
        (1) Monitor liver function tests every 6 months in high risk patients
        (2) Avoid use in patients with chronic alcohol abuse
        (3) If patients are ingesting more than 2 ounces of alcohol daily, the dose of acetaminophen should be decreased to 2.5 g per day
    c. Evidence of the potential for renal damage is also increasing
2. COX-2 selective nonsteroidal anti-inflammatory drug (NSAID) is the first choice for patients with moderate to severe pain and/or inflammation; these agents have a better safety profile (reduce but do not eliminate the risk of gastrointestinal bleeding and perforations) than nonselective NSAIDs and are not contraindicated with warfarin administration; renal toxicity, hypertension, and edema are possible adverse reactions; select one of the following:
    a. Rofecoxib (Vioxx) 25 mg QD
    b. Celecoxib (Celebrex) 200 mg QD or 100 mg BID
    c. Valdecoxib (Bextra) 10 mg QD
3. Nonselective NSAIDs should be used only if the patient is unresponsive to or unable to take COX-2 NSAIDs and/or acetaminophen
    a. Before using these agents, perform a risk analysis to ascertain that the patient is not at risk for NSAID-induced gastrointestinal complications
    b. If risk exists, then prescribe a prophylactic agent such as a proton pump inhibitor or misoprostol (Cytotec), 200 microgram tabs, one tab QID with meals and HS
4. Patients at risk for a cardiovascular event should be given a regular aspirin (between 75-160 mg per day), whether the patient is treated with a nonselective or COX-2 selective NSAID
5. Tramadol or an opioid (morphine, oxycodone, hydrocodone, or other mu agonist opioids) as a single agent or in combination with NSAIDs or acetaminophen should be considered in patients who have not responded to other pain treatments
6. Capsaicin 0.025% cream (Zostrix) is sometimes beneficial
    a. Apply thin layer over painful joints; therapeutic effect requires that cream is applied 4 times daily (ineffective if applied only when symptoms occur)
    b. Can use concurrently with other pain medications
    c. Wash hands after applying
7. Hyaluronic acid (HA) viscosupplementation or intra-articular HA injection is FDA approved for treatment of knee pain in patients who are unresponsive to other pain therapies
    a. Provides a replacement for the lubrication that has been lost due to OA
    b. Contraindicated in persons allergic to chickens or eggs
    c. Use hyaluronate sodium derivative (Synvisc): 3 injections of 2 mg/injection each week for 3 sequential weeks or hyaluronic acid (Hyalgan): 5 injections of 2 mg/injection each week for 5 sequential weeks
    d. Inform patient that it takes a few weeks to notice improvement, but relief usually lasts at least 6 months
8. Consider intra-articular injection with corticosteroids for patients who have significantly increased and inflammatory flare or extensive inflammation in one or a few joints
    a. Before injection, joints should be aspirated and fluid tested to rule-out infection (cell count, Gram's stain, culture) and gout (crystals)
    b. Injections should not be given more than 3-5 times per year in any one joint

E. Physical modalities to manage pain and improve function
   1. Local treatments of moisture, hot and cold therapy, ultrasound, and transcutaneous electrical nerve stimulation (TENS) may be beneficial
   2. Compression gloves decrease swelling in the fingers, thereby decreasing pain
   3. Elastic wrist orthoses may improve pain and hand function
   4. Collagen II, copper bracelets, gold rings, and magnet therapy have not demonstrated a consistent benefit to recommend their use

F. Surgical procedures such as total joint replacements are excellent options for patients; surgical referral should be considered early in the disease process, rather than as a last resort
   1. Patients who have disabling OA or patients whose pain is unrelieved with other treatments should be referred to orthopedic surgeon
   2. Consider surgery for patients in whom pain and functional limitations prevent the minimum amount of activity (30 minutes on most days of the week)

G. Adjunctive therapies
   1. Total hip and knee arthroplasty should be considered in patients when nonsurgical treatment becomes less effective and before deconditioning becomes severe
   2. Arthrodesis, osteotomy, bone removal procedures, and soft tissue procedures may be helpful
   3. Arthroscopic debridement and joint lavage are not supported by empirical data

H. Experimental treatments may be effective approaches in the future and include the following: Cytokine modulation, autologous chondrocyte transplants, gene therapy, and iontophoresis

I. Follow Up
   1. Schedule follow-up appointment within 2-4 weeks of initial visit
   2. Regularly monitor (i.e., every 3-6 months) CBC, electrolytes, LFTs, BUN, creatinine, and stool guaiac if on NSAIDs
   3. Return to clinic if there is a flare up of symptoms

OSTEOPOROSIS

I. Definitions:

A. Skeletal disorder characterized by compromised bone strength predisposing an individual to an increased risk of fracture; bone strength is determined by both bone density and bone quality
   1. Bone density is denoted as grams of mineral per area or volume and is quantified by peak bone mass and amount of bone loss
   2. Bone quality is related to architecture, turnover, damage accumulation, and mineralization

B. World Health Organization operational definition: Bone mineral density (BMD) more than 2.5 standard deviations below the normal bone mass of women who are less than 35 years of age; this definition is controversial because it is not clear how to apply this diagnostic criterion to children, men, and persons of different ethnic groups

II. Pathogenesis

A. May result from bone loss as one ages or may be a result of sub-optimal bone growth in childhood and adolescence

B. Primary osteoporosis (OP) occurs in both genders and results from normal aging and decreased gonadal functioning; usually after menopause in women and later in life in men

C. Secondary osteoporosis in adults is a result of medications and other diseases; in men and perimenopausal women a high percentage of osteoporotic cases are attributed to secondary causes
   1. Endocrine: Glucocorticoid excess, hyperthyroidism, hyperparathyroidism, hypogonadism, hyperprolactinism, diabetes mellitus

2. Drug induced: Glucocorticoids (most common form of drug-related osteoporosis), anticonvulsants, ethanol, tobacco, barbiturates, heparin, thyroid hormones, gonadotropin-releasing hormone agonists (Lupron, etc. for prostate cancer), and, possibly, loop diuretics
3. Other: Chronic renal failure, liver disease, chronic obstructive pulmonary disease (COPD), congestive heart failure, hematologic disorders, rheumatoid arthritis, malignancy, Cushing's syndrome, organ transplant

D. Risk factors
1. Age is the greatest risk factor for both genders; other factors include: Female gender, estrogen deficiency, Caucasian race, low weight and body mass index (BMI), family history of OP, smoking, history of prior fracture, and excessive intake of alcohol and caffeine-containing beverages
2. Past and current levels of exercise, late menarche in women, and low endogenous estrogen levels in both genders are associated with low BMD in several studies
3. Possible risk factors are excessive salt and protein intake; irregular menstrual periods in women

III. Clinical Presentation

A. Once viewed as a normal part of aging among women, today OP is regarded as a preventable disease that occurs in both genders; the most important determinant of life-long bone health is the bone mass attained in childhood and adolescence

B. OP is often considered a silent disease, because less than a third of the cases have been diagnosed

C. Postmenopausal OP
1. Bone loss is most rapid during the first postmenopausal decade
2. Patients are often asymptomatic; considerable bone loss (over 35%) can occur before complaints are present or abnormalities are detected on x-rays
3. Fractures of the vertebrae, hip, or forearm are early manifestations of OP and often occur spontaneously or with minor trauma
   a. About 50% of all postmenopausal women will have an osteoporosis-related fracture during their lives
   b. Vertebral fractures are most common and cause chronic pain and fatigue, particularly in the middle back (vertebrae T12 and L1 are most common sites)
      (1) Signs include spinal deformity (kyphosis, scoliosis) and loss of height
      (2) Arm span is longer than body height
4. Fractures of the hip cause the most morbidity and mortality; approximately 80% of hip fractures are related to osteoporotic changes; about 12-20% of patients with hip fractures die within 12 months of presentation

D. OP in men
1. Approximately 1/3 of patients with primary OP who are older than 70 years are men
2. A man's lifetime risk of hip fracture is greater than his risk of prostate cancer
3. Age-adjusted hip fracture incidence is lower in men than women, but by age 85, fracture incidence is the same in both genders
4. In men, 2/3s of cases are due to secondary causes such as corticosteroid therapy (most common), hypogonadism (common), alcoholism (common), endocrine disorders, or smoking

E. Glucocorticoid-related OP results from long-term administration of steroids for conditions such as rheumatoid arthritis, chronic obstructive pulmonary disease, or organ transplants and is associated with a high rate of fractures

IV. Diagnosis/Evaluation

A. History
1. Ascertain onset, duration, location, and characteristics of back pain
2. Question about previous fractures and falls
3. Ask whether patient has noticed loss of height
4. Ask questions to detect risk factors
   a. Determine level of physical activity
   b. Ask about smoking history and alcohol use
   c. Determine medication history, particularly use of corticosteroids
   d. Inquire about diet; explore calcium, Vitamin D, and caffeine intake

      e.   Explore whether female patients are postmenopausal, have had surgical menopause, or are amenorrheic

      f.   Obtain complete medical history, focusing on endocrine problems; in men ask about orchiectomy

      g.   Explore family history of spinal fractures and osteoporosis

      h.   Ask about protein and calcium intake, athletic activity participation, and history of eating disorders

  5.   Ask about dental health as bone loss is a risk factor for periodontal disease

B.   Physical Examination

  1.   Measure height and compare against patient's previous measurements

      a.   After achieving maximum height, most individuals will loss 1.0 to 1.5 inches of height as part of normal aging

      b.   In asymptomatic women, height loss >1.5 inches may be related to vertebral compression fractures

  2.   Observe back for dorsal kyphosis and cervical lordosis from multiple compression fractures

  3.   Palpate spine to detect any painful areas

  4.   Assess for physical abnormalities that may interfere with mobility

  5.   In adolescents, assess for secondary sex characteristics and obtain a sexual maturity rating

  6.   To detect secondary causes of OP, a complete physical examination is recommended (e.g., thyroid nodule suggests hyperthyroidism; buffalo hump suggests Cushing's syndrome; wasting suggests malignancy)

C.   Differential Diagnosis: Rule out conditions noted under Pathogenesis (II.C.)

D.   Diagnostic Tests

  1.   Bone mineral density (BMD) testing

      a.   Dual-energy x-ray absorptiometry (DEXA) is the most accurate test for measuring bone density; DEXA can confirm the diagnosis, predict future fracture risk, and help monitor the response to therapy or changes due to medical condition

      b.   DEXA of hip (femoral head) is the best predictor of hip fracture, but DEXA of the hand, wrist, forearm, and heel can also detect risk

      c.   Quantitative ultrasound of the heel can predict fractures nearly as well as DEXA; advantages are low cost and lack of ionizing radiation

      d.   BMD testing should be performed on all postmenopausal women who present with low-trauma fractures to confirm the diagnosis and determine disease severity

      e.   In patients diagnosed with OP, order every 2 years to evaluate effectiveness of treatments

      f.   Defining OP by BMD testing: A *T*-score is assigned, based on the expected distribution of BMD for "young, normal" adults of the same sex with the difference expressed as standard deviation (SD) above (+) or below (-) the mean; *T*-scores decline with aging and provide convenient cut-points for treatment decisions

g. See following tables for screening recommendations

RECOMMENDATIONS FOR BONE MINERAL DENSITY SCREENING IN WOMEN

US Preventive Services Task Force (2002)
- ✓ Women >65 years
- ✓ Women 60-64 years who are under 154 pounds and not using estrogen

North American Menopause Society (2002)
- ✓ Women >65 years
- ✓ All women with medical causes of bone loss
- ✓ Postmenopausal women <65 years with one of following risk factors for fractures: Nonvertebral fracture after menopause, low body weight (<127 lbs), or history of first-degree relative who has had a hip or vertebral fracture
- ✓ Premenopausal women who experience a low-trauma fracture or who have known secondary causes of OP

American Association of Clinical Endocrinologists (2001)
- ✓ Women >65 years
- ✓ Women >40 years who have sustained a fracture
- ✓ Women who have risk factors for fractures and are willing to consider available interventions
- ✓ Women who have x-ray finding suggesting osteoporosis
- ✓ Women beginning or receiving long-term glucocorticoid therapy or other drugs associated with bone loss
- ✓ Women with symptomatic hyperparathyroidism or other diseases or nutritional conditions associated with bone loss

American College of Obstetricians and Gynecologists (2002)
- ✓ Women >65 years
- ✓ All postmenopausal women who present with fractures
- ✓ May be recommended to postmenopausal women <65 years who have one of more risk factors for OP
- ✓ All postmenopausal women who present with fractures to confirm diagnosis and determine disease severity

---

RECOMMENDATIONS FOR BONE MINERAL DENSITY SCREENING IN MEN

- ✓ Screening for men is less standardized
- ✓ Consider in men with nontraumatic fractures or who have risk factors for fractures
- ✓ Since the incidence of fracture risks increases markedly at age 75 years, consider this a good age for initiating BMD testing

---

2. Bone markers (bone-specific alkaline phosphatase and osteocalcin; urinary levels of pyridinoline and deoxypyridinolines; and serum and urine levels of type I collagen telopeptides) identify changes in bone remodeling but do not predict bone mass or fracture risk and are not recommended in routine clinical practice

3. In patients with diagnosed osteoporosis, consider ordering the following blood tests to establish baseline conditions or to exclude secondary causes:
    a. CBC and erythrocyte sedimentation rate (ESR)
    b. Serum calcium: If elevated consider primary hyperparathyroidism, metastatic cancer, multiple myeloma; if low consider osteomalacia
    c. Urinary calcium excretion to detect calcium malabsorption or renal calcium leak
    d. Thyroid stimulating hormone (TSH), parathyroid function tests, glucose level, estrogen level to R/O endocrine disease
    e. Alkaline phosphatase (serum and 24-hr urine) may be slightly increased with a recent fracture, but if persistently elevated in absence of fracture consider osteomalacia, other bone diseases, and liver disease
    f. Serum creatinine to R/O renal impairment
    g. Albumin to detect malnutrition
    h. In men, order prostate-specific antigen

4. Primary osteoporotic patient will have normal serum levels of calcium, phosphate, vitamin D, parathyroid hormone, and alkaline phosphatase (although alkaline phosphatase may be elevated in context of a healing fracture)

5. Consider additional tests based on history and physical findings:
    a. Serum thyrotropin
    b. Serum 25-hydroxyvitamin D concentration (for possible primary or secondary hyperparathyroidism)
    c. Urinary free cortisol and other tests for possible adrenal hypersecretion
    d. Acid-base studies
    e. Serum tryptase, urine N-methylhistamine, or other tests for mastocytosis
    f. Serum or urine protein electrophoresis to R/O multiple myeloma and leukemia

g. Serum free or total testosterone and luteinizing hormone (in men, to exclude hypogonadism)

h. Bone marrow aspiration and biopsy to detect marrow-based diseases

6. In patients with known or suspected fractures or unexplained loss of height, radiography of the thoracic and lumbar spine may be indicated; radiography is unwarranted in absence of suspected fractures as detection of OP is not possible until 30-50% of skeletal mass is lost

7. Technetium-99m bone scan, computed tomography, and magnetic resonance imaging are usually recommended for detecting vertebral fractures

V. Plan/Management

A. Prevention and lifestyle approaches

1. Estimates indicate that 50% of osteoporotic hip fractures and 90% of vertebral fractures can be prevented

2. Childhood is a critical time to develop habits conducive to bone health

3. **Sufficient intake of calcium** is an important area of counseling; remember, however, that adequate calcium intake alone is not sufficient for preventing OP in most postmenopausal women

4. A high intake of calcium in childhood and throughout life increases mineral density and decreases risk (see following table for recommended calcium intake)

RECOMMENDED CALCIUM INTAKE	
Age	**Recommended Intake**
Adults 19-50 years	1,000 mg/day
Adults older than 50 years	1,200-1,500 mg/day (higher dose if not on estrogen)

Adapted from Institute of Medicine. (1997). *Dietary reference intakes: Calcium, phosphorus, magnesium, Vitamin D, and fluoride.* Washington DC: National Academy Press.

a. See following table for good sources of calcium; the preferred source of calcium is dietary

b. Inform patients that oxalic acid-containing foods such as spinach and phytate-rich grains such as wheat bran may inhibit calcium absorption

FOODS WHICH ARE GOOD SOURCES OF CALCIUM			
Food Source	**Approximate Calcium Content**	**Food Source**	**Approximate Calcium Content**
Milk (skim, 1%, 2%, whole)	300 mg/cup	Vegetarian baked beans	128 mg/cup
Ice cream	160 mg/cup	Collard greens	350 mg/cup
Oatmeal, instant (2 packages)	326 mg	Broccoli	100 mg/cup
Cottage cheese	125 mg/cup	Orange juice, fortified	350 mg/cup

Adapted from J.A.T. Pennington. (1994). *Bowes and Churche's food values of portions commonly used.* Philadelphia: Lippincott.

5. Calcium supplement may be needed; supplementation need only add to dietary intake which means that most postmenopausal women need a supplementation of 400-600 mg per day; suggest one of the following:

a. Calcium citrate is better absorbed than calcium carbonate; suggest Citracal 200 mg tabs, 1-2 tabs BID

b. Alternatively can recommend calcium carbonate, (Os-Cal) 500 mg, 1-2 tabs BID or Tums 500 mg, 1 tab, 2-3 times/day

c. All should be taken with meals, but remember that high fiber food may reduce absorption

d. Contraindications to use of supplements are hypercalciuria that cannot be controlled with a thiazide and calcium-containing renal calculus until urinary biochemical profile is assessed

6. **Vitamin D is essential** for intestinal absorption of calcium
   a. Recommend 400 IU/day for women 51-70 years and 600-800 IU/day for women >70 years
   b. Recommend 800 IU of Vitamin D daily for people >51 years who are at risk for deficiency such as persons house-bound, institutionalized, chronically ill, or who get little Vitamin D from sunlight or fortified dairy products
   c. Sources of Vitamin D include sunlight, vitamin-D fortified dairy products, fatty foods, fish oils (cod liver oil), fortified cereals and breads, and supplements (typically, a supplement of 400 IU is adequate)
7. Magnesium supplementation is not universally recommended, but may be needed in frail, elderly women with gastrointestinal disease
8. A balanced diet is also important for bone development; in general, advise patients to eat more fruits and vegetables and less saturated fats
9. For women 75 years and older, adequate protein intake may help lessen bone loss; protein supplements (20 g/day) may improve outcomes after a hip fracture
10. **Recommend daily exercise**; high impact exercise (weight training) stimulates accrual of bone mineral content in the skeleton; lower impact exercises such as walking have minimal effects on bone mineral density
11. **Avoidance of cigarette smoking, excessive alcohol intake, and caffeine** may reduce risk of osteoporosis and should be discussed
12. Recommend regular dental visits
13. **Educational interventions to prevent falls** should be implemented: Patients should rise slowly from sitting or lying, look around room before walking, wear flat, rubber-soled shoes, use proper lifting techniques, install hand grips and safety mats in tubs, remove throw rugs, keep halls and stairways well lit and free of clutter; hip padding may provide protection against hip fractures
14. See following table for patient education resources

PATIENT EDUCATION RESOURCES	
National Institutes of Health Osteoporosis and Related Bone Diseases - National Resource Center	http://www.osteo.org
National Osteoporosis Foundation	http://www.nof.org
North America Menopause Society	http://menopause.org

B. **Drug therapy in women** (also see table DRUG THERAPY: PREVENTION AND TREATMENT OPTIONS for dosages and adverse effects of specific agents)
   1. Adequate calcium and Vitamin D intake and practice of other health-promoting behaviors are needed regardless of which drug therapy is used
   2. Consider therapy in the following women (see table that follows)

CANDIDATES FOR DRUG THERAPY
• All postmenopausal women who present with vertebral or hip fractures
• All postmenopausal women with BMD *T*-scores of -2.5 and below
• Women with borderline BMD *T*-scores (e.g. *T*-scores of -1.5 or -2.0 and below) if risk factors are present
• Women in whom nonpharmacologic preventive measures are ineffective (bone loss continues)
• Consider therapy in women >70 years with multiple risk factors

DRUG THERAPY: PREVENTION AND TREATMENT OPTIONS

Therapy	Recommended for Prevention	Recommended for Treatment	Dosage	Adverse Effects
Bisphosphonates Alendronate (Fosamax) OR Risedronate (Actonel)	Postmenopausal women and patients who have received extensive corticosteroid treatment	Postmenopausal women, patients with Paget's disease of the bone, patients who have received extensive corticosteroid treatment	**Prevention:** 5 mg QD or 35 mg once weekly Glucocorticoid induced: 5 mg QD Glucocorticoid induced in postmenopausal women not on estrogen: 10 mg QD **Treatment** in men and women: 10 mg QD or 70 mg once weekly	Upper gastrointestinal irritation
Raloxifene (Evista)	Postmenopausal women	Postmenopausal women	60 mg QD	Hot flashes, leg cramps, thromboembolic disorders
Calcitonin (Miacalcin)	Not indicated for prevention	Women more than 5 years postmenopausal, with low BMD	1 spray of 200 IU/puff intra-nasally, alternating nostrils daily OR 100 units SC or IM injection every other day	Rhinitis, GI upset Site irritation, GI upset
Hormone Replacement Therapy (HRT)	Postmenopausal women, after discussion of individual risk-benefit issues	Not indicated for treatment	Varies (see section in MENOPAUSE)	Carcinoma, gallbladder disease, thromboembolic diseases, hepatic tumors, cardiovascular disease

3. There are no clear guidelines on which agent should be prescribed first; however, bisphosphonates are gaining favor as drugs of choice because they are effective for both prevention and treatment as well as have a good safety profile

4. Bisphosphonates alendronate (Fosamax) and risedronate (Actonel) inhibit osteoclast activity, decrease bone turnover, and shift the balance between bone formation and resorption toward formation; classified as resorption-inhibiting agents
   a. Found to significantly reduce vertebral, nonvertebral, and hip fractures and to increase BMD at spine and hip
   b. Effect on fetus is unknown; bisphosphonates should not be given to healthy premenopausal woman who could become pregnant
   c. Contraindicated in persons with hypocalcemia, inability to follow dosing regimen (inability to remain upright for ½ hour), and presence of esophageal abnormalities; relatively contraindicated in patients with active upper gastrointestinal disease
   d. Use cautiously for patients with creatinine clearance less than 30 mL per minute
   e. See following table for patient education

EDUCATION FOR PATIENTS TAKING ALENDRONATE (FOSAMAX) AND RISEDRONATE (ACTONEL)

1. Take drug first thing in morning, at least 30 minutes prior to eating or drinking anything other than water; must take on an empty stomach as the drug binds with food and beverages
2. Take drug with at least 6-8 ounces of plain water (not mineral) to wash drug completely through esophagus and into stomach
3. Do not lie down for a least 30 minutes after taking drug; lying down would allow drug to pool in esophagus whereas staying erect allows gravity to help drug reach stomach
4. Stop taking drug and call health care provider if any of the following symptoms develop: difficulty or pain on swallowing, chest pain, or new and/or severe heartburn
5. Important to take calcium supplementation along with drug

5. Salmon calcitonin (Calcimar, Miacalcin) inhibits activity of osteoclasts, inhibits bone resorption, and slows remodeling; classified as a resorption-inhibiting drug
   a. Effectiveness is less than bisphosphonates, but this drug has fracture-risk-reduction properties and a good safety profile
   b. Often reserved for elderly patients with low BMD levels, who are less prone to fractures, and have difficulty tolerating bisphosphonates
   c. Usually second-line drug, but because of the analgesic properties, it is the drug of choice for patients with recent fractures and pain

6. Raloxifene HCl (Evista) is a selective estrogen receptor modulator that has a mechanism of action similar to estrogen
   a. Found to be of value in prevention of early postmenopausal bone loss as well as beneficial in risk reduction of vertebral fractures in elderly postmenopausal women
   b. Less effective in increasing bone density than HRT, but, on other hand, has less adverse effects on uterus and breast than HRT
   c. Reduces total cholesterol and low-density lipoprotein cholesterol, but has no effect on high-density lipoprotein cholesterol
7. Hormone replacement therapy; estrogen inhibits osteoclast activity, possibly binds to osteoblasts; main effect is reduction in the rate of bone absorption; classified as an resorption-inhibiting drug
   a. Prevention of OP is considered a valid indication for longer-term use of HRT (defined as 5 years or more), but **only** in a select group of postmenopausal women (because HRT may influence so many conditions that affect women after menopause, women should base their decisions to use HRT on the potential risks/benefits on numerous conditions)
      (1) Substantial risk for cardiovascular disease and breast cancer must be weighed against the benefit for increases in bone mineral density and for fracture reduction in selecting HRT from available agents to prevent OP
      (2) Do not prescribe to women with the following contraindications: Unexplained vaginal bleeding, active liver disease, history of venous thromboembolism, history of endometrial cancer, history of breast cancer; relative contraindications (hypertriglyceridemia, active gallbladder disease)
      (3) Most authorities advise that HRT should not be prescribed to women who have first-degree relatives with breast cancer, a history of breast biopsy demonstrating atypia, or susceptibility genes for breast cancer, such as BRCA1 and BRCA2
      (4) Benefits: Long-term users have higher bone density than past or never users; studies found that women on HRT have reduced hip and vertebral fractures, particularly for women <60 years
   b. Prescribe oral estrogen with progesterone in women with intact uterus or prescribe estrogen only in women without uterus plus calcium supplementation (see section MENOPAUSE for dosing)
   c. Short-term use does not prevent fractures in future; women must continue taking HRT, because the beneficial effects disappear after HRT is discontinued
   d. Consider lower doses of conjugated equine estrogens (CEEs) (0.45 and 0.3 mg/day) with or without medroxyprogesterone acetate (MPA); in one clinical trial, lowered doses prevented loss of BMD and reduced bone turnover in early postmenopausal women
8. Combination of antiresorptive regimens may increase BMD of the spine and hip more than single drug regimens; although limited data are available, consider combination therapies (bisphosphonates with estrogen or with raloxifene) in patients who are not responding to single drug therapies or in patients who have exceptionally high hip fracture risk; combining calcitonin with other agents is not recommended

C. Treatment of vertebral fracture
   1. Manage pain with analgesics, heat/cold therapy, and massage
   2. To decrease spinal stress when resting on back, place thin pillows under head and legs; when resting on side, place a thin pillow between legs and keep both hips slightly flexed
   3. Early extension exercises rather than flexion exercises may be beneficial in preventing future fractures
   4. Calcitonin may provide symptomatic relief in acute stages
   5. Surgical options
      a. Vertebroplasty: A thin paste of cement is injected to fill defects and prevent exacerbations
      b. Kyphoplasty: Balloon is inflated to elevate the end plates of the vertebral body and void is filled with materials

D. Men with osteoporosis
   1. Preventive strategies should include calcium 1.0-1.5 grams per day or higher, regular exercise, 800 IU/day of Vitamin D supplementation, and avoidance of excessive alcohol and cigarette smoking
   2. For men who have fractures, are losing BMD for unknown reasons, have T scores lower than -2 SD without risk factors, or have T scores less than -1.5 with risk factors, drug therapy is beneficial
      a. Alendronate is the only FDA-approved treatment for men with low bone density
      b. Although not FDA approved, calcitonin may be beneficial for men with painful vertebral OP
      c. Testosterone 5-6mg/day as a transdermal patch is FDA approved if patient has documented hypogonadism; adverse effects include increased risk of prostate cancer and polycythemia

E. Treatment of steroid-induced osteoporosis
  1. Order DEXA at baseline, before patients begin long-term (3 months or longer) corticosteroid therapy, and then every 6 months
  2. Recommend preventive therapies
     a. Calcium and vitamin D supplementation; American College of Rheumatology recommends 1500 mg of elemental calcium per day along with 800 IU of vitamin D; daily dosage should be divided into at least three equal doses
     b. Weight-bearing exercise program
  3. Bisphosphonates, alendronate and risedronate, were found to prevent bone loss at beginning of steroid therapy and to reduce fractures in patients with established steroid-induced OP
  4. Guidelines for when to initiate bisphosphonate therapy:
     a. Patients requiring high dose steroids (>30 mg/day) for long periods of time (>6 months) should receive bisphosphonates from the beginning, regardless of their BMD levels
     b. In patients taking 7.5 mg/day of prednisone or greater or a dose equivalent for 3 months or longer, initiate bisphosphonate therapy if their *T*-scores are lower than -1 SD; also begin bisphosphonate therapy if BMD levels significantly decline after initiation of steroid therapy
     c. Thiazide diuretics and sodium restriction are helpful in reducing the hypercalciuria that accompanies corticosteroid use; reducing hypercalciuria improves calcium balance; consider prescribing hydrochlorothiazide (Thiazide) 25 mg/day

F. Adjuvant pharmacotherapies
  1. Human parathyroid hormone, teriparatide (Forteo) 20 mcg SC QD, stimulates new bone growth and has a high therapeutic potential
  2. Several additional bisphosphonates may prove effective
     a. Etidronate (Didronel) is typically prescribed in cycles of 400 mg/day for 2 weeks every 3 months); studies found increase in BMD and reduction in fractures for high-risk subgroups
     b. Two bisphosphonates given intravenously are being studied
        (1) Intravenous pamidronate is administered over a 2-hour period every 3 months; important to ascertain that patients have adequate calcium and vitamin D intake before using this therapy
        (2) Zoledronic acid (Zometa) is a potent IV bisphosphonate that takes minutes to administer; women who were given drug either once, twice, or four times in one year had increased BMD levels
  3. In studies, sodium fluoride improved BMD, but did not reduce fracture risk; disadvantage is that high doses may increase incidence of hip fractures
  4. Tamoxifen citrate (Nolvadex) is a selective estrogen reuptake inhibitor which is rarely used because of adverse effects (increases the risk of endometrial proliferation, endometrial polyp, and adenocarcinoma), but found to maintain bone mass in postmenopausal women; effects of fracture risks are uncertain
  5. Plant-derived phytoestrogens have weak estrogen-like effects, but to date, no effects on fracture reduction have been found
  6. Statins were found to inconsistently reduce fracture rates in observational studies

G. Follow Up
  1. Patients who are prescribed drug therapy for prevention of treatment should return in 1-2 months and have regular follow up visits every 3-6 months
  2. Patients on other preventive and therapeutic strategies should have annual reassessments that include complete medical examination, breast and pelvic examinations, mammograms, Papanicolaou smear if indicated
  3. BMD testing should be performed every 2 years in patients receiving drug treatment

PLANTAR FASCIITIS

I. Definition: Overuse injury of the plantar fascia (the thickened fibrous aponeurosis that originates from the medial tubercle of the calcaneus and runs forward to form the longitudinal foot arch; this structure maintains integrity of foot function and serves as a major shock absorber)

II. Pathogenesis: Caused by collagen degeneration that results from repetitive microtears of the plantar fascia

III. Clinical presentation

    A. Risk factors
        1. Overuse (most common) from running or other weight-bearing activities
        2. Anatomic conditions: Pes planus (flat feet), pes cavus (high arches), overpronation, discrepancy in leg length, excessive lateral tibial torsion, and excessive femoral anteversion
        3. Functional factors: Tightness and weakness in the gastrocnemius, soleus, Achilles tendons, and intrinsic foot muscles
        4. In elderly patients, poor intrinsic muscle strength compounded by a decrease in body's healing capacity are likely causative factors
        5. Obesity may be a predisposing factor

    B. Classic sign is heel pain that occurs with first steps in the morning and resolves or lessens with activities but then returns over the course of the day

    C. Point tenderness at the anteromedial region of the calcaneus that worsens with passive dorsiflexion of the toes or when patient stands on tips of toes is characteristic

    D. Heel spurs may or may not be present

    E. Condition is usually self-limited, but resolution of symptoms may take 6-18 months

IV. Diagnosis/Evaluation

    A. History
        1. Determine onset, severity, and characteristics of pain
        2. Question about possible risk factors such as athletic activity, frequent and prolonged standing on feet, history of anatomic problems of the structures and muscles of the feet
        3. Inquire about success of current and previous treatments
        4. Determine degree to which pain is interfering in activities of daily living

    B. Physical Examination
        1. Inspect feet and legs for anatomic abnormalities
        2. Palpate foot; tenderness is typically along the medial plantar aspect of foot, about 3 finger breadths distal to posterior heel
        3. Passively dorsiflex toes; this technique typically elicits pain
        4. Ask patient to stand on toes which usually produces pain

    C. Differential Diagnosis
        1. Entrapment syndromes such as tarsal tunnel syndrome; results in radiating, burning pain and paresthesia
        2. Calcaneal fractures and calcaneal stress fractures; history includes trauma or overuse; pain may be similar or more intense than pain related to plantar fasciitis; x-rays are abnormal
        3. Paget's disease; anatomic deformities such as bowed tibia or kyphosis are usually observable
        4. Calcaneal apophysitis; typically occurs in adolescents and causes posterior heel pain
        5. Soft tissue causes
            a. Fat pad syndrome; atrophy of the heel pad may be visible
            b. Heel bruise; patient has a history of trauma
            c. Bursitis; swelling and erythema of the heel usually occur
            d. Tendonitis; pain occurs with resisted motion
            e. Plantar fascia rupture; pain is acute and knifelike; ecchymosis may be present
        6. Neuropathy secondary to diabetes; paresthesia is usually present

7. Gout; acute onset of intense pain is typical
8. Arthritides; systemic signs of joint pain and swelling
9. Tumors present with deep bone pain and other constitutional symptoms

D. Diagnostic Tests: X-rays and additional tests are rarely needed unless there is suspicion of tumors or other serious conditions

V. Plan/Management

A. Rest and correction of the problems that place the patient at risk for plantar fasciitis are recommended initially

B. A stretching, flexibility, and strengthening exercise program should be started after the initial resting phase (see figure 17.19)

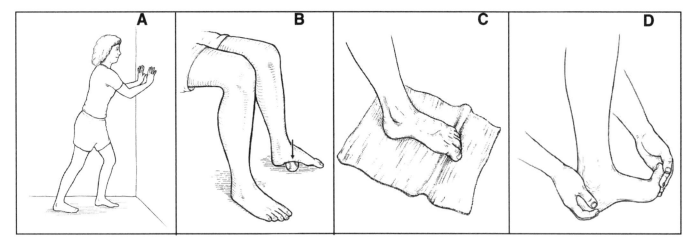

Figure 17.19: Stretching, Flexibility, and Strengthening Exercises
(A) Stretch calf muscles by performing wall exercises; (B) stretch foot muscles by rolling foot arch over a tennis ball; (C) strengthen intrinsic muscles of foot with towel curls; (D) strengthen intrinsic muscles of foot by dorsiflexing toes

C. Footwear
1. In some patients, simply changing shoes is all that is needed; shoes that are too small or worn often aggravate symptoms
2. Over-the-counter arch supports may be beneficial but simply taping the arch may be less expensive, but equally effective
3. Custom orthotics and heel cups are useful for some patients

D. Night splints may be tried to maintain the patient's ankle in a neutral position overnight

E. Nonsteroidal anti-inflammatory drugs may or may not be helpful (see section on PAIN for dosing)

F. Ice applied as an ice massage, ice bath, or an ice pack often relieves pain

G. Iontophoresis which uses electric impulses to drive topical corticosteroids into the soft tissue structures may be used as adjunct therapy

H. Cortisone injections may be prescribed in intractable cases

I. Surgical debridement of affected tissue is indicated for the most recalcitrant cases

J. Patient education: Suggest that patient avoid flat shoes, barefoot walking, and lose weight if obesity is a problem

K. Follow Up
1. Return evaluation is not needed if symptoms abate
2. Consider follow-up in 2-4 weeks for patients who continue to have pain or sooner if symptoms worsen
3. If no improvement occurs after six weeks, refer to podiatric foot and ankle surgeon

RHEUMATOID ARTHRITIS

I. Definition: A chronic, systemic, inflammatory disease which primarily affects joints but often has generalized manifestations

II. Pathogenesis

    A. Autoimmune disorder of unknown etiology, associated with various factors: Inflammatory response mechanisms, immune system responses, bone resorption mechanism, endogenous hormonal response, neuronal response mechanics, and genetic predisposition (many patients have genetic marker HLA-DR4)

    B. Inflammation of synovial membranes results in panus or thickened synovium which adheres to articular cartilage and later erodes cartilage and underlying bone; adhesions develop between opposing joint surfaces and/or cysts grow

III. Clinical Presentation

    A. Criteria for diagnosis in adults (see following table)

REVISED CRITERIA FOR CLASSIFICATION OF RHEUMATOID ARTHRITIS* (AMERICAN RHEUMATOLOGY ASSOCIATION, 1987)
• Morning stiffness -- at least one hour before maximal improvement (6 weeks)[†]
• Arthritis of 3 or more joint areas (6 weeks)[†]
• Arthritis of hand joints (wrist, metacarpophalangeal joints or proximal interphalangeal joints) (6 weeks)[†]
• Symmetric arthritis -- simultaneous involvement of same joint areas on both sides of body (6 weeks)[†]
• Rheumatoid nodules
• Rheumatoid factor in serum
• Radiologic changes (hand x-ray changes typical of RA must include erosions or unequivocal bony decalcification)

* Diagnosis of rheumatoid arthritis if satisfies 4 criteria
[†] This symptom must be present for at least 6 months to be considered a positive criterion
Adapted from Arnet, F.C. (1989). Revised criteria for classification of rheumatoid arthritis. *Bulletin on Rheumatic Diseases, 38*, 1-6.

    B. Three times more common in women than men; peak age of onset is 20-30 years

    C. Onset usually is insidious but may be acute following stress, surgery, infection, trauma, or pregnancy

    D. Course of rheumatoid arthritis (RA) is highly variable
        1. Approximately 50% of patients have a progressive disease, but only about 3% have erosive, destructive arthritis
        2. The following predict a poor prognosis: Earlier age at onset, high titer of rheumatoid factor, elevated sedimentation rate, swelling of >20 joints, and extra-articular manifestations

    E. Joint involvement
        1. Swelling is soft and spongy; not bony as in osteoarthritis
        2. May have carpal tunnel syndrome, shoulder bursitis, Baker's cyst behind knee, hallux valgus, temporomandibular joint problems, and atlantoaxial (C1-C2) subluxation

    F. Extra-articular involvement
        1. Rheumatoid nodules over extensor surfaces of elbows, forearms and hands
        2. Vasculitis, pleurisy, keratoconjunctivitis, pericarditis, peripheral neuropathy
        3. Felty's syndrome may occur in older population with rheumatoid arthritis, splenomegaly, and leukopenia
        4. Systemic symptoms may include fever, fatigue, weight loss, anorexia, sweats, and Raynaud's phenomenon

IV.   Diagnosis/Evaluation

   A.   History
      1.   Exactly determine duration, location, and characteristics of pain, tenderness, inflammation, and morning stiffness
      2.   Question about systemic symptoms such as weight loss, fever, and fatigue
      3.   Inquire about associated symptoms such as nodules, eye pain, or conjunctivitis
      4.   Ask about past medical history and medication use; comorbid conditions may be exacerbated by RA or by its treatment (infection, renal insufficiency, cardiovascular disease, chronic pulmonary disease, peptic ulcer disease, lymphoproliferative disease, and mental illness)
      5.   Inquire about family medical history
      6.   Specifically determine degree of limitation in patient's activities of daily living

   B.   Physical Examination
      1.   Measure vital signs
      2.   Count number of swollen joints, noting bilateral symmetry of joint involvement
      3.   Check for various deformities of the hand such as swan-neck deformity, mallet finger, Boutonnière deformity
      4.   Carefully palpate joints noting tenderness, temperature, and swelling
      5.   Apply traction maneuvers to determine joint stability
      6.   Assess muscular strength, particularly grip strength
      7.   A complete physical examination is often needed because of systemic problems such as pleurisy, pericarditis, splenomegaly

   C.   Differential Diagnosis (see section on JOINT PAIN)
      1.   Polymyalgia rheumatica
      2.   Reiter's syndrome
      3.   Systemic lupus erythematosus
      4.   Gouty arthritis, gonococcal arthritis, psoriatic arthritis
      5.   Lyme disease
      6.   Acute rheumatic fever
      7.   Ulcerative colitis and Crohn's disease

   D.   Diagnostic Tests
      1.   Baseline laboratory information in patients suspected of RA includes CBC with differential, erythrocyte sedimentation rate, urinalysis, rheumatoid factor titer, and C-reactive protein
      2.   Before initiating any drugs it is important to get the following: CBC, electrolytes, serum creatinine, liver function tests, hepatic panel, urinalysis, stool guaiac, and radiographs of affected joints
      3.   In selected patients, consider ordering the following:
         a.   Synovial fluid analysis to rule out other diseases; may need repeated during disease flares to rule-out septic arthritis
         b.   X-rays of selected joints; limited diagnostic value early in disease, but helpful in establishing a baseline to periodically monitor progression and response to therapy
         c.   Additional serological studies such as antinuclear antibodies (ANAs) and serum hemolytic complement (CH50) may be needed to rule-out other diseases

V.   Plan/Management: Goals are to reduce inflammation, relieve pain, preserve joint function, prevent further disease progression, and preserve ability to perform daily activities

   A.   Initially, patients are treated by specialists; consultation is also needed when patients have exacerbations or flares of their symptoms

   B.   Patient education includes discussion of chronicity of disease and ways to decrease exacerbations and prevent deformities; early referrals to a physical therapist and occupational therapist are recommended
      1.   Maintain ideal body weight
      2.   Exercise with emphasis on joint extension (physical therapy is always helpful)
      3.   Receive adequate rest with naps; balance rest therapy with an exercise plan that includes stretching, strengthening, and endurance
      4.   Perform correct body mechanics
      5.   Always use large joints, such as shoulders or hands, rather than fingers to carry pail of water, etc.
      6.   Tell patients about the Arthritis Foundation's educational resources and Web site (www.arthritis.org)

C. General management program
   1. Prescribe splints and protheses to protect joints, to keep in functional position, and to reduce pain
   2. Hot and cold therapy, ultrasound, electrical stimulation with transcutaneous nerve stimulator are often beneficial
   3. Visual imagery, massage, acupuncture, and hypnosis may be helpful
   4. Treat pain effectively because it limits joint use, interferes with ability to exercise, and is associated with depression and insomnia (see V.D.8.)
   5. Screen and, if necessary, provide early treatment for depression and insomnia

D. Drug therapy
   1. General principles
      a. An aggressive pharmacological plan is recommended today; the pyramid approach in which nonsteroidal anti-inflammatory drugs (NSAIDs) were used for at least 3-6 months and then other drugs were added is **no** longer recommended for several reasons:
         (1) NSAIDs are more toxic than previously believed
         (2) NSAIDs may provide relief from pain but do not prevent further joint damage or delay progression of disease
         (3) Disease-modifying drugs have been found to forestall progression of disease
      b. Remember that most disease-modifying drugs are relatively slow acting, with a delay of 1-6 months before response is evident
   2. A disease modifying drug should be started within 3 months for most newly diagnosed patients; disease modifying drugs are categorized as disease-modifying antirheumatic drugs (DMARDs) or biological response modifiers (BRMs)
      a. DMARDs reduce inflammation effects
      b. BRMs inhibit proinflammatory cytokines and related enzymes involved in producing joint destruction
         (1) Efficacious but are more expensive than DMARDs and must be given by injection
         (2) BRMs block cytokines which play a role in preventing infection; use cautiously in patients with a history of recurring infections or underlying conditions that may predispose to infection such as poorly controlled diabetes
         (3) Typically these drugs are given in combination with other DMARDs, particularly methotrexate, but etanercept and anakinra can be used as monotherapy
   3. Disease modifying drugs have adverse effects and need frequent monitoring (see following table, RECOMMENDED MONITORING STRATEGIES)

RECOMMENDED MONITORING STRATEGIES FOR DISEASE MODIFYING AGENTS

Drugs	Toxicities Requiring Monitoring	Baseline Evaluation, Vaccines, & Screening Tests	Monitoring and Screening Tests
Hydroxychloroquine	Macular damage	None unless patient is >40 years or has previous eye disease	Funduscopic and visual fields every 6-12 months
Sulfasalazine	Myelosuppression	CBC, AST or ALT in patients at risk, G6PD	CBC every 2-4 weeks for first 3 months, then every 3 months
Methotrexate	Myelosuppression, hepatic fibrosis, cirrhosis, pulmonary infiltrates or fibrosis	CBC, chest radiography, hepatitis B and C serology in high-risk patients, AST or ALT, albumin, alkaline phosphatase, and creatinine	CBC, platelet count, AST, albumin, creatinine every 4-8 weeks
Gold, intramuscular	Myelosuppression, proteinuria	CBC, platelet count, creatinine, urine dipstick for protein	CBC, platelet count, urine dipstick every 1-2 weeks for first 20 weeks, then at the time of each injection
Gold, oral	Myelosuppression, proteinuria	CBC, platelet count, urine dipstick for protein	CBC, platelet count, urine dipstick for protein every 4-12 weeks
D-penicillamine	Myelosuppression, proteinuria	CBC, platelet count, creatinine, urine dipstick for protein	CBC, urine dipstick for protein every 2 weeks until dosage stable, then every 1-3 months

(Continued)

Drugs	Toxicities Requiring Monitoring	Baseline Evaluation, Vaccines, & Screening Tests	Monitoring and Screening Tests
		RECOMMENDED MONITORING STRATEGIES FOR DISEASE MODIFYING AGENTS *(CONTINUED)*	
Azathioprine	Myelosuppression, hepatotoxicity, lympho-proliferative disorders	CBC, platelet count, creatinine, AST or ALT	CBC and platelet count every 1-2 weeks with changes in dosage, and every 1-3 months thereafter
Cyclophosphamide	Myelosuppression, myeloproliferative disorders, malignancy, hemorrhagic cystitis	CBC, platelet count, urinalysis, creatinine, AST or ALT	CBC and platelet count every 1-2 weeks with changes in dosage, then every 1-3 months, urinalysis and urine cytology every 6-12 months
Cyclosporine	Renal insufficiency	CBC, AST or ALT, creatinine, urinalysis, potassium	Creatinine every 2 weeks until dose is stable, CBC, AST or ALT every 3-6 months, potassium periodically
Minocycline	Hepatotoxicity	CBC, urinalysis, creatinine, AST or ALT	CBC, urinalysis, creatinine, AST or ALT every 3-6 months
Leflunomide	Hepatotoxicity, renal insufficiency, immunosuppression	CBC, AST or ALT, urinalysis, creatinine; screen for hepatitis B and C; perform pregnancy test	CBC, AST or ALT every 4-8 weeks
Etanercept	Immunosuppression, hematological abnormalities	CBC; update vaccines before initiating; screen for ANA and DNA antibodies, screen for TB with skin test	CBC every 3-6 months
Adalimumab	Immunosuppression, hematological abnormalities	CBC; update vaccines before initiating; screen for ANA and DNA antibodies, screen for TB with skin test	CBC every 3-6 months
Infliximab	Lymphoproliferative disorders, immunosuppression	CBC; TB skin test before initiating, screen for ANA and DNA antibodies	CBC every 3-6 months
Anakinra	Immunosuppression, hematological abnormalities	CBC, urinalysis, creatinine, AST or ALT	CBC monthly for first 3 months; then every 3 months up to 1 year; creatinine, AST or ALT periodically

4. For **mild disease** prescribe one of following as initial therapy:
   a. Hydroxychloroquine (Plaquenil): 200-600 mg daily in one or two divided doses
   b. Sulfasalazine (Azulfidine): Begin 500 mg QD to maximum of 1 gram BID; safest drug but can cause annoying adverse effects
   c. Minocycline (Minocin) 100 mg BID and oral gold, auranofin (Ridaura) with maximum dose of 3 mg TID may also be prescribed
5. For **moderate to severe disease**, methotrexate (Rheumatrex) is the initial recommended therapy, particularly if there is presence of RF positivity, erosions, or persistent synovitis
   a. Start orally at dosage of 7.5 mg/week. The 2.5 mg tablets should be taken in 3 separate doses, 12 hours apart once a week or take all 3 tablets in a single dose; maximum dose is 20 mg/week
   b. Methotrexate is the DMARD with the most predictable benefit and has become the cornerstone of therapy
   c Prescribe folic acid (1-2 mg/day) to help avoid many of the nuisance toxicities
6. **For moderate to severe disease that remains active or is progressing**, the following options are available:
   a. Switch from oral methotrexate to parenteral methotrexate
   b. Switch from methotrexate to one of the new biologic therapies (leflunomide or a biologic response modifier [etanercept, anakinra, adalimumab]) (see following table)
   c. Combine two or three disease modifying agents (see below for choices)
      (1) Methotrexate plus sulfasalazine plus hydroxychloroquine
      (2) Methotrexate plus leflunomide
      (3) Methotrexate plus etanercept
      (4) Methotrexate plus infliximab
      (5) Methotrexate plus adalimumab

NEW BIOLOGIC THERAPIES		
Drug	**Mechanism of Action**	**Dose**
Leflunomide (Arava)*	DMARD; pyrimidine synthesis inhibition	Loading dose: 100 mg PO QD x 3 days; maintenance of 20 mg PO QD; reduce dose or discontinue if ALT is elevated
Etanercept (Enbrel)[†]	BRM; tumor necrosis factor-α (TNF-α) antagonist	25 mg SQ injection twice weekly; 72-96 hours apart
Infliximab (Remicade)[‡]	BRM; tumor necrosis factor-α (TNF-α) antagonist	3 mg/kg at weeks 0, 2, 6, then every 8 weeks by IV infusion over at least 2 hours; may increase to 10 mg/kg or give every 4 weeks
Anakinra (Kineret)[†]	BRM; interleukin-1 (IL-1) receptor antagonist	100 mg SC QD
Adalimumab (Humira)[†]	BRM; tumor necrosis factor-α (TNF-α) antagonist	SQ every other week

* Leflunomide (Arava) is contraindicated in pregnant women and premenopausal women should use birth control
[†] Etanercept, anakinra, and adalimumab package inserts carry a strong caution on the use of this drug in patients with a history of recurring infections or underlying conditions that may predispose to infection such as poorly controlled diabetes
[‡] Infliximab must be administered with methotrexate

7. Other DMARDs that can be prescribed are the following:
   a. Gold IM is effective but is expensive, inconvenient, and needs frequent monitoring; gold sodium thiomalate (Myochrysine) and aurothioglucose (Solganal) 10-50 mg IM are given weekly up to a total dose of 1000 mg, then 25-50 mg monthly
   b. d-penicillamine (Cuprimine) has a latent onset of 8-12 weeks; begin 125-150 mg/day for 4-8 weeks and raise every 1-3 months to maximum of 750 mg/day
   c. Azathioprine (Imuran) is used only after multiple therapies have failed; 1 mg/kg daily in 1-2 divided doses; may increase by 0.5 mg/kg/day increments every 4 weeks; maximum 2.5 mg/kg/day
   d. Cyclosporine (Neoral) is used only after multiple therapies have failed; begin 2.5 mg/kg/day in 2 divided doses to a maximum of 4 mg/kg/day
8. For **symptomatic therapy,** nonsteroidal anti-inflammatory drugs (NSAIDs) are beneficial in relieving pain and swelling; remember that they do not prevent joint pain (see section on PAIN for dosing and discussion of specific NSAIDs)
   a. NSAIDs should not be used as the sole treatment
   b. NSAIDs are often prescribed as an adjuvant therapy to disease modifying agent; initially, a NSAID may be prescribed to control pain until the disease modifying agent reaches steady state
   c. Later in course of disease, NSAID may be used in combination with disease modifying agents when patients have a flare in their symptoms
   d. Select drug based on dosing regimen, efficacy, toxicity, tolerance, costs, patient's age, comorbidities, concurrent medications, and patient preference
   e. Avoid combination of two or more NSAIDs
   f. COX-2 inhibitors should be considered first for elderly patients or patients who are at risk for gastrointestinal complications
   g. If used long-term, order CBC, creatinine, AST, and ALT before initiating and then annually
9. Low-dose oral glucocorticoids and local intra-articular injections of glucocorticoids are highly effective in relieving symptoms and may slow joint damage; they can be used with disease modifying agents
   a. For uncomplicated RA, prescribe low-dose oral prednisone (do not give dosage higher than 10 mg daily) or for short courses may give 20 mg per day with rapid taper over 5 days
      (1) Beneficial during the period before disease modifying agent has gained full effect or when symptoms are severe (some patients may need maintenance therapy to control symptoms)
      (2) Limit prednisone to short course, or, if maintenance dose is needed, use at the lowest possible dosage
      (3) Even low doses of glucocorticoids can increase the risk of osteoporosis, hypertension, and hyperglycemia (monitor blood pressure regularly and order urinalysis, chemistry panel, and bone densitometry in high risk patients periodically)

      b.   Intra-articular injections can treat most symptomatic joints early in the disease and can be used to treat flares in one or more joints
- (1) Rule-out infection in joint before injecting
- (2) Do not inject joint more than once within 3 months

E. Surgery is needed if there is marked structural damage on x-ray, lack of response to medical therapy, or significant pain and loss of function

F. Follow Up
1. When initiating new drug therapies, patient should be seen every 1-2 weeks
2. Interval between follow up visits depends upon patient's condition and monitoring recommendations of medications (see table on RECOMMENDED MONITORING STRATEGIES V.D.3.)
3. Patients in remission may be seen every 6 months (see table for the American College of Rheumatology criteria)

AMERICAN COLLEGE OF RHEUMATOLOGY CRITERIA FOR REMISSION

Complete remission is defined as absence of:
- ✓ Symptoms of active inflammatory joint pain
- ✓ Morning stiffness
- ✓ Synovitis on joint examination
- ✓ Fatigue
- ✓ Progression of radiographic damage on sequential radiographs
- ✓ Elevated ESR or CRP level

Adapted from the American College of Rheumatology Ad Hoc Committee on Clinical Guidelines. (1996). Guidelines for the management of rheumatoid arthritis. *Arthritis and Rheumatology, 39*, 713-722.

SHOULDER PAIN

I. Definition: Pain in the shoulder that is either acute or chronic

II. Pathogenesis (see figure 17.20 for anatomy of shoulder)

A. Acute shoulder pain
1. Fractures, dislocations, sprains, separations, and strains are the most common causes
2. Trauma is usually responsible

B. Chronic shoulder pain
1. Subacromial impingement (SI) syndrome or rotator cuff disorders are common
    a.   The rotator cuff, the dynamic stabilizer of the glenohumeral joint, is composed of four muscles--the subscapularis, the supraspinatus, the infraspinatus, and the teres minor, along with their musculotendinous attachments
    b.   Rotator cuff injury or dysfunction occurs when the space between the undersurface of the acromion and the superior aspect of the humeral head becomes so narrowed that there is impingement of the acromion onto the rotator cuff tendons
    c.   In the younger patient, SI causes inflammation with subsequent tendinitis and bursitis that occurs during forward shoulder elevation and with repetitive overhead activities
    d.   As the patient ages, the degenerative process advances and may result in a tear; tears are primarily due to degenerative failure of the tendon, but may be a result of trauma
2. Adhesive capsulitis or frozen shoulder, is due to thickening and contraction of the capsule around the glenohumeral joint; typically results from immobility following a shoulder injury or due to a painful stimulus that causes the patient to limit movement
3. Osteoarthritis of the acromioclavicular and glenohumeral joints may be due to previous trauma, overuse, or rotator cuff tear

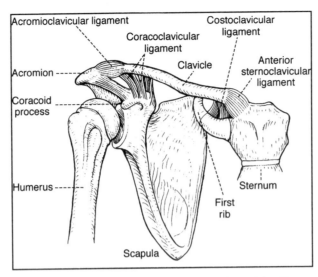

Figure 17.20. Anatomical Structures of the Shoulder Bones and Joints

III.   Clinical Presentation: Shoulder pain is one of the most common orthopedic complaints in primary care

    A.   Fractures
        1.   Fractures of the clavicle
            a.   Most common fracture that occurs in childhood; today more common in adults secondary to motor vehicle accidents and participation in contact sports
            b.   Mechanisms of injury are usually either a fall on outstretched hand or a direct blow to the shoulder
            c.   Considerable force is needed to crack the clavicle in an adult; therefore, if trauma is minor, look for an underlying cause (neoplastic disease, infection)
            d.   Patients may have concomitant dislocation of the sternoclavicular joint and disruption of the ligaments of the acromioclavicular joint
            e.   Patient usually presents with pain at the fracture site
            f.   Patient may avoid moving the arm or may angle head toward the injured side to relax the pull of the trapezius to limit pain
            g.   On examination, there is a visible and palpable deformity
        2.   Fractures of the proximal humerus
            a.   Mechanism of injury is usually a fall on an outstretched hand or a direct blow to shoulder
            b.   Incidence increases with age and women are twice as likely as men to sustain this injury
            c.   Patient typically presents with complaints of pain, tenderness, and swelling in the area of the greater tuberosity
            d.   Crepitus may or may not be present
        3.   Fractures of the scapula
            a.   Uncommon fracture that results from a direct blow to the scapular area or from extremely high-force impact elsewhere to the thorax; may be associated with multiple fractures relating to severe trauma
            b.   Patient complains of tenderness at fracture site and arm abduction is painful
            c.   Fractures are easy to diagnose because the scapula is directly beneath the skin; palpation will detect point tenderness or an obvious deformity

    B.   Dislocations make up about 25% of all shoulder injuries, with about 95% being anterior glenohumeral dislocations (following presentation pertains to anterior glenohumeral dislocations)
        1.   Occurs when the arm is forcefully elevated and pulled backwards
        2.   First-time dislocations are always the result of significant trauma; once glenohumeral instability is present, however, dislocations tend to recur
        3.   Patient usually presents with the affected arm in external rotation and abduction; a dimple in the skin beneath the acromion may be present
        4.   Shoulder is extremely painful, especially with passive range of motion
        5.   Generalized weakness of entire arm may be present; active range of motion may be very difficult due to muscle spasm

6. Shoulder is grossly deformed; shoulder appears as if deltoid muscle has disappeared; a protrusion inferior to the acromion and lateral to the coracoid (result of the head of the humerus being displaced) is usually apparent

C. Acromioclavicular (AC) joint sprain and separation
   1. Common among athletes and results from direct blow to the superior aspect of the shoulder or a lateral blow to the deltoid area; infrequently may result from falling onto outstretched hands
   2. Classification of AC joint injuries
      a. Grade I sprain: Complete congruity, or overlap, of the distal clavicle and acromion
      b. Grade II sprain: Incomplete overlap of the clavicle and acromion
      c. Grade III sprain: Clavicle and acromion are completely separated, a result of a complete tear of the AC and coracoclavicular ligaments
      d. Grades IV, V, VI are variations of the completely disrupted AC joint, with the clavicle being displaced posteriorly, superiorly, or inferiorly, respectively
   3. Patients experience point tenderness and swelling directly over the joint
   4. Localized pain with elevation of arm usually occurs
   5. Patients with tears usually have a noticeable bump at the AC joint or what is referred to as a step-off between the acromion and the distal end of the clavicle

D. Sternoclavicular joint sprain and separation
   1. Anterior sternoclavicular joint separation typically results from motor vehicle accident
      a. Medial end of clavicle is displaced anteriorly or anterosuperiorly with respect to the anterior border of the sternum
      b. Pain occurs primarily with adduction and is often exacerbated when patient is supine
      c. Localized tenderness and deformity are typically present and head may be tilted toward side of injury
   2. Posterior joint separation may be life-threatening due to compression of the trachea and great vessels of the neck

E. Shoulder strain is a diagnosis of exclusion and is reserved for muscle injury, usually involving the large deltoid muscles

F. Rotator cuff problems involve subacromial impingement syndrome; impingement syndrome is a general term that includes bursitis, tendinitis, and associated tears of the rotator cuff; the rotator cuff is the part of the shoulder that helps arm do a circular motion
   1. The most frequent cause of chronic shoulder pain is injury to the rotator cuff with pain, weakness, and loss of motion usually reported
   2. Patients typically complain of pain over the anterolateral aspect of the shoulder that does not radiate below the elbows; pain is worse when patient raises arm or lifts something above head
   3. May have a clicking or popping sensation in the affected shoulder
   4. Biceps tendonitis often accompanies syndrome; patient has discrete pain and tenderness in the area of the bicipital groove
   5. Disorder may be primary or secondary impingement
      a. Primary impingement occurs from chronic overuse and degeneration of the tendon; patient complains of anterior shoulder pain
      b. Secondary impingement is due to an underlying problem of instability; patient is typically young and complains of arm heaviness and numbness
   6. Rotator cuff impingement syndrome (and associated tears of the rotator cuff) is usually classified into three stages (see following table)

STAGES OF ROTATOR CUFF IMPINGEMENT SYNDROME	
Stage I	• Usually involves patients <25 years of age • Usually results from overuse and most often occurs in athletes, with pain developing after exercise • Pain is dull, aching, and diffuse • Rotator cuff edema and hemorrhage may by present • Process is reversible at this point
Stage II	• Typically occurs in laborers aged 25-40 • Work requires repeated and constant overhead reach for many hours during the day • Occurs both during and after activity • Pain frequently occurs at night, interfering with sleep • Pathologic changes become evident and include fibrosis and irreversible tendon changes
Stage III	• Final stage usually occurs in patients >40 years of age, but may occur to younger patients as a result of trauma • Usually, person has been a laborer or involved in repetitive overhead activities for many years • In addition to the pain described under Stage II, above, additional complaints of stiffness and weakness may be present • Patients present with a long history of shoulder problems • May also present with sudden, severe episode of pain with resultant shoulder disability from an apparently minor recent trauma • Rotator cuff is either partially or completely torn • Damage is irreversible at this stage

G. Adhesive capsulitis or frozen shoulder
   1. Occurs most commonly in individuals >40 years and women
   2. Typically involves 3 stages
      a. Freezing stage
         (1) Lasts 3-9 months with slow gradual onset of limited pain localized near the deltoid insertion; pain is achy but becomes sharp when affected shoulder reaches the extremes of its range of motion
         (2) Patient often has restricted glenohumeral elevation and external rotation
         (3) Patient may be unable to sleep on affected side
      b. Frozen stage
         (1) Lasts about 4-12 months
         (2) Involves increasing stiffness with diminishing pain
         (3) Greater than 60% loss of active and passive range of motion
      c. Thawing stage
         (1) Last 1-2 years
         (2) Pain is minimal
         (3) Gradual improvement in range of motion

H. Osteoarthritis is usually associated with pain, loss of passive motion, and stiffness

IV. Diagnosis/Evaluation

A. History
   1. Determine patient's age, dominant hand, and work or sports activities
   2. Ask about the onset (sudden or gradual), duration, location, radiation, and intensity of pain (have patient rate on a scale of 1 to 10 with 1 being no pain at all and 10 being the worst pain the patient has ever experienced) [**Note**: Gradual onset of pain is the hallmark of impingement syndrome]
   3. Ask what reduces the pain and what makes it worse
   4. Ask if the shoulder feels loose or unstable; if there is muscle weakness, catching, stiffness, or paresthesias; inquire about swelling or deformity
   5. Ask about problems with other joints, especially the neck and elbow
   6. Ask about previous treatments (including diagnostic testing, hospitalizations, surgeries, and pain management)
   7. Obtain past medical history including medication use and allergies
      a. Ask about previous surgeries and orthopedic problems
      b. Obtain complete neurologic history for the upper extremity

c. Obtain a complete ROS to detect referred, remote, or nonshoulder sources of symptoms (with a focus on respiratory, cardiovascular, gastrointestinal systems); ask about systemic symptoms including fevers, night sweats, and weight loss

8. Determine if the pain hampers normal work and recreational activities

9. Important to distinguish if problem is acute or chronic; for acute pain, determine the following:

   a. Determine whether the onset of pain was related to a single event (macrotrauma) or to a reinjury of a chronically symptomatic joint

   b. If macrotrauma was involved, ask about the activity or sport being performed at the time of the injury, the position of the arm when injured, and the exact mechanism of the injury. Ask if there was a direct blow to the shoulder or an indirect injury such as falling on the elbow or arm

   c. If macrotrauma was involved, was there immediate pain, swelling, or deformity?

   d. If reinjury of a chronically symptomatic joint is suspected, ask what activities were being engaged in when pain started (was the patient lifting overhead, pulling, throwing, or was there no apparent cause for the reinjury?) [**Note**: If no apparent cause, consider systemic arthritis, neoplasm, infection, or cardiac disease]

10. For chronic pain, determine the following:

   a. Determine if pain awakens patient from sleep and if lying on the affected shoulder is avoided because of discomfort

   b. Ask appropriate questions to grade the patient's overuse pain in terms of impact on function (from less to most impact)

     (1) Grade 1: Pain occurs only after activity (implies early inflammatory activity)

     (2) Grade 2: Pain during activity but not restricting performance

     (3) Grade 3: Pain during activity and restricting performance

     (4) Grade 4: Pain chronic and unremitting, even at rest

B. Physical Examination (see Figures 17.21 and 17.22 for specific assessment maneuvers); **Note**: Examination of the unaffected shoulder should be performed at each step of the exam for comparison with the involved shoulder

1. Inspection; patient should be properly disrobed to permit inspection of both shoulders

   a. Observe how the patient moves and carries shoulders

   b. Inspect front and back of shoulders for swelling, discoloration, asymmetry, muscle atrophy, scars, abrasions, lacerations, and any venous distention

   c. Observe the height of the shoulders and scapulae (common for the dominant shoulder to be slightly lower) and observe for deformities

     (1) Squaring of shoulders occurs with anterior dislocations

     (2) Scapular winging is associated with shoulder instability and muscle dysfunction

2. Palpation should be done with patient at rest and with shoulder movement; palpate the following: acromioclavicular and sternoclavicular joints, the cervical spine, the biceps tendon, the anterior glenohumeral joint, coracoid process, acromion, and scapula

   a. Palpate for point tenderness, snapping, grinding, and bony crepitus

   b. Palpate the area distal and proximal to the pain location

3. Assess passive and active (with and without resistance) range of motion: Forward elevation, abduction, external rotation, internal rotation

4. Perform muscle strength testing as weakness is often both the underlying cause and the result of injury (on a standard scale of 0 to 5, results of muscle testing should be in 4 to 5 range)

5. Assess for nerve injury

   a. Sensation in the arm and hand on the affected side should be evaluated

   b. Muscles that are innervated by the major nerves of the extremity should be examined for motor function

6. Assess for arterial blood flow

   a. Assess for circulatory compromise on the affected side

   b. Color, warmth, and nail bed capillary refill time should be assessed in each finger

   c. Radial, ulnar, and brachial pulses should be evaluated

7. In the absence of trauma (i.e., patient denies a precipitating event for the acute onset of shoulder pain), it is important to carefully check the neck, chest, heart, and abdomen for sources of referred pain

8.   Perform specific maneuvers (see figures that follow)

MANEUVERS TO ASSESS SHOULDER PAIN

Test	Description	Interpretation
Maneuvers to Test for Rotator Cuff Problems		
Empty Can Test (Drawing A)	• Patient attempts to elevate the arms against resistance while the elbows are extended and the thumbs are pointing downward	• Pain accompanied by weakness in the affected shoulder suggests rotator cuff problems
Neer's Test (Drawing B)	• Place the patient's arm in forced flexion with arm fully pronated; scapula should be stabilized during maneuver to prevent scapulothoracic motion	• Pain with this maneuver suggests subacromial impingement syndrome
Maneuver to Test for Acromioclavicular Joint Disease		
Cross-arm Test (Drawing C)	• Patient raises arm to 90 degrees then actively adducts arm (patient's arm crosses body so that hand grasps contralateral shoulder)	• Pain in the area of acromioclavicular joint suggests a disorder in this area
Maneuver to Test for Glenohumeral Joint Stability		
Apprehension Test (Drawing D)	• Shoulder should be in a neutral position at 90° of abduction. Examiner applies slight anterior pressure to the humerus and externally rotates the arm	• Pain or apprehension about the feeling of impending subluxation or dislocation suggests anterior glenohumeral instability

Figure 17.21

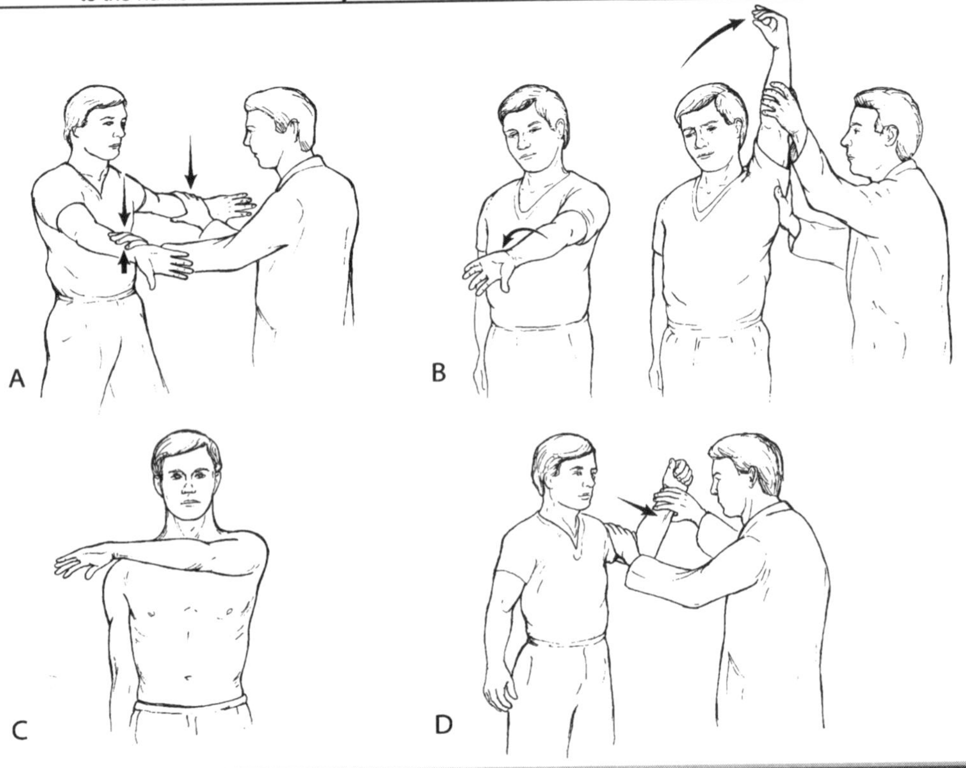

A

B

C

D

MANEUVERS TO ASSESS FOR CERVICAL SPINE PATHOLOGY AND TO TEST ROM

Maneuver to Screen for Cervical Spine Pathology

Head Compression Test
(Drawing A)

- With patient sitting on low stool, stand behind patient, lock hands together, and then apply gentle but firm downward pressure on head, using both hands locked together

- Pain localized to neck suggests disk degeneration or facet joint arthritis
- Burning pain or pain radiating to involved shoulder suggests nerve root involvement
- If test is negative (shoulder pain is not reproduced), continue with exam

Maneuvers to Test Range of Motion

Scratch Test
(Drawings B & C)

- Evaluate adduction and internal rotation by having patient place arm and hand behind back and reach toward the opposite scapula with the thumb pointed up
- Evaluate abduction and external rotation by having patient place the hand behind the neck and touch the border of the scapula on the opposite side

- Repeat with the unaffected side and compare differences
- Adhesive capsulitis reduces range of motion on the affected side

Painful Arc Test
(Drawing D)

- Patient begins test with arm held at side, and then lifts arm to position over head. At 45° of abduction, pain is felt when inflamed tissue is forced under the acromion; pain continues until the 120° point on the arc is reached; then, pain subsides as the inflamed tissue passes from beneath the acromion as the arm moves into full abduction

- This pattern of pain strongly supports impingement

Figure 17.22

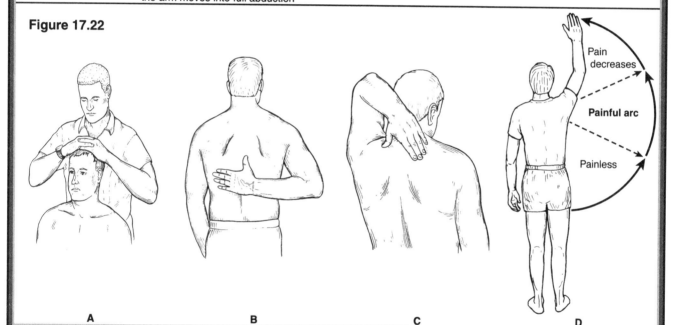

C. Differential Diagnosis
   1. Acute shoulder pain
      a. Necessary to differentiate among intrinsic causes (fracture, dislocation, strains, and sprains) and to determine if pain is being referred from areas such as the chest (myocardial infarction, thoracic outlet syndrome, diaphragmatic irritation), abdomen (gallbladder disease), or cervical spine (cervical spondylosis)
      b. Infection from osteomyelitis or septic arthritis may have an acute or more gradual onset; signs are severe pain, fever, and possibly swelling
   2. Chronic shoulder pain
      a. Septic arthritis, gout, rheumatoid arthritis, cervical radiculopathy, avascular necrosis may mimic impingement syndrome
      b. Malignant (i.e., osteosarcoma in young persons) and benign tumors may have gradual onset of pain

D. Diagnostic Tests
1. X-rays should be ordered to evaluate acute shoulder injuries
   a. Clavicle fractures: Anteroposterior (AP) view of shoulder; in patients with substantial trauma, also order x-ray of chest
   b. Humerus fractures: AP and lateral views of the humerus
   c. Scapular fractures: AP and axillary or lateral views of the shoulder; order chest film in patient with substantial trauma (rule out co-existing pneumothorax, rib fractures)
   d. Glenohumeral dislocations: AP and axillary views of the shoulder; CT scan may detect subtle dislocations
   e. Acromioclavicular joint sprain and separation: AP view of shoulder; order axillary view if Grade 4 to Grade 6 injuries are suspected
   f. Sternoclavicular joint sprain and separation: This injury is difficult to visualize on plain films; a modified radiographic view, such as a 40° cephalic tilt view, may be needed; a CT scan is often recommended
2. For patients with chronic shoulder problems, the following diagnostic testing is recommended:
   a. The routine radiograph or x-ray film should be used first before consideration of more sophisticated and expensive studies
   b. The standard views include the AP and lateral views (can disclose basic bony structures and degenerative changes that occur with osteoarthritis but are not helpful in viewing the coracoacromial arch or the glenohumeral joint)
   c. Scapular Y (outlet) view discloses the coracoacromial arch as well as the supraspinatus outlet
   d. West Point axillary view can be used to rule out dislocation and assess for avulsion fractures of the glenoid caused by dislocation
3. Consider other imaging studies (usually with consultation of a specialist)
   a. Magnetic resonance imaging is helpful in detecting adhesive capsulitis, rotator cuff tears, partial cuff tears, cuff degeneration, and chronic tendonitis
   b. Ultrasonography detects complete rotator cuff tears but is less helpful in identifying partial tears; a disadvantage is that the interpretation of this test is operator-dependent
   c. Arthrography is helpful in detecting complete rotator cuff tears or adhesive capsulitis, but is invasive and less useful in detecting partial tears

V. Plan/Management

A. Simple clavicle fractures can be treated by a trained primary care clinician; fractures with evidence of neurovascular compromise or if acromioclavicular joint is displaced more than 1 cm require orthopedic consultation
   1. Patients are often in severe pain and require analgesics
   2. Use a figure 8 strap in addition to a sling for 2-4 weeks
   3. Teach patients to be aware of possible signs and symptoms of neurovascular compromise; advise to avoid contact sports for 3 months
   4. Order a follow-up x-ray in a week to ensure adequate positioning and healing

B. Refer patients with humeral fractures; stable fractures can usually be treated with a shoulder immobilizer to prevent external rotation and abduction; surgical treatment is indicated for complex fractures

C. Simple scapular fractures can be treated by a trained primary care clinician; patients with acromial, neck, and glenoid fractures should be referred to orthopedist; for simple fractures:
   1. Apply ice, order analgesics, and use a sling for comfort
   2. Begin range-of-motion exercises as soon as acute pain resolves (usually within 2 weeks) to avoid a frozen shoulder
   3. Refer patients to a specialist if fractures are unstable or involve the articular site

D. Glenohumeral dislocations can be treated by a trained primary care clinician provided the axillary nerve has not been damaged (perform sensory test over shoulder and deltoid to rule-out)
   1. Treatment involves relocation of the humerus; several techniques are available, but should only be performed by an experienced clinician; Stimson's maneuver is one technique that can be performed
      a. Patient is placed prone on examining table with affected arm hanging over the side with a 5- to 10-pound weight strapped to affected arm
      b. If reduction does not occur within 15 minutes (light analgesia or a muscle relaxant may be helpful), place arm in sling and refer to a specialist

2. Following reduction, immobilize shoulder and elbow, and reassess neurovascular status of arm
3. Obtain postreduction x-rays; if pain persists for more than one week, repeat x-rays and refer to orthopedist
4. Apply ice every 3-4 hours during the first 2-3 days after the injury and order analgesics
5. Range-of-motion exercises should begin as soon as possible (usually within 7-10 days) to prevent frozen shoulder
6. Surgery is often needed for recurrent shoulder dislocations

E. Grade 1 and possibly Grade 2 acromioclavicular joint injuries can be treated by a trained primary care clinician; do not confuse AC joint injuries with shoulder dislocations (with shoulder dislocations the deltoid muscle looks like it has disappeared)
1. Immobilize arm in sling for 2 days to 2 weeks depending on degree of injury
2. Apply ice to painful area and give analgesics
3. As soon as possible, begin pendulum exercises (patient swings arm back and forth, side-to-side, and around); typically, refer to physical therapist
4. Gradually advance to exercises to strengthen trapezius and deltoid muscles

F. Patients with Grade 3 to Grade 6 acromioclavicular joint injuries need referral to a specialist; because a Grade 2 injury is difficult to differentiate from a Grade 3 injury, also consider referral of these patients

G. Simple sternoclavicular joint sprains can be treated with a sling or figure-eight appliance, ice, analgesics, and early, progressive range-of-motion exercises; refer more serious sprains and separations

H. Rotator cuff problems
1. Patients with Stage I impingement (pain is Grade 1 or 2 which suggests mild to moderate inflammation) can be managed conservatively with the goal of decreasing the inflammation that is compressing the subacromial space before irreversible damage occurs

---

CONSERVATIVE TREATMENT FOR STAGE I SHOULDER IMPINGEMENT
ADVICE THAT SHOULD BE GIVEN TO PATIENT

- **Rest without** immobilization
- **Use** arm and shoulder in activities that do not require overhead motion
- **Refrain** from activities that precipitated the injury
- **Apply ice** as often as desired and as long as inflammation is present (**Note:** Ice is a potent anti-inflammatory agent that can reduce both pain and muscle spasm)
- **Use** nonsteroidal anti-inflammatory drugs (NSAIDs) for 2-4 weeks
- **Visit** physical therapist for therapeutic modalities such as high-voltage electrical stimulation and ultrasound, and training in stretching and strengthening exercises
- **Exercise programs** (see figure 17.23)
- The final step is exercise training with weight machines or free weights

---

2. Patients with Stage I impingements that do not respond to conservative therapy in 4 weeks should be referred for further evaluation and possible corticosteroid injections
3. Patients with Stages II and III impingement syndrome require referral to an orthopedist
   a. Large tears require prompt surgical treatment
   b. Partial tears sometimes respond to an exercise program
   c. Repetitive steroid injections should be avoided

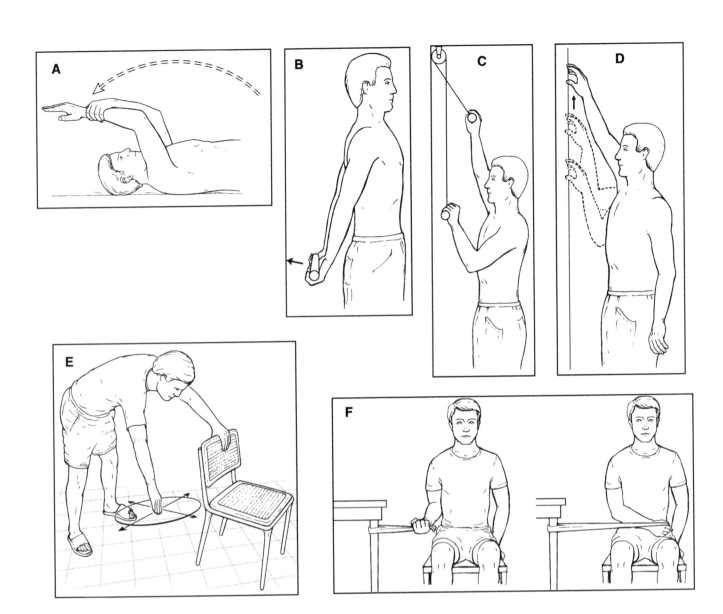

Figure 17.23. Exercise Programs

A. Forward evaluation: Grasp wrist of affected arm with unaffected hand and pull/stretch in an arc to head; repeat 5-10 times every day
B. Extension: Grasp stick with both hands behind back and push backwards; repeat 5-10 times every day
C. Pulley: Pull affected arm near pulleys and stretch; unaffected arm supplies the power; repeat 5-10 times every day
D. Wall climbing: Stand 1-2 feet from wall and slowly "walk" fingers up the wall so that stretch can be felt; increase distance walked up wall as motion improves
E. Pendulum: Lean forward, dangle affected arm, and swing arm back and forth, side-to-side, and around; increase length of swing as motion improves; repeat 5-10 times every day
F. Internal rotation: Anchor rubber tubing to solid object (table leg or doorknob); sit or stand with arm at side and elbow bent; slowly rotate arm inward toward body; hold 5-10 seconds, relax, and repeat; initially do 10 times in 1 set; try to increase number of sets per day as pain decreases

    I.   Adhesive capsulitis (frozen shoulder)
        1.   Conservative treatment with early, extensive physical therapy, analgesics; see Figure 17.23 for exercises that are recommended
        2.   Subacromial or intra-articular injections of corticosteroids may be helpful if conservative therapy fails
        3.   Capsular distension by intra-articular injection of an anesthetic, saline, corticosteroid, or air may provide pain relief
        4.   Surgical referral is needed if conservative treatment fails

    J.   Osteoarthritis is treated similarly to adhesive capsulitis (see section on OSTEOARTHRITIS)

K. Follow Up
    1. Patients with simple acute injuries (simple fractures, sprains, separations, dislocations) should be re-evaluated within 2 weeks
        a. Repeat x-rays are needed for clavicle fractures a week after injury
        b. Post-reduction x-rays are needed for shoulder dislocations
        c. For patients with acute injuries who have persistent pain, consider repeat x-rays and refer to specialist
    2. For patients with Stage I impingement syndrome (chronic pain) follow-up should be in 4 weeks to assess the efficacy of conservative management
    3. For patients with Stages II and III impingement syndrome, follow-up should be with specialist to whom patient was referred
    4. For patients with adhesive capsulitis and osteoarthritis follow-up is variable and depends on the patient's progress; typically re-evaluate patient within 2-4 weeks

WRIST PAIN

I. Definition: Chronic or recurrent pain or discomfort of the hand or wrist caused by selected common problems

II. Pathogenesis

A. Carpal tunnel syndrome
    1. An entrapment neuropathy involving the median nerve of the wrist
    2. Conditions that compromise the median nerve function due to any of the following:
        a. Decrease in the size of the carpal tunnel such as Colles' fracture, rheumatoid arthritis, osteoarthritis
        b. Enlargement of median nerve such as occurs with endoneural edema in diabetes mellitus
        c. Increase in the volume of other structures within the tunnel such as one of the following:
            (1) Tenosynovitis that is most often due to forceful repetitive wrist and hand movements
            (2) Urate deposits in gout
            (3) Fluid retention in pregnancy, premenstrual period, or with hypothyroidism

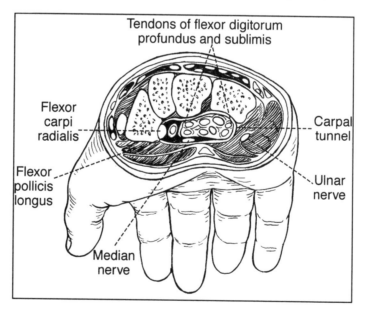

Figure 17.24. Cross Section of the Wrist Illustrating Location of the Median Nerve in the Carpal Tunnel

B. De Quervain's tenosynovitis: Subacute or chronic inflammation of the extensor tendons within the first dorsal compartment of the wrist

C. Ganglion cysts
   1. Believed to result from an out pouching of the wrist capsule; cysts contain fluid similar to joint fluid
   2. May be caused by damage to the scapholunate ligament, either from trauma or overuse

III. Clinical Presentation

A. Carpal tunnel syndrome is the most common entrapment neuropathy
   1. Affects nearly 1% of the general population in the US
   2. Most common among women 30-60 years old, industrial workers, and persons whose hobby or occupation requires forceful repetitive wrist and hand movements or the use of vibratory tools
   3. The typical presenting symptoms are pain and hand numbness or dysesthesia extending into the radial three digits of the hand and occasionally the thumb
   4. Early in the course of the disorder, pain and numbness that awaken the patient from sleep are common (shaking the hands and stretching the wrists are reported to relieve the discomfort)
   5. As the condition progresses, the patient often describes a fixed sensory loss and a feeling of loss of strength in the hand; symptoms remain relatively stable and unrelated to any specific activities at this point

B. De Quervain's tenosynovitis is one of the most commonly encountered wrist problems
   1. Most frequently occurs in middle-aged women
   2. Excessive repetitive handwork such as knitting and peeling vegetables aggravates the condition
   3. Pain is exacerbated by use of the thumb and is reproducible by having patient tuck his/her thumb into palm, making a fist, and then ulnarly deviating and palmar flexing the wrist

C. Ganglion cysts are extremely common, solitary, fluid-filled cysts found in a number of sites, most often the dorsum of the wrists between the midcarpal and radiocarpal joints
   1. In many cases, patients are unable to link the ganglia with a specific traumatic event
   2. Many ganglia are asymptomatic and resolve spontaneously; others produce mild to moderate pain
   3. The cysts are benign, feel soft to palpation, and fluctuate in size

IV. Diagnosis/Evaluation

A. History
   1. Determine onset, duration, and location of all symptoms related to the presenting problem
      a. If pain is present, ask if it disturbs sleep and if it is relieved by shaking hands and wrists
      b. If numbness is present, ask about location and whether it is constant or recurring
      c. If weakness or loss of strength in hand is present, ask patient to describe
      d. If mass on wrist is present, determine if it is painful and if it changes in size
   2. Ask about recent trauma to wrist, hand, or elbow
   3. Determine if patient engages in activities requiring repetitive movements or use of vibratory tools
   4. Obtain past medical history to determine if patient has any condition (including pregnancy) that might compromise median nerve function (see II.A.)
   5. Obtain medication history
   6. Inquire about what makes the condition better or worse (do symptoms increase with activity and improve with rest?)
   7. Ask about previous treatments and their results

B. Physical Examination
   1. Inspect hands and wrists in resting position with wrists in the neutral position; observe the bone and soft-tissue contours of the forearm, wrist, and hand, for any deviations, comparing both sides
   2. Note any muscle wasting on the thenar eminence (median nerve) or hypothenar eminence (ulnar nerve) that may indicate nerve injury
   3. Observe for any localized swellings or masses; palpate the mass to determine if it is soft and easy to manipulate (**Note**: A mass that is firm and fixed, and lies blow the level of the fascia is not likely to be a ganglia); transilluminate the mass if it is large enough (ganglia usually contain clear fluid and will often transilluminate)
   4. Palpate the proximal forearm for tenderness in the area where the median nerve passes beneath the pronator teres
   5. Palpate the forearm just proximal and radial to the anatomic "snuff box" for tenderness

6.   Perform Finkelstein test to reproduce pain characteristic of De Quervain's tenosynovitis (see Figure 17.25)

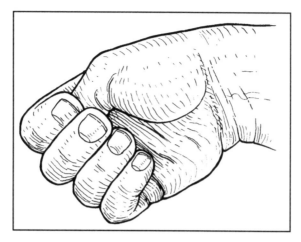

Figure 17.25. Finkelstein Test

Have patient tuck thumb into palm and make a fist as illustrated. Then ulnarly deviate and palmar flex the wrist; pain with this maneuver is a positive test

7.   To test for carpal tunnel syndrome, perform the following two tests (Figures 17.26 and 17.27)
    a.   Gently tap the carpal tunnel at and just distal to the flexor crease near the palmaris longus tendon (Tinel's sign); positive sign is a tingling sensation in the sensory distribution of the median nerve (thumb, index finger, and the middle and lateral half of the ring finger)

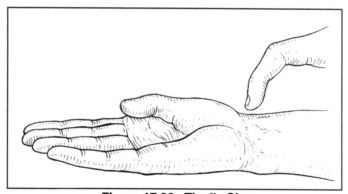

Figure 17.26. Tinel's Sign

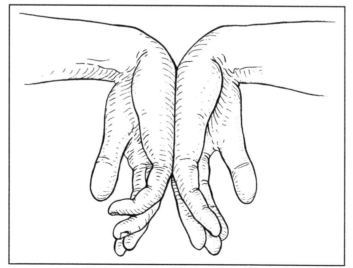

Figure 17.27. Test for Carpal Tunnel Syndrome (Phalen's Test)

b. Position the patient with elbows placed on a flat surface and the forearms held in a vertical position; the wrists are then acutely flexed. The test is positive if pain, numbness, or tingling is produced or made worse within 60 seconds (considered one of the most sensitive tests)

8. Motor evaluation: Evaluate motor function of the hand by asking patient to abduct the thumb, index, and little fingers against resistance

9. Sensory evaluation: Evaluate sensation at the dorsal web space between thumb and index finger (radial nerve), the tip of the long finger (median nerve), and the tip of the little finger (ulnar nerve)

C. Differential Diagnosis
1. Traumatic injuries such as fracture of the scaphoid or radial styloid, dislocations, and sprains
2. Nontraumatic conditions such as extensor tenosynovitis, mucous cysts, ulnar tunnel syndrome, osteoarthritis, rheumatoid arthritis
3. Infections
4. Tumors

D. Diagnostic Tests: Variable depending upon findings in history and physical examination
1. Consider wrist x-ray to rule out fractures and lesions
2. Testing is not indicated for diagnosing carpal tunnel syndrome unless the clinical findings are unclear, if the condition persists, or if patient is considering surgical intervention; definitive diagnosis can be made with electromyography (EMG) and nerve conduction studies
3. No tests are usually needed for De Quervain's tenosynovitis
4. Tests for diagnosing ganglions
   a. Needle aspiration of ganglion is the most definitive method of diagnosing a suspected ganglion (may also be therapeutic, but ganglion often returns)
   b. Although not usually indicated, AP and lateral radiographs of hand and wrist as well as ultrasonography can rule out other conditions that cause wrist swelling and lesions

V. Plan/Management

A. Carpal tunnel syndrome
1. Patients with mild symptoms (intermittent numbness, tingling, and pain in wrist and hands) are likely to respond to conservative therapy
   a. Wrist splinting with wrist in the neutral position; response to splinting is variable
   b. Use of NSAIDs is also important; splinting combined with use of NSAIDs provides relief in most patients
   c. Patients should be assisted to use proper body mechanics at work if repetitive use is believed to be part of the etiology; if possible, encourage patient to rotate jobs to reduce the amount of time spent on activities that expose the hypothenar area to vibration or pressure
2. Control of underlying systemic disorders is important
3. If conservative therapy fails to provide relief, consider corticosteroid injection of the carpal canal which has the advantage of both confirming the diagnosis and reducing the symptoms
4. Patients with more severe symptoms such as those described below should be referred for surgery without attempts at conservative management
   a. Patients with persistent symptoms that include hyperesthesia, clumsiness, and loss of dexterity and pinch strength
   b. Burning pain that increases at night and with hand use
   c. Patients with thenar muscle atrophy and motor weakness noted on physical examination

B. De Quervain's tenosynovitis
1. Conservative therapy involves rest, use of a thumb spica splint to immobilize the thumb, and oral NSAIDs
2. If conservative therapy fails to provide relief, refer the patient to an orthopedist or consider injecting corticosteroid under the pulleys of the abductor pollicis longus and the extensor pollicis brevis

C. Ganglion cyst
1. Explain to patients that the cyst is insignificant and may spontaneously drain without any treatment, but may also recur
2. Needle aspiration is another option; aspiration is both diagnostic and therapeutic, but cysts frequently return after being evacuated
3. Recurrent ganglions may best be managed surgically; refer patient to a hand surgeon who can resect ganglions arthroscopically with good results and very few recurrences

D. Follow Up: In one month to evaluate therapy and determine need for referral

REFERENCES

American Association of Clinical Endocrinologists. (2001). American Association of Clinical Endocrinologists 2001 medical guidelines for clinical practice for the prevention and management of postmenopausal osteoporosis. *Endocrine Practice, 7,* 293-312.

American College of Obstetricians and Gynecologists Committee on Gynecologic Practice. (2002). Bone density screening for osteoporosis. *ACOG Committee Opinion, 270,* 523-554.

American College of Rheumatology Ad Hoc Committee on Clinical Guidelines. (1996). Guidelines for the management of rheumatoid arthritis. *Arthritis and Rheumatology, 39,* 713-722.

American College of Rheumatology Subcommittee on Osteoarthritis Guidelines. (2000). Recommendations for the medical management of osteoarthritis of the hip and knee. *Arthritis and Rheumatism, 43,* 1905-1915.

American Pain Society. (2002). *Guideline for the management of pain in osteoarthritis, rheumatoid arthritis, and juvenile chronic arthritis.* Glenview, IL: American Pain Society.

Arcuni, S.E. (2000). Rotator cuff pathology and subacromial impingement. *The Nurse Practitioner, 25,* 58-78.

Arnet, F.C. (1989). Revised criteria for classification of rheumatoid arthritis. *Bulletin on Rheumatic Diseases, 38,* 1-6.

Austermuehle, P.D. (2001). Common knee injuries in primary care. *The Nurse Practitioner, 26,* 26-45.

Bauer, S.J., Hollander, J.E., Fuchs, S.H., & Thode, H.C., Jr. (1995). A clinical decision rule in the evaluation of acute knee injuries. *Journal of Emergency Medicine, 13,* 611-615.

Bigos, S., Bowyer, O., Braen, G., Brown, K., Deyo, R.A., Haldeman, S., et al. (1994). *Acute low back problems in adults. Clinical practice guideline No. 14.* AHCPR Publication No. 95-0642. Rockville, MD: Agency for Health Care Policy and Research, Public Health Service, U.S. Department of Health and Human Services.

Blumenthal, D.E. (2002). Hyperuricemia and gout. In R.E. Rakel, & E.T. Bope, (Eds.). *2002 Conn's current therapy.* Philadelphia: Saunders.

Bratton, R.L. (1999). Assessment and management of acute low back pain. *American Family Physician, 60,* 2299-2308.

Braunader, R., & Shelton, D.K. (2002). Radiologic bone assessment in the evaluation of osteoporosis. *American Family Physician, 65,* 1357-1364.

Browning, M.A. (2001). Rheumatoid arthritis: A primary care approach. *Journal of the Academy of Nurse Practitioners, 13,* 399-408.

Civitelli, R., & Williams, M.T. (2002). Prevention, diagnosis, and treatment of osteoporosis in men. *Federal Practitioner,* 40-48.

Committee on Menopause and Osteoporosis. (2001). The Canadian Consensus on Menopause and Osteoporosis. *Journal of Obstetrics and Gynaecolology Canada, 23,* 1198-1203.

Crandall, C. (2002). Parathyroid hormone for treatment of osteoporosis. *Archives of Internal Medicine, 11,* 2297-2309.

Cote, L.G. (2001). Management of osteoarthritis. *Journal of the Academy of Nurse Practitioners, 13,* 495-501.

Cummings, S.R., Bates, D., & Black, D.M. (2002). Clinical use of bone densitometry: Scientific review. *JAMA, 288,* 1889-1897.

Department of Veterans Affairs. (1999). Low back pain or sciatica in the primary care setting. *National Guideline Clearinghouse.*

Deyo, R.A., & Weinstein, J.N. (2001). Low back pain. *New England Journal of Medicine, 344,* 363-370.

Epperly, T.D., Moore, K.M., & Harrover, J.D. (2000). Polymyalgia rheumatica and temporal arteritis. *American Family Physician, 62,* 789-796, 801.

Evans, J. (2003). Vertebral compression fractures: Pain reduction and improvement in functional mobility after percutaneous polymethylmethacrylate vertebroplasty – Retrospective report of 245 cases. *Radiology, 226,* 366-372.

Gallagher, J.C., Rapuri, P.B., Haynatzki, G., & Detter, J.R. (2002). Effect of discontinuation of estrogen, calcitriol, and the combination of both on bone density and bone markers. *Journal of Clinical Endocrinology and Metabolism, 87,* 4914-4923.

Gates, S.J., & Mooar, P.A. (1999). *Musculoskeletal primary care.* Philadelphia: Lippincott.

Gerritsen, A.A.M., deVet, H.C.W., Scholten, R.J.P.M., Bertelsman, F.W., deKrom, M.C.J.F.M., & Bouter, L.M. (2002). Splinting versus surgery in the treatment of carpal tunnel syndrome. *JAMA, 288,* 1245-1251.

Goroll, A.H., & Mulley, Jr., A.G. (2000). Evaluation of acute monoarticular arthritis. In A.H. Goroll, & A.G. Mulley, Jr., (Eds.). *Primary care medicine,* (4th ed.). Lippincott: Philadelphia.

Goroll, A.H., & Mulley, Jr., A.G. (2000). Evaluation of polyarticular complaints. In A.H. Goroll, & A.G. Mulley, Jr., (Eds.). *Primary care medicine,* (4th ed.). Lippincott: Philadelphia.

Grossman, J.M., & MacLean, C.H. (2001). Quality indicators for the management of osteoporosis in vulnerable elders. *Annals of Internal Medicine, 135,* 722-730.

Halin, J. (2000). Treatment of rheumatoid arthritis: Etanercept, a recent advance. *Journal of American Nurse Practitioner, 12,* 433-441.

Hinton, R., Moody, R.L., Davis, A.W., & Thomas, S.F. (2002). Osteoarthritis: Diagnosis and therapeutic considerations. *American Family Physician, 65,* 841-8.

Hochberg, M.C., Altman, R.D., Brandt, K.D., Clark, B.M., Dieppe, P.A., Griffin, M.R., Moskowitz, R.W., & Schnitzer, T.J. (1995). Guidelines for the medical management of osteoarthritis, Part I: Osteoarthritis of the hip, Part II: Osteoarthritis of the knee. *Arthritis and Rheumatism, 38,* 1535-1541.

Hockenbury, R.T., & Sammarco, G.J. (2001). Evaluation and treatment of ankle sprains. *The Physician and Sportsmedicine, 29,* 57-64.

Howite, N.T. (2002). Current treatment of juvenile rheumatoid arthritis. *Pediatrics, 109,* 109-115.

Hulley, S., Furberg, C., Barrett-Connor, E., Cauley, J., Grady, D., Haskell, W., et al. (2002). Noncardiovascular disease outcomes during 6.8 years of hormone therapy: Heart and estrogen/progestin replacement study follow-up (HERS II), *JAMA, 288,* 58-66.

Institute of Medicine. (1997). *Dietary reference intakes: Calcium, phosphorus, magnesium, Vitamin D, and fluoride.* Washington DC: National Academy Press.

Jarvik, J.G., & Deyo, R.A. (2002). Diagnostic evaluation of low back pain with emphasis on imaging. *Annals of Internal Medicine, 137,* 586-597.

Johnson, M.W. (2000). Acute knee effusions: A systematic approach to diagnosis. *American Family Physician, 61,* 2391-2400.

Jupiter, J.B., & Ring, D. (2000). Approach to minor orthopedic problems of the elbow, wrist, and hand. In A.H. Goroll, & A.G. Mulley, Jr., (Eds.). *Primary care medicine,* (4th ed.). Lippincott: Philadelphia.

Kremer, J.M. (2001). Rational use of new and existing disease-modifying agents in rheumatoid arthritis. *Annals of Internal Medicine, 134,* 695-706.

Kupecz, D., & Berardinelli, C. (2002). Using anakinra for adult rheumatoid arthritis. *The Nurse Practitioner, 27,* 62-65.

Lawson, M.T. (2001). Evaluating and managing osteoporosis in men. *The Nurse Practitioner, 26,* 26, 29-36, 43-44.

Ledlie, J.T., & Renfro, M. (2003). Balloon kyphoplasty: One year outcomes in vertebral body height restoration, chronic pain, and activity levels. *Journal of Neurosurgery, 98: Spine:* 36-42.

Lindsay, R., Gallagher, J.C., Kleerekoper, J., & Picak, J.H. (2002). Effect of lower doses of conjugated equine estrogens with and without medroxyprogesterone acetate on bone in early postmenopausal women. *JAMA, 287,* 2668-2676.

Loder, R. (1998). Slipped capital femoral epiphysis. *American Family Physician, 57,* 2135-2142.

Lucasey, B. (2001). Corticosteroid-induced osteoporosis. *Nursing Clinics of North America, 36,* 455-466.

MacLean, C.H. (2001). Quality indicators for the management of osteoarthritis in vulnerable elders. *Annals of Internal Medicine, 135,* 711-721.

Manek, N.J., & Lane, N.E. (2000). Osteoarthritis: Current concepts in diagnosis and management. *American Family Physician, 61,* 1795-1804.

Mankin, K.P. (2001). Chronic orthopedic problems. In C. Green-Hernandez, J.K. Singleton, & D.Z. Aronzon, (Eds.). *Primary care pediatrics.* Philadelphia: Lippincott.

Mazzone, M.F., & McCue, T. (2002). Common conditions of the Achilles tendon. *American Family Physician, 65,* 1805-1810.

McClung, B., & McClung, M. (2001). Pharmacologic therapy for the treatment and prevention of osteoporosis. *Nursing Clinics of North America, 36,* 433-440.

Millea, P.J., & Holloway, R.L. (2000). Treating fibromyalgia. *American Family Physician, 62,* 1575-1582, 1587.

Miller, P.D. (2002). Osteoporosis. In R.E. Rakel & E.T. Bope, (Eds.). *2002 Conn's current therapy.* Philadelphia: Saunders.

Mortensen, S.E. (2002). Bursitis, tendonitis, myofascial pain, and fibromyalgia. In R.E. Rakel & E.T. Bope, (Eds.). *2002 Conn's current therapy.* Philadelphia: Saunders.

National Institutes of Health (March 27-29, 2000) Osteoporosis Prevention, Diagnosis, and Therapy: Consensus Development Conference Statement. Available at: http://adp.od.nih.gov/consensus/cons/111/111_intro.htm.

Nelson, H.D. (2002). Assessing benefits and harms of hormone replacement therapy. *JAMA, 288,* 882-884.

Nelson, H.D., Humphrey, L.L, Nygren, P., Teutsch, S.M., & Allan, J.D. (2002). Postmenopausal hormone replacement therapy: Scientific review. *JAMA 288,* 872-881.

The North American Menopause Society. (2002). Management of postmenopausal osteoporosis: Position statement of The North American Menopause Society. *Menopause, 9,* 84-101.

Owens, S., & Itamura, J.M. (2001). Differential diagnosis of shoulder injuries in sports. *Orthopedic Clinics of North America, 32,* 393-398.

Patel, A.T., & Ogle, A.A. (2000). Diagnosis and management of acute low back pain. *American Family Physician, 61,* 1779-1786, 1789-1790.

Pavelká, K., Gatterová, J., Olejarová, M., Machacek, S., Giacovelli, G., & Rovati, L.C. (2002). Glucosamine sulfate use and delay of progression of knee osteoarthritis: A 3-year, randomized, placebo-controlled, double-blind study. *Archives of Internal Medicine, 162,* 2113-2123.

Pennington, J.A.T. (1994). *Bowes and Churche's food values of portions commonly used.* Philadelphia: Lippincott.

Perron, A.D., Brady, W.J., & Keats, T.A. (2002). Management of common stress fractures. *Postgraduate Medicine, 111,* 95-106.

Rizzoli, R., Schaad, M., & Uebelhart, B. (2001). Osteoporosis in men. *Nursing Clinics of North America, 36,* 467-479.

Salerno, S.M., Browning, R., & Jackson, J.L. (2002). The effect of antidepressant treatment on chronic back pain. *Archives of Internal Medicine. 162,* 19-24.

Schroeder, B.M. (2002). American College of Foot and Ankle Surgeons: Diagnosis and treatment of heel pain. *American Family Physician, 65,* 1687-1688.

Shalaota, M.D., & Leggit, J. (2003). Adhesive capsulitis: Helping patients break free. *Federal Practitioner,* 11-20.

Smidt, N. (2002). Corticosteroid injections, physiotherapy, or a wait-and-see policy for lateral epicondylitis: A randomized controlled trial. *Lancet, 259,* 657-662.

Solomon, D.H., Simel, D.L., Bates, D.W., Katz, J.N., & Schaffer, J.L. (2001). Does this patient have a torn meniscus or ligament of the knee? *JAMA, 286,* 1610-1620.

South-Paul, J.E. (2001). Osteoporosis: Part I. Evaluation and assessment. *American Family Physician, 63,* 897-904, 908.

Stiell, I.G., Wells, G.A., Hoag, R.H., Sivilotti, M.L., Cacciotti, T.F., Verbeek, P.R., et al. (1997). Implementation of the Ottawa Knee Rule for the use of radiography in acute knee injuries. *JAMA, 278,* 2075-2079.

Tan, E.M., Cohen, A.S., Fries, J.F., Masi, A.T., McShane, D.J., Rothfield, W.F., et al. (1982). The 1982 revised criteria for the classification of systemic lupus erythematosus. *Arthritis and Rheumatism, 25,* 1275-1277.

Tandeter, H.B., Shvartzman, P., & Stevens, M.A. (1999). Acute knee injuries: Use of decision rules for selective radiograph ordering. *American Family Physician, 60,* 2599-2608.

US Preventive Services Task Force. (2002). Screening for osteoporosis in postmenopausal women: Recommendations and rationale. Available at http://www.preventiveservices.ahrg.gov

Von Korff, M., & Moore, J.C. (2001). Stepped care for back pain: Activating approaches for primary care. *Annals of Internal Medicine, 134,* 911-917.

Wolfe, F., Smythe, H.A., Yunus, M.B., Bennett, R.M., Bombadier, C., Goldenberg, D.L., et al. (1990). The American College of Rheumatology 1990 criteria for the classification of fibromyalgia. *Arthritis and Rheumatism, 33,* 160-172.

Wolfe, M.W., Uhl, T.L., & McCluskey, L.C. (2001). Management of ankle sprains. *American Family Physician, 63,* 93-104.

Woodward, T.W., & Best, T.M. (2000). The painful shoulder: Part I. Clinical evaluation. *American Family Physician, 61,* 3079-3088.

Woodward, T.W., & Best, T.M. (2000). The painful shoulder: Part II. Acute and chronic disorders. *American Family Physician, 61,* 3291-3300.

Writing Group for the Women's Health Initiative Investigators. (2002). Risks and benefits of estrogen plus progestin in healthy postmenopausal women. *JAMA, 288,* 321-333.

Young, C.C., Rutherford, D.S., & Niedfeldt, M.W. (2001). Treatment of plantar fasciitis. *American Family Physician, 63,* 467-474, 477-478.

Neurologic Problems

MARY VIRGINIA GRAHAM

Acute Facial Paresis (Bell's Palsy)

Alzheimer's Disease

Dizziness

Headache

Parkinson's Disease

Restless Legs Syndrome

Seizures and Epilepsy

Stroke and Transient Ischemic Attack

Tremor

ACUTE FACIAL PARESIS (BELL'S PALSY)

I. Definition: Acute, unilateral paresis of facial muscles due to inflammation and subsequent mechanical compression of the 7th (the facial) cranial nerve

II. Pathogenesis

    A. Believed to be a viral neuropathy caused by herpes simplex virus (HSV) type 1

    B. Most likely the herpes virus spreads from the oral cavity along the chorda tympani nerve to the geniculate ganglion where it remains dormant until reactivated by various physiologic stressors

III. Clinical Presentation

    A. Disease is common, with an incidence each year of 20 per 100,000; affects all age groups but occurs most often in young and middle-age adults

    B. Typical presentation is rapid onset of facial weakness with little or no progression beyond 48 to 72 hours
        1. There is loss of facial expression, loss of voluntary movement of facial and scalp muscles on affected side, altered ability to close one eye, and numbness of the face
        2. In addition, patient may experience loss of taste, be hypersensitive to sound, and have excessive tearing
        3. Usually, the diagnosis is established without difficulty in patients presenting with unexplained, unilateral, isolated facial weakness

    C. May have ear or facial pain (which is usually transient and may have resolved by time of presentation) on affected side for about 24 hours prior to onset of weakness

    D. Most patients recover completely without treatment within weeks to a few months, but some have residual effects
        1. Three months after initial onset of symptoms seems to be an important landmark in terms of recovery
        2. Patients whose recovery is delayed beyond this time period often experience significant sequelae

    E. Recurrent facial nerve palsy is unusual; if patient has more than two episodes of the condition, the possibility of tumor should be suspected

IV. Diagnosis/Evaluation

    A. History
        1. Question about onset of symptoms as paresis in Bell's palsy is abrupt and does not occur gradually over days or weeks (waxing and waning of symptoms suggest another cause)
        2. Ask about facial pain, particularly in area of mastoid process (not atypical to have pain in this area)
        3. Include careful questioning about neurological symptoms in other areas of face and body
        4. Ask about prior history of facial weakness (if positive, raises concern for another cause)
        5. Inquire about cerebrovascular and cardiac risk factors
        6. Ask about predisposing factors such as infection, trauma, recent outdoor activities in area endemic for Lyme disease

    B. Physical Examination
        1. Measure vital signs, noting elevations in blood pressure and temperature
        2. Observe general appearance including gait, evidence of trauma or distress
        3. Inspect skin for herpetic lesions or characteristic lesions of Lyme disease
        4. Carefully examine the head, ears, eyes, nose, and throat
        5. Special attention should be given to assessment of the cranial nerves and the neurological examination, looking for evidence of other cranial neuropathies or neurologic deficits
            a. To differentiate between Bell's palsy and a central lesion (an ominous cause of facial weakness), have patient raise eyebrows and wrinkle forehead

b. With peripheral lesions, both the upper and lower face are affected (cannot wrinkle forehead)

c. With central lesions, mainly the lower face is affected (can wrinkle forehead)

C. Differential Diagnosis: Simultaneous bilateral facial palsies, unilateral facial weakness that slowly progresses over 3 weeks with or without facial hyperkinesis, and failure of facial function to return within 6 months after acute onset suggest a diagnosis other than Bell's palsy; possible alternative diagnoses are the following

1. Benign and malignant tumors
2. Infectious processes, viral, bacterial, or spirochete (acute or chronic otitis media; Lyme disease, herpes zoster, herpes simplex type 1)
3. Trauma (temporal bone fracture)
4. Guillain-Barré syndrome (typically has symmetric bilateral weakness)

D. Diagnostic Tests

1. In patients with a classic history for Bell's palsy and a physical examination that is otherwise normal, order an audiogram in the acute phase to help rule out a lesion in cerebellopontine angle and temporal bone (this is usually the only test needed during the acute phase)
2. Obtain Lyme titer if there is a history of exposure to ticks and patient resides in geographic location where disease is prevalent
3. If there is uncertainty about the diagnosis, or if the patient has gradual progression of symptoms over the follow-up period (see below for follow-up), then refer the patient to a neurologist for further diagnostic testing
4. Additional diagnostic testing in patients with Bell's palsy usually involves tests to estimate the patient's prognosis
   a. Electrical testing during the first week or two involves use of the Hilger nerve stimulation test and electroneurography–these tests are used to determine prognosis and have little utility beyond the first 2-3 weeks after onset of symptoms
   b. Electromyography testing can be performed many weeks later (not in the early phases) to also provide information on recovery potential

V. Plan/Management

A. Explain that symptoms usually resolve in 3-4 weeks without any treatment and with no sequelae

B. Good eye care is paramount as corneal abrasion can easily occur in patients with facial paralysis; inability to close eye completely and blink, as well as decreased tearing and corneal hyperesthesia, predispose the eye to injury

1. Advise patient to use lubricant eye drops 1-2 drops every 2 hours when awake and ophthalmic ointment at night
2. Available products include HypoTears PF, Duratears Naturale, and Bion Tears, all preservative-free and available over-the-counter
3. Glasses should be worn when outdoors to protect eye from drying effects of wind
4. Affected eye may need to be patched, especially at night, to reduce eye damage; care must be taken that the lid does not open and expose the cornea to material covering the eye

C. A physical therapy referral may be beneficial; usually involves heat therapy, electrical stimulation, or massage

D. Even though the benefit of corticosteroid use in Bell's palsy has not been definitively established, steroids are safe for short-term use and are probably effective in improving facial functional outcomes in affected patients

1. Whereas some have suggested that patients with complete paralysis (not paresis) benefit most from steroids, there is little evidence that severity of facial weakness at the onset of treatment influences effectiveness of oral prednisone therapy
2. If there are no contraindications, initiate short-term treatment with oral prednisone (1.0 mg/kg/day for 3 days, 0.75 mg/kg/day for 3 days, 0.50 mg/kg/day for 3 days, and then a rapid taper over the next 4-5 days)
3. Corticosteroids should be started as soon as possible after the onset of facial paralysis/paresis
4. Initiation of therapy within 3 days is considered optimal

E.   The benefit of antiviral agents in the treatment of Bell's palsy has not been established; however, antivirals (combined with prednisone) are possibly effective in improving facial functional outcomes in affected persons; consider treatment with either famciclovir or valacyclovir for one week

F.   Follow Up
1.   Patients who present with facial weakness or paralysis believed to be due to Bell's palsy should be seen several times a week for the first 2-3 weeks to make sure that symptoms are not progressing and that the eye on the affected side is receiving proper care
2.   If symptoms are resolving at that point, and the patient is performing proper eye care, then visits can be less often (every 1-2 weeks)
3.   Patients who have delayed or incomplete recovery should be referred to a neurologist for management
4.   Patient should be referred without delay to an ophthalmologist if any eye symptoms or signs develop

ALZHEIMER'S DISEASE

I.   Definition: A syndrome of progressive and irreversible cognitive and functional decline with variable noncognitive or behavioral manifestations

II.   Pathogenesis: The core neuropathologic features of Alzheimer's disease are neuritic amyloid plaques and neurofibrillary tangles which are regionally specific, occurring most often in the hippocampus, entorhinal cortex, and association areas of the neocortex

A.   Amyloid precursor protein (APP), a normal protein produced by healthy neurons, aids in the growth and maintenance of neurons
1.   At least three enzymes–called alpha, beta, and gamma secretase–cleave APP into shorter forms; a protein called beta amyloid (A-beta) is generated which drifts away from the cell membrane; most A-beta dissolves quickly in fluid surrounding the neuron, but some of it folds into forms called fibrils which survive and cluster together forming plaques (with aging, some plaque generation is normal)
2.   Clusters of A-beta gradually expand to create large plaques which displace brain cells and may destroy them, both by triggering inflammation and by damaging the cell interiors

B.   In healthy neurons, neurites house skeletal structures known as microtubules which give the neuron its shape and also serve as its circulatory system, transporting nutrients and chemical messengers; tau proteins bind tightly to the sides of the microtubules enabling the microtubules to perform its critical tasks
1.   Enzymes loosen tau in persons with Alzheimer's disease (AD) and abnormal cells containing tau (neurofibrillary) tangles are formed; lacking tau proteins to hold them together, the microtubules begin to disintegrate, the neurites shrink, and the neuron dies
2.   Formation of tau tangles is a process that begins when amyloid plaques exert pressure against the outer surfaces of neurons, initiating a cascade of events involving chemical changes within the neuron that result in neuron destruction; there is general agreement that beta-amyloid plaques form before tau tangles

C.   Alzheimer's disease selectively damages critical clusters of neurons in the cortex and limbic structures of the central nervous system, particularly the basal forebrain, amygdala, hippocampus, and cerebral cortex
1.   These areas are associated with functions of higher learning, memory, reasoning, behavior, and emotional control
2.   There are four major alterations in these brain structures: cortical atrophy, degeneration of cholinergic and other neurons, presence of neurofibrillary tangles (NFTs), and accumulation of amyloid plaques
3.   The invariant consequence of these alterations is the death of neurons, impaired cognition, and, ultimately, brain failure and death; the process of neuronal death is termed "apoptotic" or programmed cell death to distinguish it from cell death due to ischemia or necrosis

D.   Widespread cell destruction leads to a variety of neurotransmitter deficits, with the cholinergic pathways most profoundly damaged

E. Recent research into early-onset AD has shown that mutations in at least three genes are present in persons with AD in certain families, including mutant APP and mutant presenilin-1 and presenilin-2

F. It has been established that the apolipoprotein E epsilon4 (APOE epsilon4) gene on chromosome 19 is associated with late-onset AD, the most common form of the disease; presence of the APOE epsilon4 allele is the most important genetic risk factor known for this form of AD

III. Clinical Presentation

A. The most common of the dementing disorders affecting an estimated 4 million persons in the US; this number is expected to increase to 14 million by 2050

B. Increasing age remains the primary risk factor for AD; prevalence of dementia rises dramatically with age, from 24% of those 75-79 years old to 75% in those 95 and older

C. Average duration from onset of symptoms to death is 8 to 10 years; plateaus may occur, but progression usually resumes after a period of months or a few years

D. Manifestations of AD in the early stages of the disease
   1. Memory impairment is the most prominent early symptom
      a. Effect on recent memory is most pronounced
      b. Remote memory is less affected
   2. Cognitive impairments create problems with functioning in daily life; for many patients and families, the functional impairments are the first sign that there is a problem
   3. Attention impairment occurs and is manifest by difficulty with competing stimuli and in changing mental set
   4. Visual-spatial functioning is affected and patients experience difficulty with drawing and route finding (diminishes ability to safely operate a motor vehicle)
   5. Both problem-solving and calculations are affected as abstract thinking and judgment become impaired
   6. Deficits in executive function (e.g., performing tasks involving multiple steps, such as planning and preparing a meal, organizing a shopping trip) are typically seen
   7. Personality changes or increased irritability may be exhibited
   8. Generally, there is relative preservation of motor and sensory functions until the later stages
   9. Language and social skills may be fairly well preserved so that a casual observer would be unaware that the person is experiencing cognitive impairment

E. By the middle and late stages of the disease, a number of mental and physical disabilities occur
   1. Agitation (a range of behavioral disturbances including aggression, combativeness, shouting, hyperactivity, and disinhibition) is the most commonly occurring behavioral change, with as many as 50% of patients, particularly in middle and later stages of the illness, exhibiting this behavior
   2. Psychotic symptoms (paranoia, delusions, and hallucinations) are far less frequent than agitation, but are much more dangerous to the patient and alarming to the family
   3. Patients may also develop wandering behaviors which place them in great jeopardy of injury
   4. Gait, motor disturbances, and incontinence may also occur in later stages

F. Diagnostic criteria for dementia of the Alzheimer's type as set forth in the *Diagnostic and Statistic Manual of Mental Disorders* (4th ed.) [Revised], (2000) are often used by clinicians and are contained in the following table (**Note:** Use of *DSM-IV Criteria* is recommended by the American Academy of Neurology in recently published guidelines for diagnosis of dementia [see reference at the end of this chapter])

The development of multiple cognitive deficits that is manifested by **both of the following**
- ➡ Memory impairment (both in learning new information and recalling previously learned information)
- ➡ One or more of the following cognitive disturbances
  - Aphasia (disturbance in language)
  - Apraxia (inability to carry out motor activities despite intact motor function)
  - Agnosia (inability to recognize objects despite intact sensory function)
  - Disturbances in executive functioning (planning, organizing, sequencing)

The cognitive deficits described above cause significant impairment in social or occupational functioning and represent a significant decline from previous functioning

The course is characterized by both gradual onset and continuing decline

The cognitive deficits described above are not due to any of the following
- ➡ Other central nervous system conditions that cause progressive decline in memory and cognition such as cerebrovascular disease, Huntington's disease, and Parkinson's disease
- ➡ Systemic conditions known to cause dementia such as hypothyroidism, vitamin B_{12} or folic acid deficiency, neurosyphilis, and HIV infection
- ➡ Substance-induced conditions

The deficits do not occur exclusively during the course of a delirium

The disturbance is not better accounted for by another disorder such as major depressive disorder or schizophrenia

Adapted from American Psychiatric Association. (2000). *Diagnostic and statistical manual of mental disorders,* (4th ed.) [Revised]. Washington, DC: Author.

IV. Diagnosis/Evaluation

    A. History
        1. Overview of history taking is contained in the box below

┌───┐
│ ***Overview of History Taking***   │
│   │
│ ✓ In addition to the usual components of the history, **five areas** that   │
│   require assessment (and periodic reassessment) are the following–**ability│
│   to perform activities of daily living (ADLs) and instrumental activities │
│   of daily living (IADLs), cognitive functioning, comorbid medical and   │
│   mood disorders, and caregiver status**   │
│ ✓ The history should be obtained from the patient and a **reliable informant** │
│ ✓ Validity of patient reports are often limited by memory loss and lack of │
│   insight   │
│ ✓ To increase accuracy of reporting, information from more than one family │
│   member may be helpful   │
│ ✓ Patient should be informed that others may be interviewed to help with   │
│   understanding of symptoms   │
│ ✓ Dignity of the patient should be preserved!   │
└───┘

        2. To begin the evaluation, ask the patient the following three questions in order to observe his/her general behavior, mannerisms, and determine ability to respond appropriately to simple questions
            a. How are you?
            b. What sorts of things do you like to do?
            c. What did you do yesterday?
        3. To continue the evaluation, use the *DSM-IV* criteria contained in the table above to document the presence and chronology of each of the cognitive deficits set forth in the criteria
        4. Systematically determine the presence of each of the symptom areas–memory impairment (must be present) and **at least one other** index of cognitive dysfunction–aphasia, apraxia, agnosia, or disturbances in executive functioning
            a. For the first criterion, memory impairment (which includes both recent and remote memory), Ask, "Do you (or interviewing the informant, "Does [patient's name]) have trouble remembering recent conversations, events, or appointments?" **Repeat the question relating to events in the past**
            b. Ask about onset: "Was it abrupt or gradual?"
            c. Ask about progression "Is it getting worse?" "Is it improving?"
            d. Ask about duration: "How long has this been going on?"
        5. Repeat this process for each of the other areas of the *DSM-IV*–aphasia, apraxia, agnosia, and disturbances in executive functioning with both patient and the informant

EXAMPLES OF HISTORY QUESTIONS RELATING TO **APHASIA, APRAXIA, AGNOSIA, AND EXECUTIVE FUNCTIONING ABILITY**	
Criteria	*Questions to Ask*
Aphasia	"Do you (if interviewing the informant, "Does [patient's name]) have difficulty: ✓ Finding the right word or words when having a conversation?" ✓ Writing letters/e-mails/telephone messages/grocery lists/To-Do lists?" (Select one or two to inquire about) ✓ Following directions that are given verbally?" ✓ Explaining a brief article of interest from the newspaper?"
Apraxia	"Do you (if interviewing the informant, "Does [patient's name]) have difficulty: ✓ Remembering what to do with a broom/remote control/video/seat belt?" (Select one or two to inquire about or ask about use of any common object with which persons are normally familiar)
Agnosia	"Do you (if interviewing the informant, "Does [patient's name]) have difficulty: ✓ Recognizing what something is by just feeling it?" (Ask about a specific object that patient should be able to recognize by feel; failure to recognize common object despite normal sensory function signifies agnosia)
Executive Functioning	"Do you (if interviewing the informant, "Does [patient's name]) have difficulty: ✓ Preparing a balanced meal?" ✓ Shopping for groceries?" ✓ Participating in hobbies such as sewing, playing cards, gardening?"

To meet diagnostic criteria for dementia of the Alzheimer's type as set forth in *DSM-IV*, the patient must exhibit memory impairment and at least one other cognitive disturbance (either aphasia, apraxia, agnosia, or disordered executive functioning)

6. Obtain medical history including any systemic diseases, psychiatric disorders, any known neurological disorders, history of head trauma
7. Obtain social history including alcohol, tobacco, drug use
8. Ask about occupational or recreational exposures to toxic substances
9. Determine what medications the patient is taking, including prescription products, over-the-counter drugs, and vitamin and herbal remedies
10. Obtain an in-depth family history with a focus on presence in the family of early-onset Alzheimer's disease or rare genetic conditions such as Huntington's disease
11. Assess the patient's daily functioning as described in the box below

---

Use tools such as the *Activities of Daily Living* (ADL) scale, the *Instrumental Activities of Daily Living* (IADL) scale, or the *Functional Activities Questionnaire* (FAQ)

ADL scale evaluates patient's abilities in bathing, dressing, toileting, transfer, continence, and feeding
Patients are ranked in each activity at one of 3 levels ranging from
    ✓   Completely independent
    ✓   Needs some assistance
    ✓   Almost/or completely dependent

IADL scale evaluates ability to perform 7 complex activities (e.g., managing money, shopping, traveling, using telephone) necessary for optimal independent living

FAQ evaluates performance on 10 complex, higher-order activities (a summary of the scale is contained in a table below)

These three scales are widely available and are all informant-based measure (completed by informant, not patient)

SUMMARY OF THE FUNCTIONAL ACTIVITIES QUESTIONNAIRE (FAQ)
• Bill paying
• Assembling records relating to business affairs
• Shopping alone
• Playing a game of skill
• Performing a task involving multiple steps (writing letter, stamping envelope, placing in mailbox)
• Preparing a balanced meal
• Being aware of current events
• Understanding and discussing TV program, book, newspaper article
• Remembering and keeping appointments
• Driving, arranging to take bus, or walking to familiar places
In normal persons, all 10 activities are performed; the fewer activities the person can perform independently, the more dependent he/she is
The FAQ was developed by R.I. Pfeiffer, T.T. Kurosake, & C.H. Harrah and is available in the *Journal of Gerontology*, (37), 323-329, 1982. Administration and scoring of the instrument is explained in the article

12. Screen for depression as recommended by the American Academy of Neurology (2001) in its recently published practice guidelines (see reference at end of this chapter)
   a. According to the US Preventive Services Task Force (USPSTF), asking two simple questions about mood and anhedonia may be as effective as using longer instruments
   b. "Over the past 2 weeks, have you felt down, depressed, or hopeless?" and "Over the past 2 weeks have you felt little interest or pleasure in doing things?"
   c. Positive screening tests should trigger full diagnostic interview, using standard diagnostic criteria (e.g., those from the *DSM-IV*) [see section on DEPRESSION for more information]
13. Identify the primary caregiver and assess the adequacy of family and other support systems

B. Physical Examination
   1. Measure vital signs; take blood pressure with patient supine and standing
   2. Assess vision and hearing
   3. Perform complete physical examination, with focus on cardiovascular, respiratory, and neurological systems
      a. Assess the cranial nerves, the motor system, the sensory system, and reflexes (during early stage, motor, sensory, and cerebellar portions of the exam are usually normal)
      b. Assess mental status using the *DSM-IV* criteria (an example of how to do this is contained in the table that follows), the Clock Drawing Test (CDT), a tool which has experienced popularity in assessing patients for cognitive impairment (see in table that follows) or the Mini-Mental State Examination (MMSE) [also contained in a table that follows]

MENTAL STATUS EXAMINATION USING *DSM-IV* CRITERIA

Criteria	How to Test
Memory Hold Function	Ask patient to repeat 6 or 7 digits forward and 3 or 4 digits backward. (Normally, retention of this information is only a few seconds, so give patient opportunity to repeat immediately)
Recent Memory	• Ask patient to remember a short simple story consisting of no more than 4-5 sentences; ask patient to repeat the story to make certain the information has been properly understood and held
	• After a few minutes, ask patient to repeat what he/she was asked to remember; if patient cannot remember spontaneously (due to anxiety), give hints about the story to prompt memory
Remote Memory	Ask patient about significant national and international events in the past (asking about September 11 is a convenient way to test this function)
Aphasia	
Language Production	
Verbal	Ask patient to name body parts or objects in the room
Written	Hand patient a tablet and pencil and ask him/her to write one sentence describing what he/she is wearing
Language Comprehension	
Verbal	Ask patient to follow a simple verbal command such as "Walk over to the window"
Written	Write a simple request such as "Look into your purse (pocket)" on a tablet and hand to patient
Apraxia	Ask the patient to pantomime the use of a common object such as a hammer or a toothbrush ("Pretend your (index) finger is a toothbrush–show me how you would use it")
Agnosia	Ask the patient to close his/her eyes but to keep his arms relaxed. Then say, "I'm going to put something in the palm of each hand; move it around with your fingertips and thumb and tell me what you have." Place a quarter in one hand and a dime in the other. Almost all adults familiar with US coins can identify these items without looking at them
Disturbances in Executive Functioning	Ask the patient to perform a simple task such as "Walk over to the window, close the blinds, and then open the door to this room" which is a way to evaluate ability to plan, initiate, and sequence a task

Interpretation: To meet diagnostic criteria for dementia of the Alzheimer's type as set forth in *DSM-IV*, the patient must exhibit memory impairment in hold function, recent memory, or remote memory. In addition, patient must also exhibit at least one other cognitive disturbance (either aphasia, apraxia, agnosia, or disordered executive functioning)

CLOCK DRAWING TEST

Task:	Ask the patient to draw a clock with the hands indicating either 10 minutes after 11 or 20 minutes after 8
Scoring:	Give 1 point for each of the following: Closed circle; numbers in correct position; all 12 correct numbers; and hands in correct position
	A score <4 indicates the need for further evaluation

OVERVIEW OF THE MINI-MENTAL STATE EXAMINATION

Function	Test	Maximum Score
Orientation	✓ Ask date including year, season, date, day, month	5
	✓ Ask where presently located, including state, county, city	5
Registration	✓ Ask patient to repeat the name of three objects you have just named	3
	✓ (Example--bird, ring, boat)	
Attention and Calculation	✓ Ask the patient to begin with 100 and count backwards by 7 (stop after five subtractions); alternately ask to spell "world" backwards	5
Recall	✓ Ask patient to repeat the three objects named in Registration above	3
Language	✓ Point to familiar objects like clock and pencil; ask patient to name	2
	✓ Ask patient to repeat this sentence after you "No ifs, ands, or buts"	1
	✓ Direct patient to follow a 3-stage command "Take a paper in your right hand, fold it in half, and put it on the floor"	3
	✓ Ask patient to read and obey the following statement: "Close your eyes"	1
	✓ Ask patient to write a sentence; do not dictate sentence	1
	✓ Ask patient to copy a drawing of intersecting pentagons	1

Generally, a score of <23 indicates cognitive impairment, but this is only a crude indicator of functioning (a perfect score is 30)

Assess level of consciousness along a continuum from alert, to drowsy, to stupor, to coma

The Mini-Mental State Examination was developed by M.F. Folstein, S.E. Folstein, & P.R. McHugh. A copy of the instrument including instructions for administration and scoring is available in *Journal of Psychiatric Research* (1975), Volume 12, pp. 196-198

C. In interpreting the MMSE, keep in mind that normal scores on this questionnaire vary according to age and education; cognitive measures such as the MMSE are probably **most** useful in terms of measuring change over time in the same individual

D. Differential Diagnosis

Depression. Often mistaken for dementia; screening for depression should always be included in the initial assessment for dementia (see IV.A.12. above)

Delirium. Often difficult to differentiate from dementia because both are marked by global disturbances in cognition and the conditions may occur together
Clinical course of delirium is one in which features develop over a short period of time (usually hours to days) and there are significant fluctuations in degree of cognitive impairment over the course of the day
Person who develops sudden onset of cognitive impairment, disorientation, and perceptual disturbances (such as hallucinations) is likely to have delirium
Delirium is a medical emergency requiring immediate evaluation and treatment of the underlying cause, some of which can be fatal (e.g., bacterial meningitis or hypoglycemia)

Vascular (multi-infarct) dementia. Due to the effects of strokes on cognitive function; typically an abrupt onset and course within the context of cerebrovascular disease documented by history, focal neurological signs and symptoms and imaging studies

Dementia due to Parkinson's disease. Dementia associated with Parkinson's disease (a slowly progressive condition characterized by tremor, rigidity, and bradykinesia) has an insidious onset and slow progression; other signs and symptoms of Parkinson's are present

Dementia due to Pick's disease and other frontal lobe dementias. Characterized in early stages by changes in personality, executive dysfunction, deterioration of social skills (frontal lobe changes); difficult to distinguish clinically from atypical AD; brain imaging reveals prominent frontal and/or temporal atrophy with relative sparing of parietal and occipital lobes

Dementia associated with Lewy bodies (DLB). Disorder that is clinically similar to AD, but tends to have earlier and more prominent visual hallucinations and parkinsonian features, and a more rapid evolution; positive diagnosis requires both a finding of dementia and at least one of three core symptoms: detailed visual hallucinations, parkinsonian signs, and alterations of alertness or attention

Dementia due to other causes. A number of general medical conditions can cause dementia including structural lesions, head trauma, endocrine conditions, nutritional conditions, infectious conditions, and toxic effects of long-standing substance abuse, especially alcohol

---

E. Diagnostic Tests
   1. Structural neuroimaging with either a noncontrast CT or MR scan in the routine initial evaluation of patients with dementia is appropriate
      a. Use of neuroimaging examination allows for the detection of pathology such as brain neoplasms or subdural hematomas which may be responsive to treatment
      b. Normal pressure hydrocephalus may also be detected using structural neuroimaging but it is very rare
   2. Routine screening for selected comorbid conditions should also be part of the initial assessment for dementia; screen for the following comorbidities:
      a. Depression (see IV.A.12. above)
      b. B_{12} deficiency
      c. Hypothyroidism
   3. Screening for syphilis is not recommended unless the patient has some specific risk factors or evidence of prior syphilitic infection, or resides in one of the few areas in the US with high numbers of syphilis cases
   4. Additional **routine** screening (e.g., complete blood count, serum electrolytes, liver function tests, glucose, blood urea nitrogen/creatinine, folate) is not recommended
   5. Neuropsychological testing and evaluation should be performed on all patients in whom the diagnosis remains unclear after an initial assessment

V. Plan/Management

A. As soon as possible after AD has been diagnosed, a meeting with the patient and family should be held in which the following topics are addressed
   1. The diagnosis and education about the illness and its treatment
   2. Probable course of the illness

3. Comprehensive management plans based on needs, values, and preferences of the patient and family
   a. Patient and family need to be involved in development of the plan to the degree that they are willing to make decisions
   b. Management plan should be modified as the disease progresses in order to address emerging issues
4. Availability of support groups and educational resources (see table at end of section, RESOURCES FOR PATIENTS AND FAMILIES)

B. The overall goal of care for patients with AD is to improve quality of life for both the patient and family by maximizing the patient's cognition, behavior, and mood, thereby improving or at least maintaining his/her functional ability
   1. Pharmacologic therapies to temporarily slow progression of cognitive impairment, to manage behavioral problems associated with dementia, and to improve mood in patients with comorbid depression can have a significant impact on quality of life
   2. Nonpharmacologic therapies to modulate cognitive impairment, manage behavior, and improve mood are also important
   3. Interventions of various types for family members who are caregivers are crucial as nearly half of all caregivers become depressed

C. From a management standpoint, **early diagnosis** of AD has important consequences
   1. Patient and family are better able to cope with the disease once they are provided with information, can anticipate and plan for future medical, legal, and financial challenges, and have access to formal support services
   2. Cognition enhancing drugs are more likely to be effective early rather than late in the course of the illness when neurons become severely damaged

D. **Management of mildly impaired patients and their families**
   1. A major focus at this time is dealing with loss and the perceived stigma of the illness
   2. It is important to highlight remaining abilities while assisting with specific impairments
   3. Pharmacologic therapy with cognitive and functional enhancers should be instituted at this time (see recommendations below under V.G. and H.)
   4. Nonpharmacologic strategies may help manage cognitive deficits, decrease behavioral problems, and improve mood in the patient (see recommendations below under V.J. and K.)
   5. Patients with depressive symptoms may benefit from treatment with a selective serotonin reuptake inhibitor (SSRI) as described below under V.L.
   6. Risk of driving should always be discussed; there is no consensus on this issue, but concern for the safety of the patient and others should be discussed with recommendations on how to handle this situation (see V.M.2. below)

E. **Management of moderately impaired patients and their families**
   1. A major focus at this time is on keeping the patient safe and requires working closely with the family; patients in this stage are likely to require more supervision (see V.M. below)
   2. Another focus at this time is respite care for the caregiver; home healthcare or day care should be considered for part of the day so that the caregiver is not overburdened
   3. Families should begin to consider options for care including placement in a long-term care facility
   4. Suggest the nonpharmacologic strategies listed below, if not done previously
   5. Pharmacologic therapy with cognitive and functional enhancers should be instituted at this time, if not done previously
   6. Patients with depressive symptoms may benefit from treatment with a selective serotonin reuptake inhibitor (SSRI) as described below
   7. Patients with psychosis and agitation are best managed by a specialist

F. **Management of profoundly impaired patients and their families**
   1. At this stage, patients are almost completely dependent on others for help with the activities of daily living
   2. Families typically struggle greatly when a family member is in this stage of the disease
      a. Most caregivers benefit from a frank discussion of their feelings of grief, guilt, and resentment
      b. Families should be assisted in locating additional resources during this stage; hopefully, most families will already have been involved with support services prior to this stage

      c.   The decision to continue cognitive and functional enhancing medications at this time should be made on an individual basis

      d.   Patients in this category may require referral to a specialist for management

G.   **Pharmacologic treatment of cognitive deficits** with cholinesterase inhibitors can provide *modest improvement* of symptoms, temporary stabilization of cognition, or a slowing in the rate of cognitive decline in some patients with mild to moderate AD; some improvement in behavioral symptoms may also occur

    1.   Prior to initiation of this therapy, caution patient and family to expect only modest benefit with use of this class of drugs

    2.   Review dosing schedules, side effects, and need for follow up to determine efficacy of treatment with patient and family

    3.   Consult the table below for first-line cholinesterase inhibitors used in the treatment of cognitive deficits in patients with mild to moderate AD

FIRST-LINE CHOLINESTERASE INHIBITORS FOR THE TREATMENT OF COGNITIVE DEFICITS IN PATIENTS WITH MILD TO MODERATE ALZHEIMER'S DISEASE

Medication	Starting Dose	Increase Dose as Follows	Side Effects
Donepezil (Aricept)	5 mg once daily at bedtime	If necessary, dosage can be increased to 10 mg once daily after 4-6 weeks	✓ Mild side effects, including nausea, vomiting, and diarrhea; these effects can be reduced by taking donepezil with food ✓ Initial increase of agitation in some patients; agitation typically subsides after a few weeks
Rivastigmine (Exelon)	1.5 mg twice daily (3 mg per day)	If necessary, dosage can be increased as tolerated, but no more quickly than by 1.5 mg twice daily (3 mg per day) every 4 weeks to maximum of 6 mg twice daily (12 mg per day) Twice-daily dosing is as efficacious as thrice-daily dosing and has comparable tolerability	✓ Nausea, vomiting, diarrhea, headaches, dizziness, abdominal pain, fatigue, malaise, anxiety, and agitation; these effects can be reduced by taking rivastigmine with food
Galantamine (Reminyl)	4 mg twice daily (8 mg per day) taken with morning and evening meals for 4 weeks	After 4 weeks, increase dosage to 8 mg twice daily (16 mg per day) for at least 4 weeks. Based on clinical benefit and tolerability, an increase to 12 mg twice daily (24 mg per day) can be considered	✓ Mild side effects, including nausea, vomiting, and diarrhea; these effects can be reduced by taking galantamine with food ✓ No apparent association with sleep disturbances (which can occur with other cholinergic treatments)

Consult PDR for precautions, contraindications, interactions, and complete listing of adverse reactions for these three medications

Adapted from Cummings, J.L., et al. (2002) Guidelines for managing Alzheimer's disease: Part II. Treatment. *American Family Physician, 65*, 2527.

H.   **Pharmacologic treatment of cognitive deficits** with vitamin E (1000 IU) given orally twice a day should also be considered in an attempt to slow progression of AD; as another option, some patients may benefit from selegiline, 5 mg given orally twice a day (**Note:** Use vitamin E **or** selegiline; these agents should not be combined)

I.   Use of anti-inflammatory agents, prednisone, and estrogen to prevent the progression of AD is **not recommended** by the American Academy of Neurology (2001)

J.   **Nonpharmacologic management of cognitive deficits** may be helpful in stabilization of cognition in some patients and should be used in *addition* to treatment with cholinesterase inhibitors (and vitamin E or selegiline, if prescribed)

    1.   Graded assistance (a spectrum of assistance ranging from verbal prompts to physical demonstration, physical guidance, partial [advancing to complete] physical assistance aimed at providing the least amount of help possible) supplemented by practice and positive reinforcement has been shown to improve performance in ADLs in patients with dementia

    2.   Memory training, manual/creative activities, improving sensorimotor functions, and self-management therapy have also been demonstrated to be effective in some patients

    3.   Caregivers can help with memory and orientation through encouraging patient to read newspapers and watch television programs which are educational and help link the patient with the outside world

4. The use of frequent reminders about the content of conversations, if done in a kind way, can be very helpful to the patient in social situations
5. Important family events in which reminiscence by the patient is encouraged can be positive experiences for both the patient and family

K. **Nonpharmacologic management of problem behaviors** is usually beneficial in all patients with mild to moderate AD, and is summarized here
1. Encourage caregivers to modulate the environment, guided by the principle that patients with dementia are sensitive to their environments and often do best with moderate stimulation; too much stimulation may increase agitation and confusion while too little may lead to withdrawal
2. Familiar routines are comforting to the patient through promotion of a sense of security and predictability
3. Sensory stimulation of various types (auditory, visual, tactile) can improve mood
4. Low lighting levels, music (of the patient's choice), and simulated nature sounds may be calming to some patients
5. An exercise program should be instituted that includes outdoor daily walking if possible (**Note**: The role of daily exercise in the improvement of mood and behavior [appears to reduce wandering and agitation] is critically important and cannot be overemphasized)
6. Some research indicates that pet therapy can be very helpful in improving mood

L. **Pharmacologic management of comorbid depression** should be initiated in patients who have this mood disorder; treatment may also benefit some problem behaviors that are not adequately managed via other treatments already initiated
1. Use of selective serotonin reuptake inhibitors (SSRIs) are recommended because of their safety and tolerability; compared with other SSRIs, sertraline (Zoloft) has been reported to have less effect on metabolism of other medications
2. See section on DEPRESSION for dosing recommendations
3. Consult PDR for precautions, contraindications, interactions, and side effects

M. **Address safety concerns** with all patients and their families: Wandering and operating a motor vehicle are two of the most crucial safety issues and must be discussed soon after diagnosis
1. Wandering is a major safety concern as patients may become lost or injured
   a. Sedatives and antipsychotic medications do not prevent wandering (unless patient is markedly oversedated; such an approach should not be used to control this behavior)
   b. The best approach is to provide a safe environment so the patient can wander at will; caregiver-supervised daily exercise is also important to reduce wandering
   c. All wandering patients should wear an ID bracelet or anklet and be enrolled in the Alzheimer's Association Safe Return Program (Safe Return, Box A-3956, Chicago, IL 60690)
2. Advancing AD in persons who drive is correlated with a higher risk of traffic accidents; driving an automobile is very risky and should be discontinued early in the disease
   a. Many states encourage healthcare clinicians to report persons who have conditions that may affect their ability to drive safely
   b. California is the only state with a specific public policy requiring the reporting of persons with AD
   c. Pennsylvania requires reporting of persons with any disorder that would impair their ability to drive
   d. Know the requirements in your state

N. Unfortunately, patients with AD are sometimes victims of **abuse or neglect**
1. Assess patient for abuse/neglect on each visit (see DOMESTIC VIOLENCE: ELDER ABUSE for details)
2. Reporting requirements and procedures for elder abuse can be found at www.elderabusecenter.org which provides links to individual states

O. **Interventions for caregivers** are crucially important and include **education, support, and respite care**; interventions aimed at caregivers may delay nursing home placement for patients
1. Refer the caregiver to comprehensive, psychoeducational caregiver training, if available
2. Provide the caregiver with information about support groups in the area and telephone support groups if patient is unable to attend meetings of support groups on a regular schedule
3. Give caregiver information about adult day care for patients and other respite services in the area (including availability, services, and costs)

4. For caregivers with computers and internet access, suggest the use of computer networks to provide education and support to caregivers
5. Reassess the stress level and psychological well-being of the caregiver at every visit (every 3-6 months)
6. Refer to table below for listing of resources

P. A discussion of **advance directives** should be initiated at some point early in the disease so that the patient/family will have an opportunity to determine some important issues such as the following
1. Durable power of attorney
2. Estate management
3. Advance directives for management of terminal stage of disease
4. Appointment of surrogates to make medical, financial, and legal decisions at the point when patient becomes incompetent

Q. Follow Up
1. Regular patient monitoring is important and should be at least every 2-4 weeks in early management to titrate medication dosage
2. Once patient's medication regimen is stable, follow-up every 3-6 months to determine if clinical benefit is being achieved. Reassess patient in the five areas of functioning: ADLs, IADLs, cognition, comorbid medical and mood disorders to determine efficacy of nonpharmacologic and pharmacologic interventions
3. Assess caregiver status and refer for support/counseling as indicated

---

SELECTED RESOURCES FOR PATIENTS WITH AD AND THEIR FAMILIES

Books

Keeping Busy: A Handbook of Activities for Persons with Dementia. Dowling JR. Johns Hopkins University Press; 1995

Living in the Labyrinth: A Personal Journey through the Maze of Alzheimer's. McGowin DF. Dell Publishing Company; 1994

The Loss of Self: A Family Resource for the Care of Alzheimer's Disease & Related Disorders. Revised edition. Cohen D, Eisdorfer C. Norton; 2001

Share the Car: How to Organize a Group to Care for Someone Who is Seriously Ill. Capossela C, Warnock S. Simon & Schuster; 1995

Tangled Minds: Understanding Alzheimer's Disease and Other Dementias. Gillick MR, Gallick M. Plume; 1999

The 36-Hour Day: A Family Guide to Caring for Patients with Alzheimer's Disease. Revised edition, Mace NL, Rabins PV, McHugh PR. Warner Books; 1992

Understanding Difficult Behaviors: Some Practical Suggestions for Coping With Alzheimer's Disease and Related Illnesses. Robinson A, Spencer B, White L (eds). Available through the Alzheimer's Program, PO Box 994, Ann Arbor MI 48106, or by calling 313-712-1339

The Vanishing Mind. White J, Heston L W.H. Freeman & Co; 1991

Journals

Alzheimer's Disease Review. A quarterly publication on the Internet. http://www.coa.uky.edu/ADReview

Agencies and Organizations

Alzheimer's Disease and Related Disorders Association, Inc.
919 N. Michigan Avenue, Suite 1000
Chicago IL 60611-1676   312-335-8700   Fax: 312-335-1110
Hotline for referrals, information, problem solving, and counseling assistance: 800-272-3900
Website: http://www.alz.org
The national organization provides educational material and other information on Alzheimer's and related disorders. Local chapters can help direct caregivers to local services for AD patients, and some provide respite and day-care services.

Alzheimer's Disease Education and Referral Center (ADEAR)
The ADEAR Center
Box 8250
Silver Spring MD 20907-8250
301-495-3311   Fax: 301-495-3334
Website: http://www.alzheimers.org   E-mail: adear@alzheimers.org
Sponsored by the National Institute on Aging, ADEAR acts as a national clearinghouse for information on AD, drug treatment, and new research. It can direct families to support services and does free literature searches for healthcare professionals

Local Area Agencies on Aging
These agencies have guidebooks listing local support services and residential settings for older adults. For the nearest Area Agency on Aging, consult the phone book or call the Eldercare Locator at 800-677-1116.

National Council on the Aging   National Institute on Aging
409 3rd Street SW, Suite 200   31 Center Drive
Washington DC 20024   Bethesda MD 20892
202-479-1200 Fax: 202-479-0735   800-438-4380 or 301-496-1752

(Continued)

DIZZINESS

I.   Definition: Various abnormal sensations relating to perceptions of the body's position or motion in relation to the environment

II.   Pathogenesis

    A.   There are four subtypes of dizziness–vertigo, presyncopal lightheadedness, disequilibrium, and other dizziness (does not fit into the first three categories)

    B.   **Vertigo:** Sensation that the body or environment is moving, usually spinning
        1.   Suggests disorder of the vestibular system
        2.   Systemic causes of vertigo and dizziness include certain drugs, infectious disease, endocrine disease, and vasculitis

    C.   **Presyncope:** Feeling of lightheadedness that produces the sensation of an impending faint; occurs episodically, and usually caused by diffuse temporary cerebral ischemia

    D.   **Disequilibrium:** Sense of imbalance or postural instability generally described as involving legs/trunk without a sensation in the head
        1.   Isolated symptoms of disequilibrium are usually due to some type of neurologic disorder–multiple sensory deficits are the most common cause
        2.   Imbalance that accompanies other types of dizziness is most often a secondary rather than a primary symptom

    E.   **Other dizziness:** A vague feeling of floating (patients often have difficulty describing this sensation)
        1.   Often caused by psychological disorders and often accompanied by other somatic symptoms such as headache or abdominal pain
        2.   Also, a distinct though rare form of dizziness is in this category–ocular dizziness due to rapid vision change (e.g., cataract surgery) or to a change in corrective lenses

III.   Clinical Presentation

    A.   Dizziness occurs in all age groups and is more common in women than in men

    B.   Patients who seek treatment for a complaint of "dizziness" are more likely to be in the older age groups (whereas persons younger than 65 frequently experience dizziness, they are less likely than their older counterparts to actually seek treatment for the complaint)

    C.   Many patients, particularly those >65 years of age, are unable to place their symptom of dizziness in one category; this is especially true with disequilibrium which often accompanies other kinds of dizziness and distinguishing between the primary symptom and the secondary disequilibrium if often very difficult

    D.   Critical diagnoses (conditions that can be life threatening) that clinicians must not overlook in patients who present with dizziness are listed in the table below (**Note**: Patients with acute forms of dizziness are more likely to have life-threatening illnesses than are those with chronic forms)

Acute ischemic heart disease
Acute infection (such as pneumonia)
Cardiac arrhythmia
Gastrointestinal bleeding
Intracranial mass lesion (e.g., acoustic neuroma, subdural hematoma)
Neurosyphilis
Stroke
Transient ischemic attack
Toxic exposure (e.g., anthrax, carbon monoxide poisoning)

E. **Vertigo**: About 50% of patients who present to primary care settings with a complaint of dizziness have true vertigo due to either vestibular or nonvestibular causes
   1. Vestibular problems may be **peripheral** (very common) or **central** (uncommon)
       a. Peripheral vestibular causes of vertigo are problems or conditions affecting labyrinthine structures or the vestibular nerve
       b. Central vestibular causes of vertigo are a manifestation of progressive disease of the central nervous system
   2. Nonvestibular causes of vertigo are also very common with infection, metabolic problems, and adverse effects of drugs being predominant causes

F. **Vertigo: Peripheral vestibular causes of vertigo** are characterized by isolated vertigo (i.e., without associated signs and symptoms, with the exception of tinnitus or hearing loss that is common in Ménière's syndrome). Commonly occurring peripheral vestibular problems are the following
   1. Benign paroxysmal positional vertigo (BPPV) is the most common type of vertigo and is caused by free-floating particulate matter, usually in a posterior semicircular canal, that moves within the canal with certain head movements by the patient, thereby disturbing the vestibular sensory receptors and producing vertigo
       a. Patients typically complain that position changes (lying down, rising from a recumbent position, rolling over in bed, looking up while standing, or bending forward) cause an abrupt onset of transient vertigo that always lasts less than a minute, and then resolves when the head is returned to a neutral position; may recur throughout the day
       b. Patients typically do not report tinnitus or hearing loss, but may have associated nausea and vomiting during episodes of dizziness
       c. A common problem in the elderly who often feel slightly unsteady between episodes
       d. Even though this is a "benign" disorder, can impair quality of life especially in the elderly as it often becomes chronic (may resolve in 6 months in many patients)
   2. Ménière's syndrome is believed to be caused by endolymphatic hydrops manifested by excess fluid in the cochlea and vestibular labyrinth
       a. Patients typically complain of a feeling of fullness in the ear, hearing loss, roaring tinnitus, and vertigo that is unrelated to position change
       b. Episodes are paroxysmal, last minutes to hours; tinnitus and sensorineural hearing loss often persist; over time, hearing loss which is initially reversible, becomes permanent
       c. In about 75% of cases, symptoms are unilateral
   3. Acute labyrinthitis (or vestibular neuronitis which is believed to be the same disorder without any cochlear involvement) is caused by a viral infection involving the cochlea and labyrinth
       a. Patients typically report a recent upper respiratory syndrome that was followed by onset of vertigo, tinnitus, and hearing loss (patients with vestibular neuronitis do not experience hearing loss or tinnitus–only vertigo)
       b. Usual course is for symptoms to resolve completely in 3 to 6 weeks with no sequelae

G. **Vertigo: Central vestibular causes of vertigo** are uncommon and include brainstem ischemia and infarction, intrinsic brainstem lesions, cerebellopontine angle tumor such as acoustic neurinoma, and demyelinating disease such as multiple sclerosis
   1. Patients with central vestibular disorders typically present with vertigo in association with other brainstem deficits
   2. Commonly associated neurologic symptoms and signs include diplopia and focal sensory or motor deficits

H. **Vertigo: Nonvestibular causes of vertigo** include the following
   1. Many patients with a systemic viral or bacterial infection present with dizziness, which is most likely due to postural hypotension (these patients most often experience presyncope rather than true vertigo)
   2. Metabolic problems such as hypoglycemia, hyperglycemia, electrolyte disturbances, thyrotoxicosis and anemia can cause dizziness
   3. A wide variety of drugs can cause vertigo/dizziness; examples are anticonvulsants, hypnotics, antihypertensives, alcohol, analgesics, and tranquilizers

I. **Presyncope:** Cardiac and vascular insufficiency and the resultant inadequate cerebral perfusion can cause dizziness; patients often report feeling "light-headed"
   1. Patients typically report a worsening of symptoms with standing and an improvement with lying down
   2. Postural changes in blood pressure and pulse are characteristic
   3. Patients have a history of underlying heart disease
   4. See section on PRESYNCOPE/SYNCOPE for a discussion of this topic

J. **Disequilibrium:** Multiple sensory deficits are the most common cause in this type of dizziness that patients describe as a feeling of "unsteadiness on the feet"
   1. Patients with multiple sensory deficits are usually elderly and have conditions such as diabetes mellitus that impair eyesight, sense of position, and sensory and motor function
   2. Sense of imbalance may come on with standing and can be aggravated by walking or turning
   3. Typically, symptoms worsen in the dark–because of elimination of visual positional input–and improve with use of a cane or holding onto a railing
   4. Such patients often have a history of falling

K. **Other dizziness:** Most often caused by psychological disturbances such as anxiety states, depression, or psychosis or the medications used to treat these disorders; a rare cause is ocular dizziness due to a rapid vision change
   1. Dizziness is usually ill-defined and is unrelated to position change; there is no history of underlying heart disease or conditions that would cause multiple sensory deficits
   2. Precise mechanism of the dizziness is unknown, but is believed to be related to the confusional state induced by the illnesses or by the medications used to treat them
   3. Hyperventilation can produce metabolic alkalosis, causing patients to experience light-headedness, and paresthesias

L. Most acute dizziness-related conditions are self-limited and most chronic dizziness-related conditions are generally benign; however, many patients with chronic dizziness that is considered benign report great impairment of daily activities, depressed mood, and symptom-related fears

IV. Diagnosis/Evaluation

   A. History
      1. Ask patient to describe in a few words the sensation he/she experiences; if patient's description is too vague, prompt with the following questions
         a. "Do you feel like you or the room is spinning around?" (a positive response favors vertigo)
         b. "Do you feel like you might black out?" (a positive response favors presyncope)
         c. "Do you feel unsteady on your feet, like you are about to lose your balance?" (a positive response favors disequilibrium)
      2. Guided by the patient's response, determine which of the subtypes of dizziness the patient is experiencing; determine if the symptoms are severe, moderate, or mild and ask what makes the symptoms better or worse
      3. Determine how often the dizziness occurs and what makes the dizziness better or worse
      4. Ask about associated symptoms; specifically ask about nausea and vomiting, and about auditory symptoms such as hearing impairment, tinnitus (whether pulsatile or constant), history of ear infections, sensation of aural pressure
      5. Ask about associated neurologic symptoms that suggest a central cause of dizziness; specifically ask if there is diplopia, facial numbness, weakness/numbness in arms or legs, confusion, slurring of speech, difficulty swallowing
      6. Ask appropriate questions to rule out metabolic disturbances reported to cause dizziness (Note: Beyond the scope of this book to cover this in detail)
      7. Determine if patient has (or is recovering from) a viral or bacterial infection that can present with dizziness
      8. Determine if patient has recently had cataract surgery or a change in a corrective prescription

9. Ask appropriate questions relating to the critical diagnoses listed in the box above under III.D. (Note: Beyond the scope of this book to cover this in detail)
10. Obtain past medical history including past episodes of dizziness, trauma, and risk factors for cardiovascular disease such as smoking, diabetes, hypertension, or hyperlipidemia; ask if history of falls
11. Obtain complete medication history including over the counter products and alternative therapies to determine if dizziness is drug-related

B. Physical Examination
1. Evaluation of an undifferentiated symptom such as dizziness is difficult; the steps in the physical examination below are considered most important but are not all inconclusive; findings from the history should also guide the physical examination
2. Measure vital signs; assess for orthostatic hypotension (see section on PRESYNCOPE/SYNCOPE for measurement procedure)
3. Perform a complete ear examination
4. Auscultate neck for carotid bruits
5. Perform a complete cardiovascular exam to rule out conditions that can be life threatening
6. Do a careful neurological examination to rule out multiple sensory deficits as well as conditions that can be life threatening
   a. Test sensory function, peripheral vision, and gait
   b. Test cranial nerves (**Note**: Any cranial nerve abnormality suggests a serious cause for dizziness)
   c. Test cerebellar function (tandem gait or heel-to-toe walking) and perform the Romberg test (patient stands upright with feet close together and arms folded across chest with eyes open and then closed–minimal movement or sway is normal finding)
7. Symptom reproduction with hyperventilation may be helpful if suggested by history

C. Differential Diagnosis
1. The major challenge is identifying critical diagnoses (those that are life threatening)
2. Vestibular versus nonvestibular causes (see III.E. through H. above)

D. Diagnostic Tests
1. Cost of diagnostic testing to evaluate an undifferentiated symptom such as dizziness can be great; history and physical examination should guide test selection; consultation with an expert may be warranted
2. Hearing and stimulation of the vestibular apparatus can be performed in the office and may be helpful in differentiating among the vestibular diseases
   a. If patient reports hearing loss, Weber and Rinne tests help to differentiate between conductive and sensorineural hearing loss (see section on HEARING LOSS for details on testing and interpretation); perform office audiometry if available or refer for audiometric testing
   b. Conduct the Dix-Hallpike test to help in establishing the diagnosis of BPPV (see Figure 18.1 below for illustration, description, and interpretation of the test)

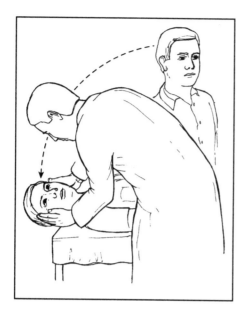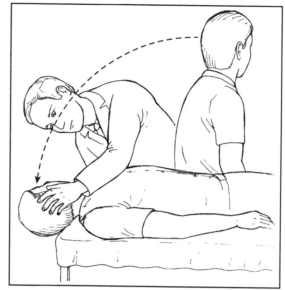

Figure 18.1. Dix-Hallpike Test

Performing the Test

✓ First, ask the patient which ear or side of head is likely to trigger dizziness (patient cannot always identify)

✓ Then, with the patient seated on the examination table, maneuver him rapidly from a sitting to a supine position with his head turned to the unaffected side as identified by the patient, and hanging over the edge of the examination table (see illustration)

✓ Symptoms should not be elicited when this initial maneuver is performed with unaffected side facing downward

✓ Next, return the patient to an upright, seated position, and repeat the maneuver with the presumed involved ear facing downward--called the provocative position (see illustration)

✓ After a delay of a few seconds, patients in the provocative position with BPPV will experience vertigo and torsional (upward and lateral) nystagmus beating toward the lower ear and lasting 10-20 seconds

✓ If this procedure is repeated, the vertigo and nystagmus will often diminish in severity (called fatigability)

Interpretation

A positive test favors a diagnosis of BPPV; however, because of the paroxysmal and fatigable nature of this disorder, patients with a history suggestive of BPPV may not exhibit vertigo and nystagmus at the time of the maneuver; thus a negative test does not rule out the diagnosis

V.   Plan/Management

    A.   Patients with a history and physical examination suggesting a life-threatening diagnosis should be immediately referred for emergent care

    B.   Management of patients with acute onset of dizziness that interferes with ability to function (but is not life-threatening) and with a cause not immediately identifiable should be referred to a specialty setting for urgent management

    C.   Management of patients with acute onset of dizziness due to an identifiable cause such as infection, metabolic problems, and adverse effects of drugs should be focused on correcting the underlying problem; short-term use of an antivertiginous drug may be helpful (see V.F. below)

    D.   Patients with a presumed diagnosis of BPPV should be referred to an otolaryngologist for further evaluation and for treatment with two specific maneuvers
        1.   Epley maneuver, a very effective physical maneuver that can be performed in the office that works by relocating free-floating debris from the posterior semicircular canal into the vestibule of the vestibular labyrinth, where it no longer causes problems with dizziness. Usually eliminates symptoms after being performed once
        2.   Positional exercises that the patient can be taught to perform at home; such exercises often lead to remission within 2 weeks but usually must be continued for many months

    E.   Patients with Ménière's disease are usually managed with salt restriction and diuretics; these patients are best referred to an otolaryngologist for further evaluation and management as permanent hearing loss can occur

F. Prolonged use of antivertiginous drugs for a vestibular disorder is not recommended as these drugs may delay adaptation of the central nervous system to a peripheral vestibular disorder; one of the following may be prescribed on a short-term basis
   1. Meclizine (Antivert) 12.5-25 PO QD or TID with dosage tapered as symptoms improve
   2. Dimenhydrinate (Dramamine) 50 mg PO, Q 4-6 hours

G. Patients with multiple sensory deficits or cerebellar dysfunction causing disequilibrium may benefit from gait training and vestibular exercises under the supervision of a trained therapist

H. Patients with psychogenic lightheadedness should be treated for the appropriate underlying cause; however, these patients frequently have significant comorbidity and disability and require an interdisciplinary evaluation; therefore, they are best referred for expert evaluation and management

I. For motion sickness, prescribe scopolamine transdermal patch (Transderm Scop) 1 disc applied behind ear at least 4 hours prior to travel; patch should be removed and replaced after 72 hours

J. Follow Up: Variable depending on diagnosis and whether the patient was referred for evaluation and management

HEADACHE

I. Definition: Diffuse pain in various parts of the head with the pain not confined to the area of distribution of a nerve

II. Pathogenesis

A. Primary headaches are caused by traction on pain sensitive structures, inflammation of vessels and meninges, vascular dilation, excessive muscle contraction, and dysregulation of the ascending brain stem serotonergic system

B. Secondary headaches are due to an underlying organic cause; fewer than 2% of patients in office and 4% of patients in emergency department settings will be found to have headaches secondary to significant pathology

III. Clinical Presentation of Primary Headache

A. The lifetime prevalence of headaches is more than 90%
   1. Nearly 25% of US adults report recurrent episodes of severe headache and 4% report daily or almost daily headache
   2. Prescription or non-prescription products are used by 9% of US adults each week, and equals that of hypertension as the primary reason for medication use

B. Recurrent headaches provoke visits to the primary care clinician when they are debilitating, frequent, or associated with worrisome symptoms

C. Primary headache disorders—migraine, tension-type, and cluster—are usually acute-recurrent and have no underlying disease process as their cause; descriptions of the three types of primary headache are contained in the box that follows

	Migraine	*Tension-type*	*Cluster*
Patient population	More common in females; episodes often begin in adolescence or early adulthood but are quite common in childhood beginning as early as age 5-6 years; often remit by age 50	Most common headache type, occurs in both genders and all age groups (in children, most commonly begins between 8-12 years of age)	More common in men (mean age of onset in late 20s); incidence diminishes with age; compared with migraine and tension-type headache, an uncommon form of primary headache
Family history	Positive	Negative	Negative
Typical time of onset	Any time of day	Later in the day	Frequently nocturnal, waking patient from sleep
Untreated duration	4 to 72 hours	30 minutes to 7 days	15 minutes to 3 hours
Characteristics	Often unilateral, throbbing head pain that is made worse by movement and physical activity	Bilateral, often slowly progressing, non-throbbing, mild to moderate pain; patient may complain of dull pressure or band-like sensation about head; physical activity does not worsen pain	Unilateral, severe, sharp, orbital, supraorbital, or temporal pain always on the same side. Distinctive temporal pattern of grouped attacks recurring over weeks or months
Associated symptoms	Nausea, vomiting, phonophobia, and photophobia	Usually none; the least distinct of the primary headache types because of the absence of associated features	At least one of the following is present on the headache side: lacrimation, conjunctival injection, nasal congestion, ptosis or eyelid swelling, and rhinorrhea
Comments	Women often report relationship between migraine and menses, with remission after menopause. Two categories: *Migraine with aura* (only about 15% of patients have this type) such as visual prodromes [flashing lights, zigzags], strange odors, or paresthesias; previously known as classic migraine. *Migraine without aura*; (most patients have this type) previously known as common migraine	Affects up to 80% of adults and accounts for more than one half of headache patients who present to primary care settings; compared with migraine headache, tension-type receives little attention in the medical literature. Rarely requires healthcare visit given the typical absence of disabling or concerning symptoms	Attacks may occur once a day or as frequently as 8 times/day; duration may be as short as 15 minutes or last more than 3 hours; occur in bouts which may last days to weeks; most patients experience one bout per year. Due to its low population prevalence, cluster headache is infrequently encountered in primary care

IV. Diagnosis/Evaluation

    A.   History (**Note:** This approach assumes the patient presents with an acute headache; if patient presents for evaluation of acute-recurrent headaches, but is not experiencing attack at time of presentation, modify history questions accordingly)

        1.   Ask patient when headache began and if onset was gradual or sudden; ask how often headaches occur

        2.   Ask where pain is located and if the pain seems to spread to any other area; if yes, determine where; ask patient to describe the pain (throbbing, stabbing, dull, other)

        3.   Ask patient to rate pain on a scale from 1 to 10 with 1 being no pain at all and 10 being the worst pain ever experienced)

        4.   Ask if this is first or worst headache (see Red Flags in table below)

        5.   Ask if headaches occur on a regular basis and if this headache is like the ones that he/she usually has or is it different; if different, ask how

        6.   Question about associated symptoms: Ask, "What symptoms do you have before the headache starts? What symptoms do you have during the headache? What symptoms are you having now?"

        7.   Ask about precipitating factors such as stress, diet, caffeine intake, physical exertion, sleep problems, or menses

        8.   Inquire about prescription and over-the-counter medication use (especially caffeine-containing analgesics); determine the frequency of medication use

        9.   Obtain past medical history and determine if any concurrent medical conditions are present

      10.   Ask about previous trauma to the head and any medical or dental procedures

      11.   Document family medical history, especially history of migraine headaches

      12.   Explore present and previous treatments and responses to treatments including prescription, over-the-counter medications, herbal remedies, and home remedies

      13.   Determine impact of headaches on patient's quality of life and daily functioning (for migraineurs, get a quick but accurate estimate about impact of temporary disability via use of the *Migraine Disability Assessment Scale (MIDAS)*, a well-validated five-item scale that is easy to use in clinical practice (for source, see Stewart et al., 1999, in reference list or access more information on MIDAS at www.migraine-disability.net)

B. Physical Examination
 1. Keep in mind that the main purpose of the examination is to identify causes of secondary headache
 2. Observe general appearance, noting signs of acute distress, anxiety, or depression
 3. Measure blood pressure, pulse, pulse pressure
 4. Palpate head and face, focusing on temporal arteries for tenderness (adults) [patients with temporal arteritis have firm, tender, enlarged arteries], sinuses, and temporomandibular joint (TMJ); examine mouth and teeth for signs of inflammation/trauma/infection
 5. Perform ophthalmoscopic assessment
 6. Perform cardiovascular assessment
 7. Perform complete neurological exam including mental status, level of consciousness, cranial nerve testing (with particular attention to detecting problems related to the optic, oculomotor, trochlear, and abducens nerves–cranial nerves II III, IV, and VI, respectively), pupillary responses, motor strength testing, deep tendon reflexes, sensation, reflexes (e.g., Babinski's sign), cerebellar function, gait testing, and signs of meningeal irritation

C. Differential Diagnosis
 1. Whereas a minority of headaches are secondary, diagnoses in this category are the most life-threatening and **must not** be missed
 2. Consult table below—Red Flags for Secondary Headache Disorders

RED FLAGS FOR SECONDARY HEADACHE DISORDERS

Red Flag	Differential Diagnosis
New onset headache beginning after age 50	Temporal arteritis, mass lesion
Sudden onset of severe headache "worst headache in life"	Subarachnoid hemorrhage, mass lesion, hemorrhage into a mass lesion or vascular malformation
Headaches increasing in frequency and severity (change or progression in headache pattern)	Mass lesion, subdural hematoma, medication overuse (rebound headache)
New-onset headache in a patient with immunosuppression, cancer, or pregnancy	Meningitis, brain abscess, metastasis
Headache with signs of systemic illness (fever, stiff neck, rash)	Meningitis, encephalitis, Lyme disease, systemic infection, collagen vascular disease
Neurological signs or symptoms of disease lasting >1 hour (other than typical aura)	Mass lesion, vascular malformation, stroke, collagen vascular disease
Headache triggered by exertion, sexual activity, or Valsalva maneuver	TIA, stroke
Headache associated with alteration in or loss of consciousness	Intracranial hemorrhage, subdural hematoma, epidural hematoma, post-traumatic headache

D. Diagnostic Tests
 1. If there is a likelihood of intracranial pathology based on abnormal findings on neurologic examination that are unexplained, the patient should be referred to a neurologist for further evaluation and possible neuroimaging
 2. Random use of laboratory testing in the evaluation of headache is not warranted; if there is diagnostic uncertainty (clinician is unable to classify patient's headache as primary or secondary, or is uncertain about type of primary), referral to a headache subspecialist is recommended

V. Plan/Management

A. Management of patients with primary headache—migraine, tension, or cluster—is outlined below, beginning with management of patients with migraine headache

B. Goals of long-term migraine treatment, both nonpharmacologic and pharmacologic, are to (1) reduce attack frequency, severity, and patient disability, (2) reduce patient reliance on poorly tolerated or ineffective medications, and (3) improve quality of life

C. The initial step, after establishing a diagnosis, is to educate the patient about his/her condition and its treatment
 1. Provide a brief overview of what the problem is and how it can best be managed
 2. Refer patient to web sites that may be helpful

D. Create a formal management plan with the patient in order to implement preventive and/or acute episodic therapy for migraine; treatment choice depends on several factors
   1. Frequency/severity of attacks
   2. Presence and degree of temporary disability
   3. Associated symptoms such as nausea and vomiting

E. General proactive counseling for all patients with migraine headache includes the following
   1. Encourage patient to keep a headache diary to assist in identifying precipitating events and risk factors and for tracking progress of treatment approaches
   2. Encourage the patient to identify and avoid triggers (examples are provided in the box below)

Common Migraine Triggers

- ✓ Disrupted sleep (not enough sleep/sleeping later than usual)
- ✓ Skipped meals
- ✓ Consumption of certain foods: Common triggers are cheese, chocolate, citrus fruits, foods containing nitrates (contained in some processed meats) and monosodium glutamate
- ✓ Alcoholic beverages (adults), especially red wine
- ✓ Stress
- ✓ Caffeine overuse (soft drinks and coffee) as well as caffeine withdrawal

---

F. Determine if patient is a candidate for preventive therapy for migraine headaches

---

Candidates for Preventive Therapy

Institution of preventive therapy should be considered for patients who:
- ✓ Have recurrent headaches that interfere with daily functioning despite treatment for acute attacks
- ✓ Exhibit a trend toward an increasing frequency of attacks as documented by patient in migraine diary
- ✓ Have contraindications to or adverse effects from acute therapy
- ✓ Experience failure/overuse of acute therapy

Rule of Thumb
If headaches occur 1-2 days per month, preventive therapy is usually not needed
If occurrence is 3-4 days per month or more, preventive therapy should be seriously considered

---

G. **Nonpharmacologic therapies for the prevention of migraine** are contained in the box that follows

---

Nonpharmacologic Preventive Therapy

These therapies may be best suited to patients who have a poor tolerance of, or poor response to drug therapy, who have contraindications to drug therapy, who have a past history or excessive use of analgesics, and for patents who are pregnant (planning to become pregnant), or nursing
- ✓ Relaxation training
- ✓ Thermal biofeedback combined with relaxation training
- ✓ Electromyographic (EMG) biofeedback
- ✓ Cognitive-behavioral therapy

H. **Drugs for treatment of migraine** can be divided into **two classes**
   1. Drugs that are taken daily whether or not headache is present to reduce the severity of attack (called preventive therapy)
   2. Drugs that are taken to treat attacks as they arise

I. **Drugs used to prevent migraine (preventive therapy)** are contained in the table that follows
   1. Initiate therapy with the lowest effective dose of the drug and increase it slowly until clinical benefits are achieved
   2. Take coexisting conditions into account; select a drug that will treat both the coexisting condition and migraine, if possible

3. Counsel patient that the prescribed medication must be given an adequate trial and that it may take 2-3 months to achieve clinical benefit

SELECTED RECOMMENDED DRUGS FOR USE IN PREVENTION OF MIGRAINE

Select one of the following:

Class/Drug	Dose	Selected Side Effects
β-Blockers		Reduced energy, tiredness, postural symptoms, contraindicated in patients with asthma
Propranolol	40-120 mg twice daily	
Timolol	10-15 mg twice daily	
Anticonvulsants		Drowsiness, weight gain, tremor, hair loss, hematologic/liver abnormalities
Divalproex sodium	400-600 mg twice daily	
Antidepressants		
Amitriptyline	25-75 mg at bedtime	Drowsiness

Adapted from Silberstein, S.D. for the US Headache Consortium. Report of the Quality Standards Subcommittee of the American Academy of Neurology. (2000). Practice parameter: Evidenced-based guidelines for migraine headache (an evidence-based review). *Neurology, 55*, p. 758.

J. **Drugs used for the acute treatment of migraine** are contained in the table that follows
   1. The approach outlined in the table is based on the stratified care model (treatment intensity is matched to headache disability) versus step care (agent selection based on cost) or staged care (milder first-line and stronger second-line agents)
   2. Efficacy of acute treatment is determined by correct choice of medication as well as the timing of intervention; most experts recommend limiting acute therapies to 2 days/week to avoid medication-overuse headache
   3. Early intervention at the outset of the headache (when pain is mild) can abort headache in most cases within 2 to 4 hours with lower headache recurrence
   4. During migraine attacks, the oral absorption of many drugs is delayed; thus, consideration should be given to use of nonoral routes with quicker onset of action

SELECTED RECOMMENDED DRUGS FOR ACUTE TREATMENT OF MIGRAINE USING THE STRATIFIED CARE MODEL

Patients with **mild to moderate headache** often respond well to **nonspecific** therapy
   ✓ Ibuprofen (Motrin, generic), 400-800 mg/dose PO Q 6 hours as needed; maximum 3200 mg/day
   ✓ Acetaminophen, aspirin, plus caffeine (Excedrin Migraine), 2 tabs PO Q 6 hours as needed; maximum 8 tabs a day for 2 days
Patients with **moderate to severe headache** often require **specific** therapy; select a nonoral route of administration for patients with associated nausea or vomiting

Class/Drug	Dosing
Serotonin receptor agonists (triptans)	
Eletriptan (Relpax)	20-40 mg PO initially; may repeat after 2 hours, max 80 mg/day
Rizatriptan (Maxalt)	5-10 mg PO initially; available in orally-disintegrating tabs (Maxalt MLT); may repeat after 2 hours, max 30 mg/day; if taking a β-blocker, use 5 mg per maximal dose up to 15 mg/day
Sumatriptan (Imitrex), available as PO, SC, IN	Oral Dose: 25-100 mg PO initially; may repeat after 2 hours, max 200 mg/day SC Dose: 6 mg SC initially; may repeat once after 1 hour, max 12 mg/day Nasal Spray Dose: 20 mg spray nasally; may repeat once after 2 hours, max 40 mg/day
Zolmitriptan (Zomig),	1.25-2.5 mg PO initially; may repeat after 2 hours, max 10 mg day
Ergot alkaloids and derivatives	
Dihydroergotamine [DHE] (Migranal) Nasal spray	0.5 mg/spray 1 spray in each nostril; may repeat in 15 minutes, max 4 sprays per 24 hours and 8/week

Use of antiemetics should not be restricted to patients who are vomiting or likely to vomit as nausea in and of itself is a very disabling symptom (consult section on NAUSEA AND VOMITING for drug selection and dosing recommendations)

Adapted from Silberstein, S.D. for the US Headache Consortium. Report of the Quality Standards Subcommittee of the American Academy of Neurology. (2000). Practice parameter: Evidenced-based guidelines for migraine headache (an evidence-based review). *Neurology, 55*, p. 759 and Abramowicz, M. (2003). Triptans for migraine. *The Medical Letter, 45*, pp. 33-36.

K.   Follow up for patients with migraine headache
1.   Monitor trends in headache frequency, severity, and response to therapies (both preventive and acute pharmacologic therapy) via a headache diary kept by patient and reviewed on every follow up visit (every 2-4 weeks in first 3 months, then every 3-6 months)
2.   If after 3-6 months, headaches are well controlled with preventive therapy, consider tapering or discontinuing treatment

L.   Referral considerations
1.   Patients who do not respond to (or fail) treatments outlined above for moderate to severe migraine should be referred to an expert for management
2.   Patients who prefer nonpharmacologic treatments (e.g., behavioral treatments [see V.G. above] or complementary therapies such as acupuncture and cervical manipulation) should be referred to experts in these modalities for management
3.   Patients with migraine headache and who are pregnant or who want to become pregnant should be referred to an expert for management

M.   **Management of patients with episodic tension-type headache** is described in the table below

---

MANAGEMENT OF PATIENTS WITH EPISODIC TENSION-TYPE HEADACHE

Nonpharmacologic
Because of the chronic nature of these headaches, nonpharmacologic approaches such as biofeedback, stress management, relaxation training, and aerobic exercise should be given a trial; provide patient with specific referral for any of these approaches that seem appropriate and that patient is willing to try

Pharmacologic
The following OTC medications are usually effective; use should be limited to 2-3 days per week to avoid medication-overuse headache
- ✓ Ibuprofen, 400-600 mg every 4-6 hours; maximum 3200 mg/day
- ✓ Acetaminophen, 650 mg every 4 hours OR 1000 mg every 12 hours
- ✓ Aspirin, 650 mg every 4 hours
- ✓ Acetaminophen, 250 mg/aspirin, 250 mg/caffeine, 65 mg (Excedrin Extra Strength), 2 tabs PO at start of attack; up to 8 per day

---

N.   Educate patient about overuse of analgesics which can lead to rebound headaches; patients who take analgesics several times a day for 3 or more days a week are prone to rebound headache

O.   **Management of patients with cluster headache** (an uncommon disorder) includes both preventive therapy and acute therapy and is described in the table below

---

MANAGEMENT OF PATIENTS WITH CLUSTER HEADACHE

The brevity of cluster headache attacks precludes most oral acute-relief therapies

First-line treatment is oxygen delivered at 7-12 L/min for 15 min; repeat as needed

Triptans are very efficacious using the subcutaneous or nasal spray routes of administration
    Sumatriptan (Imitrex), 6 mg SC initially; may repeat in 1 hour, max 12 mg/day; the nasal spray dose is 5-20 mg spray nasally; may repeat after 2 hours, max 40 mg/day

Preventive therapy for cluster headache is indicated when there is high attack frequency
    Verapamil (Calan), 80-120 mg PO TID is effective and usually well tolerated (Not FDA approved for this indication)

If this medication proves to be ineffective or poorly tolerated, refer patient for expert care (surgical procedures are available for refractory cases)

P.   Follow Up
1.   Patients with migraine headaches, as outlined above under V.N.
2.   Patients with tension or cluster headache, follow up is necessary within 2-4 weeks after patient is placed on therapy to determine efficacy

PARKINSON'S DISEASE

I.   Definition: Chronic, degenerative, and progressive central nervous system movement disorder

II. Pathogenesis

    A.   Etiology of Parkinson's disease (PD) remains unclear, but it is likely the result of the cumulative effects of genetic and environmental factors in a given patient

        1.   The majority of cases of PD probably result from a complex interaction among many genes and proteins that differ among individuals

        2.   A cascade of pathophysiologic events occurs leading to abnormal protein aggregation and eventual cell death by an apoptotic mechanism (apoptosis is a gradual form of cell death characterized by fragmentation of DNA with relative absence of inflammation)

        3.   Many factors have been implicated in pathogenesis of PD including oxidative stress, excitotoxicity, mitochondrial dysfunction, calcium dysregulation, and inflammation

    B.   Degeneration of specific neuronal populations in the brain, most notably the dopaminergic neurons of the substantia nigra pars compacta is believed to be responsible for the clinical findings that characterize the disease; symptoms appear when 70-80% of dopamine is lost

III. Clinical Presentation

    A.   PD is the second most common neurodegenerative disorder, affecting 1-2% of the population over the age of 65; main risk factors for developing PD include advancing age and family history suggesting it is an age-dependent genetic disorder, at least in a subset of patients

    B.   Prevalence of PD is estimated at 100 to 200/100,000 population; with an average age of onset of 60 years; about 80% of affected persons are between the ages of 60 and 79

    C.   As a progressive disorder, PD results in significant disability 10-15 years after onset

    D.   The onset of PD is insidious with nonspecific symptoms such as easy fatigability, generalized malaise, and subtle personality changes

    E.   Over time (sometimes years), the 3 cardinal features of PD appear—tremor, rigidity, and bradykinesia

---

Tremor

✓ Most visible manifestation, present in 75% of patients at some point in their disease

✓ Typically a resting tremor which is more prominent when patient is sitting and relaxed and attempts an activity such as holding and reading a newspaper

✓ Initially (in many patients), the tremor is an internal tremor, that is, patients feel that they are shaking, but there is no visible tremor; over time, the tremor becomes evident to an observer

✓ Can begin in any extremity, but in most cases, it begins in one arm, affecting the hand initially or even a single finger, then spreading up the arm

✓ Often described as "pill-rolling" for the rhythmic movements made by the index finger as it flexes and extends against the thumb repetitively

✓ Over time, tremor may develop on the contralateral side or in the ipsilateral leg

✓ Can affect the chin, lips, and tongue, but typically does not involve the head

✓ Appears intermittently, disappearing during sleep, and increasing when the patient is stressed, either emotionally or physically

✓ Whereas tremor is often the most noticeable sign of PD, it is usually the **least disabling** because purposeful movement has a dampening effect on the tremor

---

Rigidity

✓ Defined as resistance to passive movement that occurs in both flexors and extensors throughout range of motion (ROM)

✓ Often has a *cogwheel* quality when the extremity is passively moved, i.e., there is resistance that stops and starts in quick repetitive sequence as the extremity is moved through ROM–believed to be due to tremor combined with altered muscle tone

✓ Almost always present to some extent from the onset of disease and lack of arm swing on one side of the body (rigidity, like tremor, usually beings **unilaterally**) may be the first indication

✓ Symptoms may remain unilateral for some time before progressing and becoming symmetric

Bradykinesia

✓ Defined as the diminished ability to initiate movement, with akinesia being the extreme form

✓ The **most disabling** symptom of PD–patients complain of inability to rise from a chair and to begin walking from a standing position

✓ Many patients have difficulty describing the symptom and usually use global terms such as "being weak or tired"

✓ Facial masking is usually first noticed by family members who describe the patient as having a blank look on his/her face; blink frequency is reduced so that patient seems to stare

✓ Speech becomes slower and is often slurred; swallowing becomes slowed and results in the pooling of saliva in the mouth–as the disease progresses, saliva may leak from the mouth (sialorrhea), initially occurring more prominently at night (patient awakens with wet pillow) but eventually occurring throughout the day

E. Other clinical features of PD include the following
    1. Postural instability presents as changes in gait and balance
        a. Usually a later sign of PD
        b. Slow, shuffling gait with a tendency toward propulsion or retropulsion
        c. Loss of postural "righting" reflexes which leads to development of a stooped or "simian" posture, with flexion of the knees, trunk, elbows, wrists, and metacarpophalangeal joints
        d. Lacking the autonomic righting reflex, the patient may unconsciously drift sideways or backward when sitting or standing
        e. Turning requires several steps
    2. Motor symptoms such as intermittent immobility or "freezing" and difficulty at halting steps while walking, termed "festination"
    3. Autonomic dysfunction which results in seborrhea and excessive perspiration, orthostatic blood pressure changes, sexual disturbances, bladder and anal sphincter dysfunction, and constipation
    4. Mental status changes including confusion, dementia, and depression
        a. Depression can potentially be more disabling than motor dysfunction
        b. Dementia is estimated to be present in 15-30% of patients with PD

IV. Diagnosis/Evaluation

    A. History: Keep in mind that diagnosis is based on clinical criteria
        1. Explore onset and progression of signs and symptoms, with focus on tremor, rigidity, dyskinesia, postural instability, manifestations related to autonomic dysfunction, and mental status changes
        2. Determine patient's functional disability (degree to which symptoms interfere with motor function and activities of daily living [ADLs])
            a. The Unified Parkinson's Disease Rating Scale (UPDRS) is a useful way to initially assess patient and to perform interval assessments of functional status
            b. The ADL component of the UPDRS evaluates speech, salivation, swallowing, handwriting, cutting food, handling utensils, hygiene, turning in bed, falling, freezing, walking, tremor, and sensory symptoms
            c. Careful questioning, using the ADL component as a framework, can provide insight into the degree of disability and helps to assess change over time
            d. Copies of the UPDRS can be obtained from We Move, 204 West 84th Street, 3rd Floor, New York, NY 10024, or it can be downloaded from www.wemove.org
        3. Assess for depression using the 2-question screening method recommended by the US Preventive Services Task Force (USPSTF) [2002]
            a. To assess mood, ask, "Over the past 2 weeks, have you felt down, depressed, or hopeless?"
            b. To assess anhedonia, ask, "Over the past 2 weeks, have you felt little interest or pleasure in doing things?"

4. Ask the patient which symptoms of PD are the most bothersome (for example, is his or her job in jeopardy)
5. Carefully question about medication history, focusing on neuroleptic, gastrointestinal, and antihypertensive medications
6. Inquire about occupational, recreational, and environmental history to uncover exposure to toxins such as carbon monoxide, manganese or cyanide, licit and illicit drugs
7. Obtain complete past medical history, social history, and family history with a focus on any dementing illnesses or hereditary disorders

B. Physical Examination: Keep in mind that diagnosis is based on clinical criteria
1. (**Note**: Obtaining a history and physical examination on a PD patient requires TIME and PATIENCE; bradykinesia causes patient to respond slowly to commands, and bradyphrenia causes the patient to require more time to process questions and respond)
2. Observe for characteristic posture (simian) and gait (difficulty turning, absent arm swing, slow, shuffling gait, tendency toward propulsion or retropulsion)
3. Elicit signs of PD—tremor, rigidity, and bradykinesia—to help verify the diagnosis (consult box below for specific examination techniques)
4. Perform orthostatic blood pressure and pulse readings to assess for autonomic dysfunction
5. Perform mental status exam (see section on ALZHEIMER'S DISEASE for details on assessment of cognitive functioning)
6. Assess cranial nerves
   a. Sense of smell is often lost
   b. Blink reflex often is reduced
   c. Extraocular movements are normal except for impairment in upward gaze (disturbance in ocular motility suggests progressive supranuclear palsy)
7. Test motor and extrapyramidal systems
   a. Passively move limbs, noting characteristic rigidity
   b. Observe for hand and foot posturing which is common
8. Check reflexes which are usually normal but may be slightly hyperactive or difficult to elicit due to tremor and rigidity
9. Examine sensory system for common peripheral neuropathies
10. Examine skin for scaly, greasy lesions characteristic of seborrhea

---

Tremor

Test for the presence of tremor at rest

- Tremor of PD is inhibited during movement and sleep
- Ask patient to rest hands on lap and observe for a slow, rhythmical, involuntary, oscillatory movement

Rigidity

Test for resistance to passive movement of the limbs

- With the patient in a relaxed position, place thumb across the antecubital fossa with one hand while passively flexing and extending the elbows several times with the other hand
- Rigidity usually increases with repeated flexion and extension movements
- With cog wheeling, alternate periods of resistance and relaxation may be felt with the examining hands
- With lead-pipe rigidity, smooth but increased muscle tone throughout passive flexion and extension may be felt with the examining hands
- Whereas rigidity and cog wheeling may be felt in other, larger joints, if detected in the arms, further examination is unnecessary

Bradykinesia

Perform maneuvers to detect bradykinesia—decrease in speed and amplitude of complex movements

- Clearly explain each maneuver to the patient and then observe his/her performance before moving on to the next maneuver
  - ✓ *Tapping the fingers*—sequential tapping of the 4 fingers of each hand on a firm surface; hands are placed in front of patient, supported on a table—forearms are resting on table and fingers are raised in air. Fingers are then tapped in sequence beginning with the little finger of both hands, and moving to the index fingers for several repetitions (see illustration)
  - ✓ *Pinching and circling*—consists of 3 movements, repeated with both hands: (1) Pinching using opposing thumb and index finger with right hand, then left hand; (2) Circling or moving the hand in a circle—index finger extended, other fingers in flexion. Patient should perform with right hand, then left hand; (3) Pinching with the right hand while simultaneously circling with the left and then reversing the process (pinching with left hand/circling with right) [see illustration]
  - ✓ *Tapping with heel*—patient seated or standing, with foot flat on floor. Foot is raised on toes and then heel is brought down to tap the floor with heel in a repeated fashion; test both feet, one at a time (see illustration)
- Poor performance on these maneuvers is easily detectable

Adapted from Rao, G, Fisch, L., Srinivasin, S., D'Amico, F., Okada, T., Eaton, D., & Robbins, C. (2003). Does this patient have Parkinson disease? *JAMA, 289*, 347-353.

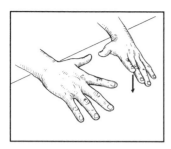 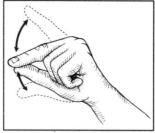 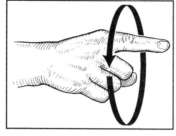 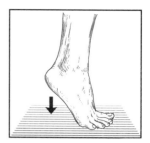

Tapping fingers   Pinching   Circling   Tapping heel

Figure 18.1. Maneuvers to Detect Bradykinesia

C. Differential Diagnosis
1. Essential tremor (patients usually have positive family history and an action tremor)
2. Neuroleptic-induced parkinsonism due to medication intake (bilateral onset; reversible) [it is important to distinguish between PD and parkinsonism—the latter refers to <u>any</u> clinical syndrome in which 2 or more features are present such as tremor, rigidity. PD is a form of primary or idiopathic parkinsonism]
3. Progressive supranuclear palsy which usually has impaired vertical neck extension (axial rigidity) and early dysarthria and dysphagia
4. Infarcts and tumors in the basal ganglia (distinguished on basis of clinical and laboratory criteria)
5. Wilson's disease, which occurs in younger persons and is characterized by copper accumulation throughout the body

D. Diagnostic Tests
1. Neuroimaging techniques are not required in patients with straightforward PD; diagnosis is made on the basis of clinical criteria
2. Referral to a neurologist for neuroimaging is indicated when diagnosis is not straightforward; positron emission tomography (PET) and single photon emission computerized tomography (SPECT) can be used to assess the integrity of the nigrostriatal system and metabolic activity within the basal ganglia
3. The history and physical examinations should guide decisions to order testing to rule out other conditions; in general, a CBC, chemistry profile, and urinalysis are ordered on all patients
4. Genetic testing may become more important in the future

V. Plan/Management

A. Consultation with a neurologist is recommended when the diagnosis of PD is made so that the neurologist can confirm the diagnosis and develop a treatment plan; the primary care clinician can then follow the patient and refer to neurologist when difficulties in management occur (**Note:** The classic presentation of PD usually poses few problems in diagnosis, but some presentations are more difficult to recognize)

B. The management recommendations that are outlined here are based on the most recent practice parameters released by the American Academy of Neurology (2001, 2002); definitive management of a particular patient should be planned in consultation with a neurologist

C. Early treatment of PD consists of **nonpharmacologic therapies** and **initial symptomatic treatment**

D. Nonpharmacologic therapies have a fundamental role in the management of PD; recommendations are outlined in the table that follows

NONPHARMACOLOGIC THERAPIES FOR PATIENTS DIAGNOSED WITH PARKINSON'S DISEASE

Education
- ✓ Keep in mind that education of the patient/family is not a one-time occurrence; rather, it is an on-going process
- ✓ Provide patient/family with facts about the disease at initial and subsequent visits
- ✓ Provide ample opportunities for questions/discussion at every visit
- ✓ Recognize that providing patient with only written material is inadequate

Support
- ✓ Maintain an empathetic approach to patient/family as adjustment to the diagnosis is made
- ✓ Refer patient/family to support groups in the area as these groups can offer psychological and social benefits to both patients and families; in addition, practical tips on how best to deal with specific problems are often shared in such groups

Exercise
- ✓ Educate patient about the many benefits of exercise including positive impact on mobility and mood
- ✓ Goals of exercise are to improve/maintain flexibility and strength
- ✓ A reasonable goal is 20 minutes of exercise of some type 3 times a week
- ✓ Emphasize to patient that the type of exercise is not as important as engaging in the activity on a regular basis
- ✓ Recommend exercise such as walking and stretching activities; many patients find tai chi and yoga programs helpful and enjoyable
- ✓ Write an exercise prescription and ask patient to keep a log of exercises; review log at every visit (**Note**: All of these factors serve to emphasize the importance of exercise)

Nutrition
- ✓ Patients with PD are at risk for poor nutrition, unintended weight loss, and loss of muscle mass
- ✓ To counteract this, emphasize a healthy diet; no specific diet is required (refer to the section on CHILD, ADOLESCENT, AND ADULT NUTRITION for counseling recommendations)
- ✓ Because constipation is frequently a problem, emphasize a high fiber intake and adequate fluid intake
- ✓ Emphasize that in generally healthy persons, nutritional needs can be readily met by diet alone; however, persons with chronic diseases such as PD are at risk for suboptimal vitamin intake; therefore, recommend that the patient take one multivitamin daily; discourage the patient from taking vitamins in harmful doses

Caregiver Support/Respite care
- ✓ Providing care for the caregiver is all important and should not be ignored
- ✓ Take the time to assess the caregiver's emotional and physical status while examining the PD patient
- ✓ Inquire about recent difficulties with care, and be attentive to nonverbal signals that the caregiver is overwhelmed
- ✓ Suggest the caregiver join a support group
- ✓ Give specific information about groups in the area to increase the likelihood that the caregiver will join

E. **Initial symptomatic treatment** of patients with early or newly diagnosed PD when symptoms are present but not yet particularly troublesome
   1. Consider prescribing selegiline with the aim of providing mild, symptomatic benefit prior to the initiation of dopaminergic therapy
   2. Whereas there is insufficient evidence to recommend the use of selegiline to confer neuroprotection in patients with PD, its use to confer "mild, symptomatic benefit" is currently recommended for consideration
   3. Selegiline (Eldepryl) is a relatively selective MAO-B inhibitor
      a. Dose of selegiline should not exceed 10 mg/day, divided into two doses, with the first dose in AM and the second dose at noon
      b. A single 5 mg dose in AM may be sufficient for many patients; the drug has a long half-life, and the stimulatory effect of the drug may produce insomnia in some persons
      c. Patients taking selegiline do not have to be on an MAO inhibitor diet so long as the dose does not exceed 10 mg day (tyramine-containing foods can cause hypertensive crisis in patients taking MAO inhibitors); patients cannot take meperidine while taking this drug because of risk of severe adverse events

F. **Once functional impairment occurs**, patients require dopaminergic treatment – either a dopamine agonist or levodopa
   1. Definition of functional impairment must be considered on individual basis
   2. If no symptoms were present, the patient would not have sought medical attention; thus the issue is not whether impairment is present, but rather whether the impairment represents a source of disability
   3. Impairment that one patient considers minor may represent a major impairment to another patient (most often related to job performance requirements)
   4. In most early PD patients, symptoms are predominantly unilateral, and the degree of functional impairment often depends on whether there is dominant-hand involvement
   5. Use the UPDRS to assess functional disability (see under IV.A. above)

G. Important considerations for choosing the initial dopaminergic therapy for a particular patient are outlined in the box below

Factor	Considerations
Age	Older patients (those more than 70 to 75 years of age) may be less likely to develop levodopa-induced motor complications because life expectancy at that age is relatively short; thus levodopa rather than a dopamine agonist is probably a more reasonable choice; for patients less than 70, and certainly for patients in their 40s and 50s, drug of choice for initiation of therapy is a dopamine agonist
Mental Status	Patients with mental impairment should be treated with levodopa as this drug seems more efficacious in this group of patients; however, drug is often poorly tolerated by such patients
Comorbidities	Presence of comorbidities can impact treatment choice due to drug interactions
Cost	If cost is a factor, levodopa is less expensive than are the dopamine agonists

H. In the past, levodopa has been considered the gold standard for symptomatic treatment of PD because it is more effective than dopamine agonists in treating the motor and activities of daily living (ADL) features of PD; the role of dopamine agonists has been to supplement levodopa when the patient began to develop dyskinesias or motor fluctuations; unfortunately, once motor complications have developed, they are difficult to control with medical therapies and surgical intervention is often required

I. The American Academy of Neurology (2001, 2002), recommends that symptomatic therapy be initiated with a dopamine agonist; the addition of levodopa as a supplement is indicated when dopamine agonist monotherapy no longer provides satisfactory clinical control
    1. This is especially true for patients <70 who are at high risk for development of motor complications
    2. Dopamine agonists are associated with a reduced risk for inducing motor complications when compared with levodopa
    3. Motor complications represent a major source of disability to the majority of PD patients and frequently lead to surgical intervention
    4. Further, dopamine agonists have putative neuroprotective effects
    5. Thus, use of a dopamine agonist is a major therapeutic advantage for most patients

J. **Initiating dopaminergic treatment** once symptoms begin to interfere with daily activities: a dopamine agonist is recommended for most patients
    1. Risks and benefits of symptomatic management should be discussed with the patient
    2. Cabergoline, ropinirole, and pramipexole are equally effective in ameliorating motor and ADL disability in patients with PD who require dopaminergic therapy
    3. Unlike the older dopamine agonists (pergolide and bromocriptine), these drugs are non-ergot derivatives and are relatively selective in stimulating D_2 and D_3 receptors
    4. Dopamine agonist monotherapy can provide therapeutic effects comparable to those of levodopa in the early stages of PD and these effects can be sustained for up to 5 years with a lower incidence of dyskinesia even when L-dopa rescue becomes necessary
    5. (**Note**: Starting therapy with levodopa is still preferred in PD patients with cognitive impairment who may not tolerate dopamine agonists and in the elderly who have a reduced likelihood of developing motor complications)
    6. Dosing of these drugs is contained in the table that follows (Note: Cabergoline has not been promoted for the treatment of PD in the US, but it is marketed for this indication in some European countries and in Japan)

DOPAMINE AGONISTS USED FOR SYMPTOMATIC THERAPY

Ropinirole (Requip): Initiate with 0.25 mg TID for the first week, gradually increasing dose at weekly intervals to a usual therapeutic dose of 3-12 mg per day, in divided doses, TID

Pramipexole (Mirapex): Must be dosed based on creatinine clearance results with the starting dose (usually 0.125 mg, TID for first week) gradually increased to therapeutic levels at intervals of 5-7 days (usual maintenance dose is 3 mg per day, in divided doses, TID)
  ✓ Dopamine agonists should be introduced at a low dose and gradually titrated to optimal clinical benefit over the course of several weeks to months; use the lowest maintenance dose that provides adequate benefit
  ✓ Dopamine agonists are less likely than levodopa to cause adverse motor effects, but more likely to cause neuropsychiatric effects
  ✓ Use with caution in older patients and in all patients with a history of psychiatric disorders

---

K. When dopamine agonists no longer provide satisfactory clinical control, the addition of levodopa to the treatment regimen is necessary
   1. Levodopa with or without COMT inhibitor (used to extend its elimination half-life) is added and dopamine agonist is continued
   2. Either sustained release or immediate-release levodopa may be used
   3. The rule of thumb is to use the lowest dose that controls symptoms rather than the highest dosage that the patient can tolerate
   4. Levodopa is combined with carbidopa which blocks the peripheral conversion of L-dopa to dopamine, thus increasing the amount of L-dopa transported to the brain
   5. Carbidopa/levodopa is available in both standard release (Sinemet) and controlled-release form (Sinemet CR)
      a. Usual starting dose of Sinemet (standard form) is one-half to one tablet of 25/100 mg QD increasing by 25/100 mg per day each week until TID dosing is achieved (slowly titrate to 300-400 mg of L-dopa per day)
      b. Alternatively, Sinemet CR may be used; usual starting dose is one-half tablet of 50/200 mg QD increasing slowly to one tablet BID (**Note:** There is no difference in the rate of motor complications between immediate-release levodopa and sustained-release levodopa)
      c. Not every symptom responds equally as well, with bradykinesia and rigidity responding best, and tremor responding least
      d. After 3 or more years of treatment, approximately one-third of patients receiving this drug begin to develop involuntary movements and to have very short-duration responses to the medication (wearing off)
   6. COMT inhibitors may or may not be added to levodopa therapy; there is a lack of consensus on this therapy; COMT inhibitors block peripheral levodopa metabolism, thereby enhancing its brain availability
      a. COMT inhibitors reduce "off" time in fluctuating PD patients, increase duration of benefit, and enhance motor response and activities of daily living in nonfluctuating patients
      b. The usual starting and maintenance doses of tolcapone (Tasmar) is 100 mg TID (requires monitoring of liver enzymes weekly for the first 6 months of therapy)

L. Because of the complexity in management of patients with advanced PD requiring levodopa therapy, referral to a neurologist is recommended at this point (if not done previously)
   1. Management of side effects of levodopa therapy including nausea and vomiting (early effect), orthostatic hypotension, motor fluctuations, dyskinesias (all later effects) is very complex and if not done correctly, greatly compromises the patient's quality of life
   2. Patients in this category frequently have comorbidities which increase the risk of adverse events and drug interactions
   3. Over time, response fluctuations begin to occur so that there is a wearing off or end-of-dose failure in response to a previously adequate dose of levodopa
   4. The "offs" tend to be mild at first, but progress to become deeper with more severe parkinsonism and the duration of the "on" response becomes shorter
   5. Many patients who develop response fluctuations also develop abnormal involuntary movements
   6. Frequent evaluation and medication adjustments are needed as loss of dopamine response occurs

M. Potential of surgical therapies to provide benefit for PD patients who can no longer be satisfactorily controlled with available medical therapies is a major advance in modern therapy
   1. Pallidotomy can provide relief for refractory dyskinesias
   2. Deep brain stimulation procedures are effective for refractory tremor
   3. Fetal transplantation continues to be an area of research

N. Depression is a common nonmotor symptom in PD; it is unknown whether depression is endogenous, exogenous, or both
   1. Endogenous depression may occur as a result of the monoamine deficiency that characterizes PD
   2. Exogenous depression is likely to occur in anyone with a chronic, debilitating disease; further, older patients are likely to encounter many losses which can also contribute to depression
   3. Unless the patient suffers from profound depression, treatment of PD should be given the first priority
   4. Once the patient is stabilized with adequate antiparkinsonian therapy, the patient should be re-evaluated to determine if psychotherapy, antidepressants, or in more extreme cases, ECT is indicated

5. Major treatment options are the tricyclic antidepressants (TCAs) and the selective serotonin reuptake inhibitors (SSRIs)
   a. SSRIs avoid the anticholinergic side effects associated with the TCAs and are generally preferred in treatment of PD patient
   b. However, keep in mind that SSRIs in general, and fluoxetine in particular, can be activating which may be desirable in patients who are apathetic or withdrawn but undesirable in agitated patients
   c. Dosing of SSRIs used to treat depression in PD patients is the same as for other causes of depression in the general population (see section on DEPRESSION)
   d. If a TCA is selected for treatment, (for example, in a patient with insomnia), nortriptyline, and desipramine have less anticholinergic activity than the tertiary amines and are cleared more rapidly; thus, they are the preferred agents in this class of drugs
   e. For purposes of facilitating sleep, nighttime doses of nortriptyline, 20-40 mg, or desipramine, 25-50 mg, can be helpful

O. Referrals to physical, speech, or occupational therapists are often needed

P. Follow up is variable depending on involvement of the neurologist, patient's degree of disability, and the need to monitor adverse events and renal functioning in patients on certain medications

RESTLESS LEGS SYNDROME

I. Definition: A neurologic movement disorder characterized by the following clinical features: dysesthesias, or unpleasant sensations in the extremities that are made worse by inactivity (as occurs at night when the patient goes to bed) and relieved with movement of the legs which the individual feels compelled to do in an attempt to minimize the discomfort

II. Pathogenesis

   A. Vascular, systemic, peripheral nervous system, central nervous system, and genetic etiologies have all been proposed

   B. The primary lesion is probably in the spinal cord

   C. Secondary causes of RLS include pregnancy, chronic renal failure, diabetes mellitus, iron or folic acid deficiency, and drug induced (examples are tricyclic antidepressants, selective serotonin reuptake inhibitors (SSRIs), lithium, and dopamine antagonists)

   D. Certain behavioral conditions have also been implicated as aggravating or increasing the symptoms of RLS; these include tobacco use, obesity, sedentary lifestyle, and caffeine use

III. Clinical Presentation

   A. RLS is a common disorder, and as many as 15% of otherwise healthy individuals may experience RLS symptoms which cause discomfort, sleep disturbances, and daytime fatigue thereby affecting occupational functioning, social activities, and family life

   B. Symptoms generally exhibit a circadian pattern, occurring most commonly between 10 PM and 4 AM with symptoms almost always abating before dawn

   C. Prevalence increases with age with as many as 25% of persons over age 65 experiencing symptoms; prevalence is also increased among patients with secondary causes listed in II. C. above

   D. Patients most often report an irresistible urge to move their legs that occurs when they go to bed—this urge to move is prompted by sensations described as "creepy-crawly" and "like worms under the skin," that are experienced in the extremities, usually the legs and less often in the arms or elsewhere
      1. Symptoms are bilateral and originate in the calves and are associated less with the skin of the legs than with muscles and bones

2. Patients may attempt to relieve the unpleasant sensations by moving the legs, stretching or rubbing the legs, or getting out of bed and walking
3. Thus sleep is disturbed and becomes difficult for patients with mild to moderate disease, and even impossible for untreated patients with severe disease

E. Whereas symptoms are most likely to follow a circadian rhythm and occur at night, patients may also experience symptoms of RLS when sitting for long periods of time, so that riding in a car, on an airplane, or going to the theatre or attending church services may be uncomfortable

F. RLS commonly occurs concomitantly with periodic limb movement disorder (PLMD), a similar condition characterized by involuntary stereotyped, repetitive flexions of the limbs (usually legs)
1. Movement occur **only** during sleep—the most common movement is a dorsiflexion of the ankles and flexion of the knees or hips
2. Frequently occurs among individuals with sleep apnea
3. Whereas many patients with RLS also develop PLMD, most persons with PLMD no not experience RLS; in general patients with PLMD do not complain of sensory discomfort and patients with RLS almost always do

G. Clinical criteria for the diagnosis of RLS are contained in the table below

---

DIAGNOSTIC CRITERIA FOR THE RESTLESS LEGS SYNDROME

➡ Unpleasant sensation in the legs at night or difficulty in falling asleep
➡ Disagreeable sensations of "creeping" inside the calves of the legs, often associated with generalized aches and pains in the legs
➡ Discomfort is relieved somewhat by limb movements
➡ Polysomnographic monitoring demonstrates limb movements at rest
➡ No evidence of a medical or mental disorder that can account for symptoms
➡ Other sleep disorders may be present but do not account for symptoms

---

Adapted from American Sleep Disorder Association (1997). *International classification of sleep disorders, revised: Diagnostic and coding manual.* Rochester, MN, p. 65.

IV. Diagnosis/Evaluation

A. History
1. Ask patient to describe sensations in legs (or arms) and when this occurs (time of day)
2. Determine how long this has been occurring and what, if anything, relieves the sensations (i.e., moving, rubbing the legs, stretching, getting out of bed)
3. Obtain past medical and medication history with a focus on secondary causes of RLS
4. Determine if onset of symptoms is associated with a change in medication
5. Always ask patient about tobacco use and document response in the chart; ask about caffeine use, drug and alcohol use, and use of supplements of any sort

B. Physical Examination
1. Obtain vital signs
2. Perform neurologic examination, with a focus on **motor system, sensory system, and muscle stretch reflexes**—particularly in the lower extremities to rule out other causes for symptoms

Motor system: Lower extremity function can best be assessed by having patient stand, walk, hop, and walk on tiptoe (More detailed examination on the basis of an observed abnormality may be required, e.g., movement against the examiner's resistance may be needed to test both upper and lower extremities)

Sensory system: Light touch, pain, vibration, and position sense are tested—usually tested are the face, both the radial and ulnar aspect of the hand, and the feet; when testing position sense, make certain patient understand precisely how to respond

Testing Position Sense

✓ Examiner holds toe laterally within the patient's view

✓ Examiner moves the toe in very small degrees in an irregular fashion—up or down—while asking the patient to tell which direction the toe is being moved (patient is looking at direction of movement)

✓ Once it is certain that patient understands how to appropriately respond to questions relating to toe movements, ask him/her to close eyes and then to indicate whether the movement of the toe is up or down (or if not certain, to respond, "I don't know")

✓ If small movements of the toe cannot be detected by the patient, increase the degree of the movement to the point that the patient's responses are correct (or it is obvious that the patient's position sense is impaired)

Muscle Stretch Reflexes: Should be completed after motor and sensory testing

Testing Muscle Stretch Reflexes

✓ Examiner places finger across tendon of muscle to be tested, and then hits finger with the reflex hammer (repeatedly) to determine the least intensity of the blow that can produce a barely perceptible contraction

✓ Advantages of method: Allows examiner to feel the tension of the muscle, monitor intensity of the blow and detect the least degree of contraction **and** does not subject patient to direct hammer blows

✓ Best to test one reflex repeatedly and then test the homologous reflex in the other extremity

    3.   Always perform a vascular exam to rule out vascular disorders

    4.   Additional physical examination should be based on patient history to rule out conditions associated with RLS

C.   Differential Diagnosis

    1.   Polyneuropathy (Not necessarily worse at night, not relieved by movement, distal predominance, neurologic abnormality)

    2.   Radiculopathy (Usually unilateral, neurologic abnormalities)

    3.   Claudication (Worse with walking, not with rest)

    4.   Periodic limb movement disorder (In this disorder, there are repetitive, highly stereotyped limb muscle movements—for example, extension of big toe with partial flexion of ankle, knee, and sometimes hip. Polysomnographic monitoring shows repetitive episodes (0.5-5 second duration) of muscle contraction every 20-40 seconds; movements are involuntary and occur during sleep, not while the individual is attempting to go to sleep

D.   Diagnostic Testing

    1.   Diagnosis is clinical, based primarily on careful history

    2.   Serum folate and ferritin levels should be measured to rule out folate/iron deficiency

    3.   Consider other diagnostic testing (e.g., serum chemistries) to rule out secondary causes of RLS based on patient history

    4.   Because RLS and PLMD often occur concomitantly, overnight sleep testing should also be considered, if the sleep disorder is the major complaint and a sleep laboratory is readily available (**Note**: A sleep study (polysomnography) is not routinely indicated in the workup of RLS but if there is diagnostic uncertainly, it should be considered)

V.   Plan/Management

A.   Patients with RLS need validation and support as many such patients have delayed seeking healthcare for months and even years after symptom onset

B.   If a specific medication is implicated as the cause, consider changing the medication to another class, or to a different drug in the same class to determine if there is improvement in the RLS

C.   If a medical conditions is implicated as the cause, the underlying condition should be treated or referred to an expert for management

D. For patients diagnosed with primary RLS, treatment begins with nonpharmacologic interventions that may control symptoms and improve sleep quality as well as quality of life in general

---

NONPHARMACOLOGIC TREATMENT FOR RESTLESS LEGS SYNDROME

Provide educational resources—the following sources provide a great deal of information which can be very reassuring to the patient and family

Internet Connections

✓ The Restless Legs Syndrome Foundation, Inc.   http://www.rls.org/main.asp

✓ National Institutes of Health
National Center for Sleep Disorders Research   http://www.nhlbi.nih.gov/about/nscdr/

Books
Sleep Thief: Restless Legs Syndrome by Virginia N. Wilson, David Buchholz, & Arthur S. Walkers, Galaxy Books, Inc. (1996)

E. Anecdotal reports of relief of symptoms with moderate daily activity (all adults without contraindications should engage in 60 minutes of physical activity each day—see section on NUTRITION for more information), massage, caffeine and alcohol avoidance, vitamins (see section on NUTRITION for recommendations related to multivitamin intake in preventing chronic diseases), and hot baths
   1. Patients should be advised that these interventions sometimes relieve symptoms, but that they are not evidence-based
   2. Counseling related to physical activity, proper nutrition, maintaining a healthy weight, and multivitamin intake (as well as smoking cessation, if patient uses tobacco) should be incorporated into every visit if possible
   3. Patients should also be counseled in sleep hygiene (see section on INSOMNIA for specific recommendations

F. If nonpharmacologic interventions provide only partial symptom relief, initiate pharmacologic therapy

---

PHARMACOLOGIC TREATMENT FOR RESTLESS LEGS SYNDROME

No medication has been approved specifically for use in patients with RLS; thus use of any pharmacologic agent is an "off-label" use. The table below lists some of the commonly used drugs for mild to moderate symptoms of RLS.
Consult PDR for precautions, contraindications, interactions, side effects, and laboratory monitoring requirements prior to prescribing these or any other drugs

Dopaminergic Agents	
Carbidopa/levodopa (Sinemet)	Start with one-half of 25/100 mg tab at bedtime; titrate to 25/100-50/200 mg
Pramipexole (Mirapex)	0.125 mg titrated to 0.75 mg at bedtime
Anticonvulsants	
Gabapentin (Neurontin)	300 mg at bedtime; can increase to TID
Carbamazepine (Tegretol)	200 mg at bedtime; can increase to TID
Benzodiazepines	
Clonazepam (Klonopin)	0.5 mg at bedtime

G. For patients with severe, unrelenting symptoms, referral to an expert is warranted; opioids can be used on an intermittent basis, but carry the risk of addiction

H. Follow Up
   1. Patients who are treated with nonpharmacologic interventions should be evaluated in 1-3 months for treatment efficacy, and then every 6 months for 1 year
   2. Patients who fail nonpharmacologic therapy should be placed on pharmacologic therapy and monitored closely at appropriate intervals for adverse events. Consult PDR for precautions, contraindications, interactions, side effects, and laboratory monitoring requirements before prescribing the medications in the above table
   3. Patients who remain symptomatic after both nonpharmacologic and pharmacologic interventions should be referred to an expert for management

SEIZURES AND EPILEPSY

I.   Definitions

    A.   Seizures: Behavioral changes resulting from abnormal paroxysmal neuronal discharge and are a symptom of an underlying brain problem

    B.   Epilepsy: Recurrent unprovoked seizures with few other systemic or neurologic symptoms

II. Pathogenesis

    A.   Initiated by electrochemical abnormalities in brain such as alterations in concentration of excitatory or inhibitory neurotransmitter

    B.   Abnormal electrical discharge from one site is rapidly transmitted to other parts of the brain, producing disturbances in perception, motor control, attention, and consciousness

    C.   Major causes of seizure by age group are as follows:

Infancy and childhood	✓ Birth trauma, congenital malformations ✓ Inborn errors of metabolism ✓ Idiopathic
Adolescents	✓ Idiopathic ✓ Trauma ✓ Infection
Early adulthood	✓ Idiopathic ✓ Trauma ✓ Tumor ✓ Alcohol or drug related
Late life	✓ Vascular disease ✓ Tumor ✓ Degenerative disease ✓ Infection

III. Clinical Presentation

    A.   Approximately 2 million persons in US have epilepsy; about 100,000 new cases are diagnosed each year

    B.   In addition to idiopathic seizures, adults are likely to have seizures secondary to a pre-existing known condition such as vascular disorders, tumors, or related to drug or alcohol use
        1.   Alcohol and drug related seizures occur via a number of mechanisms
            a.   Alcohol can cause seizures due to malnutrition, increased risk of head trauma, and during withdrawal
            b.   Cocaine and other stimulants are associated with increased risk of seizure; withdrawal from barbiturates can also cause seizures
        2.   Tumors (both benign and malignant), are responsible for a significant number of seizures in older adults
            a.   Patients often have a history of malignancy
            b.   Focal findings on neurologic examination and documentation of mass or masses via neuroimaging help make the diagnosis
        3.   Vascular disease can cause seizures
            a.   In older adults, circulatory abnormalities account for many seizures
            b.   Hypoxemia in pulmonary disease and metabolic disorders such as occur in uremia, hypoglycemia, and liver failure can cause seizures

    C.   Seizure disorders increase in incidence and prevalence after the age of 60 years

D. Principal types of seizures and their clinical features are listed in the table that follows:

PRINCIPAL TYPES OF SEIZURES	
Type of Seizure	*Clinical Features*
Partial Seizures	
Simple partial seizures (focal)	**No alteration/impairment of consciousness occurs** ✓ Signs and symptoms may be motor, sensory, autonomic, or psychic ✓ With motor symptoms, movements often begin in single muscle group and spread to entire side of body ✓ With sensory symptoms, sensory changes may involve paresthesia, or visualization of flashing lights ✓ With autonomic symptoms, patient experiences symptoms such as tachycardia, loss of bowel/bladder control ✓ With psychic symptoms, patients may report hallucinatory experiences, déjà vu, or a dreamlike state
Complex partial seizures *(Temporal lobe or psychomotor)*	**Impairment of consciousness occurs** ✓ Seizure may begin without warning or with motor, sensory, autonomic, or with psychic signs or symptoms ✓ Automatisms (automatic acts about which patient has no recollection) may occur ✓ Seizure is often followed by period of confusion
Secondarily generalized partial seizures *(tonic-clonic or grand mal)*	**Impairment of consciousness occurs** ✓ Seizures may begin with motor, sensory, autonomic, or psychic signs/symptoms ✓ A tonic increase in muscle tone occurs with subsequent rhythmic (clonic) jerks that slowly subside ✓ Seizure duration is one minute or longer and there is increased muscle tone during the event ✓ After seizure, patient is comatose and slowly recovers ✓ Tongue biting and incontinence may occur
Generalized Seizures	
Absence seizures	**Impairment of consciousness occurs** ✓ Very brief, frequent periods of nondistractible staring (average ~10 seconds) occurring primarily in children (age at first seizure is 3-20 years); recovery is rapid ✓ Increased or decreased muscle tone may also occur as well as automatisms or mild clonic movements (atypical absence seizures) [petit mal]
Primarily generalized tonic-clonic *seizures (grand mal)*	**Loss of consciousness occurs** ✓ Patient loses consciousness (without warning or is preceded by myoclonic jerks) ✓ Clinical features are similar to those of secondarily generalized partial seizure

Adapted from Brown, T.R., & Holmes, G.L. (2001). Epilepsy. *New England Journal of Medicine, 344*, p. 1146.

IV. Diagnosis/Evaluation

A. History: Initial step is to determine whether patient does or does not have seizures; next step is to determine type of seizure (by classifying it as focal or generalized in onset) and etiology (if identifiable)
   1. Important to question family members and witnesses as well as patient (for much of the history, witnesses are better sources than patients, but patients are the best source for presence and type of aura)
   2. Explore precipitating factors
   3. Describe the focal onset, duration, and seizure characteristics
   4. Inquire about the setting in which episode occurred
      a. Determine whether the patient completely lost consciousness and/or was incontinent
      b. Determine if there was an aura, antegrade amnesia, or postictal period
   5. Determine if this was a first seizure or if patient has history of minor types of seizures (e.g., myoclonic or absence seizures) [**Note**: History of minor types of seizures in a person presenting with a possible tonic-clonic seizure helps establish the diagnosis of a seizure disorder]
   6. Obtain past medical history including history of head trauma, birth complications, febrile convulsions, middle ear or sinus infections, alcohol or drug use, or symptoms of cancer
   7. Obtain medication history
   8. Inquire about possible toxic exposures (related to occupation or recreational pursuits)
   9. Determine if there is a family history of epilepsy
   10. For patients with known epilepsy who present with seizures, determine the following:
      a. Precipitating factors
      b. Similarity and differences between these seizures and ones in the past
      c. Medications currently taking and adherence with regimen
      d. If the seizures are occurring more frequently

B. Physical Examination
1. Assess vital signs and evaluate for orthostatic hypotension
2. Perform a complete physical examination with a focus on signs of disorders associated with seizures
   a. HEENT–look for signs of head trauma, infections of ears/sinuses
   b. Cardiovascular system
   c. Neurologic–assess pupils, fundi, cranial nerves, sensory, motor and reflexes exam (**Note**: A normal neurologic exam is often found in persons with idiopathic seizure disorder)

C. Differential Diagnosis
1. Most common causes of seizures are listed under II.C. above and must be considered
2. Syncope does not cause seizures but is often confused with this disorder
   a. Whereas patients with syncope may exhibit repetitive clonic, myoclonic, or dystonic movements, these movements rarely last beyond 5-10 seconds and do not exhibit the organized progression from tonic to clonic phase seen in convulsive seizures
   b. Incontinence does not occur with syncope but may occur with seizures
   c. Tongue biting does not occur with syncope but may occur with seizures
   d. A few minutes of confusion immediately following the event is not likely with syncope but is likely with seizures
3. TIAs are sometimes confused with seizures (TIAs cause focal negative phenomena such as weakness, aphasia, ataxia; seizures usually cause positive phenomena such as jerking, automatisms, or movements)
4. Pseudoseizures must be differentiated from seizures; pseudoseizures are more likely to be long in duration, may involve bizarre or unusual movements, and may be precipitated by stressful events

D. Diagnostic Tests
1. Basic laboratory evaluation to determine cause of a newly diagnosed seizure disorder includes the following
   a. CBC with differential and chemistry profile
   b. Liver function tests in adults (not routinely performed in children)
   c. Electroencephalography in waking and sleeping states
   d. Magnetic resonance imaging (MRI) or computed tomography (CT), with MRI being the preferred test because it is more likely to reveal small tumors
   e. Toxicology screening should be performed if there is any question of drug exposure or substance abuse
   f. Lumbar puncture if infection or cancer is suspected
   g. Additional diagnostic testing may be needed based on findings from the history and physical examinations
2. American Academy of Neurology practice guidelines for neuroimaging studies in patients who have had a first seizure are outlined in the box below

> Neuroimaging should be performed **immediately** in patients who may have a serious structural lesion, including those with
> ✓ New focal deficits
> ✓ Persistently altered mental status (with or without intoxication)
> ✓ Fever
> ✓ Recent trauma
> ✓ Persistent headache
> ✓ History of cancer
> ✓ History of anticoagulation therapy
> ✓ AIDS

V. Plan/Management

A. Data from the history, physical examination, and laboratory studies are usually sufficient to diagnose a seizure disorder
1. If presence of seizure disorder or type of disorder cannot be established, additional data should be collected (e.g., additional information about the event from other witnesses, repeated electroencephalogram)
2. Referral to an expert for this additional evaluation is recommended

B. Some seizures are from correctable etiologies and the underlying problem must be identified and corrected in those cases

C.	Once the type of seizure disorder has been established, an antiepileptic drug (AED) appropriate for the type seizure should be prescribed in adult patients who have had two or more seizures; patients who have had a single seizure are usually monitored but are not treated with AEDs
	1.	Candidates for antiepileptic drug therapy include patients with recurrent seizures, onset of seizure presenting as status epilepticus, or a clear structural predisposition for seizures
	2.	In certain circumstances, patients who have had a single seizure are treated; refer patient to neurologist to make this determination

D.	Goal of treatment of patients with epilepsy is to provide optimal control of seizures without producing unacceptable side effects; thus the selection and adjustment of medications are important therapeutic decisions
	1.	Begin treatment with an average dose of a first line antiepileptic drug appropriate for the patient's type of epilepsy
	2.	Select one that best fits the patient based on both patient and medication characteristics including side-effect profile
	3.	Make incremental changes that will enhance effectiveness and tolerability
	4.	A general rule of thumb is to initiate therapy with one-fourth to one-third of the anticipated maintenance dose and increase the dose to maintenance level over a 3-4 week period
	5.	Most side effects are experienced at the initiation of therapy and can be minimized by starting with a low enough dose
		a.	Sedation, dizziness, ataxia, headache, and nausea are common dose-related side effects
		b.	These side effects can be managed by reducing the dose by 25 to 50% and then waiting 2 weeks for tolerance to develop before gradually increased doses can be resumed
	6.	In addition to dose-related side effects, idiosyncratic reactions to AEDs can also occur; these reactions, some of which are potentially fatal, do not correlate with the dose of medication and occur unpredictably, most often early in the course of treatment
		a.	Many AEDs can cause a rash during the first weeks of therapy which in some cases progresses to Stevens-Johnson syndrome or other serious conditions; rashes are usually erythematous, maculopapular or morbilliform eruptions, often beginning on trunk, face, or upper arms
			(1)	Patients should immediately be evaluated at the onset of any new rash, especially rashes that blister, peel, bleed, or involve the mucous membranes, palms, or soles
			(2)	Fever, dry cough, symptoms common with viral syndromes can be the initial features of Stevens-Johnson syndrome
		b.	Liver dysfunction and bone marrow suppression can also occur
			(1)	Protracted vomiting, lethargy, easy bruisability, protracted bleeding from minor cuts, or persistent infection may indicate liver dysfunction or bone marrow suppression
			(2)	Routine measurement of blood chemistry profile, liver function tests, and complete blood count every 3-6 months are standard practice but are not likely to identify potentially life-threatening conditions until late in the course of the condition
		c.	Patients must be educated to recognize the warning signs of idiosyncratic reactions so that early intervention can occur

E.	First-line antiepileptic drugs according to seizure type are listed in the table that follows:

FIRST-LINE ANTIEPILEPTIC DRUGS ACCORDING TO SEIZURE TYPE	
Seizure Type	First-Line Drugs
Generalized Seizures Absence seizures (petit mal)	Ethosuximide, divalproex sodium
Primarily generalized tonic-clonic seizures (grand mal)	Divalproex sodium, phenytoin
Partial Seizures Simple (focal) and complex (temporal lobe or psychomotor) partial seizures	Carbamazepine, divalproex sodium, oxcarbazepine, phenytoin
Secondarily generalized partial seizures	Carbamazepine, divalproex sodium, oxcarbazepine, phenytoin

G. Patients must be monitored closely for adverse effects, drug interactions, poor seizure control, and toxicity
1. If adequate seizure control is attained with the average dose of a first-line drug and the side effects are tolerable, no adjustment in dosing is needed
2. If the seizures are not controlled with the average dose of a first-line drug, and if there is no evidence of serious toxicity, there are two options to consider: The dose of the drug can be systematically increased until the seizures are controlled or until side effects preclude further increases in the dose OR a second AED can be added

---

If the maximal tolerated dose of the first-line AED does not control the seizures, one option is to substitute another first-line AED for use as monotherapy
✓ Start a second drug and taper the first. As the dosage of the new medication is titrated, the first medication is gradually tapered until monotherapy with the new agent is achieved. If control is not obtained with monotherapy with a second drug, then refer to a neurologist
✓ Never abruptly withdraw any drug; gradually taper
A second option when the first AED does not control the seizures is to add another first-line (or second-line) AED while continuing the first
✓ Until very recently, therapy with 2 or more AEDs was used only after two or more first-line drugs given as monotherapy had been ineffective
✓ Since most of the newer AEDs for partial seizures (the most common types of seizures) are approved by the FDA only as adjunctive therapy, there has been an increased use of two-drug regimens that consist of one first-line drug and one of the newer second-line drugs approved for adjunctive therapy
✓ Selected adjunctive medications for use in patients with partial seizures are listed in the box below

> ### *Selected adjunctive medications for partial seizures*
>
> Divalproex sodium (Depakote) [approved for monotherapy or adjunctive therapy]
> Gabapentin (Neurontin)
> Levetiracetam (Keppra)
> Oxcarbazepine (Trileptal) [approved for monotherapy or adjunctive therapy]
> Tiagabine (Gabitril)

H. Patient's age, seizure type, daily activities, and economic considerations should influence selection of AED
1. Oxcarbazepine may have less initial toxicity than carbamazepine and phenytoin and may be particularly useful in patients with poor tolerance of side effects which tends to reduce compliance
2. Phenytoin is a poor first choice for young adults because of the consequences of long-term use that may include coarsening of the facial features, gingival hyperplasia, hirsutism, and enlargement of the lips
3. For some patients, phenytoin and phenobarbital (which has fallen out of favor as an AED) are attractive choices because of once-daily dosing and low cost
4. Elderly patients are likely to be taking multiple medications; gabapentin is very desirable because it is very well tolerated and has no pharmacokinetic interactions
5. Potential teratogenicity is an important consideration for women with potential to become pregnant; rate of mild birth defects appears to be the same for all older (conventional) AEDs, but valproate frequently causes neural tube defects

I. The newer AEDs include tiagabine, gabapentin, lamotrigine, levetiracetam, oxcarbazepine, zonisamide, and topiramate; these drugs are used primarily as adjunctive therapy in refractory patients

J. Usual dosages of commonly prescribed AEDs
1. Carbamazepine: Tegretol, 100, 200 mg scored tabs and chewable tabs; Tegretol suspension, 100 mg/5 mL
   a. Starting dose is 200-400 mg/day divided into 2 doses; increase dose by 200 mg/day at 1-wk intervals
   b. Maintenance dose is 800-2800 mg/day, divided in 2-3 doses
   c. Tegretol-XR: 100, 200, 400 mg tabs: Same beginning dose and weekly rate of increase as described above for adults **except** dosing should remain at twice a day for this extended release product
   d. Carbamazepine interacts with many other drugs
2. Phenytoin: Dilantin, 30, 100 mg caps, and 50 mg chewable tabs; Dilantin suspension, 125 mg/5 mL
   a. Begin with 200 mg/day, in a once daily dose; increase dose by 100 mg/day at 4-wk intervals (adjustments in maintenance dose >300 mg should be made in 25-30 mg increments)
   b. Maintenance dose is 300-400 mg/day in a single dose or divided into 2 doses
   c. Patients who develop hypersensitivity reactions to phenytoin are often susceptible to similar reactions with carbamazepine and phenobarbital
   d. Phenytoin may interfere with cognitive function related to learning

    e. Interacts with many other drugs
   3. Ethosuximide: Zarontin 250 mg caps; Zarontin suspension, 250 mg/5 mL
    a. Starting dose is 500 mg/day, divided into two doses; increase dose by 250 mg/day at 1-wk intervals
    b. Maintenance dose is 750-1500 mg/day, divided into 2 doses
    c. Used only for absence seizures, thus uncommonly used in adults as few adults have this seizure type
   4. Divalproex sodium (Depakote) [monotherapy or adjunctive medication], 125, 250, 500 mg tabs; Depakote Sprinkle, 125 mg
    a. Dosing is by weight. Starting dose is 10-15 mg/kg/day (for most adults, 250-500 mg/day), divided in 1 or 2 doses; increase weekly by 5-10 mg/kg/day until optimal response
    b. Maintenance dose is usually 750-3000 mg/day (maximum 60 mg/kg/day) divided into 2-3 doses
    c. Effective and usually well tolerated; fatal liver failure can occur
   5. Phenobarbital
    a. Starting dose is 30-60 mg/day, in a once daily dose; increase dose by 30 mg/day at 4-wk intervals
    b. Maintenance dose is 90-180 mg/day, once daily or BID
    c. Interacts with many drugs
   6. Gabapentin (Neurontin) [adjunctive medication], 100, 300, 400 mg caps; 600, 800 mg tabs; oral solution, 250 mg/5 mL
    a. Starting dose is 900 mg/day, divided into 3 doses; increase dose by 300 mg/day at 24-hour intervals
    b. Maintenance dose is 1200-3600 mg/day, divided into 3 doses
    c. Gabapentin is not metabolized and is almost completely excreted by the kidneys; dosage adjustment required in patients with renal function impairment
    d. Generally well tolerated and there are few drug interactions
   7. Oxcarbazepine (Trileptal) [monotherapy or adjunctive medication], 150, 300, 600 mg tabs; oral solution, 300 mg/5 mL
    a. Starting dose is 300-600 mg/day, divided into 2 doses; increase dose by 300 mg/day at 1-wk intervals
    b. Maintenance dose is 900-2400 mg/day, divided into 2 or 3 doses
    c. Drug interactions are minor
   8. Levetiracetam (Keppra) [adjunctive medication], 250, 500, 750 mg scored tabs
    a. Starting dose is 500-1000 mg/day, divided into 2 doses; increase dose by 1000 mg/day at 2-wk intervals
    b. Maintenance dose is 1000-3000 mg/day, divided into 2 or 3 doses
    c. No life-threatening adverse effects have been reported
   9. Tiagabine (Gabitril) [adjunctive medication], 2, 4, 12, 16 mg tabs
    a. Starting dose is 4 mg/day divided into 2 doses for one week; increase by 4-8 mg weekly to clinical response
    b. Maintenance dose is 32-56 mg/day, divided into 3-4 doses
    c. Should be taken with food to minimize abdominal pain and nausea

K. For drugs with established therapeutic range of plasma concentrations, titrate dosage to achieve adequate concentrations, recognizing that this is only a rough guide for determining the appropriate dosage
  1. Treat the patient, not the plasma drug concentration
  2. Plasma drug concentrations within the therapeutic range may have toxic effects
  3. Seizures may be controlled in some patients with plasma drug concentrations below the therapeutic range
  4. Titration of dose of phenytoin must be done with great caution because of its nonlinear pharmacokinetics

L. Once AED therapy is initiated, it is maintained for 2 or more years, even if the patient is seizure free
  1. If after 2 years of therapy, the patient remains free of seizures, withdrawal of the AED should be considered
  2. Disadvantages of continuing therapy include the risks of side effects, drug interactions, and teratogenicity (in women) as well as the costs of therapy
  3. Withdrawal of therapy should be gradual (with dose tapering over time) and at a mutually agreed upon time with the patient

4. Risk of recurrent seizures is 25% among patients without risk factors and about 50% in patients with such factors

5. About 80% of recurrences occur within 4 months after a regimen of tapering of dosage has been begun and 90% occur within the first year

6. Caution patients about driving and operating machinery for at least the first 4 months after the start of drug withdrawal

M. Patient education is summarized below
1. Understanding the disorder and the prescribed medications by both the patient and family is of the utmost importance; non-adherence to the medication regime has been identified as the single most common reason for treatment failure
   a. Teach patient regarding dosing, actions, side effects, and drug interactions of the particular AED that is being prescribed
   b. For women of childbearing age or who are taking oral contraceptives, emphasize that AEDs are teratogenic and that they also reduce the effectiveness of oral contraceptives
   c. Patient education must be continuous and must be addressed at every visit
2. Instruct families regarding the fundamentals of emergency management of seizures

N. Review the law in your state concerning operating a motor vehicle by persons with seizure disorders
1. In most states, drivers are required to self-report a seizure disorder to the Department of Motor Vehicles at the time of diagnosis; healthcare clinicians may not report a patient's condition without a written release of information from the patient (there are exceptions to this, however)
2. Six states (CA, DE, NV, NJ, OR, and PA) require mandatory provider reporting of patients with seizures to regulatory authorities
3. Recognize that whereas regulating driving privileges of epileptic patients may seen beneficial, it actually is unnecessary and may hinder medical management
   a. The relative risk for MVAs involving epileptic drivers is comparable to or lower than those of more prevalent conditions not subject to similar mandatory reporting requirements
   b. Only about 25% of epileptic drivers experiencing a seizure in the past 12 months report the seizure to their healthcare clinician for fear of being reported to the licensing authorities
4. A summary of requirements for each state is available from the Epilepsy Foundation at http://www.efa.org

O. Refer the patient and family to the Epilepsy Foundation of American (EFA), an organization dedicated to countering societal misconceptions and prejudices about epilepsy as well as improving the quality of life for persons affected by seizures
1. The national office can be contacted by writing EFA, 4351 Garden City Drive, Landover, MD 20785-2267 or by calling 301-459-3700 or 1-800-EFA-1000; the website is listed above
2. Most states have local affiliates which provide community outreach programs, support groups, information and referral, employment services, respite care for families, and help with living arrangements

P. Follow Up
1. Follow-up visits should be weekly during period of adjusting medication dose, then every 3 months for the next 6 months, and then every 6 months thereafter
2. Monitoring of plasma drug concentrations for therapeutic range is indicated for many of the AEDs and should be done on a regular basis and with any medication adjustment
3. Periodic monitoring of blood cell counts and hepatic enzyme levels—every 3-6 months is recommended with many of the medications (consult package inserts for monitoring requirements for all medications prescribed)

STROKE AND TRANSIENT ISCHEMIC ATTACK

I.   Definitions

    A.   Stroke: An episode of focal cerebral ischemia that causes cerebral infarction in a vascular territory relevant to the patient's symptoms

    B.   Transient ischemic attack (TIA): A neurologic deficit lasting <24 hours that is attributed to cerebral or retinal ischemia
        1.   This standard definition of TIA is currently being reconsidered; a new definition has been proposed that preserves the concept of the TIA, but replaces the arbitrary 24-hour criterion for the maximal duration of symptoms with a criterion that more closely matches the typical duration of a TIA
        2.   The proposed definition of a TIA is as follows: A brief episode of neurologic dysfunction caused by focal brain or retinal ischemia, with clinical symptoms typically lasting less than one hour and without evidence of acute infarction (TIA Working Group [Albers, et al.], 2002)

II.   Pathogenesis

    A.   Ischemia is the most frequent cause of cerebrovascular dysfunction; approximately 70% of all strokes are ischemic strokes
        1.   Atherosclerosis is the underlying process resulting in ischemic cerebrovascular disease in most patients
            a.   Larger vessels at base of brain and in neck at bifurcations are most commonly affected
            b.   Narrowed sites in the affected vessels collect atherosclerotic plaque, cholesterol debris, and platelet-fibrin material, a process that over time leads to significant stenosis and cerebral ischemia
            c.   Lacunar events are small infarcts caused by thrombotic occlusion of the small, deep penetrating vessels in the deeper, subcortical parts of the cerebrum and brain stem
        2.   Embolic strokes occur when a thrombus is released from a proximal site and lodges in a distal vessel, compromising blood flow; the most common sources of emboli are the heart and major vessels (carotid and vertebral arteries) with stenotic lesions
            a.   Cardiac sources of emboli include myocardial infarction, valvular heart disease, ventricular septal defects with thrombus formation, and arrhythmias, especially atrial fibrillation which accounts for 65% of all embolic strokes
            b.   Rare causes of emboli include endocarditis and fat emboli secondary to long bone fractures

    B.   The causes of true transient ischemic attacks are identical to those of ischemic stroke; stroke and TIA are both on the spectrum of serious conditions involving brain ischemia

    C.   Hemorrhage is the other main type of cerebrovascular dysfunction and results from leakage of blood outside normal vessels
        1.   In a subarachnoid hemorrhage, bleeding occurs within the surrounding membranes and cerebrospinal fluid
        2.   An intracerebral hemorrhage occurs when bleeding is directly into the cerebral parenchyma; the majority of cases of intracerebral hemorrhage are associated with chronic hypertension
        3.   Hemorrhagic transformation of an ischemic stroke can occur after large infarctions or with heparin or tPA therapy

III. Clinical Presentation

    A.   Stroke is the most common cause of major neurologic disability and third most common cause of death in the US among persons ≥65 years of age

    B.   Cerebrovascular disorders including TIAs and stroke occur most often in those >65 years of age with risk factors of hypertension (the major risk factor), atherosclerosis, smoking, and hyperlipidemia; male gender and diabetes mellitus are also important risk factors

    C.   Nearly all thrombotic strokes are preceded by a TIA affecting the same region as the ensuing stroke; after a first TIA, 10-20% of patients have a stroke in the next 90 days, and in 50% of these patients, the stroke occurs in the first 24-48 hours after the TIA

D. The occurrence of a TIA provides an opportunity to prevent stroke in a group at very high risk
   1. Factors associated with an increased risk of stroke after a TIA include advanced age, diabetes mellitus, symptoms for more than 10 minutes, weakness, and impaired speech
   2. The cause of true TIAs (e.g., atrial fibrillation, carotid-artery disease, and large- and small-artery disease in the brain) are identical to those of stroke; thus strategies to prevent further attacks are similar to those for stroke

E. TIAs and ischemic stroke are characterized by sudden onset (over seconds to minutes) of neurologic deficits such as weakness, anesthesia, incontinence, loss of vision, aphasia, and dysarthria; occasionally headache or vertigo may occur

F. Hemorrhagic events usually have abrupt onset with deficits rapidly evolving
   1. Subarachnoid hemorrhages often occur in a younger population (50% of patients are under age 55) and the first symptom may be a sudden, severe headache followed by nausea, vomiting, and altered consciousness
   2. Symptoms and signs of intracerebral hemorrhage are variable, and may range from minor focal problems to coma; loss of function, headache, nausea and vomiting are common

G. Hemorrhagic stroke cannot be accurately differentiated from ischemic stroke without CT scanning

IV. Diagnosis/Evaluation: Patients who present to primary care settings and report **on-going** symptoms suggesting a TIA or stroke as well as those patients who report that such symptoms were experienced within **hours or days prior to presentation** but have since apparently resolved, should be immediately sent to the emergency department (ED) for initial evaluation as even a short delay in treatment can have important consequences. Patients who present within weeks of the event can be evaluated in the primary care setting as described below

A. History
   1. Patients presenting with possible TIAs several weeks after the event: Determine severity, duration, and frequency of symptoms
   2. Inquire about symptoms indicating neurologic impairment such as transient blindness, double vision, dizziness, headache, sensory deficiencies, speech problems, motor difficulties, and weakness/numbness
   3. Question about risk factors such as hypertension, smoking, hyperlipidemia, cardiac disease, diabetes mellitus, and heredity
   4. Involve family members in history taking because patient is often unaware of the total clinical presentation (it is not reasonable to base the diagnosis on recollections of the patient who was neurologically impaired during the event)

B. Physical Examination
   1. Blood pressure readings both in lying and sitting positions
   2. Ophthalmoscopic examination to detect ocular plaques in retinal artery branches
   3. Gently palpate and auscultate carotid arteries for bruits
   4. Complete cardiovascular exam including palpation and auscultation of peripheral pulses
   5. Perform complete neurological examination to identify any persistent deficits
   6. Complete a mental status examination using the Mini-Mental State Exam (see section on ALZHEIMER'S DISEASE)

C. Differential Diagnosis: Migraine, seizure, vasovagal syncope, arrhythmia, compressive neuropathy, anxiety, and conversion disorder

D. Diagnostic Tests
   1. For patients who present with a history suggestive of a transient ischemic attack that occurred several weeks prior to presentation, order CBC, platelet count, erythrocyte sedimentation rate, serum glucose, lipid panel, creatinine, sodium, and potassium levels; also measure homocysteine, serum folate, and vitamin B_{12} (purpose is to identify causes of TIA that would require specific therapy and to assess modifiable risk factors)
   2. An electrocardiogram (ECG) is recommended for all patients
   3. Brain imaging is recommended in all patients; whereas MRI has greater sensitivity than CT for the identification of acute ischemic lesions and for differentiating infarcts of varying ages, it is more expensive and less widely available

4. To assess suspected carotid lesions, prompt ultrasonography, magnetic resonance angiography, or CT angiography is recommended
5. Neurologic consultation is appropriate for determining the optimal diagnostic evaluation and establishing the diagnosis

V. Plan/Management

A. See IV. above for management of patients who present with on-going symptoms suggesting a TIA or stroke as well as patients who report that such symptoms were experienced (but have now resolved) within hours or days prior to presentation

B. All patients who present with a history of continuing TIAs despite ongoing therapy with aspirin or another antiplatelet agent should be referred for emergent care

C. Patients who present with a remote (>1 month since event) **history** of TIAs and who are not presently receiving antiplatelet therapy should be managed as follows
1. Aspirin 81 mg to 325 mg is the first-line therapy for secondary prevention of TIAs and subsequent strokes
2. Clopidogrel (Plavix) 75 mg QD is an acceptable option for patients who are intolerant of aspirin
3. Another option is aspirin (25 mg)/dipyridamole (200 mg) [Aggrenox], one tab BID
   a. Consult PDR for precautions, contraindications, interactions, and monitoring requirements before prescribing these or any other medications
   b. Ticlopidine (Ticlid) can cause life-threatening hematological adverse reactions so its use as an antiplatelet agent has declined

D. In addition to the initiation of antiplatelet therapy in patients after a TIA, treatment of risk factors for CVD to prevent subsequent TIAs should be implemented
1. For patients with atrial fibrillation, anticoagulation with warfarin should be initiated
2. Hypertension must be appropriately controlled (maintain systolic blood pressure below 140 mm Hg and diastolic blood pressure below 90 mm Hg; for patients with diabetes, heart failure, or chronic renal failure maintain systolic blood pressure below 130 mm Hg and diastolic blood pressure below 85 mm Hg); ACE inhibitors are effective in preventing stroke in patients with diabetes
3. For patients with diabetes mellitus, maintain fasting blood glucose levels below 126 mg/dL (7.0 mmol/dL)
4. Inadequate physical activity and obesity should also be addressed in patients who require such interventions (see section on OBESITY for latest recommendations on goals and counseling)
5. Patients with elevated lipid levels should receive appropriate dietary counseling, weight management counseling (see section on OBESITY), and placement on lipid-lowering drugs if indicated; statins appear to reduce the risk of stroke and cardiovascular events in patients with CAD, even when dyslipidemia is absent, and gemfibrozil seems to be effective in patients with low levels of both high-density and low-density cholesterol
6. Tobacco use is a major risk factor for stroke; see section on TOBACCO USE AND SMOKING CESSATION for details on management of patients who use tobacco

E. Patients in whom carotid disease is confirmed should be considered for carotid endarterectomy (CEA)
1. Carotid endarterectomy is beneficial in patients with internal-carotid-artery stenosis of 70-90% who have had a stroke or a TIA attributable to the stenosis
2. The procedure is marginally beneficial in selected patients with stenosis of 50-69%
3. Benefits are highly dependent on the surgical experience of the treatment center; thus caution should be used in referring patients for this procedure

F. Follow Up
1. Patients should be evaluated every 3-6 months to determine response to treatment outlined above
2. Patients who continue to experience TIAs in spite of the intervention should be referred to a specialist for management

TREMOR

I.   Definition: Visible, involuntary, rhythmic oscillatory movements of a body part

II.   Pathogenesis

    A.   Tremor is produced by repetitive patterns of involuntary muscle contractions and relaxation

    B.   All humans exhibit a physiologic tremor of the hands; even though not visible to the naked eye, this physiologic tremor is detectable with the use of electrophysiological techniques such as quantitative accelerometry
       1.   Stressful events such as fatigue, anger, or fear may produce transient enhancement of physiologic tremor
       2.   Endocrine disorders such as hyperthyroidism and substances such as caffeine, cigarettes, and certain medications such as lithium, prednisone, levothyroxine, beta-adrenergic bronchodilators, valproate, and selective serotonin-reuptake inhibitors can result in enhanced physiologic tremor
       3.   With enhancement, a physiologic tremor may become visible to the naked eye

    C.   Tremors can be classified according to their specific clinical features--resting tremor, action tremor (also called postural tremor), and intention tremor

    D.   **Resting tremor** is most commonly due to one of the following
       1.   Parkinson's disease (most common cause of resting tremor)
       2.   Secondary parkinsonism: postencephalitic, toxic (e.g., carbon monoxide), tumor, trauma
       3.   Heterogeneous disorders with parkinsonian features such as Wilson's disease

    E.   **Action tremor** is most commonly due to one of the following
       1.   Essential tremor (a so-called benign tremor) is by far the most common action tremor
       2.   Enhanced physiologic tremor is also a common type of action tremor
       3.   Parkinson's disease can also cause an action tremor although resting tremor is much more common

    F.   **Intention tremor** is most commonly due to one of the following
       1.   Cerebellar disease
       2.   Multiple sclerosis

III. Clinical presentation of common tremors

    A.   **Resting tremor** occurs when the limb is relaxed and stationary, for example, in the hand when a person is walking or standing still; resting tremor of Parkinson's disease often begins with a "pill-rolling" tremor of one hand (see section on PARKINSON'S DISEASE)

    B.   **Action tremor** occurs during sustained extension of the arm and hand during such activities as writing or pouring a liquid from a container
       1.   Most prevalent clinical type of tremor
       2.   Because it occurs when the hands are in active use, can be very disabling
       3.   **Most common action tremor** is essential tremor, a tremor of the hands that may also affect the head, voice, trunk, and legs; a distal tremor (amplitude greatest at wrist joint and least at shoulder), that is slightly asymmetric (an average of 30% difference between sides)
          a.   Prevalence of essential tremor in general population is estimated at between 0.4-6%
          b.   Highest prevalence is in persons over 65 years of age
          c.   About 15-25% of affected persons retire prematurely, and up to 60% elect not to apply for a job or promotion because of uncontrollable shaking of their hands
       4.   The **second most common action tremor** is enhanced and sustained physiologic tremor
          a.   Physiologic tremor can be enhanced and sustained by an identifiable cause such as stressful circumstances, endocrine disorders (e.g., hyperthyroidism), and certain substances and medications
          b.   Cause of the tremor may not be readily identifiable
          c.   Tremor is fine, barely visible, and rapid, often occurring when hands are outstretched

C. **Intention tremor** is a coarse terminal tremor that occurs as the arm approaches a target, for example, during the finger-to-nose maneuver; often accompanied by ataxic gait and other signs of cerebellar disease

D. Clinical criteria for essential tremor are contained in the table below

CLINICAL CRITERIA FOR ESSENTIAL TREMOR
Definite Essential Tremor

➡ Moderate amplitude action tremor is present in at least one arm while performing at least four of the following tasks
   ✓ Pouring water
   ✓ Drinking water
   ✓ Using a spoon to drink water
   ✓ Performing finger-to-nose maneuver
   ✓ Drawing a spiral

➡ Tremor interferes with at least one activity of daily living (ADL)
➡ Tremor is not caused by medications, hyperthyroidism, alcohol use, and other neurological disorders
Probable Essential Tremor
➡ Moderate amplitude action tremor present in at least one arm during at least four of tasks listed above, or head tremor is present
➡ Tremor is not caused by medications, hyperthyroidism, alcohol use, and other neurological disorders

Adapted from Louis, E.D. (2001). Essential tremor. *New England Journal of Medicine, 345*, 887-891.

IV. Diagnosis/Evaluation

A. History
1. The first step is to characterize the tremor by asking whether tremor occurs during rest, activity, or when the hand approaches a target (patient reaches for an object)
2. Determine age of onset, type, and rate of progression
3. Ask about presence of associated signs and symptoms with a focus on neurologic and endocrine-related symptoms
4. Inquire about family history of tremor
5. Obtain medication history; inquire about substance use including alcohol, caffeine, tobacco, and illicit substances
6. Determine the impact of tremor on performing activities of daily living and work-related activities

B. Physical Examination
1. Assess the characteristics of the tremor by asking the patient to perform certain activities
   a. Observe hands resting in patient's lap and with arms outstretched
   b. Observe patient during performance of finger-to-nose and heel-to-shin maneuvers, rapid alternating movements, and handwriting
2. Assess functional competence—observe patient pour water, drink from cup, apply lip balm
3. Perform a complete neurological examination

C. Differential Diagnosis
1. In Parkinson's disease, both resting and action tremor may be present but resting is much more common; other signs of Parkinson's disease are usually present (rigidity, flexed posture, slow finger taps, minimal arm swing)
2. In Wilson's disease, both resting and action tremor are present; a wing-beating tremor is seen; other neurologic abnormalities are present (dystonia, dysarthria); age is <40 years
3. In cerebellar disease, ataxic gait, nystagmus, and slurred or scanning speech are common findings in addition to intention tremor
4. Motor tics often begin in childhood and are differentiated from tremor by their lack of rhythmicity, and by their complexity of movement, and associations with vocalizations and behavioral disturbances
5. In enhanced physiologic tremor (an action tremor), tremor is usually present equally in the outstretched arms and legs, and signs/symptoms of the underlying cause often become evident based on history and physical examination
6. In essential tremor (an action tremor), the tremor is distal with the greatest movement at the wrist joint and the least at the shoulder; most often mildly asymmetric with an average of 30% difference between sides; neurologic exam is normal. Reliable clinical criteria for essential tremor are presented in the table above (see III.D.)

D. Diagnostic Tests
    1. If enhanced physiologic tremor is suspected, appropriate tests based on findings from history and physical examination should be performed to diagnose the underlying cause (most often hyperthyroidism)
    2. If essential tremor is diagnosed based on history and physical examination, no tests are needed
    3. In patients with action tremor who are <40 years of age, possibility of Wilson's disease should be explored with measurement of serum ceruloplasmin
    4. Patients with abnormal neurologic findings on physical examination should be referred to a neurologist for further diagnostic testing

V. Plan/Management

A. Management of patients with enhanced physiologic tremor depends on the underlying cause; if no cause is identified, refer to expert for evaluation and management

B. Patients with essential tremor who are dysfunctional or impaired by the tremor require pharmacotherapy in order to improve function and reduce embarrassment associated with the tremor
    1. Most current medications were found to be useful as a result of serendipity rather than through an understanding of the mechanisms of the disease, which remain unclear
    2. Medications used in the management of essential tremor are contained in the following table

PHARMACOLOGIC MANAGEMENT OF ESSENTIAL TREMOR*

Medication	Usual Starting Dose (mg/day)	Usual Therapeutic Dose (mg/day)
First-Line Agents		
Propranolol	30	160-320
Primidone	62.5	62.5-1000
Second-Line Agents		
Gabapentin	300	1200-3600
Alprazolam	0.75	0.75-2.75

Comments

Propranolol
Dose of at least 120 mg/day results in significant reduction in severity of tremor; contraindications include asthma, sinus bradycardia, 2nd or 3rd degree AV block, heart failure, cardiogenic shock; slowly advance to therapeutic dose and avoid abrupt cessation! Long acting propranolol usually produces better compliance (once-daily dosing). Consult PDR for precautions, interactions, adverse reactions

Primidone
Dose of up to 750 mg/day can be effective in reducing tremor; increase dose every 3 days as needed to reach therapeutic dose; tolerability is a common problem with sedation, nausea, vomiting, ataxia, frequent side effects; even though initial tolerability is problematic, long-term tolerability is better. Consult PDR for contraindications, precautions, interactions

Gabapentin
In doses of 1200 to 3600 mg/day, tremor reduction may be similar to that of propranolol; titrate dose over several days and avoid abrupt cessation; well tolerated. Consult PDR for contraindications, precautions, interactions, adverse reactions

Alprazolam
The only benzodiazepine shown to be effective in essential tremor in controlled trials; drowsiness and sedation are significant problems and risk of dependence is also an important concern. Consult PDR for contraindications, precautions, interactions, adverse reactions

*None of the medications listed here are FDA approved for this indication
Adapted from Louis, E.D. (2001). Essential tremor. *New England Journal of Medicine, 345,* 887-891.

C. Patient education prior to prescribing medication to control tremor should include a discussion of the fact that, in most cases, tremor may be reduced in severity but not totally eliminated

D. Response to medications is variable; a trial of several agents may be necessary and management by a neurologist is recommended if patient response to medication is poor

E. There are currently two surgical approaches to tremor reduction that are available for patients who are severely disabled by essential tremor; referral for surgery should be a joint decision by the patient and the neurologist

F.   Follow Up
1.   Patients diagnosed with enhanced physiologic tremor should return on a regular schedule to monitor the underlying cause of the tremor
2.   Patients diagnosed with essential tremor and treated with medications should have first return visit scheduled in 2 weeks after initiation of treatment to determine effectiveness; other return visits should be scheduled based on patient need

REFERENCES

Abramowicz, M. (2003). Drugs for epilepsy. *Treatment Guidelines from the Medical Letter, 1*, 57-64.

Abramowicz, M. (2003). Triptans for migraine. *The Medical Letter, 45*, pp. 33-36.

Adler, C.H. (2001). Diagnosing and treating restless legs syndrome. *Women's Health in Primary Care, 4*, 224-230.

Albers, G.W., Caplan, L.R., Easton, J.D., Fayad, P.B., Mohr J.P., Saver, J.L., et al. (TIA Working Group) (2002). Transient ischemic attack— proposal for a new definition. *New England Journal of Medicine, 347*, 1713-1716.

American Sleep Disorders Association. (1997). *International classification of sleep disorders, revised: Diagnostic and coding manual.* Rochester, MN. Author.

Bahra, A., May, A., & Goadsby, P.J. (2002). Cluster headache: A prospective clinical study with diagnostic implications. *Neurology, 58*, 354-361.

Bendadis, S.R., & Tatum, W.O. (2001). Advances in the treatment of epilepsy. *American Family Physician, 64*, 91-98.

Breslau, N., & Rasmussen, B.K. (2001). The impact of migraine. *Neurology, 56*, S4-S12.

Brown, T.R., & Holmes, G.L. (2001). Epilepsy. *New England Journal of Medicine, 344*, 1145-1151.

Clark, C.M., & Karlawish, J.H.T. (2003). Alzheimer disease: Current concepts and emerging diagnostic and therapeutic strategies. *Annals of Internal Medicine, 138*, 400-410.

Clinch, C.R. (2001). Evaluation of acute headaches in adults. *American Family Physician, 63*, 685-692.

Colcher, A., & Simunia, T. (1999). Clinical manifestations of Parkinson's disease. *Medical Clinics of North America, 83*, 327-345.

Cummings, J.L., Frank, J.C., Cherry, D., Kohatsu, N.E., Kemp, B., Hewett, L., & Mittman, B. (2002). Guidelines for managing Alzheimer's disease: Part I. Assessment. *American Family Physician, 65*, 2263-2272.

Cummings, J.L., Frank, J.C., Cherry, D., Kohatsu, N.E., Kemp, B., Hewett, L., & Mittman, B. (2002). Guidelines for managing Alzheimer's disease: Part II. Treatment. *American Family Physician, 65,* 2525-2534.

Diaz-Arrastia, R., Agnostini, M.A., & Van Ness, P.C. (2002). Evolving treatment strategies for epilepsy. *Journal of the American Medical Association, 287*, 2917-2922.

Dodick, D.W. (2003). Diagnosing headache: Clinical clues and clinical rules. *Advanced Studies in Medicine, 2*, 87-92.

Doody, R.S., Stevens, J.C., Beck, C., Dubinsky, R.M., Kay, J.A., Gwyther, L., et al. for the Quality Standards Subcommittee of the American Academy of Neurology. (2001). Practice parameter: Management of dementia (an evidence-based review). *Neurology, 56*, 1154-1166.

Epley, J.M. (1992). The canalith repositioning procedure for treatment of benign paroxysmal positional vertigo. *Otolaryngology, Head & Neck Surgery, 107*, 399-405.

Fago, J.P. (2001, January 15). Dementia: Causes, evaluation, and management. *Hospital Practice*, 59-69.

Folstein, M.F., Folstein, S.E., & McHugh, P.R. (1975). Mini-mental state: A practical method for grading the cognitive state of patients for the clinician. *Journal of Psychiatric Research, 12*, 189-198.

Fountain, N.B. (2002). Seizures and epilepsy in adolescents and adults. In R.E. Rakel, & E.T. Bope (Eds.), *Conn's current therapy* (pp. 884-893). Philadelphia: Saunders.

Furman, J.M., & Cass, S.P. (1999). Benign paroxysmal positional vertigo. *New England Journal of Medicine, 341*, 1590-1598.

Goadsby, P.J., Lipton, R.B., & Ferrari, M.D. (2002). Migraine—Current understanding and treatment. *New England Journal of Medicine, 346*, 257-269.

Goroll, A.H., & Mulley, Jr., A.G. (2002). *Primary care medicine recommendations.* Philadelphia: Lippincott Williams & Wilkins.

Hotson, J.R., & Baloh, R.W. (1998). Acute vestibular syndrome. *New England Journal of Medicine, 339,* 680-685.

Johnston, S.C. (2002). Transient ischemic attack. *New England Journal of Medicine, 347,* 1687-1687.

Kaniecki, R. (2003). Headache assessment and management. *JAMA, 289,* 1430-1433.

Kapoor, W. N. (2000). Syncope. *New England Journal of Medicine, 343,* 1856-1862.

Karlawish, J.H.T., & Clark, C.M. (2003). Diagnostic evaluation of elderly patients with mild memory problems. *Annals of Internal Medicine, 138,* 411-419.

Katz, S., Ford, A.B., Moskowitz, R.W., Jackson, B.A., & Jaffe, M.W. (1963). Studies of illness in the aged: The index of ADL, a standardized measure of biological and psychosocial function. *Journal of the American Medical Association, 185,* 914-919.

Knopman, D.S., DeKosky, S.T., Cummings, J.L., Chui, H., Corey-Bloom, J., Relkin, N., et al. for the Quality Standards Subcommittee of the American Academy of Neurology. (2001). Practice parameter: Diagnosis of dementia (an evidence-based review). *Neurology, 56,* 1143-1153.

Kraus, G.L., Ampaw, L., & Krumholz, A. (2001). Individual state driving restrictions for people with epilepsy in the US. *Neurology, 57,* 1780-1785.

Lambert, P.R. (2002). Acute facial paralysis (Bells' palsy). In R.E. Rakel, & E.T. Bope (Eds.), *Conn's current therapy* (pp. 948-950). Philadelphia: Saunders.

Lawton, M.P., & Brody, E.M. (1969). Assessment of older people: Self-maintaining and instrumental activities of daily living. *Gerontologist, 9,* 179-186.

Lipton, R.B., Stewart, W.F., & Stone, A.M. (2000). Stratified care versus step care strategies for migraine. *JAMA, 284,* 2599-2605.

Llinas, R., Aldrich, E., & Wityk, R. (2003). Update on stroke prevention and treatment. *Advanced Studies in Medicine, 3,* 93-101.

Logemann, G.D., & Ranking, L.M. (2000). Newer intranasal migraine medications. *American Family Physician, 61,* 180-186.

Louis, E.D. (2001). Essential tremor. *New England Journal of Medicine, 345,* 887-891.

Martin, C.O. (2002). Neurology. In M.A. Graver & M.L. Lanternier (Eds). *The family practice handbook* (pp. 337-390). St. Louis: Mosby.

Millea, P.J., Brodie, J.J. (2002). Tension-type headache. *American Family Physician, 66,* 797-804.

Miyasaki, J.M., Martin, W., Suchowersky, O., Weiner, W.J., & Lang, A.E. for the Quality Standards Subcommittee of the American Academy of Neurology. (2002). Practice parameter: Initiation of treatment for Parkinson's disease: An evidence-based review. *Neurology, 58,* 11-17.

Morey, S.S. (2000). Guidelines on migraine: Part 2. General principles of drug therapy. *American Family Physician, 62,* 1915-1918.

Morey, S.S. (2000). Guidelines on migraine: Part 3. Recommendations for individual drugs. *American Family Physician, 62,* 2145-2152.

Morey, S.S. (2000). Guidelines on migraine: Part 4. General principles of preventive therapy. *American Family Physician, 62,* 2359-2364.

Morey, S.S. (2000). Guidelines on migraine: Part 5. Recommendations for specific prophylactic therapy. *American Family Physician, 62,* 2359-2364.

Morey, S.S. (2000). Headache consortium releases guidelines for use of CT or MRI in migraine. *American Family Physician, 62,* 1699-1702.

Mouradian, M.M. (2002). Recent advances in the genetics and pathogenesis of Parkinson disease. *Neurology, 58,* 179-185.

National Heart, Lung, and Blood Institute, National Center on Sleep Disorder Research and Office of Prevention, Education, and Control. (2000). *Restless legs syndrome: Detection and management in primary care.* Bethesda, MD: Author.

Nordli, D.R. (2002). Medical treatment of the child with epilepsy. In. F.D. Burg, J.R. Ingelfinger, R.A. Polin, & A.A. Gershon (Eds.), *Gellis & Kagan's current pediatric therapy* (pp. 446-453). Philadelphia: Elsevier Science.

Oas, J.G. (2002). Episodic vertigo. In R.E. Rakel, & E.T. Bope (Eds.), *Conn's current therapy* (pp. 912-917). Philadelphia: Saunders

Olanow, C.W., Watts, R.L., & Koller, W.C. (2001). An algorithm (decision tree) for the management of Parkinson's disease: Treatment guidelines. *Neurology, 56* (Suppl 4) S1-S88.

Paulson, G.W. (2000). Restless legs syndrome: How to provide symptom relief with drug and nondrug therapies. *Geriatrics, 55,* 35-48.

Petersen, R.C., Stevens, J.C., Ganguli, M., Tangalos, E.G., Cummings, J.L., & DeKosky, S.T. for the Quality Standards Subcommittee of the American Academy of Neurology. (2001). Practice parameter: Early detection of dementia: Mild cognitive impairment (an evidence-based review). *Neurology, 56,* 1133-1142.

Phillips, B.A. (2001, May) Restless legs syndrome: What is it? *Hospital Practice,* 53-57.

Prusiner, S.B. (2001). Neurodegenerative diseases and prions. *New England Journal of Medicine, 344,* 1516-1526.

Radtke, A., Neuhauser, H., von Breven, M., & Lempert, T. (1999). A modified Epley's procedure for self-treatment of benign paroxysmal positional vertigo. *Neurology, 53,* 1358-1360.

Rao, G., Fisch, L., Srinivasan, S., D'Amico, F., Okada, T., Eaton, C., & Robbins, C. (2003). Does this patient have Parkinson disease? *JAMA, 289,* 347-353.

Rehman, H. (2000). Diagnosis and management of tremor. *Archives of Internal Medicine, 160,* 2438-2444.

Rothdach, A.J., Trenkwalder, C., & Haberstock, J. (2000). Prevalence and risk factors of RLS in an elderly population: The MEMO study: Memory and morbidity in Augsburg elderly. *Neurology, 54,* 1064-1068.

Santacruz, K.S., & Swagerty, D. (2001). Early diagnosis of dementia. *American Family Physicians, 63,* 703-713.

Silberstein, S.D., for the US Headache Consortium. Report of the Quality Standards Subcommittee of the American Academy of Neurology. (2000). Practice parameter: Evidenced-based guidelines for migraine headache (an evidence-based review). *Neurology, 55,* 754-762.

Sloane, P.D., Coeytaux, R.R., Beck, R.S., & Dallara, J. (2001). Dizziness: State of the science. *Annals of Internal Medicine, 134,* 823-832.

Stewart, W.F., Lipton, R.B., Kolodner, K., Liberman, J., & Sawyer, J. (1999). Reliability of the migraine disability assessment score in a population-based sample of headache sufferers. *Cephalalgia, 19,* 107-114.

Tatum, W.O., Galvez, R., Benbadis, S., & Carrazana, E. (2000). New antiepileptic drugs. *Archives of Family Medicine, 9,* 1135-1141.

Tinetti, M.E., Williams, C.S., & Gill, T.M. (2000). Dizziness among older adults: A possible geriatric syndrome. *Annals of Internal Medicine, 132,* 337-344.

US Preventive Services Task Force. (2002). Screening for depression: Recommendations and rationale. *Annals of Internal Medicine, 136,* 760-764.

Velez, L., & Selwa, L.M. (2003). Seizure disorders in the elderly. *American Family Physician, 67,* 325-332.

Warshaw, G. (2002). Alzheimer's disease. In R.E. Rakel & E.T. Bope (Eds.), *Conn's current therapy* (pp. 867-872). Philadelphia: Saunders.

Young, M.G. (2001, February 15). Providing care for the caregiver. *Patient Care,* 68-74.

Young, R.R. (2002). What is a tremor? *Neurology, 58,* 165-166.

Hematologic Problems

MARY VIRGINIA GRAHAM

Anemia of Chronic Disease

Iron Deficiency Anemia

Megaloblastic Anemia

ANEMIA OF CHRONIC DISEASE

I. Definition: A hypoproliferative anemia associated with infectious, inflammatory, or neoplastic disorders that lasts >1-2 months

II. Pathogenesis

   A. The cause of anemia of chronic disease (ACD) is uncertain but the result is a decreased RBC life span as well as a reduction in the production or action of erythropoietin

   B. The basic defect is in the iron utilization for erythropoiesis
      1. For unknown reasons the delivery of iron from the reticuloendothelial iron stores to the developing red cell is blocked (defect in release mechanism)
      2. Consequently, the red cells are deficient in iron, whereas the body stores have abundant iron

   C. When the primary disease is controlled, the anemia is reversible

III. Clinical Presentation

   A. Clinical presentation is similar to that of iron deficiency anemia, but physical findings depend more on the nature of the underlying disease than on the anemia; anemia is usually mild and asymptomatic

   B. Laboratory findings are as follows:
      1. Usually, the peripheral blood smear shows a normochromic, normocytic picture, but in advanced states, the appearance may be hypochromic and microcytic (though not as severe as with iron deficiency anemia)
      2. Anemia is usually moderate, and if hematocrit is <25%, another explanation should be sought
      3. Serum iron and total iron-binding capacity (TIBC) are low; low TIBC helps differentiate this disorder from iron deficiency anemia
      4. Serum ferritin is normal or increased; use this point to discriminate between ACD and iron deficiency anemia since serum ferritin values are low in iron deficiency states

IV. Diagnosis/Evaluation

   A. History
      1. Determine onset, duration of symptoms
      2. Obtain complete medical history and medication history to determine if chronic disorder present

   B. Physical Examination: Guided by the history since numerous inflammatory processes, chronic infections, and malignant neoplasms can produce the anemia; **always** obtain stool for occult blood

   C. Diagnostic Tests

   ┌──┐
   ➡ CBC with peripheral smear should be ordered (or repeated since many patients will present because of abnormal hemoglobin/hematocrit on previous CBC)
   ➡ Test **first** for iron deficiency by ordering serum ferritin (test of choice for iron deficiency)
      • If iron deficiency identified, see IRON DEFICIENCY ANEMIA section for more information
      • If iron deficiency ruled out, assess for thalassemia (Mediterranean extraction, family history of anemia or thalassemia, characteristic findings of RBC indices and peripheral smear [target cells, teardrops, RBC count, reduced MCHC])
   ➡ Once iron deficiency and thalassemia have been ruled out
      • Review serum ferritin (usually normal or increased) and obtain transferrin saturation (iron/TIBC) to help differentiate anemia of chronic disease (ferritin normal or slightly increased, transferrin saturation low to normal, TIBC and serum iron decreased) from sideroblastic anemia (ferritin high, transferrin saturation high)
   ➡ At this point, should also order appropriate tests to determine underlying cause (based on findings from history and physical exam) or can wait for results of CBC and iron studies before proceeding
   └──┘

D. Differential Diagnosis
    1. Must be differentiated from other types of anemia with most common types in differential being iron deficiency, α-thalassemia, β-thalassemia, and sideroblastic anemia
    2. Numerous underlying causes including chronic infection, inflammatory processes, and malignant neoplasms

V. Plan/Treatment

   A. No specific therapy for ACD; successful treatment of the underlying disease leads to resolution of the anemia

   B. Consult specialist regarding use of erythropoietin (EPO) to stimulate erythropoiesis; patients with ACD have a relatively impaired response to erythropoietin and treating with EPO may not be successful

   C. Red cell transfusions are effective, but should be limited to situations in which oxygen transport is inadequate due to other medical problems

   D. Follow Up: Variable depending on underlying disorder causing the anemia

IRON DEFICIENCY ANEMIA

I. Definition: Anemia characterized by small, pale RBCs, and depletion of iron (Fe) stores

II. Pathogenesis

   A. Iron loss exceeds intake so that storage iron is progressively depleted

   B. As storage Fe is depleted, a compensatory increase in absorption of dietary Fe and in the concentration of transferrin occurs

   C. Iron stores are no longer able to meet the needs of the erythroid marrow; the plasma-transferrin level increases, the serum Fe concentration declines, resulting in a decrease in Fe available for RBC formation

   D. In adults, iron deficiency usually occurs as a result of bleeding

   E. In early childhood and adolescence, poor dietary intake and increased demand are common causes

III. Clinical Presentation

   A. In adults, the most common cause of iron deficiency anemia by far is blood loss
      1. In adult men and in postmenopausal women, bleeding is usually from the GI tract
      2. In women of childbearing age, menstrual loss is often the underlying mechanism, but other sites of bleeding must always be considered

   B. Other causes of IDA in adults include increased demand (as often occurs with pregnancy), inadequate absorption of iron from the gastrointestinal tract (as can occur with malabsorption syndromes, postgastrectomy states, or unrelenting diarrhea) and uncommonly from dietary deficiencies (for example, in vegetarians, food faddists, or anorectics)

   C. Iron deficiency anemia is usually slow in onset, allowing for compensatory mechanisms to develop so that symptoms may be minimal until significant anemia develops

   D. Clinical presentation depends on severity, age, and ability of the cardiovascular and pulmonary systems to compensate for decreasing oxygen carrying capacity of the blood

   E. There are few symptoms when hematocrit (HCT) is 30 or above in otherwise healthy individuals and anemia is frequently discovered during routine health maintenance visits; as HCT falls, dyspnea and mild fatigue with exercise as well as nonspecific complaints of headache, poor concentration, palpitations, and anorexia may occur

F.   Signs of anemia include pallor, best seen in the conjunctiva; in very severe anemia, atrophic glossitis, cheilitis, and koilonychia may appear

G.   Laboratory indices that reflect an iron-deficient state: mean corpuscular volume (MCV) is low, serum ferritin level is reduced, serum iron level is reduced, and serum iron-binding capacity is increased

H.   In mild forms of IDA, the laboratory values of iron-deficiency and iron-sufficiency may overlap considerably, thus presenting a diagnostic challenge

IV.   Diagnosis/Evaluation

A.   History
1.   Inquire about onset and duration of symptoms
2.   Ask if there has recently been an unintended weight loss
3.   Obtain a careful history of gastrointestinal complaints that might suggest gastritis, peptic ulcer disease, or other conditions that might produce gastrointestinal bleeding
4.   Ask if there has been change in stool patterns or color and if there are hemorrhoids present (**Note:** Black tarry stools usually indicate an upper GI source of bleeding, while stool streaked with red blood is more often associated with colorectal bleeding [or bleeding from hemorrhoids])
5.   In menstruating women, ask about blood loss during menses
6.   Ask about dietary intake of iron rich foods and pica
7.   Obtain medication history, particularly use of aspirin and other NSAIDs; ask about past history of GI bleeding

B.   Physical Examination
1.   Obtain weight and compare with previous weight
2.   Observe for pallor, particularly the conjunctiva
3.   Examine tongue, corners of mouth, and nails for characteristic changes
4.   Perform abdominal exam for tenderness on palpation and enlargement of the spleen
5.   Auscultate heart for systolic flow murmurs
6.   Obtain stool for occult blood

C.   Differential Diagnosis: Any condition that causes acute or chronic blood loss; inadequate intake of iron

D.   Diagnostic Tests

Basic Laboratory Studies
➡ CBC and peripheral smear should be used to confirm a low hemoglobin or hematocrit test and to classify the anemia
➡ Serum ferritin level is considered the single most powerful test for the diagnosis of iron deficiency anemia (after bone marrow aspiration)
   •   The earliest laboratory change associated with IDA is decreased serum ferritin
   •   The absence of storage iron, as defined as a serum ferritin level below 20 µg per liter in any patient with microcytic anemia is **conclusive evidence** of IDA
➡ Menstruating women who are found to have microcytic anemia with reticulocytopenia and there is no reason to suspect GI blood loss usually do not require additional evaluation

Additional Evaluation is Needed for Adult Men and Postmenopausal Women
➡ Consider iron studies which include measurement of serum iron, total iron-binding capacity, transferrin saturation, and serum ferritin
➡ In those patients who are asymptomatic (no weight loss, abdominal pain, or report of black, tarry stools or frank blood in stools), obtain stool for occult blood x 6; patient is directed to collect two samples of stools on each of 3 days during which specific dietary, medication use, sample collection, and storage guidelines are followed
➡ In those patients who are symptomatic or in whom occult blood is found in the stool, either colonoscopy or endoscopy of the upper GI tract is indicated (based on history) to look for the source of bleeding
➡ Urinalysis for blood loss from the urinary tract (a much less common source of bleeding) should also be performed

V.   Plan/Treatment

A.   In 1998, the CDC updated the criteria for defining anemia in a healthy reference population; see the following table for diagnosing anemia based on hemoglobin and hematocrit levels for men and women

MAXIMUM HEMOGLOBIN CONCENTRATION AND HEMATOCRIT VALUES FOR ANEMIA*		
Sex/Age, Years	Hemoglobin, < g/dL	Hematocrit, < %
Males ≥18	13.5	39.9
Females ≥18	12.0	35.7

* Age- and sex-specific cutoff values for anemia are based on the 5th percentile from the third National Health and Nutrition Examination Survey (NHANES III)

Adapted from Centers for Disease Control and Prevention (1998). Recommendations to prevent and control iron deficiency in the United States. *MMWR 47* (RR-3), 1-29.

B. The World Health Organization hemoglobin (Hb) and hematocrit (HCT) cut-points for diagnosing anemia in adults have been widely adopted and differ somewhat from values set by the CDC
   1. In men, anemia is defined as an Hb level of <13 g/dL or HCT level of <41%
   2. In menstruating women, anemia is defined as an Hb level of <12 g/dL or HCT of <36%

C. Cigarette smokers and adults living at high altitudes (>3000 feet) have higher Hb and HCT levels and therefore anemia cut-points are increased (consult CDC guidelines for more information [see reference list at the end of this chapter])

D. A therapeutic trial of oral iron therapy is justified for menstruating women who are determined to have mild to moderate anemia based on the values listed above and whose low hemoglobin or hematocrit test result has been confirmed by a CBC
   1. The most widely recommended oral iron agent is ferrous sulfate, which is inexpensive, well absorbed, and well tolerated
   2. In menstruating women with anemia, iron deficiency anemia is treated with 200 mg of elemental iron daily

---

- For maximum cost-effectiveness, prescribe generic ferrous sulfate tablets
- Start with 300 mg/day and build to 900 mg/day to minimize GI upset (300 mg ferrous sulfate = 60 mg of elemental iron)
   o Iron should be taken between meals for better absorption
   o Vitamin C containing juice boosts absorption
   o Iron preparations should not be taken within one hour of substances that may inhibit iron absorption (e.g., dairy products, antacids, calcium supplements, coffee, tea, bran, and whole grains)
- Avoid use of time-release and enteric coated preparations because they may be less effectively absorbed (dissolve slowly and may bypass duodenum where iron absorption mainly occurs)

E. Counsel the patient about adequate dietary intake of iron-rich foods (see section on NUTRITION, p. 23)

F. In men, non-menstruating, and non-pregnant women, source of bleeding must be identified: See Diagnostic Tests in section IV.D. above

G. Follow Up: Menstruating women
   1. In 3-4 weeks for repeat examination and hemoglobin
      a. A hemoglobin response of ≥1 g/dL over a 4-week period confirms the diagnosis of IDA
      b. Restoration of iron stores is the goal of iron replacement therapy; the time required to accomplish this goal varies from patient to patient; in general, approximately 3 months of therapy is necessary
      c. CBC or hemoglobin/hematocrit should be repeated 6 months after successful treatment
   2. A reticulocytosis occurs within 7-10 days after initiation of iron therapy, but a reticulocyte count is not usually ordered unless there are concerns about the diagnosis; if the patient does not develop reticulocytosis, the diagnosis should be re-evaluated
   3. Common causes of treatment failure include noncompliance with therapy, misdiagnosis, and malabsorption
   4. The therapeutic trial should not be continued beyond 1 month if the hemoglobin concentration has not increased appropriately and the patient has been compliant with the treatment regimen; referral to an expert for further evaluation is indicated

H. Follow up in men and postmenopausal women is variable depending on cause of anemia (source of blood loss, cause of malabsorption, or dietary deficiency)

MEGALOBLASTIC ANEMIAS

I. Definition: A group of disorders characterized by the presence of hypersegmented neutrophils and oval macrocytes in the blood or presence of megaloblasts in bone marrow; most common cause is deficiency of either vitamin B_{12} (cobalamin) [Cbl] or folate

II. Pathogenesis

A. Folic acid and vitamin B_{12} are cofactors for the pyrimidine synthesis of DNA

B. The deficiency of these factors alters the synthesis of DNA, resulting in a decreased rate of cellular duplication

C. Abnormal amounts of DNA and proteins are produced resulting in the morphologic changes of megaloblastosis

OVERVIEW OF VITAMIN B_{12} (COBALAMIN) DEFICIENCY

Vitamin B_{12} deficiency can result from inadequate intake, decreased absorption, or inadequate utilization; however, it is **almost always** an absorptive problem

Most Common Cause	Pernicious anemia (PA) is the most common cause of vitamin B_{12} deficiency PA is an autoimmune disease characterized by production of autoantibodies to gastric parietal cells and their secretory product, intrinsic factor (necessary for absorption of B_{12} in the terminal ileum)
Other Causes	✓ Other conditions that interfere with absorption and utilization include Crohn's disease, Whipple's disease, sprue, and gastrectomy ✓ Poor intake is extremely rare, but can occur in strict vegetarians ✓ Many drugs interfere with cobalamin-folate-dependent metabolic pathway, especially chemotherapeutic agents (e.g., methotrexate, fluorouracil) ✓ If gastric production of acid is greatly reduced, for example, as occurs in patients undergoing prolonged treatment with proton pump inhibitors, cobalamin (Cbl) absorption from food may be impaired
Food Sources	Animal products are the primary dietary source of vitamin B_{12}
Recommended Dietary Allowance	2 µg/day
Amount Provided in Average Diet	Average Western diet provides an excess of the vitamin (5-15 µg/day) which is stored mainly in the liver
Storage Amount	Body stores a large amount of Cbl (2-5 mg) relative to daily requirements; thus it takes 2 to 5 years to develop cobalamin deficiency even in the presence of severe malabsorption

OVERVIEW OF FOLATE DEFICIENCY

Folate deficiency may result from inadequate intake, deceased absorption, hyperutilization, or inadequate utilization; however, it is **almost always** caused by inadequate intake

Most Common Cause	Inadequate intake, usually encountered in those with very poor diets such as elderly, chronically ill, food faddists, and alcoholics
Other Causes	✓ Hyperutilization of folic acid may occur in physiologic states (such as pregnancy, and the growth spurts seen in infancy and adolescence) and in disease states such as malignancy, chronic inflammatory disorders such as Crohn's disease, and rheumatoid arthritis ✓ Less common causes include malabsorption syndromes such as tropical and nontropical sprue and drugs that interfere with the cobalamin-folate-dependent metabolic pathway, especially chemotherapeutic agents such as methotrexate and fluorouracil
Food Sources	Leafy green vegetables, wheat bran, beans, grains, and liver
Recommended Dietary Allowance	200 µg/day with increased requirements in pregnancy and other physiologic states
Amount Provided in Average Diet	Average Western diet supplies 200-300 µg of folate daily
Storage Amount	Body stores (5-10 mg) are small relative to daily requirements; thus folate deficiency can develop quickly with dietary deficiency and increased folate demand

III. Clinical Presentation

    A. Vitamin B_{12} deficiency is almost always due to malabsorption; pernicious anemia is most common cause
        1. Onset is insidious, usually occurring in fifth and sixth decades of life with the median age at diagnosis being 60 years
        2. Slightly more women than men are affected
        3. Earlier studies suggested that the disorder was largely restricted to Northern Europeans; more recent studies have reported the disease in African-American and Latin-American persons with an earlier age of onset in African-American women
        4. The patient most often presents because of the presence of unexplained anemia, macrocytosis, or neurologic symptoms
        5. The most common neurologic symptoms are paresthesias, numbness, and ataxia
            a. Dementia and psychosis may also occur, but much less often
            b. Hematologic abnormalities often develop before the onset of neurologic disease (about 75% of the time)
            c. Up to 25% of patients with neurologic manifestations of cobalamin deficiency have either a normal hematocrit (HCT) or a normal mean corpuscular volume (MCV) and sometimes both values are normal
        6. Gastrointestinal manifestations include several abnormalities
            a. A smooth and beefy red tongue due to atrophic glossitis is a common finding
            b. Megaloblastosis of the epithelial cells of the small intestine may produce malabsorption and diarrhea

    B. Folic acid deficiency is almost always due to a dietary deficiency
        1. The patient most often presents because of the presence of unexplained anemia or macrocytosis
        2. Elderly, alcoholics, and indigents may have inadequate intake due to poor diet
        3. Neuropsychiatric manifestations are not present; if they are, likely to be caused by coexisting cobalamin deficiency or other disorders

IV. Diagnosis/Evaluation

    A. History
        1. Inquire about onset, duration of symptoms
        2. If gastrointestinal complaints, inquire about presence of red, burning tongue, abdominal complaints, presence of diarrhea or constipation
        3. If neurologic complaints, inquire about presence of pins-and-needles paresthesia and weakness, unsteadiness due to proprioceptive difficulties, and memory loss
        4. Inquire about dietary intake, using 24-hour recall
        5. Ask about alcohol consumption
        6. Obtain medication history with a focus on drugs commonly implicated in interference with absorption or utilization of cobalamin or folate
        7. Obtain past medical history, specifically if history of gastrectomy, resection of ileum

    B. Physical Examination
        1. Examine oral cavity for characteristic red, shiny tongue
        2. Perform abdominal exam for tenderness, organomegaly
        3. Perform neurologic exam with a focus on uncovering abnormal findings described under III.A.5. above

    C. Differential Diagnosis
        1. The many causes of anemia should be grouped according to the red cell indices into microcytic, normochromic-normocytic, and macrocytic as a beginning point
        2. Once the patient is determined to have macrocytosis, the primary differential diagnostic approach is the identification of vitamin B_{12} or folate deficiency

    D. Diagnostic Tests
        1. CBC and peripheral smear should be done (or repeated since many patients will present because of previous finding of macrocytosis after undergoing automated complete blood cell counts) to determine classification of anemia
        2. Value of a peripheral blood smear is questionable as it seldom avoids the need for use of less observer-dependent tests in the evaluation of macrocytosis

3. The most common method of establishing B$_{12}$ deficiency is by measurement of serum B$_{12}$ level (lower limit of normal is variable; usually set at about 148 pmol/L [200 pg/mL])
   a. Vitamin B$_{12}$ deficiency as the cause of megaloblastic anemia is established by a low serum B$_{12}$ concentration and normal folate level
   b. A Shilling test will confirm that the vitamin B$_{12}$ deficiency is a result of intestinal malabsorption due to intrinsic factor deficiency versus other malabsorptive states
   c. Measurement of serum levels of methylmalonic acid (MMA) and total homocysteine (Hcy) may also be used in equivocal cases (these amino acids are both increased in cobalamin-deficient states because enzymes responsible for their conversion are cobalamin dependent)
4. The most common method of establishing folate deficiency is by measurement of either serum or red blood cell (RBC) folate levels
   a. Sensitivity of serum folate measurement for diagnosis of folate deficiency is uncertain; serum folate levels increase with feeding, and the use of fasting determinations has been recommended
   b. Determination of RBC folate levels has been advocated as a more sensitive measure
   c. Differentiation of Cbl and folate deficiencies can also be made based on measurement of methylmalonic acid (MMA) and homocysteine (Hcy) as described above; whereas both MMA and Hcy are expected to be increased with Cbl deficiency, only Hcy level is expected to be increased in patients with folate deficiency
5. The accurate diagnosis of Cbl and folate deficiency is complex; if diagnostic uncertainty exists, referral to a hematologist is advisable

V. Plan/Management

A. Initial treatment of vitamin B$_{12}$ (cobalamin) deficiency is directed toward minimizing the risk of permanent neurologic damage and correcting the anemia; the maintenance treatment is aimed at maintaining therapeutic levels and prevention of relapse

---

TREATMENT OF VITAMIN B$_{12}$ (COBALAMIN) DEFICIENCY

- There are numerous replacement regimens, all of which are adequate. Select **one**
  - ➡ Begin with 100 to 1000 µg/day IM cyanocobalamin for 1-2 weeks, repeated 2 times a week for one month; then monthly for remainder of the patient's life **OR**
  - ➡ Administer a series of seven 100 µg injections of cyanocobalamin every other day over a period for 2 weeks; then continue with weekly injections over the next 4 weeks to ensure replacement of the vitamin stores; then, continue monthly for life **OR**
  - ➡ Administer IM cyanocobalamin, 1000 µg per week for 6 weeks and then 1000 µg IM every month for life
- With any of these regimens, the initial treatment should be adequate to saturate B$_{12}$ stores and resolve clinical manifestations of the deficit
- Cyanocobalamin is both the least expensive and most widely used vitamin B$_{12}$ in the US; hydroxocobalamin is more physiologic (also more expensive) and has a longer half-life than cyanocobalamin because it is better bound to serum proteins and less rapidly excreted
- If hydroxocobalamin is used, it may be given by IM injection every 3 months instead of every month because of longer half-life

---

B. Treatment of folic acid deficiency is aimed at reversal of the anemia, replenishment of folate stores, and improving dietary intake of folate to ensure adequacy of diet

---

TREATMENT OF FOLATE DEFICIENCY

- To replenish stores, therapy should be initiated with 1-2 mg of folic acid PO QD for 4-5 weeks; replenishment of folate stores can be achieved within several weeks of oral therapy
- Maintenance therapy is not indicated if the underlying cause can be reversed; however, when underlying cause persists and cannot be corrected (e.g., malabsorption, malignancy, hemodialysis), continue treatment with 1 mg of folic acid PO QD indefinitely
- Patients with alcohol problems should be counseled according to guidelines contained in ALCOHOL PROBLEMS
- Dietary counseling regarding foods high in folic acid should be provided (important sources are liver, wheat bran, leafy green vegetables, beans, grains); refer to nutritionist for intensive counseling

---

C. With both types of anemia, treatment brings about the following results
1. A rapid reticulocytosis following treatment (peaks in 5-8 days)
2. A rise in hematocrit and hemoglobin values in 1 week
3. In uncomplicated cases, hematocrit should reach normal levels within two months

D. Follow Up
1. Patients with vitamin B_{12} deficiency must be seen in 2 weeks to determine response to treatment
    a. Patient should experience an increased sense of well being and appetite in 2-3 days and a diminution in neurologic signs/symptoms
    b. Increased reticulocyte count and increased hematocrit as described above should also occur
    c. The patient should be followed monthly for B_{12} injections; patients (or family members) can also be taught self-administration of injections in which case they can be seen less often for monitoring
2. Patients with folic acid deficiency must be seen in 2 weeks to determine response to treatment, and then monthly until condition stabilizes; symptomatic improvement as evidenced by increased alertness, appetite, and cooperation are often noted early during the course of treatment

REFERENCES

Bergin, J.J. (2002). Anemia: A strategy for the workup. *Consultant, 63*, 869-882.

Blackwell, S., & Hendrix, P.C. (2001). Common anemias: What lies beneath. *Clinician Reviews, 11*, 53-62.

Centers for Disease Control and Prevention. (1998). Recommendations to prevent and control iron deficiency in the United States. *MMWR, 47,* RR-3, 1-36.

Chen, K., & Graber, M.A. (2002). Anemia. In M.A. Graber & M.L. Lanternier (Eds.), *University of Iowa: The family practice handbook* (pp. 216-223). St. Louis: Mosby.

Goroll, A.H., & Mulley, A.G. (2002). *Primary care recommendations.* Philadelphia: Lippincott Williams & Wilkins.

Hamilton, C.W. (1998). Hematologic disorders. In B.G. Wells, J.T. DiPiro, T.L. Schwinghammer, & C.W. Hamilton (Eds.), *Pharmacotherapy handbook* (pp 367-375). Stamford, CT: Appleton & Lange.

Izaks, G.J., Westendorp, R.G., & Knook, D.L. (1999). The definition of anemia in older persons. *Journal of the American Medical Association, 281,* 1714-1717.

McLaren, G.D., & Gordeuk, V.R. (2002). Iron deficiency. In R.E. Rakel & E.T. Bope (Eds.), *Conn's current therapy* (pp. 366-369). Philadelphia: Saunders.

Sacher, R.A. (2002). Pernicious anemia and other megaloblastic anemias. In R.E. Rakel & E.T. Bope (Eds.), *Conn's current therapy* (pp. 355-359). Philadelphia: Saunders

Snow, C.F. (1999). Laboratory diagnosis of vitamin B_{12} and folate deficiency. *Archives of Internal Medicine, 159*, 1289-1298.

Minor Emergencies

CONSTANCE R. UPHOLD & MARY VIRGINIA GRAHAM

AVULSED TOOTH

I. Definition: A total displacement of a tooth out of its socket, usually due to trauma

II. Pathogenesis: Teeth not fully erupted have loosely structured periodontal ligaments; thus these are the teeth most likely to be displaced when trauma to mouth occurs

III. Clinical Presentation

    A. An upper central incisor is the most frequently avulsed tooth

    B. Children are more likely to have avulsed teeth, but avulsion can also occur in adults

IV. Diagnosis/Evaluation

    A. Primary teeth should not be replanted because they often ankylose or fuse to the bone

    B. Immediate replanting of a secondary tooth is necessary to maintain vitality of the tooth (each minute the tooth remains out if its socket greatly reduces the likelihood that replantation will be successful); thus, assess for fractures of the teeth and alveolar ridge while simultaneously performing steps to preserve tooth

V. Plan/Treatment

    A. The avulsed tooth should be replanted immediately if possible
        1. If the tooth was displaced from the mouth and has collected debris from the ground or floor, rinse gently with sterile water holding the tooth by the crown. (DO NOT TOUCH ROOT SURFACE)
        2. Holding the tooth by the crown, gently tease it back onto the socket and cover with gauze; instruct patient to gently bite down on gauze during transport to dentist's office
        3. If the avulsed tooth cannot be placed into socket for transport, store tooth in physiologic medium to preserve vitality of tooth
            a. Best medium is a commercially available kit containing Hank's balanced salt solution (Sav-A-Tooth)
            b. Cold milk is also a good storage medium
            c. Saline and saliva are acceptable as storage media, and are certainly preferable to allowing the tooth to become dry
            d. If milk, saline, or Hank's balanced salt solution is not available, and placement back into socket cannot be done, placement of the tooth under the patient's tongue or in the buccal vestibule between gums and teeth is better than allowing to air dry which is destructive to the tooth (irreversible damage to the periodontal cells occurs in 30 minutes of air drying)
        4. Transport to the dentist must be immediate

    B. Antibiotic prophylaxis with penicillin is often prescribed

    C. Administer tetanus vaccine if patient has not received one in the past 5 years

    D. Follow Up: By dentist to whom the patient was referred for replantation

BITE WOUNDS

I.   Definition: Mechanical trauma to skin and/or underlying tissue from bite of an animal or human

II.   Pathogenesis

    A.   Transmission of bacteria from animal's or human's mouth into wound may produce infection
        1.   *Pasteurella multocida* is the causative agent in 20-50% of infections from dog bites and 80% of infections from cat bites
        2.   Dog and cat bites also become infected with *Staphylococcus aureus*, streptococci, anaerobes, *Capnocytophaga, Moraxella, Corynebacterium, Neisseria*
        3.   Enteric gram-negative bacteria and anaerobes are likely to cause infections from reptile bites
        4.   Rat and mice bites may become infected from *Streptobacillus moniliformis*
        5.   Streptococci, *Staphylococcus aureus*, *Eikenella corrodens,* or anaerobes are likely to cause infections from human bites
        6.   Hepatitis B and human immunodeficiency virus (HIV) can be transmitted by human bites; especially consider if the biter is within a high-risk group

    B.   Rabies, an acute viral illness, may be transmitted to human beings by infected saliva or other secretions after an animal bite or by licking mucosa of an open wound; airborne transmission has been reported in bat-infested caves

III. Clinical Presentation

    A.   Dog bites account for over 90% of mammal bites

    B.   Most bites are minor and may include scratches, abrasions, lacerations, and puncture wounds

    C.   Potential complications of bites include to the following:
        1.   Infection is the most common problem
            a.   Cat bites become infected more frequently than dog bites because they are often deep puncture wounds; approximately 50% of all cat bites and 15-20% of all dog bites become infected
            b.   Bites on the hand have the highest infection rates; bites on the face have the lowest rates
            c.   Cellulitis and abscesses are common; infections of tendons, periosteum, and joint spaces can be devastating infections
        2.   Rabies may occur after a bite; transmission is more likely if the bite was unprovoked
            a.   Rabies in small rodents is rare
            b.   Rabies in domestic animals has been decreasing, but rabies in wild animals is on the increase
            c.   Skunks, bats, raccoons, bobcats, coyotes, and foxes may harbor the virus and may also bite and infect domestic dogs, cats, horses, and cows
            d.   Incubation period in humans averages 4-6 weeks, but ranges from 5 days to more than one year
            e.   Infection with rabies produces an acute febrile illness with central nervous system problems (anxiety, dysphagia, seizures) and death if untreated
        3.   Bites of large dogs and other animals may produce crush injuries, avulsions, and fractures
        4.   Human bites: "Clenched-fist" injuries that occur during fistfights can cause potential tendon or joint capsule injuries and often require hospitalization

IV.   Diagnosis/Evaluation

    A.   History
        1.   Inquire about type of animal that bit patient
        2.   Ask if attack was provoked or unprovoked
        3.   If animal is known to the patient, obtain name and telephone number(s) of owner
        4.   Ask about condition of animal: Was the animal acting strangely or did the animal appear ill?
        5.   Determine the amount of time that elapsed since the bite
        6.   If patient receives a human bite, determine whether the biter is HIV infected or has hepatitis B or if biter is from a high risk group

7. Inquire about all self-treatments of injury
8. Determine immune status of the animal or human biter
9. Inquire about tetanus immunization status and prior rabies immunizations
10. Inquire about patient's past medical history, especially diseases such as diabetes mellitus and immunodeficiencies which would place patient at risk for infection and other complications

B. Physical Examination
1. Check distal to the injured site for neurovascular status and motor function
2. Assess range of motion of affected joint
3. Determine extent and depth of wound; check for foreign body
4. In patients with old wounds, check for signs of infection
5. Diagrams and photographs are useful

C. Differential Diagnosis: See Pathogenesis

D. Diagnostic Tests
1. Order x-rays if bony injury or presence of a foreign body such as tooth is suspected
2. Obtain wound cultures in following cases:
    a. If wound is ≥8 hours and <24 hours from time of injury
    b. All cases in which there are signs of infections regardless of time from injury
3. To determine if an animal is rabid, brain tissue can be examined by fluorescent microscopy

V. Plan/Management

A. Wound care
1. Sponge away visible dirt
2. Irrigate wound with copious amounts of sterile saline; do not irrigate puncture wounds
    a. Irrigate under pressure with either an 18 gauge needle and a 35 mL syringe or a Water-Pik
    b. Use at least 500-1000 mL of solution for irrigation and direct stream at all surfaces of wound
    c. Do not use antibiotic or anti-infective solutions as they may increase tissue irritation
3. Scrub the surrounding area
4. Débride all wounds to reduce risk of infection unless they are small and superficial
5. Trim jagged edge of wound

B. Open-wound management versus sutures
1. Do not suture wounds that are likely to become infected such as the following:
    a. Hand bites
    b. Bites that are older than 8 hours
    c. Deep or puncture bites
    d. Bites with extensive injury
2. See section on WOUNDS for suturing procedure

C. Antibiotic prophylaxis of bite wounds to prevent infection
1. Following type of wounds need prophylaxis:
    a. All wounds with signs of infections
    b. Moderate or severe wounds, especially if edema or crush injury is present
    c. Puncture wounds, especially if bone, tendon sheath, or joint penetration occurred
    d. Facial bites
    e. Hand and foot bites
    f. Genital area bites
    g. Wounds in immunocompromised and asplenic persons

2. Selection of antimicrobial agent is based on organism likely to cause infection and should be modified after receiving culture results (see following table for antibiotics)

ANTIBIOTICS FOR ANIMAL OR HUMAN BITE WOUNDS			
	Dog/Cat	Reptile	Human
Oral Route	Amoxicillin-clavulanate*	Amoxicillin-clavulanate*	Amoxicillin-clavulanate*
Oral Alternatives for Penicillin-Allergic Patients**	Extended spectrum cephalosporin or trimethoprim-sulfamethoxazole **PLUS** clindamycin	Extended spectrum cephalosporin or trimethoprim-sulfamethoxazole **PLUS** clindamycin	Trimethoprim-sulfamethoxazole **PLUS** clindamycin
Intravenous Route	Ampicillin-sulbactam[†]	Ampicillin-sulbactam[†] **PLUS** gentamicin	Ampicillin-sulbactam[†]
Intravenous Alternative for Penicillin-Allergic Patients**	Extended spectrum cephalosporin or trimethoprim-sulfamethoxazole **PLUS** clindamycin	Clindamycin **PLUS** gentamicin	Extended spectrum cephalosporin or trimethoprim-sulfamethoxazole **PLUS** clindamycin

*Prescribe amoxicillin/clavulanate (Augmentin) 250-500 mg every 8 hours for 3-7 days or 40 mg/kg/day in 3 divided doses
**In patients with history of allergy to penicillin or one its many congeners, a cephalosporin or other β-lactam class drug may be acceptable. However, these drugs should not be used in patients with an immediate hypersensitivity (anaphylaxis) to penicillin because approximately 5% to 15% of penicillin-allergic patients also will be allergic to the cephalosporins
[†]Ticarcillin-clavulanate may be used as an alternative

Adapted from American Academy of Pediatrics. (2000). Bite wounds. In L.K. Pickering (Ed.). *Red book: Report of the Committee on Infectious Diseases* (25th ed., pp. 156-157). Elk Grove Village, IL: American Academy of Pediatrics.

D. Prescribe appropriate tetanus prophylaxis; see WOUND section for guidelines

E. If there is a high risk or known exposure to hepatitis B after a human bite, provide passive prophylaxis with hepatitis B immune globulin (HBIG) 0.06 mL/kg intramuscularly and begin hepatitis B vaccination three-shot series

F. Consult infectious disease specialist if there is a high risk or known exposure to HIV after a human bite

G. Control measures related to rabies
   1. Contact personnel in local health department who can provide information on the risk of rabies in a particular area for each species of animals (unprovoked attack is more suggestive of rabid animal than provoked attack; properly immunized domestic animals have only a minimal chance of developing rabies)
   2. A suspected domestic animal should be caught, confined, and observed by a veterinarian for 10 days; if animal develops signs of rabies it should be killed and its head removed and shipped to laboratory for examination. No treatment is necessary if examination of brain is negative
   3. A suspected wild animal should be killed and its brain examined for evidence of rabies. No treatment is necessary if examination of brain is negative
   4. Patients with bites from bats and wild carnivores need rabies prophylaxis (see V.H.) if the offending animal cannot be caught; because the injury inflicted by a bat bite or scratch may be small and not visibly evident, prophylaxis is indicated for situations in which the bat was physically present unless prompt testing of bat excludes rabies infection

H. Care of patients exposed to rabies (consult with local health department); after local wound care, use both passive and active immunoprophylaxis as soon as possible after exposure, ideally within 24 hours, but even patients who have been exposed >24 hours should still be given therapy
   1. Active immunization: Human diploid cell vaccine (HDCV), rabies vaccine absorbed (RVA), or purified chick embryo cell (PCEC) 1.0 mL is given intramuscularly in the deltoid or anterolateral aspect of thigh on first day of treatment, and repeat doses are administered on days 3, 7, 14, and 28
   2. Passive immunization: Rabies immune globulin (Human) (RIG) should be used simultaneously with first dose of HDCV or RVA; recommended dose is 20 IU/kg of body weight; approximately one half of RIG is infiltrated into wound and the remainder is given intramuscularly

I.   Patient Education
     1.   Teach patient to watch for signs of infection
     2.   Educate about bite prevention
          a.   Caution against approaching unknown dogs, cats, and wild animals and avoid contact when animals are eating
          b.   Secure garbage containers so that raccoons and other animals will not be attracted to home
          c.   Chimneys and other potential portals of entry for wild animals should be identified and covered
          d.   Teach to avoid running and screaming in the presence of a dog; best to remain calm and avoid eye contact when threatened by a dog

J.   Referral/consultation is needed in the following cases:
     1.   Bites of ears, face, genitalia, hands, and feet
     2.   Large, contaminated wounds

K.   Follow Up: Inspect wound for signs of infection within 48 hours

BURNS, MINOR

I.   Definition: Lesions caused by heat or other cauterizing agents; the following burns are considered minor if they do not involve the eyes, ears, face, hands, feet, genitalia

     A.   Partial-thickness burns <15% total percentage of body surface area (TBSA) in adults 10-50 years of age

     B.   Partial thickness burns <10% TBSA in adults >50 years

     C.   Full-thickness burns ≤2% TBSA

II. Pathogenesis

     A.   Cellular protein coagulation and destruction of enzyme systems occur as a result of excessive heat energy which is transferred into the skin

     B.   Burns impair the skin's ability to retain water and heat, thereby increasing the risk of infection

     C.   Common agents causing burns include the following:
          1.   Scalds or burns from wet heat
          2.   Direct burns from flames; matches and cigarettes are common sources; irons and ovens are other sources
          3.   Chemicals
          4.   Electricity
          5.   Radiation; burns caused by exposure to sunlight

III. Clinical Presentation

     A.   Approximately 95% of burns are minor and can be managed in the ambulatory care setting

     B.   Depth of burn depends on the intensity of the burning agent and the amount of time the burning agent was in contact with skin; the traditional classification of first-, second-, and third-degree burns has been replaced (see below)
          1.   Superficial (first degree) burns have minimal epithelial damage and cause no skin loss
               a.   Skin has slight erythema, blanches with pressure, and sometimes has small, dry blisters
               b.   Heals without scarring or contractures in about 7-14 days
               c.   Burns are very painful
          2.   Partial thickness (superficial second degree) burns involve the upper layers of the epidermis, but spare epidermal appendages such as hair follicles, nails, sweat and sebaceous glands, and sensory nerve cells
               a.   Present with tender, erythematous, weeping skin and blisters
               b.   Skin blanches with pressure

    c. Wounds are painful as sensory function is preserved

    d. Heal within 14-21 days with minimal scarring and no contractures; changes in pigmentation may last for months or throughout life

  3. Deep dermal partial thickness (deep second degree) burns typically have patchy areas of injury varying from superficial partial thickness to full thickness; wounds may progress to full thickness

    a. Epidermal appendages are usually spared

    b. Appear pale and waxy with patchy red areas and may have large blisters

    c. No blanching with pressure

    d. Decreased pinprick sensation but pressure sensation is intact

    e. Healing may take more than 21 days

    f. May have contracture formation and hypertrophic scarring

  4. Full thickness (third degree) burns involve the entire thickness of the skin; may involve subcutaneous fat, connective tissue, muscle, and even bone

    a. Skin is charred or whitish in appearance

    b. Sensation is absent

    c. Unless burn is very small, the dermal elements needed to regenerate new skin are destroyed and surgical management with excision and grafting is needed

C. Scalds are the most common type of burn injury and generally result in superficial skin loss

D. Burns from flames are the second most common cause of burns; burns in which clothing catches on fire are almost always third degree and serious

E. The severity of chemical burns depends on the type of chemical, its concentration, and the contact time; cement and phenol are common sources

F. Electricity burns often cause small, punctate, deep burns at the entry point; electrical burns across the chest can cause cardiac problems

G. Radiation burns due to sun exposure are always superficial but can be extensive, painful, and result in hospitalization

H. Minor burns do not result in systemic problems (shock, acute renal failure, hypothermia, and severe depression of the immune system) which may occur with severe burns

I. Other injuries may accompany minor burns and include trauma and smoke inhalation; singed facial or nasal hairs, facial burns, change in voice, or altered mental status suggest an inhalation injury

J. Carbon monoxide and cyanide poisoning do not usually occur with minor burns, but should be considered in more extensive burns

K. Bacterial infection is a complication of minor burns

IV. Diagnosis/Evaluation

A. History

  1. Ask what caused the burn or how the burn was acquired

  2. Query about length of time the skin was in contact with the burning agent

  3. Determine how much time has elapsed from burn occurrence to seeking treatment

  4. Question about occurrence of smoke inhalation

  5. Ask about associated injuries

  6. When chemicals are involved ask the name and concentration of the chemical

  7. Ask patients with electrical injury about the amount of voltage involved and whether there was loss of consciousness at time of injury

  8. Ask about tetanus status

  9. Ask about past medical history, particularly cardiac valvular disease (pre-existing medical problems can adversely affect healing of burns)

  10. Inquire about history of alcohol and narcotic abuse; this information is important in managing the patient's pain

  11. Ask about recent streptococcal infection

  12. Because of possibilities of abuse and neglect, ask about prior injuries and burns; documentation of quotes should be recorded

B. Physical Examination; important to remove all clothing, dressings, jewelry, dentures and prostheses to thoroughly assess burns and any associated injuries
    1. Remember that it may require 3-5 days of serial examinations and debridement to determine whether partial-thickness wound is superficial or deep or has progressed to a full-thickness injury
    2. Observe general appearance for distress
    3. Observe for any signs that suggest abuse such as scald burns consistent with "dipping" injuries of the buttocks or arms and legs, cigarette burns, and iron burns
    4. Measure vital signs
    5. Estimate the area of burn from Lund-Browder burn charts (see figure that follows); surface area of the patient's palm can be used to estimate the extent of small or patchy burns (palm represents 0.4 percent of TBSA and entire hand represents 0.8 percent of TBSA)

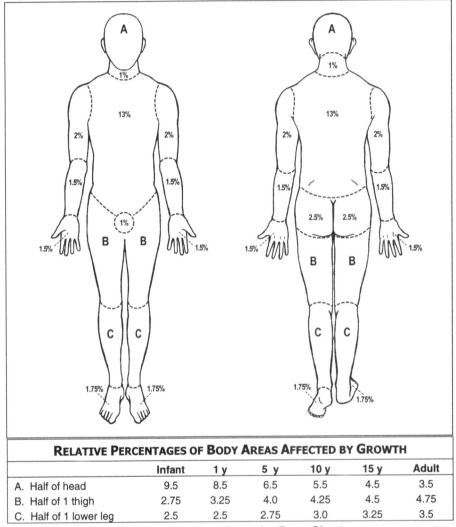

RELATIVE PERCENTAGES OF BODY AREAS AFFECTED BY GROWTH						
	Infant	1 y	5 y	10 y	15 y	Adult
A. Half of head	9.5	8.5	6.5	5.5	4.5	3.5
B. Half of 1 thigh	2.75	3.25	4.0	4.25	4.5	4.75
C. Half of 1 lower leg	2.5	2.5	2.75	3.0	3.25	3.5

Figure 20.1. Lund-Browder Burn Chart

    6. Determine depth of burn
    7. Assess sensation in the burn area by using a blunt sterile needle or pin
    8. Check distal to the burn site for neurovascular status and motor function
    9. Perform a complete exam of the lung and heart
    10. Other body systems should be examined depending on location and extent of burn and to determine any associated injuries such as fractures and dislocations from jumping from windows in house fires
    11. Assess for signs of infection

C. Differential Diagnosis:
    1. Always consider possibility of abuse or neglect, particularly if location of burn is inconsistent with the history
    2. Burn injuries may be the initial presentation of an alcohol or drug abuse problem

D.   Diagnostic Tests: None usually needed
1.   If inhalation injury is suggested, order chest radiograph and arterial blood gases
2.   Consider other studies based on coexisting trauma such as complete blood count, blood type and screen, x-rays

V.   Plan/Management

A.   Refer to a burn center patients who meet the following criteria:
1.   Age 11-49 years with partial-thickness burns ≥15-20% TBSA
2.   Age <10 years and/or >50 years with partial-thickness burns ≥10% TBSA
3.   Any age with full-thickness burns ≥2-5% TBSA
4.   Partial- or full-thickness burns to hands, feet, face, eyes, ears, perineum, and/or major joints
5.   Circumferential burns to the chest or extremities
6.   Electrical injuries, including lightning injuries
7.   Significant burns from caustic chemicals
8.   Burns complicated by multiple trauma in which the burn poses the greatest risk of morbidity
9.   Significant inhalation injury
10.   Co-morbid conditions that could complicate the management
11.   Lack of social or emotional support and/or long-term rehabilitative support
12.   Suspected family violence

B.   Emergency treatment of severe burns while waiting transport of the patient to a burn center or an emergency department includes prompt IV fluid resuscitation with lactated Ringer's solution, elevating the burned areas, and administering 100% oxygen if inhalation injury is present

C.   First aid
1.   Remove the burning agent, maintain patent airway, and resuscitate if needed
2.   Remove all clothing, jewelry, and shoes before swelling develops
3.   Keep patients covered with blanket to prevent hypothermia
4.   Lavage burned area with cool water or normal saline; chemical burns require extensive lavaging (at least 15 minutes)

D.   Outpatient treatment of superficial burns from all causes except radiation
1.   Apply cool water- or saline-soaked gauze to burn (do not apply ice or immerse wound in fluid)
2.   Cleanse with water or saline with or without mild soap; do **not** use agents such as hydrogen peroxide or alcohol; even Hibiclens and Betadine are discouraged because they can delay healing
3.   May use topical anesthetic such as dibucaine (Nupercainal) cream or benzocaine (Americaine) spray 3-4 times a day as needed for pain
4.   Infection prophylaxis and dressings are not needed

E.   Outpatient treatment of partial-thickness burns from all causes except radiation
1.   Cool burn with water- or saline-soaked gauze; because of risk of hypothermia, exercise caution in cooling extensive burns
2.   Cleanse burned areas with saline or tap water and mild soap (may need to sedate patient before cleansing and debridement or use local or regional anesthesia [do not apply anesthesia topically to burn or inject directly into wound])
3.   Tar and asphalt residues should be removed with a mixture of cool water and mineral oil, but never débrided; application of polymyxin B-bacitracin zinc ointment over several days should emulsify and remove residual tar
4.   Manually débride or use whirlpool to remove necrotic tissue to minimize infection
5.   Leave intact all blisters that are clean with clear fluid unless they are large and thin-walled and likely to rupture (may use sharp debridement or use sterile aspiration with a 19-gauge hypodermic needle to remove fluid if likely to rupture)
6.   Remove blistered skin that is almost detached and other devitalized skin
7.   For small burns on face cover with bacitracin ointment and leave open; for other small burns cover with bacitracin and apply nonadherent dressing and a bulky dressing to absorb drainage from burn
8.   For larger burns:
a.   Bacitracin is gaining favor as topical prophylactic antibiotic of first choice; this agent should always be used around mucous membranes and on the face
b.   Silver sulfadiazine 1% cream (Silvadene) can be used; cover burned area with a thin layer; do not use if patient is allergic to sulfa drugs or is pregnant

833

        c.   Biologic dressings are expensive but effective; apply within first 6 hours after the burn; dressings gradually peel of as skin epithelializes

        d.   Bismuth-impregnated petroleum gauze and Biobrane dressings are other effective agents; both are applied as single layer over burn and covered with a bulky dressing that should be changed every other day

        e.   For burns not treated with biologic dressings, apply nonadherent gauze and bulky dressing to absorb drainage from burn; to reduce circulatory impairment apply nonadherent dressing in successive strips rather than wrapping around extremity

            (1)   Dressings should be changed twice daily to once a week

            (2)   Remove dressing whenever it becomes soaked with exudate

            (3)   At each dressing change, completely clean wound with gentle washings

        f.   Splinting hands with burns is not usually recommended as it impedes patients in regaining range of motion

F.   For mild sunburns use cool compresses and topical dexamethasone aerosol spray every 3 hours; most effective if treatment is started within 12 hours of injury

G.   Pain management of all types of burns is important; recommend regular use of acetaminophen or a nonsteroidal anti-inflammatory drug

      1.   During dressing changes or increased physical activity a narcotic may be needed

      2.   Patient's worst pain score should be less than 5 on a scale from zero to 10

H.   Tetanus prophylaxis is needed if the patient has not received either a course of immunizations or a booster within 10 years; see guidelines for tetanus prophylaxis in the WOUND section

I.   Systemic antibiotics are given only if patient has a valvular disease or a concomitant streptococcal infection

J.   Patient Education

      1.   Teach patient to clean burned area completely with gentle soap and water, dry burn well, and reapply ointment or cream and dressing

      2.   Keep dressing and/or burn clean and dry

      3.   Increase fluid intake

      4.   Elevate affected parts

      5.   Maintain active range of motion of all joints with overlying burns

      6.   Teach signs and symptoms of infection and need to return to clinician if they occur

K.   Follow Up

      1.   Patients should be re-evaluated in 24 hours to assess pain control, evidence of infection, and to change dressing

      2.   At least once a week, partial-thickness burns should be assessed for signs of complications

      3.   Wounds that have not healed in 3 weeks in adults have a high incidence of hypertrophic scarring and these patients should be referred to surgeon

CORNEAL ABRASION

I.   Definition: Partial or complete removal of a focal area of epithelium on the cornea

II.   Pathogenesis

      A.   The cornea is composed of three principal layers: epithelium (the outer layer), stroma, and endothelium

      B.   Disruption of the epithelium on the cornea by mechanical or chemical factors results in corneal abrasion

      C.   Because the epithelium is richly innervated with sensory nerve endings, even the tiniest injuries are painful

III. Clinical Presentation

    A.   Corneal injuries are very painful, with the degree of pain generally related to the amount of epithelial disruption; motion of the eyeball and blinking increase the pain and foreign body sensation

    B.   Patients usually complain of a scratchy, gritty sensation (foreign body sensation) that develops suddenly and worsens with blinking

    C.   Redness of the eye follows corneal insult due to the reactive conjunctival vasodilation (injection)

    D.   Photophobia is often present and occurs because the disruption in the optical surface causes light to be scattered within the eye rather than focused so that bright light sources have a glaring appearance

IV. Diagnosis/Evaluation

    A.   History
        1.   Ask which eye is injured
        2.   Determine how, when, and where the eye was injured
        3.   Ascertain if eye pain or vision loss is present
        4.   Ask if any eye protection was being used at time of injury and if anyone witnessed the injury
        5.   Ask if contact lenses are being worn (or were being worn at time of injury)
        6.   Ask about tetanus immunization status

    B.   Physical Examination
        1.   Measure visual acuity (**Note**: Even in the case of trauma, it is critically important to know visual ability is present; if patient is unable to read chart, acuity may be grossly evaluated by finger counting)
        2.   Evert the eyelids and examine the conjunctival fornices for foreign body. The presence of a foreign body under the upper lid should **always** be looked for in the presence of a suspected corneal abrasion
        3.   Using a bright hand-held light and oblique illumination, inspect the cornea; an abrasion may be apparent by noting that an obvious shadow is cast on the iris from a surface defect illuminated when the light strikes the cornea
        4.   If trained and experienced in the technique of corneal staining with fluorescein, examine cornea using this technique which makes identification of abrasions much easier

---

CORNEAL STAINING WITH FLUORESCEIN TO ASSESS EPITHELIAL INTEGRITY

Technique

✓   Instill 1 or 2 drops of a rapid onset and short duration topical anesthetic (e.g., proparacaine HCl 0.5% [Ophthetic])

✓   Moisten the sterile fluorescein strip with sterile normal saline (can also touch strip to the tear film in the lower cul de sac of affected eye)

✓   Touch moistened fluorescein strip to lower conjunctiva of the eye being inspected (If tear film was used to moisten strip, this step is unnecessary as dye has already been placed in eye)

✓   Ask patient to blink eye

✓   Illuminate the eye with cobalt blue light and inspect for patterns of fluorescence

✓   Remove excess dye with sterile saline and remind patient not to rub eye

Interpretation

✓   If the corneal epithelium has been disturbed, fluorescein will pool within these areas and stain the hydrophilic stroma; the resultant brighter fluorescence of these pools will delineate the corneal abrasion from surrounding intact epithelium

✓   The size and pattern of the defect depends on nature and extent of injury

✓   A characteristic pattern that suggests the presence of a foreign body trapped underneath the upper lid is a faint vertically-oriented pattern on the cornea

---

    C.   Differential Diagnosis
        1.   Corneal foreign body
        2.   Viral keratitis
        3.   Corneal laceration

    D.   Diagnostic Tests: None indicated beyond corneal staining with fluorescein described above (consider referral to an ophthalmologist for this test)

V.   Plan/Management

A.   Instill an antibiotic ointment such as erythromycin ophthalmic ointment (Ilotycin) OR gentamicin ophthalmic ointment (Garamycin) into the affected eye

B.   Instruct patient to close injured eye and then apply a two-pad pressure dressing over the closed lids of the affected eye
1.   The patch must be firm and tight such that the eye cannot be opened beneath it
2.   Leave pad in place for 24 hours
3.   Instruct patient to return after 24 hours for removal of dressing
4.   After removal of the dressing, a topical antibiotic ointment such as listed above, or drops such as sulfacetamide sodium solution (Sulamyd) should be continued for 5 days after the injury as protection against infection. Small amount of ointment or 2-3 drops of solution should be used 4 x/day
5.   Administer tetanus immunization if indicated

C.   If the type of injury sustained is chemical, thermal, or a mechanical injury that has qualities of both blunt and sharp trauma, immediate transport to an ophthalmologist is required because of threat to vision

D.   Follow Up: In 24 hours to remove patch and evaluate healing

HEAD TRAUMA, MINIMAL AND MILD

I.   Definition: Trauma to the head; simple linear skull fractures and concussions are the most common examples of minor head injuries

A.   Simple linear skull fractures: Small break in skull that is not associated with depressed bone fragments and underlying brain injury

B.   Concussion: Trauma-induced alteration in mental status that may or may not involve loss of consciousness (previously, to be diagnosed with a concussion, the patient had to have a loss of consciousness)

C.   Classification of head injuries

CLASSIFICATION OF HEAD INJURIES		
Minimal	**Mild**	**Moderately or Potentially Severe**
All of the following: ✓ No loss of consciousness or amnesia ✓ Glasgow Coma Scale score of 15 ✓ Normal alertness and memory ✓ No focal neurologic deficit ✓ No palpable depressed skull fracture	Any of the following: ✓ Brief (<5 min) loss of consciousness ✓ Amnesia for the event ✓ Glasgow Coma Scale score of 14 ✓ Impaired alertness and memory	Any of the following: ✓ Prolonged (>5 min) loss of consciousness ✓ Glasgow Coma Scale score of <14 ✓ Focal neurologic deficit ✓ Post-traumatic seizure ✓ Intracranial lesion detected on CT scan

Adapted from Smith, E.E. (1993). Minor head injury: A proposed strategy for emergency management. *Annals of Emergency Medicine, 22,* 1193-1196.

II.   Pathogenesis:

A.   Common causes of traumatic head injuries
1.   In adults, auto accidents, falls, and assaults are causative factors
2.   In the elderly, falls are the most common cause

B. Outcomes following head trauma:
1. Seriousness of the head injury is related to the nature and extent of the cerebral injury rather than the damage to the overlying scalp or skull structures
2. Clinical course is dependent on the degree of acute injury to brain at the time of the accident (primary brain injury) and to delayed neurochemical and metabolic changes that result during the initial hours and days after the injury (secondary brain injury)
3. Even minimal head injuries can result in a secondary brain injury which involves tissue injury, swelling, and ischemia
   a. Delayed cerebral edema may occur within 8-12 hours
   b. Maximal cerebral edema occurs within 48-72 hours after the injury
4. "Second impact syndrome" occurs when a person (particularly an athlete) has a second concussion without recovering from the first; may lead to massive acute-brain swelling and ultimately death; multiple head injuries can result in chronic impairment of brain function

III. Clinical Presentation

A. Epidemiology
1. Head injury is the most common cause of traumatic mortality in the US
2. Most patients with head injuries are between 15-24 years of age
3. Males are 2-3 times more likely to have a head injury than females
4. In 50-60% of adult cases with head injuries, a positive blood alcohol is detected

B. Simple or linear skull fractures
1. Patients with linear fractures are usually asymptomatic, but any fracture requires close observation because the force required to fracture a skull is significant
2. Skull fractures with underlying lacerations may predispose the patient to meningitis

C. Concussion
1. Hallmarks are confusion and amnesia which occur immediately after injury or several minutes later
2. Early symptoms (first few minutes or hours) include headache, dizziness or vertigo, lack of awareness of surroundings, and nausea and vomiting
3. Postconcussive syndrome may occur and includes low-grade headaches, light-headedness, poor attention and concentration, memory dysfunction, reduced energy levels, intolerance of bright lights and noise, sleep disturbances, and irritability and depression; symptoms may last as long as 3 months post injury
4. A grading scale based on severity of the injury follows:

SCALE FOR GRADING THE SEVERITY OF CONCUSSION		
Grade 1	**Grade 2**	**Grade 3**
✓ Transient confusion ✓ No loss of consciousness ✓ Concussion symptoms or mental status abnormalities on examination **resolve in less than 15 minutes**. Grade 1 concussion is the most common yet the most difficult form to recognize	✓ Transient confusion ✓ No loss of consciousness ✓ Concussion symptoms or mental status abnormalities on examination **last more than 15 minutes**. Grade 2 symptoms (greater than 1 hour) warrant medical observation	✓ Any loss of consciousness either brief (seconds) or prolonged (minutes). Grade 3 concussion is usually easy to recognize--the patient is unconscious for any period of time

Adapted from American Academy of Neurology, Quality Standards Subcommittee: Practice parameter. (1997). The management of concussion in sports (summary statement). *Neurology, 48,* 581-585.

IV. Diagnosis/Evaluation

A. History: Important to obtain information from the patient as well as a person at the scene of the injury as the patient may be amnestic or confused
1. Determine how the injury occurred and the incidents surrounding the injury; explore possibility of alcohol or illicit drug use
2. Ask whether the patient had a loss of consciousness and amnesia
3. Inquire about symptoms after the injury such as vomiting, headaches, confusion, drowsiness, or abnormal behaviors
4. Determine if there is any neck pain or pain in other areas of the body
5. Inquire about other injuries

6. Ask about self treatments
7. Always ask about previous head injuries, particularly in athletes, to determine "second impact syndrome"

B. Physical Examination
   1. To quickly rule out a serious injury which needs immediate intervention, perform the following:
      a. Assess airway patency, breathing, and circulation
      b. Assess level of consciousness
      c. Measure vital signs
      d. Stabilize neck and check for signs of neck injury which often accompany head trauma
      e. Assess the thorax for hemothorax and pneumothorax
      f. Examine abdomen for signs of bleeding such as fullness and rigidity
      g. Signs of increased intracranial pressure are listed in the following table

SIGNS OF INCREASED INTRACRANIAL PRESSURE[†]	
Papilledema	Decreased pulse
Elevated systolic pressure	Slow respirations
Wide pulse pressure	

[†] In young children a full fontanelle (even when upright) and separation of cranial sutures are signs

   2. A rapid system for evaluating athletes who suffer injuries during an event is presented in the following table

QUICK EVALUATION OF ATHLETES WITH HEAD INJURIES DURING THE SPORTS EVENT	
Mental Status Testing	
Orientation	Time, place, person, and situation (circumstances of injury)
Concentration	Digits backward (e.g., 3-1-7, 4-6-8-2, 5-3-0-7-4) Months of the year in reverse order
Memory	Names of teams in prior contest; recall of 3 words and 3 objects at 0 and 5 minutes Recent newsworthy events; details of the contest (plays, moves, strategies, etc)
External Provocative Testing	40-yard sprint; 5 push ups; 5 sit ups; 5 knee bends (any appearance of associated symptoms is abnormal, e.g., headaches, dizziness, nausea, unsteadiness, photophobia, blurred or double vision, emotional lability, or mental status changes)
Neurologic Tests	
Pupils	Symmetry and reaction
Coordination	Finger-nose-finger, tandem gait
Sensation	Finger-nose (eyes closed) and Romberg

Adapted from McCrea, M., Kelly, J.P., Kluge, J., Ackley, B., & Randolph, C. (1997). Standardized assessment of concussion in football players. *Neurology, 48,* 586-588.

3. After determining that the patient is not in acute distress, perform the following at frequent intervals:
    a. Use the Glasgow coma scale to assess mental status which can be used later to evaluate the patient's progress (see following table)

GLASGOW COMA SCALE*
Eye-Opening Response

Score

Score	
4	Spontaneous
3	To verbal command
2	To pain
1	None

Motor Response

Score

Score	
6	Obeys commands
5	Localizes pain
4	Withdraws from pain
3	Displays abnormal flexion to pain (decorticate rigidity)
2	Displays abnormal extension to pain (decerebrate rigidity)
1	None

Verbal Response

Score

Score	
5	Is oriented and converses
4	Conversation is confused
3	Words are inappropriate
2	Sounds are incomprehensible
1	None

* Score of less than 8 denotes severe head injury

Adapted from Simon, J. (1992). Accidental injury and emergency medical services for children. In R.E. Behrman (Ed.). *Nelson textbook of pediatrics.* Philadelphia: WB Saunders.

    b. Observe gait
    c. Examine the eyes
        1) Evaluate pupillary size, equality, and reaction to light
        2) Perform funduscopy to detect retinal hemorrhage and papilledema
    d. Carefully inspect and palpate head, noting wounds, indentations
    e. Examine nasopharynx and ears for evidence of fresh blood
4. Palpate abdomen for signs of bleeding
5. Perform a complete neurologic examination including assessment of cranial nerves, reflexes, motor functioning, sensory functioning, and coordination
6. Assess mental status
7. Assess memory

C. Differential Diagnosis: Crucial to identify persons who are at risk for development of complications such as intracranial mass lesions, intracranial edema, and delayed neurological deterioration
    1. Age, co-morbidity, and mechanism of the injury are potential risk factors for severe head injuries (see following table)

RISK FACTORS FOR SEVERE HEAD INJURIES		
Mechanism	**Age**	**Medical Condition**
✓ High speed motor vehicle accident	✓ Greater than 65 years	✓ Long-term anticoagulant therapy
✓ Fall of more than 8 feet		✓ Presence of cerebrovascular malformation
✓ Injury with extensive damage to other areas of body		

Adapted from Marion, D.W. (1998). Acute head injuries in adults. In R.E. Rakel (Ed.), *1998 Conn's current therapy.* Philadelphia: WB Saunders.

2. Common causes of serious head trauma include the following:
    a. Basilar skull fractures
        (1) Bruising around the eye (raccoon sign), blood in external auditory canal (Battle's sign), cerebrospinal fluid leakage in the ear or nose, and cranial nerve palsies often occur
        (2) Fractures may not be present on plain x-rays, but are apparent on computed tomography (CT)
    b. Cerebral contusion or laceration results from edema, hemorrhage, and possibly necrosis
        (1) Associated with trauma directly beneath the site of blunt or penetrating injury (coup) or may result from indirect trauma contralateral to the injury (contré coup)
        (2) Typically, the patient has loss of consciousness for >2 minutes
        (3) May result in death or severe residual neurologic deficits such as post-traumatic epilepsy
    c. Acute epidural hemorrhage results from a tear in the meningeal artery, vein, or dural sinus and is usually associated with a skull fracture
        (1) Several hours after injury the patient may have a headache, confusion, somnolence, seizures, or focal deficits
        (2) Without treatment, coma, respiratory arrest, and death follow
    d. Acute subdural hematoma is due to a tear in veins from cortex to superior sagittal sinus or from cerebral laceration
        (1) More common injury than acute epidural hemorrhage
        (2) The symptoms and complications are similar to an epidural hemorrhage but the interval before onset of symptoms is longer
    e. Cerebral hemorrhage develops immediately after the injury with symptoms of intracranial pressures and distress; a hematoma is usually visible on CT scan
3. Typical characteristics of severe head injuries include the following:
    a. Loss of consciousness associated with one or more neurologic deficits
    b. Glasgow Coma Scale score of less than 8
    c. Alterations in mental status
    d. Prolonged memory deficit
    e. Persistent vomiting and severe headache
    f. Seizures
    g. Signs of primary brainstem injury include coma, irregular breathing, fixation of pupils to light, and diffuse motor flaccidity
4. Child abuse or family violence should always be included in differential diagnosis

D. Diagnostic Tests:
1. No tests are needed in patients with minimal head trauma (see classification system in I.C.) who have no abnormal neurological signs but monitoring for neurological abnormalities should extend for at least 48 hours after the injury
2. Consider head CT for the following patients: Those with headaches, vomiting, age >60 years, drug or alcohol intoxication, deficits in short-term memory, physical evidence of trauma above the clavicle, or seizure
3. Patients with mild head injuries who present 6 hours after the trauma, who have a normal clinical examination, and who have a head CT scan that does not show any acute injury can be safely sent home; patients with a responsible third party can go home earlier
4. Always consider ordering cervical spine films or other radiographs for any patient depending on the mechanism and circumstances surrounding the injury
5. Consider ordering blood alcohol

V. Plan/Management

A. Hospitalization
    1. For patients with simple fractures and concussions without abnormal neurologic signs and symptoms, hospitalization is not required
    2. Hospitalization is recommended in the following situations:
        a. Suspicion of family violence
        b. All head injuries categorized as mild, moderate, or severe
        c. Injuries accompanied by a neurologic deficit
        d. Any mechanism severe enough to cause concern of secondary brain injury

B. For patients who are not hospitalized, monitoring for delayed abnormal signs and symptoms is essential; careful assessment of the caregiver's anticipated compliance with instructions and abilities to care for patient (i.e., adequate transportation) is crucial; patient education includes the following:
    1. Provide printed information and teach family members that there is a need for thorough, frequent observation and precautions for at least 48 hours after the injury; recommend the following:
        a. Check whether pupils are equal and react to light
        b. Determine arousability and coherence by waking patient every 4 hours
        c. Time respiratory rate and check whether respiratory pattern is regular
    2. Call health care provider for any of the following:
        a. Headaches which worsen
        b. Vomiting becomes more frequent
        c. Pupils are unequal or do not react to light
        d. Symptoms such as seizures, neck pain, drowsiness, confusion, difficulty walking, talking, or visualizing occur
    3. Instruct family members that patient should be observed for the development of complications for at least 2 weeks after the injury; signs of complications include drowsiness, vomiting, gait disturbance, or severe headache
    4. Emphasize to family members of athletes that repeat head injuries can lead to permanent brain damage

C. Guidelines for the management of sports-related concussions were developed by the American Academy of Neurology
    1. Initial management following the head injury depends on the grade of the concussion (see III.D.4.)
        a. Athletes with Grade 1 injuries may return to play the same day if the following are met: Normal on-site evaluation (see IV.B.2) while at rest and with exertion, including a normal, detailed mental status examination
        b. Athletes with Grade 2 and Grade 3 injuries must have a complete neurologic examination and may not return to play the same day
    2. Decisions on when to return to play after removal from the athletic event are based on grade of the concussion and whether previous head injuries have occurred (see table that follows)

RECOMMENDATIONS ON ATHLETE'S RETURN TO PLAY	
Grade of Concussion	**Time Until Return to Play***
Multiple Grade 1 concussion	1 week
Grade 2 concussion	1 week
Multiple Grade 2 concussions	2 weeks
Grade 3--brief loss of consciousness (seconds)	1 week
Grade 3--brief loss of consciousness (minutes)	2 weeks
Multiple Grade 3 concussions	1 month or longer, based on clinical decision of evaluating health care provider

*Only after being asymptomatic with normal neurologic assessment at rest and with exercise

Adapted from American Academy of Neurology, Quality Standards Subcommittee: Practice parameter. (1997). The management of concussion in sports (summary statement). *Neurology, 48*, 581-585.

D. Prevention of head injuries
   1. Remind patients to wear safety belts in motor vehicles and helmets when riding a bike or motorcycle
   2. Proper safety equipment is needed for even recreational sports
   3. Measures to prevent falls in the household such as removing loose carpets and maintaining uncluttered, well-lit walkways are important

E. Follow Up
   1. Frequent monitoring of all head injuries is important
   2. Communicate with family members within first 4-12 hours after the injury and then periodically depending on the clinical condition of the patient

INSECT STING AND BROWN RECLUSE SPIDER BITE

I. Definition: A sting or bite in which there is secretion of venom into skin by insect or spider

II. Pathogenesis

A. Insect Sting
   1. Honeybees, wasps, hornets, and yellow jackets of the order Hymenoptera embed a firm, sharp stinger in the skin; venom is secreted
   2. Honeybees leave their stingers in the skin (with venom sac attached; other stinging insects of the order have a retractable stinger and thus may sting many times)
   3. The injected venoms are proteins with enzyme activity that can cause local or general reactions, or both; reactions are classified as toxic or allergic

B. Brown Recluse Spider Bite
   1. Of the 50 or so species known to bite humans, the brown recluse spider (*Loxosceles reclusa*) is one of two species in the US (black widow is the other) capable of producing severe reactions
   2. The brown recluse is the most widespread, well-studied, and clinically important of the *Loxosceles* species in North America
   3. Brown recluse spider is small (1.5 cm or less) light brown, and lives in dark areas such as closets, under porches, or in basements; usually found in river country of mid-America, most commonly in the south-central US
      a. Endemic range of this spider is southeastern Nebraska through Texas, east to Georgia and southernmost Ohio
      b. Several additional species of this spider are native to the southwestern deserts, but are rarely found inside urban houses
   4. Spider venom is composed of enzyme-spreading factor hyaluronidase, and a toxin distributed by the enzyme
   5. The venom of the spider is antigenic and once a person has been bitten, subsequent bites are not severe
   6. Spider bite can cause local or general reactions, but does not cause allergic reactions

III. Clinical Presentation

A. Insect Sting
   1. A sharp, pinprick sensation is felt at the instant of stinging followed by burning pain at site
   2. A red papule or weal appears, enlarges, then subsides within hours
   3. Multiple stings can cause a toxic reaction producing symptoms such as syncope, dizziness, vomiting, diarrhea, and headache because of the large toxin load
   4. Allergic reactions may be localized or systemic
   5. Systemic reactions begin 2-60 minutes after sting and range from a few hives to anaphylaxis; 40% of persons with generalized allergic reactions have a previous history of similar reaction
   6. Anaphylaxis symptoms include generalized itching, hypotension, shortness of breath, throat tightness, dizziness, and wheezing which may subside spontaneously or progress to edema of upper airway, causing obstruction and death

B. Brown Recluse Spider Bite
1. *Loxosceles* spiders are very shy creatures that are reticent to bite; bites typically occur when spider is accidentally trapped against human skin
2. Bite may feel sharp, or it might cause little or no pain; subsequent minor swelling and erythema at site often occur
3. Severity of local reaction appears to depend on site of bite with fatty areas of body developing more severe reactions
4. Tissue necrosis in bite area may develop as early as four hours after bite
5. Cutaneous changes at the site include a blue-gray, macular halo around puncture site; emergence of pustule or vesicle/bulla at site; widening of macule and sinking of center of lesions producing a "sinking infarct"; sloughing of tissue leaves a deep ulcer which takes weeks or months to heal
6. In rare cases, within 12 hours after bite, systemic symptoms of fever, chills, nausea, vomiting, and generalized weakness may appear; rarely, severe systemic reactions of generalized hemolysis, disseminated intravascular coagulation, and renal failure occur (usually only in children)
7. There are no proven US fatalities involving brown recluse spider bites in which the spider bite was witnessed, and the spider was collected and identified by an expert
8. Throughout the US, dermonecrotic wounds of uncertain etiology are often (incorrectly) attributed to the brown recluse spider

IV. Diagnosis/Evaluation

A. History
1. Quickly question regarding type of bite or sting, time of occurrence, and location of bite/sting
2. If sting, quickly determine if allergic reaction is present (generalized itching, shortness of breath, throat tightness, urticaria, or wheezing)
3. If sting, question about history of previous allergic reactions

> ***** **ALERT** *****
> **If allergic reaction is present or anticipated based on history,**
> **go immediately for treatment**

4. If bite is suspected, attempt to determine the following: Whether anyone witnessed the bite; whether spider was collected; and whether spider can be identified or described
5. If bite is suspected, determine if dermonecrotic wound is present, and ask about the timing and progression of changes at the site of the suspected bite
6. If bite is suspected, ask about presence of systemic symptoms such as fever, chills, nausea, vomiting, and weakness

B. Physical Examination
1. If history suggests an anaphylactic reaction is imminent, do not complete exam or wait for symptoms to develop, institute treatment immediately (See V.B. below)
2. If sting with no systemic allergic reaction evident or anticipated based on history, take pulse, respirations, and blood pressure
3. Examine site of bite or sting for characteristic erythema and edema or localized allergic reactions
4. Examine site of suspected spider bite for presence of characteristic dermonecrotic wound (not present until hours or days after event)

C. Differential Diagnosis
1. Vasovagal attacks: May follow pain or upset and be accompanied by nausea, diaphoresis and hypotension; lasts only a few minutes and relieved by lying down
2. Hyperventilation episodes: Accompanied by tachypnea, perioral tingling, but BP is maintained and other signs of anaphylaxis are absent
3. Necrotic wounds may be caused by infectious (e.g., Lyme disease, cutaneous anthrax) or neoplastic processes; in general, brown recluse spider bite has been overdiagnosed as the cause of necrotic lesions and other, more likely causes of the wound should be considered
4. Of recent interest, a 7 month-old child in New York who contracted cutaneous anthrax was initially diagnosed as having a brown recluse spider bite as the cause of the necrotic wound (the state of New York is outside the endemic range of the brown recluse and has no populations of the spider)
5. The many causes of necrotic wounds should be considered before attributing such wounds to spider bites without any corroborating evidence

D.   Diagnostic Tests: None indicated for bites or stings without systemic symptoms

V.   Plan/Treatment

    A.   Treatment of anaphylactic reactions is based on type of reaction which can range from mild to life-threatening; in all cases, epinephrine is the drug of choice

    B.   Treatment of mild anaphylaxis is outlined in the table that follows

---

TREATMENT OF MILD ANAPHYLAXIS

For mild symptoms of pruritus, erythema, urticaria, and wheezing, treat with epinephrine injected via the intramuscular route (now the recommended route rather than subcutaneous), followed by diphenhydramine, hydroxyzine, or other antihistamine given orally or parenterally

Epinephrine, 1:1000 (aqueous) 0.01 mL/kg per dose. Usual dose: 0.3-0.5 mL

Repeat in 10-20 minutes up to 3 doses; monitor patient's condition constantly, and monitor BP every 5 minutes

Antihistamine: Give **one** of the following:
    Hydroxyzine, oral or IM: Give 0.5-1 mg/kg/dose (100 mg maximum single dose) Q 4-6 hours PRN
    Diphenhydramine, oral or IM: Give 1-2 mg/kg/dose (100 mg maximum single dose) Q 4-6 hours PRN

Ice: Immediately apply ice to the site of the sting

Also, give oral antihistamines for next 24 hours; see dosing above

Observe patient in office for several hours (a period of 4-6 hours is considered reasonable in patients who are responding well to initial therapy) before discharging to home. Instruct patient to continue to apply ice to site of insect sting and elevate the affected extremity to control local reaction

Advise patient to immediately seek emergency care if difficulty in breathing develops

Follow Up: By telephone in 12-24 hours.

Adapted from American Academy of Pediatrics. (2003). Active and passive immunization. In L.K. Pickering (Ed.), *2003 red book: Report of the Committee on Infectious Diseases*, 26th ed. Elk Grove Village, IL: Author, pp. 64-65.

    C.   For severe and potentially life-threatening systemic anaphylaxis (bronchospasm, laryngeal edema, hypotension, shock, and cardiovascular collapse) institute the following and call 911 for immediate transport

---

TREATMENT OF SEVERE ANAPHYLAXIS

Promptly institute airway maintenance and oxygen therapy. Give Intravenous (IV) epinephrine

An initial bolus of intravenous epinephrine is given to patients not responding to intramuscular epinephrine using a dilution of 1:10 000 rather than a dilution of 1:1000. This dilution can be made using 1 mL of the 1:1000 dilution in 9 mL of physiologic saline solution. The dose is 0.01 mg/kg or 0.1 mL/kg of the 1: 10 000 dilution. A continuous infusion should be started if repeated doses are required. For a continuous infusion, add one milligram (1 mL) of 1:1000 dilution of epinephrine to 250 mL of 5% dextrose in water, resulting in a concentration of 4 µg/mL; initially infuse at a rate of 0.1 µg/kg/minute and increase gradually to 1.5 µg/kg/minute to maintain blood pressure

If bronchospasm is prominent, inhaled β_2 agonist: Albuterol (Ventolin) should be administered via nebulizer
Usual dose: 2.5 mg (0.5 cc of 0.5% solution) in 3 cc saline

Transport to emergency department

Adapted from American Academy of Pediatrics. (2003). Active and passive immunization. In L.K. Pickering (Ed.), *2003 red book: Report of the Committee on Infectious Diseases*, 26th ed. Elk Grove Village, IL: Author, pp. 64-65.

D.   Prevention of recurrence in patients with mild to severe anaphylactic reactions
    1.   Refer for allergy testing to identify the venom responsible for sensitization
    2.   Five Hymenoptera venoms are commercially available for this purpose: honeybee, yellow jacket, yellow hornet, white-faced hornet, and Polistes wasps
    3.   If skin tests produce ambiguous results, serologic methods (RAST) can be performed to detect IgE antibody to venoms
    4.   Immunization with insect venom can prevent future systemic reactions in patients with a previously documented reaction

E.   Emergency treatment kits (available by prescription) for self-treatment before reaching medical help should be obtained by all persons at risk for anaphylaxis from insect stings
    1.   Patients should be prescribed 3 kits: one for home, one for car, and one to carry; detailed information regarding when and how to use the kit should be given to patient
    2.   Ana-Kit (Hollister-Stier, Spokane, WA) contains a preloaded syringe
    3.   Epi-Pen (Dey Laboratories, Napa, CA) is a spring-loaded automatic injector for individuals reluctant to perform self-injection

F.   Patients should also wear a medical alert tag and should be counseled to take special precautions such as the following:
    1.   Avoid eating outdoors, going barefoot outdoors, and mowing the lawn; nesting areas should be avoided or eliminated
    2.   Insect repellents do not seem to prevent stings and thus should not be relied upon

G.   For insect stings which are localized with mild urticaria
    1.   Remove stinger if present using forceps, or by scraping out (do not attempt to squeeze out)
    2.   Wash the wound thoroughly and immediately apply ice packs
    3.   Prescribe oral antihistamines (see above for dosing of hydroxyzine and diphenhydramine) to relieve local reaction and discomfort
    4.   Recommend continued use of ice packs and elevation for the next 8-12 hours

H.   For moderate localized swelling, the interventions outlined above should be used. In addition, a burst of oral prednisone (40 mg on day 1, tapering over 4-7 days) is also recommended

I.   Diagnosis of brown recluse spider bite should be made only after corroborative evidence is sought; other, more likely causes of necrotic wounds should be sought in cases where no spider is recovered and identified by an expert

J.   Treatment of brown recluse bite is controversial; there are no conclusively established guidelines
    1.   All experts recommend the following conservative treatment
        a.   Gently cleanse with soap and water
        b.   Apply ice and elevate
        c.   Avoid strenuous exercise
        d.   AVOID APPLICATION OF HEAT
        e.   Monitor the patient closely for the first 72 hours
        f.   Give tetanus toxoid if indicated

2. Controversy surrounds which drugs, if any, are indicated
   a. No drug treatments are indicated, according to most experts (excellent outcomes usually occur without any pharmacologic interventions)
   b. If systemic signs and symptoms are present, refer patient to an expert for management

K. Follow Up
   1. Stings: In 12-24 hours (may be by telephone) for patients with anaphylactic symptoms; none indicated for those with localized reactions only
   2. Brown recluse spider bite: No follow up is needed, but patients must be instructed to report any systemic problems such as headache, myalgia, fever, chills, gastrointestinal complaints, rash and darkening of urine (the presentation of hemolysis is within the first weeks); complications of wound healing may occur at any time until resolution and patients must be instructed in signs and symptoms of wound infection

OCULAR FOREIGN BODY

I. Definition: Presence of a foreign body in the cul-de-sacs and under the upper lid or on the cornea

II. Pathogenesis

   A. A foreign body of the conjunctiva occurs when particles become entrapped under the upper lid or in the cul-de-sacs

   B. Most often occurs with blowing dirt or sand; there is usually no trauma involved

   C. A foreign body of the cornea occurs when substances become embedded in the corneal epithelium, most often due to some traumatic event

   D. A sudden event such as an explosion, or an accident involving metal grinding may scatter small fragments onto the cornea

III. Clinical Presentation

   A. The most common conjunctival foreign bodies are dust, sand, and contact lenses

   B. The most common foreign bodies found on the cornea are metallic, often rusty particles

   C. Foreign bodies may be single or multiple, easily seen without magnification or barely detectable with slit-lamp examination

   D. Symptoms are photophobia, lacrimation, and foreign body sensation

IV. Diagnosis/Evaluation

   A. History
      1. Ask which eye is injured
      2. Determine how, when, and where the eye was injured
      3. Ascertain if eye pain or vision loss is present
      4. Ask if any eye protection was being used at time of injury and if anyone witnessed the injury (important for medicolegal reasons)
      5. Ask if contact lenses are in place (or were in place at time of injury)
      6. Ask about tetanus immunization status
      7. Note: Based on history, if foreign body is result of explosion, blunt or sharp trauma, (i.e., if **corneal** foreign body is suspected) eye should be protected from further damage by placing eye shield over eye (or if shield not available, a paper cup to prevent rubbing eye); at this point, arrangements should be made to transport the person for emergency care by an ophthalmologist

B. Physical Examination
1. Measure visual acuity (**Note**: Even in the case of trauma, it is critically important to know visual ability is present; if patient is unable to read chart, acuity may be grossly evaluated by finger counting)
2. Evert the eyelids and examine for foreign body
3. Technique for everting the eyelid is as follows:

EVERSION OF THE UPPER LID

✓ Instill 1 or 2 drops of a rapid onset, short duration topical ophthalmologic anesthetic such as proparacaine HCl (Ophthetic, 0.5%) into the affected eye

✓ Ask patient to look down

✓ Grasp the lashes with one hand and apply gentle pressure on the lid above the tarsal plate with a cotton-tip applicator with the other hand

✓ Foreign bodies such as soft contact lenses and grit are often found in superior temporal cul-de-sac of the orbit

---

4. Examine the inferior cul-de-sac by having the person look up while the lower lid is pulled down

V. Plan/Management

A. When foreign body is visualized, sweep sterile cotton-tipped swab moistened with topical anesthetic across conjunctival area to remove the object
1. If there is difficulty with removal or if patient complains of severe pain, attempts should be discontinued
2. Refer to ophthalmologist

B. After removal of conjunctival foreign body (or if conjunctival foreign body cannot be located), determine if corneal abrasion present (See CORNEAL ABRASION)
1. If no corneal abrasion present, prescribe topical antibiotic ointment or drops such as sulfacetamide sodium (Sulamyd); apply small amount of ointment or 2-3 drops to affected eye 4 x/day x 5 days
2. If corneal abrasion present, see CORNEAL ABRASION for treatment recommendations
3. Provide tetanus immunization if indicated

C. Follow Up: In 24 hours

SUBCONJUNCTIVAL HEMORRHAGE

I. Definition: A flat, bright-red hemorrhage under the conjunctiva

II. Pathogenesis

A. May occur spontaneously, with raised venous pressure from a forced Valsalva maneuver (as in coughing, sneezing)

B. May occur with major, minor, or no detectable trauma to the front of the eye

III. Clinical Presentation

A. Presents as a striking flat, deep-red hemorrhage under the conjunctiva and may become sufficiently severe to cause a "bag of blood" to protrude over lid margin

B. Subconjunctival hemorrhage is usually asymptomatic

IV. Diagnosis/Evaluation

    A. History
        1. Determine which eye affected and how, when, and where the injury occurred
        2. Ascertain if eye pain, discharge of secretions, or vision loss is present
        3. Ask if patient has had previous symptoms or complaints similar to the current complaint

    B. Physical Examination
        1. Measure visual acuity
        2. Examine lids and the adnexa for symmetry, swelling, abnormal discharge, and erythema
        3. Palpate the soft tissue of the orbit, lids, and zygoma
        4. Inspect the conjunctiva and sclera for localized swelling, signs of hemorrhage
        5. Examine pupils for size, shape, reaction to light, and perform funduscopic exam

    C. Differential Diagnosis
        1. Conjunctivitis
        2. Conjunctival laceration

    D. Diagnostic Tests: None indicated

V. Plan/Management

    A. With no other signs and symptoms, no treatment is required; the patient should be reassured that the blood will clear over a 2-3 week period

    B. If trauma with a sharp object is suspected, or if there is impaired vision, eye pain, foreign body sensation, discharge of secretions from the eye, change in the appearance of the globe, patient should be referred to an ophthalmologist for evaluation

    C. Follow Up: None required; for patients with signs and symptoms described under V.B. above, follow-up should be by the ophthalmologist to whom the patient was referred

---

WOUNDS

I. Definition: Breach in the external surface of the body

II. Pathogenesis

    A. Wounds such as lacerations and abrasions typically heal through a 3-stage process: Clotting, inflammatory, and proliferative stages

    B. Devitalized tissue, oral secretions, toxic solutions, soil and dirt, and injurious forces can impede the healing process and possibly cause infection

    C. *Staphylococcus aureus* and *β-hemolytic streptococcus* are the most common pathogens causing wound infection

    D. Tetanus can also occur due to multiplication of *Clostridium tetani*, producing a toxin which can block motor neurons

III. Clinical Presentation

    A. Mechanism of injury is important in determining likelihood of infection and tissue damage
        1. Sharp objects often make smooth cuts which can penetrate deep structures
        2. Crushing injuries often damage underlying tissues and can result in fractures
        3. Human bites have the greatest risk of bacterial infection and can also transmit hepatitis B and possibly human immunodeficiency virus (HIV)

B. Location or environment in which the wound occurred suggests potential problems; wounds which occur in dirty soil such as farmyards are at risk for contamination with spores of *Clostridium tetani*

C. The time interval between when the wound first occurred to when the patient received appropriate care affects the chances of infection; if 6 hours have elapsed, bacterial multiplication is likely

D. Site of the wound influences rate of healing and potential for complications:
   1. Due to rich vascular supply, wounds on face heal rapidly, but may create future cosmetic problems
   2. Hands are used extensively; wounds on hands have increased risk for reinjury and infection

E. Certain types of wounds may be problematic
   1. Dirty wounds are more at risk for infection
   2. Deep wounds can cause underlying tissue destruction and also have increased risk of contamination
   3. Wounds with untidy edges often heal slowly and may heal with disfigurement
   4. Wounds with tissue necrosis have potential for infection and delayed healing

F. Characteristics of the patient are also factors in wound healing; patients who are elderly, undernourished, who have underlying illness, and who are taking corticosteroids and chemotherapeutic agents are at greatest risk for adverse sequela from wounds

G. Tetanus is a rare but dangerous complication of a wound and is characterized by trismus and severe muscular spasms

IV. Diagnosis/Evaluation

A. History
   1. Ask patient to explicitly describe how the wound occurred
   2. Determine where the injury was sustained
   3. Question how much time has elapsed since the wound occurred
   4. Ascertain tetanus immunization status
   5. Ask about allergies to drugs, dressings, and local anesthetics
   6. Ask about current medication use, especially steroid and anticoagulant therapy
   7. Inquire about past medical history to determine if patient has underlying illness such as immunodeficiency which could affect healing process
   8. Ask whether the patient has a tendency to form keloids, because this could result in a poor scar

B. Physical Examination: Always use sterile technique when examining wounds; it may be necessary to apply local or regional anesthesia prior to the examination
   1. Measure wound
   2. Assess depth of wound
   3. Explore wound for foreign bodies
   4. Fully examine underlying structures
   5. Assess circulation, sensation, and movement distal to wound
   6. Palpate underlying bone
   7. Assess range of motion and strength against resistance of all body parts surrounding wound site
   8. Test tendon function against resistance; if function is intact but there is pain, suspect a partial tendon laceration
   9. Examination of the patient with an old wound includes the following:
      a. Carefully inspect wound and surrounding area
      b. Palpate for local lymphadenopathy
      c. Measure patient's temperature

C. Differential Diagnosis: Always consider the possibility of non-accidental injury (see following table)

INDICATORS OF POSSIBLE NON-ACCIDENTAL INJURY
✓ Delay between injury and seeking treatment
✓ The history of the accident does not match the observed injury
✓ The history changes
✓ Other injuries, especially if at different stages of healing
✓ Signs of general neglect or failure to thrive
✓ Signs of family tension or indications of alcohol or drug abuse

Adapted from Wardrope, J., & Smith, J.R.R. (1992). *The Management of wounds and burns.* New York: Oxford.

D. Diagnostic Tests
   1. Order x-rays for crushing and deep penetrating wounds
   2. Obtain wound swabs for culture on any wound which is slow to heal; fresh wounds do not require a culture

V. Plan/Management

A. The following wounds should be managed by a clinician with extensive experience in wound management
   1. Wounds involving nerve, tendon, or bone damage
   2. Wounds with full thickness skin loss
   3. Facial and hand wounds (small, superficial wounds, however, may be treated in outpatient setting)

B. Wound-cleansing is the first step of wound care (consider using anesthesia before cleansing)
   1. Irrigate wound with one of the following:
      a. Normal saline is an economical and effective irrigant
      b. Povidone-iodine, hydrogen peroxide, and other detergents can cause tissue toxicity and should not be used
      c. Use high-pressure irrigation which can be achieved with a 35- or 65-ml syringe and a 16- or 19- gauge needle; higher pressure may result in tissue trauma and should be reserved for highly contaminated wounds
      d. Alternatively, a plastic disposable splashguard (Zerowet) can be substituted for the needle to give high-pressure irrigation; avoids inadvertent exposure to blood-contaminated fluid
   2. Apply mechanical force to clean wound: May use a fine-pore sponge such as an Optipore with a surfactant such as poloxamer 188 (Shur Clens)

C. Preparation of the wound site is next
   1. Debridement of devitalized tissue is important
   2. Clip, do not shave, surrounding hair as close to skin surface as possible; never shave an eyebrow

D. After appropriately preparing the wound, the next step is to decide whether to apply sutures; the following wounds require open-wound management:
   1. Abrasions and superficial lacerations
   2. Wounds with a great deal of tissue damage
   3. Wound which have a low risk for infection of >12-24 hours of age
   4. Wounds which have a high risk for infection of >6 hours of age
   5. Wounds contaminated by feces, human or animal saliva, or large amounts of soil or dirt
   6. Abrasions or wounds involving large superficial denudement of skin

E. Wound dressings: Best environment for wounds which are not sutured is a moist one; the following occlusive or semiocclusive dressings can promote a moist environment and all are effective
   1. Occlusive dressings such as DuoDERM, Telfa, and OpSite can be used
   2. Hydrocolloid dressing is another possible choice (good for leg ulcers and pressure sores)
   3. Hydrogel dressing such a Vigilon may be selected
   4. Foam dressings are another choice

F. Closure of the wound with tape (Steri-strip) is appropriate if the wound is superficial, has little tension, the edges are well approximated, and the injured area has full range of motion; strips can be left in place until they fall off on their own

G. Other wounds require sutures
1. Anesthesia
a. Topical anesthetics such a mixture of lidocaine 4% plus epinephrine 1:1000 plus tetracaine 0.5% (LET) are safe, effective, and inexpensive; put 3 mL on cotton ball and firmly place in wound for 15 minutes; before suturing assess effectiveness of anesthesia
b. Alternatively inject plain lidocaine (Xylocaine) solution buffered by adding 1 mL of sodium bicarbonate solution to every 9-10 mL of lidocaine and allow to reach body temperature before use
c. For crush injuries and lacerations with fractures, inject 0.25% bupivacaine (Marcaine) which has a slower onset, but longer duration of action; do not exceed dose of 3 mg/kg
d. Do not use any anesthetic containing epinephrine in an area in which circulation is easily compromised such as fingers, toes, nose, penis, or ears
e. Subdermally inject anesthesia slowly inside the cut margin of wound, avoiding piercing intact skin
f. Use regional blocks to minimize distorting tissue or where there is no loose areolar tissue to infiltrate, such as the finger tip
2. Wound edge approximation should be achieved with little or no tension to the surrounding area. Tension would be indicated by puckering of the skin
a. In patients with a history of keloid formation, close skin with minimal tension and consider applying a pressure dressing for 3-6 months
b. Many different suture techniques are available; suturing technique will depend on site and extent of injury
c. Different suture materials are available
(1) Skin is usually closed with nonabsorbable suture material such as nylon, Prolene, or silk
(2) Subcutaneous tissue and mucosal surfaces are usually closed with absorbable material, such as Dexon, Vicryl, or plain or chromic gut
(3) Rapidly dissolving suture forms may be used to close the skin in some patients to avoid the discomfort associated with follow up suture removal
3. Delayed primary closures with sutures
a. This technique is used for wounds that cannot be closed initially because of gross contamination, potential injury to joints or other deep structures, retained foreign bodies, host immune status, or an inability to adequately cleanse the wound
b. Consider closing wound in 3-5 days when the risk of infection decreases
4. Care of wound after suturing
a. For simple lacerations, place gauze over suture line and cover with occlusive dressing for 24-48 hours. For more complex lacerations, immobilize injured body part for 5-7 days and apply bulky dressing; some advocate wound closure tape directly over the sutures
b. Splint sutured wounds which are over or around a joint
c. Instruct patient to keep wound clean and dry for at least 48 hours

H. Cyanoacrylate tissue adhesives can be used for skin closure of short (<6-8 cm), low tension (≤0.5 cm gap between wound edges), clean edged, straight or curved lacerations
1. Dry wound edges are approximated with fingers or forceps; approximated edges are painted with adhesive using short brush strokes in a multilayering fashion, allowing 15 seconds to elapse between layers (usually about four layers are applied)
2. At end of process, edges are held together for 30-60 seconds to dry
3. Adhesives act as their own dressings and have antimicrobial effects against gram-positive organisms; a dry gauze dressing may or may not be applied
4. Ointments and creams should not be used
5. Suture removal is not necessary as adhesives slough off in 7-14 days
6. Patients may shower and gently bathe wound, but should avoid prolonged wetness that occurs with swimming, scrubbing, or soaking
7. Advantages: Less pain, decrease in time to perform procedure, reduction in risk of needlestick to health care workers, decrease in need for instruments and supplies, no need for follow-up suture removal, and good antibacterial effect
8. Disadvantages: Adhesives have lower tensile strength than sutures and may break over high-tension areas such as joints; adhesive may drip into uninvolved areas; improperly applied adhesive may delay healing and have poor cosmetic results

I. Certain types of wounds require different therapy
1. Puncture wounds should have very high-powered irrigation with saline; do not close puncture wounds with sutures
2. Flap wounds which have edges which are not approximated should be cleaned, non-viable fat should be removed, and Steri-Strips should be applied to appose but not close the wound
3. For small scalp lacerations, consider skin staples

J. Topical antibiotic ointments can be applied to open or sutured wounds; limit prophylactic ointments to high-risk wounds
1. Polysporin, bacitracin, and mupirocin are appropriate choices
2. Avoid Neosporin because it may cause allergies

K. Oral antibiotics are sometimes used for prophylactic purposes to prevent infection
1. Prophylactic antibiotics should be given in the following cases:
   a. Most mammal bites (see section on BITE WOUNDS)
   b. Puncture wounds in which cleansing was difficult
   c. Patients with valvular disease or implants who are at risk for bacteremia
2. Also, consider prophylactic antibiotics in the following cases:
   a. Heavily contaminated wounds
   b. Wounds with delayed treatment
   c. Wounds with tissue necrosis
3. Choose one of the following antibiotics for prophylaxis
   a. Amoxicillin-clavulanate (Augmentin); prescribe 250-500 mg every 8 hours or 40 mg/kg/day in 3 divided doses
   b. For patients with penicillin allergies, prescribe erythromycin (Ery-Tab) 250 mg QID for 7-10 days or 30-50 mg/kg/day in 4 divided doses

L. Prevention of tetanus is important (following table provides guidelines on tetanus prophylaxis)

GUIDE TO TETANUS PROPHYLAXIS IN WOUND MANAGEMENT				
History of Tetanus Immunization (doses)	Clean, Minor Wounds		All Other Wounds*	
	dT[†]	TIG	dT[†]	TIG
Uncertain or <3	Yes	No	Yes	Yes
3 or more[‡]	No[¶]	No	No[§]	No

*Such as, but not limited to, wounds contaminated with dirt, feces, soil, and saliva; puncture wounds; avulsions; wounds resulting from missiles, crushing, burns, and frostbite
[†] For adults, dT is recommended. dT indicates adult-type diphtheria and tetanus toxoids; TIG, tetanus immune globulin (human)
[‡] If only 3 doses of fluid toxoid have been received, a fourth dose of toxoid, preferably an adsorbed toxoid, should be given
[¶] Yes, if >10 years since the last dose
[§] Yes, if >5 years since the last dose. More frequent boosters are not needed and can accentuate adverse effects
Adapted from American Academy of Pediatrics. (2000). Tetanus. In L.K. Pickering (Ed.), *2000 red book: Report of the Committee on Infectious Disease*. 25th ed. Elk Grove Village, IL: Author.

M. Patient Education
1. Teach patient to return if wound is increasingly painful, if there is significant discharge, or if there is spreading of redness around wound, or a red streak developing from the wound in the direction of the heart
2. Inform patient that appearance of the wound and subsequent scar will change substantially during the year after the injury; thus, decisions for scar revision should be made after one year
3. Advise patients to avoid sun exposure of their wounds to reduce the risk of developing hyperpigmentation

N. Follow Up
1. On return visits evaluate and consider hospitalization or aggressive antimicrobial therapy if signs and symptoms of pyogenic abscess, cellulitis, and ascending lymphangitis (red line spreading proximally on a limb) are present
2. Return for re-evaluation, dressing change, and/or suture removal in 2 days

3. Time to remove sutures depends on wound location; apply surgical adhesives or tape after sutures are removed
   a. Facial wounds: 3-5 days
   b. Scalp wounds: 7-10 days
   c. Hand wounds: 10-14 days
   d. Lower legs: 14 days
   e. Other: 7-21 days

REFERENCES

American Academy of Neurology, Quality Standards Subcommittee: Practice parameter. (1997). The management of concussion in sports (summary statement). *Neurology, 48,* 581-585.

American Academy of Pediatrics. (2000). Bite wounds. In L.K. Pickering (Ed.), *2000 red book: Report of the Committee on Infectious Diseases* (25th ed., pp. 155-159). Elk Grove Village, IL: Author.

American Academy of Pediatrics. (2000). Rabies. In L.K. Pickering (Ed.), *2000 red book: Report of the Committee on Infectious Diseases* (25th ed., pp. 475-482). Elk Grove Village, IL: Author.

American Academy of Pediatrics. (2000). Tetanus. In L.K. Pickering (Ed.), *2000 red book: Report of the Committee on Infectious Diseases* (25th ed., pp. 563-568). Elk Grove Village, IL: Author.

American Academy of Pediatrics (2003). Active and passive immunization. In L.K. Pickering (Ed.), *2003 red book: Report of the Committee on Infectious Diseases* (26th ed., pp. 1-93). Elk Grove Village, IL: Author.

American Burn Association. (1996). *Guidelines for transfer of patients in burn centers.* New York: Author.

Bower, M.G. (2001). Managing dog, cat, and human bite wounds. *The Nurse Practitioner, 26,* 36-45.

Buttaravoli, P., & Stair, T. (2000). *Minor emergencies: Splinters to fractures.* Mosby: St. Louis.

Doody, D.P. (1999). Lacerations and abrasions. In R.A. Dershewitz (Ed.), *Ambulatory pediatric care.* Philadelphia: Lippincott.

Douglass, A.B., & Douglass, J.M. (2003). Common dental emergencies. *American Family Physician,67,* 511-516.

Golden, D.B. (2002). Allergic reactions to insect stings. In R.E. Rakel & E.T. Bope (Eds.), 2002 *Conn's current therapy* (pp. 768-771). Philadelphia: Saunders.

Jagoda, A.S. (2002). Clinical policy: Neuroimaging and decision making in adult mild traumatic brain injury in the acute setting. *Annals of Emergency Medicine, 40,* 231-240.

Kushner, D.S. (2001). Concussion in sports: Minimizing the risk for complications. *American Family Physician, 64,* 1007-1014.

Leclerc, S., Lassonde, M., & Delaney, J.S. (2001). Recommendations for grading of concussion in athletes. *Sports Medicine, 31,* 629-636.

Lewis, D.P. (2001). Burns: Initial management and outpatient follow-up. *Family Practice Recertification, 23,* 19-34.

Marion, D.W. (1998). Acute head injuries in adults. In R.E. Rakel (Ed.), *1998 Conn's current therapy.* Philadelphia: WB Saunders.

McCrea, M., Kelly, J.P., Kluge, J., Ackley, B., & Randolph, C. (1997). Standardized assessment of concussion in football players. *Neurology, 48,* 586-588.

Morgan, E.D., Beldsoe, S.C., & Barker, J. (2000). Ambulatory management of burns. *American Family Physician, 62,* 2015-2026.

Osterhoudt, K.C., Zaortis, T., & Zorc, J.J. (2002). Lyme disease masquerading as brown recluse spider bite. *Annals of Emergency Medicine, 39,* 558-561.

Pavan-Langston, D. (2002). Burns and trauma. In D. Pavan-Langston (Ed.), *Manual of ocular diagnosis and therapy* (5th ed., pp. 31-46). Philadelphia: Lippincott Williams & Wilkins.

Pavan-Langston, D. (2002). Cornea and external disease. In D. Pavan-Langston (Ed.), *Manual of ocular diagnosis and therapy* (5th ed., pp. 67-129) Philadelphia: Lippincott Williams & Wilkins.

Presutti, R.J. (2001). Prevention and treatment of dog bites. *American Family Physician, 63,* 1567-1572, 1573-1574.

Simon, J. (1992). Accidental injury and emergency medical services for children. In R.E. Behrman (Ed.). *Nelson textbook of pediatrics.* Philadelphia: WB Saunders.

Singer, A.J., Hollander, J.E., & Quinn, J.V. (1997). Evaluation and management of traumatic lacerations. *New England Journal of Medicine, 337,* 1142-1148.

Smith, E.E. (1993). Minor head injury: A proposed strategy for emergency management. *Annals of Emergency Medicine, 22,* 1193-1196.

Sorrentino, A., & Monroe, K. (2002). Insect stings In F.D. Burg, J.R. Ingelfinger, R.A. Polin, & A.A. Gershon (Eds.), *Gellis and Kagan's current pediatric therapy* (pp. 1052-1054). Philadelphia: Saunders.

Valadka, A.B. (2002). Acute head injuries in adults. In R.E. Rakel & E.T. Bope (Eds.). *2002 Conn's current therapy* (pp. 967-971). Saunders: Philadelphia.

Vetter, R.S., & Bush, S.P. (2002). The diagnosis of brown recluse spider bite is overused for dermonecrotic wounds of uncertain etiology. *Annals of Emergency Medicine, 39,* 544-546.

Wardrope, J., & Smith, J.R.R. (1992). *The management of wounds and burns.* New York: Oxford.

Index

Rabies, 827-830
Refractive errors, 280
Reiter's syndrome, 323, 702, 703
Renal calculi, 532
Renal osteodystrophy, 522
Restless legs syndrome, 795-798
    Diagnostic criteria, 796
Rheumatic fever, 317
Rheumatoid arthritis, 740-745
    Biological response modifiers (BRMs), 742
    Classification of RA, 740
    Criteria for remission, 745
    Diagnostic tests, 741
    Plan/Management, 741
        Drug therapy, 742
        Patient education, 741
Rhinitis, allergic, 301-308
    Allergen immunotherapy, 307
    Diagnosis/Evaluation, 303
    Environmental control in the home, 304
    Management, 303
    Patient information websites, 304
Rhinitis, non-allergic, 301-308
    Diagnosis/Evaluation, 303
Rhinosinusitis. *See* Sinusitis
Ringworm. *See* Dermatophyte infections or Tinea
Rinne test, 287
Rocky Mountain spotted fever, 192-193
    Diagnosis/Evaluation, 192
    Pathogenesis, 192
    Plan/Management, 193
Rosacea, 210-213
    Diagnostic criteria, 211
    Dry eye syndrome, 213
    Environmental and lifestyle factors, 212
    Patient resource, 212
Rotator cuff disorders, 745-755
Rubella, 193-195
    Control procedures, 195
    Diagnosis/Evaluation, 194
    Enteroviral infections, 194
    Pathogenesis, 193
    Postnatal rubella, 194
    Treatment of exposed persons, 195
Rubeola, 195-197
    Case definition, 196
    Diagnosis/Evaluation, 196
    Pathogenesis, 195
    Plan/Management, 196
    Treatment of exposed persons, 196

Safe Return, 777
Salivary gland disorders, 328
Salmonella, 460
Salt, 26
    Decreasing intake, 26
Scabicide, 241
Scabies, 239-241
Scabies, Norwegian, 240
Scarlet fever, 317
Scleroderma, 493, 702
Sebaceous hyperplasia, 206
Seborrheic dermatitis, 226-228
    HIV infection, 227
    Treatment
        Facial involvement, 227
        Intertriginous involvement, 227
        Scalp involvement, 227
Seborrheic keratosis, 206
Second impact syndrome, 837
Seizures. *See* Epilepsy
Serous otitis media, 299
Shigella, 460
Shin splints, 719-725

Shingles, 254-258
Shoulder pain, 745-755
    Acute shoulder pain, 745
    Chronic shoulder pain, 745
    Diagnosis/Evaluation, 748
    Diagnostic tests, 752
    Differential diagnosis, 751
    Physical examination, 749
        Maneuvers to assess shoulder pain, 750
    Plan/Management, 752
        Exercise program, 754
Silent (lymphocytic) thyroiditis, 157
Sinusitis, 311-316
    Antibiotics, 314
    Diagnosis/Evaluation, 313
    Diagnostic predictors of bacterial rhinosinusitis, 312
    Pathogenesis, 311
    Patient education, 315
    Treatment
        Acute sinusitis due to dental infection, 315
        Chronic sinusitis, 315
        Fungal infections, 315
Skin cancer
    Screening, 20
Skin care, 203-205
    Dry skin, 203
    Lactic acid-containing lotions, 204
    Moisturizers, 204
    Oily skin, 203
    Urea creams and lotions, 204
Skin lesions, 205-207
Skull fractures, 836-42
Slipped capital femoral epiphysis, 720, 721, 724, 725
Smallpox, 182, 198
Smoking cessation, *See* Tobacco use
Solar lentigo, 206
Soy foods, 603
    Recipes, free guide, 603
    Types of supplements, 603
Spermicides, 582
Spinal stenosis, 711-719
Spirometry, 336, 349
Spondylolisthesis, 712, 713, 717
Spondylolysis, 712, 713, 717
Squamous cell carcinoma, 208
Staphylococcus aureus, 462
Sternoclavicular joint sprain and separation, 747-755
Stomach cancer, risk reduction 30
Stomatitis. *See* Aphthous stomatitis
Streptococcal pharyngitis, 319
    Treatment, 320
        Carriers, 320
        Recurrent, 320
Stress fractures, 719-725
Stroke, 806
Stucco keratosis, 206
Stye. *See* Hordeolum
Subacromial impingement (SI) syndrome, 745-755
Subacute thyroiditis, 157-159, 162
Subclavian steal syndrome, 437-439
Subclinical hyperthyroidism, 158-159, 162
Subclinical hypothyroidism, 164
    Treatment, 167
Subconjunctival hemorrhage, 847
Subdural hematoma, 840
Suicide, 103
    Suicide risk assessment, 103
Supraglottitis.   Epiglottitis
Syncope, 435-439
    Carotid sinus hypersensitivity, 436
    Diagnostic tests, 438
    Drug-induced syncope, 436
    Orthostatic hypotension, 436

864

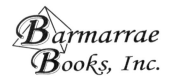

Barmarrae Books, Inc.